Practice Considerations for the Adult-Gerontological Acute Care Nurse Practitioner

Thomas W. Barkley, Jr., PhD, ACNP-BC, FAANP

Professor
Director of Nurse Practitioner Programs
California State University, Los Angeles
School of Nursing
and
President, Barkley & Associates
Los Angeles, California

Charlene M. Myers, DNP, ACNP-BC, CNS

Associate Clinical Professor
Adult Acute Care Nurse Practitioner Program Coordinator
University of South Alabama
College of Nursing
Mobile, Alabama

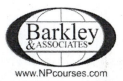

Barkley
& ASSOCIATES

www.NPcourses.com

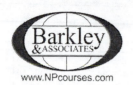

www.NPcourses.com

P.O. Box 69901
West Hollywood CA 90069

PRACTICE CONSIDERATIONS FOR ADULT-GERONTOLOGICAL
ACUTE CARE NURSE PRACTITIONERS
Copyright ©2014 by Barkley & Associates

ISBN 978-0-578-14831-1

Notice

Knowledge and best practices are subject to change, as new research and further experience expand knowledge. Changes in practice, treatment, and drug therapy may be warranted or appropriate. It is recommended that readers verify the most up-to-date information regarding procedures featured or check the manufacturers of administered products, so as to verify the recommended dose, formula, methods of administration, and contradindications. It is the duty of practitioners, relying on their experience and knowledge of the patient's circumstances, to determine dosages and the best treatment for each patient, while taking all safety precautions. To the fullest extend of the law, neither the Publisher nor the Editors and Authors assume any liability for any injury and/or damage to persons or property arising out of or related to any use of the content in this book.

The Publisher

International Standard Book Number: 978-0-578-14831-1

Managing Editor: Charlie Wang
Assistant Editor: Taylor Spining
Project Manager: Austin Butler
Staff Coordinator: Azadouhi Garabedian

PREFACE

Practice Considerations for Adult Gerontology Acute Care Nurse Practitioners is a comprehensive textbook for advanced practice nurses. The text is organized in a systematic fashion, addressing over 350 of the most common conditions experienced by adult patients in acute care. Using an easy-to-read outline format, coverage of each condition includes defining terms, incidence/predisposing factors, subjective and physical examination findings, diagnostic tests, and management strategies.

The text has been written to provide the practitioner with a thorough overview of evidence-based practice guidelines. In this light, the text builds on previous knowledge of anatomy, physiology, and pathophysiology concepts that have not been separately emphasized. Although many practitioners may be highly specialized, this text was designed as a useful tool for the entire scope of acute care nursing practice, including settings such as clinics, emergency departments, medical/surgical departments in hospitals, as well as critical care units. Although this text was developed based on research and expertise, we also feel strongly that collaborative practice with other experts and clinicians is essential to successfully meeting patient goals.

Thomas W. Barkley, Jr.

Charlene M. Myers

ACKNOWLEDGMENTS

We gratefully acknowledge the previous authors of the first and second editions of *Practice Guidelines for Acute Care Nurse Practitioners* whose knowledge and dedication provided the foundation for the expansion of this textbook. We would additionally like to thank the outstanding contributors and reviewers of this text. Without the expertise of these scholars, this work would not have been possible.

We also thank the following people at Barkley and Associates:

Pharmacology Editor: Robert Fellin

Editing Manager: Charlie Wang

Assistant Editing Manager: Taylor Spining

Project Coordinator: Austin Butler

Office Manager: Azadouhi Garabedian

Cover Design: Andres Morgan

whose combined efforts have produced what we believe is a state-of-the art, evidence-based, excellent resource for the profession.

Thomas W. Barkley, Jr.

Charlene M. Myers

Distinguished Contributors

Bimbola F. Akintade, PhD, ACNP-BC, MBA, MHA
Assistant Professor
Organizational Systems and Adult Health
Specialty Director
Adult Gerontology Acute Care Nurse Practitioner/Clinical Nurse Specialist
Program
University of Maryland
Baltimore, Maryland
23. Measures of Oxygenation and Ventilation, 31. Pneumothorax, 86.
Managing the Surgical Patient

Kimberly Alva, MSN, ACNP-BC, CCRN
Acute Care Nurse Practitioner
Neurosurgical Intensive Care Unit
Cedars Sinai Medical Center
Los Angeles, California
4. Neurologic Trauma

Susan J. Appel, PhD, ACNP-BC, FNP-BC, CCRN, FAHA
Professor
The University of Alabama
Capstone College of Nursing
Tuscaloosa, Alabama
47. Diabetes Mellitus, 48. Diabetes-Related Emergencies

Amita Avadhani, DNP, DCC, ACNP-BC, ANP-BC, APN, CCRN
Assistant Professor
Track Coordinator
Adult Gerontology Acute Critical Care Nurse Practitioner Program
Rutgers School of Nursing
Rutgers Biomedical and Health Sciences University
Newark, New Jersey
Critical Care Nurse Practitioner-Adult ICU
Saint Peters University Hospital
New Brunswick, New Jersey
22. Diagnostic Concepts of Oxygenation and Ventilation, 35. Mechanical Ventilatory Support

Thomas W. Barkley, Jr., PhD, ACNP-BC, FAANP
Professor
Director of Nurse Practitioner Programs
California State University, Los Angeles
School of Nursing
President, Barkley & Associates
Los Angeles, California
3. Peripheral Neuropathies, 11. Cardiovascular Assessment, 12. Hypertension, 13. Coronary Artery Disease and Hyperlipidemia, 14. Angina and Myocardial Infarction, 15. Adjunct Equipment/Devices, 16. Peripheral Vascular Disease, 17. Inflammatory Cardiac Diseases, 18. Heart Failure, 19. Valvular Disease, 20. Cardiomyopathy, 21. Arrhythmias, 24. The Chest X-Ray, 25. Pulmonary Function Testing, 26. Obstructive (Ventilatory) Lung Diseases, 27. Restrictive (Inflammatory) Lung Diseases, 28. Pulmonary Hypertension and Pulmonary Vascular Disorders, 29. Chest Wall and Secondary Pleural Disorders, 30. Respiratory Failure, 31. Pneumothorax, 32. Lower Respiratory Tract Pathogens, 33. Obstructive Sleep Apnea, 34. Oxygen Supplementation, 35. Mechanical Ventilatory Support, 47. Diabetes Mellitus, 48. Diabetes-Related Emergencies, 49. Thyroid Disease, 50. Cushing's Syndrome, 51. Primary Adrenocortical Insufficiency (Addison Disease) and Adrenal Crisis, 52. Pheochromocytoma, 53. Syndrome of Inappropriate Antidiuretic Hormone, 54. Diabetes Insipidus, 67. HIV/AIDS and Opportunistic Infections Among Older Adults, 68. Autoimmune Diseases, 69. Integumentary Disorders, 70. Ectopic Pregnancy and STIs, 71. Eye, Ear, Nose, and Throat Disorders, 72. Headache, 73. Fever, 74. Pain, 76. Management of the Patient in Shock, 77. Nutritional Considerations, 78. Fluid, Electrolyte, and Acid-Base Imbalances, 79. Poisoning and Drug Toxicities, 80. Wound Management, 81. Infections, 82. Trauma Considerations, 83. Solid Organ Transplantation, 84. Burns, 85. Hospital Admission Considerations, 86. Managing the Surgical Patient, 87. Guidelines for Health Promotion and Screening, 89. Immunization Recommendations

Catherine Blache, MSN, RN, CCRC
Owner/Director of Research
Precision Clinical Research, LLC
Mobile, Alabama
80. Wound Management, 84. Burns

Bob Blessing, DNP, ACNP-BC
Consulting Associate Professor
Duke University
School of Nursing
Durham, North Carolina
Lead Nurse Practitioner
Neuroscience Critical Care Unit
Duke University Health System
Durham, North Carolina
3. Peripheral Neuropathies, 76. Management of the Patient in Shock

Kelly Blessing, MSN, FNP-BC
Neurology Provider
Duke University Health System
Durham, North Carolina
Family Nurse Practitioner
Cerebrovascular Center
Duke University Health System
Durham, North Carolina
3. Peripheral Neuropathies

Lorris J. Bouzigard, DNP, ACNP-BC, ANP-C, DCC
Acute Care Nurse Practitioner
Internal Medicine Clinic
Louisiana Heart Hospital Medical Group
Lacombe, Louisiana
Adjunct Clinical Instructor
University of South Alabama
Mobile, Alabama
73. Fever

Travis Bradley, MSN, ACNP-BC, CEN
Acute Care Nurse Practitioner
Neuro-Surgical Intensive Care Unit
Cedars-Sinai Medical Center
Los Angeles, California
1. Cerebrovascular Accidents: Brain Attack, 2. Structural Abnormalities

Steven W. Branham, PhD, RN, ACNP-BC, FNP-BC, FAANP, CCRN
Assistant Professor
Acute Care Nurse Practitioner Program
Texas Tech University
College of Nursing
Lubbock, Texas
43. Acute Kidney Injury and Chronic Kidney Disease

Barbara Ann Shelton Broome, PhD, RN, CNS, FAAN
Dean
Kent State University
College of Nursing
Kent, Ohio
88. Major Causes of Mortality in the United States

Fredrick Carlston, MSN, ACNP-BC
Acute Care Nurse Practitioner
Cardiovascular Medicine
Keck Hospital of USC
Los Angeles, California
Acute Care Nurse Practitioner
Cardiology Nuclear Medicine
Cedars-Sinai Medical Center
Los Angeles, California
21. Arrhythmias

Jennifer Coates, MSN, ACNP-BC, MBA, ACNPC
Assistant Clinical Professor
Adult Gerontology Acute Care Nurse Practitioner Program
Drexel University
College of Nursing & Health Professions
Philadelphia, Pennsylvania
29. Chest Wall and Secondary Pleural Disorders, 33. Obstructive Sleep Apnea

Marla Couture, MSN, ACNP-BC, CCRN
Clinical Instructor
Acute Care Department
The University of Alabama at Birmingham
School of Nursing
Birmingham, Alabama
46. Nephrolithiasis

R. Michael Culpepper, MD
Professor
Chief Division of Nephrology
University of South Alabama
College of Medicine
Mobile, Alabama
78. Fluid, Electrolyte, and Acid-Base Imbalances

Rita A. Dello Stritto, PhD, ACNP-BC, CNS, ENP
Associate Professor
Texas Woman's University
Nelda C. Stark College of Nursing
Houston, Texas
49. Thyroid Disease, 50. Cushing's Syndrome, 51. Primary Adrenocortical Insufficiency (Addison Disease) and Adrenal Crisis, 54. Diabetes Insipidus

Lisa Evans, DNP, ACNP-BC
Hospitalist Nurse Practitioner
Director of Skilled Nursing Facility Services
Pulmonary Consultants & Primary Care Physicians
Orange, CA
Lecturer
Adult Gerontology Acute Care Nurse Practitioner Program
California State University, Los Angeles
Los Angeles, California
61. Anemias, 62. Sickle Cell Disease/Crisis, 63. Coagulopathies

Robert Fellin, PharmD, BCPS
Pharmacist
Cedars-Sinai Medical Center
Los Angeles, California
Faculty
Barkley & Associates
Los Angeles, California
9. Parkinson's Disease, 12. Hypertension, 18. Heart Failure, 19. Valvular Disease, 21. Arrhythmias

Alison Forbes, MSN, ACNP-BC, CCRN
Acute Care Nurse Practitioner
Division of Neurocritical Care, Department of Surgery
Harbor UCLA Medical Center
Torrance, California
Lecturer
Adult Gerontology Acute Care Nurse Practitioner Program
California State University, Los Angeles
Los Angeles, California
81. Infections, 82. Trauma Considerations

Catherine L. Fung, MSN, ACNP-BC
General Surgery Acute Care Nurse Practitioner
Division of Upper GI and General Surgery
Keck Hospital of USC
Los Angeles, California
40. Anatomic Intestinal Disorders

Donna Gullette, PhD, ACNP-BC, APRN
Professor
Director of Master of Nursing Science Programs
Associate Dean for Practice
University of Arkansas for Medical Sciences
College of Nursing
Little Rock, Arkansas
69. Integumentary Disorders, 72. Headache

Haley Hoy, PhD, ACNP-BC
Interim Associate Dean, Graduate Programs
University of Alabama Huntsville
Huntsville, Alabama
Acute Care Nurse Practitioner
Lung Transplantation
Vanderbilt Medical Center
Nashville, Tennessee
25. Pulmonary Function Testing, 28. Pulmonary Hypertension and Pulmonary Vascular Disorders

Alicia Huckstadt, PhD, APRN, FNP-BC, GNP-BC, FAANP
Professor
Director of Graduate Programs
Wichita State University
School of Nursing
Wichita, Kansas
36. Peptic Ulcer Disease, 89. Immunization Recommendations

Lisa A. Johnson, DrNP, CRNP, ACNP-BC
Assistant Professor
Director, AGACNP Program
De Sales University
Department of Nursing and Health
Center Valley, Pennsylvania
39. Inflammatory Gastrointestinal Disorders, 68. Autoimmune Diseases

Joan E. King, PhD, ACNP-BC, ANP-BC, FAANP
Professor
Adult-Gerontology Acute Care Nurse Practitioner Program Director
Vanderbilt University
School of Nursing
Nashville, Tennessee
11. Cardiovascular Assessment, 13. Coronary Artery Disease and Hyperlipidemia, 14. Angina and Myocardial Infarction, 18. Heart Failure

Honore Kotler, MSN, ACNP-BC
Lead Acute Care Nurse Practitioner
Comprehensive Transplant Center
Cedars Sinai Medical Center
Los Angeles, California
83. Solid Organ Transplantation

Victoria Ku, MSN, ACNP-BC, CCRN
Acute Care Nurse Practitioner
Thoracic Surgery
Keck Hospital of USC,
Los Angeles, California
Clinical Instructor
West Coast University
Ontario, California
24. The Chest X-Ray

Judi Kuric, DNP, ACNP-BC, CNRN
Assistant Professor
University of Southern Indiana
College of Nursing and Health Professions
Evansville, Indiana
Acute Care Nurse Practitioner
Neurosurgical Private Practice
Louisville, Kentucky
5. Central Nervous System Disorders, 8. Multiple Sclerosis, 9. Parkinson's Disease, 10. Amyotrophic Lateral Sclerosis, 85. Hospital Admissions Considerations

Patrick A. Laird, DNP, ACNP-BC, APRN
Assistant Professor of Clinical Nursing
Adult-Gerontology Acute Care Nurse Practitioner Program Director
The University of Texas Health Science Center at Houston
School of Nursing
Houston, Texas
6. Seizure Disorders

Monique Lambert, DNP, ACNP-BC
Director of the Advanced Practice Institute
RUSH University Medical Center
Chicago, Illinois
52. Pheochromocytoma, 53. Syndrome of Inappropriate Antidiuretic Hormone

Paula McCauley, DNP, ACNP-BC, APRN, CNE
Assistant Clinical Professor
Associate Dean for Academic Affairs
University of Connecticut
School of Nursing
Storrs, Connecticut
Acute Care Program Coordinator
University of Connecticut
School of Nursing
Storrs, Connecticut
77. Nutritional Considerations

Sheila Melander, PhD, ACNP-BC, FCCM, FAANP
Professor
University of Kentucky
College of Nursing
Lexington, Kentucky
15. Adjunct Equipment/Devices, 17. Inflammatory Cardiac Diseases, 20. Cardiomyopathy

Helen Miley, PhD, ACNP-BC. AGACNP-BC
Clinical Associate Professor
Specialty Director
Adult Geriatric Acute Care Nurse Practitioner Program
Rutgers, The State University of New Jersey
Newark, New Jersey
Adult Geriatric Acute Care Nurse Practitioner
Medical Intensive Care Unit
Robert Wood Johnson University Hospital
New Brunswick, New Jersey
12. Hypertension, 87. Guidelines for Health Promotion and Screening

David A. Miller, MD, FCCP
Associate Professor
Family Nurse Practitioner Program
Texas A&M University-Corpus Christi
College of Nursing and Health Sciences
Corpus Christi, Texas
27. Restrictive (Inflammatory) Lung Diseases, 30. Respiratory Failure, 32. Lower Respiratory Tract Pathogens, 67. HIV/AIDS and Opportunistic Infections Among Older Adults, 71. Eye, Ear, Nose, and Throat Disorders

Charlene M. Myers, DNP, ACNP-BC, CNS
Associate Clinical Professor
Adult Acute Care Nurse Practitioner Program Coordinator
University of South Alabama
College of Nursing
Mobile, Alabama
1. Cerebrovascular Accidents: Brain Attack, 2. Structural Abnormalities, 4. Neurologic Trauma, 5. Central Nervous System Disorders, 6. Seizure Disorders, 7. Dementia, 22. Diagnostic Concepts of Oxygenation and Ventilation, 23. Measures of Oxygenation and Ventilation, 25. Pulmonary Function Testing, 29. Chest Wall and Secondary Pleural Disorders, 34. Oxygen Supplementation, 35. Mechanical Ventilatory Support, 36. Peptic Ulcer Disease, 37. Liver Disease, 38. Biliary Dysfunction, 39. Inflammatory Gastrointestinal Disorders, 40. Anatomic Intestinal Disorders, 41. Gastrointestinal Bleeding, 42. Urinary Tract Infections, 43. Acute Kidney Injury and Chronic Kidney Disease, 44. Benign Prostatic Hyperplasia, 45. Renal Artery Stenosis, 46. Nephrolithiasis, 71. Eye, Ear, Nose, and Throat Disorders, 72. Headache, 73. Fever, 74. Pain, 76. Management of the Patient in Shock, 77. Nutritional Considerations, 78. Fluid, Electrolyte, and Acid-Base Imbalances, 80. Wound Management, 86. Managing the Surgical Patient, 87. Guidelines for Health Promotion and Screening, 89. Immunization Recommendations

Marcie Nomura, MSN, ACNP-BC, CCRN
Acute Care Nurse Practitioner
Hepatobiliary Surgery
Cedars-Sinai Medical Center
Comprehensive Transplant Center
Los Angeles, California
74. Pain

Michalyn Pelphrey, MSN, ACNP-BC, CCTC
Acute Care Nurse Practitioner
Liver Transplant
Cedars-Sinai Medical Center
Los Angeles, California
37. Liver Disease, 38. Biliary Dysfunction

Nicole Perez, MSN, ACNP-BC,CCRN
Critical Care Intensivist Nurse Practitioner
Harbor UCLA Medical Center
Torrance, California
Lecturer
Adult Gerontology Acute Care Nurse Practitioner Program
California State University, Los Angeles
Los Angeles, California
41. Gastrointestinal Bleeding

Tobias P. Rebmann, MSN, ACNP-BC, CCRN
Acute Care Nurse Practitioner
Trinity Clinic Cardiothoracic Surgery
Louis and Peaches Owen Heart Hospital
Cardiothoracic Intensive Care Unit
Tyler, Texas
26. Obstructive (Ventilatory) Lung Diseases, 27. Restrictive (Inflammatory) Lung Diseases

Jacqueline Rhoads, PhD, APRN-BC, CNL-BC, PMHNP-BE, FAANP
Professor
Tulane University
School of Tropical Medicine
Center of Applied Environmental Public Health
New Orleans, LA
64. Leukemias

Ivan Robbins, MD
Professor
Director, Pulmonary Vascular Center
Vanderbilt Medical Center
Nashville, Tennessee
28. Pulmonary Hypertension and Pulmonary Vascular Disorders

Jennifer Javier Roberg, MSN, ACNP-BC
Staff Education
Research & Consulting
Kaiser Permanente South Bay
Harbor City, California
44. Benign Prostatic Hyperplasia

Jenna Rush, MSN, ACNP-BC, CCTC
Heart Transplant Coordinator
Cedars-Sinai Medical Center
Comprehensive Transplant Center
Los Angeles, California
65. Lymphoma

Valerie K. Sabol, PhD, ACNP-BC, GNP-BC
Associate Professor
Specialty Director
Adult-Gerontology Acute Care Nurse Practitioner Master's Program
Duke University
School of Nursing
Durham, North Carolina
76. Management of the Patient in Shock

Angela Starkweather, PhD, ACNP-BC, CNRN
Associate Professor and Chair
Department of Adult Health and Nursing Systems
Virginia Commonwealth University
School of Nursing
Richmond, Virginia
7. Dementia, 70. Ectopic Pregnancy and STIs

Michele Talley, MSN, ACNP-BC
Clinical Instructor
Specialty Track Coordinator
Adult-Gerontology Acute Care Nurse Practitioner Program
University of Alabama at Birmingham
School of Nursing
Birmingham, Alabama
42. Urinary Tract Infections, 45. Renal Artery Stenosis

Carol Thompson, PhD, DNP, ACNP-BC, FNP-BC
Professor
University of Kentucky
College of Nursing
Lexington, Kentucky
34. Oxygen Supplementation

Elizabeth A. VandeWaa, PhD
Professor
Adult Health Nursing Department
University of South Alabama
College of Nursing
Mobile, Alabama
79. Poisoning and Drug Toxicities

Paula K. Vuckovich, PhD, PMHCNS-BC
Associate Professor
Psychiatric Mental Health Graduate Option Coordinator
Doctor of Nursing Practice Program Coordinator
California State University, Los Angeles
School of Nursing
Los Angeles, California
75. Psychosocial Problems in Acute Care

Theresa M. Wadas, PhD, DNP, ACNP-BC, FNP-BC, CCRN
Assistant Professor
University of Alabama
Captone College of Nursing
Tuscaloosa, Alabama
16. Peripheral Vascular Disease, 19. Valvular Disease

Colleen R. Walsh, DNP, ACNP-BC, ONC, ONP-C, CS
Contract Assistant Professor of Graduate Nursing
University of Southern Indiana
College of Nursing and Health
Evansville, Indiana
55. Arthritis, 56. Subluxations and Dislocations, 57. Soft Tissue Injury, 58. Fractures, 59. Compartment Syndrome, 60. Back Pain Syndromes, 66. Other Common Cancers

Distinguished Reviewers

Laura Kierol Andrews, PhD, ACNP-BC
Assistant Professor
Yale University
School of Nursing
Orange, Connecticut
Senior Acute Care Nurse Practitioner
Department of Critical Care Medicine
Hospital of Central Connecticut
New Britain, Connecticut

Susan J. Appel, PhD, ACNP-BC, FNP-BC, CCRN, FAHA
Professor
The University of Alabama
Capstone College of Nursing
Tuscaloosa, Alabama

Kelly Arashin, MSN, ACNP-BC
Associate Professor of Graduate Nursing
Armstrong Atlantic State University
School of Nursing
Savannah, Georgia
Acute Care Nurse Practitioner
Critical Care Clinical Nurse Specialist
Hilton Head Hospital
Apollo, Maryland

Melanie Schwartz Binshtok, MS, ACNP-BC, AACC
Adjunct Faculty
Virginia Commonwealth University
School of Nursing
Richmond, Virginia
Inpatient Cardiology Nurse Practitioner
Bon Secours Richmond Health System
Richmond, Virginia

Valeria K. Bisig, MSN, ACNP-BC, FNP-BC
Acute Care Nurse Practitioner
TriHealth Corporate Health
Cincinnati, Ohio

Jennifer M. Blake, MSN, ACNP-BC, CNRN
Neuroscience Nurse Practitioner
Seton Brain and Spine Institute
Austin, Texas

Shari W. Bryant MSN, ACNP-BC, AOCNP
Adjunct Faculty
Acute Care Nurse Practitioner
Program
University of Southern Indiana
College of Nursing and Health
Evansville, Indiana
Hospitalist Acute Care Nurse Practitioner
St. Mary's Medical Center
Evansville, Indiana

Megan M. Butts, MSN, ACNP-BC
Neuro Critical Care Nurse Practitioner
Neuroscience Intensive Care Unit
The University of Mississippi Medical Center
Jackson, Mississippi

Sandra K. Callaghan, MSN, NP-C
Family Nurse Practitioner
Specialty in Neurosurgery and Pain
Management
Antelope Valley Neuroscience
Medical Group
Lancaster, California
Owner
Universal Pain Management
CEO, Callaghan, Inc.
Palmdale, California

Jaime Cannon, MSN, ACNP- BC
Acute Care Nurse Practitioner
Montgomery Pulmonary Consultants
Montgomery, Alabama

Melanie A. Caustrita, MSN, ACNP-BC
Hospitalist Nurse Practitioner
Miami Valley Hospital
Dayton, Ohio
Locum Tenens Nurse Practitioner
StaffCare, Inc.
Irving, Texas

Grace Courreges, MSN, ACNP-BC
Acute Care Nurse Practitioner
Sierra Medical Center
El Paso, Texas

Patricia Cunningham, DNSc, PMHNP-BC, PMHCNS-BC, FNP-BC
Associate Professor
Coordinator of the Psychiatric
Mental Health Doctor of Nursing
Practice Program
University of Tennessee Health
Science Center
College of Nursing
Memphis, Tennessee

Caroline Lloyd Doherty, MSN, AGACNP-BC, AACC
Associate Program Director
Adult-Gerontology Acute Care
Nurse Practitioner and
Adult-Gerontology Clinical Nurse
Specialist Programs
University of Pennsylvania
School of Nursing
Philadelphia, Pennsylvania

Lisa Evans, DNP, ACNP-BC
Hospitalist Nurse Practitioner
Director of Skilled Nursing Facility
Services
Pulmonary Consultants & Primary
Care Physicians
Orange, California
Lecturer
Adult Gerontology Acute Care
Nurse Practitioner Program
California State University, Los
Angeles
Los Angeles, California

Mary Franklin, PhD, ACNP-BC
Clinical Assistant Professor
Wayne State University
College of Nursing
Detroit, Michigan

**Connie L. Leonard Geimer, MSN,
ACNP-BC, CRNP, CCRN**
Acute Care Nurse Practitioner
Pegasus Emergency Group
Gadsden Regional Medical Center
Gadsden, Alabama

**Donna L. Gerber, PhD, ACNP-
BC, AOCN**
Acute Care Nurse Practitioner
Department of Sarcoma
University of Texas M.D. Anderson
Cancer Center
Houston, Texas

Darla Gowan, DNP, FNP-BC
Assistant Professor
Division of Graduate Studies in
Nursing
Family Nurse Practitioner Program
Indiana Wesleyan University
School of Nursing
Marion, Indiana

**Laura Griffin, DNP, ACNP-BC,
CCRN**
Adjunct Professor
Adult-Gerontology Acute Care
Nurse Practitioner Program
Texas Woman's University
School of Nursing
Denton, Texas
Chief Nurse Executive/Chief Clini-
cal Officer
Kindred Sugar Land Hospital
Sugar Land, Texas
Acute Care Nurse Practitioner
Houston Methodist Sugar Land
Hospital
Sugarland, Texas

**Tonja M. Hartjes, DNP, ACNP-
BC, CCRN, CSC**
Clinical Associate Professor
Adult-Gerontology Acute Care
Nurse Practitioner Program
University of Florida
College of Nursing
Gainesville, Florida

**Constance W. Hartman, MSN,
ACNP-BC, CCRN**
Pulmonary and Sleep Nurse Practi-
tioner
Central Ohio Pulmonary Disease,
Inc
Columbus, Ohio

**Melissa Hill, MSN, ACNP-BC,
APRN, CNRN, CCRN, SCRN**
Clinical Instructor
Acute Care Nurse Practitioner
Neuroscience Intensive Care Unit
Medical University of South Caroli-
na
Charleston, South Carolina

Susan Hunt, MSN, ACNP-BC
Adjunct Assistant Professor
Adult-Gerontology Acute Care
Nurse Practitioner Program Coordinator
Indiana University
School of Nursing
Indianapolis, Indiana

Lindsay Iverson, DNP, ACNP-BC
Assistant Professor
Adult-Gerontology Acute Care
Nurse Practitioner Program Coordinator
Creighton University
College of Nursing
Omaha, Nebraska

Carolyn I. Johnson, MSN, ACNP-BC, ARNP-BC
Post-Acute Rehabilitation Nurse
Practitioner
Advanced Registered Nurse Practitioner Manor Care Post-Acute
Rehabilitation
Waterloo, Iowa

Karin Jonczak, MSN, ACNP-BC, CRNP, CNRN
Neurovascular Nurse Practitioner
Neurovascular Associates of Abington
Neurosciences Institute
Comprehensive Stroke Center
Abington Memorial Hospital
Abington, Pennsylvania

Vanessa M. Kalis, DNP, ACNP-BC, PNP, CNS
Assistant Professor
Director of the Adult-Gerontologic
Acute Care Doctor of Nursing Practice Program
Brandman University
Irvine, California

Kimberly J. Langer, MSN, ACNP-BC
Associate Professor and Program
Coordinator
Acute Care Nurse Practitioner
Program
Winona State University
Rochester, Minnesota
Mayo Clinic
Division of Blood and Marrow
Transplant
Rochester, Minnesota

Beatrice K. Launius, MSN, ACNP-BC, CCRN
Adjunct faculty
Coordinator Adult-Gerontology
Acute Care Nurse Practitioner
Program
Northwestern State University
Shreveport, Louisiana
Clinical instructor
Chief Nurse Practitioner Division
of Trauma and Critical Care Surgery
Louisiana State University Health
Sciences Center Shreveport
Shreveport, Louisiana

Gail Ann Lis, DNP, ACNP-BC
Professor
Madonna University
College of Nursing and Health
Livonia, Michigan

Lisa Marchetti, MSN, ACNP-BC
Nurse Practitioner
Surgical Intensive Care Unit
William Beaumont Hospital
Royal Oak, Michigan

Tara McEnany, DNP, ACNP-BC, FNP-BC
Assistant Professor
Allen College
Unity Point Health
Waterloo, Iowa

Taylor A. Mercier, MSN, ACNP-BC, FNP-BC
Acute Care Nurse Practitioner
Emergency Care Specialist
Spectrum Health Butterworth
Emergency Department
Grand Rapids, Michigan

Deidre Meyer, MSN, ACNP-BC
Acute Care Nurse Practitioner
ProMedica Physicians Group
The Toledo Hospital
Toledo, Ohio

Rebecca L. Mogensen, MSN, ACNP-BC, APNP
Acute Care Nurse Practitioner
Division of Hospital Medicine
University of Wisconsin Medical Foundation
University of Wisconsin Hospital and Clinics
Madison, Wisconsin

S. Lori Neal, MSN, ACNP-BC, FNP-BC
Trauma Nurse Practitioner
Erlanger Trauma Services
Chattanooga, Tennessee

Jeni Page, MSN, ACNP-BC
Acute Care Nurse Practitioner
Neurosurgery
Swedish Neuroscience Institute
Seattle, Washington

Elizabeth Palermo, MSN, ACNP-BC, ANP-BC
Assistant Professor of Clinical Nursing
Acute Care Nurse Practitioner Program Specialty Director
University of Rochester
School of Nursing
Rochester, New York
Acute Care Nurse Practitioner
Hospital Medicine Division
Strong Memorial Hospital
Rochester, New York

Carmen Paniagua, EdD, ACNP-BC, AGACNP-BC, APNG-BC, FAANP
Clinical Instructor
Department of Emergency Medicine
University of Arkansas for Medical Sciences
College of Medicine
Little Rock, Arkansas
Adult Acute Care Nurse Practitioner and Adult-Gerontology Acute Care Nurse Practitioner
Gastroenterology Associates of Southeast Arkansas (GASA)
Pine Bluff, Arkansas

Patty Pawlow, MSN, ACNP-BC
Lecturer
Course Director
Adult Gerontology Acute Care Nurse Practitioner Program
University of Pennsylvania
School of Nursing
Philadelphia, Pennsylvania

Leslie Karns Payne, PhD, ACNP-BC, FNP
Assistant Professor
Baylor University Louise Herrington
School of Nursing
Dallas, Texas

Daniel J. Rauh, MSN, AGACNP-BC, CCRN, EMT-P
Emergency Department Nurse Practitioner
Good Samaritan Hospital
Cincinnati, Ohio

Rosalyn R. Reischman, PhD, ACNP-BC
Adult-Gerontology Acute Care Nurse Practitioner Program Coordinator
University of Florida
College of Nursing
Gainesville, Florida

Patti Renaud, MSN, ACNP-BC
Acute Care Nurse Practitioner
Hepatobiliary and Transplant Surgery
Henry Ford Health System
Detroit, Michigan

Molly K. Rothmeyer, DNP, APRN, FNP-BC, PNP-AC, Fellow NAPNAP
Adjunct Faculty
Graduate Nursing Program
Maryville University
Catherine McAuley School of Nursing
College of Health Professions
St. Louis, Missouri
Adjunct Faculty
Graduate Nursing Program
Brandman University
Marybelle and S. Paul Musco School of Nursing and Health Professions
Irvine, California

Lori Rubio, DNP, ACNP-BC, MBA, HCM
Acute Care Nurse Practitioner
University Medical Center
Ysleta Clinic
El Paso, Texas

Kara Rumley, MSN, ACNP-BC
Vascular Surgery Acute Care Nurse Practitioner
Regional Hemodialysis Access Coordinator
Evansville Surgical Associates
Evansville, Indiana

Alexandra E. Saborio, MSN, ACNP-BC
Acute Care Nurse Practitioner
Inpatient Specialty Program
Cedars-Sinai Medical Center
Los Angeles, California

Kristine Anne Scordo, PhD, ACNP-BC, FAANP
Professor and Director
Adult-Gerontology Acute Care
Nurse Practitioner Program
Wright State University
College of Nursing
Dayton, Ohio

Julie Settles, MSN, ACNP-BC, CEN
Clinical Research Scientist
Indianapolis, Indiana

Michelle R. Smith, MSN, AGACNP-BC
Hospitalist Nurse Practitioner
Indiana University Health Ball
Memorial Hospital
Hospitalist Department
Muncie, Indiana

Mary Beth Tombes, MSN, ACNP-BC, CCRC
Clinical Research Nurse Practitioner
Virginia Commonwealth University
Massey Cancer Center
Richmond, Virginia

Colleen R. Walsh, DNP, ACNP-BC, ONC, ONP-C, CS
Contract Assistant Professor of
Graduate Nursing
University of Southern Indiana
College of Nursing and Health
Evansville, Indiana

Marjorie G. Webb, DNP, ACNP-BC
Associate Professor
Interim Department Chair
Community and Professional Studies
Metropolitan State University
School of Nursing, College of Health
Saint Paul, Minnesota

Brett Whaley, MSN, ACNP-BC
Adjunct Professor
Evolution Health Transitional
Care and Urgent Care Program Developer, Manager, and Clinician
Texas Woman's University
College of Nursing
Denton, Texas

Julie L. Yerke, MSN, ACNP-BC
Acute Care Nurse Practitioner
Floyd Medical Center
Rome, GA

Sheila Zielinski, DNP, ACNP-BC, FNP-BC, CCRN, CEN
Intensive Care Unit Nurse Practitioner
Indiana University Health Physicians, Pulmonary & Critical Care
Indiana University Health – Methodist
Indianapolis, Indiana

Table of Contents

SECTION **TWO**

Management of Patients with Cardiovascular Disorders

SECTION **THREE**

Management of Patients with Pulmonary Disorders

SECTION **FOUR**

Management of Patients with Gastrointestinal Disorders

SECTION **FIVE**

Management of Patients with Genitourinary Disorders

SECTION **SIX**

Management of Patients with Endocrine Disorders

SECTION **SEVEN**

Management of Patients with Musculoskeletal Disorders

SECTION **EIGHT**

Management of Patients with Hematologic Disorders

SECTION **NINE**

Management of Patients with Oncologic Disorders

SECTION **TEN**

Management of Patients with Immunologic Disorders

SECTION **TWELVE**

Common Problems in Acute Care

SECTION **THIRTEEN**

Health Promotion

Management of Patients With Neurologic Disorders

CHAPTER 1

Cerebrovascular Accidents: Brain Attack

TRAVIS BRADLEY • CHARLENE MYERS

TRANSIENT ISCHEMIC ATTACK

I. **Definition**
   A. Classic definition: sudden or rapid onset of neurologic deficit caused by focal ischemia that lasts for a few minutes and resolves completely within 24 hr
   B. It has been found that with more widespread use of modern imaging techniques for the brain, up to one third of patients with symptoms lasting less than 24 hr actually have a small infarct.
   C. Updated definition: a transient episode of neurological dysfunction caused by focal brain, spinal cord, or retinal ischemia, without acute infarction

II. **Incidence/prevalence**
   A. Incidence is 160/100,000; prevalence is 135/100,000

III. **Etiology**
   A. Atherosclerotic disease
      1. Aorta
      2. Carotid arteries
      3. Vertebral arteries
      4. Intracranial atherosclerosis
   B. Cardiac emboli as seen in arrhythmia (atrial fibrillation), myocardial infarction (MI), congestive cardiomyopathy, and valvular disease
   C. Vasculitis conditions such as moyamoya disease, fibromuscular dysplasia, lupus, and others
   D. Hematologic causes
      1. Red blood cell (RBC) disorders
         a. Increased sludging
         b. Decreased cerebral oxygenation such as in severe anemia

    c. Polycythemia, sickle cell anemia

  2. Platelet disorders

    a. Thrombocytosis

    b. Thrombocytopenia

  3. Increased viscosity/hypercoagulable conditions

    a. Antiphospholipid antibody syndrome (e.g., lupus anticoagulant, anticardiolipin antibody)

    b. Oral contraceptive and/or estrogen use

    c. Antithrombin III deficiency

    d. Protein S and C deficiency

    e. Tissue-type plasminogen activator (t-PA) and plasminogen deficiencies

    f. Patients particularly at risk for a hypercoagulable state:

      i. Older than 45 years

      ii. History of thrombolytic event

      iii. History of spontaneous abortion

      iv. Related autoimmune conditions (e.g., lupus)

      v. Stroke of unknown cause

      vi. Family history of thrombotic events

  4. Myeloproliferative disorders, leukemia with white blood cell count greater than 150,000

E. Intracranial causes

  1. Brain tumor

  2. Focal seizure

  3. Hemorrhage

    a. Subdural hematoma (SDH)

    b. Subarachnoid hemorrhage (SAH)

    c. Intracerebral hemorrhage (ICH), which may cause cerebrovascular dysfunction due to leakage of blood outside the normal vessels

F. Subclavian steal syndrome

  1. Localized stenosis or occlusion of a subclavian artery proximal to the source of the vertebral artery, so that blood is stolen from that artery

  2. Blood pressure (BP) is significantly lower in the affected arm than in the opposite arm.

G. Others

  1. Transient hypotension

  2. Osteophytes that cause compression of neck vessels

  3. Cocaine abuse

  4. Hypoglycemia

  5. Migraines

IV. **Risk factors**

A. A transient ischemic attack (TIA) is an important predictor of stroke.

  1. The 90-day risk of stroke after a TIA is as high as 17%

   2. The greatest risk is within the first week
   3. Approximately one third of stroke patients have a history of TIA
B. Hypertension
C. Cardiac disease, such as the following:
   1. Mitral valve disease
   2. Anterior wall MI
   3. Congestive myopathy
   4. Arrhythmia (e.g., atrial fibrillation)
D. Smoking
E. Obesity
F. Hyperlipidemia
G. Elevated homocysteine levels in the elderly
H. Advanced age
I. Diabetes
J. Alcohol and recreational drug abuse

V.   **Clinical manifestations**
A. Carotid artery syndrome
   1. Hemianopia, ipsilateral monocular blindness (amaurosis fugax) described as similar to a shade coming down over one eye
   2. Visual field cut
   3. Paresthesia/weakness of contralateral arm, leg, and face (may be episodic)
   4. Dysarthria, transient aphasia
   5. Confusion
   6. Gait disturbance
   7. Carotid bruit may be present
   8. Microemboli, hemorrhage, and exudate may be visualized in the ipsilateral retina
B. Vertebrobasilar artery syndrome
   1. Visual bilateral disturbances (blurred vision, diplopia, and complete blindness)
   2. Vertigo and ataxia
   3. Nausea and/or vomiting
   4. Sudden loss of postural tone in all extremities while consciousness remains intact (drop attacks)
   5. Dysarthria
   6. Facial paresthesia
   7. Gait instability

VI.   **Diagnostics/laboratory findings**
A. Laboratory evaluation may include the following:
   1. Complete blood count (CBC), platelet count, prothrombin time (PT), partial thromboplastin time (PTT), and international normalized ratio (INR) to detect these conditions:
      a. Anemia
      b. Polycythemia

        c. Leukemia

        d. Thrombocytopenia

        e. Hypercoagulopathy

2. Electrolytes, glucose to detect the following:

        a. Hyponatremia

        b. Hypokalemia

        c. Hypoglycemia

        d. Hyperglycemia

3. Lipid profile

        a. Detects hyperlipidemia

4. In selected patients, antinuclear antibody, Venereal Disease Research Laboratory (VDRL) test, and toxicology screen

5. Sedimentation rate, to detect these conditions:

        a. Vasculitis

        b. Infective endocarditis

        c. Hyperviscosity

        d. Giant cell arteritis

6. Homocysteine level

        a. An amino acid

        b. Elevated plasma level associated with increased risk of vascular events

7. Anticardiolipin antibodies (immunoglobulin [Ig]G, IgM, and IgA) and assay for lupus anticoagulant for suspected antiphospholipid antibody syndromes

8. Assays for antithrombin III, proteins S and C, plasminogen, and t-PA

B. Computed tomographic (CT) scan of the head

    1. May reveal "silent" ischemia or ischemic images, as well as hemorrhage or infarct and SDH

C. Magnetic resonance imaging (MRI), particularly diffusion-weighted imaging, and perfusion-weighted imaging

    1. More sensitive than CT scan to early pathologic changes of ischemic infarction because of its excellent detection of brain edema

    2. MRI is also preferred for the detection of lacunar or vertebrobasilar TIAs, or when vascular territory is not well defined.

    3. Up to one third of patients with TIAs have an infarct in the territory relevant to their symptoms

D. Duplex ultrasonography

    1. 85% sensitivity and 90% specificity

    2. Useful in identifying hemodynamically significant carotid stenosis

E. CT angiography (CTA)

    1. Evaluation of neck and brain vessels

    2. Requires use of contrast material

        a. Normal renal function

        b. Adequate intravenous access

F. Magnetic resonance angiography (MRA)

    1. Alternative to ultrasound or CT studies

    2. No contrast medium is needed

    3. Can be obtained at the same time as an MRI scan

    4. Good means for assessment of extracranial and intracranial vessels

G. Echocardiography and a 24-hr Holter monitor are used to evaluate for a cardiac source of emboli.

H. Transesophageal echocardiography (TEE) to evaluate the aortic arch, left atrium, and for patent foramen ovale

I. Cerebral angiography for patients whose symptoms suggest involvement of the carotid circulation and who are candidates for carotid endarterectomy (CEA)

J. Chest x-ray for enlarged heart

K. Blood cultures to monitor for infective endocarditis

L. Temporal artery biopsy to detect giant cell arteritis

M. Cardiac enzymes to detect an acute MI

N. Electroencephalography indicated in patients suspected of having a seizure disorder associated with stroke, as well as an underlying toxic-metabolic disorder that may cause seizure activity

VII. **Management**

A. Address the following underlying risk factors:

    1. Hypertension

    2. Diabetes mellitus (DM)

    3. Obesity

    4. Hyperlipidemia

    5. Smoking

B. Carotid TIAs

    1. Greater than 70%–80% obstruction: intervention is indicated for those who are a good surgical risk

    2. Controversy exists about patients who have 50%–69% obstruction but are symptomatic; should be evaluated on a case-by-case basis by a vascular specialist.

    3. Less than 50% obstruction: surgery is not indicated

    4. Carotid angioplasty and stenting (CAS) is an alternative to CEA

    5. Several recent trials such as the Stenting and Angioplasty with Protection in Patients with High Risk for Endarterectomy (SAPPHIRE) and the Carotid Revascularization Endarterectomy versus Stent Trial (CREST) reveal that CAS is safe and effective.

        a. Determination of CAS versus CEA is largely based on availability of trained personal and institutional expertise

C. Anticoagulation if caused by a cardioembolic event from atrial fibrillation or paroxysmal atrial fibrillation

    1. May prevent recurrent cardioembolic events

2. Traditional treatment has been a bridging of heparin to warfarin (Coumadin). Although with newer-generation anticoagulants, the heparin bridge may not be necessary.
3. Begin with heparin, 12 units/kg/hr
4. Target PTT should be 1.5–2.5 times patient's baseline value
5. Follow with warfarin, 5–10 mg PO (orally), which is indicated for the following:
   a. TIA caused by embolism arising from a mural thrombus after an MI
   b. TIA caused by embolus in patients with mitral stenosis or prosthetic heart valves
   c. Recurrent TIAs despite platelet antiaggregant agents
   d. INR of 2–3 is considered therapeutic
D. Common antiplatelet therapy
1. Aspirin (acetylsalicylic acid) decreases incidence of subsequent stroke by 15%–30% in male patients with TIAs; dose of 81–325 mg/day is as effective as higher doses and causes fewer adverse effects
2. Clopidogrel (Plavix)
   a. Indicated for secondary prevention of ischemic stroke, MI, and other vascular events in patients who cannot tolerate aspirin, or in patients who were taking aspirin at the time of the event
   b. Dosage is 75 mg/day PO
   c. May cause thrombotic thrombocytopenia purpura during the first 2 weeks of treatment
3. Aspirin, 25 mg/extended-release dipyridamole, 200 mg (Aggrenox)
   a. Both drugs suppress platelet aggregation but do so through different mechanisms
   b. Combination treatment is more effective than either drug alone
   c. Recommended dose is one capsule PO twice a day
   d. Significantly more expensive than aspirin therapy
   e. Main side effect is headache

STROKE/BRAIN ATTACK

I. **Definition**
A. Rapid onset of a neurologic deficit involving ischemia to a certain vascular territory and lasting longer than 24 hr
B. A stroke in evolution is an enlarging infarction manifested by neurologic defects that increase over 24–48 hr
C. Because of advances in early recognition and treatment, stroke dropped from being the third leading cause of death to the fourth. It remains the leading cause of disability.

  D. Stroke can be classified as ischemic and hemorrhagic

  E. Eighty percent of strokes are caused by blood clots that produce ischemic areas in the brain; remaining 20% of strokes are caused by ICH

II. **Etiology and risk factors**

  A. Same as for TIA

  B. Cocaine-related stroke is increasingly common

  C. Women who use oral contraceptives and who smoke are at high risk

  D. Hyperlipidemia raises the risk of ischemic stroke

  E. Low cholesterol increases the risk of hemorrhagic stroke

III. **Public education**

  A. Need to increase public awareness of the warning signs of stroke to facilitate early treatment

  B. Five "suddens" of stroke:

   1. Sudden weakness

   2. Sudden speech difficulty

   3. Sudden visual loss

   4. Sudden dizziness

   5. Sudden severe headache

  C. Need to call 9-1-1 and/or active emergency medical systems (EMS) to expedite best chance of meeting treatment window limits

  D. Should be treated like a heart attack; "brain attack" may become new nomenclature

IV. **Prehospital stroke management**

  A. Implementation strategies for emergency medical services within stroke systems of care policy statement:

   1. Dispatched to highest level of care available in the shortest possible time

   2. Time between call and dispatch of response team less than 90 seconds

   3. EMS response time less than 8 min

   4. On-scene time less than 15 min barring extenuating circumstances

   5. Travel time equivalent to trauma or acute MI calls

V. **Stroke systems of care**

  A. Goals of creating stroke systems of care include stroke prevention, community stroke education, optimal use of EMS, effective acute and subacute stroke management, rehabilitation, and performance review of stroke care delivery.

  B. Hospitals with the capacity and commitment to deliver acute stroke care in the emergency department and stroke unit are essential to effective stroke care.

  C. Transporting patients to stroke centers optimizes their chance of timely therapy and decreases the morbidity and mortality associated with stroke.

VI. Primary stroke center
- **A.** Established in 2004 by The Joint Commission (TJC); currently more than 800 primary stroke centers exist
- **B.** Have dedicated and organized stroke resources that lead to increased rates of intravenous t-PA administration, increased lipid profile testing, improved deep vein thrombosis prophylaxis, and better clinical outcomes

VII. Comprehensive stroke center
- **A.** Criteria established in 2011 by the American Stroke Association
- **B.** Ability to offer 24/7 state-of-the-art care on the full spectrum of cerebrovascular disease
- **C.** Neurocritical care units and interventional radiology for cerebral interventions essential
- **D.** Can be part of a "hub and spoke" model of care to maximize stroke care
- **E.** Even patients with a large infarct, but outside intervention window, should be admitted to a neurocritical care unit for complication management.

ISCHEMIC STROKE

I. Etiology
- **A.** Caused by a thrombus that occludes a blood vessel in the head or neck (30%)
    1. Progression of symptoms over hours to days, or can be sudden
    2. Patients often have a history of TIA.
    3. Predisposing factors:
        - **a.** Atherosclerosis
        - **b.** Hypertension (HTN)
        - **c.** DM
        - **d.** Hyperlipidemia
        - **e.** Vasculitis
        - **f.** Hypotension
        - **g.** Smoking
        - **h.** Connective tissue disorders
        - **i.** Trauma to the head and neck
- **B.** Caused by embolism (25%)
    1. Very rapid onset
    2. History of TIA
    3. Predisposing factors:
        - **a.** Atrial fibrillation
        - **b.** Mitral stenosis and regurgitation
        - **c.** Endocarditis
        - **d.** Mitral valve prolapse

II. Clinical manifestations (depending on the cerebral vessel involved)
- **A.** Middle cerebral artery

1. Hemiplegia (involves upper extremity and face more often than lower extremity)
2. Hemianesthesia
3. Hemianopia (blindness of half the field of vision)
4. Eyes may deviate to the side of the lesion
5. Aphasia if dominant hemisphere is involved
6. Neglect syndrome
7. Occlusions of various branches of the middle cerebral artery may cause different findings (involvement of the anterior division may cause expressive aphasia, and involvement of the posterior branch may produce receptive aphasia).

B. Anterior cerebral artery
1. Hemiplegia (lower extremity more often than upper extremity)
2. Primitive reflexes
3. Confusion
4. Abulia
5. Bilateral anterior infarction may cause behavioral changes and disturbance in memory.

C. Vertebral and basilar arteries
1. Decreased level of consciousness (LOC)
2. Vertigo
3. Dysphagia
4. Diplopia
5. Ipsilateral cranial nerve findings
6. Contralateral (or bilateral) sensory and motor deficits

D. Deep penetrating branches of major cerebral arteries (lacunar infarction)
1. Most common: less than 5 mm in diameter
2. Associated with poorly controlled HTN or diabetes
3. Contralateral pure motor or sensory deficits
4. Ipsilateral ataxia with crural (pertaining to the leg or thigh) paresis
5. Dysarthria with clumsiness of the hand

III.   Diagnostics/laboratory findings

A. CT scan of the head without contrast should be done initially
1. Preferable to MRI in the acute stage to rule out cerebral hemorrhage as MRI is usually not as readily available, especially for patients who present with stroke symptoms and are on anticoagulation therapy; also will rule out abscess, tumor, and SDH
2. Appears as an area of decreased density
3. Lacunar infarcts appear as small, punched-out, hypodense areas.
4. Initial CT scan may be negative, and the infarct may not be visible for up to 24 hr

B. Chest radiography
1. May reveal cardiomegaly or valvular calcification

2. Neoplasm may suggest metastasis rather than stroke as the cause of neurologic deficits

3. Dilated aorta may reveal aortic dissection.

C. CBC, sedimentation rate, blood glucose, VDRL, lipid profile, INR, PTT prior to anticoagulation, blood urea nitrogen/serum creatinine (Cr) to evaluate renal function before contrast media may be given, homocysteine level, drug screen, and blood alcohol level

D. Electrocardiogram (ECG) (if unrevealing, may place patient on cardiac monitor/Holter monitor)

E. Blood cultures if endocarditis is suspected

F. Echocardiography with bubble study

G. TEE to detect dysfunction of left atrium (thrombus)

H. Carotid duplex ultrasonography

I. MRI/MRA: Diffusion-weighted MRI is more sensitive than conventional MRI in detecting cerebral ischemia.

J. CTA
  1. Can provide information regarding vascular anatomy with three-dimensional reconstruction (requires the use of contact dye)
  2. May allow for rapid evaluation and diagnosis in hospitals without MRI capability
  3. Can be used to image the carotid arteries instead of duplex ultrasonography, and will show internal carotid artery structure
  4. CT perfusion can also be performed as part of the CTA, which can provide evidence of salvageable tissue (penumbra) or an already completed infarct, and may affect the treatment plan.

K. Cerebral angiography continues to be the gold standard for complete evaluation of intracranial and extracranial vessels

L. Lumbar puncture (LP)
  1. Not always necessary but may be helpful if the cause of stroke is uncertain
  2. Obtain a CT scan first to rule out cerebral hemorrhage or any expanding mass that could lead to herniation if LP is performed

IV. **Management**

A. Correct treatment depends on a correct diagnosis of stroke type; therefore, it is imperative that diagnostic tests be completed quickly. A report from the National Institute of Neurological Disorders and Stroke advocates the following goals, which are based on time of arrival:
  1. Perform an initial emergency department evaluation within 10 min
  2. Notify the stroke team or neurologist within 15 min
  3. Start a CT scan within 25 min
  4. Obtain a CT scan interpretation within 45 min
  5. Administer thrombolytics, if appropriate, within 60 min
  6. Transfer the patient to an inpatient bed within 3 hr

B. BP control

1. Acute lowering of systemic BP is not recommended because it may lead to further damage in the ischemic penumbra, in which autoregulation may be defective, and may clinically worsen the stroke.

2. Most patients with acute cerebral infarction have an elevated BP, which usually returns to baseline within 48 hr without any special treatment.

3. BP control may be warranted, however, in the following conditions:

   a. Systolic BP (SBP) exceeds 220 mmHg, and diastolic BP (DBP) exceeds 120 mmHg (malignant hypertension)

   b. Hypertensive encephalopathy is present

   c. Vital organs are compromised

   d. Aortic dissection

   e. Symptomatic cardiac disease

   f. Patient is receiving t-PA therapy

      i. Some experts recommend decreasing BP in those who are receiving intravenous heparin therapy as well, although this is not universally accepted.

   g. In patients who are candidates for t-PA, BP should be lowered to SBP less than 185 and DBP less than 110 prior to t-PA administration. After t-PA administration, SBP should be maintained less than 180 and DBP less than 105.

4. When indicated, BP should be lowered by approximately 15% and closely watched for neurological deterioration related to decreased perfusion.

5. The current 2013 Stroke Guidelines recommend the use of either labetalol, 10–20 mg IV push over 1–2 min, can repeat once; or nicardipine, intravenous drip titratable from 2.5–15 mg/hr for BP management.

6. An alternative is esmolol (Brevibloc), 2.5 grams/250 ml NS or 2 grams/100 ml NS continuous infusion titrated to desired BP; maximum dose should not exceed 300 mcg/kg/min.

C. Anticoagulation

   1. Intravenous heparin has historically been used as a treatment for acute stroke. However, it does not reduce the severity of a stroke that has occurred and is no longer routinely recommended. The decision to even consider the use of heparin in the acute management of stroke should be determined by a neurology expert.

   2. It may be used in patients with stroke in evolution and in hypercoagulable states, or in patients with very high-risk or recurrent emboli.

3. Heparin may increase the risk of transformation from ischemic stroke to hemorrhagic stroke and, therefore, is not recommended for massive stroke.

4. No loading dose of heparin is recommended as the potential risk of hemorrhagic transformation is high. A maintenance infusion of 12 units/kg/hr (max 1000 units/hr) can be started. PTT should be 1.5–2.5 patient's baseline value.

5. Heparin followed by warfarin (5–10 mg/day PO) is indicated as secondary prevention in suspected cerebral embolism resulting from the following:

   a. Mural thrombus

   b. Mitral stenosis

   c. Atrial fibrillation

   d. Mechanical heart valves

6. Several newer anticoagulants are now on the market and targeted at stroke prevention for patients with atrial fibrillation or paroxysmal atrial fibrillation.

   a. Dabigatran (Pradaxa) is a direct thrombin inhibitor. Originally used to prevent thromboembolic events after orthopedic procedures, the randomized evaluation of long-term anticoagulation therapy (RE-LY) study demonstrated that dabigatran had benefit compared with warfarin for prevention of stroke in patients with atrial fibrillation.

      i. Food and Drug Administration approved in 2010 at 150 mg BID, or 75 mg BID in renally-impaired patients.

   b. Apixaban (Eliquis) is a factor Xa inhibitor also recently approved for stroke prevention in patients with atrial fibrillation. Standard dose is 5 mg BID or 2.5 mg BID for patients greater than 80 years of age, body weight 60 kg or less, or Cr greater than 1.5 mg/dl.

   c. Rivaroxaban (Xarolto) is a factor Xa inhibitor approved for stroke prevention in patients with atrial fibrillation. Standard dose is 20 mg daily with evening meal for patients with creatinine clearance greater than 50 ml/min, or 15 mg daily with evening meal for patients with creatinine clearance 15–50 ml/min. Avoid use when CrCl less than 15 mL/min.

   d. Because of the mechanism of action of the above three drugs, no routine lab draws of PTT or INR are necessary for ongoing treatment and may facilitate better patient compliance.

   e. If acute hemorrhage develops, holding anticoagulants or use of activated charcoal may reverse bleeding. Empiric fresh frozen plasma, factor VII, or factor IX complex may be attempted in emergency situations.

      f. The decision to use one of the newer anticoagulants should be determined after a thorough discussion between the neurologist, cardiologist, patient, and/or family has occurred. The risks and benefits should be carefully examined.

    7. CT scan may be necessary after 48 hr to determine whether any hemorrhaging has occurred.

    8. Anticoagulation is contraindicated if CT scan or LP suggests cerebral hemorrhage, tumor, abscess, SDH, or epidural hematoma.

    9. Use cautiously in patients with a history of GI bleeding, bleeding tendencies, severe HTN, or a large cerebral infarct

  10. May be used after a completed stroke if embolization is determined to be the cause

D. Antiplatelet therapy may be used for non-cardioembolic stroke patients not due to vertebral or carotid dissection.

    1. Aspirin, 81–325 mg/day PO

        a. Continues to be the least expensive and most widely used antiplatelet medication

    2. Clopidogrel (Plavix), 75 mg PO daily

    3. Aggrenox (aspirin, 25 mg immediate release, and dipyridamole, 200 mg extended release), 1 tablet BID (1 in the morning and 1 at night)

        a. Approved for stroke prevention

        b. Study has shown that this combination may reduce stroke by 22% compared with aspirin therapy alone

E. Mannitol and/or hypertonic saline can be used for cerebral edema that may occur on the second or third day.

        a. Mannitol (0.25–1 gram/kg IV every 4–6 hr) may help decrease elevated intracranial pressure (ICP) by overall osmotic diuresis. Side effects can include acute kidney injury. Serum osmolality should be monitored.

        b. Hypertonic saline (23.4%) can be administered as an intravenous push through a central line in the event of an acute decompensation. Standard dose is 30 ml IV administered over greater than 30 min; subsequent doses dependent on ICP

        c. Hypertonic saline (3%) can be administered as an intravenous drip to maintain a higher sodium level at the discretion of the intensivist. Standard dose is initial bolus of 250–300 ml IV over 60 min, followed by continuous infusion titrated to treatment goals including 145–155 mEq/L and serum osmolality 310–320 mOsm/L. Recommend checking sodium levels every 6 hr and adjusting drip PRN.

F. Corticosteroids are used to reduce vasogenic cerebral edema related to tumor burden but are not recommended for cytotoxic edema from strokes. Hypertonic solutions are used to reduce cytotoxic edema associated with cerebral infarct.

G. t-PA is now being used, if appropriate conditions are met, as thrombolytic therapy for acute stroke when the patient is brought in within 3–4.5 hr after the stroke. The traditional window of 3 hr has been expanded to 4.5 hr with certain criteria listed below. Such conditions include the following:

1. Availability of a physician with appropriate expertise to diagnose the stroke
2. 24-hr availability of CT scanning to assess for hemorrhage
3. Capability of facility to manage intracranial hemorrhage or transfer to higher level of care
4. Patients must seek help early and have a well-defined onset of symptoms.
    a. Commonly called "last known well time"
5. Patient's condition must be carefully examined for contraindications, such as the following:
    a. Previous and/or current hemorrhage
    b. Previous stroke or head trauma within 3 months
    c. Major surgery within 14 days
    d. Urinary or GI hemorrhage within 24 days
    e. Seizure at stroke onset
    f. Arterial puncture at noncompressible site within 7 days
    g. Elevated PTT and PT (longer than 15 seconds)
    h. Oral anticoagulants or heparin with elevated PTT within 48 hr
    i. Serum glucose level less than 50 or greater than 400 mg/dl
    j. SBP greater than 185 mmHg or DBP greater than 110 mmHg
    k. Active internal bleeding within 22 days
6. Additional criteria for patients within the 3- to 4.5-hr window
    a. Inclusion:
        i. Ischemic stroke causing measurable deficit
        ii. Onset of symptoms within 3–4.5 hr
        iii. Age greater than 18 years
    b. Exclusion:
        i. Age greater than 80 years
        ii. Severe stroke (National Institutes of Health Stroke Scale greater than 25)
        iii. Taking an oral anticoagulant regardless of international normalized ratio
        iv. History of both diabetes and prior ischemic stroke
        v. SBP greater than 185 mmHg or DBP greater than 110 mmHg
7. Dose: 0.9 mg/kg (maximum dose of 90 mg) given over 60 min, with 10% of the calculated dose given as an initial bolus over one min
    a. Admit to stroke unit

      b. Vital signs and neuro checks every 15 min during and for 2 hr after administration, then every 30 min for 6 hr, then hourly until 24 hr after t-PA onset

H. Surgery and CEA may be indicated for those with high-grade extracranial carotid artery disease (greater than 70%) if not at high risk

I. Rehabilitation should take a multidisciplinary approach

J. Additional treatment options

    1. Mechanical reperfusion

      a. There are numerous devices available that are used to mechanically retrieve a clot from within a cerebral artery.

      b. Examples include the MERCI device, the Solitaire device, the Trevo device, and the Penumbra device

      c. Use is largely determined by the experience and expertise of the user and the institution

    2. Combined intra-arterial (IA) and intravenous thrombolysis

      a. The Interventional Management of Stoke (IMS) study evaluated the use of IA t-PA in patients who received standard intravenous t-PA but displayed little or no improvement by the end of the t-PA administration.

      b. The initial IMS and then IMS trial two showed good rates of recanalization of the occluded artery with comparable safety data to t-PA alone; however, the IMS trial three was stopped early for reported futility. Although the artery was recanalized, it has been reported that overall outcomes were not significantly better. Further study is warranted.

HEMORRHAGIC STROKE

I. **Definition**

    A. Condition resulting from bleeding into the subarachnoid space or brain parenchyma

    B. Accounts for approximately 14% of all cerebral infarctions

II. **Etiology**

    A. SAH

      1. Ruptured saccular aneurysm (85%)

      2. Arteriovenous malformation (AVM) (8%)

      3. Cryptogenic

    B. ICH

      1. Usually associated with HTN

      2. Predisposing factors

        a. HTN

        b. Use of anticoagulants or thrombolytics

        c. Use of illicit street drugs (e.g., cocaine)

        d. Heavy use of alcohol

        e. Hematologic disorders

III.   Clinical manifestations
- **A.** SAH
    1. Sudden headache of intense severity that radiates into the posterior neck region and is worsened by neck and head movements; often described as a "thunderclap headache" or "worst headache of my life"
    2. Grading scales: standardized way to describe SAH patients among providers
        - **a.** Hunt and Hess classification (clinical assessment)
            - **i.** Grade I: asymptomatic or slight headache
            - **ii.** Grade II: moderate to severe headache, stiff neck, no focal signs other than cranial nerve palsy
            - **iii.** Grade III: drowsy, mild focal deficit, or confusion
            - **iv.** Grade IV: stupor, hemiparesis
            - **v.** Grade V: deep coma, decerebration
        - **b.** Fisher grade (based on CT findings)
            - **i.** Grade I: no blood detected
            - **ii.** Grade II: diffuse or vertical layers less than 1 mm thick
            - **iii.** Grade III: localized clot and/or vertical layer $\geq$ 1 mm
            - **iv.** Grade IV: intracerebral or intraventricular clot with diffuse or no SAH
- **B.** ICH
    1. Elevation in BP, often to very high levels (90% of patients)
    2. Headache (40%)
    3. Vomiting is an important diagnostic sign, particularly if the hemorrhage lies in the cerebral hemisphere (49%).
    4. Sudden onset of neurologic deficits that can rapidly progress to coma or death, depending on area involved (50%)
    5. Basal ganglia hemorrhage
        - **a.** Conjugate deviation of eyes to the side of the lesion
        - **b.** Decreased LOC
        - **c.** Contralateral hemiplegia
        - **d.** Hemisensory disturbance
    6. Thalamic hemorrhage
        - **a.** Downward deviation of the eyes, looking at the nose
        - **b.** Pupils pinpoint with a positive reaction
        - **c.** Coma is common
        - **d.** Flaccid quadriplegia
    7. Cerebellar hemorrhage
        - **a.** Ipsilateral lateral conjugate gaze paresis
        - **b.** Pupils equal, round, reactive to light (PERRL)
        - **c.** Inability to stand or walk
        - **d.** Facial weakness
        - **e.** Ataxia of gait, limbs, or trunk
        - **f.** Vertigo and dysarthria

IV.   Diagnostics/laboratory findings

A. SAH

1. CT scan of the head will assist in differentiating between an ischemic and a hemorrhagic stroke.

a. Sensitivity of CT in the first 3 days after an aneurysmal SAH is very high (close to 100%). After 5–7 days, the rate of a negative CT scan increases, and LP should be considered.

b. Aneurysms less than 3 mm in size are unreliably demonstrated on CTA

c. Depending on site, size, CT scan quality, and whether or not fine cuts were obtained, aneurysm itself may be seen in 50% of cases when contrast material is given.

2. LP if CT scan is unavailable or negative and suspicion is high

a. Contraindicated in any expanding mass because it may cause herniation

b. A funduscopic examination must be performed prior to the procedure to rule out papilledema if no CT available

c. Cerebrospinal fluid (CSF) will be uniformly grossly bloody, although this may not occur if the bleed is small. In a true SAH, the LP reveals 103–106 RBCs/mm

d. Opening pressure may be elevated.

e. Xanthochromia is present.

  i. Yellowish discoloration of CSF produced by blood breakdown products

  ii. Xanthochromia appears no earlier than 2–4 hr after bleeding occurs

  iii. Cerebral angiography

   (a) Used to determine source of bleed, presence of an aneurysm, and best source of treatment (medical or surgical)

   (b) May demonstrate vasospasm

   (c) Should be performed after the patient has been stabilized

3. CTA is beneficial in patients who are too unstable to undergo cerebral angiography or in an emergent setting prior to surgical evacuation of clot.

B. ICH

1. CT scan without contrast

a. To confirm a bleed and determine the size and site

b. May reveal structural abnormalities such as aneurysms, AVMs, or brain tumors that may have caused the bleed, as well as complications such as herniation, intraventricular hemorrhage, or hydrocephalus

2. Cerebral angiography may be performed

a. To determine whether the source is an aneurysm or an AVM

  b. Should be considered for all patients without a clear cause of hemorrhage who are surgical candidates, particularly young, normotensive patients who are clinically stable

  c. Timing depends on the patient's clinical state and the neurosurgeon's judgment about the urgency of surgery, if needed

3. MRI and MRA may be useful for detecting structural abnormalities (i.e., AVMs and aneurysms). Gradient recalled echo MRI may be useful in detecting hemorrhage

4. CTA may be used to allow noninvasive imaging of large and medium-sized vessels

5. CBC, platelet count

6. Electrolytes

7. ECG

8. Chest x-ray

9. Bleeding time

10. PT/PTT

11. Liver enzymes

12. Renal studies

13. LP is contraindicated: may cause herniation in the presence of a large hematoma

V. **Management**

 A. SAH

  1. Basic ABCs first; many patients may need to be intubated if unable to protect airway

  2. External ventricular drain (EVD) placement if hydrocephalus seen on CT scan; relieving the pressure from acute hydrocephalus may dramatically improve a patient's LOC

  3. Strict bed rest in a quiet, stress-free environment

  4. Cardiac monitoring

  5. Treat symptomatically for headache or anxiety (acetaminophen and/or escalating opiates). Avoid use of nonsteroidal anti-inflammatory drugs due to bleeding risk.

  6. Have the patient avoid all forms of straining and exertion.

  7. Order stool softeners and laxatives (docusate [Colace], 100–200 mg PO/NG twice a day)

  8. Seizure prophylaxis

   a. Up to 26% of patients with SAH will experience seizures

   b. Short-term seizure prophylaxis is used to prevent seizures in the acutely ill patient and prevent spikes in BP and possible rebleeding of the aneurysm.

   c. Commonly used medications include:

    i. Phenytoin sodium (Dilantin), 100 mg IV every 8 hr, titrate to blood level 10–20 mcg/ml for 7 days

    ii. Levetiracetam (Keppra), 500 mg IV or PO twice a day for 7 days
       (a) Alternative to phenytoin; there is limited literature to support use for this indication and is not approved as monotherapy for seizures

  d. If the patient has a seizure during the acute phase, consider continuing antiepileptic therapy for a longer duration.

9. Acute hypertension can contribute to aneurysm re-rupture and should be aggressively managed.
  a. Maintain SBP less than 160 mmHg
  b. Consider intravenous titratable nicardipine drip or
  c. Labetalol, 10 mg intravenous push
  d. Hydralazine, 10–20 mg IV push if patient has bradycardia

10. Cerebral edema can be reduced with mannitol and/or hypertonic saline solutions.
  a. Mannitol, 0.25–1 gram/kg IV every 4–6 hr
  b. Saline, 3% solution, loading dose of 250–300 ml IV over 60 minutes, followed by continuous infusion titrated to treatment goals, including 145–155 mEq/L and serum osmolality of 310–320 mOsm/L
  c. Saline, 23.4% solution, 30 ml IV administrated over 30 min or longer, subsequent doses dependent on ICP

11. Surgical clipping or endovascular coiling should be performed as early as possible. Interventional choice of aneurysm obliteration is dependent on the size and location of the aneurysm, the patient's age and clinical condition, and the neurosurgeon's experience.

12. Coil embolization and/or stent placement for ruptured aneurysm: performed by trained neurovascular surgeon or neuroradiologist.
  a. Nonsurgical procedure involving the threading of tiny coils through a microcatheter into the aneurysm
  b. May be used when bleeding is in a difficult-to-reach area of the brain

13. Cerebral vasospasms
  a. Vasospasms occur in approximately 30% of patients. It is most frequent between days 7 and 10 after aneurysm rupture and usually resolves after 21 days. It may be associated with the presence of a thick clot in the subarachnoid space.
  b. Symptoms, which include confusion, decreased LOC, localizing neurological deficits, headache, and increased ICP, may or may not be present. Cerebral infarction can occur with severe vasospasm.

c. Calcium channel blockers (nimodipine) may be used to treat cerebral blood vessel spasm after SAH from ruptured aneurysms (60 mg PO/NGT every 4 hr for 3 weeks). Recent studies demonstrate improved neurological outcomes by processes other than preventing large vessel narrowing.

d. If symptomatic vasospasm occurs, the patient is usually treated with IVF loading. Traditional "triple H" therapy has been modified to euvolemia maintenance and induced hypertension.

   i. Aim for a hematocrit of approximately 30% (although optimal hemoglobin levels are still to be determined)

   ii. Monitor cardiac output and central venous pressure if necessary

   iii. The goal is to optimize the low shear rate viscosity of the whole blood and to ensure cerebral perfusion pressure (CPP) that is adequate to restore regional cerebral blood flow in perfusion areas beyond the vasospastic vessels

e. Treatment is less risky if the aneurysm has been clipped

f. Balloon angioplasty or IA vasodilators may be used for vasospasms resistant to the preceding treatments

g. Daily transcranial Doppler ultrasounds should be performed to monitor for vasospasm

14. Rebleeding

   a. Rebleeding is unpredictable but often occurs between days 2 and 19 after initial rupture and is thought to originate from fibrinolysis of the clot at the site of the ruptured aneurysm.

   b. Forty percent of patients rebleed, and approximately half of these rebleeds are fatal; therefore, efforts to seal off an aneurysm should be made as soon as possible.

   c. Neurologic deterioration is generally abrupt

   d. A repeat CT scan, and occasionally a repeat LP, is needed to confirm rebleeding

   e. The use of antifibrinolytic agents (aminocaproic acid, tranexamic acid) to prevent rebleeding and decrease mortality in patients with subarachnoid hemorrhage is controversial. Use of these agents has been associated with an increase in cerebral ischemia and no significant decrease has been noted in mortality rate or in degree of disability among survivors.

   f. For patients with an unavoidable delay in obliteration of aneurysm, a significant risk of rebleeding, and no compelling medical contraindications, short term (less than 72 hr) therapy with tranexamic acid or aminocaproic acid is reasonable to reduce the risk of every aneurysm rebleeding.

15. Cerebral salt wasting

   a. Hyponatremia develops after aneurysmal SAH.

      b. Excessive secretion of natriuretic peptides that causes hyponatremia from excessive natriuresis and volume contraction

      c. Crystalloid fluid replacement to maintain euvolemia

      d. Three percent saline solution to correct hyponatremia

      e. Consider fludrocortisone to aid in correction of hypovolemia and hyponatremia and to maintain euvolemia

16. Fever

      a. Most common medical complication in aneurysmal SAH

      b. The presence of fever that is noninfectious (central) has been associated with severity of injury, amount of hemorrhage, and development of vasospasm

      c. May be a marker of a systemic inflammatory state

      d. Fever often associated with worse cognitive outcomes

      e. Aggressive fever management is recommended

B. ICH

   1. Initial management should be directed toward the basic airway, breathing, and circulation and toward focal neurologic deficits.

   2. Intubation is indicated for insufficient ventilation, for hypoxia (partial pressure of oxygen [Po_2] less than 60 mmHg or partial pressure of carbon dioxide [Pco_2] greater than 50 mmHg), and for obvious risk of aspiration.

   3. Oxygen should be administered to all patients with possible ICH

   4. Control severe HTN

      a. Should be achieved through short-acting agents like nicardipine that are titratable

      b. The goal is to decrease the risk of ongoing bleeding from ruptured small arteries and arterioles.

      c. Overaggressive treatment of HTN may decrease CPP and, therefore, worsen brain injury, particularly in the setting of increased intracranial pressure.

      d. However, recent studies demonstrate that SBP kept above 140–150 mmHg was associated with more than double the risk of subsequent death or dependency.

      e. Further study is still warranted, but current evidence suggests that acute lowering of SBP to 140 mmHg is probably safe.

      f. Patients should be carefully monitored during the BP lowering phase, and if neurological exam deteriorates, consider increasing the BP goal to improve cerebral perfusion

   5. CPP (Mean arterial pressure[MAP]-ICP) should be kept at 50–70 mmHg

   6. Some suggested medications for elevated BP include the following:

      a. Labetalol (Trandate), 5–10 mg IV push

    b. Nicardipene (Cardene), intravenous titratable drip, 2.5–15 mg/hr

    c. Esmolol (Brevibloc), maintenance, 50–300 mcg/kg/min

7. If BP falls to less than 90 mmHg, pressors should be given (dopamine, 2–20 mcg/kg/min; phenylephrine, 0.5–5 mcg/kg/min (50–400 mcg/min); epinephrine, 0.01–0.2 mcg/kg/min (1–10 mcg/min); or norepinephrine [Levophed], 0.01–0.5 mcg/kg/min (1–40 mcg/min).

8. Maintain ICP at less than 20 mmHg and CPP at greater than 50–70 mmHg

    a. Mannitol for cerebral edema (0.25–1 gram/kg of a 20% solution) given intravenously every 4–6 hr

        i. Because of its rebound phenomenon, mannitol is recommended for 5 days or less

        ii. Serum osmolality should be measured BID for those receiving osmotherapy and should be kept at no greater than 320 mOsm/L. Watch renal function carefully and fluid balance status.

    b. Hypertonic saline may also be used to treat cerebral edema

        i. Three percent saline infusions may be started with sodium checks every 6 hr. Administer loading dose of 250–300 ml IV over 60 minutes, followed by continuous infusion titrated to treatment goals. Goal sodium levels of up to 145–155 mEq/L and serum osmolality of 310–320 mOsm/L are at the discretion of the intensivist.

        ii. Twenty-three percent saline may be given in an acutely decompensating patient as an emergency measure to treat elevated ICP. Administer as 30 ml IV over 30 min or longer; subsequent doses dependent on ICP.

    c. Ventricular drain for secondary hydrocephalus

        i. Use should not exceed 7 days because of possible infectious complications

        ii. Intravenous antibiotic prophylaxis may be used if ventricular catheter is non-antibiotic coated

    d. If hyperventilation is used, PCO2 should be maintained at 30–35 mmHg

    e. Steroids are not recommended

9. Supportive measures

    a. IVFs (normal saline fluid of choice)

        i. Excessive administration can worsen cerebral edema.

        ii. Goal is euvolemia.

        iii. Fluid balance is calculated by measuring daily urine production and adding 500 ml for insensible losses plus 300 ml per degree in febrile patients.

   b. Phenytoin (Dilantin), 100 mg every 8 hr, titrate to blood level
   10–20 mcg/ml
      i. Levetiracetam (Keppra), 500 mg IV/PO twice a day, as
         an alternative to phenytoin
   c. Nutritional support
   d. Maintain body temperature with acetaminophen (Tylenol),
   650 mg for temperature greater than 101.3°F (38.5°C).
   e. Physical therapy
   f. Skin care/turning
10. Surgery
   a. Indicated for patients with cerebellar hemorrhage greater than
   3 cm in diameter
   b. Indicated for those with surgically accessible cerebral
   hematoma generally extending to within one cm of the cortical
   surface
   c. Patients with a hemorrhage greater than 1 cm from the cortical
   surface or with a GCS score of 8 or less tended to do worse
   with surgical removal as compared with medical management.
   d. Must take into account age and overall prognosis when
   considering a surgical intervention

BIBLIOGRAPHY

Adams, H. P., Jr. (2009). Secondary prevention of atherothrombotic events after ischemic stroke. *Mayo Clinic Proceedings, 84*(1), 43–51.

Bederson, J. B., Connolly, E. S., Batjer, H. H., Dacey, R. G., Dion, J. E., Diringer, M. N., ... Rosenwasser, R. H. (2009). Guidelines for the management of aneurysmal subarachnoid hemorrhage: A statement for healthcare professionals from a special writing group of the Stroke Council, American Heart Association. *Stroke, 40*(3), 994–1025.

Broderick, J. P. (2004). William M. Feinberg lecture: Stroke therapy in the year 2025: Burden, breakthrough, and barriers to progress. *Stroke, 35*(1), 205–211.

Connolly, E. S., Rabinstein, A. A., Carhuapoma, J. R., Derdeyn, C. P., Dion, J., Higashida, R. T., . . . Vespa, P. (2012). Guidelines for the management of aneurysmal subarachnoid hemorrhage: A guideline for healthcare professionals from the American Heart Association/American Stroke Association. *Stroke, 43*(6), 1711–1737.

Diringer, M. N., Scalfani, M. T., Zazulia, A. R., Videen, T. O., & Dhar, R. (2011). Cerebral hemodynamic and metabolic effects of equi-osmolar doses mannitol and 23.4% saline in patients with edema following large ischemic stroke. *Neurocritical Care, 14*(1), 11–17.

Easton, J. D., Saver, J. L., Albers, G. W., Alberts, M. J., Chaturvedi, S., Feldmann, E., . . . Sacco, R. L. (2009). AHA/ASA scientific statement: Definition and evaluation of transient ischemic attack. *Stroke, 40,* 2276–2293.

Elliott, J., & Smith, M. (2010). The acute management of intracerebral hemorrhage: A clinical review. *Anesthesia & Analgesia, 110*(5), 1419–1427.

Ferrero, E., Ferri, M., Viazzo, A., Gaggiano, A., Ferrero, M., Maggio, D., ... Nessi, F. (2010). Early carotid surgery in patients after acute ischemic stroke: Is it safe? A retrospective analysis in a single center between early and delayed/deferred carotid surgery on 285 patients. *Annals of Vascular Surgery, 24*(7), 890–899.

Ferri, F. F. (2010). *Practical guide to the care of the medical patient* (8th ed.). St. Louis, MO: Mosby.

Frontera, J. A., Fernandez, A., Schmidt, J. M., Claassen, J., Wartenberg, K. E., Badjatia, N., . . . Mayer, S. A. (2009). Defining vasospasm after subarachnoid hemorrhage. What is the most clinically relevant definition? *Stroke, 40*, 1963–1968.

Furie, K. L., Kasner, S. E., Adams, R. J., Albers, G. W., Bush, R. L., Fagan, S. C., . . . Wentworth, D. (2011). Guidelines for the prevention of stroke in patients with stroke or transient ischemic attack: A guideline for healthcare professionals from the American Heart Association/American Stroke Association. *Stroke, 42*(1), 227–276.

Harrigan, M. R., Rajneesh, K. F., Ardelt, A. A., & Fisher III, W. S. (2010). Short-term antifibrinolytic therapy before early aneurysm treatment in subarachnoid hemorrhage: Effects on rehemorrhage, cerebral ischemia, and hydrocephalus. *Neurosurgery, 67*(4), 935–940.

Jamieson, D. G. (2009). Diagnosis of ischemic stroke. *The American Journal of Medicine, 122*(4), S14–S20.

Jauch, E. C., Saver, J. L., Adams, H. P., Jr., Bruno, A., Connors, J. J., Demaerschalk, B. M., . . . Yonas, H. (2012). Guidelines for the early management of patients with acute ischemic stroke: A guideline for healthcare professionals from the American Heart Association/American Stroke Association. *Stroke, 44*(3), 870–947.

Kwon, W. K., Park, D. H., Park, K. J., Kang, S. H., Lee. J. H., Cho, T. H., & Chung, Y. G. (2014). Prognostic factors of clinical outcome after neuronavigation-assisted hematoma drainage in patients with spontaneous intracerebral hemorrhage. *Clinical Neurology and Neurosurgery, 123*, 83–89.

Lansberg, M. G., O'Donnell, M. J., Khatri, P., Lang, E. S., Nguyen-Huynh, M. N., Schwartz, N. E., . . . Aki, E. A. (2012). Antithrombotic and thrombolytic therapy for ischemic stroke. *Chest, 141*(2 Suppl), e601S–e636S.

Lu, A. Y., Ansari, S. A., Nyström, K. V., Damisah, E. C., Amin, H. P., Matouk, C. C., ... Bulsara, K. R. (2014). Intra-arterial treatment of acute ischemic stroke: The continued evolution. *Current Treatment Options in Cardiovascular Medicine, 16(*2), 1–10.

Manno, E. M. (2010). Update on intracerebral hemorrhage. *Critical Care Neurology, 18*(3), 598–610.

Martinez-Vila, E., & Sieira, P. I. (2010). Current status and perspectives of neuroprotection in ischemic stroke treatment. *Cerebrovascular Diseases, 11*(1), 60–70.

Mlynash, M., Olivot, J. M., Tong, D. C., Lansberg, M. G., Eyngorn, I., Kemp, S., ... Albers, G. W. (2009). Yield of combined perfusion and diffusion MR imaging in hemispheric TIA. *Neurology, 72*(13), 1127–1133.

Morgenstern, L. B., Hemphill, J. C., III, Anderson, C., Becker, K., Broderick, J. P., Connolly, E. S., Jr., . . . Tamargo, R. J. (2010). Guidelines for the management of spontaneous intracerebral hemorrhage: A guideline for healthcare professionals from the American Heart Association/American Stroke Association. *Stroke, 41*(9), 2108–2129.

National Institute of Neurological Disorders and Stroke (NINDS). (2004). *Stroke: Hope through research. (NIH Publication No. 99-2222).* Retrieved from http://www.ninds.nih.gov/disorders/stroke/detail_stroke.htm

Overview of hemorrhagic stroke. (2014). In R. S. Porter & J. L. Kaplan (Eds.), *The Merck Manual Home Health Handbook.* Retrieved from http://www. merckmanuals.com/home/brain_spinal_cord_and_nerve_disorders/stroke_cva/ overview_of_hemorrhagic_stroke.html

Papadakis, M. A., & McPhee, S. J., (Eds.) (2014). *Current medical diagnosis and treatment* (53rd ed.). New York, NY: McGraw Hill Education.

Seevinck, P. R., Deddens, L. H., & Dijkhuizen, R. M. (2010). Magnetic resonance imaging of brain angiogenesis after stroke. *Angiogenesis, 13,* 101–111.

Vijayaraghavan, K., & Deedwania, P. (2011). Renin-angiotensin-aldosterone blockade for cardiovascular disease prevention. *Cardiology Clinics, 29*(1), 137–156.

CHAPTER **2**

Structural Abnormalities

TRAVIS BRADLEY • CHARLENE M. MYERS

ANEURYSM

I.   **Definition**
  A. Abnormal dilatation of an arterial wall in which the intima bulges outward
  B. Usually caused by abnormal weakening
  C. Usually occurs with a sudden increase in systolic blood pressure that is caused by events such as straining or sexual intercourse, which may precipitate a rupture

II.   **Types**
  A. Berry (saccular)—congenital aneurysm of a cerebral vessel
    1. Tends to occur at arterial bifurcations
    2. More common in adults
    3. Frequently multiple
    4. Usually asymptomatic
    5. May be associated with polycystic kidney disease or coarctation of the aorta
  B. Fusiform—aneurysm that is tapered at both ends and spindle shaped; all walls of the blood vessel dilate more or less equally, creating tubular swelling
    1. More common in the vertebrobasilar system
  C. Mycotic—caused by or infected by microorganisms (bacterial)
  D. Traumatic

III.   **Location**
  A. Most intracranial aneurysms, 85%–95%, are located in the carotid system.
    1. 30% occur in the anterior communicating artery
    2. 25% occur in the posterior communicating artery

   3. 20% occur in the middle cerebral artery
B. Some intracranial aneurysms, 5%–15%, occur in the posterior
   circulation.
   1. 10% occur in the basilar artery
   2. 5% occur in the vertebral artery
C. Multiple intracranial aneurysms, usually two or three in number, are
   found in 20%–30% of patients.
D. Rupture results in the following:
   1. Subarachnoid hemorrhage (SAH)—most common (see
      Cerebrovascular Accidents: Brain Attack)
   2. Intraventricular hemorrhage—13%–28%
   3. Intracerebral hemorrhage—less common (see Cerebrovascular
      Accidents: Brain Attack)
   4. Subdural hematoma—rare (see Neurologic Trauma)

IV.   **Risk factors**
A. Evidence supports the association of intracranial aneurysm with
   heritable connective tissue disorders (e.g., polycystic kidney disease,
   Ehlers–Danlos syndrome type IV, neurofibromatosis type I, Marfan
   syndrome) and their familial occurrence.
B. Some of the patients with aneurysmal SAH, 7%–20%, have a first- or
   second-degree relative with a confirmed intracranial aneurysm.
C. Cigarette smoking is an environmental factor.
   1. The risk of an aneurysmal SAH is approximately three to ten times
      higher among smokers.
   2. Risk increases with the number of cigarettes smoked.
   3. Smoking decreases the effectiveness of α1-antitrypsin, the main
      inhibitor of proteolytic enzymes (protease), such as elastase;
      the imbalance between protease in smokers may result in the
      degradation of a variety of connective tissues including the arterial
      wall.
D. Risk is higher among women than among men older than 50 years.
   1. Suggests a role for hormonal factors
   2. Premenopausal women have a low risk of aneurysmal SAH.
   3. Postmenopausal women have a relatively high risk.
   4. Postmenopausal women receiving hormone replacement therapy
      have an intermediate risk.
E. A moderate to high level of alcohol consumption is an independent risk
   factor for aneurysmal SAH. Recent heavy use of alcohol, in particular,
   appears to increase the risk of SAH.
F. Aneurysm size of 7 mm or greater has a higher risk of rupture.
G. Incidence:
   1. Overall estimates in the United States are 14.5 aneurysmal SAH
      per 100,000 adults.
   2. Incidence increases with age; the typical age at onset is greater
      than 50 years. It is rare in children.

3. Women have a 1.24 times greater risk than men.
4. African Americans and Hispanics have higher incidence than Caucasians.

V. **Signs/symptoms**

A. Most aneurysms are asymptomatic until they rupture, at which time, SAH results (see signs and symptoms of SAH in Cerebrovascular Accidents: Brain Attack).

B. Some focal neurologic deficits may be related to compression of adjacent structures.

C. Small amounts of blood from the aneurysm ("warning leaks") may precede the major hemorrhage by a few hours or days. These may cause the patient to have headaches, nausea, and neck stiffness.
   1. Often referred to as a "sentinel" headache

D. Ophthalmologic examination may reveal unilateral or bilateral subhyaloid hemorrhages in approximately one fourth of patients with aneurysmal SAH. These hemorrhages are venous in origin, are located between the retina and the vitreous membrane, and are convex at the bottom and flat on the top.

E. Some aneurysms have a mass effect, causing the patient to become symptomatic. These aneurysms are generally large or giant (25 mm or larger).
   1. The most common symptom of mass effect is headache.
   2. The most common sign is palsy of cranial nerve III (pupils).
   3. Brain stem dysfunction, visual field defects, trigeminal neuralgia, cavernous sinus syndrome, seizures, and hypothalamic–pituitary dysfunction may also occur, depending on the location of the aneurysm.
   4. These aneurysms carry a high risk of rupture (approximately 6% per year).

VI. **Laboratory/diagnostics**

A. A computed tomography (CT) scan or a magnetic resonance angiography can be performed to obtain a baseline value for ventricular size and to rule out infarct/hemorrhage. These studies are noninvasive and carry a lower complication rate than is associated with conventional catheter angiography.
   1. CT scans are sensitive in detecting acute hemorrhage, and they show the presence of SAH in almost 100% of patients who undergo scanning within the first 24 hr after hemorrhage.
   2. The sensitivity of CT scanning decreases sharply after 5–7 days because blood is cleared rapidly from the subarachnoid space.
   3. CT scans are also useful in detecting any associated intracranial hemorrhage or hydrocephalus, and the distribution of blood may offer important clues about the location of the ruptured aneurysm.

B. Cerebral angiography can be ordered to discern the size, shape, location, and number of aneurysms, as well as the occurrence of arterial spasm. The risk of permanent neurologic complications is lower than previously recognized, and cerebral angiography has a high level of diagnostic accuracy. Angiography provides superior spatial resolution and lacks the flow-related artifacts that may affect magnetic resonance angiography.

C. Magnetic resonance imaging (MRI) angiography does not require contrast material and can be used to detect intracranial aneurysms as small as 2–3 mm in diameter.

D. Standard MRI is the best method for detecting the presence of a thrombus within the aneurysmal sac.

E. CT angiography with a 64-slice scanner is an accurate tool for detecting and characterizing aneurysms and can aid in the decision to clip or coil an aneurysm. Helical CT angiography has the ability to demonstrate the relation of the aneurysm to bony structures of the skull base; it can be performed safely in patients who have been treated with ferromagnetic clips, which are a contraindication to MRI angiography.

F. Lumbar puncture: If the CT scan is negative but a strong clinical suspicion of SAH persists, then a lumbar puncture should be performed. Herniation may occur if intracranial pressure is increased (see Cerebrovascular Accidents: Brain Attack).

G. Elevations in white blood cell count and sedimentation rate are indicators of a ruptured aneurysm.

VII.   Management

   A. Surgery

     1. Choosing surgery for patients with an unruptured intracranial aneurysm involves weighing the risk of intracranial rupture against the risks associated with brain surgery.

     2. Size, location, and previous SAH are the most important features for predicting aneurysmal rupture.

       a. As noted in the Cooperative Study of Intracranial Aneurysms and Subarachnoid Hemorrhage, which involved 6,038 ruptured aneurysms, the critical size for rupture is 7–10 mm. Many studies support the critical size as larger than 10 mm.

       b. Major compressive symptoms (e.g., headache and neurologic signs and symptoms) should lead to consideration of surgery.

       c. Coexisting medical problems or factors that favor the need for surgery must be considered (e.g., hypertension and poorly controlled hypertension) to prevent the risk of bleeding.

     3. Early (within 72 hr of the bleed) surgery is desirable for eliminating the risk of rebleed and for allowing aggressive treatment for vasospasm, should it occur.

     4. Late: after 7 days post bleed

     5. Methods

        a. Clipping

        b. Wrapping

        c. Embolization

        d. Endovascular treatment: Soft metallic coils are inserted within the lumen of the aneurysm. The goal is complete obliteration of the aneurysmal sac.

B. Medical management if surgery is not feasible, as outlined for SAH in Cerebrovascular Accidents: Brain Attack, is continued for approximately six weeks.

VIII. Possible complications

A. Vasospasm

    1. It occurs several days to 3–4 weeks after treatment.

    2. Calcium channel blockers (nimodipine, 60 mg every 4 hr for 21 days) have been shown to improve outcomes.

    3. Intravascular volume expansion, induced hypertension, or transluminal balloon angioplasty of involved cranial vessels may also be used after the aneurysm has been obliterated.

B. Rebleeding

    1. It is greatest within 2–24 hr of the first hemorrhage.

    2. Approximately 20% of patients will have further bleeding within 2 weeks, and 40% within 6 months.

    3. Prevent hypertensive episodes (see Cerebrovascular Accidents: Brain Attack)

    4. Antifibrinolytic agents: Aminocaproic acid or tranexamic acid, used during the first 2 weeks after hemorrhage, has been shown to reduce the risk of rebleeding.

        a. Short-term therapy (less than 72 hr) indicated for patients with unavoidable delay in obliteration of aneurysm, significant risk of rebleeding, and no significant medical contraindications to reduce risk of early aneurysm bleeding

        b. The use of antifibrinolytic agents (e.g., aminocaproic acid, tranexamic acid) to prevent rebleeding and decrease mortality in patients with subarachnoid hemorrhage is controversial. It has been associated with an increase in cerebral ischemia and no significant decrease has been noted in mortality rate or in degree of disability among survivors.

C. Hydrocephalus (see Communicating Hydrocephalus)

    1. Caused by interference in the flow of cerebrospinal fluid (CSF)

    2. Acute hydrocephalus occurs in 15%–87% of patients with aneurysmal SAH.

    3. Chronic hydrocephalus requiring shunt placement occurs in 8.9%–48% of patients with aneurysmal SAH.

    4. Acute hydrocephalus is usually managed by the placement of an external ventricular drain or lumbar drain.

D. Seizures

E. Increased intracranial pressure

OTHER ABNORMALITIES

I. **Arteriovenous malformations (AVMs)**
    A. AVMs are the condition of dilated arteries and veins with dysplastic vessels, no capillary bed, and no intervening neural parenchyma.
    B. In adults, AVMs are medium to high pressure and high flow.
    C. AVMs usually present with hemorrhage.
    D. AVMs are congenital lesions with a lifelong risk of bleeding of approximately 2%–4% per year.
    E. Treatment options are as follows: embolization, stereotactic radiosurgery, and/or surgical excision.

II. **Dural arteriovenous fistula**
    A. It is different from an AVM, more of a direct fistula.
    B. It is an arteriovenous shunt contained within the leaflets of the dura matter exclusively supplied by the branches of the carotid or vertebral arteries before they penetrate the dura.
    C. Evidence suggests these are not congenital but acquired lesions, usually resulting from collateral revascularization after thrombosis of a venous sinus.
    D. It usually presents with tinnitus, headache, or visual changes.
    E. Treatment options are as follows: embolization, stereotactic radiosurgery, and/or surgical excision.

III. **Chiari malformation**
    A. It is a heterogeneous group of conditions with a common factor of CSF flow disruption through the foramen magnum; some are congenital, and some are acquired.
    B. There are four types, although types 1 and 2 most common.
    C. Cerebellar tonsillar herniation is the most common type.
    D. Surgery is usually the treatment of choice.

HYDROCEPHALUS

I. **Definition**
    A. Hydrocephalus is a condition in which an excessive amount of CSF accumulates within the cerebral ventricles.
        1. The human brain makes approximately 500 ml of CSF per day, most of which is generated by the choroid plexus within the ventricular system.
            a. CSF circulates around the brain and spinal cord and is reabsorbed in the venous system.
    B. Hydrocephalus is a common neurosurgical problem that leads to changes in cerebral blood flow caused by displacement, deformation, stretching, or decrease in the caliber of cerebral vessels.
        1. Change in the vessels causes a change in vascular resistance and cerebral perfusion pressure, which is important for cerebral microcirculation.

C. Normal pressure hydrocephalus is an unusual cause of dementia.
   1. Although the cause is often idiopathic, it may occur as a late complication of intracerebral infection, Alzheimer's disease, or SAH. CSF opening pressure is usually 5–18 mmHg (70–245 mm H_2O).
   2. The syndrome develops subacutely for a few weeks; in some patients, no predisposing reason is identified.

II. **Etiology**
   A. Oversecretion/overproduction of CSF
   B. Obstruction of CSF (lesions or tumors)
   C. Impaired absorption
   D. Normal pressure hydrocephalus may follow head injury, SAH, or meningoencephalitis.

III. **Classification**
   A. Communicating
      1. Ventricles are patent; obstruction occurs beyond the fourth ventricle.
      2. Caused by impaired absorption or overproduction
      3. Usually occurs 4–20 days after aneurysmal rupture, although it may occur at any time
   B. Noncommunicating
      1. Obstruction occurs within or next to the ventricular system, preventing CSF made in the lateral and third ventricles from circulating normally; thus, this fluid no longer communicates with the subarachnoid space.
      2. It is related to lesions or tumors

IV. **Signs/symptoms (adults)**
   A. Acute hydrocephalus
      1. Papilledema
      2. Headache
      3. Nausea and vomiting
      4. Gait change
      5. Upgaze
   B. Normopressure hydrocephalus
      1. Classic triad
         a. Dementia
         b. Gait disturbance
         c. Urinary incontinence

V. **Management**
   A. Acute: external ventricular drain
   B. Chronic: ventricular shunt

C. Endoscopic third ventriculostomy (Mixter surgery) has been used in noncommunicating hydrocephalus to enable the surgeon to control the condition without the need for ventricular shunting and without long-term complications associated with shunts.

    1. The advantage of endoscopic surgery is that, when feasible, it can be performed with minimal disruption of neural tissue, thus frequently allowing patients to become mobilized rapidly, resulting in shorter hospitalizations and reduced costs.

SPACE-OCCUPYING LESIONS (BRAIN TUMORS)

I.   Definition

    A. Brain tumors consist of primary neoplasms (originating in the brain) or secondary neoplasms (originating from sites other than the brain, such as the lung, the breast, the genitourinary tract, and the gastrointestinal tract) located within the intracranial vault.

    B. Glioblastoma multiforme is the most common primary tumor, followed by meningioma and astrocytoma.

    C. The cause is unknown; however, genes and viruses may be associated with these lesions.

II. Types and characteristics

Table 2.1	Primary intracranial tumors	
Tumor	**Clinical Features**	**Treatment and Prognosis**
Glioblastoma multiforme	Commonly nonspecific, and complaints of increased intracranial pressure. As the tumor grows, focal deficits develop.	Course is rapidly progressive, with poor prognosis. Total surgical removal is usually not possible and response to radiation therapy is poor.
Astrocytoma	A glioma whose presentation is similar to that of glioblastoma multiforme, but its course is more protracted, often extending for several years. Cerebellar astrocytoma, especially in children, may have a more benign course.	Prognosis is variable. By the time of diagnosis, total excision is usually impossible; tumor often is not radiosensitive. In cerebellar astrocytoma, total surgical removal is often possible.
Medulloblastoma	A glioma is seen most frequently in children. Generally arises from roof of fourth ventricle and leads to increased intracranial pressure accompanied by brain stem and cerebellar signs. May seed subarachnoid space.	Treatment consists of surgery combined with radiation therapy and chemotherapy.

Table 2.1	Primary intracranial tumors	
Tumor	**Clinical Features**	**Treatment and Prognosis**
Ependymoma	A glioma arising from the ependyma of a ventricle, especially the fourth ventricle; leads to early signs of increased intracranial pressure. Arises also from central canal of spinal cord.	Tumor is not radiosensitive and is best treated surgically, if possible.
Oligodendroglioma	A slow-growing glioma. Usually arises in cerebral hemisphere in adults. Calcification may be visible on skull x-ray.	Treatment is surgical and is usually successful.
Brain stem glioma	Occurs during childhood with cranial nerve palsies and then with long-tract signs in the limbs. Signs of increased intracranial pressure occur late.	Tumor is inoperable; treatment is by irradiation and with a shunt for increased intracranial pressure.
Cerebellar hemangioblastoma	Presents with disequilibrium, ataxia of trunk or limbs, and signs of increased intracranial pressure; sometimes familial. May be associated with retinal and spinal vascular lesions, polycythemia, and hypernephromas.	Treatment is surgical.
Pineal tumor	Manifests with increased intracranial pressure; sometimes associated with impaired upward gaze (Parinaud's syndrome) and other deficits indicative of midbrain lesion.	Ventricular decompression by shunting is followed by surgical approach to tumor; irradiation is indicated if tumor is malignant. Prognosis depends on histopathologic findings and extent of tumor.
Craniopharyngioma	Originates from remnants of the Rathke pouch above the sella, depressing the optic chiasm. May occur at any age but usually in childhood, with endocrine dysfunction and bitemporal field deficits.	Treatment is surgical, but total removal may not be possible.

Table 2.1	Primary intracranial tumors	
Tumor	**Clinical Features**	**Treatment and Prognosis**
Acoustic neuroma	Ipsilateral hearing loss is the most common initial symptom. Subsequent symptoms may include tinnitus, headache, vertigo, facial weakness or numbness, and long-tract signs (may be familial and bilateral when related to neurofibromatosis). Most sensitive screening tests are MRI and brain stem auditory evoked potential.	Treatment is excision by translabyrinthine surgery, craniectomy, or a combined approach. Outcome is usually good.
Meningioma	Originates from the dura mater or arachnoid; compresses, rather than invades, adjacent neural structures. Increasingly common with advancing age. Tumor size varies greatly. Symptoms vary with tumor site (e.g., unilateral exophthalmos [sphenoidal ridge], anosmia, and optic nerve compression [olfactory groove]). Tumor is usually benign and is readily detected by CT scan; may lead to calcification and bone erosion visible on plain x-rays of skull.	Treatment is surgical. Tumor may recur if removal is incomplete. If removal is incomplete, patients may undergo radiation to decrease the risk of recurrence.
Primary cerebral lymphoma	Associated with AIDS and other immunodeficient states. Presentation may occur with focal deficits or with disturbances of cognition and consciousness. May be indistinguishable from cerebral toxoplasmosis.	Treatment is by whole brain irradiation; chemotherapy may have an adjunctive role. Prognosis depends on CD4 count at diagnosis.

III.   **Signs/symptoms**
   A. Vary—depending on the type, location, and growth of the tumor; most symptoms do not develop until the tumor is well advanced
   B. Progressive neurological deficit, 68%, usually motor deficit
   C. Headache, 54%
   D. Seizures, 26%

E. Other signs and symptoms can include:
   1. Hydrocephalus
   2. Dysphagia
   3. Confusion
   4. Lethargy
   5. Vision changes
   6. Endocrine disturbances

IV.   Laboratory/diagnostics

A. MRI is the procedure of choice for imaging all types of brain tumors because of its high sensitivity, capacity to delineate small tumors in sites near bone, sensitivity to tissue edema, and inherent multiplanar capability that allows an accurate localization of tumors and the identification of their relation to normal structures.

B. CT scan may be useful for screening patients with known cancers elsewhere in the body and patients with atypical headache. Contrast medium may be needed. If CT scan is negative but suspicion is strong, an MRI should be performed. CT scan is effective for following the progression of a diagnosed tumor.

C. Cerebral angiography can facilitate the assessment of the vascularity of lesions and/or their proximity to blood vessels.

D. Electroencephalography can detect the presence and location of seizure activity.

E. Open brain biopsy (craniotomy) or CT- or MRI-directed stereotactic needle biopsy provides a definitive diagnosis.

F. Metastatic workup is necessary.
   1. Chest x-ray
   2. Mammogram
   3. Bone scan
   4. Prostate examination
   5. Chest/abdominal/pelvic CT

V.   Management

A. Referral to oncologist, as pharmacologic therapy is determined by the hematologist or oncologist

B. Chemotherapy, depending on the type and stage of tumor
   1. Carmustine (BCNU), lomustine (CCNU), cisplatin, and procarbazine are the agents most commonly used for malignant glioma in adults.

C. Radiation therapy, depending on the type of tumor
   1. Malignant gliomas are not radiosensitive; however, radiation increases the survival rate in affected patients.

D. Corticosteroids
   1. Dexamethasone (Decadron)
      a. Preferred over methylprednisolone
      b. Standard dose at initiation of therapy is 4–10 mg IV/PO four times a day.

        c. Monitor for adverse effects

        d. Taper slowly, and discontinue if possible

        e. Patients with incompletely treated tumors may not tolerate the decrease in dosage (e.g., they continue to show neurologic deterioration/cerebral edema) and, therefore, may require long-term steroid usage during their last months of life.

        f. Prescribe a concurrent H_2 blocker to prevent gastric irritability associated with steroid use: ranitidine (Zantac), 150 mg PO BID; or famotidine (Pepcid), 20 mg PO BID.

        g. Watch for hyperglycemia-related to steroid use

    2. Methylprednisolone (Solu-Medrol), 120–200 mg IV in 4–6 divided doses (although optimal dosing not well defined) to reduce tumor-associated edema

E. For patients with severe cerebral edema, or in situations where intracranial pressure becomes life threatening, an osmotic diuretic may be necessary. Mannitol (Osmitrol) in the usual dose of 0.25–2 grams/kg of a 20% solution IV for 3–5 minutes can reduce intracranial pressure.

F. In patients with recurrent seizures caused by tumor location and/or edema, anticonvulsants may be necessary.

    1. The agent of choice for many practitioners is phenytoin (Dilantin), 1 gram IV or PO as a loading dose, followed by 300 mg/day in divided doses as a maintenance dose.

    2. Levetiracetam (Keppra) may also be used, with a starting dose of 500 mg IV or PO BID.

G. Brachytherapy (the stereotactic implantation of interstitial radionuclide sources [wafer]) may have a positive effect on survival in patients with glioblastoma.

H. The modified linear accelerator used with stereotactic guidance, the gamma knife, and the proton beam are other noninvasive stereotactic radiosurgical methods that have produced some successful results.

I. If obstructive hydrocephalus is present, surgical shunting can produce dramatic benefit.

BIBLIOGRAPHY

Aminoff, M. J., & Kerchner, G. A. (2014). Nervous system disorders. In. M. A. Papadakis & S. J. McPhee (Eds.), *Current Medical Diagnosis & Treatment* (53rd ed., p. 954). New York, NY: McGraw-Hill Education.

Armstrong, T. S. (2009). *Head's up on the treatment of malignant glioma patients. Oncology Nursing Forum, 36*(5), E232-E240. doi:10.1188/09.ONF.E232-E240

Bederson, J. B., Sander Connoly, E., Hunt Batjer, H., Dacey, R. G., Dion, J. E., Diringer, M. N., . . . Rosenwasser, R. H.(2009). Guidelines for the management of aneurysmal subarachnoid hemorrhage. A statement for healthcare professionals from a special writing group of the Stroke Council, American Heart Association. *Stroke*. Advance online publication. doi:10.1161/ STROKEAHA.108.191395

Connolly, E. S., Rabinstein, A. A., Carhuapoma, J. R., Derdeyn, C. P., Dion, J., Higashida, R. T., . . . Hoh, B. L. (2012). Guidelines for the management of aneurysmal subarachnoid hemorrhage: A guideline for healthcare professionals from the American Heart Association/American Stroke Association. *Stroke, 43*(6), 1711-1737. doi:10.1161/STR.0b013e3182587839

Dea, N., Borduas, M., Brendan, K., Fortin, D., Mathieu, D. (2010). Safety and efficacy of gamma knife surgery for brain metastases in eloquent locations. *Journal of Neurosurgery, 113*, 79-83. doi:10.3171/2010.8.GKS10957

Ferri, F. F. (2011). *Practical guide to the care of the medical patient* (8th ed.). St. Louis, MO: Mosby/Elsevier.

Gagliano, N., Costa, F., Cossetti, C., Pettinari, L., Bassi, R., Chiriva-Internati, M., . . . Pluchino, S. (2009). Glioma-astrocyte interaction modifies the astrocyte phenotype in a co-culture experiment model. *Onocology Reports, 22*, 1349-1356. doi: 10.3892/or_00000574

Gallagher, R., Osmotherly, P., Chiarelli, P. (2014). Idiopathinc normal pressure hydrocephalus, what is the physiotherapist's role in assessment for surgery? *Physical Therapy Reviews, 19*(4), 245-251.

Greenberg, M. (2010). *Handbook of neurosurgery* (7th ed.). New York, NY: Thieme.

Hickey, J. V. (2011). *Clinical practice of neurological and neurosurgical nursing* (2nd ed.). Philadelphia, PA: Lippincott Williams & Wilkins.

Jauch, E. C., Saver, J. L., Adams, H. P., Jr., Bruno, A., Connors, J. J., Demaerschalk, B. M., . . . Yonas, H. (2013). Guidelines for the early management of patients with acute ischemic stroke: A guideline for healthcare professionals from the American Heart Association/American Stroke Association. *Stroke, 44*, 870-947. doi:10.1161/STR.0b013e318284056a

Kernan, W. N., Ovbiagele, B., Black, H. R., Bravata, D. M., Fang, M. C., Fisher, M., . . . Wilson, J. A. (2014). Guidelines for the prevention of stroke in patients with stroke and transient ischemic attack: A guideline for healthcare professionals from the American Heart Association/American Stroke Association. *Stroke, 45*, 2160-2236. doi:10.1161/STR.0000000000000024

Kondziella, D., & Waldemar, G. (2013). *Neurology at the bedside*. New York, NY: Springer Publishing.

Longo, D., Fauci, A., Kasper, D., & Hauser, S. (2011). *Harrison's principles of internal medicine: Volumes 1 and 2* (18th ed.). New York, NY: McGraw-Hill Education.

Lynn-McHale Wiegand, D. J. (2011). *AACN procedure manual for critical care* (6th ed.). Philadelphia, PA: Elsevier/Saunders.

McPhee, S. J., Papadakis, M. A., & Tierney, L. M. (Eds.). (2014). *Current medical diagnosis and treatment* (53rd ed.). New York, NY: McGraw-Hill/Appleton & Lange.

Proust, F., Matinaud, O., Gérardin, E., Derrey, S., Levèque, S., Bioux, S., . . . Fréger, P. (2009). Quality of life and brain damage after microsurgical clip occlusion or endovascular coil embolization for ruptured anterior communicating artery aneurysms: Neuropsychological assessment. *Journal of Neurosurgery, 110*, 19-29. doi:10.3171/2008.3.17432

Tisell, M., Tullberg, M., Hellström, P., Edsbagge, M., Högfeldt, M., Wikkelso, C. (2011). Shunt surgery in patients with hydrocephalus and white matter changes. *Journal of Neurosurgery, 114*(5), 1432-1438. doi:10.3171/2010.11.JNS10967

Wyckoff, M., Houghton, D., & LePage, C. (2009). *Critical care: Concepts, role, and practice for the acute care nurse practitioner*. New York, NY: Springer Publishing.

Zaidi, H., Del Guerra, A. (2011). An outlook on future design of hybrid PET/MRI systems. *Medical Physics, 38*(10), 5667-5689. doi:10.1118/1.3633909

CHAPTER 3

Peripheral Neuropathies

ROBERT BLESSING • KELLY BLESSING • THOMAS W. BARKLEY, JR.

GUILLAIN–BARRÉ SYNDROME

I. **Definition**
   A. Guillain–Barré syndrome (GBS) is an acute, usually rapidly progressive, form of inflammatory demyelinating radiculoneuropathy; typically motor greater than sensory.
   B. Characterized by a monophasic course of muscular weakness, mild distal sensory loss, and autonomic dysfunction, with the majority of patients reporting an antecedent infection
      1. The maximum deficit is usually attained by week 4.
   C. Most frequently acquired demyelinating neuropathy

II. **Etiology**
   A. Unknown, although an autoimmune basis is probable
   B. Majority of cases are triggered by an antecedent infection, suggesting a response involving antibodies cross-reacting with both humoral and cellular immunity with peripheral nerve gangliosides
   C. Frequent antecedent infections include the following: upper respiratory infections, *Campylobacter jejuni* enteritis, cytomegalovirus infection, EpsteinBarr virus infection, hepatitis infection, HIV, and mycoplasma infection
   D. Immunological response may vary between subtypes.
      1. In cases of *C. jejuni* exposure, ganglioside antibodies, such as GM1, lead to the formation of membrane-attacking complexes damaging axons and disturbing nerve conduction in muscles.
      2. In cases of acute inflammatory demyelinating polyneuropathy, the most common subtype of GBS, T cells initiate complement and macrophage activity, leading to myelin destruction.

III. **Significance**
- A. Incidence/prevalence in the United States
  1. 1.3–3 cases/100,000 annually
  2. Nonseasonal, nonepidemic in nature
  3. Incidence increases with age
     a. 0.8 cases/100,000 at age 18
     b. 3.2 cases/100,000 at age 60
- B. Systems affected: nervous, endocrine/metabolic
- C. Predominant age/sex
  1. All ages
  2. Men affected more frequently (1.25:1)
  3. Bimodal peaks of occurrence in the 15- to 35-year-old group and the 50- to 75-year-old group

IV. **Signs/symptoms**
- A. May differ somewhat between subtypes of the disease
- B. Usually symmetric, rapidly progressive distal muscle weakness and paresthesia, beginning in the legs and ascending rapidly to the arms, face, and oropharynx
  1. Progression to total motor paralysis can ensue, leading to death from respiratory failure; therefore, this condition is considered a medical emergency.
- C. Demyelinating neuropathy occurs in most patients, but approximately 5% of cases present with a primary axonopathy. This subtype, called the Miller Fisher variant, may present with descending paralysis and often involves eye muscles on presentation.
  1. The Miller Fisher variant may also include a triad of symptoms, including ophthalmoplegia, ataxia, and areflexia.
- D. Deep tendon reflexes are often significantly reduced or absent on presentation, although this may take days to develop.
- E. Weakness is more prominent than sensory signs and symptoms and may be more prominent proximally.
- F. Sensory involvement can present early, but usually without the objective signs of sensory dysfunction (e.g., stocking distribution sensory loss).
  1. Patient may have hyperesthesia, which may make the touch of a hand or a bed sheet very painful
  2. Perception of joint position, vibration, and temperature may diminish
- G. Bulbar involvement: bilateral facial and oropharyngeal paresis
- H. Difficulty swallowing (may have cranial nerve involvement)
- I. Urinary retention
- J. Respiratory paralysis (involvement of intercostal muscles)

K. Autonomic dysfunction often presents as a hyper-sympathetic state with unexplained tachycardia, but may include bradycardia, blood pressure fluctuations, inappropriate antidiuretic hormone secretion, cardiac arrhythmias, and pupillary changes.

L. Most patients will have a good outcome without sequelae after appropriate treatment and management, but approximately 5% will die from complications.

V. Laboratory/diagnostics

A. Cerebrospinal fluid

1. Albuminocytologic dissociation or elevation in cerebrospinal fluid protein (especially immunoglobulin [Ig]G) without pleocytosis (lack of nucleated cells)

2. Normal values may be seen on presentation.

3. Elevation may not occur until the second week of illness.

4. Protein elevation may be very high (greater than 1000 mg/dl) but may not be elevated until symptoms have been present greater than 1 week.

B. Complete blood count: Early leukocytosis may be seen with a left shift that resolves during the course of illness.

C. If diagnosis is strongly suspected, a repeat lumbar puncture may be indicated.

VI. Pathological findings

A. Segmental demyelination of peripheral nerves and axonal degeneration

B. Inflammatory lesion: lymphocyte and macrophage invasion of myelin sheath

C. Presence of antibodies depending on subtypes (i.e., GM1 or anti-GQ1b)

D. Special tests: motor and sensory nerve conduction studies and needle electromyography, which reveals slowed conduction velocities and prolonged motor, sensory, and F-wave latencies or absent F-waves; decreased nerve conduction related to demyelination

VII. Management

A. There is no known cure for Guillain–Barré syndrome. However, there are therapies that lessen the severity and accelerate recovery in many patients.

B. Refer to neurology—treatment is usually determined by a specialist, rather than general practitioner. Most therapies outside of intravenous immunoglobulin (IVIG) and plasmapheresis are not FDA-labeled.

C. Severe acute polyneuropathy is a medical emergency. Initiate therapy as soon as possible following diagnosis. Delayed therapy, even 2 weeks after first motor symptoms, may prove to be ineffective.

D. Admit to the intensive care unit for constant monitoring and vigorous support of vital functions

E. Measure vital capacity and arterial blood gases

1. Intubation with mechanical ventilation may be indicated for the following: vital capacity less than 12–15 ml/kg, partial pressure of oxygen in arterial blood (PaO_2) less than 70, negative inspiratory force weaker than negative 20 cm H2O or rapidly worsening, difficulty clearing secretions, and/or concerns of aspiration

F. Anticipate respiratory support by mechanical ventilation.

G. Monitor patients with autonomic dysfunction (bradyarrhythmias, tachyarrhythmias, orthostatic hypotension, systemic hypertension, and hypotension) PRN, as dysautonomia is a leading cause of mortality in patients with GBS.

H. Immunomodulating treatment with IVIG and plasmapheresis are both considered first-line therapy and deemed equivalent in efficacy.

1. Combination of therapies does not offer additional benefit.

2. Corticosteroids are not indicated for patients with GBS.

   a. IVIG
      i. Has been used traditionally as an alternative to plasmapheresis (0.4 grams/kg/d IV for 5 consecutive days)
      ii. The major component is the IgG molecule and is derived from healthy donated blood-neutralizing pathogenic antibodies and limiting activation of the complement system.
      iii. Recommended within 2 weeks (possibly 4 weeks) of symptom onset
      iv. Decision to use this over plasmapheresis is usually determined by available resources and comorbidities increasing potential complications such as heart disease, renal insufficiency, and IgA deficiency

   b. Plasmapheresis
      i. Recommended as first-line treatment, especially for patients with severe symptoms such as impaired independent walking or ventilator dependency
      ii. Mechanically removes antibodies and activated complements from the blood
      iii. The routine frequency is five times (approximately 50 ml/kg) every other day for acute severe cases.
      iv. Shorter courses of therapy have been reported for less severe cases or chronic conditions.
      v. Although data are limited, plasmapheresis may reduce time on ventilator.
      vi. The decision to use this over IVIG is usually determined by available resources and comorbidities increasing potential complications such as labile blood pressure, unstable angina, septicemia, and venous access difficulties.

        c. Other potential agents
- i. Interferons
  - (a) Inhibitory glycoproteins that act as cellular immunomodulators that may inhibit antigen presentation and tumor necrosis factor secretion
  - (b) May decrease T-cell proliferation, increase anti-inflammatory cytokine production, and modulate macrophage activity

I. Prevention of thromboembolic events
1. Thromboembolic events are a leading cause of mortality in patients with GBS.
2. Heparin (5,000 units SQ every 8 hr) or low-molecular weight heparin along with sequential compression devices is indicated.
3. Therapeutic anticoagulation may be considered in patients without contraindications and determined by risk factors other than those derived from GBS.

J. Pain management
1. Pain may be significant in GBS, especially during the reinnervation phase.
2. Suitable analgesics range from nonsteroidal anti-inflammatory agents to opioids.
3. Neuropathic pain medications may be beneficial (e.g., gabapentin and pregabalin)

K. Stress ulcer prevention, especially in those receiving ventilatory support
1. Ranitidine, 150 mg PO/NG every 12 hrs or 50 mg IV every 8 hrs
2. Famotidine, 20 mg PO/NG/IV every 12 hrs
3. Cimetidine, 300 mg PO/NG/IV every 6 hrs or 37.5–50 mg/hr via continuous infusion

L. Encourage fluid intake to maintain adequate urine output

M. Monitor serum electrolytes

N. Maintain skin integrity, protect skin from trauma and pressure, reposition frequently

O. Apply moist heat to relieve pain and to permit early physical therapy

P. Range of motion
1. Perform passive range-of-motion exercises immediately
2. Perform active range-of-motion exercises when acute symptoms subside
3. Prevention of joint contractures is very important

Q. Nutrition management
1. Assess pharyngeal function
2. If patient has difficulty swallowing, initiate enteric or parental nutrition.

R. Emotional support and social counseling

S. Interdisciplinary care team is necessary to provide the complex care needed for patients and families

VIII. **Follow-up**
   A. Patient will require physical rehabilitation to regain strength
   B. Subsequent development of chronic course: chronic inflammatory demyelinating polyradiculoneuropathy
      1. Chronic inflammatory demyelinating polyradiculoneuropathy has an insidious onset after GBS and may continue for years.
      2. Plasmapheresis benefits one third of patients, as do immunosuppressive agents (azathioprine).

IX. **Expected course and prognosis**
   A. Weakness and paralysis progress during a 2-week period, stabilize, and then gradually improve. Improvement for a period of months is common.
   B. 10%–23% of patients require ventilatory support
   C. 7%–22% of patients are left with mild disability, mild weakness, or reflex loss
   D. Approximately 10% of patients—those with a more prolonged course— may have severe residual defects.
   E. Axonal regeneration requires 6–18 months.
   F. Mortality occurs at a rate of approximately 5%.

MYASTHENIA GRAVIS

I. **Definition**
   A. Disorder of the neuromuscular junction resulting in a pure motor syndrome; characterized by weakness that may fluctuate most notably after prolonged muscle use, particularly of the extraocular, pharyngeal, facial, cervical, proximal limb, and respiratory musculature
   B. Caused by an autoimmune attack on the acetylcholine receptor (AChR) complex at the postsynaptic membrane of the neuromuscular junction, resulting in AChR dysfunction and jeopardizing normal muscular transmission
   C. Onset may be sudden or severe (myasthenic crisis) but typically is mild and intermittent for many years.

II. **Significance**
   A. The reported prevalence is 14–20 cases per 100,000 population with 10–20 new cases per million.
   B. Predominant age is 20–40 years, but it can occur at any age (1–80 years). The incidence in women peaks in the third decade, in men in the fifth and sixth decades.
      1. Bimodal distribution
      2. May be under recognized in elderly patients
   C. Female-to-male ratio of 2:1 in early adulthood, but it becomes more equally distributed later in life

III.   **Signs/symptoms**

    A. Ptosis—ocular muscles are affected initially in 40% of patients and eventually in 80%

    B. Diplopia

    C. Facial weakness

    D. Fatigue from chewing

    E. Bulbar muscle weakness resulting in dysphagia and dysarthria

    F. Dysphonia

    G. Neck weakness

    H. Fatigue after exercise

    I. Proximal limb weakness with upper limbs more noticeable than lower

    J. Respiratory weakness

    K. Generalized weakness

    L. Sensory modalities and deep tendon reflexes remain normal

    M. Severe generalized quadriparesis may develop, especially in relapse

IV.   **Myasthenic crisis**

    A. Myasthenia crisis, defined by respiratory failure, is an emergency that occurs in up to 20% of MG patients and requires mechanical ventilation.

    B. It weakens oropharyngeal and laryngeal muscles, causing airway obstruction.

    C. It affects 10%–15% of patients with the greatest risk within 2–3 years of diagnosis.

    D. Increasing muscle weakness and diplopia may be seen prior to onset of crisis.

    E. Patients with muscle-specific kinase (MuSK) antibody-positive are more likely to have crisis.

    F. Common precipitating factors include:

        1. Infections

        2. Stress (trauma and surgery)

        3. Rapid introduction, escalation, or tapering of steroids

        4. Withdrawal of cholinesterase inhibitors

        5. Exposure to drugs

            a. Neuromuscular blocking agents

            b. Antibiotics including macrolides, aminoglycosides, and fluoroquinolones

            c. Cardiovascular agents, including β-blockers, calcium channel blockers, procainamide, and quinidine

            d. Quinine

            e. Magnesium

            f. Iodinated contrast agents

            g. Botulinum toxin

            h. Chemotherapeutic agents such as cisplatin

V. Laboratory/diagnostics

   A. Strategy for diagnostic testing based on clinical, serological, and electrodiagnostic findings and may include edrophonium testing

   B. Antibody testing: AChR and MuSK

      1. AChR is positive in 80%–85% of generalized myasthenia patients.

      2. MuSK antibodies are present in nearly half of those negative for AChR.

      3. Seronegative (approximately 10%) may have antibody-clustered AChRs.

   C. Electrodiagnostics

      1. Repetitive nerve stimulation: A decremental response occurs after maximal voluntary contraction; this is seen more frequently in the proximal, cervical, or facial muscles and is considered positive if motor response declines more than 10%.

      2. Single-fiber electromyography: highly sensitive but less specific, technically difficult to perform, and limited availability

         a. Single-fiber electromyography assesses temporal variability between two muscle fibers within the same motor unit (jitter). MG is a condition in which jitters are increased.

   D. Edrophonium (Tensilon) test: short duration (less than 5 minutes); used in MG for differentiating between myasthenic and cholinergic crises

      1. Requires objective improvement in a testable muscle

      2. Administer 2 mg IV as a test dose, while monitoring electrocardiogram for changes in heart rate or rhythm (cholinergic side effects may include increased salivation, sweating, flushing urgency, and periorbital fasciculations)

      3. After observing for approximately two minutes, additional dosing may be required up to a total of 10 mg.

      4. In MG, a sudden, brief improvement in muscle function occurs, whereas those in cholinergic crises worsen

      5. Dangerous cardiorespiratory depression may occur, and atropine and equipment to maintain respiration must be available during the test.

   E. MRI or CT scan of the anterior mediastinum may document an associated thymoma.

   F. Laboratory data that may be present with MG:

      1. Thyroid function test: Patients with MG have a greater incidence of thyroid disease.

      2. Vitamin B12 levels may be low because of associated pernicious anemia.

      3. Antinuclear antibodies, antithyroid antibodies, and rheumatoid arthritis factor are often present.

      4. Lumbar puncture is typically normal

VI.   Management

A. Typically outpatient, but focus will be on inpatient management

B. Inpatient care includes symptomatic and immunosuppression management of MG as well as myasthenic crisis.

C. General measures: management is difficult and should be carried out by a neurologist who specializes in neuromuscular disease

D. Symptomatic management

1. Cholinesterase inhibitors: pyridostigmine bromide (Mestinon)
   a. First-line therapy for general management
   b. Slows down degradation, thereby increasing availability of acetylcholine at the neuromuscular junction
   c. Dosing: tailored to individual requirements throughout the day
      i.   30–60 mg PO every 4–6 hr initially, with a maximum daily dose of 360 mg
      ii. Average daily dose: 600 mg/day
      iii. Mild MG: 60–360 mg/day
      iv. Severe MG: maximum daily dose as high as 1500 mg
   d. Onset of effect is 30 minutes, duration 4 hr
   e. Longer-acting preparation is available for patients on stable dosing.
   f. Monitor patient for cholinergic adverse effects, such as nausea, vomiting, diarrhea, increased salivation, bronchial secretions, and cramps. These adverse effects can be controlled with propantheline (15 mg may be given 15–30 minutes prior to administration of pyridostigmine).

2. Drugs to try to avoid in patients with MG include:
   a. Ketolides
   b. Aminoglycosides
   c. Polypeptides (when not used topically)
   d. Glycopeptides
   e. Lincosamide
   f. Class 1 antiarrhythmics

E. Immunomodulating therapy: necessary for patients with MG and may require lifelong therapy (IVIG and plasmapheresis for rapid immunomodulating therapies, see myasthenic crisis)

1. Prednisone
   a. Should be administered to those who have responded poorly to anticholinesterase drugs and, if indicated, have already undergone thymectomy
   b. Dose is determined on an individual basis
   c. High initial dose can gradually be tapered to a lower maintenance dose
   d. Continue to taper very slowly, attempting to establish the minimum dosage necessary to maintain remission

2. Azathioprine
    a. Widely used as a nonsteroidal immunosuppressant and can be used as monotherapy
    b. Dose is started at 50 mg/day, titrated up to 2–3 mg/kg PO per day if well tolerated
    c. May cause macrocytosis and lymphopenia (drug should not be discontinued for this effect)
    d. If remission not achieved, refer to specialist for other immune modulating therapies (e.g., methotrexate, cyclosporin, mycophenolate, or tacrolimus)
F. Management of impending myasthenic crisis
    1. Airway and ventilatory management
        a. Patients with bulbar weakness, declining vital capacity (less than 20 ml/kg), maximal inspiratory force of negative 30 cm H_2O, or weak or ineffective cough that increases work of breathing, should be admitted to an intensive care unit to monitor for possible intubation and mechanical ventilation.
        b. Vital capacity may not be reliable in patients having difficulty maintaining a seal around a spirometer mouthpiece.
    2. Rapid immunomodulating therapies (IVIG and plasmapheresis are equivocal in efficacy in myasthenic crisis)
        a. IVIG
            i. Therapy that has been used traditionally as an alternative to plasmapheresis
            ii. Dosing: 1 gram/kg/day IV for 2 days or 400 mg/kg/day IV for 5 days, for a total of 1–2 grams/kg IV for 2–5 days
            iii. Major component is IgG molecule and is derived from healthy donated blood-neutralizing pathogenic antibodies and limiting activation of the complement system
            iv. Decision to use over plasmapheresis usually determined by available resources and comorbidities increasing potential complications, such as heart disease, renal insufficiency, and IgA deficiency
        b. Plasmapheresis
            i. Mechanically removes antibodies and activated complements from the blood
            ii. Routine frequency is five times (approximately 50 ml/kg) every other day for acute severe cases.
            iii. Shorter courses of therapy have been reported for less severe cases or chronic conditions.
            iv. Decision to use over IVIG usually determined by available resourcets and comorbidities increasing potential complications such as labile blood pressure, unstable angina, septicemia, venous access difficulties

VII. **Associated conditions**
   A. Thymoma (present in 10%–15% of patients with MG)
      1. CT scan is indicated to assess for presence
      2. Thymectomy may result in long-term improvement in patients with suspected thymoma
      3. Thymectomy is generally delayed if patient is in acute respiratory failure
   B. Thymic hyperplasia
   C. Thyrotoxicosis
   D. Other autoimmune disease

BIBLIOGRAPHY

Barth, D., Nabavi Nouri, M., Ng, E., Nwe, P., & Bril, V. (2011). Comparison of IVIG and PLEX in patients with myasthenia gravis. *Neurology, 76,* 2017–2023.

Cavaicante, P., Bernasconi, P., & Mantegazza, R. (2012). Autoimmune mechanisms in myasthenia gravis. *Current Opinion in Neurology, 25*(5), 621–629.

Chhibber, V., & Weinstein, R. (2012). Evidence-based review of therapeutic plasma exchange in neurological disorders. *Seminars in Dialysis, 25,* 132–139.

Jacob, S., Stuart, V., Lashley, D., & Hilton-Jones, D. (2009). Myasthenia gravis and other neuromuscular junction disorders. *Practical Neurology, 20,* 364–371.

Huan, M., & Smith, A.G. (2012). Weakness (Guillain-Barré syndrome). In K. L. Roos (ed.), *Emergency Neurology* (211-234). New York, NY: Springer Science and Business Media.

Hui, D. (2011) *Approach to Internal Medicine: A Resource Book for Clinical Practice* (3rd ed.). New York, NY: Springer Science and Business Media.

Kieseier, B. C., Lehmann, H. C., & Meyer, G. (2012). Autoimmune diseases of the peripheral nervous system. *Autoimmunity Reviews, 11,* 191–195.

Maggi, L., & Manteegazza, R. (2011). Treatment of myasthenia gravis, focus on pyridostigmine. *Clinical Drug Investigation, 13*(10), 691–701.

Myasthenia Gravis Association. *Myasthenia Gravis Medication List.* Retrieved from http://mgakc.org/wp-content/uploads/2011/07/MGA-Medication-List-12–1-12.pdf

Patwa, H. S., Chaudhry, V., Katzberg, H., Rae-Grant, A. D., & So, Y. T. (2012). Evidenced-based guideline: Intravenous immunoglobulin in the treatment of neuromuscular disorders: Report of the therapeutics and technology assessment subcommittee of the American Academy of Neurology. *Neurology, 78,* 1009–1015.

Spillane, J., Higham, E., & Kullmann, D. (2012). Easily missed? Myasthenia gravis. *BMJ, 345.* doi:10.1136/bmj.e8497

Vincent, J. L., Abraham, E., Moore, F. A., Kochanek, P. M., & Fink, M. P. (2011). *Textbook of critical care* (6th ed.). Philadelphia, PA: Elsevier Saunders.

Xiao, J., Simard, A. R., Shi, F., & Hao, J. (2013). New strategies in the management of Guillain–Barre Syndrome. *Clinical Reviews in Allergy and Immunology.*

Yuebing, L. (2013). Myasthenia gravis: Newer therapies offer sustained improvement. *Cleveland Clinic Journal of Medicine, 80*(11), 711–721.

CHAPTER 4

Neurologic Trauma

KIMBERLY ALVA · CHARLENE M. MYERS

HEAD TRAUMA/TRAUMATIC BRAIN INJURY

I.   Head trauma accounts for two thirds of all casualties of motor vehicle accidents.
  A. Head trauma is the leading cause of death in all trauma cases.
  B. Anatomic structures and physiologic functions of the head provide protection for the brain.
    1. Scalp
    2. Skull
    3. Cerebral meninges (pia mater, arachnoid, and dura mater)
    4. Cerebrospinal fluid (CSF)
  C. The brain is dependent on glucose (25%) and oxygen (20%) for functioning.

II.   Mechanism of injury
  A. Acceleration/deceleration
  B. Deformation
  C. Blunt trauma
  D. Penetrating injury
    1. High-velocity object
    2. Low-velocity object
  E. Coup-contrecoup injuries: brain tissue injury directly at the site of impact (coup) and at the pole opposite of the site of impact (contrecoup) that may be caused by movement of cranial contents within the skull

III.   Categories of injury
  A. Primary head injury
    1. Scalp laceration
      a. The most common head injury

    b. May result in profuse bleeding caused by the great vascular supply to the scalp (monitor for signs and symptoms of hypovolemia, such as increased heart rate and decreased blood pressure)

    c. Apply direct pressure to control bleeding (first assess for skull fracture)

    d. Suture/staple laceration after thorough examination and cleansing

        i. Lidocaine 1% with epinephrine should be used on scalp lacerations to help control bleeding.

        ii. Do not use lidocaine with epinephrine on lacerations located on the nose or ears.

2. Skull fracture

    a. Simple: no displacement of bone

        i. Observe for scalp laceration; protect the cervical spine

        ii. May indicate underlying brain injury

    b. Depressed: bone fragment depressing the thickness of the skull

        i. Patients often have a scalp laceration

        ii. Patient may be asymptomatic or may have an altered level of consciousness

        iii. Surgery is often required to elevate and debride the wound.

        iv. Prophylactic broad-spectrum antibiotics should be initiated

        v. Tetanus toxoid, if indicated

        vi. Institute seizure precautions

    c. Basilar: fracture in the floor of the skull

        i. Raccoon eyes—periorbital ecchymosis

        ii. Battle sign—mastoid ecchymosis

        iii. Otorrhea and/or rhinorrhea (positive Dextrostix test result, halo or target sign, and salty taste in mouth); do not obstruct the flow

        iv. Prophylactic antibiotic coverage

        v. Oral intubation and oral gastric tube are indicated in place of nasal intubation and nasogastric tube

3. Brain injury

    a. Concussion: transient, reversible alteration in brain functioning

        i. Brief loss of consciousness and amnesia of events

        ii. Lethargy, headache, nausea, and dizziness

        iii. Do not give opioids or other sedating medications. Evaluate for changes in the level of consciousness.

        iv. May need to admit to hospital if unconsciousness lasts longer than 2 minutes

   b. Contusion: bruising to the surface of the brain with varying degrees of edema; contrecoup injury

    i. Most commonly seen in the frontal or temporal regions; the skull is rough and jagged, and the brain may be damaged as it moves across underlying structures

    ii. Variable levels of consciousness and amnesia

    iii. Nausea, vomiting, and/or dizziness

    iv. Visual disturbances

    v. Institute seizure precautions

    vi. Brain stem contusion: posturing, variable temperature, and variable vital signs

B. Hematoma

 1. Epidural hematoma (EDH): most commonly seen in the temporal/parietal region; associated with skull fracture resulting in arterial injury, causing bleeding into the epidural space between the skull and the dura mater

   a. Brief loss of consciousness

   b. "Lucid interval"

   c. Deterioration—may be rapid

    i. Obtundation

    ii. Contralateral hemiparesis

    iii. Ipsilateral pupil dilatation

   d. Evaluation and treatment

    i. Obtain CT scan (noncontrast)

    ii. Medical therapy based on Brain Trauma Foundation (BTF) if EDH is less than 15 mm thick, has a midline shift less than 5 mm, and the patient has a Glasgow coma score (GCS) greater than 8; serial CT scans and close neurological assessments

    iii. Surgical intervention if an EDH is greater than 30 cm; should be evacuated regardless of GCS

 2. Subdural hematoma: most commonly caused by tearing of bridging veins, causing bleeding between the dura mater and the brain tissue

   a. Most frequently seen type of intracranial bleeding

   b. Acute: develops over minutes to hours

    i. Drowsiness, agitation, and confusion

    ii. Headache

    iii. Unilateral or bilateral pupil dilatation

    iv. Late hemiparesis

    v. Obtain CT scan (noncontrast)

        vi. If subdural hematoma meets surgical criteria, surgery is indicated immediately (surgical indications: greater than 10 mm thickness with greater than 5 mm midline shift regardless of GCS, or in a patient with deteriorating GCS less than 9 despite the size of the hematoma).

    c. Chronic: develops over days or weeks, generally occurs in elderly patients

        i. Headache

        ii. Memory loss

        iii. Personality changes

        iv. Incontinence

        v. Ataxia

        vi. Obtain CT scan (noncontrast)

        vii. Surgery is usually required (burr holes or craniotomy), but close monitoring may be sufficient if the hematoma is small.

C. Infection

  1. Meningitis

  2. Brain abscess

D. Cerebral edema/elevated intracranial pressure (ICP)/herniation

  1. Clinical manifestations

    a. Decrease in the level of consciousness

    b. Herniation—indicated by pupillary dilation; "blown pupil"

    c. Cushing triad—present in combination in only about one third of patients, indicates increasing ICP and impending cerebral herniation

        i. Hypertension: Widening pulse pressure (systolic blood pressure will increase in attempts to maintain a constant cerebral perfusion pressure [CPP]); CPP = mean arterial pressure (MAP) - ICP

        ii. Decreased respiratory rate

        iii. Bradycardia

E. Neurologic examination

  1. AVPU (A—awake; V—responds to verbal stimuli; P—responds to painful stimuli; U—unresponsive)

  2. GCS (range: 3–15) used to assess the level of consciousness; a score of 8 or below is considered comatose

  3. Posturing

    a. Decorticate: flexion of arms, wrists, fingers; adduction of arm against thorax; extension, internal rotation, and/or plantar flexion with lower extremities

    b. Decerebrate: stiff extension, adduction, and internal rotation of upper extremities (palms pronated); stiff extension and plantar flexion of lower extremities (clenched teeth and hyperextended back, more of the brain stem is involved)

F. Electrolyte disturbances in brain injury
1. Hyponatremia—most common electrolyte disturbance in brain injury
   a. Syndrome of inappropriate antidiuretic hormone
   b. Cerebral salt wasting (CSW): The differentiation of CSW from the syndrome of inappropriate antidiuretic hormone is imperative as the treatment differs significantly.
2. Hypernatremia
   a. Diabetes insipidus: increased urinary output with specific gravity of 1.005 or less; may cause severe hypernatremia if left untreated
      i. Often seen in herniation syndromes
   b. Use of osmotic (mannitol) and thiazide diuretics

IV. **Management of traumatic brain injury**
A. Consult a neurosurgeon
B. Limit secondary injury
C. Prevent hypotension and hypoxemia
1. Both may increase morbidity and mortality from traumatic brain injury
2. According to BTF guidelines, resuscitation should be aimed at maintaining a systolic blood pressure greater than 90 mmHg and a partial pressure of arterial oxygen (PaO_2) greater than 60 mmHg.
3. The administration of blood is another way to improve tissue perfusion to the brain by optimizing the oxygen-carrying capacity of intravascular fluid. The goal is to maintain hematocrit at 30%–33%.

D. Treating cerebral edema/elevated ICP/herniation
1. Hyperventilation/hyperoxia
   a. Hyperventilation ($PaCO_2$ [partial pressure of carbon dioxide in arterial blood], 25–30 mmHg) has been used for decades to cause cerebral vasoconstriction and thereby lower ICP. Cerebral vasoconstriction caused by hyperventilation has also been known to cause cerebral ischemia.
   b. Experts now recommend that hyperventilation should not be used routinely, especially during the first 24 hr after injury, unless ICP is severely high or the patient requires suctioning.
      i. BTF guidelines specifically recommend that hyperventilation should be undertaken to bring $PaCO_2$ to less than 35 mmHg only if a measured increase in ICP is reported, or if increased ICP is suspected because of physical signs, while intracranial hypertension is refractory to other interventions.
      ii. Other methods known to control ICP (e.g., elevating the head of the bed, sedation, paralysis, mannitol, CSF drainage) should be instituted first.

E. Sedation and analgesia
   1. Opioid sedatives help lower ICP by reducing metabolic demand and relieving anxiety and pain.
   2. Short-acting opioids are the best choices
      a. IV fentanyl (2 mcg/kg test dose; 2–5 mcg/kg/hr continuous infusion) or sufentanil (Sufenta) (10–30 mcg test dose; 0.05–2 mcg/kg/hr continuous infusion)
         i. Fentanyl and sufentanil have the potential to slightly raise ICP
         ii. Morphine may be used in this setting, but is longer acting.
      b. These may be supplemented with propofol (Diprivan) (0.5 mg/kg test dose; 20–75 mcg/kg/min continuous infusion [not to exceed 5 mg/kg/hr]) or benzodiazepines, such as diazepam (Valium [2.5–10 mg]) or lorazepam (Ativan [0.5–2 mg]), if the patient remains agitated or ICP remains elevated.
   3. Neuromuscular blocking agents—use removes the ability to perform a neurological assessment; should only be given after consultation with the neurologist or neurosurgeon
      a. Vecuronium (Norcuron) or cisatracurium (Nimbex)
         i. Dosage should be individualized and a peripheral nerve stimulator or train-of-four (TOF) monitor should be used to measure neuromuscular function during administration.
         ii. Cisatracurium, 0.1–0.2 mg/kg bolus, followed by 1–10 mcg/kg/min continuous infusion; titrate to TOF
      b. Can be used to help lower ICP in patients in whom confusion, posturing, or severe agitation is interfering with treatment or diagnostic testing
      c. Patient must be sedated and intubated with an adequate set rate on the ventilator
      d. Paralytic agents also may be needed to help oxygenate and ventilate the patient
F. Steroids
   1. Corticosteroids in multiple studies, including the CRASH trial, have shown to increase morbidity and mortality.
      a. The BTF highly recommends that steroids not be used in traumatic brain injury.
G. Hyperosmolar therapy
   1. Mannitol—drug of choice in an emergency situation when brain herniation is pending
      a. Creates an osmotic gradient across the blood-brain barrier that pulls water from the central nervous system into the intravascular space

       b. May enhance cerebral oxygen delivery via decreased blood viscosity, increased CPP, or both

       c. May also provide some cytoprotective effects through oxygen-free radical scavenging

       d. Administer as a bolus (0.25–1 grams/kg) or continuous infusion

       e. Results are quick, occurring usually within 10–20 min, and can last up to 6 hr

       f. May need to avoid use in patients with renal failure

       g. Monitor serum osmolarity. Maintain serum osmolarity less than 320 mOsm

       h. Monitor electrolytes, especially serum sodium

       i. Monitor blood pressure closely

          i. Hypotension is an adverse effect that results from dehydration caused by diuresis.

          ii. The goal is to attain beneficial effects without inducing dehydration.

       j. Volume replacement may be necessary to keep the patient euvolemic and to prevent hypotension (e.g., replace urinary with isotonic crystalloids).

       k. An indwelling urinary catheter should be in place and urine output recorded each hour.

   2. Hypertonic saline (3% or 23% NaCl)

       a. The effect is on the osmotic mobilization of fluid across the blood-brain barrier, similar to mannitol

       b. May exacerbate pulmonary edema in patients with cardiac or pulmonary issues

       c. May be given as a bolus or a continuous infusion

H. ICP monitoring

   1. ICP monitoring is appropriate for the following:

       a. Comatose patients (GCS score of 3–8) with an abnormal CT scan

       b. Comatose patients with a normal CT scan and two of the following:

          i. Older than 40 years of age

          ii. Unilateral or bilateral motor posturing

          iii. Hypotension

   2. ICP monitoring is not routinely appropriate for patients with mild or moderate head injury.

   3. Ventricular catheter allows the practitioner to measure ICP and to drain CSF

   4. If the ICP is greater than 20–25 mmHg for greater than 5 minutes, treatment should be initiated to lower ICP.

   5. Monitoring of ICP allows the practitioner to calculate CPP (CPP = MAP − ICP).

6. Ideally, CPP should be maintained at a minimum of 60 mmHg.

I. Seizure prophylaxis in traumatic brain injury

    1. It is recommended that anticonvulsants such as phenytoin (Dilantin) may be used to prevent early posttraumatic seizures in those at high risk after a head injury.

        a. IV loading dose of 15–20 mg/kg, followed by maintenance dose 5 mg/kg/day

    2. Levetiracetam (Keppra) is used for prophylaxis of both early and late seizures after trauma

        a. Easier to use and better side effect profile compared to phenytoin; however, further research is needed to ascertain that levetiracetam may be an acceptable alternative to phenytoin

        b. Treatment protocols range from 7–30 days; may be administered in daily doses of 1000 mg, 2000 mg, and 3000 mg, given as twice-daily dosing

    3. Prophylactic use is not recommended for preventing late posttraumatic seizures.

    4. Prophylactic seizure treatment is not suggested to be used longer than 7 days.

J. DVT/VTE prophylaxis

    1. Use graduated compression stockings or intermittent pneumatic compression (IPC) stockings until patients are ambulatory

    2. Low molecular weight heparin (LMWH) or unfractionated heparin (UFH) should be used in combination with mechanical prophylaxis.

        a. Note an increased risk for expansion of intracranial hemorrhage

    3. There is insufficient evidence for precise recommendations concerning the preferred agent, dose or timing of pharmacologic prophylaxis for DVT.

K. Neurological assessment and management of traumatic brain injury (TBI) patient

    1. It is an ongoing process

    2. GCS score may be necessary every 30–60 minutes for the first 24 hr

        a. Note whether the patient is receiving sedation and/or paralytics; cannot assess GCS while on paralytics

    3. Pupil size and reaction

    4. Vital signs

    5. All patients with head injury are presumed to have a cervical spine injury until proven otherwise. Once the patient's condition has stabilized, a cervical spine series should be ordered.

6. Avoid any condition (e.g., fever, pain, and shivering) that increases metabolic rate and therefore increases the demand for O_2 and glucose.

L. Hypothermia
  1. Possibly improves clinical outcomes by controlling ICP
     a. Lowering the temperature to 89.6°F–91.4°F
     b. There is no evidence that hypothermia improves mortality. Some studies have shown improved GCS. Currently, it is not recommended by national guidelines but may be used in practice.

M. Decompressive craniectomy
  1. Surgical intervention where part of the skull is removed (placed in the abdomen, stored, or discarded) to allow swelling of the brain
  2. Used in patients with increased ICP refractory to treatment
     a. It is considered for those who have failed to respond to conservative therapy.
     b. Studies have shown that ICP normalizes after a craniectomy.

N. Brain oxygenation monitoring
  1. Prevention of secondary brain injury relies on providing adequate oxygen and metabolic substrate to the brain.
  2. Brain tissue oxygen monitoring allows the clinician to gauge the adequacy of oxygen delivery to the brain.
  3. Different ways to monitor:
     a. Jugular venous oxygen saturation ($SjvO_2$) provides global O_2 saturation within the brain; normal value is 55%–70%.
     b. Brain tissue oxygen monitoring ($PbrO_2$): Levels lower than 15 mmHg during the resuscitation phase of TBI predict poor outcome.

V. Brain death

A. A condition where the patient has sustained irreversible cessation of all functions of the entire brain, including the brainstem

B. The Uniform Determination of Death Act has been adopted by most states to assist in determining death in all situations.

C. A patient cannot be declared brain dead as a result of the following conditions:
  1. Hypothermic (temperature less than 32°C)
  2. Drug intoxication or poisoning
  3. Severe electrolyte, acid base, or endocrine disturbance

D. Examination to determine brain death
  1. No spontaneous movement
  2. Absence of brain stem reflexes
     a. Fixed and dilated pupils
     b. No corneal reflexes
     c. Absent doll's eyes
     d. Absent gag reflex

      e. Absent vestibular response to caloric stimulation
    3. Absence of breathing drive (apnea)—must perform apnea test
    4. Must have absence of all of the above before making consideration of brain death
  E. Ancillary tests for brain death
    1. Electroencephalography
    2. Cerebral angiography
    3. Transcranial doppler
    4. Cerebral blood flow study
    5. CT angiogram of brain

SPINAL CORD TRAUMA

I.   **Mechanisms of injury**
  A. Motor vehicle accidents account for the largest number of spinal cord injuries (SCIs) (40%)
  B. Falls or falling objects (10%–20%)
  C. Acts of violence (15%)
  D. Sports-related injuries (13%)
  E. Penetrating wounds (12%)

II. **Spinal cord injuries**
  A. Rapid acceleration/deceleration
    1. Hyperextension
      a. Usually occurs as the result of a fall onto the face, forehead, or chin
      b. Rear-end collisions may result in rupture of the anterior longitudinal ligament
      c. Hyperextension may cause the cord to stretch, resulting in central cord syndrome (see Section IX. Spinal cord lesions [syndromes], C)
    2. Hyperflexion: greatest stress occurs at C5-C6, causing bilateral facet dislocations
    3. Vertical column loading (compression)
      a. Occurs in diving accidents or falls, when the patient lands on the feet or buttocks
      b. Vertebral body is compressed and/or shattered, resulting in a "burst" fracture, and bone fragments may become embedded in the cord.
      c. Injuries commonly occur at the level of C1 with diving accidents
    4. Whiplash: sudden hyperextension of the spine that stretches the ligaments as a result of the force of the lower body moving forward and the backward and downward movement of the head
  B. Distraction injuries: result from hanging
  C. Penetrating trauma
    1. Gunshot wound

    2. Stab wound

    3. Bony fragments

  D. Hematoma

  E. Pathologic fractures: occur in patients with osteoporosis or metastatic disease

III. **Epidemiology**

  A. Incidence

    1. Sixty percent of SCIs involve the cervical spine

    2. Approximately 8,000 SCIs occur each year, or 32.1 per million

    3. Approximately 40% of patients with SCI die before they reach the hospital or during the initial resuscitation phase.

    4. Average hospital costs: $80,200 for quadriplegics and $72,000 for paraplegics

    5. Average lifetime care costs of a young adult with an SCI exceed $1 million

IV. **Age**

  A. More common in young men (82%)

  B. More common in younger persons (80% younger than 40 years, and 50% between 15 and 25 years of age)

V. **Anatomy and physiology**

  A. 33 vertebrae

    1. Cervical spine (C1-C7)

      a. Highly flexible in nature, small in diameter

      b. Therefore, many fractures occur

    2. Thoracic spine (T1-T12)

      a. Articulates with the ribs

      b. Less common site for fracture because of its stability

    3. Lumbar spine (L1-L5)

      a. Highly mobile, yet large in diameter

      b. Requires a greater amount of force to fracture

    4. Sacral spine (S1-S5)

    5. Coccygeal vertebrae (3–5 coccyges)

  B. Spinal cord

    1. Gray matter

    2. White layer

    3. Meningeal layer (pia mater, arachnoid, and dura mater)

VI. **Assessment**

  A. History

    1. Mechanism of injury, such as the following:

      a. Speed of impact

      b. Blunt versus penetrating forces

      c. Flexion, extension, rotation, or distraction to the spine

      d. Height of fall

      e. Use of restraints or deployed airbag

      f. Extent of vehicular damage

        g. Position of patient in vehicle
   2. Patient complaints, such as the following:
        a. Back pain
        b. Neck pain
        c. Numbness
        d. Paresthesia
   3. Motor/sensory response
   4. Prehospital treatment

B. Physical assessment
   1. Problems with airway, breathing, and circulation and life-threatening injuries are treated first
   2. Pulmonary complications account for most of the early deaths that occur after acute traumatic quadriplegia
   3. Assess respiratory ability
        a. Chest excursion
        b. Use of intercostal muscles or diaphragm
        c. Cervical cord injury above C3 results in respiratory arrest
        d. C5-C6 injuries spare the diaphragm, and diaphragmatic breathing occurs
        e. T1-L2 lesions cause loss of intercostal muscle use
   4. Intubation if necessary
        a. Jaw thrust maneuver
        b. Apnea
        c. Breathing difficulty
        d. Diaphragmatic fatigue
   5. Arterial blood gases should be monitored closely
   6. Monitor for pneumonia, pulmonary edema, and pulmonary emboli

C. Motor assessment
   1. Inability to perform the functions listed here indicates that the lesion is above the level indicated
        a. Deltoids (C4): apply pressure to shoulders and ask patient to shrug shoulders
        b. Biceps (C5): have patient flex arm (gravity), then apply pressure by trying to straighten the arm. Tell patient not to let you straighten it (resistance)
        c. Wrist (C6): have patient hyperextend the wrist (gravity) and apply pressure by trying to straighten the wrist; tell the patient not to let you push down (resistance)
        d. Triceps (C7): have patient extend arm (gravity) and try to pull arm up to the flexed position; tell patient not to let you bend arm (resistance)
        e. Intrinsic (C8): have patient abduct (fan) fingers and try to push them together
        f. Hip flexion: have patient bend knee and apply pressure to determine resistance (L2-L4)

    g. Knee extension: while hip is flexed and knee bent, have patient try to extend the knee (L2-L4)

2. Grade strength using the following scale:
   a. 5: normal movement against gravity and full resistance
   b. 4: full range of motion against moderate resistance and gravity
   c. 3: full range of motion against gravity, not against resistance
   d. 2: extremity can move, but not against gravity (can roll but not lift)
   e. 1: muscle contracts, but extremity cannot move
   f. 0: no visible or palpable muscle contraction or movement of extremity (flaccid)
3. All motor groups must be comprehensively assessed
4. Complete lesion
   a. Patient lacks sensory function, proprioception, and voluntary motor activity below the level of spinal cord damage
   b. Worse prognosis for recovering neurologic function
5. Incomplete lesion
   a. Parts of the spinal cord at the level of the lesion are intact.
   b. Sacral sparing occurs
   c. Note sensory perception and voluntary contraction of the anus around the examiner's finger

D. Sensory function
1. Begin at the area of no feeling and proceed to the area of feeling
2. Assess response to pain
   a. Great toe: L4
   b. Back of leg: S1-S3
   c. Perianal area: S4-S5
   d. Umbilicus: T10
   e. Nipple line: T4
   f. Ring and little fingers: C8
   g. Middle finger: C7
   h. Thumb: C6
   i. Top of shoulder: C4
3. If the patient is unable to feel pain, the lesion is at or above the spinal nerve level indicated

E. Evaluate the patient's back
1. Perform a well-coordinated log-roll maneuver
2. Maintain in-line spinal stabilization
3. Gently palpate spine for pain, tenderness, or gaps between spinous processes
4. Observe for entrance/exit wounds, impaled objects, and other signs of injury

VII. **Key signs of various levels of injury**
    A. C2-C3
        1. Respiratory paralysis (breathing center-C3)

        2. Flaccid paralysis

        3. Areflexia (deep tendon reflexes [DTRs])

        4. Loss of sensation below the mandible

    B. C5-C6

        1. Diaphragmatic breathing

        2. Paralysis of intercostal and abdominal muscles

        3. Quadriplegia

        4. Anesthesia below the clavicle and the ulnar half of the arms

        5. Areflexia (with possible exception of the biceps reflex)

        6. Fecal and urinary retention

        7. Priapism (spontaneous erection)

    C. T12-L1

        1. Paraplegia

        2. Anesthesia in the legs

        3. Areflexia in the legs

        4. Fecal and urinary retention

        5. Priapism (spontaneous erection)

    D. L1-L5

        1. Flaccid paralysis to partial flaccid paralysis

        2. Abdominal and cremasteric reflexes present

        3. Ankle and plantar reflexes absent

VIII. **Multisystem impact of SCIs**

    A. Cardiovascular

        1. Hypotension

            a. Caused by loss of sympathetic tone in patients with high thoracic or cervical injury with pooling of blood into the periphery

            b. If associated with a neurologic deficit, normal or decreased heart rate, and warm, vasodilated extremities, spinal shock is suspected.

            c. For initial fluid resuscitation, use 2–3 L of Lactated Ringer's solution. (Do not overload. Possible loss of cardiac contractility puts the patient at risk for congestive heart failure and pulmonary edema.)

            d. Rule out hypovolemia as a cause of hypotension.

            e. Vasopressors (dopamine) and hemodynamic monitoring may be indicated if patient is unresponsive to intravenous fluids

        2. Bradycardia

            a. Caused by sympathetic blockade and may lead to arrhythmia (junctional or ventricular escape)

            b. Be alert for conditions that promote bradycardia in patients with SCIs: hypoxia, hypothermia, and vagal stimulation

            c. Be sure the patient is well oxygenated

            d. Maintain body temperature at greater than 96.8°F

      e. Administer atropine for symptomatic bradycardia (decreased level of consciousness, urinary output, and blood pressure)

  3. Vasovagal reflex

      a. Induced by straining, coughing, or bearing down

      b. Frequently induced by suctioning, which leads to hypoxia, and by vagal stimulation (bradycardia—cardiac arrest)

      c. Oxygenate and hyperventilate with 100% O_2 prior to suctioning

      d. Limit suctioning to 10 seconds

      e. Monitor cardiac rate and rhythm

  4. Poikilothermy

      a. Patient's temperature is dependent on the temperature of the environment; this association is the result of interruption of the sympathetic pathways to the temperature-regulating centers in the hypothalamus

      b. Maintain temperature of the environment

  5. Venous thrombosis

      a. A venous stasis in the legs and pelvis resulting from decreased blood flow and flaccid paralysis

      b. Administer deep venous thrombosis prophylaxis (low-dose heparin, 5,000 units subcutaneously BID, or low molecular weight heparin [Lovenox], 30–40 mg subcutaneously BID); use antiembolic stockings, range of motion, and vena cava filters

      c. Measure thighs and calves for swelling from deep venous thrombosis

  6. Orthostatic hypotension

      a. Occurs when patients move from supine to sitting position; it is related to venous pooling in the legs and abdomen caused by loss of skeletal muscle pump and impaired sympathetic nervous system control

      b. Use thigh-high stockings and abdominal binders to promote venous return

      c. Raise the head of the bed gradually, and monitor blood pressure closely

B. Gastrointestinal

  1. Abdominal injuries resulting from trauma

      a. Difficult to diagnose in SCI because abdominal pain and muscular rigidity—telltale signs of internal bleeding—are absent if the patient has sensory and motor deficits.

      b. Assess patient for abdominal distention; monitor hematocrit and hemoglobin and blood volume

      c. Perform diagnostic peritoneal lavage

  2. Curling's ulcer

    a. Patients with central nervous system injury may have this type of stress ulcer as a result of vagally stimulated gastric production and/or release of adrenocorticotropic hormone.

    b. Assess gastric pH, and administer H_2 antagonists (ranitidine, 150 mg PO quarterly for 12 hr) for prevention and treatment

    c. Warm and cold water lavage may be used to treat bleeding

    d. Monitor patient for coagulation defects

    e. Gastrectomy may be necessary in severe cases

  3. Gastric atony and ileus

    a. Related to loss of central control

    b. Leads to severe gastric distention that in turn can lead to respiratory compromise, vomiting, and aspiration

    c. Place a nasogastric tube to lower wall suction, note amount and quality of aspirate

  4. Loss of bowel function

    a. Patient cannot sense when the bowel is full or cannot perform the Valsalva maneuver to aid in evacuation

    b. May lead to obstruction or autonomic dysreflexia

    c. Initiate a bowel program—suppository same time every day, AM or PM

C. Genitourinary

  1. Autonomic dysreflexia

    a. Distended bladder is the most common cause, although it can result from any noxious stimuli (e.g., distended bowel, wrinkled sheets, pressure ulcers, constrictive clothing, constrictive devices such as foot splints, and shoes that are tied too tightly).

    b. Hypertensive crisis that may result from a noxious stimulus in injuries above T6—the sympathetic outflow level

    c. SCI may result in denervation of the bladder, which may become overdistended.

    d. Noxious stimulus below the level of injury triggers the sympathetic nervous system, causing massive release of catecholamines.

    e. Result of catecholamine release is vasoconstriction

    f. Vasodilatation occurs above the site of injury—red, flushed, warm skin, as well as headache, vasocongestion, and diaphoresis.

    g. Piloerection occurs below the level of injury

    h. Place a urinary catheter to monitor urinary output and to decompress the bladder

    i. Do not drain bladder rapidly if cardiovascular system suggests autonomic dysreflexia (no more than 600 ml at a time)

  2. Urinary tract infection

    a. May result from urinary retention or catheterization

  b. Intermittent catheterization is recommended

  c. Early detection is essential to prevent sepsis or prolonged spinal shock.

D. Musculoskeletal

 1. Impaired skin integrity related to abnormal nerve supply and poor circulation

 2. Paralysis

  a. Muscle atony and wasting

  b. Contractures

  c. Perform passive range of motion and positioning, and use hand splints and boots to prevent foot drop

E. Psychological devastation

 1. Effects on the patient

  a. Disturbance of self-concept

  b. Ineffective coping

  c. Feelings of powerlessness

  d. Denial, anger, and depression

 2. Practitioner's response

  a. Be honest with a positive attitude

  b. Include patient in his or her care

  c. Set limits of behavior, and be consistent with care

  d. Take an interdisciplinary approach, including the following:

   i. Social services

   ii. Psychiatry

   iii. Physical therapy

   iv. Occupational therapy

   v. Pastoral care

IX. **Spinal cord lesions (syndromes)**

A. Anterior cord syndrome

 1. Probably the most devastating of the syndromes

 2. Disruption of blood flow through the anterior spinal artery

 3. Flexion injuries

 4. Weakness or paralysis with loss of sense of pain and temperature

 5. Proprioception intact

B. Posterior cord syndrome

 1. Rare injury resulting from disruption of the posterior column

 2. Decrease in touch proprioception and vibration

C. Central cord syndrome

 1. Hyperextension injuries with stretching of the cord and subsequent hemorrhaging in the center of the cord

 2. Greater motor loss and sensation in the upper extremities than in the lower extremities because the upper extremities are controlled by the central portion of the cord

D. Brown-Séquard syndrome

1. Stab wounds, gunshot wounds, fractures of the vertebral process, and spinal cord tumors
2. One side of the spinal cord is damaged
3. Ipsilateral motor loss and contralateral loss of pain and temperature sensation
4. Extremities that can move have no feeling, and those that have feeling cannot move

X. **Laboratory/diagnostics**
  A. Cervical vertebrae
   1. Cross-table lateral position first; all seven vertebrae must be seen; to do so, the following may be required:
       a. Firmly pulling the patient's shoulders down
       b. Lateral swimmer's view
   2. Obtain anteroposterior x-ray if lateral x-ray is abnormal
   3. Obtain open-mouth odontoid x-ray for conscious patient for visualization of C2
   4. Failure to obtain basic radiographic studies is the primary reason for missed diagnosis of cervical spine injury.
  B. Thoracic vertebrae
   1. Perform lateral and anteroposterior x-rays
   2. View all 12 vertebrae
  C. Lumbar vertebrae
   1. Perform lateral and anteroposterior views
   2. View all five lumbar vertebrae
  D. CT may be helpful for clear identification of normal cervical spine anatomy or the presence of bony fragments.
  E. Films in flexion/extension position or oblique films at times for further delineation of suspected fractures
  F. Myelogram detects compression of the cord by herniated disks, bone fragments, or foreign matter, which requires surgical intervention.
  G. MRI can provide further information regarding cord impingement, hematomas, and infarcts. Cord contusion or hemorrhage cannot be visualized by any other technique.

XI. **Management**
  A. Consult neurosurgeon
  B. Airway maintenance
   1. Perform nasotracheal intubation or cricothyrotomy, if necessary
   2. Do not hyperextend or rotate the neck
   3. Administer oxygen
  C. Immobilization
   1. Use protective devices (e.g., cervical collar and spine board)
   2. Do not remove device until x-rays have been obtained and cleared
   3. Perform log roll only (will require more than two people)
  D. Intravascular fluids (limit to appropriate levels)

1. Distinguish neurogenic shock (warm, dry extremities; bradycardia) from hypovolemic shock (cool, clammy skin; tachycardia)

E. Monitor blood pressure very closely because perfusion to the spinal cord is crucial
   1. Hypotension must be avoided to prevent ischemia caused by decreased blood flow and perfusion to the spinal cord, which may produce neuronal injury and neurologic deficit.
   2. Attempts should be made to maintain MAP at 85–90 mmHg

F. Bladder catheterization

G. Nasogastric intubation

H. Corticosteroids (controversial)
   1. It may be useful in the early treatment (within the first 8 hr) of patients with acute, nonpenetrating SCI to reduce swelling.
      a. Reduce damage to cellular membranes that contributes to neuronal death after injury
      b. Reduce inflammation near the injury
      c. Suppress activation of immune cells that appear to contribute to neuronal damage
   2. Improvement is noted 6 weeks to 6 months after injury
   3. Monitor patient for elevation in blood glucose levels
   4. Monitor patient for other adverse effects, such as the following:
      a. Immunosuppression
      b. Fluid and electrolyte disturbances
      c. Adrenocortical insufficiency
      d. Impaired wound healing
      e. Gastrointestinal disturbances

I. Preliminary clinical trials of another agent, GM-1 ganglioside
   1. Although evidence does not support a significant clinical benefit, may potentially be useful in acute SCI for preventing secondary damage caused by the following:
      a. Oxidative free radicals
      b. Calcium-mediated damage
      c. Proteases
      d. Cytoskeletal dysfunction
      e. Excitotoxicity
      f. Immune reactions
      g. Apoptosis
      h. Necrosis
   2. Studies suggest that it may also improve neurologic recovery from SCI during rehabilitation.

J. Antibiotics for penetrating injuries

K. Maintain room temperature; avoid poikilothermy

L. Provide meticulous skin care: Order rotating bed for respiratory therapy (postural drainage) and skin therapy

M. Prepare for insertion of skeletal tongs and traction (Stryker frame, kinetic bed, or halo vest) used to assist in restoration of the spine to a normal position (reduction)
  1. At least 10 lb of weight is initially applied.
  2. Weight is applied on the basis of 5 lb per interspace (i.e., a C5-C6 injury would require 25–30 lb of traction).
  3. Muscle relaxants are helpful
  4. Lateral x-rays are taken to assess vertebral alignment as weights are applied.
  5. Too much weight can pull the spine apart, resulting in distraction injury
  6. If paralytics are needed, weight may have to be reduced.
N. Fixation: involves stabilizing vertebral fracture with wires, plates, and other types of hardware
O. Fusion: involves attaching injured vertebrae to uninjured vertebrae with bone grafts and steel rods
P. Surgery may be indicated to remove bony fragments or to drain hematomas that compress the cord
Q. Rehabilitation begins upon admission; follow an interdisciplinary approach
R. Electrical stimulation devices or neural prostheses were recently approved by the FDA but are still experimental. These can be implanted in the body to allow some hand movement and bladder/bowel control; some may also assist with breathing.

BIBLIOGRAPHY

Adams, J. P., Bell, D., & McKinlay, J. (Eds.). (2010). *Neurocritical care: A guide to practical management*. London, UK: Springer-Verlag London Limited.

Aarabi, B., & Yukuwa, Y. (2011). Emergency room evaluation of the spinal injury patient including assessment of spinal shock. *Spine and Spinal Cord Trauma: Evidence-Based Management*.

Aries, M. J., Czosnyka, M., Budohoski, K. P., Steiner, L. A., Lavinio, A., Kolias, A. G., . . . Smielewski, P. (2012). Continuous determination of optimal cerebral perfusion pressure in traumatic brain injury. *Critical Care Medicine, 40*(8), 2456–2463.

Brain Trauma Foundation. (2007). Guidelines for the management of severe traumatic brain injury (3rd ed.), *Journal of Neurotrauma, 24*(Suppl 1), S1–S106.

Burns, S. (2014). *AACN Essentials of Critical Care Nursing* (3rd ed.). New York, NY: McGraw-Hill.

Fehlings, M. G., Rabin, D., Sears, W., Cadotte, D. W., & Aarabi, B. (2010). Current practice in the timing of surgical intervention in spinal cord injury. *Spine, 35*(21S), S166–S173.

Ferri, F. F. (2014). *Practical guide to the care of the medical patient* (9th ed.). St. Louis, MO: Mosby.

Greenberg, M. S. (2010). *Handbook of neurosurgery* (7th ed.). New York, NY: Thieme.

Gupta, R., Bathen, M. E., Smith, J. S., Levi, A. D., Bhatia, N. N., & Steward, O. (2010). Advances in the management of spinal cord injury. *Journal of the American Academy of Orthopaedic Surgeons, 18*(4), 210–222.

Haddad, S. H., & Arabi, Y. M. (2012). Critical care management of severe traumatic brain injury in adults. *Scand J Trauma Resusc Emerg Med, 20*(12). Retrieved from http://www.ncbi.nlm.nih.gov/pmc/articles/PMC3298793/

Hartings, J. A., Vidgeon, S., Strong, A. J., Zacko, C., Vagal, A., Andaluz, N., . . . Bullock, M. R. (2014). Surgical management of traumatic brain injury: A comparative-effectiveness study of 2 centers. *Journal of Neurosurgery, 120*(2), 434–446.

Hickey, J. V. (2011). *The clinical practice of neurological & neurosurgical nursing* (6th ed). Philadelphia, PA: Lippincott Williams & Wilkins.

Krassioukov, A., Eng, J. J., Claxton, G., Sakakibara, B. M., & Shum, S. (2010). Neurogenic bowel management after spinal cord injury: A systematic review of the evidence. *Spinal Cord, 48*, 718–733.

Mulligan, R. P., Friedman, J. A., Mahabir, R. C. (2010). A nationwide review of the associations among cervical spine injuries, head injuries, and facial features. *Journal of Trauma-Injury Infection & Critical Care, 68*(3), 587–592.

Oddo, M., Levine, J. M., Frangos, S., Carrera, E., Maloney-Wilensky, E., Pascual, J. L., . . . LeRoux, P. D. (2009). Effect of mannitol and hypertonic saline on cerebral oxygenation in patients with severe traumatic brain injury and refractory intracranial hypertension. *J Neurol Neurosurg Psychiatry, 80*, 916–920.

Olson, D. A. (2013). In S. A. Berman (Ed.), *Head injury*. Retrieved from http://emedicine.medscape.com/article/1163653-overview

Papadakis, M. A., McPhee, S. J., & Rabow, M. W. (2013). *Current medical diagnosis and treatment* (53rd ed.). New York, NY: McGraw Hill/Appleton & Lange.

Park, S., Roederer, A., Mani, R., Schmitt, S., LeRoux, P. D., Ungar, L. H., . . . Kasner, S. E. (2011). *Neurocritical Care, 15*(3), 469–476.

Paul, P. & Williams, B. (2009). *Brunner & Suddarth's textbook of Canadian medical-surgical nursing*. Philadelphia, PA: Lippincott Williams & Wilkins.

Rabchevsky, A. G., & Kitzman, P. H. (2011). Latest approaches for the treatment of spasticity and autonomic dysreflexia in chronic spinal cord injury. *Neurotherapeutics, 8*(2), 274–282.

Rangel-Castilla, L., Lara, L. R., Gopinath, S., Swank, P. R., Valadka, A., & Robertson, C. (2010). Cerebral hemodynamic effects of acute hyperoxia and hyperventilation after severe traumatic brain injury. *Journal of Neurotrauma, 27*(10), 1853–1863.

Roy, R. R., Harkema, S. J., & Edgerton, V. R. (2012). Basic concepts of activity-based interventions for improved recovery of motor function after spinal cord injury. *Archives of Physical Medicine and Rehabilitation, 93*(9), 1487–1497.

Skandsen, T., Kvistad, K. A., Solheim, O., Strand, I. H., Folvik, M., & Vik, A. (2010). Prevalence and impact of diffuse axonal injury in patients with moderate and severe head injury: A cohort study of early magnetic resonance imaging findings and 1-year outcome. *Journal of Neurosurgery, 113*(3), 556–563.

Spiotta, A. M., Stiefel, M. F., Gracias, V. H., Garuffe, A. M., Kofke, W. A., Maloney-Wilensky, E., . . . Le Roux, P. D. (2010). *Journal of Neurosurgery, 113*(3), 571–580.

Stein, M. B., & McAllister, T. W. (2009). Exploring the convergence of posttraumatic stress disorder and mild traumatic brain injury. *The American Journal of Psychiatry, 166*(7).

Urbano, L. A., & Oddo, M. (2012). Therapeutic hypothermia for traumatic brain injury. *Current Neurology and Neuroscience Reports, 12*(5), 580–591.

Walker, J. (2009). Spinal cord injuries: Acute care management and rehabilitation. *Nursing Standard, 23*(42), 47–56.

Wyckoff, M., Houghton, D., & LePage, C. (Eds.). (2009). *Critical Care: Concepts, Role, and Practice for the Acute Care Nurse Practitioner*. New York, NY: Springer.

CHAPTER **5**

Central Nervous System Disorders

JUDI KURIC • CHARLENE M. MYERS

MENINGITIS

I. **Definition**
   A. Inflammation of the arachnoid, dura mater, and/or pia mater of the brain or spinal cord (also known as the meninges), which is caused by viral, bacterial, or fungal infections
II. **Etiology/predisposing factors**
   A. Predisposing factors for the development of meningitis include sinusitis, otitis media, mastoiditis, pneumonia, trauma, and congenital malformations.
   B. Bacterial meningitis
      1. Profound and life threatening; may be fatal within hours
      2. Bacteria that are present in the meninges attract inflammatory cells and cytokines, causing a breach in the blood brain barrier, which allows white blood cells (WBCs), fluids, and other infection-fighting particles to enter the meninges.
      3. Neutrophils gather in the area and begin making exudates within the subarachnoid space.
      4. Exudates cause the cerebrospinal fluid (CSF) to thicken and decrease the flow of CSF through the brain and the spinal cord.
         a. *Streptococcus pneumoniae* (pneumococcal meningitis)
            i. Most common and most serious bacterial meningitis that may cause neurologic damage ranging from deafness to severe brain damage
            ii. Occurs frequently in infants (younger than 2 years), adults with weakened immune systems, and the elderly

        iii. Rates in children younger than 2 years have decreased since the pneumococcal 7-valent conjugate vaccine (Prevnar) has been available.

   b. *Neisseria meningitidis* (meningococcal meningitis)

        i. May occur in schools, colleges, and other group settings

        ii. Spreads through contact with drainage of the nasopharynx or with blood

        iii. High-risk groups include infants younger than 1 year, people with suppressed immune systems, travelers to foreign countries where the disease is endemic, and college students (freshman in particular) who reside in dormitories.

   c. *Haemophilus influenzae*

        i. At one time, this was the most common cause of acute bacterial meningitis.

        ii. *H. influenzae B* (Hib) vaccine has greatly reduced the number of cases in the United States.

        iii. Children most at risk are those in daycare and children who do not have access to the vaccine.

   d. *Escherichia coli* and *Enterobacter*, *Klebsiella*, and *Proteus*

        i. May occur in infants, the elderly, and immunosuppressed patients

   e. Atypical bacterial meningitides (less common)

        i. *Listeria monocytogenes*

        ii. Staphylococci (*Staphylococcus aureus* and *Staphylococcus epidermidis*)

        iii. *Mycobacterium tuberculosis*

        iv. Streptococci

   f. Meningitis may follow an upper respiratory tract infection or head trauma.

C. Aseptic or viral meningitis

   1. Pia and arachnoid space are filled with lymphocytes but not with exudate forms.

   2. Much more benign and self-limited than bacterial meningitis

   3. Most viral meningitis occurs in late summer and early fall.

   4. Transmission usually occurs via cough, saliva, and fecal matter of an infected person.

   5. Caused by viruses

      a. Enterovirus (most common)

      b. Arbovirus

      c. Mumps

      d. Varicella zoster

      e. Herpes simplex types 1 and 2

      f. Measles

      g. Rubella

        h. Cytomegalovirus

        i. Influenza

        j. Epstein-Barr virus

        k. Human immunodeficiency virus (HIV)

    6. Fungal

        a. Most common in immunocompromised (particularly in patients with AIDS through inhalation and bloodstream spread)

        b. *Candida albicans*

        c. *Coccidioides immitis*

        d. *Cryptococcus neoformans* (most common fungal meningitis; found in bird droppings)

        e. *Histoplasma capsulatum*

        f. *Aspergillus*

  D. Syphilis

III. **Clinical manifestations**

  A. Severe headache

  B. Stiff neck (nuchal rigidity) related to meningeal irritation (meningismus)

  C. Photophobia, may have diplopia

  D. Fever of 101°F–103°F (38°C–40°C); toxic appearance

  E. Altered mental status

  F. Cranial nerve palsy

  G. Seizures

  H. Chills, myalgias

  I. Kernig's sign

    1. Flex the patient's leg at the knee, then at the hip, to a 90° angle, and then extend the knee

    2. In a patient with meningitis, this maneuver will trigger pain and spasms of the hamstring muscles caused by inflammation of the meninges and spinal nerve roots.

  J. Brudzinski's sign

    1. Flex the patient's head and neck to the chest.

    2. The legs will flex at the hips and at the knees in response to this movement.

  K. Nausea and vomiting

  L. Purpura or petechiae may be seen with meningococcal meningitis.

    1. Located on the trunk, lower extremities, mucous membranes, conjunctiva

    2. Patients with rapidly evolving rash, indicative of poor outcome, require emergent care

  M. Vertigo

  N. Exaggerated deep tendon reflexes

Table 5.1	Comparison of cerebrospinal fluid in bacterial versus viral meningitis	
	Bacterial	**Viral**
Appearance	Cloudy	Clear (occasionally cloudy)
Opening pressure	Elevated (greater than 180 mm H_2O)	Normal (less than 200 mm H_2O)
Cells	Increased white blood cells (100–5,000 mm) Most are polymorphonuclear	Increased white blood cells (50–1,000 mm) Most are mononuclear
Total protein	Increased (100–500 mg/dl)	Normal or slightly increased (less than 200 mg/dl)
Glucose	Decreased (5–40 mg/dl or 0.3 times blood glucose level)	Normal (greater than 45 mg/dl)
Culture	Bacteria present on Gram stain	No bacteria present

IV.   Laboratory findings/diagnostics

   A. Lumbar puncture (LP) should be performed as soon as a diagnosis is suspected.

   1. CT scan of the head should be completed prior to the LP in patients with altered level of consciousness, papilledema, neurologic deficits, new-onset seizures, immunocompromised state, or history of central nervous system (CNS) disease

   B. LP in bacterial meningitis (see table 5.1)

   1. Appearance of CSF: cloudy
   2. Opening pressure: elevated (greater than 180 mm H_2O)
   3. Cells: increased WBCs (100–5,000/mm; most are polymorphonuclear cells)
   4. Total protein: increased (100–500 mg/dl [normal, 15–45 mg/dl])
   5. Glucose: decreased (5–40 mg/dl or 0.3 times blood glucose level [normal 45–80 mg/dl or 0.6 times blood glucose level])
   6. Culture: bacteria present on Gram stain and culture

   C. LP in viral meningitis

   1. Appearance of CSF: clear, occasionally cloudy
   2. Opening pressure: usually normal (less than 180 mm H_2O)
   3. Cells: increased WBCs (50–1,000/mm; most are mononuclear cells)
   4. Total protein: normal or slightly increased (less than 200 mg/dl)
   5. Glucose: normal (greater than 45 mg/dl)
   6. Culture: no bacteria present; demonstration of virus requires special technique

   D. CT scan of the head is indicated in patients with focal neurologic signs or diminished level of consciousness.

E. In patients who have signs, symptoms, and CSF findings typical of bacterial meningitis but in whom no organisms are found, follow-up CT scans should be obtained, even if clinical improvement occurs, because such patients may have a brain abscess and may require neurosurgical intervention.

F. An additional maneuver in assessing for meningitis is to elicit jolt accentuation of the patient's headache by asking the patient to turn his or her head horizontally at a frequency of two to three rotations per second.

   1. Worsening of a baseline headache is a positive sign.

   2. Include examination of the cranial nerves, motor and sensory systems, and reflexes, as well as testing for Babinski's reflex

G. Assess the ears, sinuses, and respiratory system.

H. Obtain blood and sputum cultures, nasopharyngeal specimen.

I. Obtain complete blood count (CBC), electrolytes, coagulation profiles, and liver/renal panel.

J. Chest, skull, and sinus films or chest CT scan may be necessary to facilitate detection of primary infection

K. Serology (antigen tests)

   1. Latex agglutination tests

      a. Can detect antigens of encapsulated organisms such as *S. pneumoniae, H. influenzae, N. meningitidis,* and *C. neoformans*

      b. Rarely used, beneficial in patients who have been pretreated with antibiotics and who have a negative Gram stain and CSF

   2. Polymerase chain reaction testing of CSF

      a. Has been employed to detect bacteria (*S. pneumoniae, H. influenzae, N. meningitidis, M. tuberculosis, Borrelia burgdorferi,* and *Tropheryma whippelii*) and viruses (herpes simplex, varicella-zoster, cytomegalovirus, Epstein-Barr virus, and enterovirus) in patients with meningitis

      b. Test results are rapid and are obtained within hours.

   3. Enzyme linked immunosorbent assay (ELISA)

      a. Detects immunoglobulin (Ig)M early in the infection and IgG as the disease progresses

   4. HIV/AIDS testing

V.   Management

A. Consult infectious disease specialist, particularly for cases in which the preferred therapy cannot be used or when the pathogens/organism is resistant to usual therapy

B. Antibiotics must be initiated immediately in those suspected to have meningitis. See table 5.2 for empiric treatment.

Table 5.2	Empiric Treatment for Suspected Meningitis	
	Common Pathogens	**Drugs of First Choices**[a]
2–50 years	*N. meningitidis, S. pneumoniae, H. influenzae*	Vancomycin weight based dose to achieve vancomycin trough level of 15–20 mg/L PLUS Ceftriaxone 2 grams IV every 12 hr or Cefotaxime 2 grams IV every 4–6 hr
Older than 50 years	*S. pneumoniae, N. meningitidis, H. influenzae, L. monocytogenes,* aerobic gram-negative bacilli	Vancomycin weight based dose to achieve Vancomycin trough level of 15–20 mg/L PLUS Ampicillin 2 grams IV every 4 hr PLUS Ceftriaxone 2 grams IV every 12 hr or cefotaxime 2 grams IV every 4–6 h
Neurosurgery or Head Trauma	*S. aureus, Enterobacteriaceae,* Resistant gram negative bacilli, *S. pneumoniae*	Cefepime 2 grams IV every 8 hr PLUS Vancomycin weight based dose to achieve vancomycin trough level of 15–20 mg/L

[a]In those allergic to penicillin and third-generation cephalosporin, consult with infectious disease specialist or pharmacist for alternative therapy.

C. Meningococcal meningitis: patients 18–60 years of age with penicillin-susceptible infection: aqueous penicillin G (4 million units IV every 4 hr); continue until 5–7 days after the patient becomes afebrile
   1. If penicillin-intermediate sensitivity: ceftriaxone, 2 grams IV every 12 hr, or cefotaxime, 2 grams IV every 4–6 hr
D. *H. influenzae* meningitis that is β-lactamase negative: ampicillin, 2 grams IV every 4 hr
   1. If β-lactamase positive: third-generation cephalosporin (ceftriaxone [Rocephin], 2 grams IV every 12 hr or cefotaxime, 2 grams IV every 4 hr)
E. Aseptic meningitis: supportive therapy
   1. Treat the severely ill empirically with antibiotics.
F. Tuberculosis: isoniazid (INH), 5 mg/kg/day (maximum, 300 mg/day) plus pyridoxine, 50 mg PO daily; rifampin (RIF), 600 mg IV/PO daily; pyrazinamide (PZA), 15–30 mg/kg once daily (maximum, 2000 mg/day); ethambutol (EMB), 15–25 mg/kg once daily (maximum, 1600 mg/day)

G. If *S. Pneumonia* is suspected, add dexamethasone, 0.15 mg/kg IV every 6 hr for 2–4 days

   1. Should be administered prior to, or with, first antibiotic dose, not after regimen has already been started.

H. Anticonvulsants (lorazepam or diazepam) for acute seizure control

I. Acetaminophen, 325–1000 mg every 4 hr PRN for pain/fever (not to exceed 3000 mg/24 hr)

J. Intravenous hydration with lactated Ringer's solution or normal saline; avoid hypotonic solutions and dextrose 5% in water

CEREBRAL ABSCESS

I. **Definition/etiology**

  A. Infected space-occupying lesion containing pus, cells, and other materials in the brain

  B. Usually due to bacterial or fungal infection from a different primary source, generally in or near the brain

    1. Otitis media

    2. Mastoid infection

    3. Sinusitis

    4. Oral surgery (rare)

  C. Other sources for abscess

    1. Lung infection/empyema

    2. Skin infection

    3. Bacterial endocarditis

    4. Bronchiectasis

    5. Congenital heart disease

    6. Penetrating trauma, skull fracture, intracranial procedures

II. **Clinical manifestations (symptoms depend on location in the brain)**

  A. General: ill appearance, lethargic

  B. Elevated body temperature may or may not be present

  C. Signs of increased intracranial pressure: nausea, vomiting, altered level of consciousness, focal neurologic deficit

  D. Neurologic: speech and visual disturbances, hemiparesis, seizures, headache

  E. Patients go through two phases of symptoms with cerebral abscess

    1. Stage I: initial formation of abscess

      a. Headache, chills, fever, malaise

      b. Confusion, drowsiness, speech disorder

    2. Stage II: due to expanding cerebral mass

      a. Vague signs and symptoms of brain tumor: recurrent headache of increased severity, confusion, drowsy, stupor, flulike symptoms

III. **Diagnosis/treatment**

  A. Laboratory studies

1. Elevated WBC count, elevated sedimentation rate
2. LP (need CT prior to procedure)—elevated opening pressure, mild increase in protein level
3. CT scan of the head—identify space-occupying lesion with contrast enhancement
   a. Multiple lesions possible
4. Magnetic resonance imaging (MRI) of the head: similar to CT; more information on necrosis versus edema

B. Treatment: identification of pathogen and primary infection source are key to successful treatment; long-term (6–12 weeks) antibiotic treatment is given

C. Surgical removal and debridement is considered in abscesses that are greater than 2.5 cm and easily accessible.

D. Outcome is directly related to neurologic status of patient at the time of diagnosis

ENCEPHALITIS

I.   **Definition**

A. Acute inflammation of the brain caused by virus, bacteria, fungus, or parasite; viral encephalitis is most common

II.   **Etiology**

A. Herpes simplex virus (HSV) encephalitis
   1. Most common cause of acute sporadic viral encephalitis in the United States

B. Mumps, measles, varicella-zoster virus

C. Possible influenza

D. Tick infestation
   1. Lyme disease
   2. Rocky Mountain spotted fever
   3. Eastern equine encephalitis
   4. Japanese encephalitis (1 year after travel to Asia)
   5. La Crosse encephalitis
   6. St. Louis encephalitis (3,000 cases/year)
   7. Western equine encephalitis
   8. West Nile virus
      a. Transmission of West Nile virus
         i. Mosquitoes become infected when they feed on infected birds.
         ii. The mosquito circulates the virus in the blood for several days.
         iii. During this time, the mosquito can infect humans and other animals by biting to take blood.
         iv. The virus is injected into the human or animal, where it multiplies and may cause illness.

E. Toxoplasmosis

        1. Commonly seen in patients with AIDS

    F. Enteroviruses, polioviruses

    G. Rabies

    H. Cytomegalovirus (CMV), HIV, rubella virus

III. **Signs and symptoms (vary based on organism and area involved)**

    A. General: anxious, lethargic, possibly comatose

    B. Vital signs: unstable if advanced CNS infection, fever

    C. Eyes: nystagmus, ocular paralysis, photophobia

    D. Gastrointestinal: nausea/vomiting

    E. Musculoskeletal: nuchal rigidity

    F. Neurologic: severe headache, altered level of consciousness, ataxia, dysphagia, hemiparesis, stupor progressing to coma, confusion, olfactory or gustatory hallucinations, seizures, aphasia, cranial nerve deficit, Babinski reflex

IV. **Diagnostic testing**

    A. Standard laboratory tests

        1. Complete blood count

        2. Chemistry

        3. Liver function tests

        4. Culture of body fluids: blood, urine, stool, nasopharynx, sputum

    B. LP

        1. Elevated WBC count

        2. Red blood cell count normal (elevated with HSV)

        3. Protein: normal or slightly elevated

        4. Glucose: normal or slightly elevated

    C. Possible open brain biopsy to identify treatable causes

V. **Specific diagnostic testing**

    A. Electroencephalogram (EEG): abnormal with slowing or epileptiform activity; temporal lobe abnormalities suggest HSV infection

    B. Measurement of IgM antibody in serum and CSF

        1. Collect within 8 days; use the IgM antibody capture enzyme-linked immunosorbent assay (MAC-ELISA)

    C. IgM does not cross the blood-brain barrier; if it is present in the CSF, a CNS infection (likely, encephalitis) is suggested.

VI. **Imaging diagnostics**

    A. CT scan

    B. MRI

    C. Brain scan

    D. Usually normal initially; later, nonspecific abnormalities are identified

    E. If temporal lobe disease exists, a diagnosis of HSV infection is suggested.

VII. **Treatment for encephalitis**

    A. Admit to the intensive care unit; most treatment is supportive

    B. Intravenous fluids

    C. Respiratory support

    D. Circulatory support

    E. Prevention of secondary infection

    F. Anticonvulsants (lorazepam or diazepam for acute seizure treatment)

    G. Monitor for cerebral edema.

    H. Monitor for syndrome of inappropriate antidiuretic hormone secretion.

VIII. Specific treatments

    A. Consult an infectious disease specialist

    B. Acyclovir, 10 mg/kg IV every 8 hr for adults, is used for herpes simplex virus—administer as early as possible, adjust dose for renal impairment

        1. Acyclovir should be initiated in all patients with suspected encephalitis, pending results of diagnostic studies

    C. Other empirical antimicrobial agents should be initiated on basis of specific epidemiologic or clinical factors, including appropriate therapy for presumed bacterial meningitis, if clinically indicated

    D. No specific antiviral therapy is available for other causes.

    E. Supportive care

IX. Reporting encephalitis

    A. The Centers for Disease Control and Prevention has devised standards for reporting cases of encephalitis in humans, mosquitoes, and birds.

    B. Each state has specific guidelines regarding human, mosquito, and bird notification.

    C. Guidelines are available for handling dead birds and mosquitoes at www.cdc.com.

ENCEPHALOPATHY

I. Definition

    A. Dysfunction of the brain caused by a disease or disease process

II. Etiology

    A. Hepatic

    B. Hypertensive

    C. Metabolic (lactic acidosis, metabolic acidosis)

    D. Electrolytes (hyponatremia, hypoglycemia, hypercalcemia)

    E. Uremic

    F. Anoxic-ischemic

    G. Hypercapnic

    H. Endocrine (hyperparathyroidism, Cushing's disease)

    I. AIDS

    J. Thiamine deficiency (Wernicke disease)

III. Clinical manifestations

    A. Depends on cause and may include the following:

        1. Headache

        2. Inattentiveness, impaired judgment

        3. Motor incoordination

      4. Drowsiness

      5. Confusion

      6. Stupor

      7. Coma

      8. Altered mental status or personality changes

IV. Diagnosis

  A. Depends on clinical event

      1. Physical presentation

      2. Serum laboratory analysis (ammonia)

      3. CSF analysis

      4. EEG activity

      5. MRI

V. Management

  A. ABCs of emergency care (airway, breathing, and circulation)

  B. Correction of underlying cause

      1. Specific treatment determined by underlying cause (i.e., hepatic = lactulose, anoxia = oxygen, hypoperfusion of CNS = vasopressors)

  C. Prevention of irreversible neurologic injury

  D. Anticonvulsant therapy for seizures (lorazepam or diazepam for treatment of acute seizures), if clinically indicated

BIBLIOGRAPHY

Bader, M. K., & Littlejohn, L. R. (2010). *AANN core curriculum for neuroscience nursing* (5th ed.). Glenview, IL: American Association of Neuroscience Nurses.

Bamberger, D. (2010). Diagnosis, Initial Management, and Prevention of Meningitis. *Am Fam Physician, 82*(12), 1491–1498.

Centers for Disease Control. (2010). *St. Louis encephalitis*. Retrieved from http://www.cdc.gov/sle/

Centers for Disease Control. (2010). *Eastern equine encephalitis*. Retrieved from http://www.cdc.gov/EasternEquineEncephalitis/

Centers for Disease Control. (2013). *Japanese encephalitis*. Retrieved from http://www.cdc.gov/japaneseencephalitis/

Centers for Disease Control. (2013). *West Nile virus: information for health care providers*. Retrieved from http://www.cdc.gov/westnile/healthCareProviders/

Ferri, F. F. (2010). *Practical guide to the care of the medical patient* (8th ed.). St. Louis, MO: Mosby.

Hasbun, R., & Bronze, M. S. (2014). *Meningitis*. Retrieved from http://emedicine.medscape.com/article/232915-overview

Ibrahim, S. I., Cheang, P. P., & Nunez, D. A. (2010). Incidence of meningitis secondary to suppurative otitis media in adults. *Journal of Laryngology and Otology, 124*(11), 1158–1161.

Longo, D., Fauci, A., Kapser, D., & Hauser, S. (2011). *Harrison's principles of internal medicine* (18th ed.). New York, NY: McGraw Hill/Appleton & Lange.

Molyneux, E., Nizami, S. Q., Saha, S., Huu, K. T., Azam, M., Bhutta, Z. A., . . . Qazi, S. A. (2011). 5 versus 10 days of treatment with ceftriaxone for bacterial meningitis in children: A double-blind randomised equivalence study. *Lancet, 377*(9780), 1837–1845.

Papadakis, M. A., McPhee, S. J., & Tierney, L. M. (Eds.). (2013). *Current medical diagnosis and treatment* (52nd ed.). New York, NY: McGraw Hill/Appleton & Lange.

Thigpen, M. C., Whitney, C. G., Messonnier, N. E., Zell, E. R., Lynfield, R., Hadler, J. L., . . . Schuchat, A. (2011). Bacterial meningitis in the United States, 1998–2007. *New England Journal of Medicine, 364*(21), 2016–2025.

Thwaites, G. E. (2012). The mangement of suspected encephalitis. *British Medical Journal, 344*, e3489. doi: 10.1136/bmj.e3489

Waghdhare, S., Kalantri, A., Joshi, R., & Kalantri, S. (2010). Accuracy of physical signs for detecting meningitis: A hospital-based diagnostic accuracy study. *Clinical Neurology and Neurosurgery, 112*(9), 752–757.

CHAPTER **6**

Seizure Disorders

PATRICK A. LAIRD • CHARLENE M. MYERS

I. Definition

  A. Seizure disorders are transient disturbances of the cerebral function caused by an abnormal paroxysmal neuronal discharge within the brain; epilepsy is the term used to describe recurrent, unprovoked seizures

II. Etiology

  A. Cause may be unknown

  B. Metabolic disorders

    1. Acidosis

    2. Electrolyte imbalance (e.g., hyponatremia, hypocalcemia)

    3. Hypoglycemia

    4. Hypoxia

    5. Alcohol or barbiturate withdrawal are the most common causes of new-onset seizures in adults

  C. Central nervous system (CNS) infection

  D. Head trauma

  E. Tumors and other space-occupying lesions

  F. Vascular disease (common with advancing age and the most common cause of onset of seizure disorder at age 60 or older)

  G. Degenerative disorders, such as Alzheimer's disease in later life

  H. The most common cause of seizures is noncompliance with a drug regimen on the part of a patient in whom epilepsy has been diagnosed.

III. Clinical manifestations

  A. Focal seizures: cortical discharges localized within one cerebral hemisphere

1. Focal seizures without dyscognitive features
   a. Consciousness is preserved; rarely lasts longer than 1 minute
   b. Jacksonian march movements: convulsive jerking or paresthesias/tingling that spreads to different parts of the limb or body
   c. Todd's paralysis: localized paresis in the involved region lasting minutes to hours
   d. Sensory symptoms
      i. Flashing lights
      ii. Simple hallucinations
      iii. Alterations in taste
      iv. Olfactory changes (intense smells)
      v. Paresthesias
      vi. Buzzing
   e. Autonomic symptoms
      i. Abnormal epigastric symptoms
      ii. Pallor
      iii. Sweating
      iv. Flushing
      v. Pupillary dilatation
      vi. Piloerection
   f. Speech arrest or vocalization
   g. Nausea
   h. May have an aura: subjective events not directly observable
   i. Psychic symptoms
      i. Déjà vu
      ii. Dreamy states
      iii. Fear
      iv. Distortion of time perception
2. Focal seizures with dyscognitive features
   a. Most common seizure in epileptics
      i. Any simple partial seizure onset followed by impairment of consciousness
   b. Automatisms may occur
      i. Lip smacking
      ii. Chewing
      iii. Swallowing
      iv. Sucking
      v. Picking at clothes
   c. May begin with a stare at the time consciousness is impaired
   d. Frequently begin with an aura
B. Generalized seizures—originates in all areas of cortex simultaneously
   1. Typical absence seizures

      a. Sudden loss of consciousness (5–30 seconds), with eyes fluttering or muscles spasms occurring at a rate of 3 per second; begins and ends so quickly that it may not be apparent

      b. Common in children (ages 6–14 years)

      c. Occasionally accompanied by mild clonic, tonic, or atonic components

      d. Autonomic components (enuresis)

      e. Can accompany automatisms

      f. If the seizure occurs during conversation, the patient may miss a few words or may break off for a few seconds.

      g. Frequently occur several times a day, often when the patient is sitting quietly; infrequent during exercise

  2. Atypical absence seizures

      a. Alteration in consciousness typically longer

      b. Often accompanied by obvious motor signs

      c. May be associated with structural abnormalities of the brain

      d. Less responsive to anticonvulsants

  3. Generalized tonic-clonic seizures: Neuronal discharge spreads throughout the entire cerebral cortex.

      a. Often begins abruptly followed by an outcry (caused by air being forced out of the lungs due to generalized muscle tonicity)

      b. Loss of consciousness and falling

      c. Respiration is arrested.

      d. Tonic (muscle rigidity) then clonic (synchronous muscle jerks) contractions of the muscles of the extremities, trunk, and head

      e. Commonly with urinary incontinence

      f. Usually lasts 2–5 minutes

      g. May be preceded by a prodromal mood change and followed by a postictal state

         i. Deep sleep

         ii. Headache

         iii. Muscle soreness

         iv. Amnesia of events

         v. Nausea

         vi. Confusion

         vii. Combination of any of the above

C. Status epilepticus: a series of seizures lasting longer than 5 minutes with the patient never returning to baseline between seizures

  1. Aggressive treatment is required for a patient with continuing seizures lasting 5–10 minutes or seizures without intervening consciousness.

  2. Status epilepticus is a medical emergency requiring immediate treatment.

3. The longer the seizure activity lasts, the more difficult it is to control the seizure.

IV. **Diagnosis**

A. Obtain a thorough history from the patient, the family, and/or the observers of the event

B. Twenty-four-hour continuous EEG is an important test for supporting the diagnosis of epilepsy, differentiating between types of seizures, and providing a guide to prognosis.
1. Focal abnormalities indicate partial seizures
2. Generalized abnormalities indicate primary generalized seizures
3. A normal EEG does not rule out a seizure

C. CT scan or MRI of the head—performed for all new-onset seizures, especially after age 30 years, because of the possibility of an underlying neoplasm
1. MRI preferred over CT scan to identify specific lesions in non-emergent cases

D. Lumbar puncture (if indicated) is performed to assess for an infectious process after CT scan or MRI has been used to rule out expanding mass that may increase intracranial pressure (ICP).

E. Twenty-four-hour EEG to document seizure activity

F. Blood analysis
1. Complete blood count
2. Glucose, liver, and renal function tests
3. Venereal Disease Research Laboratory test
4. Electrolytes
5. Magnesium
6. Calcium
7. Antinuclear antibody
8. Erythrocyte sedimentation rate
9. Arterial blood gases

G. Urinalysis, drug screen

H. Serum prolactin rises two to three times above normal for 10–60 minutes after occurrence of 80% of tonic-clonic or complex partial seizures

V. **Management**

A. Initial management is supportive

B. Most seizures are self-limiting
1. Maintain open airway
2. Place patient in left lateral decubitus position
3. Protect the patient from injury
4. Administer oxygen if the patient is cyanotic
5. Do not force airways or objects (e.g., tongue blade) between the teeth until the muscles have relaxed because this may cause the tongue to occlude the airway or teeth to break off and cause a partial obstruction

6. Start with intravenous (IV) normal saline
7. Perform ECG, and monitor respiration and blood pressure

C. For status epilepticus:
1. Benzodiazepines are first-line treatment, as these are able to rapidly control seizures
2. Lorazepam (Ativan), 0.1 mg/kg (4–8 mg with a maximum dose of 10 mg) at 2 mg/minute; IV diazepam (Valium), 0.1 mg/kg at 5 mg/minute (maximum, 20 mg); or midazolam (Versed), 0.1–0.3 mg/kg IV for a maximal dose of 10 mg (if IV lorazepam is not available)
3. If IV access is not available, nurse practitioner may prescribe midazolam 10 mg IM in patients greater than 40 kg or 5 mg IM for body weight between 13 and 40 kg
4. Monitor for respiratory depression after medications are given; intubation may become necessary
5. Increase normal saline if the patient becomes hypotensive
6. Phenytoin (Dilantin) should be administered simultaneously with lorazepam or diazepam and saline at 50 mg/minute until a loading dose of 20 mg/kg is reached
   a. Fosphenytoin (Cerebyx) does not irritate the veins and can be given with all common IV solutions; it may be administered more quickly than phenytoin (150 mg/minute vs. 50 mg/minute) without risk of cardiovascular collapse
      i. It is also more expensive
7. If the above measures to abort status epilepticus are unsuccessful, intubate and administer phenobarbital (Luminal), 100 mg/minute IV to a maximum of 20 mg/kg.
8. If still unsuccessful after 60 minutes, consider general anesthesia with propofol (Diprivan), loading dose of 3–5 mg/kg, followed by an infusion of 30–100 mcg/kg/min.

D. Clinical pharmacology of the antiepileptic drugs (AEDs) (Table 6.1)
E. Drugs for specific types of seizures (Table 6.2)
F. Titrate dosages to achieve adequate serum levels. If a first drug partially controls seizures at a maximal therapeutic level, add a second drug to achieve therapeutic levels. Evaluation of serum phenytoin may require additional correction based on serum albumin level and/or current renal function; consult pharmacist for appropriate correction of phenytoin levels to avoid unnecessary dosage adjustments.
G. If the patient is seizure-free, monitor the patient, not the levels.
H. One should never abruptly withdraw an anticonvulsant from a patient; these drugs should be tapered.

Table 6.1	Clinical pharmacology of antiepileptic drugs				
Drug	**Product name**	**Dosing schedule**	**Daily maintenance dosage in adults, mg**	**Target serum level, mcg/ml**	**Induces hepatic drug metabolism**
Traditional antiepileptic drugs					
Carbamazepine	Tegretol	3 times daily	600–1800	4–12	Yes
	Epitol	3 times daily			
	Tegretol-XR	2 times daily			
	Carbatrol	2 times daily			
	Equetro	2 times daily			
Ethosuximide	Zarontin (generic)	1–2 times daily	750	40–100	No
Phenobarbital		1–2 times daily	60–120	15–45	Yes
Phenytoin	Dilantin-125	2–3 times daily	200–300	10–20	Yes
	Dilantin Infatab	2–3 times daily			
	Phenytek	1 time daily			
	Dilantin (ER capsules)	1 time daily			
Primidone	Mysoline	3–4 times daily	500–750	5–15[d]	Yes
Valproic acid	Depakene	3–4 times daily	750–3000	40–100	No
	Depakote	3–4 times daily			
	Depakote ER	2 times daily			
	Stavzor	2–3 times daily			
Additional antieplileptic drugs					
Gabapentin	Neurontin	3 times daily	1200–3600	ND	No
Lacosamide	Vimpat	2 times daily	200–400	ND	No
Lamotrigine	Lamictal, Lamictal ODT	2 times daily	400[bc]	ND	No

Table 6.1   Clinical pharmacology of antiepileptic drugs

Drug	Product name	Dosing schedule	Daily maintenance dosage in adults, mg	Target serum level, mcg/ml	Induces hepatic drug metabolism
	Lamictal XR	1 time daily			
Levetiracetam	Keppra	2 times daily	2000–3000	ND	No
Oxcarbazepine[a]	Trileptal	2 times daily	900–2400	3–40	No
Pregabalin	Lyrica	2–3 times daily	150–600	ND	No
Rufinamide	Banzel	2 times daily	3200	ND	Yes[e]
Tiagabine	Gabitril	2–4 times daily	16–32	ND	No
Topiramate	Topamax	2 times daily	100–400	ND	No
Vigabatrin	Sabril	2 times daily	3000–6000	ND	Yes
Zonisamide	Zonegran	1–2 times daily	200–400	ND	No

Note. To avoid serious adverse effects, all anticonvulsant medications must be tapered up or down while drug levels and other pertinent diagnostic test results (laboratory and radiologic) are monitored. Patients should be maintained at the lowest effective dose. ND = not determined; ER = extended release; XR = extended release; ODT = orally disintegrating tablet. Adapted with permission from "Drugs for Epilepsy," by R.A. Lehne, 2013, *Pharmacology for Nursing Care, 8th Edition*, p. 232. Copyright 2013 by WB Saunders.

[a]Oxcarbazepine does not induce enzymes that metabolize antiepileptic drugs, but it does induce enzymes that metabolize other types of drugs. [b]Dosages must be decreased in patients taking valproic acid. [c]Dosages must be increased in patients taking drugs that induce hepatic drug-metabolizing enzymes. [d]Target serum levels are 5–15 mcg/ml for primidone itself and 15–40 mcg/ml for phenobarbital derived from primidone. [e]Rufinamide produces mild induction of CYP3A4.

I. Vagus nerve stimulation is used in conjunction with medications by patients with severe, uncontrolled seizures. Stimulation is typically applied for 30 seconds every 5 minutes. When the vagus is stimulated, resultant impulses in some way interrupt or prevent abnormal neuronal firing.

Table 6.2 Drugs for specific types of seizures		
Seizure Type	**Traditional AEDs**	**Newer AEDs**
Focal Seizures **With and without** **dyscognitive features**	Carbamazepine Phenytoin Valproic Acid Phenobarbital Primidone	Ezogabine Oxcarbazepine Gabapentin Lacosamide Lamotrigine Levetiracetam Pregabalin Topiramate Tiagabine Vigbatrin Zonisamide
Generalized **Tonic-clonic**	Carbamazepine Phenytoin Valproic Acid Phenobarbital Primidone	Lamotrigine Levetiracetam Topiramate
Absence **Typical and atypical**	Ethosuximide Valproic Acid	Lamotrigine
Myoclonic	Valproic Acid	Lamotrigine Levetiracetam Topiramate

Note. To avoid serious adverse effects, all anticonvulsant medications must be tapered up and down while drug levels and other pertinent diagnostic test results (laboratory and radiologic) are carefully monitored. Patients should be maintained at the lowest effective dose. AED=anti-epileptic drug. Adapted from "Drugs for Epilepsy," by Richard A. Lehne, 2013, *Pharmacology for Nursing Care, 8*[th] *Edition*, p. 228. Copyright 2013 by WB Saunders, with permission.

BIBLIOGRAPHY

Aminoff, M. J., & Kerchner, G. A. (2014). Nervous system disorders. In M. A. Papadakis, S. J. McPhee, M. W. Rabow, & T. G. Berger (Eds.), *CURRENT Medical Diagnosis & Treatment 2014*. New York, NY: McGraw-Hill.

Bothamley, J., & Boyle, M. (2009). *Medical conditions affecting pregnancy and childbirth*. Oxford: Radcliffe Pub.

Engel, J. (2013). *Seizures and epilepsy*. Oxford, UK: Oxford University Press.

Foreman, B., & Hirsch, L. J. (2012). Epilepsy emergencies: Diagnosis and management. *Neurologic Clinics, 30*(1), 11–41.

French, J. A., & Pedley, T. A. (2009). Initial management of epilepsy. *New England Journal of Medicine, 359*(2), 166–176.

Holtkamp, M., & Meierkord, H. (2011). Nonconvulsive status epilepticus: A diagnostic and therapeutic challenge in the intensive care setting. *Therapeutic Advances in Neurological Disorders, 4,* 169–181.

Kwan, P., Schachter, S. C., & Brodie, M. J. (2011). Current concepts: Drug-resistant epilepsy. *New England Journal of Medicine, 365*(10): 919–926.

Lee, K. (Ed.). (2012). *The NeuroICU book*. New York, NY: McGraw-Hill.

Lehne, R. A. (2013). *Pharmacology for nursing care* (8th ed.). St. Louis, MO: WB Saunders.

Lowenstein, D. H. (2012). Seizures and epilepsy. In A. S. Fauci, E. Braunwald, D. L. Kasper, S. L. Hauser, D. L. Longo, J. L. Jameson, et al. (Eds.), *Harrison's principles of internal medicine* (18th ed.). New York, NY: McGraw Hill.

Loscalzo, J. (Ed.). (2012). *Harrison's principles of internal medicine* (18th ed., pp. 3251–3270). New York, NY: McGraw-Hill.

Marik, P. E., & Varon, J. (2004). The management of status epilepticus. *Chest, 126*(2), 582–591.

Marx, J. A., Hockberger, R. S., & Walls, R. M. (2014). *Rosen's emergency medicine: Concepts and clinical practice* (8th ed., expert consult premium edition). Philadelphia, PA: Elsevier.

Shorvon, S., Guerrini, R., Cook, M., & Lhatoo, S. (2012). *Oxford textbook of epilepsy and epileptic seizures*. Oxford, UK: Oxford University Press.

Silbergleit, R., Durkalski, V., Lowenstein, D., Conwit, R., Pancioli, A., Palesch, Y., & Barsan, W. (2012). Intramuscular versus intravenous therapy for prehospital status epilepticus. *New England Journal of Medicine, 366*(7), 591–600.

CHAPTER 7
Dementia

ANGELA STARKWEATHER • CHARLENE M. MYERS

I. Definition

A. Dementia is a broad (global) acquired impairment of intellectual function (cognition) that is usually progressive and interferes with normal social and occupational activities.

B. The key features of dementia consist of an intact arousal state and impairment of memory, intellect, and personality.

C. The disorder is characterized by one or more of the following:
  1. General decrease in level of cognition
  2. Behavioral disturbance
  3. Interference with daily function and independence

D. It causes loss of mental functions such as thinking, memory, and reasoning.

E. It is not a disease but rather a group of symptoms caused by various diseases.

F. Refer to Psychosocial Problems in Acute Care chapter for ways to differentiate dementia from delirium.

II. Etiology

A. As many as 50 known causes of dementia

B. Develops when parts of the brain that are involved with learning, memory, and decision making are affected by various infections or diseases

C. Alzheimer's-type dementia (AD)
  1. AD is the most common form of dementia in the elderly.
  2. It accounts for 60%–80% of dementia cases.
  3. Neuronal damage in AD is irreversible; therefore, the disease cannot be cured.

4. The histopathology of AD is characterized by neuritic plaques, neurofibrillary tangles, and degeneration of cholinergic neurons in the hippocampus and cerebral cortex.
5. β-amyloid is present in high levels in AD; this may contribute to neuronal injury
6. AD results in cerebral atrophy

D. Diseases that cause degeneration or loss of nerve cells in the brain
1. Alzheimer's disease
2. Parkinson's disease
3. Huntington's disease

E. Vascular
1. Multi-infarct dementia
2. Stroke
3. Arteritis (15%–20%)

F. Infectious
1. HIV
2. Syphilis
3. Meningitis
4. Encephalitis
5. Abscess
6. Creutzfeldt-Jakob disease

G. Postencephalitic syndrome, central nervous system anoxia (drug overdose, cardiac arrest)

H. Nutritional deficiencies
1. Vitamin B12 deficiency
2. Folate deficiency
3. Other vitamin deficiencies

I. Toxic reactions
1. Chronic alcoholism
2. Drug toxicity

J. Subdural hematoma

K. Hydrocephalus

L. Chronic seizures

M. Illness other than in the brain
1. Kidney
2. Liver
3. Congestive heart failure
4. Hypercapnia
5. Hypoxemia
6. Rhythm disturbance
7. Acute myocardial infarction
8. Hypothyroidism/hyperthyroidism

N. Hearing loss

O. Blindness

P. Lewy body dementia

Q. Electrolyte imbalance
III. Signs/symptoms
    A. Onset may be slow, continuing over a period of months or years
    B. Confusion and memory deficits (usually short term in nature: asking the same question, repeatedly forgetting that the question was already answered)
    C. Misplacing things: putting an iron in the refrigerator
    D. Problems with language: forgetting simple words or using wrong words
    E. Impaired abstract reasoning: unable to balance a checkbook because of forgetfulness about what the numbers are and what to do with them
    F. Higher cognitive functions may be impaired.
        1. Aphasia: language difficulties that may be cognitive or receptive
        2. Apraxia: inability to perform previously learned purposeful movements (i.e., previously learned tasks) or to use objects properly
        3. Agnosia: loss of comprehension of auditory, visual, or other sensations, although the sensory sphere is intact; inability to recognize objects, shapes, persons, sounds, smells, and so forth
        4. Impaired executive functioning (abstracting/organizing)
    G. Disorientation: patients may become easily lost, even in familiar surroundings, or may wander
    H. Patients may have difficulty with learned tasks, such as dressing or cooking.
    I. Poor judgment: patients may forget that they are watching a child and may leave the child at home
    J. Loss of initiative: becoming passive; not wanting to go places or see other people
    K. Emotional problems such as depression, lability, or flattened affect
    L. Changes in mood: fast mood swings, calm to tears to anger in minutes
    M. Agitation, anxiousness, and sleeplessness
    N. Drastic personality changes: irritable, suspicious (paranoid ideation), and fearful
    O. Patients often lose insight into their deficits
    P. Difficulty recognizing family and friends
    Q. Severe symptoms include the following:
        1. Loss of speech
        2. Loss of appetite
        3. Weight loss
        4. Loss of bowel and bladder control
        5. Total dependence on caregiver
    R. Clouding of consciousness and orientation does not occur until the terminal stages.
IV. Laboratory/diagnostics
    A. History

1. Preferably with family members available to give adequate history of cognitive and behavior changes
2. Often, the spouse or other informant brings the problem to the practitioner's attention.
3. Self-reported memory loss does not usually correlate with dementia.

B. Physical examination
  1. Neurologic examination
  2. Cognitive testing
     a. Attempt the Folstein Mini-Mental State Examination to screen for dementia
        i. The maximum score is 30
        ii. A score of 23 or less indicates cognitive impairment
        iii. LOCAM-LT—mnemonic for Folstein components
            (a) Level of consciousness
            (b) Orientation
            (c) Concentration/calculation
            (d) Attention
            (e) Memory
            (f) Language
            (g) Thought process
     b. Document the progression of disease over time by repeating testing at 3- to 6-month intervals
  3. Examination should include observations of memory, thinking, concentration, attention, judgment, insight, and behavior
  4. Mini-cognitive test: recall of three unrelated words, clock-drawing task

C. Screening laboratory examination
  1. Glucose
  2. Electrolytes
  3. Magnesium
  4. Calcium
  5. Liver tests
  6. BUN/creatinine
  7. Thyroid function tests
  8. Vitamin B12 level, folate
  9. Venereal Disease Research Laboratory test
  10. HIV (selected patients)
  11. Complete blood count with differential, clotting studies
  12. Arterial blood gases
  13. Cultures: blood, urine, and sputum
  14. Serum levels of ingested drugs
  15. Illicit drugs and alcohol levels in selected patients
  16. Albumin

D. Other tests, depending on patient history and findings of physical examination

    1. CT of the head/MRI

        a. Note: for tumor, subdural hematoma, infarction, hemorrhage, hydrocephalus, and atrophy

    2. PET scan—may be useful in differentiating dementia types or pathologic processes in which clinical symptoms are similar

    3. Lumbar puncture—to rule out neurosyphilis, chronic meningitis, and normal pressure hydrocephalus

    4. Electroencephalography

    5. Chest X-ray—to rule out congestive heart failure, chronic lung disease, pulmonary embolus, and infection

    6. Electrocardiogram

E. Identification of treatable causes is very important.

    1. Drug induced

    2. Depression

    3. Hypothyroidism/hyperthyroidism

    4. Hypoglycemia

    5. Vitamin B12 or folate deficiency

    6. Subdural hematoma

    7. Liver failure

    8. Normal pressure hydrocephalus

    9. Stroke

    10. CNS infection

    11. Generalized infection

    12. Cerebral neoplasm

    13. Renal failure

    14. Alcohol abuse

    15. Hypoxia

    16. Hypercalcemia

    17. Vasculitis

    18. Cardiopulmonary disorder

    19. Anemia

F. Diagnostic and Statistical Manual of Mental Disorders (5th ed.; DSM-V; American Psychiatric Association; 2013) criteria for dementia

    1. Memory impairment

    2. At least two of the following:

        a. Aphasia

        b. Apraxia

        c. Agnosia

        d. Disturbances in executive functioning

    3. Disturbance in one or two of the above significantly interferes with work, social activities, or relationships.

    4. Disturbance does not occur exclusively during delirium.

V. Management

A. Supportive care: consult social services or other resources for transitioning between acute and home or skilled nursing care

B. Treat underlying precipitating illnesses

C. Attempt to withdraw, reduce, or stop all nonessential medications

D. Maintain nutrition: dietary consult

E. Avoid restraints, except for safety

F. Speech therapy/physical therapy

G. Address safety issues: coordinate appropriate safety measures with the patient's caregiver to prevent injury from falls, wandering, cooking, driving, and so forth

H. Because a cholinergic deficiency is present in Alzheimer's disease, cholinesterase inhibitors modestly improve cognition, behavior, and function, and they slightly delay disease progression.

I. In patients with Alzheimer's-related dementia, the clinical benefit of pharmacologic therapy is often modest and temporary.

J. Treatment for mild to moderate Alzheimer's-type dementia includes the following:

1. Donepezil (Aricept), 5 mg PO once daily at bedtime; titrate to 10 mg orally once daily at 4–6 weeks; if suboptimal clinical response, may increase to maximum dose of 23 mg PO once daily at 3 months
   a. Well tolerated with convenient dosing; drug of choice
   b. It may cause syncope, bradycardia, and arteriovenous (AV) block; provide caregiver education and obtain baseline electrocardiogram before starting therapy
   c. Monitor for AV block, syncope, bradycardia and seizures
   d. Nausea and weight loss may occur

2. Rivastigmine (Exelon): initial dose, 1.5 mg PO BID; maximum dose, 6 mg BID
   a. It should be administered with food to enhance absorption
   b. Similar to other cholinesterase inhibitors, it can cause peripheral cholinergic adverse effects
   c. Monitor for hypotension, syncope
   d. Significant weight loss (7% of initial weight) occurs in 19%–26% of patients
   e. Rivastigmine transdermal patch daily: start with 4.6 mg once a day for 4 weeks, then 9.5 mg once a day for 4 weeks, then maximum of 13.3 mg once a day

3. Galantamine hydrobromide (Razadyne): Begin at 4 mg PO BID for a minimum of 4 weeks, after which the dosage may be increased to 8 mg BID. Four weeks later, the dosage may be increased again to 12 mg BID. Maximum dose is 24 mg/day; however, for patients with moderate renal or hepatic impairment, the maximum dose is 16 mg daily.

    a. In those with severe renal and hepatic impairment, this drug should be avoided. Caution should be used in patients with cardiac conduction defects.

    b. Monitor for sinus bradycardia, AV block, and syncope

K. Treatment for moderate to severe dementia includes the following:

    1. N-methyl-d-aspartate receptor antagonist

        a. Memantine (Namenda)

            i. Used to prevent the progression of Alzheimer's disease

            ii. Blocks pathologic stimulation of N-methyl-d-aspartate receptors and protects against further damage in patients with vascular dementia

            iii. Initiate with 7 mg PO once daily; titrate in 7-mg increments at intervals of least 1 week as tolerated to a target dose of 28 mg once daily; MAX, 28 mg/day

                (a) Low creatinine clearance (CrCl): reduce dosage to 14 mg PO once daily

            iv. May demonstrate greater efficacy when paired with cholinesterase inhibitors such as donepezil

            v. Monitor closely at initiation of therapy for Stevens-Johnson syndrome

L. Medications that affect serotonin have been useful in controlling aggression and agitation; use remains controversial.

    1. Atypical antipsychotics are the preferred treatment for dementia-related aggression and agitation in elderly patients.

        a. Examples

            i. Olanzapine (Zyprexa): initiate with 2.5 mg PO daily; titrate up to 5 mg BID MAX

            ii. Quetiapine (Seroquel): initiate with 25 mg PO at bedtime; titrate up to 75 mg BID MAX

            iii. Risperidone (Risperdal): initiate with 0.25–1 mg PO daily; dosage may be adjusted, not to exceed 1.5–2 mg daily

            iv. Ziprasidone (Geodon): initiate with 10 mg IM every 2 hr or 20 mg IM every 4 hr; switch to PO when possible

        b. Used for short periods and in low doses

        c. May produce considerable side effects, such as tardive dyskinesia and/or extrapyramidal and anticholinergic symptoms

    2. Studies show typical antipsychotics do not provide much benefit to dementia patients, except haloperidol (Haldol) in treating aggression

        a. Administer 0.5–10 mg IV/IM or PO initially, and observe patient for 20–30 minutes

       i. If the patient's condition remains unmanageable and the patient has had no adverse reactions to haloperidol, double the dose and continue to monitor

  3. Lithium (do not start lithium at a facility that cannot monitor levels; rarely used due to narrow therapeutic index)

  4. Buspirone (not used frequently due to delayed onset of action)

M. Benzodiazepines often preferred when controlling agitation and aggression

  1. Clonazepam (Klonopin): initiate 0.25 mg PO BID; increase by 0.125–0.25 mg BID every three days; target dose is 1 mg daily, 4 mg daily MAX

    a. Use cautiously; may cause paradoxical agitation or increase risk of falls or injury

  2. Lorazepam (Ativan), 1 mg IV every hour, may also be administered if needed

N. Emotional lability has been decreased by either of the following medication in some cases:

  1. Imipramine (Impril), 25–50 mg PO at bedtime; if tolerated, may increase to maximum 100 mg daily

    a. Tricyclic antidepressants such as imipramine usually avoided due to anticholinergic effects

  2. Sertraline (Zoloft): initiate at 25 mg PO daily; after one week, increase to 50 mg based on response and tolerance; 200 mg daily MAX

  3. Citalopram (Celexa): initiate at 20 mg PO daily; maximum dosage, due to risk of QT prolongation

O. Depression responds to the usual doses of tricyclic antidepressants, as well as to selective serotonin reuptake inhibitors, which have fewer anticholinergic adverse effects.

P. Other possible treatments under investigation but currently not supported by results of clinical trials include the following:

  1. Vitamin E and selegiline (Carbex) because of their antioxidant properties; use with caution in heart failure as high-dose therapy may be associated with increased mortality; currently not recommended as evidence to support vitamin E is mixed

  2. Nonsteroidal anti-inflammatory drugs because of properties in lowering plaque-producing amyloidogenic proteins; caution advised as these agents may raise rate of cardiovascular events; risks currently outweigh potential benefits

  3. Ginkgo biloba; investigated on grounds of increased cholinergic transmission; evidence is inconsistent at this time

  4. Antibiotics to treat chlamydia pneumonia, on grounds of association between *Chlamydia pneumoniae* and vascular dementia

5. In vitro studies have shown that rifampin and tetracyclines interfere with accumulation of β-amyloid peptide.
6. Statins may reduce amyloid peptides due to association between cholesterol in the brain and amyloid processing.

BIBLIOGRAPHY

American Psychological Association. (2013). *Diagnostic and statistical manual of mental disorders* (5th ed.). Washington, DC: APA Press.

Birks, J. & Evans, J.G. (2009) Gingko balboa for cognitive impairment and dementia. *Cochrane Database of Systematic Reviews,* (1). doi: 10.1002/14651858.CD003120.pub3.

Gaugler, J. E., Kane, R. L., Johnson, J. A., & Sarour, K. (2013). Sensitivity and specificity of diagnostic accuracy in Alzheimer's disease: A synthesis of existing evidence. *American Journal of Alzheimers Disease and Other Dementias, 28*(4), 337–347.

Harris, J. (2013). Cognitive approaches to early Alzheimer's disease diagnosis. *Medical Clinics of North America, 97*(3), 425–438.

Harrison-Dening, K. (2013). Dementia: Diagnosis and early interventions. *British Journal of Neuroscience Nursing, 9*(3), 131–137.

Landreville, P., Voyer, P., & Carmichael, P. (2013). Relationship between delirium and behavioral symptoms of dementia. *International Psychogeriatrics, 25*(4), 635–643.

McGuinness, B., O'Hare, J., Craig, D., Bullock, R., Malouf, R., & Passmore, P. (2010). Statins for the treatment of dementia. *Cochrane Database of Systematic Reviews*, (8). doi:10.1002/14651858.CD007514.pub2.

Papadakis, M., & McPhee, S. (2013). *Current medical diagnosis & treatment* (52nd ed., pp. 1005–1010). New York, NY: McGraw-Hill.

Schwarz, S., Froelich, L., & Burns, A. (2012). Pharmacological treatment of dementia. *Current Opinion in Psychiatry, 25*(6), 542–550.

Teipel, S. J., Grothe, M., Lista, S., Toschi, N., Garaci, F. G., & Hampel, H. (2013). Relevance of magnetic resonance imaging for early detection and diagnosis of Azheimer disease. *Medical Clinics of North America, 97*(3), 399–424.

van de Glind, E., Van Enst, W. A., Van Muster, B. C., Olde-Rikkert, M. G. M., Scheltens, P. . . . Hooft, L.(2013). Pharmacological treatment of dementia: A scoping review of systematic reviews. *Dementia and Geriatric Cognitive Disorders, 36*(¾), 211–228.

Yamamoto, H., Watanabe, T., Miyazaki, A., Katagiri, T., Idei, T. . . . Kamajima, K. (2005). High prevalance of *Chlamydia pneumoniae* antibodies and increased high-sensitive C-reactive protein in patients with vascular dementia. *Journal of the American Geriatrics Society, 53*(4), 583–589. doi: 10.1111/j.1532–5415.2005.53204.x

CHAPTER 8

Multiple Sclerosis

JUDI KURIC

I.   **Definition**
  A. Demyelinating disease of the central nervous system
  B. An acquired, immune-mediated disease
  C. Neurological symptoms can be caused by isolated inflammation, demyelination, and axonal damage leading to nerve conduction delays, alterations, or complete blocks.
  D. Characterized by relapses (attacks or exacerbations) and remissions (recovery or improvements)

II.   **Etiology/predisposing factors**
  A. Increased prevalence in populations living a greater distance from the equator
  B. Women have a 2–3 times higher incidence than men
  C. Onset of disease is earlier in women than men.
  D. Caucasians have highest risk
     1. African Americans have half the occurrence rate as Caucasians in the same geographic region.
     2. Northern Europeans, especially Scandinavians, are more likely to develop multiple sclerosis (MS).
  E. Risk in non-Caucasians can increase with movement from a low-risk to high-risk geographic region
  F. Seventy to 80% of persons with MS have onset in their 20s-40s.
  G. Approximately 10%–20% of MS patients have an afflicted family member.
  H. Patients with MS have a 5- to 7-year shorter life expectancy.
  I. No clear etiology but thought to have a multifactorial cause
     1. Viral infection is a precursor to exacerbation
     2. No identified link to several proposed viruses
        a. Measles

       b. Distemper

       c. Herpes

       d. Chlamydia

       e. Epstein-Barr

       f. Retrovirus

    3. No specific genetic association

III.   **Clinical manifestations**

    A. Classification of disease

       1. Relapsing-remitting (RR-MS)

          a. Clear and defined episodes of relapses and recovery

             i. Recovery can be full or there can be some residual deficit.

          b. There is no clinical progression between the relapse episodes.

          c. Usual initial presentaetion of 85%–90% with MS

       2. Secondary progressive (SP-MS)

          a. Usually initiates with RR-MS, followed by deterioration or progression of the disease

          b. Clinical progression noted between relapsing episodes

          c. Patients usually do not return to baseline after relapsing episode.

       3. Primary progressive (PP-MS)

          a. Continued disease progression from the initial neurologic episode

          b. Some plateaus and minor temporary improvements

          c. Most commonly occurs in patients with onset after 40 years of age

          d. Occurs in about 10%–15% of MS patients

       4. Progressive relapsing (PR-MS)

          a. Progressive disease from the onset with clear relapses after onset

          b. Recovery from the relapses may be full or partial.

          c. Continued progression of the disease between relapses

          d. Neurological status does not return to baseline after the relapse

          e. Occurs in about 5% of MS patients

       5. Malignant MS

          a. Very rapid onset and progressive deterioration

          b. Significant disability and death with short period of time

       6. Benign MS

          a. No deterioration after 10 years following onset of disease

          b. Unable to predict, identified only in historical review of the patient's disease process

    B. Subjective neurological symptom that lasts at least 24 hr, resulting in increased disability

       1. Motor weakness, spasticity, or stiffness

2. Sensory alterations of numbness, burning, tingling, tightness, and pain
3. Brain stem symptoms of double vision, dysarthria, dysphasia, dysphagia, and vertigo
4. Visual deficits: field defect, decreased acuity, impaired color perception, and pain with eye movement
5. Cerebellar symptoms: gait ataxia, intention tremor, and uncoordinated movements
6. Cognitive dysfunction: short-term memory, slowed processing, and difficulty with higher level problem solving
7. Fatigue: overall fatigue and limb fatigue
   a. Present in 90% of patients
8. Sleep disorders
9. Bladder, bowel, and sexual dysfunction
   a. Bladder urgency, frequency, and incontinence
   b. Frequent UTIs
   c. Constipation
   d. Erectile dysfunction
10. Seizure
11. Tonic spasms

C. Objective examination findings
1. Sensory track disturbances, present in 20%–50% of patients
   a. Decreased vibratory sense
   b. Decreased position sense
   c. Decreased pinprick perception
   d. Decreased temperature sensation
2. Reflex alterations
   a. Abnormal deep tendon reflexes
   b. Positive Babinski sign
   c. Positive Hoffman sign
   d. Spastic limb weakness
3. Brain stem alterations
   a. Nystagmus
   b. Hearing loss
   c. Tinnitus
4. Cerebellar
   a. Ataxia
   b. Tremor
   c. Lack of coordination
5. Visual facial
   a. Optic neuritis (initial symptom in 25% of patients)
   b. Optic disk pallor
   c. Pupil defect
   d. Visual field defect
   e. Trigeminal neuralgia

      6. Frontal lobe
         a. Cognitive dysfunction
         b. Emotional lability or disinhibition

IV. **Laboratory findings/diagnostics**
  A. Complete neurological exam with noted deficits
  B. MRI
     1. Demonstrates white mater lesions in brain
     2. Demonstrates lesions in spinal cord
     3. Demonstrates T2-weighted lesions in periventricular white matter of brain and spinal cord
     4. Gadolinium enhancement on T1 imaging
     5. Hypodensities (black holes) on T1 imaging
     6. Cerebral atrophy
  C. Cerebrospinal fluid (CSF) analysis
     1. Consistent with MS if there is elevated IgG and oligoclonal bands in CSF, but not serum
        a. Bands present in about 70% of MS-positive patients
        b. Presence indicates MS; absence does not rule out the disease
  D. Evoked potentials
     1. Evidence of slowed conduction or prolonged evoked response
     2. Used less frequently; not conclusive, supports other diagnostics
  E. McDonald Diagnostic Criteria (2010)
     1. Applied after clinical evaluation of the patient
     2. A new T2 and /or gadolinium-enhancing lesion on follow-up MRI, with reference to a baseline scan regardless of the timing of the baseline MRI
     3. Simultaneous presence of asymptomatic gadolinium-enhancing and nonenhancing lesions at any time
  F. No better explanation for these neurologic events
     1. Specific MRI findings, abnormal CSF findings, and abnormal evoked potentials
     2. One of three outcomes: MS, possible MS, or not MS

V. **Management**
  A. Referral to neurology
  B. Mild acute exacerbations that do not produce functional decline may not require treatment.
  C. Acute intervention for relapse
     1. Glucocorticoids, oral or intravenous
        a. High dose (500–1000 mg/day), usually with IV methylprednisolone; duration is dependent on clinical response
     2. Thought to promote early recovery from exacerbation but does not have any long-term effect
     3. Short-term pulse therapy preferred to prevent long-term steroid effects

D. Disease modification medications
1. Reduces relapse, delays disability, and reduces MRI lesion burden (volume)
2. Initiate early once diagnosis is established
   a. Immunomodulators
      i. Fingolimod (Gilenya)
         (a) Relapsing forms
         (b) Dose: 0.5 mg orally once daily
         (c) Observe for 6 hr after first dose for bradycardia
         (d) Adverse effects: first dose bradycardia, atrioventricular block, infection, macular edema, cough, headache, diarrhea, elevation of liver enzymes, increased blood pressure
      ii. Interferon beta-1b
         (a) Betaseron or Extavia
            1. Relapsing form
            2. 0.0625 mg SQ every other day; increase every 2 weeks by 0.0625 mg to recommended dosage of 0.25 mg SQ every other day
            3. Depression/suicidality
            4. Injection site necrosis
            5. Lymphopenia
      iii. Interferon beta-1a
         (a) Avonex
            1. Relapsing form
            2. 30 mcg IM once weekly or 7.5 mg IM each week until 30 mcg once weekly is reached
            3. Influenza-like symptoms
            4. Fatigue
            5. Myalgia
            6. Depression
         (b) Rebif
            1. Relapsing form
            2. Titration to 22 mcg dose: 4.4 mcg SQ 3 times a week for weeks 1 and 2; increase to 11 mcg SQ 3 times a week for weeks 3 and 4, then 22 mcg SQ 3 times a week
            3. Titration to 44 mcg dose: 8.8 mcg SQ 3 times a week for weeks 1 and 2; increase to 22 mcg SQ 3 times a week for weeks 3 and 4, then 44 mcg SQ 3 times a week
            4. Influenza-like symptoms (slightly less than Avonex)
            5. Fatigue
            6. Leukopenia

      iv. Glatiramer acetate (Copaxone)

          (a) RR-MS form

          (b) 20 mg SQ daily or 40 mg SQ 3 times a week at least 48 hr apart on the same 3 days each week

          (c) Injection site reaction

          (d) Flushing

          (e) Nausea

      v.   Natalizumab (Tysabri)

          (a) Restricted use; relapsing form that is intolerant to other agents; only available through TOUCH® Prescribing Program to prescribers, infusion centers, and pharmacies associated with infusion centers

              1. Only prescribed to patients who are enrolled/meet all of the requirements; contact 1–800–456–2255 for details/enrollment

          (b) 300 mg IV infused over 1 hr; given in 4 week intervals

          (c) Infusion reaction (potential anaphylaxis)

          (d) Fatigue

          (e) Black box warning: natalizumab increases the risk of progressive multifocal leukoencephalopathy (PML), an opportunistic viral infection of the brain that usually leads to death or severe disability

  b. Immunosuppressant agents

      i.   Mitoxantrone (Novantrone)

          (a) Secondary progressive, progressive relapsing, or worsening relapsing-remitting

          (b) 12 mg/m^2 IV every 3 months

          (c) Should not be administered to patients who have received a cumulative dose of 140 mg/m^2 or greater

          (d) Cardiotoxicity: left ventricular ejection fraction and electrocardiogram evaluation are required prior to administration of each dose; if signs/symptoms of congestive heart failure develop, do not exceed maximum allowable lifetime cumulative dose

          (e) Adverse effects: alopecia, diarrhea, nausea, vomiting

          (f) Black box warning: increases risk of developing secondary acute myeloid leukemia

      ii. Off-label immunosuppressants

          (a) Methotrexate

          (b) Cyclophosphamide

          (c) Mycophenolate mofetil

    E. Symptom management for common complications

1.	Spasticity	**6.**	Incontinence
2.	Fatigue	**7.**	Cognitive effects
3.	Mood disorders	**8.**	Gait disturbances
4.	Immobility	**9.**	Sexual dysfunction
5.	Seizures		

BIBLIOGRAPHY

Bader, M. K., & Littlejohn, L. R. (2010). *AANN core curriculum for neuroscience nursing* (5th ed.). Glenview, IL: AANN.

Langer-Gould, A., Brara, S., Beaber, B., & Zhang, J. (2013). Incidence of multiple sclerosis in multiple racial and ethnic groups. *Neurology, 80*(19), 1734–1739. doi:10.1212/WNL.0b013e3182918cc2

Luzio, C., & Keegan, B. (2014, January 29). *Multiple sclerosis*. Retrieved from http://emedicine.medscape.com/article/1146199-overview

Maloni, H. (2013). Multiple sclerosis: Managing patients in primary care. *Nurse Practitioner, 38*(4), 24–36.

Perrin Ross, A., Halper, J., & Harris, C. J. (2012). Assessing relapses and response to relapse treatment in patients with multiple sclerosis. *International Journal of MS Care, 14*(3), 148–159.

Polman, C., Reingold, S., Banwell, B., Clanet, M., Cohen, J., Filippi, M., . . . Wolinski, J. (2011). Diagnostic criteria for multiple sclerosis: 2010 revisions to the McDonald criteria. *Annuals of Neurology, 69*(2), 292–302. doi:10.1002/ana.22366

Rice, C. M. (2014). Disease modification in multiple sclerosis: An update. *Practical Neurology, 14*(1). doi:10.1136/practneurol-2013–000601

Rice, C., Cottrell, D., Wilkins, A., & Scolding, N. (2013). Primary progressive multiple sclerosis: Progress and challenges. *Journal of Neurology, Neurosurgery, and Psychiatry, 84*(10), 1100–1106.

Ross, A., & Thrower, B. W. (2010). Recent developments in the early diagnosis and management of multiple sclerosis. *Journal of Neuroscience Nursing, 42*(6), 342–353.

Rovira, A., Auger, C., & Alonzo, J. (2013). Magnetic resonance monitoring for lesion evolution in multiple sclerosis. *Therapeutic Advances in Neurological Disorders, 6*(5), 298–310. doi:10.1177/1756285613484079

Ruto, C. (2013). Special needs populations: Care of patients with multiple sclerosis. *AORN Journal, 98*(3), 281–293. doi:10.1016/j.aorn.2013.07.002

CHAPTER 9

Parkinson's Disease

JUDI KURIC · ROBERT FELLIN

I. **Definition**
    A. A neurodegenerative disorder caused by the depletion of dopamine-producing cells in the midbrain (substantia nigra)
    B. Cardinal symptoms of resting tremor, rigidity, and slowness of movement

II. **Etiology/predisposing factors**
    A. Approximately 60,000 new cases diagnosed annually in the United States
    B. Average age of onset is 60 years
    C. Incidence is slightly higher among men than women
    D. Caucasians have a slightly higher prevalence
    E. No single cause has been identified
    F. Environmental and genetic factors suggested as causative factors
        1. Multiple gene mutations have been identified, including the PARK1 gene, which is identified in Italian and Greek families.
        2. Occupational exposure to heavy metals, such as copper and manganese, has been associated with an increased risk.

III. **Clinical manifestations**
    A. Classic triad
        1. Resting tremor, most commonly of the arm and leg
        2. Rigidity: arms, legs, and neck stiffness with restricted range of motion
        3. Bradykinesia: slow movements in a deliberate manner
    B. Additional motor symptoms
        1. Postural instability: slumped posture and loss of posture reflexes

2. Pull test: patient steps backwards to recover from a slight tug from behind

3. Falls develop late in the disease process as a result of instability, gait problems, and diminished reflexes.

C. Gait—classic attributes
   1. Diminished arm swing
   2. Shuffling steps; related to short, restricted steps
   3. Bent forward posture: fast, short steps; tendency for forward acceleration
   4. "Frozen" gait: patient gets stuck or frozen while ambulating

D. Neuropsychiatric manifestations
   1. Depression
   2. Dementia
   3. Anxiety
   4. Psychosis
   5. Apathy
   6. Sleep disturbances
   7. Disinhibition

E. Autonomic dysfunction (medications used to treat Parkinson's disease [PD] also have autonomic side effects)
   1. Urinary incontinence
   2. Sexual dysfunction
   3. Constipation
   4. Orthostatic hypotension
   5. Impaired thermoregulation
   6. Sensory abnormalities (pain and paresthesia)

F. Craniofacial abnormalities
   1. Masked face: expressionless, fixed, and immobile face; staring eyes with mouth slightly open
   2. Dysphagia
   3. Involuntary closure of the eye lid
   4. Impaired sense of smell
   5. Excessive drooling
   6. Dysarthria

IV. **Laboratory findings/diagnostics**
   A. History and physical exam are the basis for diagnosis
      1. Physical exam findings of tremor, rigidity, impaired balance, and gait alterations are the central findings that suggest PD.
   B. CT scan and MRI are usually normal in PD but may be useful in assessing a differential diagnosis
   C. Positron emission tomography scans are used primarily in research and are not specific for diagnosis
   D. Clinical ratings scales, such as the Unified Parkinson's Disease Rating Scale, provide a standard evaluation and measure of the disease and its progression.

V.   Treatment (see Table 9.1)

    A. Referral to neurologist

    B. Pharmacological intervention provides symptom relief and can improve functioning

        1. Carbidopa-levodopa combination (Sinemet) is the standard treatment

        2. Dopamine agonists (ropinirole and pramipexole) may reduce the risk of developing motor complications and alleviate symptoms

        3. Anticholinergics (trihexyphenidyl and benztropine mesylate) are helpful in treating tremors, but may cause confusion; use cautiously

        4. Amantadine (Symmetrel) is used early in the disease, helpful with dyskinesias

        5. MAO-B inhibitors (rasagiline and selegiline) may be helpful in the treatment of motor symptoms

    C. "On-off" phenomena described when the medication is working, then stops working. This is characterized by motor function fluctuations. The addition of catechol-O-methyltransferase prevents the breakdown of dopamine and helps with these phenomena.

    D. Neuroprotective agents have been investigated to prevent degeneration of neurons. The findings have been conflicting and more research is progressing in this area.

    E. Deep brain stimulation surgery has replaced ablative procedures (e.g., pallidotomy and thalamotomy)

        1. Mechanism is unknown; the outcome of deep brain stimulation surgery enables near normal motor function. Patient selection and screening are essential for the positive outcomes of this treatment.

        2. Consult neurology/neurosurgery for evaluation

    F. Adequate nutrition

    G. Exercise

        1. Physical and occupational therapy may improve mobility, stiffness, balance, and gait

    H. Management of neuropsychiatric comorbidities

Table 9.1 Pharmacologic Agents for Parkinson's Disease			
Agent	**Initial Dosage**	**Adverse Effects**	**Comments**
Dopaminergic Agents			
Carbidopa/ levodopa (Sinemet): 10 mg/100 mg, 25 mg/100 mg, 25 mg/250 mg Sinemet CR: 25 mg/100 mg, 50 mg/200 mg	IR: 25/100 PO TID CR: 50/200 PO BID	GI upset, arrhythmias, dyskinesias, on-off and wearing-off phenomena, confusion, dizziness, headache, hallucinations	• Most effective drug for the symptomatic treatment of PD • Use with COMT/ MAO-B inhibitors prolongs duration of effect • Sinemet is available as immediate release and sustained release
Dopamine Agonists			
Bromocriptine (Parlodel)	1.25 mg PO BID	Nausea, vomiting, postural hypotension, dyskinesias, confusion, impulse control disorders, sleepiness	• Can be used as monotherapy (mild disease) or in combination with levodopa/carbidopa • Reduce the frequency of "off periods" and may allow reduction of levodopa/carbidopa dose Pramipexole: • Requires slow titration • Adjust dose for renal dysfunction Ropinirole: • Many drug-drug interactions • Contraindicated in patients with a history of psychotic illness or recent MI or active peptic ulceration
Pramipexole (Mirapex, Mirapex ER)	IR: 0.125 mg PO TID ER: 0.375 mg PO daily		
Ropinirole (Requip, Requip XL)	IR: 0.25 mg PO TID Requip XL: 2 mg PO daily		

Table 9.1 Pharmacologic Agents for Parkinson's Disease			
Agent	**Initial Dosage**	**Adverse Effects**	**Comments**
Monoamine Oxidase Inhibitors			
Rasagiline (Azilect)	0.5–1 mg PO daily	Orthostatic hypotension, rash, weight loss, GI upset, arthralgia, ataxia, dyskinesia, headache	• Adjunct therapy only • Provides modest improvements in motor function • Rasagiline is more potent than selegiline. • May cause serotonin syndrome: avoid TCADs, SSRIs Selegiline: • BBW: increases the risk of suicidal thinking and behavior in children, adolescents, and young adults • Many drug interactions: avoid meperidine, tramadol, methadone, propoxyphene, cyclobenzaprine, OTCs
Selegiline (Eldepryl)	5 mg PO BID		
COMT Inhibitors			
Entacapone (Comtan)	200 mg PO with each dose of levodopa/ carbidopa	Diarrhea, abdominal pain, orthostatic hypotension, sleep disturbances, orange discoloration of the urine	• Adjunct therapy with levodopa/carbidopa only • Extends the effects of levodopa and alleviates "wearing off" phenomenon • Reduce dose of levodopa by 30% upon initiation of treatment. Entacapone: • Available as combination product with carbidopa/levodopa = Stalevo Tolcapone: • Liver toxicity, requires signed patient consent, monitor LFT's • BBW: risk of potentially fatal, acute fulminant liver failure
Tolcapone (Tasmar)	100 mg PO TID with each dose of levodopa/ carbidopa		

Table 9.1 Pharmacologic Agents for Parkinson's Disease			
Agent	**Initial Dosage**	**Adverse Effects**	**Comments**
Anticholinergic Agents			
Benztropine (Cogentin)	0.5–1 mg PO every bedtime	Sedation, nausea, constipation, dry mouth, blurred vision, drowsiness, dizziness, tachycardia, hypotension, nervousness, urinary retention	• May improve tremor and rigidity; have little effect on bradykinesia
Biperiden (Akineton)	2 mg PO TID		• Increase dose gradually until benefit occurs
Trihexyphenidyl (Artane)	1 mg PO daily		• Taper dose when withdrawing therapy • Use of anticholinergic agents is limited due to the development of intolerable side effects, necessitating dosage reduction or drug discontinuation
Miscellaneous			
Amantadine (Symmetrel)	100 mg PO BID	Restlessness, depression, irritability, insomnia, agitation, excitement, hallucinations, confusion, headache, heart failure, postural hypotension, urinary retention, anorexia, nausea, constipation, dry mouth	• Less efficacious than levodopa • Provides modest symptomatic benefit for tremor as well as rigidity and bradykinesia • Benefit is limited as duration of efficacy may last only few weeks • Reduce dose for renal impairment • May cause livedo reticularis

Note. IR = immediate release; CR = controlled release; ER = extended release; BBW = black box warning.

BIBLIOGRAPHY

Bader, M. K., & Littlejohn, L. (2010). *AANN core curriculum for neuroscience nursing* (5th ed.). Glenview, IL: AANN.

Exercise and physical therapy. Retrieved from http://pdcenter.neurology.ucsf.edu/patients-guide/exercise-and-physical-therapy

Hickey, J. (Ed.). (2013). *The clinical practice of neurological and neurosurgical nursing* (7th ed.). Baltimore, MD: Lippincott.

Longo, D., Fauci, A., Kasper, D., Hauser, S., Jameson, J., & Loscalzo, J. (Eds.). (2012). *Harrison's manual of medicine* (18th ed.). New York, NY: McGraw-Hill.

Oertel, W., Berardelli, A., Bloem, B., Bonuccelli, U., Burn, D., Deuschl, G., . . . Trenkwalder, C. (2011). Late (complicated) Parkinson's disease. In N. Gilhus, M. Barnes, & M. Brainin (Eds.), *European handbook of neurological management* (2nd ed., Vol. 1, pp. 237–267). Oxford, UK.

Oertel, W., Berardelli, A., Bloem, B., Bonuccelli, U., Burn, D., Deuschl, G., . . . Trenkwalder, C. (2011). Early (uncomplicated) Parkinson's disease. In N. Gilhus, M. Barnes, & M. Brainin (Eds.), *European handbook of neurological management* (2nd ed., Vol. 1, pp. 217–236). Oxford, UK.

Papadakis, M. A., McPhee, S. J., & Tierney, L. M. (Eds.). (2013). *Current medical diagnosis and treatment* (52nd ed.) New York, NY: McGraw Hill/Appleton & Lange.

CHAPTER 10

Amyotrophic Lateral Sclerosis

JUDI KURIC

I.   **Definition**
A. Disease of the motor neurons causing asymmetric weakness
B. Symptom presentation largely occurs with weakness in the upper or lower extremity
C. Symptoms less likely to present with dysarthria and dysphagia or respiratory weakness

II.   **Etiology/predisposing factors**
A. Mean age of disease onset is 50 years
B. Men are slightly more likely to develop amyotrophic lateral sclerosis (ALS) than women, although the numbers equalize when women approach menopause.
C. Familial ALS is an inherited autosomal dominant trait that accounts for 5%–10% of cases.
D. Remainder of causes unknown

III. **Clinical manifestations**
A. Classification of disease—El Escorial criteria
   1. Classified by the presence of upper motor neuron (UMN) and lower motor neuron (LMN) symptoms in regions—brain stem, cervical, thoracic, and lumbosacral
   2. Categories
      a. Possible—UMN and LMN signs in one region
      b. Probable—UMN and LMN signs in two regions
      c. Probable lab supported—UMN signs in one or more regions and electromyogram (EMG) positive denervation in two or more limbs

        d. Definite—UMN and LMN signs in bulbar region plus two
          spinal regions
  B. Progressive weakness over weeks to months
  C. Sensation intact in all areas
  D. Muscle atrophy
  E. Small muscle fasciculations
  F. Abnormal reflexes (hyperreflexia)
  G. Spasticity

IV. **Laboratory findings/diagnostics**
  A. Serum CK may be slightly elevated
  B. EMG—denervation
  C. Muscle biopsy
    1. Small regions grouped with atrophic muscle fibers
  D. MRI—no abnormality that can explain UMN alterations

V. **Management**
  A. Supportive treatment and consult to palliative care—average survival
    is 2–5 years after diagnosis
    1. Immobility
    2. Altered respiratory function may be managed with non-invasive
      ventilation, suction, etc.
    3. Dysphagia and poor nutrition may be managed with altering food
      consistency, nutritional supplements, etc.
    4. Pain—refer patient to pain management specialist
    5. Anxiety (refer to Psychosocial Problems in Acute Care chapter for
      anti-anxiety agents)
    6. Communication deficits
    7. Medication: riluzole (Rilutek), 50 mg PO every 12 hr has been
      shown to extend survival rate by months but is not curative.
      Recommended by the American Association of Neuroscience
      Nursing to be offered to slow disease progression in patients with
      ALS

BIBLIOGRAPHY

Bader, M. K., & Littlejohn, L. (2010). *AANN core curriculum for neuroscience nursing* (5th ed.). Glenview, IL: AANN.

Gordon, P., Cheng, B., Katz, I., Mitsumoto, H., & Rowland, L. (2009). Clinical features that distinguish PLS, upper motor neuron-dominant ALS, and typical ALS. *Neurology, 72*(22), 1948–1952.

Hickey, J. (2013). *The clinical practice of neurological and neurosurgical nursing* (7th ed.). Baltimore, MD: Lippincott.

Longo, D., Fauci, A., Kasper, D., Hauser, S., Jameson, J., & Loscalzo, J. (Eds.). (2012). *Harrison's manual of medicine* (18th ed.). New York, NY: McGraw-Hill.

McClellan, F., Washington, M., Ruff, R., & Selkirk, S. (2013). Early and innovative symptomatic care to improve quality of life of ALS patients at Cleveland VA ALS Center. *Journal of Rehabilitation Research and Development, 50*(4), vii–xvi.

Miller, R., Jackson, C., Kasarskis, E., England, J., Forshew, D., Johnston, W., . . . Woolley, S. (2009). Practice parameter update: The care of the patient with amyotrophic lateral sclerosis: Drug, nutritional, and respiratory therapies (an evidence-based review). *Neurology, 73*(15), 1218–1226.

Miller, R., Jackson, C., Kasarskis, E., England, J., Forshew, D., Johnston, W., . . . Woolley, S. (2009). Practice parameter update: The care of the patient with amyotrophic lateral sclerosis: Multi-disciplinary care, symptom management, and cognitive/behavioral impairment. *Neurology, 73*(15), 1227–1233.

Papadakis, M., McPhee, S., & Tierney, L.(Eds.). (2013). *Current medical diagnosis and treatment* (52nd ed.). New York, NY: McGraw Hill/Appleton & Lange.

Sreedharan, J. H. (2013). Amyotrophic lateral sclerosis: Problems and prospects. *Annals of Neurology, 74*(3), 309–316.

Van den Berg, J. P., Kalmijn, S., Lindeman, E., Veldink, J. H., de Visser, M., Van der Graaff, M. M., . . . Van den Berg, L. H. (2005). Multidisciplinary ALS care improves quality of life in patients with ALS. *Neurology, 65*(8), 1264–1267.

Management of Patients With Cardiovascular Disorders

CHAPTER 11

Cardiovascular Assessment

JOAN KING • THOMAS W. BARKLEY, JR.

I. **Cardiac cycle review**
  A. Systole
    1. Atrioventricular (AV) valves (tricuspid and mitral valves) close
    2. Semilunar valves (aortic and pulmonic valves) open
  B. Diastole
    1. Aortic/pulmonic valves close
    2. Tricuspid and mitral valves open
    3. Rapid ventricular filling (75% filling of the ventricles)
    4. Atrial contraction (atrial kick) (25% filling of the ventricles)

II. **Auscultatory areas of the precordium—characterized by location at which valvular activity is heard best**
  A. Aortic—second right intercostal space (ICS) at the right sternal border (S2 heart sound louder than S1)
  B. Pulmonic—second left ICS at the left sternal border (S2 louder than S1)
  C. Erb's point—third ICS at the left sternal border
  D. Tricuspid—left lower sternal border at the fifth ICS (closure of AV valves)
  E. Mitral—fifth ICS midclavicular line (S1 louder than S2)

III. **S1 heart sound**
  A. Denotes closure of the mitral and tricuspid (AV) valves
  B. Occurs almost simultaneously with apical and carotid impulses
  C. Coincides with the R wave on ECG
  D. More easily heard than S2 at the apex

IV. **S2 heart sound**
  A. Denotes closure of the aortic and pulmonic (semilunar) valves

B. Occurs at the onset of diastole (note that diastole is between S2 and S1)

C. Heard louder than S1 at the base of the heart

V.   Split S2 heart sound

    A. Transient split occurs on inspiration because of late closure of the pulmonic valve and early closure of aortic valve.

    B. Late closure of the pulmonic valve is associated with increase in venous return to the right ventricle with inspiration.

    C. Early closure of the aortic valve is associated with a decrease in venous return to the left ventricle related to an increase in pulmonary capacity during inspiration.

    D. Heard best in the pulmonic auscultatory area

    E. S2 returns to a single sound during expiration.

    F. If the patient holds his or her breath, the sounds will disappear.

    G. Normal physiological finding in children and young adults

    H. May occur approximately every fourth heartbeat

VI.   S3 heart sound

    A. Referred to as a ventricular gallop

    B. Caused by passive filling of blood into a noncompliant left ventricle

    C. Heard early in diastole (0.12–0.16 seconds after S2) at the left lower sternal border (apex)

    D. Heard best with the bell of the stethoscope

    E. Occurs with such conditions as heart failure and cardiomyopathy when fluid overload is present

    F. Normal sound associated with pregnancy (i.e., hyperdynamic state of increased volume)

    G. Sounds like the word "Ken-tuc-ky"

VII.   S4 heart sound

    A. Referred to as an atrial or presystolic gallop

    B. Produced by blood entering a noncompliant left ventricle during atrial contraction

    C. Associated with increased ventricular diastolic pressures

    D. Heard late in diastole; immediately before S1

    E. Most clearly heard at the left lower sternal border (apex) with the bell of the stethoscope

    F. Occurs with such conditions as myocardial infarction, hypertension, left ventricular hypertrophy, and heart failure

    G. Sounds like the word "Ten-ne-ssee'"

    H. It is not heard if the patient is in atrial fibrillation secondary to a loss of atrial kick.

VIII.   Summation gallop

    A. S3 and S4 heard together

    B. Highly suggestive of severe myocardial failure

IX.   Murmurs

    A. "Blowing" or "swooshing" sound that results from turbulent blood flow; identified by the following variables:

1. Timing—is the murmur systolic or diastolic, pansystolic or holosystolic, pandiastolic or holodiastolic?
2. Loudness—graded I through VI
   a. Grade I/VI—barely audible
   b. Grade II/VI—clearly audible but faint
   c. Grade III/VI—moderately loud, easily heard
   d. Grade IV/VI—loud, associated with a thrill
   e. Grade V/VI—very loud; heard with one corner of stethoscope off the chest wall
   f. Grade VI/VI—loudest: no stethoscope needed
3. Pitch—is the pitch high, low, or medium? Is it crescendo, decrescendo, plateau, or crescendo-decrescendo (diamond shaped murmur)?
4. Quality—is the quality musical, blowing, rumbling, or harsh?
5. Location—in what area is the murmur best heard?
6. Radiation—is the murmur heard at other auscultatory areas (e.g., neck, back, left axilla)?
7. Posture—does the murmur disappear or become louder with changes in posture?

B. Early diastolic murmurs—due to incompetent semilunar valves (e.g., aortic or pulmonic regurgitation)
   1. Decrescendo quality (diminishes in intensity)
   2. High pitch (heard best with the diaphragm of the stethoscope)
   3. Aortic regurgitation (aortic insufficiency)—sound intensifies if patient sits forward and holds their breath
   4. Pulmonic regurgitation—low to medium pitched murmur

C. Diastolic rumbling murmurs—due to mitral stenosis and tricuspid stenosis
   1. Mitral stenosis
      a. Low-pitched; heard best with the bell of the stethoscope
      b. Decrescendo-crescendo quality
      c. Heard best at the apex; better in the left lateral position
      d. Murmur follows an opening snap
      e. Heard early in diastole but extends through diastole as patient's condition worsens
      f. Does not radiate
      g. Associated with rheumatic heart disease, myxomas or congenital malformation
   2. Tricuspid stenosis
      a. Mid-diastolic murmur heard louder with inspiration
      b. Heard best along the left sternal border

D. Midsystolic ejection murmurs—due to obstruction of forward flow through semilunar valves
   1. Aortic stenosis

      a. Harsh crescendo-decrescendo murmur that radiates to the carotids

      b. Heard best with the diaphragm over the aortic area

      c. Associated with aortic valve sclerosis in older adults, rheumatic heart disease, hypertrophic cardiomyopathy

   2. Pulmonic stenosis

      a. Medium-pitched

      b. Crescendo-decrescendo (diamond shaped)

      c. Radiates

  E. Pansystolic regurgitant murmurs—due to backward flow

   1. Mitral regurgitation

      a. Holosystolic high pitched blowing sound

      b. Heard best at the apex and radiates to left axilla

      c. Lateral position intensify the sound

      d. Associated with endocarditis, rheumatic heart disease and rupture of the papillary muscles after an acute myocardial infarction

   2. Tricuspid regurgitation

      a. Soft systolic blowing sound

      b. Heard best at the left lower sternal border

      c. Intensifies during inspiration

X.   **Clicks**

  A. Midsystolic click

   1. Most common type

   2. Associated with mitral valve prolapse

  B. Aortic ejection click

   1. Related to stenosis

   2. Occurs during early systole

   3. Audible at apex and base of the heart

  C. Pulmonic ejection click

   1. Occurs during early systole

   2. Audible at the base of the heart only

XI.   **Friction rub**

  A. "Scratchy," high-pitched sound

  B. Classic sound of pericarditis (inflammation)

  C. Usually heard best at the apex with the patient leaning forward

  D. Remains audible if the patient holds their breath

XII.   **Peripheral pulse amplitude**

  A. Graded on a scale from 0–4

   1. Bounding: +4

   2. Full: +3

   3. Normal: +2

   4. Diminished: +1

   5. Absent: 0

XIII. **Electrocardiographic changes associated with electrolyte disturbances**

    A. Hyperkalemia

        1. Tall, peaked T waves

        2. Widening of the QRS complex

        3. Prolongation of the P wave/PR interval

        4. Increased levels of K+ decrease ventricular depolarization and slow AV conduction.

    B. Hypokalemia

        1. Premature ventricular contractions (PVC's) both unifocal and multifocal

        2. U waves which follow the T wave and are of lower amplitude

        3. Less common changes include bradycardia, atrial flutter, and AV block

        4. Potentiated effects of digitalis toxicity

    C. Hypercalcemia

        1. AV blocks, bundle branch block, and bradycardia related to increased contractility of the heart and shortening of the QT interval (period of ventricular repolarization)

        2. Potentiated effects of digitalis toxicity

    D. Hypocalcemia

        1. Bradycardia, ventricular ectopy and asystole because low calcium levels decrease contractility

        2. Decreased cardiac output and hypotension

        3. Decreased efficacy of digitalis

    E. Hypermagnesemia

        1. Rarely evident in the acute care setting

        2. Usually related to renal failure or over-administration of magnesium during replacement therapy

    F. Hypomagnesemia

        1. Changes similar to those associated with hypokalemia and hypocalcemia

            a. Appearances of U wave

            b. Prolonged PR/QT intervals

            c. Widened QRS complexes

            d. Flattened T waves

            e. Supraventricular tachycardia (SVT)

            f. Ventricular arrhythmia

            g. Torsades de pointes

        2. Note: Hypomagnesemia may cause hypertension and coronary/systemic vasospasm.

        3. Hypomagnesemia usually must be corrected before replacement therapy for hypokalemia and hypocalcemia can be effective.

XIV. Cardiovascular changes with the elderly
   A. Heart valves—become more fibrous and rigid
   B. Conduction—decrease in number of cells in SA node and AV node
   C. Rhythm—decrease in rate both average rate and maximal rate
      1. Takes longer for heart rate to return to resting rate when stressed
      2. Tachyarrhythmias are poorly tolerated because of reduced ventricular compliance.

XV. Assessment of jugular venous distension (as an indication of central venous pressure)
   A. Patient sitting at 45° angle
   B. Assess for pulsation of the internal jugular vein
   C. Measured in centimeters from the angle of Louis
   D. The angle of Louis is approximately 5 cm right of atrium
   E. Measure vertically in centimeters from the angle of Louis to where height of pulsation is seen
   F. Add measurement to 5 cm for total; 7–9 cm is considered normal
   G. Higher than 9 cm is indication of volume overload

BIBLIOGRAPHY

Bonow, R., & Mann, D. (2012). *Braunwald's Heart Disese: A Textbook of Cardiovascular Medicine* (9th ed.). Philadelphia, PA: Elsevier.

Foreman, M, Milisen, K., & Fulmer, T. (2009). *Critical care nursing of older adults*. New York, NY: Springer Publishing Company.

Hall, J. (2010). *Guyton and Hall textbook of medical physiology* (12th ed.). Philadelphia, PA: W.B. Saunders Elsevier.

Marino, P. (2014). *The ICU book*. Philadelphia, PA: Wolters Kluwer Health/ Lippincott, Williams & Wilkins.

Siedel, H, Ball, J., Dains, J., & Flynn, J. (2010). *Mosby's guide to physical examination* (7th ed.). Philadelphia, PA: Mosby Elsevier.

Urden, L. D., Stacy, K., & Lough, M. E. (2013). *Critical care nursing: diagnosis and management* (7th ed.). St. Louis, MO: Mosby.

CHAPTER 12

Hypertension

THOMAS W. BARKLEY, JR. • HELEN MILEY • ROBERT FELLIN

I. Definition

A. Sustained elevation of systolic blood pressure (SBP) of 140 mmHg or above, or diastolic blood pressure (DBP) of 90 mmHg or above on numerous occasions

B. Includes individuals currently taking antihypertensive pharmacologic agents

C. Previous expert opinions, such as the JNC 7, identified BP as based on the average of two or more properly measured seated BP readings on each of two or more office visits. (see table 12.1)

D. In contrast to JNC 7, JNC 8 emphasizes treatment thresholds.

Table 12.1	JNC 7 blood pressure thresholds		
Classifications	**Systolic BP**		**Diastolic BP**
Normal	< 120	and	< 80
Prehypertension	120 to 139	or	80 to 89
Hypertension			
Stage 1	140 to 159	or	90 to 99
Stage 2	≥ 160	or	≥ 100

II. Incidence/predisposing factors

A. Affects 20%–30% of African Americans

B. Affects 10%–15% of Caucasians in the U.S.

C. Affects approximately 60 million Americans

D. Hypertension (HTN) is a leading risk factor for coronary artery disease, stroke, congestive heart failure, renal failure, and retinopathy.

III.   Types and theories

    A. Primary—referred to as "essential" or "idiopathic"

        1. Cause is unknown

        2. Represents 95% of all cases of HTN

        3. Onset is usually between ages 25 and 55

        4. Exacerbating factors

            a. Obesity

            b. Excessive alcohol consumption (more than two drinks a day)

            c. Cigarette smoking

            d. Use of nonsteroidal anti-inflammatory drugs

        5. Theories of etiology include the following:

            a. Genetic and environmental factors

            b. Elevated intracellular calcium and sodium levels

            c. Sympathetic nervous system hyperactivity

            d. High renin-angiotensin activity causing vascular dysfunction

    B. Secondary—related to other known causes or disease processes

        1. Represents 5% of all cases of HTN

        2. Etiology includes the following:

            a. Estrogen use (via oral contraceptives or hormone replacement therapy)

            b. Renal disease

            c. Pregnancy

            d. Endocrine disorders, such as pheochromocytoma

    C. Isolated systolic HTN—common with aging

        1. Generally defined as a systolic BP greater than 140 and a diastolic BP less than 90

        2. Widening pulse pressure is a good indication and the Framingham point scale is a good predictor.

        3. Poorly understood

        4. May account for 65%–75% of HTN in the elderly

        5. Effectively treated with diuretics and long-acting calcium channel blockers, among others

IV.   Subjective and physical examination findings

    A. Often none; known as the "silent killer"

    B. Elevated blood pressure (140/90 mmHg or higher)

    C. May complain of classic suboccipital "pulsating" headache, usually in the early morning and resolving throughout the day

    D. May complain of epistaxis, light-headedness, and visual disturbances, among others

    E. S4 heart sound may be present, related to left ventricular hypertrophy

    F. Retinal changes are present with severe, chronic disease.

    G. Rare findings, such as hematuria

V.   Diagnostics/laboratory testing

    A. Laboratory data are usually unremarkable with uncomplicated disease.

    B. Consider ordering the following:

1. CBC and electrolytes with hemoglobin levels (establish baseline)
2. Urinalysis
3. Blood urea nitrogen and creatinine concentrations
4. Fasting glucose level
5. Lipid panel
6. Electrocardiogram (establish baseline, and rule out arrhythmias)
7. Chest X-ray (rule out cardiomegaly, for example)
8. Echocardiogram (if left ventricular, hypertrophy is suspected)
9. Angiotensin-converting enzyme (ACE) inhibitor (Captopril) stimulation test (if indicated, to rule out renovascular HTN)
10. Overnight 1-mg dexamethasone suppression test (if indicated, to rule out Cushing's syndrome)
11. Aldosterone level (if indicated, to rule out aldosteronism)
12. Plasma catecholamine level (if indicated, to rule out pheochromocytoma)

VI. **Goal of treatment based on JNC 8 (see table 12.2)**
VII. **Classification for initial hypertensive measurements (see table 12.3)**

Table 12.2	JNC 8 Hypertension Treatment Recommendations	
	Population	**Goal BP**
Recommendation 1	Adults $\geq$ 60 years of age	SBP $\leq$ 150 mmHg or DBP < 90 mmHg (Grade A)
Recommendation 2	Adults < 60 years of age	DBP < 90 mmHg (Grade A)
Recommendation 3	Adults < 60 years of age	SBP < 140 mmHg (Grade E)
Recommendation 4	Adults $\geq$ 18 with CKD	SBP < 140 mmHg or DBP < 90 mmHg (Grade E)
Recommendation 5	Adults $\geq$ 18 with DM	SBP < 140 mmHg or DBP < 90 mmHg (Grade E)
Recommendation 6	Non-African-American	Thiazide type diuretic CCB ACEI ARB (Grade B)
Recommendation 7	African-American	Thiazide diuretics CCB (Grade B) (Grade C for patients with DM)
Recommendation 8	Adults over 18 Adults with CKD	ACEI ARB (Grade B) Regardless of race or other medical conditions

Table 12.2	JNC 8 Hypertension Treatment Recommendations	
	Population	Goal BP

Treatment Goal

Recommendation 9	• Treatment goal for initial treatment is 1 month • Increase dose or add second drug • Continue to assess monthly until goal is reached • Do not use and ACEI and ARB together • Refer to hypertensive specialist if 3 or more drugs are needed

Note. JNC = Joint National Committee; BP = blood pressure; SBP = systolic blood pressure; DBP = diastolic blood pressure; CKD = chronic kidney disease; DM = diabetes mellitus; CCB = calcium channel blockers; ACEI = Angiotensin converting enzyme inhibitor; ARB = angiotensin receptor blocker. Grade A = strong recommendation; Grade B = moderate recommendation; Grade C = weak recommendation; Grade E = expert opinion but insufficient evidence for recommendation.

Table 12.3	Blood pressure classification and treatment recommendations for adults age 18 and older	
Category	Systolic, mmHg	Diastolic, mmHg
Normal for patients ≥ 60	< 150	< 90
Normal for patients < 60	< 140	< 90

Table 12.4	Common Oral Hypertensive Agents	
	Agent	Usual Dose/Frequency
Diuretics: **Thiazide**	chlorothiazide (Diuril) chlorthalidone (Hygroton) hydrochlorothiazide indapamide (Lozol) metolazone (Zaroxolyn)	250–500 mg BID 12.5–25 mg daily 12.5–50 mg daily 1.25–2.5 mg daily 2.5–10 mg daily or BID
Loop	bumetanide (Bumex) ethacrynic acid (Edecrin) furosemide (Lasix) torsemide (Demadex)	0.5–2 mg daily or BID 25–100 mg daily 10–40 mg daily 5–10 mg daily
Potassium sparing	eplerenone (Inspra) spironolactone (Aldactone)	50–100 mg daily 25–50 mg daily
Arterial Vasodilators	hydralazine (Apresoline) minoxidil (Loniten)	10–100 mg BID or four times a day 5–100 mg daily or BID

Table 12.4	Common Oral Hypertensive Agents	
	Agent	**Usual Dose/Frequency**
Direct Renin Inhibitor	aliskiren (Tekturna)	150–300 mg daily
β-adrenergic Blocking Agents	acebutolol (Sectral)	25–100 mg daily
	atenolol (Tenormin)	25–100 mg daily
	betaxolol (Kerlone)	5–20 mg daily
	bisoprolol (Zebeta)	2.5–10 mg daily
	carvedilol (Coreg)	12.5–50 mg BID
	labetalol (Normodyne)	200–800 mg BID
	metoprolol (Lopressor)	50–100 mg daily or BID
	nadolol (Corgard)	40–120 mg daily
	pindolol (Visken)	10–40 mg BID
	propranolol (Inderal)	10–120 mg BID
	timolol (Blocadren)	20–40 mg BID
ACE Inhibitors	benazepril (Lotensin)	10–40 mg daily
	captopril (Capoten)	12.5–100 mg BID or TID
	enalapril (Vasotec)	5–40 mg daily or BID
	fosinopril (Monopril)	10–40 mg daily
	lisinopril (Zestril)	5–40 mg daily
	moexipril (Univasc)	7.5–30 mg daily
	perindopril (Aceon)	4–8 mg daily
	quinapril (Accupril)	10–80 mg daily
	ramipril (Altace)	2.5–20 mg daily
	trandolapril (Mavik)	1–4 mg daily
Angiotensin II Receptor Antagonists	candesartan (Atacand)	8–32 mg daily
	eprosartan mesylate (Teveten)	400–800 mg daily or BID
	irbesartan (Avapro)	75–300 mg daily
	losartan (Cozaar)	25–100 mg daily
	olmesartan (Benicar)	20–40 daily
	telmisartan (Micardis)	20–80 mg daily
	valsartan (Diovan)	40–320 mg daily or BID
Calcium Channel Blocking Agents	verapamil IR	80–320 mg twice or TID
	verapamil (Calan SR)	120–240 mg daily or BID
	diltiazem IR	45–270 mg BID
	diltiazem (Dilacor XR)	180–360 mg daily
	amlodipine (Norvasc)	2.5–10 mg daily
	felodipine (Plendil)	2.5–20 mg daily
	isradipine (Dynacirc)	2.5–10 mg BID
	nicardipine (Cardene SR)	60–120 mg BID
	nifedipine (Adalat CC)	30–90 mg daily
	nisoldipine (Sular)	10–40 mg daily
Peripheral α_1-Antagonists	prazosin (Minipress)	1–10 mg BID
	terazosin (Hytrin)	1–10 mg daily or BID
	doxazosin (Cardura)	1–16 mg daily
Central α_2-Agonists	clonidine (Catapres)	0.1–0.6 mg BID
	methyldopa (Aldomet)	250–500 mg TID

Table 12.5	Prevention and treatment of hypertension recommendations
Blood pressure measurement	• Patient should do the following: • Be seated with feet flat on floor, back and arm supported, and arm at heart level • Rest for 5 minutes before measurement • Wear short sleeves • Not drink coffee or smoke cigarettes 30 min before having blood pressure taken • Go to the bathroom before the reading; having a full bladder can change your blood pressure reading • Clinician should do the following: • Use a cuff of appropriate size for the patient; the (cuff) bladder should encircle at least 80% of the upper arm • Use calibrated or mercury manometer
Primary prevention	• Quit smoking to reduce cardiovascular risk • Maintain a healthy weight; lose weight if needed • Restrict sodium intake to no more than 100 mmol/day • Limit alcohol intake to no more than 1–2 drinks per day • Be active; get at least 30–45 minutes of aerobic activity on most days • Maintain adequate potassium intake of about 90 mmol per day • Maintain adequate intakes of calcium and magnesium for general health
Goal	• Set a clear goal of therapy based on patient's risk. Control blood pressure to the levels below: • Less than 140/90 mmHg for patients
Treatment	• Begin with lifestyle modifications for all patients • Be supportive! • Add pharmacologic therapy if blood pressure remains uncontrolled/out of goal • Start with a thiazidetype diuretic, but also consider ACE inhibitor, angiotensinreceptor blocker, calcium channel blocker, or combination • If no response, try a drug from another class or add a second drug from a different class.
Adherence	• Encourage lifestyle modifications. Be supportive! • Educate the patient and family about the disease. Involve them in measurement and treatment • Maintain communication with patient • Empathy promotes adherence, trust, and motivation • Keep care inexpensive and simple • Consider cultural beliefs, practices, and individual attitudes when treating

Note. Adapted from "The seventh report of the Joint National Committee on prevention, detection, evaluation, and treatment of high blood pressure," by the National Institutes of Health National Heart, Lung, and Blood Institute, NIH Publication No. 04-5230, 2004.

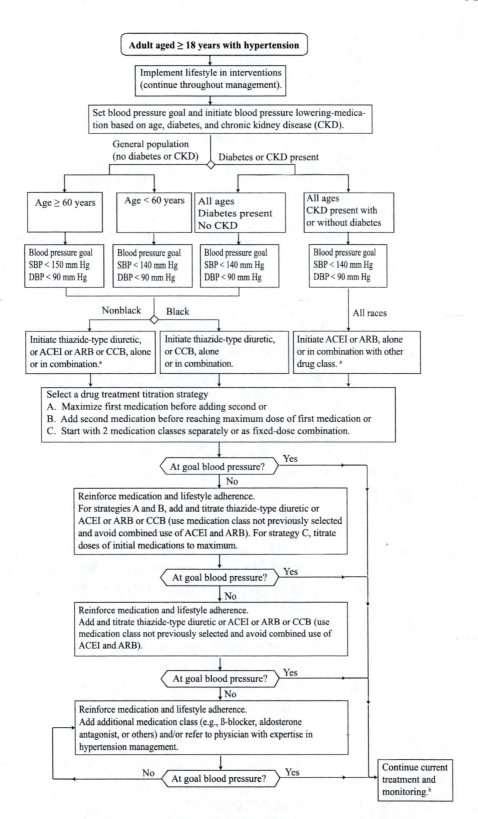

Figure 12.1. 2014 Hypertension Guideline Management Algorithm. SBP = systolic blood pressure; DBP = diastolic blood pressure; ACEI = angiotensin-converting enzyme; ARB = angiotensin receptor blocker; CCB = calcium channel blocker. Adapted with permission from "2014 Evidence-Based Guideline for the Management of High Blood Pressure in Adults," by P. A. James, S. Oparil, B. L. Cater, W. C. Cushman, C. D. Hummelfarb, J. Handler . . . E. Ortiz, 2014, *The Journal of the American Medical Association, 311*(5). Copyright 2014 by the American Medical Association.

[a]ACEIs and ARBs should not be used in combination.

[b]If blood pressure fails to be maintained at goal, reenter the algorithm where appropriate based on the current individual therapeutic plan.

VIII. Management
    A. Principle—in sequential order
        1. Analyze baseline studies
        2. See algorithm for the treatment of HTN (Figure 12.1)
        3. Use nonpharmacologic strategies
        4. Employ pharmacologic measures
    B. Nonpharmacologic strategies
        1. Restriction of dietary sodium (no more than 100 mmol per day—2.4 grams sodium or 6 grams salt)
        2. Weight loss, if overweight
        3. Adopt a DASH (Dietary Approaches to Stop Hypertension) diet (rich in fruits, vegetables, and low-fat dairy products, with reduced saturated and total fat)
        4. Exercise (aerobic exercise 30–40 min each day on most days of the week)
        5. Stress management planning
        6. Reduction or elimination of alcohol consumption (fewer than two drinks daily for men, or one drink daily for women and lighter-weight persons)
        7. Smoking cessation
        8. Maintenance of adequate potassium, calcium, and magnesium intake
    C. Pharmacologic measures (refer to Table 12.4 for specific drug names and dosages)
        1. Based on degree of blood pressure elevation and/or the presence of end-organ damage, cardiovascular disease, or other risk factors
        2. Goal of therapy—to prescribe the least number of medications possible at the lowest dosage to attain acceptable blood pressure, thereby decreasing cardiovascular and renal morbidity and mortality
        3. Thiazide diuretics, first-line drug of choice for hypertension:
            a. Increase excretion of sodium and water
            b. Reduce morbidity and mortality
            c. Screen for sulfa allergy before administering
            d. May cause hypokalemia, hypomagnesemia, hyperglycemia, hyponatremia, hypercalcemia, etc.
        4. ACE inhibitors:
            a. Cause vasodilation and block sodium and water retention
            b. Do not initiate if potassium is greater than 5.5 mEq/L.
            c. Contraindicated in pregnancy
            d. Do not use in combination with ARB
            e. May cause cough, rash, taste disturbances, hyperkalemia, renal impairment, etc.
        5. Angiotensin II-receptor blockers; reserved for patients intolerant to ACE inhibitors:

a. Cause vasodilation and block sodium and water retention
b. Do not initiate if potassium is greater than 5.5 mEq/L
c. Contraindicated in pregnancy
d. Do not use in combination with ACE inhibitor
e. May cause cough, hyperkalemia, headache, taste disturbances, renal impairment, etc.

6. Calcium channel blocking agents:
   a. Monitor heart rate, especially when administering verapamil and diltiazem
   b. May be used for angina, arrhythmias, and migraines
   c. May cause headache, flushing, bradycardia, etc.

7. Beta-blocking agents:
   a. Directly relax the heart
   b. May also be used for angina and arrhythmias
   c. Monitor heart rate and avoid use in patients with asthma/COPD
   d. Not first-line therapy
   e. May cause dizziness, bradycardia, heart block, fatigue, insomnia, nausea, etc.

8. Peripheral alpha-1 antagonists:
   a. Cause vasodilation
   b. Take first dose at bedtime
   c. Primarily used as adjunct therapy
   d. May be used for benign prostatic hyperplasia
   e. May cause first-dose syncope, dry mouth, orthostasis, dizziness, headache, nausea, etc.

9. Central alpha-2 agonists:
   a. Prevent vasoconstriction, cause vasodilation, and slow the heart rate
   b. Methyldopa is the drug of choice in pregnancy, clonidine is available as a transdermal patch
   c. Do not discontinue use abruptly, as it may cause withdrawals and rebound hypertension
   d. Primarily used as adjunct therapy
   e. May cause dry mouth, sedation, depression, headache, bradycardia, etc.

10. Arterial vasodilators:
    a. Directly relax the vascular smooth muscle resulting in arterial vasodilation
    b. Reduce frequency in renal dysfunction
    c. May cause reflex tachycardia
    d. Used primarily as adjunct therapy and is available intravenously
    e. May cause nausea, flushing, dizziness, orthostatic hypotension, etc.

Table 12.6	Select drug interactions with antihypertensive therapy		
Drug class	**Increase efficacy**	**Decrease efficacy**	**Effect on other drugs**
Diuretics	• Diuretics that act at different sites in the nephron (e.g., furosemide + thiazides)	• Resin-binding agents • NSAIDs • Steroids	• Diuretics raise serum lithium levels. • Potassium-sparing agents may exacerbate hyperkalemia caused by ACE inhibitors.
β-blockers	• Cimetidine (hepatically metabolized β-blockers) • Quinidine (hepatically metabolized β-blockers) • Food (hepatically metabolized β-blockers)	• NSAIDs • Withdrawal of clonidine • Agents that induce hepatic enzymes, including rifampin and phenobarbital	• Propranolol hydrochloride induces hepatic enzymes to promote clearance of drugs with similar metabolic pathways. • β-blockers may mask and prolong insulin-induced hypoglycemia. • Heart block may occur with nondihydropyridine calcium antagonists. • Sympathomimetics cause unopposed αadrenoceptor-mediated vasoconstriction. • β-blockers enhance angina-inducing potential of cocaine.
ACE inhibitors	• Ghlorpromazine or clozapine	• NSAIDs • Antacids • Food decreases absorption (moexipril)	• ACE inhibitors may raise serum lithium levels. • ACE inhibitors may exacerbate effect of potassium-hyperkalemic sparing diuretics.
α-blockers			• Prazosin may decrease clearance of verapamil hydrochloride.

Table 12.6 Select drug interactions with antihypertensive therapy			
Drug class	**Increase efficacy**	**Decrease efficacy**	**Effect on other drugs**
Central α_2-agonists and peripheral neuronal blockers		• Tricyclic antidepressants (and probably phenothiazines) • Monoamine oxidase inhibitors • Sympathomimetics or phenothiazines antagonize guanethidine monosulfate or guanadrel sulfate • Iron salts may reduce methyldopa absorption	• Methyldopa may increase serum lithium levels. • Severity of clonidine hydrochloride withdrawal may be increased by β-blockers. • Many agents used in anesthesia are potentiated by clonidine hydrochloride.
Calcium antagonists	• Grapefruit juice (some dihydropyridines) • Cimetidine or ranitidine (hepatically metabolized calcium antagonists)	• Agents that induce hepatic enzymes, including rifampin and • phenobarbital	• Cyclosporine levels increase[a] with iltiazem hydrochloride, verapamil hydrochloride, mibefradil dihydrochloride, or nicardipine hydrochloride (but not with felodipine, isadipine, or nifedipine). • Nondihydropyridines increase levels of other drugs metabolized by the same hepatic enzyme system, including digoxin, quinidine, sulfonylureas, and theophylline. • Verapamil hydrochloride may lower serum lithium levels.

Note. NSAIDs = nonsteroidal anti-inflammatory drugs; ACE = angiotensin-converting enzyme. Adapted from "The sixth report of the Joint National Comittee on prevention, detection, evaluation, and treatment of high blood pressure," by the National Institutes of Health National Heart, Lung, and Blood Institute, NIH Publication No. 98-4080, 1997.

[a]This is a clinically and economically beneficial drug-drug interaction because it retards the progression of accelerated atheroscelrosis in heart transplant recipients and reduces the required daily dose of cyclosporine.

11. Direct renin inhibitors:
    a. Inhibits renin, which decreases plasma renin activity (PRA) and inhibits the conversion of angiotensinogen I to angiotensin I
    b. Does not offer advantage over any other available regimens and is expensive
    c. Teratogenic, avoid use in pregnancy
    d. May cause diarrhea, dizziness, headache, hyperkalemia, etc.
12. Adrenergic antagonists:
    a. Depletes catecholamine stores to decrease blood pressure; depression of sympathetic nerve function
    b. Reserpine reserved for third-line therapy and is contraindicated in renal failure
    c. Guanethidine dose should be adjusted for patients with renal failure
    d. Rarely used due to significant adverse effects, such as drowsiness, nasal stuffiness, depression, and atrial fibrillation/arrhythmia
13. Special considerations
    a. Neither age nor gender usually affects agent responsiveness.
    b. Thiazide-type diuretics are usually recommended for first-line treatment.
    c. Beta blockers, ACE inhibitors, adrenergic receptor blockers, and calcium channel blockers are also useful alone or in combination therapy.
14. Refer to examples of commonly prescribed preparations in table 12.4
15. Follow guidelines regarding blood pressure measurement, primary prevention, goals of therapy, and treatment and adherence in the JNC 8 (Eighth Report of the Joint National Committee on Prevention, Detection, Evaluation, and Treatment of High Blood Pressure) Guide to Prevention and Treatment of Hypertension Recommendations (Table 12.2).
16. Refer often to the algorithm for treatment of HTN (see Figure 12.1)
17. Consider drug interactions with antihypertensive therapy (Table 12.6)

IX. **Hypertensive urgencies and emergencies**
    A. Hypertensive urgencies
       1. Characterized by severe elevations in blood pressure of 180/110 mmHg or higher without progressive target organ dysfunction
       2. Majority of patients present as noncompliant or inadequately treated hypertensive individuals, often with little or no evidence of target organ damage

3. Parenteral therapy is rarely required for such asymptomatic patients

4. May or may not be associated with severe headache, shortness of breath, epistaxis, or severe anxiety

5. Oral therapy may include the following:
   a. Clonidine (Catapres)
      i. Alpha-adrenergic stimulant
      ii. Dosage is 0.2 mg PO, then 0.1 mg every hour until BP is controlled or total of 0.8 mg is given
      iii. Patient may experience sedation
      iv. Rebound HTN is possible if drug is discontinued after chronic use
   b. Captopril (Capoten)
      i. ACE inhibitor
      ii. Dosage is 12.5–25 mg PO

B. Hypertensive emergencies
   1. Situations associated with severe elevations in blood pressure of 180/120 mmHg or higher. May occur at a lower blood pressure if complicated by evidence of impending or progressive target organ dysfunction
   2. Examples:
      a. Hypertensive encephalopathy
      b. Intracerebral hemorrhage
      c. Acute myocardial infarction
      d. Acute left ventricular failure with pulmonary edema
      e. Unstable angina pectoris
      f. Dissecting aortic aneurysm or eclampsia
   3. Require immediate blood pressure reduction to prevent or limit target organ damage
   4. Acute management possibilities for hypertensive emergencies
      a. Critical care unit nursing care and an arterial line are indicated
      b. Blood pressure should be lowered to 160–180 mmHg systolic or to less than 105 mmHg diastolic (no more than 25% within minutes to 1–2 hr), and then gradually lowered over several days with oral therapy to prevent additional complications such as coronary, cerebral, or renal ischemia.
      c. Nicardipine: first drug of choice
         i. Dosage is 2.5–15 mg/hr IV
      d. Sodium nitroprusside (Nipride): second drug of choice
         i. Dosage is 0.25–10 mcg/kg/min IV
         ii. May cause rapid, profound hypotension
         iii. Do not give for longer than 72 hr because of the risk of cyanide poisoning

    e. Nitroglycerin: used especially in patients with ischemia
       i. Dosage is 5–200 mcg/min IV
    f. Esmolol hydrochloride (Brevibloc)
       i. Dosage is 500 mcg/kg IV given over 1 min; maintenance dosage is 50–300 mcg/kg/min
          (a) No bolus unless heart rate is above 100
    g. Labetalol hydrochloride (Normodyne, Trandate)
       i. Used especially with hypertension associated with pregnancy
       ii. Start with 10–20 mg, then
       iii. 20–80 mg IV bolus over 10 min, or continuous infusion of 0.5–2 mg/min
    h. Hydralazine (Apresoline)
       i. Dosage is 5–20 mg IV and may be repeated in 20 min
       ii. Contraindicated in patients with coronary artery disease and aortic dissection
    i. Fenoldopam (Corlopam)
       i. Dosage is 0.03–0.1 mcg/kg/min IV; increase or decrease by 0.05–0.1 mcg/kg/min no sooner than every 15 min
          (a) Administer for up to 48 hr
       ii. May cause reflex tachycardia, hypotension, and increased intraocular pressure

BIBLIOGRAPHY

Barkley, T. W., Jr. (2014). *Acute care nurse practitioner certification review manual*. West Hollywood, CA: Barkley & Associates.

Czernichow, S., Zanchetti, A., Turnbull, F., Barzi, F., Ninomiya, T., Kengne, A. P., . . . Bruce, N. (2011). The effects of blood pressure reduction and of different blood pressure-lowering regiments on major cardiovascular events according to baseline blood pressure: Meta-analysis of randomized trials. *Journal of Hypertension, 29*(1), 4–16.

Ferri, F. F. (2011). *Ferri's clinical advisor:Instant diagnosis and treatment* (8th ed.). Philadelphia, PA: Elsevier.

Haro, J. D., Bleda, S., Florez, A., Varela, C., Esparza, L., & Acin, F. (2010). Ms481 long-term pleiotropic effect of statins upon nitric oxide and C-reactive protein levels in patients with peripheral arterial disease. *Atherosclerosis Supplements, 11*(2), 206–207.

Himmelfarb, J., & Sayegh, M. H. (2010). *Chronic kidney disease, dialysis, and transplantation companion to Brenner & Rector's the kidney* (3rd ed.). Philadelphia: Saunders/Elsevier.

Hudnut, F. (2013). Comment on "Beyond medications and diet: Alternative approaches to lowering blood pressure: A scientific statement from the American Heart Association". *Hypertension, 63*(1), e3.

James, A., Oparil, S., Carter, B., Cushman, W. C., Dennison-Himmelfarb, C., Handler, J., . . . Ortiz, E. (2014). 2014 evidence-based guideline for the management of high blood pressure in adults report from the panel members appointed to the Eighth Joint National Committee (JNC 8). *Journal of the American Medical Association, 311*(5), 507–20.

Kaplan, N. M., & Weber, M. A. (2010). *Hypertension essentials* (2nd ed.). Sudbury, MA: Physicians' Press.

Kaplan, N. M., Aronson, M. D., Bakris, G. L., & Forman, J. P. (2013). Perioperative management of hypertension. *UptoDate*. Waltham, MA: UpToDate. Retrieved from http://www.uptodate.com/contents/perioperative-management-of-hypertension

Mancia, G., Fagard, R., Narkiewicz, K., Redon, J., Zanchetti, A., Bohm, M., . . . Wood, D. A. (2013). 2013 ESH/ESC guidelines for the management of arterial hypertension: The task force for the management of arterial hypertension of the European Society of Hypertension (ESH) and of the European Society of Cardiology (ESC). *European Heart Journal, 34*(28), 2159–2219.

McPhee, S. J., Papadakis, M. A., & Tierney, L. M. (Eds.). (2014). *Current medical diagnosis and treatment* (46th ed.). New York, NY: McGraw Hill/Appleton & Lange.

Ogihara, T., Saruta, T., Raguki, H., Matsuoka, H., Shimamoto, K., Shimada, K., . . . Valsartain in Elderly Isolated Systolic Hypertension Study Group. (2010). Target blood pressure for treatment of isolated systolic hypertension in the elderly: Valsartan in elderly isolated systolic hypertension study. *Hypertension, 56*(2), 196–202.

Phillips, R. A. (2012). Controversies in blood pressure goal guidelines and masked hypertension. *Annals of the New York Academy of Sciences, 1254*(1), 115–122.

Strom, B. L. (2013). *Sodium intake in populations: Assessment of evidence.* Washington DC: National Academies Press.

Thelan, L. A., Urden, L. D., & Lough, M. E. (2009). *Critical care nursing: Diagnosis and management* (5th ed.). St. Louis, MO: Mosby.

CHAPTER 13

Coronary Artery Disease and Hyperlipidemia

JOAN KING • THOMAS W. BARKLEY, JR.

I. **Definition of Coronary Artery Disease (CAD)**

  A. Partial or complete blockage or narrowing of the coronary arteries, usually as the result of atherosclerosis; coronary vasospasm is also a cause

II. **Incidence/predisposing factors/risk factors**

  A. Heart disease continues to be the leading cause of death for men and women in the U.S.

  B. Coronary heart disease costs the United States $108.9 billion each year.

  C. Responsible for approximately 646,000 emergency department visits each year

  D. Accounts for 4.4 million cardiac procedures annually and 6.4 million hospital discharges

  E. Non-modifiable risk factors

    1. Age: increasing age increases risk

    2. Gender: men are six to eight times more likely to have CAD than premenopausal women; the incidence in postmenopausal women who are unprotected by estrogen is approximately equal to the incidence in men

    3. Race: white men die more frequently from CAD than do men of other ethnic backgrounds; women of other ethnic backgrounds die from CAD slightly more frequently than Caucasian women

    4. Heredity: family history of CAD increases risk

  F. Modifiable risk factors

    1. Smoking

      a. Increases in low-density lipoproteins (LDLs) and decreases in high-density lipoproteins (HDLs)

      b. Smokers have a two to six times greater risk of death from CAD than do nonsmokers

  2. Hypertension—risk of CAD is three times greater when BP exceeds 160/95 mmHg

  3. Diabetes: CHD risk equivalent—uncontrolled diabetes increases risk

  4. Obesity (visceral body fat) (BMI greater than 30) and/or sedentary lifestyle

  5. Increased stress and type A personality

  6. Use of oral contraceptives (especially if the woman is older than 35 years of age)

  7. Hyperlipidemia

      a. Elevations in triglyceride level, LDLs, and very low density lipoproteins (VLDLs) are associated with increased risk of CAD

      b. Low HDL levels are also associated with increased risk

III. **Laboratory/diagnostic testing**

  A. A1c is closely tied with elevated triglycerides (TG)

  B. For patients with suspected CAD who present with intermittent chest pain, do the following:

    1. 12-lead ECG

    2. See Angina and Myocardial Infarction chapter—management of angina/acute MI

    3. Stress testing (exercise stress test or thallium/Lexiscan stress test)

    4. Hemoglobin A1c as a corollary of triglycerides

  C. 12-lead ECG/stress testing

    1. Controversy exists regarding screening of asymptomatic patients in terms of resting ECG or stress testing and calcium scoring.

    2. Studies have not shown significant differences between asymptomatic individuals with and without CAD.

  D. Patients should be screened for hypertension every time they seek any health care.

  E. Pulse pressure (systolic pressure minus the diastolic pressure)

    1. Studies have correlated an increase in pulse pressure with higher mortality.

    2. Recent studies have suggested that the higher the pulse pressure, the greater the risk for CAD.

  F. Cholesterol screening that uses a fasting lipoprotein profile (total cholesterol, LDL, HDL, and TG levels) should be employed for all adults beginning at age 20 and at least every 5 years thereafter in accordance with the National Cholesterol Education Program.

  G. Plasma lipoprotein testing after a 9- to 12-hour fast

    1. Total cholesterol

      a. Desirable: less than 200 mg/dl

      b. Borderline high: 200–239 mg/dl

      c. High: 240 mg/dl or greater

  2. VLDLs contain mostly triglycerides and 10%–15% of total serum cholesterol

      a. Normal triglyceride level: less than 150 mg/dl

      b. Borderline high: 150–199 mg/dl

      c. High: 200–499 mg/dl

      d. Very high: 500 mg/dl or greater

  3. LDLs contain 60%–70% of total serum cholesterol in combination with HDLs; level is inversely correlated with HDL levels. Primary target of therapy is as follows:

      a. Optimal: less than 100 mg/dl

      b. Near optimal/above optimal: 100–129 mg/dl

      c. Borderline high: 130–159 mg/dl

      d. High: 160–189 mg/dl

      e. Very high: 190 mg/dl or greater

  4. HDLs contain 20%–30% of total cholesterol; level is inversely correlated with LDL levels and directly correlated with risk of coronary disease

      a. Low: less than 40 mg/dl

      b. High: 60 mg/dl or greater

  5. Historically, goals for patients with diabetes or documented coronary artery disease:

      a. LDL less than 70

      b. HDL greater than 40

      c. TG less than 150

IV. **Lifestyle changes to modify risk factors**

  A. Initiate therapeutic lifestyle changes (TLCs) if LDL is above optimal goal.

    1. TLC diet

      a. Saturated fat less than 5%–6% of calories

      b. Cholesterol less than 200 mg/day

      c. Consider increased viscous (soluble) fiber (10–25 grams/day) and plant stanols/sterols (2 grams/day) as therapeutic options to enhance LDL lowering.

    2. Weight management

    3. Increased physical activity

  B. Smoking cessation

  C. Control of hypertension—see Hypertension chapter

  D. Control of diabetes, including metabolic syndrome—see Diabetes Mellitus chapter

  E. Stress management

  F. Discontinuance of oral contraceptives for women at risk for CAD who are older than age 35; consider other means of contraception

G. Estrogen therapy may play a role in limiting CAD; however, estrogen therapy is not recommended as a prevention method for postmenopausal women.

H. Control of cholesterol through modifiable means or via pharmacologic therapy—see section hereafter

V. **Management of high blood cholesterol in adults**

A. Acquire a fasting lipoprotein profile after a 9- to 12-hour fast.

B. Identify total cholesterol, TGs, and LDL and HDL parameters.

C. Identify the presence of clinical atherosclerotic disease that confers high risk for coronary heart disease (CHD) events (CHD risk equivalent):

1. Clinical CHD

2. Symptomatic carotid artery disease

3. Peripheral arterial disease

4. Abdominal aortic aneurysm

5. Diabetes

D. Determine the presence of major risk factors (other than LDL) that modify LDL goals:

1. Cigarette smoking

2. Hypertension (BP 140/90 mmHg or higher, or patient is on antihypertensive medication)

3. Low HDL (less than 40 mg/dl). Note: HDL of 60 mg/dl or greater counts as a "negative" risk factor; thus, its presence removes one risk factor from the total count.

4. Family history of premature CHD (CHD in male first-degree relative younger than age 55; CHD in female first-degree relative younger than age 65)

5. Age (men age 45 or older; women age 55 or older)

6. Note: in the Adult Treatment Panel (ATP) III national guidelines, diabetes is regarded as a CHD risk equivalent

E. The latest American College of Cardiology and the American Heart Association (ACC/AHA) guidelines recommend using the new Pooled Cohort Risk Assessment Equations developed by the Risk Assessment Work Group to estimate the 10-year atherosclerotic cardiovascular disease (ASCVD) risk (defined as first occurrence nonfatal and fatal MI, and nonfatal and fatal stroke) for the identification of candidates for statin therapy.

1. The estimated risk of ASCVD is based on:

a. Age

b. Sex

c. Race

d. Total cholesterol

e. HDL cholesterol

f. Systolic blood pressure

g. Diabetic status

   h. Smoking status
   2. To estimate more closely the total burden of ASCVD, the current guideline recommends a comprehensive assessment of the estimated 10-year risk for an ASCVD event that includes both CHD and stroke. This is in contrast to the use of an estimated 10-year risk for hard CHD (defined as nonfatal MI and CHD death).
   3. To support the implementation of these guidelines, the new Pooled Cohort Equations CV Risk Calculator and Prevention Guideline Tools (web-based) are available at http://my.americanheart. org/cvriskcalculator and http://www.cardiosource.org/science- and-quality/practice-guidelines-and-quality-standards/2013- prevention-guideline-tools.aspx. In addition, links to download apps for mobile-based devices are also available.
F. Identify individuals who may benefit from statin therapy:
   1. Individuals with clinical evidence of ASCVD
   2. Individuals with elevated LDL-C of 190 mg/dl or higher
   3. Diabetics between ages of 40–75 with LDL-C between 70–189 mg/dl but without clinical evidence of ASCVD
   4. Individuals without ASCVD or diabetes with LDL-C between 70–189 mg/dl but with an estimated 10-year risk ASCVD of 7.5% or higher
G. Initiate TLC (everyone)
   1. Heart healthy lifestyle habits are the foundation of ASCVD prevention. Recalculate estimated 10-year ASCVD risk every 4–6 years for individuals with all of the following criteria:
      a. Age 40–75 years
      b. Not receiving cholesterol-lowering drugs
      c. Without clinical ASCVD or DM
      d. With LDL-C 70–189 mg/dl
H. Initiate drug therapy (adults greater than 21) (see Tables 13.1 & 13.2)
   1. High-intensity statin therapy should be initiated/continued as first-line therapy in women and men ≤ 75 years of age who have clinical ASCVD, unless contraindicated.
      a. Moderate-intensity statin therapy should be used when high-intensity statin therapy is contraindicated/statin- associated adverse effects are present.
      b. Individuals with clinical ASCVD who are 75 years of age or older, it is reasonable to evaluate the potential for ASCVD risk-reduction benefits and for adverse effects, drug-drug interactions, and to consider patient preferences when initiating a moderate or high-intensity statin.

2. Adults 21 years of age or older with primary LDL-C of 190 mg/dl or greater should be treated with statin therapy (10-year ASCVD risk estimation not required). Use high-intensity statin therapy unless contraindicated.

   a. Individuals unable to tolerate high-intensity statin therapy, use the maximum tolerated statin.

   b. Reasonable to intensify statin therapy to achieve at least a 50% LDL-C reduction

   c. After the maximum intensity of statin therapy has been achieved, addition of a non-statin drug may be considered to further lower LDL-C.

3. Moderate-intensity statin therapy should be initiated or continued for adults 40–75 years of age with DM.

   a. High-intensity statin therapy is reasonable for adults 40–75 years of age with DM with a 7.5% or higher estimated 10-year ASCVD risk unless contraindicated.

   b. Adults with DM, who are less than 40 or greater than 75 years of age, it is reasonable to evaluate the potential for ASCVD benefits and for adverse effects, for drug-drug interactions, and to consider patient preferences when deciding to initiate, continue, or intensify statin therapy.

4. The Pooled Cohort Equations should be used to estimate 10-year ASCVD risk for individuals with LDL-C 70–189 mg/dl without clinical ASCVD to guide initiation of stain therapy for the primary prevention of ASCVD.

   a. Adults 40–75 years of age with LDL-C 70–189 mg/dl without clinical ASCVD or diabetes and an estimated 10-year ASCVD risk 7.5% or higher should be treated with moderate to high-intensity statin therapy.

   b. Reasonable to offer treatment with a moderate-intensity statin to adults 40–75 years of age, with LDL-C 70–189 mg/dl, without clinical ASCVD or diabetes and an estimate 10-year ASCVD risk of 5%–7.5%

Table 13.1	Indications for statin therapy	
High-Intensity Statin Therapy	**Moderate-Intensity Statin Therapy**	**Low-Intensity Statin Therapy**
Daily dose lowers LDL-C on average, by greater than 50%	Daily dose lowers LDL-C on average, by approximately 30 to less than 50%	Daily dose lowers LDL-C on average, by less than 30%
atorvastatin 40–80 mg rosuvastatin 20–40 mg	atorvastatin 10–20 mg rosuvastatin 5–10 mg simvastatin 20–40 mg pravastatin 40–80 mg lovastatin 40 mg fluvastatin 80 mg pitavastatin 2–4 mg	simvastatin 10 mg pravastatin 10–20 mg lovastatin 20 mg fluvastatin 20–40 mg pitavastatin 1 mg

I. Identify metabolic syndrome, and treat if present after 3 months of TLC.

   1. Clinical identifications of metabolic syndrome is defined by any three of the following five criteria:

      a. Abdominal obesity: A simple measure of waist circumference is recommended to identify the body weight component of metabolic syndrome.

         i. In men, greater than or equal to 101.6 cm (40 inches)

            (a) Some men with marginally increased waist sizes (e.g., 37–39 inches) may have a strong genetic predisposition to insulin resistance and therefore, may develop multiple metabolic risk factors.

            (b) These patients should benefit from TLC similar to those men with waist sizes greater than 40 inches.

         ii. In women, larger than 88.9 cm (35 inches)

      b. Triglycerides: defining level, 150 mg/dl or above or on drug treatment for elevated triglycerides

      c. HDL: defining levels

         i. Men: less than 40 mg/dl

         ii. Women: less than 50 mg/dl

      d. BP: defining levels

         i. 130 mmHg or greater systolic or

         ii. 85 mmHg or greater diastolic or

         iii. On antihypertensive drug treatment in patient with a history of hypertension

      e. Fasting glucose: defining level, hemoglobin A1c, or on drug treatment for elevated glucose

         i. 100 mg/dl or greater

   2. Treatment of metabolic syndrome; lifestyle interventions and pharmacotherapy, if necessary, should be used to achieve hemoglobin A1c less than 7.

      a. Treat underlying causes (overweight/obesity and physical inactivity):

         i. Intensify weight management

         ii. Increase physical activity

      b. Treat lipid and nonlipid risk factors if they persist despite these lifestyle therapies

         i. Treat hypertension

         ii. Use aspirin for patients with CHD to reduce prothrombotic states

         iii. Treat elevated triglycerides and/or low HDL (as shown below)

J. Treat elevated triglycerides

   1. Treatments for triglycerides of 150 mg/dl or greater:

      a. Primary aim is to reach LDL goal

Table 13.2. Commonly used medications

Agents	Usual Dose	Lipid/lipoprotein Effects	Common Adverse Effects	Comments
Fibrates				
gemfibrozil (Lopid)	600 mg PO BID with/before meals	Decreases TG	Mild abdominal bloating, N/V/D, gallstones, altered taste, rash	Several drug-drug interactions Contraindicated severe hepatic/ renal impairment Concurrent use with statins = increased risk of myositis, rhabdomyolysis and hepatotoxicity Monitor LFT's
fenofibrate (Tricor)	48–145 mg PO daily with or without food	Slightly decreases LDL		
fenofibric Acid (Trilipix)	45–135 mg PO daily with or without food	Possibly increases HDL		
Cholesterol Absorption Inhibitor				
ezetimibe (Zetia)	10 mg PO daily	Decreases LDL	Diarrhea, abdominal pain, fatigue, arthralgia	Primary role will be _in combination_ with a statin in patients unable to achieve/ sustain target LDL levels with statin alone or in patients with contraindication/intolerance to statins Outcome data ??
Niacin				
immediate-release	500–2000 mg grams PO 2–3 times daily MAX 6 grams/day	Decreases LDL Decreases TG Increases HDL	Flushing, pruritus, hyperglycemia, hyperuricemia, ulcers, HA, dizziness, nausea, hepatotoxicity	Take aspirin 30 minutes before dose to reduce flushing Monitor LFT's Combination therapy with statins or in patients intolerant of statins
extended-release	500–2000 mg PO QHS MAX 2 grams/day			

Table 13.2. Commonly used medications

Agents	Usual Dose	Lipid/lipoprotein Effects	Common Adverse Effects	Comments
HMG-CoA reductase inhibitors (statins)				
atorvastatin (Lipitor)	See table 13.1	Decreases LDL	Myopathy/myositis, hepatic dysfunction, N/V/D, abdominal pain, HA, insomnia, rhabdomyolysis, diabetes	Many drug-drug interactions Monitor LFT's Consider decreasing when 2 consecutive LDL-C less than 40 mg/dL
fluvastatin, (Lescol)		Modestly decreases TG		
lovastatin (Pravachol)				
pitavastatin (Livalo)				
pravastatin (Pravachol)				
rosuvastatin (Crestor)				
simvastatin (Zocor)				
Bile Acid Sequestrants				
cholestyramine (Questran)	4 grams PO BID to QID	Modestly decrease LDL	Constipation, dyspepsia, bloating, stomach cramps, abdominal distension, obstruction	Several drug-drug interactions Used as adjunct therapy Contraindicated when TG greater than 300 mg/dL Malabsorption of vitamins A, D, E & K
colesevelam (Welchol)	875 mg PO BID or 3750 mg PO daily with a meal	Increases TG		
colestipol (Colestid)	2–16 grams PO daily or in divided doses			

Note. HMG-CoA = 3-hydroxy-3-methylglutaryl-coenzyme A; LDL = low-density lipoprotein; TG = triglycerides; N/V/D = nausea/vomiting/diarrhea; HA = headache; LFT = liver function tests; PO = per os; BID = two times a day

    b. Intensify weight management

    c. Increase physical activity

    d. Intensify/optimize treatment of DM

    e. Restriction/avoidance of alcohol

    f. If triglyceride level is 200 mg/dl or greater after LDL goal is reached, set a secondary goal for non-HDL cholesterol (total cholesterol minus HDL cholesterol) that is 30 mg/dl higher than the LDL goal.

        i. CHD and CHD risk equivalent (10-year risk for CHD greater than 20%)

            (a) LDL goal: less than 100 mg/dl

            (b) Non-HDL goal: less than 130 mg/dl

        ii. Multiple (two or more) risk factors and 10-year risk of 20% or less

            (a) LDL goal: less than 130 mg/dl

            (b) Non-HDL goal: less than 160 mg/dl

        iii. Zero or one risk factor

            (a) LDL goal: less than 160 mg/dl

            (b) Non-HDL goal: less than 190 mg/dl

    g. If triglyceride level is 200–499 mg/dl after LDL goal is reached, despite aforementioned measures, consider adding a drug if needed to reach non-HDL goal.

        i. Intensify therapy with LDL-lowering drug, OR

        ii. Add nicotinic acid or fibrate to further lower VLDL level

        iii. Because of the increased risk of myositis, rhabdomyolysis and hepatotoxicity, use caution when adding a fibrate with a statin.

    h. If triglyceride level is 500 mg/dl or greater, first lower triglycerides to prevent pancreatitis

        i. Very low-fat diet (15% or less of calories from fat)

        ii. Weight management and physical activity

        iii. Treatment of primary hypertriglyceridemia: fibrates, niacin, or omega-3 fatty acids (see above for risks associated with fibrates and statins)

            (a) Patients not on a statin: gemfibrozil (Lopid) or fenofibrate (Tricor) are the agents of choice

        iv. When triglycerides are less than 500 mg/dl, turn to LDL-lowering therapy.

K. Treat low-HDL cholesterol level (less than 40 mg/dl) if present

    1. First, reach LDL goals, then

    2. Intensify weight management and increase physical activity

L. Treat triglyceride levels:

    1. If triglyceride level is 200–499 mg/dl, achieve non-HDL goal

    2. If triglyceride level is less than 200 mg/dl (isolated low HDL) in CHD or CHD equivalent, consider nicotinic acid or fibrate

M. Complications of CAD—see specific complications

N. Angina—see Angina and Myocardial Infarction chapter

O. Myocardial infarction—see Angina and Myocardial Infarction chapter

P. Congestive heart failure—see Heart Failure chapter

Q. Peripheral vascular disease—see Peripheral Vascular Disease chapter

R. Hypertension—see Hypertension chapter

BIBLIOGRAPHY

Baron, R. (2012). In S. J. McPhee, M. A. Papadakis, M. & Rabow, M. (Eds.), *Current medical diagnosis and treatment* (51st ed.). New York, NY: McGraw Hill.

Berglund, L., Brunzell, J. D., Goldberg, A. C., Goldberg, I. J., Sacks, F., Murad, M. H., & Stalenhoef, A. F. H. (2012). Evaluation and treatment of hypertriglyceridemia: An Endocrine Society clinical practice guideline. *The Journal of Clinical Endocrinology & Metabolism, 97*(9), 2969–2989.

Boumaiza, I., Omezzine, A., Romdhane, M., Rejeb, J., Rebhi, L., Bouacida, L., . . . Bouslama, A (2014). Metabolic syndrome according to three definitions in Hamman-Sousse Sahloul Heart Study: A city based Tunisian study. *Advances in Epidemiology.* Retrieved from http://www.hindawi.com/journals/aep/2014/891297/

Bueche, J.L. (2010). Special topics in adult nutrition: chronic disease nutritional assessment. In J. Sharlin, & S. Edelstein (Eds.), *Essentials of Life Cycle Nutrition* (197–217). Sudbury, MA: Jones & Bartlett Publishers.

Foss-Freitas, M.C., Gomes, P.M., Andrade, R.G.G., Figueiredo, R.C., Pace, A.E., Dal Fabbro, A.L., . . . Foss, M.C. (2013). Prevalance of the metabolic syndrome using two proposed definitons in a Japanese-Brazilians community. *Diabetology & Metabolic Syndrome, 4*(38). doi:10.1186/1758–5996–4–38

Foster, J., & Prevost, S. (Eds). (2012). *Advanced practice nursing of adults in acute care.* Philadelphia, PA: F. A. Davis Company.

Gerstein, H.C., & Punthakee, Z. (2011). Dysglycemia and the risk of cardiovascular events. In S. Yusuf., J. Cairns, J. Camm, E.L. Fallen, & B.J. Gersh (eds.), *Evidence-Based Cardiology* (3rd ed.). Hoboken, NJ: John Wiley and Sons.

Godara, H., Hirbe, A., Nassif, M., Otepka, H., & Rosenstock, A. (Eds.). (2014). *The Washington manual of medical therapeutics* (34th ed.). Philadelphia, PA: Wolters Kluwer/Lippincott Williams & Wilkins.

Griffin, B., Callahan, T., & Memon, V. (Eds.). (2013). *Manual of cardiovascular medicine* (4th ed.). Philadelphia, PA: Wolters Kluwer/Lippincott Williams & Wilkins.

Gunder, L., & Martin, S. (2011). *Essentials of Medical Genetics for Health Professionals.* Sudbury, MA: Jones and Bartlett Publishers.

Ramos, L. M. (2014). Cardiac diagnostic testing: What bedside nurses need to know. *Critical Care Nurse, 34*(3), 16–26.

Stone, N., Robinson, A., Lichtenstein, C., Merz, N. B., Blum, C., Eckel, R.., . . . Wilson, P. (2013). ACC/AHA Guideline on the treatment of blood cholesterol to reduce atherosclerotic cardiovascular risks in adults: A report of the American College of Cardiology/American Heart Association Task Force on Practice Guidelines. Retrieved on December 15, 2013 from http://circ. ahajouurnals.org

CHAPTER 14

Angina and Myocardial Infarction

JOAN KING • THOMAS W. BARKLEY, JR.

I. **Definition/etiology**
   A. Angina means "squeezing and choking of the chest" related to ischemia
   B. Myocardial infarction (MI) is necrosis of myocardial tissue
   C. Pathology—supply/demand mismatch: the demand for myocardial oxygen is greater than the ability of the coronary arteries to supply oxygen

II. **Incidence/predisposing factors/general comments**
   A. Incidence
   1. Heart disease is the leading cause of death in the United States.
   2. One of every six deaths in the United States is caused by coronary heart disease.
   3. Approximately 10 million people in the United States have angina.
   4. Approximately 635,000 Americans will have a new MI each year, and 280,000 will have a recurrent attack.
   5. Each year, approximately 150,000 Americans will have a "silent" MI.
   6. 80% of deaths related to MI occur among individuals older than 65 years
   7. Classically, MI is precipitated by events that increase myocardial oxygen demand:
      a. Physical exertion (e.g., exercise and sex)
      b. Extreme weather conditions
      c. Consumption of a heavy meal (increases the risk by 4 times within a 2-hr period)
      d. Stressful events

B. Predisposing factors
1. Coronary artery disease/hyperlipidemia
2. Hypertension
3. Metabolic syndrome with increase in measured visceral fat
4. Obesity (body mass index [BMI] greater than 30 kg/m^2)
5. Cigarette smoking
6. Diabetes (type 1 and type 2)
7. Male gender (more prevalent until age 65 years, then incidence is equal in men and women)
8. Family history
9. Sedentary lifestyle
C. General comments
1. For ST elevation myocardial infarction (STEMI), national recommendations stipulate that all emergency departments should treat patients with acute MI within 30 min (door to fibrinolytics) and 90 min (door to angioplasty) upon arrival at a hospital.
2. The occurrence of MI and sudden cardiac death peaks between 6:00 a.m. and noon. A significant number of deaths related to MI also occur between 4:00 a.m. and 6:00 a.m.

III. **Types of angina**
A. Stable (chronic or classic)
1. Intermittent chest pain or discomfort with a predictable pattern: the same onset, intensity, and duration
2. Usually induced by exercise, exertion, or emotional upset
3. Pain at rest is unusual. Pain usually lasts 1–5 min, with a maximum duration of 10–20 min
4. May radiate to upper chest, epigastrium, arm, jaw, neck, or back
5. ECG at the time of the angina may show ST segment depression (ischemia)
6. Results from atherosclerotic blockage (plaques) over time
7. Nitroglycerin usually relieves pain. Rest may also relieve symptoms.
8. Angina may be controlled through lifestyle changes (e.g., weight loss, cholesterol control, blood pressure control, and smoking cessation) and medications such as nitrates, β-blockers, or calcium channel blockers. Angina may be controlled without severe complications.
B. Prinzmetal's (variant angina)
1. Precipitating event is coronary artery spasms caused by an increase in intracellular calcium levels
2. Pain often occurs at rest and may last up to 30 min
3. Pain is not usually precipitated by an increase in oxygen demand.
4. Pain may, and commonly occurs in the absence of atherosclerosis.
5. ECG usually shows ST segment elevation at time of the event.
6. Calcium channel blockers are prescribed to manage coronary artery spasms

   C. Unstable (preinfarction, rest or crescendo, and acute coronary syndrome [ACS])
      1. Chest pain lasts longer than 20–30 min.
      2. Pain may be new onset or more severe than with stable angina, and may occur at rest or with low activity levels
      3. Pattern of attacks usually progresses with increased frequency, duration, and intensity
      4. Pain may radiate to chest, epigastrium, arm, jaw, neck, or back.
      5. ECG may show ST segment depression
      6. Nitrates are usually insufficient to relieve pain
      7. Management includes adherence to ACS protocols
      8. Increased incidence of MI within 6 months after onset of angina
   D. Microvascular angina (syndrome X/metabolic syndrome)
      1. Chest pain mimics angina
      2. Exercise stress test is positive
      3. No evidence of abnormal angiogram or coronary spasm
      4. Postulated defective mechanism resulting in dilatation of the coronary microcirculation

IV.   **"P-Q-R-S-T" method of pain assessment**
      1. P = Provocative: What activities elicit pain?
      2. Q = Quality: What does the pain feel like? Do other symptoms occur simultaneously?
      3. R = Region/radiation: Where is the pain? Does the pain radiate? If so, to where?
      4. S = Severity: Rate the pain on a scale of 0–10. (Some institutions now use a 0–5 scale.)
      5. T = Timing/treatment: When did the pain begin? How long does it last? What did you do to relieve the pain? Were such measures effective?

V.   **Pain of angina versus MI**
   A. Generally, anginal pain is more diffuse and vague than pain resulting from MI.
   B. With MI, pain may be described as "vise-like"—"crushing" substernal pressure that may or may not radiate to the jaw and/or left arm.
   C. Pain from MI may radiate to the jaw, back, shoulders, arms, or abdomen.
   D. Other descriptors that patients may use include aching, cramping, grinding, burning, stinging, soreness, tearing, or gnawing.
   E. Approximately 15% of patients who experience MI have no pain. Lack of pain is particularly common among diabetic patients and the elderly, secondary to neuropathies.
   F. Generally, women who experience angina/MI complain of more gastrointestinal-like symptoms than are reported by men, or complain of pain radiating to the back.

1. Because women present differently, unstable angina (UA) or MI should be considered appropriate differentials requiring a complete cardiac workup
2. If the origin of the pain is related to acute GI causes such as esophagitis, gastritis, and gastric/duodenal ulcers, the administration of a "GI cocktail" consisting of Maalox or Mylanta, viscous lidocaine, and Donnatal should provide immediate relief.

VI. **ACS: three subclassifications**
   A. UA: new onset of symptoms, or change in pattern or frequency of symptoms
   B. Non-ST segment elevation MI (NSTEMI)
      1. May present with angina, or may be a "silent MI"
      2. Elevated enzymes
      3. No ST segment elevation on 12-lead ECG
   C. ST segment elevation MI (STEMI)
      1. Chest pain or angina that is not relieved with nitroglycerin
      2. Elevated enzymes
      3. ST segment elevation on 12-lead ECG

VII. **Subjective/physical examination findings of ACSs (UA, NSTEMI, and STEMI)**
   A. Note: Patient history and physical examination findings are very important for early detection and diagnosis.
   B. Nausea
   C. Vomiting
   D. Diaphoresis
   E. Cool, clammy skin
   F. Chest pain, usually substernal; in MI, not relieved by nitroglycerin
   G. Dyspnea
   H. Feeling of impending doom

VIII. **Diagnostics/laboratory findings of ACSs**
   A. Twelve-lead ECG changes
      1. UA and NSTEMI may present with ST segment depression (ischemia)
      2. STEMI will present with ST segment elevation (injury pattern)
      3. Signs of MI progression:
         a. Heightening or peaking of T waves
         b. ST segment elevation
         c. Inversion of T waves
         d. Formation of Q waves
         e. Diminished height of R waves
      4. Note: approximately 30% of patients who experience MI show no immediate 12-lead ECG changes
      5. Hallmarks of ischemia versus injury versus infarction include the following:

    a. Ischemia—T-wave inversion, peaked T waves, and ST segment depression. Note: With angina, cardiac changes usually do not persist once pain has been alleviated.

    b. Injury—ST segment elevation greater than 1 mm above baseline

    c. Infarction—may produce Q waves (pathologic) greater than 25% of QRS complex height or more than 1 mm wide (0.04 s)

  6. Expected site of MI based on ECG changes

    a. Inferior: leads II, III, and aVF; diaphragmatic involving the right coronary artery (80%–90%) or the left circumflex artery (10%–20%)

    b. Inferolateral: leads II, III, aVF, V5, and V6; site = left circumflex artery

    c. Anterior: V3 and V4; site = left anterior descending artery

    d. Anterolateral and lateral: leads I, aVL, V5, and V6; site = left anterior descending artery or left circumflex artery

    e. Anteroseptal: V1, V2, and V3; site = left anterior descending artery

    f. Posterior: Reciprocal changes noted in V1 and V3, broad or tall R waves, and ST depression without T-wave inversion may be seen; site = right coronary artery or left circumflex artery

    g. Right ventricular: V4R to V6R (right-sided lead tracing), also associated with inferior infarction pattern and posterior infarction pattern

B. Serum cardiac enzymes (Table 14.1)

  1. Troponin is myocardial specific and is the preferred biomaker for ACS, with Troponin I rising slightly faster than Troponin T (3 hr vs. 6 hr)

  2. Other biomakers include creatine kinase isoenzyme MB (CK-MB) and myoglobin, with myoglobin rising within 1–2 hr and CK-MB rising 4–12 hr

  3. Because of the variability of the enzymes rising, serial enzyme testing is needed every 6–8 hr

C. Laboratory analyses

  1. High levels of C-reactive protein (CRP) or high-sensitivity CRP (hs-CRP) in patients with UA and acute MI are indicators of future coronary events. Higher hs-CRP levels also are associated with lower survival rates; recent studies suggest that higher rates are associated with the reclosure of coronary arteries after angioplasty.

    a. Low risk: hs-CRP level less than 1 mg/L

    b. Average risk: hs-CRP level 1–3 mg/L

    c. High risk: hs-CRP level greater than 3 mg/L

Table 14.1	Serum cardiac enzymes			
Serum marker	Earliest increase, hours	Peak, hours	Duration	Other causes of elevation
Troponin T	4–6	10–24	14–21 days	Regenerative muscular disorders, unstable angina
Troponin I	4–6	10–24	5–7 days	100% specific for myocardial necrosis
Myoglobin	2–3	6–9	3–15 hr	Regenerative muscular disorders, unstable angina
CK-MB	4–8	15–24	48–72 hr	Post cardioversion, cardiac myocardial involvement and acute pericarditis with procedures, myocarditis, contusion, cardiac surgical
Total CK	3–6	24–36	18–30 hr	Smooth muscle injury, nonspecific
LD$_1$	8–12	72–144	7–12 days	Hemolytic and megaloblastic anemias, acute renal infarction, hemolysis, and testicular cancer
Total LD	10–12	48–72	10–14 days	Smooth muscle injury, nonspecific

Note: CK-MB = creatine kinase isoenzyme MB; CK = creatine kinase; LD1 = human heart LD1 isoenzyme;LD = human lactate dehydrogenase isoenzyme. Adapted with permission from "2010 American Heart Association Guidelines for Cardiopulmonary Resuscitation and Emergency Cardiovascular Care, Part 10: Acute Coronary Syndromes," by R.E. O'Connor, W. Brady, S.C. Brooks, D. Diercks, J. Egan, C. Ghaemmaghami, V. Menon, B.J. O'Neil, A.H. Travers, and D. Yannopoulos, 2010, *Circulation, 122*, Supple. 3 S787-S817. doi: 10.1161/CIRCULATIONAHA.110.971028. Accessed http://circ.ahajournals.org/content/122/18_suppl_3/S787/T.expansion.html , December 16, 2013. Copyright 2013 by the American Heart Association.

Table 14.2	ST segment elevation or new or presumably new LBBB: evaluation for reperfusion
Step 1	**Assess time and risk**

Time since onset of symptoms
Risk of STEMI
Risk of fibrinolysis
Time required to transport to skilled PCI catheterization suite

Step 2	**Select reperfusion (fibrinolysis or invasive) strategy**

If presentation less than 3 hr and no delay for PCI, then no preference for either strategy

Fibrinolysis generally preferred if:	An invasive strategy generally preferred if:
Early presentation (3 hr or less from symptom onset)	Late presentation (symptom onset longer than 3 hr ago)
Invasive strategy not an option (e.g., lack of access to skilled PCI facility or difficult vascular access) or would be delayed	Skilled PCI facility available with surgical backup
Medical contact-to-balloon or door-to-balloon is longer than 90 minutes	Medical contact-to-balloon or door-balloon is less than 90 minutes
(Door-to-balloon) minus (door-to-needle) is longer than 1 hr	(Door-to-balloon) minus (door-to-needle) is less than 1 hr
No contraindications to fibrinolysis	Contraindications to fibrinolysis, including increased risk of bleeding and ICH High risk from STEMI (CHF, Killip class is > 3) Diagnosis of STEMI is in doubt

Note. LBBB = left bundle branch block; STEMI = ST elevation myocardial infarction; PCI = percutaneous coronary intervention; ICH = intracerebral hemorrhage; CHF = congestive heart failure. Adapted with permission from "2010 American Heart Association Guidelines for Cardiopulmonary Resuscitation and Emergency Cardiovascular Care, Part 10: Acute Coronary Syndromes," by R.E. O'Connor, W. Brady, S.C. Brooks, D. Diercks, J. Egan, C. Ghaemmaghami, V. Menon, B.J., O'Neil, A.H. Travers, and D. Yannopoulos, 2010, *Circulation, 122*, Suppl. 3 S787-S817. Copyright 2010 by the American Heart Association.

2. Elevated levels of B-type natriuretic peptide are strongly correlated with myocardial ischemia/damage and may serve to predict severity of future cardiac complications, including heart failure and mortality.
   a. Normal B-type natriuretic peptide levels vary with age and sex, with women having slightly higher normal values.
   b. Mean levels

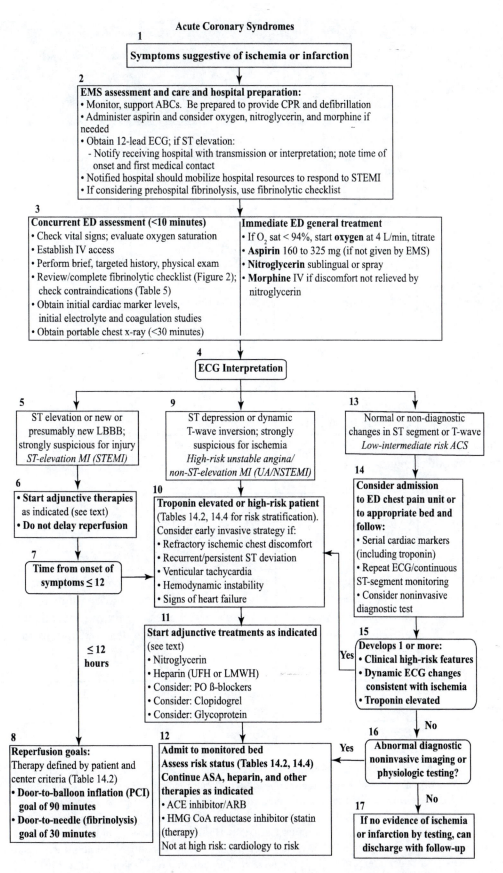

Figure 14.1. Acute cornoary syndromes algorithm. Adapted from "2010 American Heart Association Guidelines for Cardiopulmonary Resuscitation and Emergency Cardiovascular Care Science," by R.E. O'Connor, W. Brady, S. C. Brooks, D. Diercks, J. Eganm, C. Ghaemmaghami, . . . D. Yannopoulos, 2010, Circulation, 122.

Table 14.3	Likelihood of ischemic etiology and short term risk		
Part I	Chest pain patients without ST segment elevation: likelihood of ischemic etiology		
	A. High likelihood	B. Intermediate likelihood	C. Low likelihood
	High likelihood that chest pain is of ischemic etiology if patient has any of the findings in the column below.	Intermediate likelihood that chest pain is of ischemic etiology if patient has NO findings in column A and any of the findings in the column below.	Low likelihood that chest pain is of ischemic etiology if patient has NO findings in column A or B. Patients may have any of the findings in the column below.
History	Chief symptom is chest or left arm pain or discomfort plus current pain reproduces pain of prior documented angina and known CAD, including MI	Chief symptom is chest or left arm pain or discomfort Older than age 70 Male sex Diabetes mellitus	Probable ischemic symptoms Recent cocaine use
Physical examination	Transient mitral regurgitation	Extracardiac vascular disease	Chest discomfort reproduced by palpation
	Hypotension - Diaphoresis - Pulmonary edema or rales	Palpitation	Diaphoresis
ECG	New (or presumed new) transient ST deviation (0.5 mm or more) or T-wave inversion (2 mm or more) with symptoms	Fixed Q waves Abnormal ST segments or T waves that are not new	Normal ECG or T-wave flattening or T-wave inversion in leads with dominant R waves
Cardiac markers	Elevated troponin I (or T)	Any finding in column B above PLUS:	Normal
	Elevated CK-MB	Normal	

Note: If High (A) or Intermediate (B) Likelihood of Ischemia. CABG = coronary artery bypass graft; CAD = coronary artery disease; CK-MB = creatine kinase isoenzyme MB; MI = myocardial infarction; ECG = electrocardiography; VT = ventricular tachycardia; S3 = third heart sound. Adapted with permission from "2010 American Heart Association Guidelines for Cardiopulmonary Resuscitation and Emergency Cardiovascular Care, Part 10: Acute Coronary Syndromes," by R.E. O'Connor, W. Brady, S.C. Brooks, D. Diercks, J. Egan, C. Ghaemmaghami, V. Menon, B.J. O'Neil, A.H. Travers, and D. Yannopoulos, 2010, *Circulation, 122*, Suppl. 3 S787-S817. doi: 10.1161/ CIRCULATIONAHA.110.971028. Accessed http://circ.ahajournals.org/content/122/18_suppl_3/ S787/T.expansion.html , December 16, 2013. Copyright 2010 by the American Heart Association.

Table 14.3	Likelihood of ischemic etiology and short-term risk—cont'd		
Part II	Risk of death or nonfatal MI over the short term in patients with chest pain and high or intermediate likelihood of ischemia (column A or B in part I)		
	High risk	**Intermediate risk**	**Low risk**
	Risk is high if patient has any of the following findings.	Risk is intermediate if patient has any of the following findings.	Risk is low if patient has NO high-or intermediate-risk features; may have any of the following.
History	Accelerating tempo of ischemic symptoms over prior 48 hr	Prior MI or Peripheral artery disease or Cerebrovascular disease or CABG, prior aspirin use	
Character of pain	Prolonged, continuing (longer than 20 mintues) rest pain	Prolonged (longer than 20 minutes) rest angina is now resolved (moderate to high likelihood of CAD) Rest angina (less than 20 minutes) or relieved by rest or sublingual nitrates Older than age 70	New-onset functional angina (Class III or IV) in past 2 weeks without prolonged rest pain (but with moderate or high likelihood of CAD)
Physical examination	Pulmonary edema related to ischemia New or worse mitral regurgitation murmur Hypotension, bradycardia, tachycardia S_3 gallop or new or worsening rales Older than age 75		
ECG	Transient ST segment deviation (0.5 mm or more) with rest angina New or presumably new bundle branch block Sustained VT	T-wave inversion 2 mm or greater Pathologic Q waves or T waves that are not new	Normal or unchanged ECG during an episode of chest discomfort
Cardiac markers	Elevated cardiac troponin I or T Elevated CK-MB	Any of the above findings PLUS: Normal	Normal

Table 14.4	TMI risk score for patients with unstable angina and non-ST-segment elevation MI: predictor variables	
Predictor Variable	**Point value of variable**	**Definition**
Age 65 or older	1	
3 or more risk factors for CAD	1	Risk factors Family history of CAD Hypertension Hypercholesterolemia Diabetes Current smoker
Aspirin use in last 7 days	1	
Recent, severe symptoms of angina	1	2 or more anginal events in last 24 hr
Elevated cardiac markers	1	CK-MB or cardiac-specific troponin level
ST deviation 0.5 mm or greater	1	ST depression 0.5 mm or greater is significant; transient ST > 0.5 mm for < 20 minutes is treated as ST segment depression and is high risk; ST elevation 1 mm or greater for longer than 20 minutes places these patients in the STEMI treatment category
Prior coronary artery stenosis 50% or greater	1	Risk predictor remains valid even if this information is unknown
Calculated TIMI risk score	**Risk of 1 or more primary end points[a] in 14 days or less**	**Risk Status**
0 or 1	5%	Low
2	8%	
3	13%	Intermediate
4	20%	
5	26%	High
6 or 7	41%	

Note: MI, Myocardial infarction; CAD, Coronary artery disease; CK-MB, Creatine kinase isoenzyme MB; STEMI, ST elevation myocardial infarction; TIMI, Thrombolysis in myocardial infarction. Adapted with permission from "2010 American Heart Association Guidelines for Cardiopulmonary Resuscitation and Emergency Cardiovascular Care, Part 10: Acute Coronary Syndromes," by R.E. O'Connor, W. Brady, S.C. Brooks, D. Diercks, J. Egan, C. Ghaemmaghami, V. Menon, B.J. O'Neil, A.H. Travers, and D. Yannopoulos, 2010, Circulation, 122, Suppl. 3 S787-S817. Copyright 2010 by the American Heart Association.[a]Primary end points: death, new or recurrent MI, and need for urgent revascularization.

       i. Ages 55–64 years: 26 pg/ml

       ii. Ages 65–74 years: 31 pg/ml

       iii. Ages 75 years and older: 63 pg/ml

    c. Expected levels associated with MI: 100–400 pg/ml

  3. Complete blood count

  4. Prothrombin time (PT) and partial thromboplastin time (PTT)

  5. Basic metabolic panel (BMP)

  6. Lipoprotein profile

IX. **Management of ACSs**

  A. See figure 14.1 for ACS treatment algorithm. See Table 14.2, 14.3, 14.4 for ACS treatment considerations

  B. Emergency management of ACS with or without PCI

    1. Aspirin, 162–325 mg PO; chew and swallow

      a. If the patient is allergic to aspirin, consider clopidogrel as a substitution.

    2. Nitroglycerin, sublingual 0.4 mg (1 every 5 min); intravenous nitroglycerin may subsequently be used after narcotic administration (e.g., morphine), yet it should be used with extreme caution in patients with inferior MI because hypotension related to dramatic preload changes may occur.

    3. Supplemental oxygen at 2–4 L/min per nasal cannula

    4. Bedside monitor: evaluate potentially life-threatening arrhythmias

    5. Intravenous access: blood for cardiac enzymes and other laboratory values may be drawn at this time

    6. Continuous pain assessment

    7. Pulse oximetry

    8. Twelve-lead ECG within 10 min of presentation

    9. If pain is not relieved, consider morphine (0.1 mg/kg) IV, 2–4 mg, to relieve chest pain or anxiety, and may repeat with 2–8 mg every 5–15 min until pain is relieved unless other adverse effects occur. This completes adherence to national recommendations for the use of morphine, oxygen, nitroglycerin, and aspirin (MONA) in the emergent pharmacological management of ACS.

    10. Admit the patient to the coronary care unit or 23-hr observation unit to rule out NSTEMI or STEMI, pending the results of cardiac enzymes

    11. If diagnosis of ACS is made or suspected, continue immediately as follows:

      a. For hemodynamically stable patients, institute β-blocker therapy. Current guidelines recommend starting oral β-blockers within the first 24 hr of admission. ACC/AHA no longer recommends routinely using intravenous β-blockers.

i. β-blockers such as metoprolol (Lopressor) can be started at 25–50 mg PO and then titrated slowly based on hemodynamics. Maintenance dosage is 50–100 mg BID.

ii. If β-blocker therapy must be stopped, taper dosage over 1–2 weeks before ending therapy.

iii. Consider heparin continuous intravenous drip (e.g., 60 units/kg IV bolus followed by 12 units/kg/hr continuous infusion) to maintain PTT between 1.5 and 2.

(a) Note: The emergency antagonist for heparin is protamine sulfate. Low molecular weight heparin (e.g., enoxaparin [Lovenox], 1 mg/kg every 12 hr subcutaneously for 2–8 days) may be used as an alternative to unfractionated heparin, especially indicated in patients with NSTEMI and patients with UA. PTT should be monitored for unfractionated heparin and for both unfractionated heparin and Lovenox platelets should be monitored.

b. Consider the administration of an antiplatelet agent glycoprotein IIb/IIIa inhibitor, such as tirofiban (Aggrastat), in combination with heparin for patients with NSTEMI. Initial dose should be 0.4 mcg/kg/min IV for 30 min and continued at 0.1 mcg/kg/min. Dosing should be continued through angiography and for 12–24 hr after angioplasty. Monitor for bleeding.

i. Other preparations include abciximab (for PCI only, not ACS) (ReoPro), 0.25 mg/kg IV bolus, followed by 0.125 mcg/kg/min (maximum 10 mcg/min) for 12 hr; or eptifibatide (Integrilin), 180 mcg/kg IV (maximum, 22.6 mg) over 1–2 min, then 2 mcg/kg/min (maximum 15 mg/hr) by continuous infusion for up to 72 hr. If the patient is to undergo percutaneous coronary intervention (PCI), reduce infusion to 0.5 mcg/kg/min and continue for 20–24 hr after the procedure for up to 96 hr of therapy.

c. Consider continuous nitroglycerin intravenous drip if pain is not relieved by sublingual nitroglycerin and morphine. Begin at 5–10 mcg/min nitroglycerin and titrate up by 5–10 mcg/min every 5 min until either pain is relieved, or if the patient becomes hypotensive (i.e., systolic blood pressure less than 90 mmHg).

12. Consider fibrinolytic/thrombolytic therapy for STEMI (see Fibrinolytic/Thrombolytic Therapy section below)

13. Consider the need for cardiac catheterization/percutaneous transluminal coronary angioplasty (PTCA)/PCI, or coronary artery bypass graft (CABG) surgery

14. Admit to critical care unit for continuous monitoring
15. Following emergent therapy, consider the steps presented in the following section.

C. After an acute ischemic event, consider additional testing.

1. Exercise/stress test: the use of a treadmill to monitor ECG changes for signs of ischemia as well as heart rate and BP

   a. Usually requires 10–15 min

   b. A maximal test requires that the patient exercise until at least 85% of the maximum heart for the patient's age is achieved.

   c. Exercise continues until chest pain, fatigue, or other adverse effects are experienced, including the following:

      i. Extreme weakness
      ii. Severe dyspnea
      iii. Syncope or dizziness
      iv. Ataxia
      v. Claudication
      vi. Appearance of S3 or S4 heart sounds
      vii. ST segment elevation or depression of 1 mm or greater
      viii. Systolic BP above 250 mmHg
      ix. Decrease in systolic BP greater than 10 mmHg
      x. Rise in diastolic BP to higher than 90 mmHg or by more than 20 mmHg over the patient's baseline measurement
      xi. "Glassy-eyed" appearance, cold sweats, or confusion

   d. Submaximal tests are usually conducted on patients 4–7 days after MI. Identify patients with reversible ischemia. The stress test is stopped once the patient reaches a specific calculated target heart rate. Usually, the targeted heart rate (THR) is calculated with use of this formula: (220 - age) × 0.85 = THR.

   e. Abnormal results/positive stress test: downsloping or flat ST segment of 1 mm or greater than 1 mm from an originally depressed ST segment.

2. Thallium stress test: use of a radionuclide to detect perfusion of the myocardium

   a. Test is conducted similarly to the treadmill test

   b. During the final portion of the test, a radionuclide, such as thallium 201, or other tracing preparation, such as technetium-99m teboroxime (Cardiotec) or technetium-99m sestamibi (Cardiolite), is intravenously injected.

   c. Patient is then placed on a nuclear imaging scanner, where the myocardium is scanned for distribution of the radionuclide/tracing agent

   d. Scan is repeated in 3–4 hr

    e. Abnormal results: Light distribution indicates decreased or absent perfusion on the first scan. Defects depicted on the first scan, but not on the second, indicate reversible ischemia. Defects on both scans indicate areas of scar tissue that have resulted from MI.

3. Pharmacological stress test: use of pharmacological agents to increase coronary blood flow in patients who are unable to exercise to the point of reaching their target heart rates.

    a. Drugs of choice to increase coronary artery perfusion include dipyridamole (Persantine) and adenosine (Adenocard). Dobutamine (Dobutrex) is given primarily to increase cardiac output rather than to increase coronary blood flow (i.e., perfusion); subsequently, coronary blood flow will increase.

    b. If dipyridamole (Persantine) is used, thallium 201 is administered approximately 5 min after the intravenous dose, followed by a nuclear scan. Aminophylline, 50–125 mg, is given to reverse the adverse effects of dipyridamole, which may include chest pain, nausea, dizziness, or headache. Two to three hours later, administer a second dose of thallium, then conduct a second scan.

    c. Abnormal results/positive test: downsloping or flat ST segment 1 mm or greater for longer than 0.08 seconds, or greater than 1 mm depression from an initial ST segment depression of the patient's baseline measurement.

4. Ultrasonographic testing—consider the use of the following:

    a. Echocardiogram

    b. Doppler echocardiogram

    c. Color flow Doppler imaging

    d. Transesophageal echocardiogram

D. Outpatient management of stable angina

1. Nitrates—encourage the use of sublingual or buccal spray (0.4 mg) 5 min before exertion that may cause angina. Consider long-acting preparations such as the following:

    a. Isosorbide dinitrate (Isordil), 5–40 mg PO three times a day (most common)

    b. Isosorbide mononitrate (Imdur, Ismo)

        i. Imdur: 30–120 mg daily

        ii. Ismo: 20 mg PO BID (separated by 7 hr)

    c. Nitroglycerin sustained release, 2.5–6.5 mg every 8–12 hr

    d. Nitroglycerin transdermal patches (Nitro-Dur; Nitro-Derm), which deliver 5–40 mg every 24 hr

        i. Teach patient to take the patch off each morning for a nitrate-free interval—12–14 hr patch-on and 10–12 hr patch-off

2. β-blockers: preparation/initial dose (dosage range)
   a. Metoprolol (Lopressor), initial dosage: 50 mg in two doses daily, then 100 mg in two or three doses for angina; Toprol XL, 50–100 mg PO each day in one dose
   b. Carvedilol (Coreg), 6.25 mg PO BID, titrating to 25 mg PO BID
   c. Nadolol (Corgard), 20 mg daily; titrate to 40–80 mg daily; maximum dosage is 240 mg daily
   d. Atenolol (Tenormin), 25 mg daily; titrate to 100 mg daily
   e. Propranolol starting dose: 40 mg, and titrate to 180–240 mg per day in divided dosages (TID or QID)
   f. Major contraindications: bradyarrhythmias, severe bronchospastic disease, and heart failure
3. Calcium channel blockers are not first-line drugs for patients with ACS. They are recommended only for patients who have normal left ventricular function along with recurrent chest pain but cannot tolerate β blockers.
   a. Diltiazem (Cardizem SR), 90 mg BID (180–360 mg in two doses)
   b. Diltiazem (Cardizem CD), 180 mg daily (180–360 mg daily)
   c. Diltiazem (Dilacor XR), 180 or 240 mg daily (180–540 mg daily)
   d. Diltiazem (Tiazac SA), 240 mg daily (180–540 mg daily)
   e. Verapamil (Calan SR, Isoptin SR, and Verelan), 180 mg daily (180–480 mg in one or two doses)
   f. Dihydropyridine calcium channel blockers (e.g., amlodipine) may be used as adjunct therapy with β-blockers.
      i. Specifically, amlodipine and felodipine are used frequently for angina syndromes as these cause much less reflex tachycardia compared to other dihydropyridine CCBs and appear to preferentially vasodilate the coronary vasculature.
4. Ranolazine (Ranexa) 500–1000 mg PO BID; adjunct therapy for refractory angina with inadequate response to other antianginal drugs (amlodipine, β-blockers, and/or nitrates)
5. If the patient is unresponsive to a single agent, use an alternative classification of agent before progressing to combination therapy.
6. If the patient remains symptomatic, the use of either a β-blocker and a long-acting nitrate combination or a β-blocker and a calcium channel blocker (other than verapamil) combination is most effective.
7. Low-dose aspirin therapy (81–325 mg daily)
8. For patients who do not tolerate aspirin: clopidogrel (Plavix), 75 mg PO daily

9. For UA and NSTEMI, a combination of aspirin plus clopidogrel for 12 months

E. Post-MI outpatient management
   1. See patient for follow-up PRN immediately after discharge
   2. Future visits after initial follow-up should be scheduled every 2–6 months
   3. Consider stress testing 3–4 weeks after MI
   4. Repeat ECG at 3 months, then every 1–2 years thereafter
   5. Continue pharmacological therapy
      a. β-blocker, 50 mg once daily (e.g., metoprolol succinate [Toprol XL])
      b. Continue aspirin therapy, 81 mg daily, indefinitely
      c. ACE inhibitor in patients with left ventricular dysfunction and most patients with Q-wave MI for remodeling (e.g., captopril, 25–50 mg three times a day) is particularly recommended for patients with ejection fractions less than 40% beginning 3–16 days after infarction
   6. Cardiac rehabilitation as indicated
   7. Monitor lipoprotein profiles
   8. Statin therapy-atorvastatin (Lipitor), 80 mg once daily; rosuvastatin (Crestor), 20–40 mg once daily

FIBRINOLYTIC/THROMBOLYTIC THERAPY

I. **Definition**
   A. Pharmacological process in which agents are used to restore myocardial blood flow through the lysing of clots within the coronary arteries (90% of all STEMI involve a thrombus)
   B. Indications
      1. Preferred mode of treatment for STEMI if PCI is not available within 90 min
      2. Unrelieved chest pain of recent onset (longer than 30 min, but less than 6 hr); variations of this indication have been used, such as administration up to, but not beyond, 24 hr after initiation of pain
      3. ECG changes—ST segment elevation (in two contiguous leads; 1-mm elevation in limb leads, or 2 mm elevation in precordial leads), Q waves, or bundle branch block
      4. Greatest benefit occurs within 1–3 hr of onset of pain; mortality may be reduced by 50%
   C. Contraindications (see Table 14.5)
   D. Major complication: hemorrhage including intracranial hemorrhage
      a. Twofold increase in risk of intracranial hemorrhage in patients older than 75 years
      b. Increased risk of intracranial hemorrhage for patients weighting less than 70 kg, or patients with severe hypertension
   E. Preparations

Table 14.5	Contraindications and Cautions for Fibrinolytic Therapy in STEMI

Absolute contraindications

Any prior ICH

Known structural cerebral vascular lesion (e.g., arteriovenous malformation)

Known malignant intracranial neoplasm (primary or metastatic)

Ischemic stroke within 3 months (except acute ischemic stroke within 4.5 hr)

Suspected aortic dissection

Active bleeding or bleeding diathesis (excluding menses)

Significant closed-head or facial trauma within 3 months

Intracranial or intraspinal surgery within 2 months

Severe uncontrolled hypertension (unresponsive to emergency therapy)

For streptokinase, prior treatment within the previous 6 months

Relative contraindications

History of chronic, severe, poorly controlled hypertension

Significant hypertension on presentation (SBP > 180 mmHg or DBP > 100 mmHg)

History of prior ischemic stroke > 3 months

Dementia

Known intracranial pathology not covered in absolute contraindications

Traumatic or prolonged (> 10 minutes) CPR

Major surgery (< 3 weeks)

Recent (within 2 to 4 weeks) internal bleeding

Noncompressible vascular punctures

Pregnancy

Active peptic ulcer

Oral anticoagulant therapy

Note. Viewed as advisory for clinical decision making and may not be all-inclusive or definitive. CPR=cardiopulmonary resuscitation; DBP=diastolic blood pressure; ICH=intracranial hemorrhage; SBP=systolic blood pressure; STEMI=ST-elevation myocardial infarction. Adapted from "2010 American Heart Association Guidelines for Cardiopulmonary Resuscitation and Emergency Cardiovascular Care, Part 10: Acute Coronary Syndromes," by R.E. O'Connor, W. Brady, S.C. Brooks, D. Diercks, J. Egan, C. Ghaemmaghami, V. Menon, B.J., O'Neil, A.H. Travers, and D. Yannopoulos, 2010, *Circulation, 122*, Suppl. 3 S787-S817. Copyright 2010 by the American Heart Association.

1. Tissue plasminogen activator (t-PA) offers less risk of bleeding because it is fibrin specific and will not deplete clotting factors. This can be repeated later in life and is especially effective in the following types of patients:
   a. Patients with large/anterior wall MI
   b. Patients who have undergone previous CABG surgery
   c. Young patients
2. Reteplase (rPA) is an agent very similar to t-PA, but it has a longer half-life.
3. Tenecteplase (TNKase) binds to fibrin and converts plasminogen to plasmin
4. Streptokinase is a synthetic protein derived from group C β-hemolytic streptococci that combines with plasminogen to activate the fibrinolytic process. It can be administered only once in a lifetime because of the development of antibodies, and it is especially effective in the following types of patients:
   a. Patients with small MI
   b. Patients at high risk for stroke
   c. Late treatment (more than 6 hr following onset of pain)
   d. Advanced patient age (older than 75 years)
   e. Young patients

F. Select fibrinolytic/thrombolytic choices (see Table 14.6)
G. Considerations during administration
   1. Observe for signs of tissue reperfusion.
      a. Abrupt pain relief
      b. ECG normalization and/or appearance of Q waves
      c. Reperfusion arrhythmias, especially accelerated idioventricular rhythm, sinus bradycardia, ventricular tachycardia, and ventricular fibrillation
      d. Improved capillary refill and oxygen saturation
   2. Monitor neurologic status for changes related to possible cerebrovascular accident.
   3. Monitor the patient for bleeding (e.g., gums, urine, and bruising), and check therapeutic coagulation values
H. Post-fibrinolytic/thrombolytic treatment
   1. Ensure adequate pain relief via the use of morphine, 4–8 mg IV
   2. For patients who are hypertensive, tachycardic or have ongoing ischemia, consider the short-term use of intravenous β-blockers immediately after infarction, followed by oral treatment when possible.
   3. Nitroglycerin is given for recurrent chest pain; routine administration as a single agent is not recommended
   4. Consider ACE inhibitors after thrombolysis and the use of β-blockers in patients with continuing ischemia despite the use of nitrates

Table 14.6	Fibrinolytic therapy			
	Alteplase; tissue plasminogen activator (t-PA)	Streptokinase	Reteplase (r-PA)	Tenecteplase (TNKase)
Peak effect	45 min	20 min–2 hr	NA	NA
Duration	6 hr–2 days	6–24 hr	NA	Half-life 20 min
Fibrin specific	Yes	No	Yes	Yes
Dosage/Infusion	15-mg bolus followed by 50 mg over 30 min, then 35 mg over 1 hr (not to exceed 100 mg)	750,000 units over 20 min, followed by 750,000 units over 40 min	10-unit bolus over 20 min, repeated in 30 min	Give IV bolus over 5 seconds, using body weight; not to exceed 50 mg Less than 60 kg: 30 mg (6 ml) 60–70 kg: 35 mg (7 ml) 70–80 kg: 40 mg (8 ml) 80–90 kg: 45 mg (9 ml) More than 90 kg: 50 mg (10 ml)
Anticoagulation following administration	Aspirin, 325 mg every day; heparin, 5000-unit bolus followed by 1000-unit/hr infusion (maintain PTT 1.5–2 × control)	Aspirin, 325 mg every day; no evidence shown to improve outcome with use of heparin	Aspirin, 325 mg every day; heparin 5000-unit bolus followed by 1000-unit/hr infusion (maintain PTT 1.5–2 × control)	Baby aspirin, 160 mg + heparin, 5000 units IV, followed by 750–1000 mg continuous IV infusion
Allergic reactions	No	Yes	No	
Reocclusion	10%–30%	5%–20%	Unknown	5%–20%

Note. APSAC = asinoylated plasminogen streptokinase activator complex; PTT = partial thromboplastin time.

PERCUTANEOUS TRANSLUMINAL CORONARY ANGIOPLASTY (PTCA)/PERCUTANEOUS CORONARY INTERVENTION (PCI)

I. **Definition**
   A. PTCA/PCI is an invasive procedure whereby a narrow catheter with an inflatable balloon tip is inserted percutaneously into the aorta and up into the coronary arteries under fluoroscopy.
   B. The balloon is temporarily inflated to compress atherosclerotic plaque against the arterial wall, resulting in dilatation of the lumen of the coronary artery.
   C. PCIs, including intracoronary arterial stents (both bare metal and drug-eluting stents), are commonly used in conjunction with PTCA with the goal of restoring myocardial blood flow (Thrombolysis in myocardial infarction grade 3 [TIMI 3]).
      1. Bare metal stenosis stents are typically used for patients who are at high risk for bleeding, may require surgical procedures within the next 12 months, or are unlikely to be compliant with 12 months of dual antiplatelet therapy.
      2. Drug-eluting stents require 12 months of dual antiplatelet therapy (aspirin and clopidogrel)

II. **Indications/criteria for use/incidence**
   A. PTCA is the preferred mode of treatment for MI only when immediately available to patients (i.e., less than 90 min of arrival in the emergency department), or when fibrinolytics are contraindicated
   B. ECG changes, including ST segment depression or elevation, or onset of left bundle branch block (LBBB)
   C. Evolving MI
   D. Angina (recent onset, or condition is stable yet unresponsive to medical treatment)
   E. Adequate ventricular function and collateral circulation
   F. Relatively proximal, noncalcified lesions
   G. Lesions less than 10 mm in length
   H. Lesions not involving a major bifurcation
   I. It is estimated that at least 400,000 PTCAs are performed annually in the United States.

III. **Laboratory/diagnostics**
   A. Hemoglobin (Hgb), hematocrit (Hct), and platelets
   B. Basic metabolic panel electrolytes
   C. Coagulation profile
   D. Type and cross match 2 units of packed red blood cells in case CABG surgery is necessary

IV. **Special considerations**
   A. Patient teaching
      1. Chance of necessary CABG surgery if complications occur

Table 14.7	Therapeutic coagulation values	
Coagulation test	**Normal values, seconds**	**Therapeutic values**
International normalized ratio (INR)	0.8–1.2	MI or mechanical heart valve: 2.5–3.5 × normal Chronic atrial fibrillation: 2.0–3.0 × normal, or less than 2.5 × normal if patient is older than age 70 Deep vein thrombosis or pulmonary embolus treatment: 2.0–3.0 × normal
Activated coagulation time (ACT)	70–120	150–190 seconds, or longer than 300 seconds after PTCA/stent application
Activated partial thromboplastin time (APTT)	28–38	1.5–2.5 = normal
Prothrombin time (PT)	11–16	1.5–2.5 = normal
Partial thromboplastin time (PTT)	60–90	1.5–2.5 = normal

Note. MI = myocardial infarction; PTCA = percutaneous transluminal coronary angioplasty.

   2. The patient will remain awake, receive local anesthesia to the groin, and must lie still.
   3. The procedure is not painful
   4. NPO after midnight (unless emergency)
   5. The patient must keep the leg straight, and a pressure bandage may be used after the procedure has been performed (follow hospital protocol).
   6. The patient will be walking within 4–6 hr after the procedure has been completed.
 B. Observe for signs of reperfusion
   1. ECG changes
   2. Pain relief
   3. Other signs of improving clinical status
 C. Monitor therapeutic coagulation values after the procedure has been performed (may vary depending on laboratory). Many institutions are monitoring only activated coagulation time (ACT) after PTCA for sheath removal (e.g., ACT less than 175); follow hospital protocol (see table 14.7)
 D. Observe for complications
   1. Restenosis may occur in 30%–40% of patients. This is indicated by angina, ST segment elevation per 12-lead ECG, and/or arrhythmias. Emergency repeat PTCA or CABG surgery is warranted in this case.

2. Contrast dye allergy (evidenced by signs of anaphylaxis; feeling warm or somewhat flushed during PTCA is normal)
3. Hematoma formation at the groin site
4. Coronary artery perforation/rupture, embolism, spasms of coronary arteries, and MI are possible

CORONARY ARTERY BYPASS GRAFT (CABG) SURGERY

I.   **Definition**
   A. Procedure in which ischemic areas of the heart are revascularized through a grafting approach from the aortic root to a point distal to the ischemic lesion, using one of the following for the graft:
     1. Internal mammary artery (better for long-term patency)
     2. Saphenous vein
     3. Radial artery
     4. Gastroepiploic artery

II. **Indications**
   A. Refractory UA
   B. MI
   C. Failure of PTCA
   D. Greater than 50% left main coronary artery occlusion
   E. Triple-vessel coronary artery disease
   F. Left ventricular failure related to heart failure or cardiogenic shock

III. **Expectations in the immediate postoperative period**
   A. Continuous cardiac monitoring: Atrial fibrillation occurs in 20%–30% of patients, warranting consideration of anticoagulation if it persists longer than 24 hr
   B. Mechanical ventilation: extubation within 2–6 hr, or less in most patients
   C. Pulmonary artery catheter to measure hemodynamic profile
   D. Arterial line for continuous BP readings and laboratory analyses
   E. Pulmonary capillary wedge pressure, maintained slightly higher than normal (e.g., 18–20 mmHg)
   F. Hypotension: If warm cardioplegia was used, maintain BP and mean arterial pressure by volume loading with crystalloids, colloids, or packed red blood cells. Autotransfusion may also be used.
   G. Serum potassium level maintained in the high-to-normal range (e.g., 4.5–5.0 mEq/L; some protocols prefer higher ranges after CABG)
   H. Serum magnesium level maintained at approximately 2.0 mEq/L to assist in preventing arrhythmias
   I. Clotting factors: administering fresh frozen plasma and platelets as indicated for depletion

J. Mediastinal chest tubes x 2: As a general rule, if output exceeds 400 ml within 2 consecutive hr or 300–500 ml within 1 hr, re-exploratory surgery is indicated. Chest tubes are commonly removed within 24 hr postoperatively as long as significant decreases in bleeding/output are noted.

K. Epicardial pacing wires x 2 may be used if heart rate drops to below 80 bpm

L. Nasogastric (NG) tube to lower wall suction for gastric decompression

M. Foley catheter to ensure adequate (more than 30 ml/hr) urinary output, or per protocol

N. Common vasopressors, inotropes, vasodilators and antiarrhythmic agents

  1. Vasopressors:

    a. Dopamine (Intropin): used for blood pressure support/hypotension

    b. Norepinephrine (Levophed) is a vasoconstrictor used for severe shock

  2. Inotropes:

    a. Dobutamine (Dobutrex): used to increase cardiac output, thereby increasing blood pressure

    b. Milrinone (Primacor): used to increase contractility and decrease preload and afterload via vasodilatation

  3. Vasodilators

    a. Nitroprusside (Nipride): used for transient hypertension resulting from vasoconstriction related to hypothermia during surgery

    b. Nitroglycerin (Tridil): used for coronary and systemic vasodilatation to decrease preload and myocardial oxygen consumption

  4. Antiarrhythmics:

    a. Amiodarone: class II antiarrhythmic, prolongs the conduction through AV node; may be used for rate control in atrial fibrillation (AF) or converting AF to sinus rhythm

    b. Esmolol (Brevibloc): β-blocker used for tachycardia and afterload reduction

    c. Diltiazem (Cardizem): calcium channel blocker used for tachycardia

O. Monitoring for neurologic changes: Cerebrovascular accidents may occur in 5%–10% of patients. Increased risk is seen in the following types of patients:

  1. Advanced age

  2. African American men

  3. Hypertension

  4. Obesity

  5. Diabetes mellitus

  6. Atrial rhythm disorders

  7. Cardiopulmonary bypass lasting longer than 2 hr

P. Monitoring for infection: postoperative fever 101.3°F (38°C) or higher warrants suspicion for culture and sensitivity testing of blood, wound, urine, and sputum. Provide antibiotic therapy as indicated (see Infections chapter).

IV. Potential complications of MI

A. Arrhythmias—see Ectopy and Arrhythmia Emergencies chapter

B. Heart failure—see Heart Failure chapter

C. Pulmonary edema—see Restrictive (Inflammatory) Lung Diseases and Congestive Heart Failure chapter

D. Cardiogenic shock—most common fatal complication of MI (see Management of the Patient in Shock chapter)

E. Pericarditis—see Inflammatory Cardiac Diseases chapter

F. Infection—especially leg wound, sternotomy, or systemic (see Infections chapter)

CARDIAC TAMPONADE

I. Definition

A. Accumulation of blood and/or fluid in the pericardial space, resulting in a life-threatening decrease in cardiac output

II. Etiology/incidence/predisposing factors

A. Blunt/penetrating trauma to the upper chest

B. Postoperative cardiac surgical patients or following cardiac catheterization

C. Patients with pericarditis

D. Acute MI

E. May be caused by viral, bacterial, or fungal infections

III. Subjective findings—unremarkable

IV. Physical examination findings

A. Beck's triad

    1. Jugular venous distention—rarely present with traumatic injury related to hypovolemia

    2. Narrowing pulse pressure

    3. Distant heart tones

B. Tachycardia

C. Pulsus paradoxus

D. Changes in level of consciousness (e.g., anxiety and confusion)

E. Oliguria

F. Other signs of shock

V. Diagnostics/laboratory findings

A. Echocardiogram is used to confirm diagnosis

B. Chest x-ray may show widening mediastinum

VI. Management

A. Pericardiocentesis

B. Symptomatic treatment of shock (e.g., oxygen, fluid resuscitation, and inotropic agents) (see Management of the Patient in Shock chapter)

IMPLICATIONS FOR THE ELDERLY

I.   General Implications

    A. The majority of elderly patients presenting with an acute MI either have nondiagnostic ECG changes, or they present with an NSTEMI

    B. Individuals older than 75 years are more likely to have a silent MI

    C. Individuals older than 85 years are more likely to present with LBBB or signs of heart failure

    D. Clopidogrel dose is 75 mg for individuals older than 75 years and who are to receive fibrinolytic therapy rather than the normal clopidogrel loading dose of 300 mg

II.   Management

    A. Individuals older than 75 years have better outcomes with PCI than with thrombolytic therapy

    B. The risk of a hemorrhagic stroke following thrombolytic therapy is greater for individuals older than 85 years

BIBLIOGRAPHY

American College of Cardiology Foundation/American Heart Association. (2012, December 17). 2013 ACCF/AHA guideline for the management of ST-elevation myocardial infarction: Executive summary. *Circulation, 127*, 529–555. Retrieved December 15, 2013, from http://circ.ahajournals.org/content/127/4/529.full

American Heart Association. (2010, November 2). 2010 American Heart Association guidelines for cardiopulmonary resuscitation and emergency cardiovascular care science. Part 10: Acute coronary syndromes. *Circulation, 122*(Suppl 3), S787-S817. Retrieved December 16, 2013, from http://circ.ahajournals.org/content/122/18_suppl_3/S787.full

Bonow, R., Mann, D. L., Zipes, D.P., & Libby, P. (2011). *Braunwald's heart disease: A textbook of cardiovascular medicine* (9th ed.). Philadelphia, PA: Elsevier Saunders.

Brady, W., Brooks, S.C., Diercks, D., Egan, J., Ghaemmaghami, C., Menon, V., O'Neill, B.J., Travers, A.H., & Yannopoulos, D. (2010). 2010 American Heart Association guidelines for cardiopulmonary resuscitation and emergency cardiovascular care, part 10: acute coronary syndromes. In Robert E O'Connor (Chair), *Circulation 122, Suppl. 3,*S787-S817. doi: 10.1161/CIRCULATIONAHA.110.971028.

Chisholm-Burns, M., Wells, B., Schwinghammer, T., Malone, P., Kolesar, J., & DiPiro, J. (2013). *Pharmacotherapy: Principles and practice* (3rd ed.). New York, NY: McGraw Hill Medical.

Foreman, M., Milisen, K., & Fulmer, T (Eds.). (2009). *Critical care nursing of older adults, best practices* (3rd ed.). New York, NY: Springer Publishing Company.

Foster, J., & Prevost, S. (Eds.). (2012). *Advanced practice nursing of adults in acute care*. Philadelphia, PA: F.A. Davis Company.

Godara, H., Hirbe, A., Nassif, M., Otepka, H., & Rosenstock, A. (Eds.). (2014). *The Washington manual of medical therapeutics* (34th ed.). Philadelphia, PA: Wolters Kluwer Health/Lippincott, Williams & Wilkins.

Goldman, L., & Schafer, A.I. (2012). *Goldman's Cecil medicine* (24th ed.). Philadelphia, PA: Elsevier Saunders.

Griffin, B., Callahan, T., & Menon, V. (Eds.). (2012). *Manual of cardiovascular medicine* (4th ed.). Philadelphia, PA: Wolters Kluwer Health/Lippincott, Williams & Wilkins.

Guy, Jeffrey. (2012). *Pharmacology for the prehospital professional* (Rev. Ed.). Sudbury, MA: Jones and Bartlett Publishers.

Judge, E. P., Phelan, D., & O'Shea, D. (2010). Beyond statin therapy: a review of the management of residual risk in diabetes mellitus. *Journal of the Royal Society of Medicine, 103*(9), 357–362.

Marini, J.J., & Wheeler, A.P. (2009). *Critical care medicine: The essentials* (4th ed.). Philadelphia, PA: Wolters Kluwer Health/Lippincott, Williams & Wilkins.

Marino, P. (2013). *The ICU book* (4th ed.). Philadelphia, PA: Wolters Kluwer Health/Lippincott, Williams & Wilkins.

McPhee, S. J., Papadakis, M. A., & Rabow, M. W. (Eds.). (2012). *Current medical diagnosis and treatment* (51st ed.). New York, NY: McGraw Hill.

Mittleman, M. A., & Mostofsky, E. (2011). Physical, psychological, and chemical triggers of acute cardiovascular events: Preventive strategies. *Circulation, 124,* 346–354.

Parrillo, J. E., & Delllinger, R. P. (2013). *Critical care medicine: Principles of diagnosis and management in the adult* (4th ed.). Philadelphia, PA: Mosby Elsevier Saunders.

Seiden, S. W. (2009). Evaluating patients with persistent chest pain and no obstructive coronary artery disease. *Journal of the American Medical Association, 302*(6).

Urden, L. D., Stacy, K. M., & Lough, M. E. (2009). *Critical care nursing: Diagnosis and management* (6th ed.). St. Louis, MO: Mosby Elsevier Saunders.

CHAPTER 15

Adjunct Equipment/Devices

SHEILA D. MELANDER · THOMAS W. BARKLEY JR.

INTRA-AORTIC BALLOON PUMP (IABP)

I. **Overview**
   A. Introduced in late 1960s, primarily for patients with cardiogenic shock
   B. Classified as an assist device and designed to do the following:
      1. Increase coronary artery perfusion
      2. Decrease oxygen consumption

II. **Indications**
   A. Preinfarction angina refractory to pharmacological therapy
   B. Acute myocardial infarction
   C. Refractory ventricular arrhythmias related to ischemia
   D. Severe mitral valve regurgitation
   E. Severe ventriculoseptal defect
   F. Before or after heart surgery
   G. Low cardiac output states, such as septic shock

III. **Contraindications**
   A. Absolute
      1. Aortic aneurysm
      2. Bypass grafting from the aorta to peripheral vessels
      3. Aortic insufficiency
   B. Relative
      1. Peripheral or central atherosclerosis
      2. Bleeding disorders
      3. History of embolic event
      4. Ethical considerations (e.g., advanced age, severe left ventricular failure, and multisystem failure), weighing the benefits of intra-aortic balloon pump therapy against quality-of-life issues

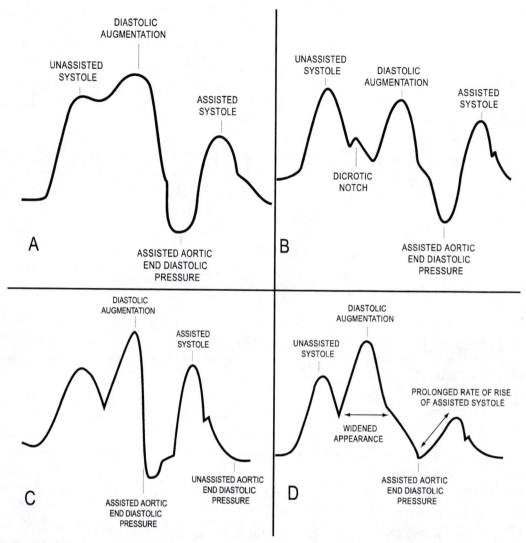

Figure 15.1. Wave form characteristics. (A) Waveform characteristics: inflation of IAB before dicrotic notch; diastolic augmentation encroaches onto systole, may be unable to distinguish. Physiological effects: potential premature closure of the aortic valve, potential increase in LVEDV and LVEDP or PCWP, increased LV wall stress or afterload, aortic regurgitation, and increased MVO2 demand. (B) Waveform characteristics: inflation of IAB after the dicrotic notch, absence of a sharp V. Physiological effects: suboptimal coronary artery perfusion. (C) Waveform characteristics: deflation of IAB is seen as a sharp decrease after diastolic augmentation, suboptimal diastolic augmentation, assisted aortic end-diastolic pressure may be equal to or less than the unassisted aortic end-diastolic pressure, and assisted systolic pressure may increase. Physiological effects: suboptimal coronary perfusion, potential for retrograde coronary and carotid blood flow, suboptimal afterload reduction, and increased MVO2 demand. (D) Waveform characteristics: Assisted aortic end-diastolic pressure may be equal to the unassisted aortic end-diastolic pressure, rate of increase of assisted systole is prolonged, and diastolic augmentation may appear widened. Physiological effects: afterload reduction is essentially absent, increased MVO2 consumption because of the left ventricle ejecting against a greater resistance and a prolonged isovolumetric contraction phase, and IAB may impede LV ejection and increase the afterload. Reproduced with permission from Datascope®. Adapted with permission from "Principles of Intra-aortic Balloon Pump Counterpulsation," by Krishna, M., & Zacharowski, K. (2009). Continuing Education in Anaesthesia, *Critical Care and Pain, 9*(1), pp. 24–28.

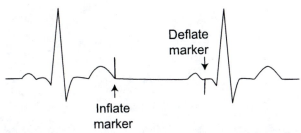

Figure 15.2. Use of timing markers as a reference on th electrocardiogram (ECG) tracing. Adapted with permission from *Introduction to Critical Care Nursing* (4th ed.), by M. L. Sole, D. Klein, and M. Moseley, 2004. Copyright 2004 by Saunders Elsevier.

IV.   Components

    A. Consists of a thin, polyurethane balloon mounted on a catheter

    B. The catheter is surgically or percutaneously inserted into the patient's aorta by threading it up through the femoral artery into the descending aorta. Note that the coronary arteries originate from the aorta immediately above the aortic valve.

    C. The catheter is connected to a bedside console that shuttles helium into and out of the balloon "in concert" with the cardiac cycle.

V.   Therapeutic effects

    A. The IABP improves coronary artery perfusion, reduces afterload, and improves perfusion to vital organs.

    B. Inflation and deflation of the balloon are automatically timed with the cardiac cycle.

    C. The IABP inflates during diastole (when the aortic valve is closed). This displaces blood backward, which increases perfusion to the coronary arteries, and also displaces blood forward, which increases perfusion to vital organs.

    D. The balloon deflates just before contraction (systole—when the aortic valve opens). This sudden deflation reduces the pressure in the aorta, decreases afterload, and reduces myocardial oxygen demand. These, in turn, assist the heart during systole.

VI.   Management considerations

    A. Vital signs and hemodynamics should be frequently monitored.

    B. Ensure accurate timing/pump operation based on any of the following:

        1. R-wave of the ECG (Figure 15.2)

        2. Upstroke (dicrotic notch) of the arterial line tracing

        3. Spike from a pacemaker

        4. Waveform on the balloon pump (Figure 15.3); the following checklist may be used to ensure optimal balloon inflation/deflation:

            a. Inflated at the dicrotic notch

            b. Should see a clear V at the inflation point

            c. Peak diastolic pressure should be greater than or equal to the peak systolic pressure

            d. Should see a clear U reflecting the balloon aortic end-diastolic pressure (BAEDP)

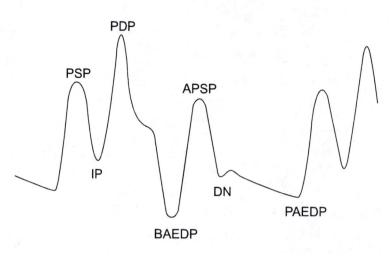

Figure 15.3. Timing the waveform to check for proper timing of counter pulsation. PSP = peak systolic pressure; PDP = peak diastolic pressure; APSP = assisted peak systolic pressure; IP = inflation point; BAEDP = balloon aortic end-diastolic pressure; DN = diacrotic notch; PAEDP = patient end-diastolic pressure. Reproduced with permission from Datascope Corp. Copyright 2013 by Datascope Corp.

      e. Ensure that the BAEDP is 5–15 mmHg less than the patient's aortic end-diastolic pressure (PAEDP)

      f. Note that the assisted peak pressure is less than the peak systolic pressure

      g. Calculate the end-diastolic dip to reflect the decreased workload of the heart: BAEDP – PAEDP = 5–15 mmHg

      h. Involved leg must be kept straight

C. Head of the bed should be elevated only slightly

D. Monitor for complications

    1. Lower extremity ischemia related to occlusion of the femoral artery by the catheter or by emboli from catheter thrombus formation

    2. Displacement of the catheter related to patient movement

    3. Balloon perforation

    4. Infection

E. Weaning parameters: hemodynamically stable vital signs, including the following:

    1. Normal cardiac index (2.5 L/minute or greater)

    2. Normal mean arterial pressure (MAP), greater than 70 mmHg

    3. Normal pulmonary capillary wedge pressure (6–12 mmHg)

    4. Absence of chest pain

    5. Absence of other signs of inadequate perfusion

F. Weaning method: either

    1. Decrease the volume in the balloon with each inflation (e.g., in periods of 25% reduction), or

    2. Decrease the frequency of inflation (e.g., from every cardiac sequence to every other, to every third)

VII. Complications
   A. Balloon rupture
   B. Embolus
   C. Arterial occlusion
   D. Destruction of red blood cells caused by the pump
   E. Inability to wean the patient from the pump

PACEMAKERS

I. Definition
   A. Electronic devices that deliver stimuli (i.e., impulses) to the cardiac muscle in an effort to maintain adequate heart rate and cardiac output when the patient's intrinsic pacemaker becomes insufficient
   B. May be used for single (atrial or ventricular) or dual (atrial, ventricular, or atrioventricular [AV]-sequential) biventricular (right and left ventricle) chamber pacing

II. Primary indications—with symptomatic patients or those refractory to pharmacological therapy
   A. Bradyarrhythmias
   B. Heart block
   C. Sick sinus syndrome
   D. Asystole
   E. Atrial tachyarrhythmias
   F. Ventricular tachyarrhythmias

III. Components
   A. The pacing system consists of a power source, called the pulse generator, which senses the patient's intrinsic cardiac activity and delivers stimuli to the cardiac muscle on the basis of the patient's intrinsic cardiac activity.
   B. The pacemaker contains a unipolar or bipolar lead/electrode catheter that is placed in the right atrium or right or left ventricle, in contact with the endocardium.
   C. The tip of the lead/electrode makes contact with the cardiac muscle and is responsible for transferring electrical stimuli from the pulse generator to the heart.
   D. Temporary pacemakers usually have a pulse generator that is external to the body, but the pulse generator of permanent pacemakers is usually internal.

IV. Operational definitions
   A. Capture—a process that occurs when the pulse generator's delivered impulse/stimulus is adequate to depolarize cardiac muscle
      1. A single-chamber pacemaker will depolarize the atrium or the ventricle, resulting in a large P-wave (atrial) or a large QRS complex (ventricular), following the respective pacing artifact (Figure 15.4).

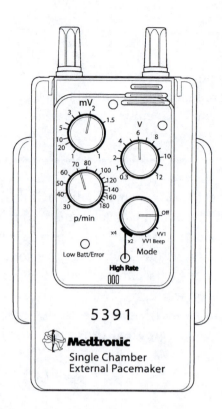

Figure 15.4. Medtronic single-chamber pacemaker, model 5391. Adapted with permission. Copyright 2014 by Medtronic.

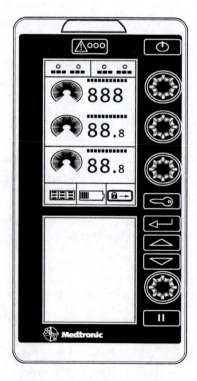

Figure 15.5. Medtronic dual-chamber pacemaker, model 5392. Adapted with permission. Copyright 2014 by Medtronic.

2. A dual-chamber pacemaker will depolarize the right atrium and the right ventricle as needed (Figure 15.5).

B. Spike/artifact—vertical line that is seen before the P-wave or the QRS complex, indicating pacemaker firing (i.e., before the P-wave [atrial pacemaker] and before the QRS complex [ventricular pacemaker])

C. Sensing—activity that occurs when the pacemaker recognizes intrinsic electrical activity of the heart; the pacemaker then "resets" the timing mechanism, resulting in inhibition of the pacing stimulus

1. Sensing is designed to prevent potentially life-threatening competition between the artificial pacemaker and the patient's intrinsic pacemaker.

D. Rate responsiveness—refers to a special modulation that enables the pacemaker to increase or decrease the rate of firing as needed

E. Programmability—ability to painlessly and noninvasively change pacemaker settings or parameters on the basis of the patient's needs

F. Programmable settings/parameters—it is possible to program three settings/parameters in all pacemakers

1. Rate—number of times each minute that the pacemaker will fire if the patient's intrinsic rate drops to less than the set rate

2. Energy output (mA)—strength of electrical current needed to depolarize the myocardium, usually set at 2–3 times the pacemaker threshold

3. Sensitivity (mV)—adjustment of the amplitude of myocardial electrical impulses that the pacemaker can detect; reflects the ability of the pacemaker to detect the patient's intrinsic cardiac activity; usually set at a low number (e.g., 2–3 mV); the lower the number, the more sensitive the pacemaker

G. Additional settings/parameters for dual-chamber pacemakers

1. AV interval—milliseconds of time between the beginning of atrial depolarization and the beginning of ventricular depolarization caused by the pacemaker; the usual setting is 120–200 ms

2. Maximum rate—upper limit of how fast the ventricle can be paced to accompany atrial activity

3. Atrial refractory period—millisecond interval denoting when the pacemaker will not respond to the patient's atrial activity

V. **Types of pacemakers**

A. Four basic types of pacemakers are available:

1. Transcutaneous—external pacemaker used to produce ventricular pacing; indicated in cardiac emergencies such as severe bradycardia and asystole; temporary

   a. An anterior and a posterior electrode (pad) are placed on the thorax.

   b. Sedation is warranted because of painful chest wall stimulation

   c. Rate, energy output, and sensitivity are programmable

Table 15.1	Five-Position Generic (NASPE/BPEG) Pacemaker Code			
I. Chamber Paced	II. Chamber Sensed	III. Mode of Response	IV. Programmable Functions	V. Special Tachyarrhythmia Functions
O—none	O—none	O—none	O—none	O—none
A—atrium	A—atrium	T—triggered	P—simple programmable	P—pacing
V—ventricle	V—ventricle	I—inhibited	M—multiprogrammable	S—shock
D—dual	D—dual	D—dual	C—communicating R—rate modulation	D—dual

Note. NASPE = North American Society of Pacing and Electrophysiology; BPEG = British Pacing and Electrophysiology Group. Adapted with permission from *Introduction to Critical Care Nursing* (4th ed.), by M. L. Sole, D. Klein, and M. Moseley, 2004. Copyright 2004 by Saunders Elsevier.

2. Transthoracic—temporary ventricular pacemaker used only as a "last resort" during cardiac emergencies such as asystole; requires a subxiphoid insertion via a long needle into the right ventricle, through which a pacing wire is threaded to the endocardium
3. Transvenous—most common type of pacemaker used permanently, yet may be used temporarily; produces atrial, ventricular, or AV-sequential pacing.
   a. The pulse generator is implanted under the skin, usually in the upper chest; the lead is inserted via the subclavian vein into the right atrium and the right ventricle.
4. Epicardial—commonly used after cardiac surgery; leads are sewn lightly to the epicardium and appear externally on the chest through puncture sites; leads are "grounded" with the use of some form of rubber, such as a glove or a glass test tube with a rubber cap
   a. Use is discontinued several days after cardiac surgery is performed
B. Description codes—each type of pacemaker is programmed by means of a five-position generic code, although the first three letters are most commonly used. Each letter in the code has a special meaning (Table 15.1).
   1. I: chamber paced
   2. II: chamber sensed
   3. III: mode of response
   4. IV: programmable functions
   5. V: special tachyarrhythmia functions
      a. AAI: atrial pacing, atrial sensing, and inhibited by atrial activity (i.e., P-waves)

Table 15.2	Pacemaker Settings to be Checked for Each Type of Pulse Generator or Pacing Mode	
Type of Pulse Generator	**Common Pacing Mode(s)**	**Controls/Relevant Settings**
Single chamber	Ventricular demand (VVI)	Rate Output/mA Sensitivity—should be on a low number, not on asynchronous
Dual chamber	Atrial asynchronous (AOO)	AV interval Ventricular rate (will reflect atrial rate in this mode) Atrial output Ventricular output—should be set at minimum level (0.1 mA), as the ventricle is not paced in this mode Ventricular sensitivity—not relevant for this mode
	Ventricular demand (VVI)	Ventricular rate Ventricular sensitivity—should be set on a low number Ventricular output Atrial output—should be set at minimum level (0.1 mA), as the atrium is not placed in this mode AV interval—Note: should be set at minimum level (0 ms), as the atrium is not paced in this mode.
DDD	Atrial demand pacing (AAI)	Base pacing rate Atrial output Atrial sensitivity Atrial refractory (automatic set at 200 ms)
	Ventricular demand pacing (VVI)	Base pacing rate Ventricular output Ventricular sensitivity
	AV-sequential demand (DVI)	Base pacing rate Ventricular output Ventricular sensitivity
	Physiologic pacing (DDD)	Base pacing rate Maximum pacing rate Atrial output Ventricular output Atrial sensitivity Ventricular sensitivity Atrial refractory AV interval

Note. AV = atrioventricular. Adapted with permission from *Critical Care Skills: A Clinical Handbook* (2nd ed.), by B. C. Mims, M. K. Roberts, K. H. Toto, J. D. Brock, L. E. Leuke, and T. E. Tyner. Copyright 2004 by Saunders Elsevier.

        b. VVI: ventricular pacing, ventricular sensing, and inhibited by ventricular activity (i.e., QRS complexes)

        c. DDD: atrial and ventricular pacing, atrial and ventricular sensing, and inhibited by responses from the atria or the ventricles

VI. **Operation and threshold measurement**

    A. Pacemaker settings—Table 15.2 shows settings that should be checked for each type of pulse generator or pacing mode

    B. Measuring the pacing threshold—to ascertain the smallest number of milliamperes needed for depolarization

        1. The rate should be set on demand mode and at approximately 10 beats per minute faster than the patient's intrinsic rate

        2. Check the ECG for 1:1 capturing (i.e., QRS complex and T-wave after every pacemaker spike)

        3. Check the pace indicator on the pulse generator—it should be flashing at the set rate

        4. Decrease the milliampere output slowly until a loss of capture occurs (i.e., spike occurs without a QRS complex or T-wave following it)

        5. Then slowly increase the milliampere output until capturing returns, and note the setting at that time

        6. The resulting setting is indicative of the pacing threshold

        7. Increase the milliampere output to two to three times the pacing threshold

        8. Return the rate to the original setting

        9. Repeat this process to determine the atrial pacing threshold by changing the atrial mA output setting; capture will be seen by a P-wave following the atrial pacemaker spike

    C. Measuring the sensing threshold—to ascertain a measurement of the smallest electrical impulse (millivolt) that the pacemaker can detect

        1. The sensing threshold is measured to ensure that the pacemaker will sense intrinsic beats and will not fire at the same time.

            a. Adjust the sensitivity to the lowest millivolt number (i.e., most sensitive setting)

            b. Adjust the rate to 10 pulses less than the patient's intrinsic rate

                i. Note: do not perform this procedure if the patient's intrinsic rate is unsatisfactory

            c. The pacemaker should not be firing at this time, and the patient's intrinsic activity should be visible on the monitor.

            d. Ensure that the patient can tolerate the new rate

            e. Check the sense indicator on the pulse generator—it should be flashing in concert with each intrinsic beat

            f. Increase the millivolts slowly (i.e., decreasing the sensitivity) until a loss of sensing is indicated, evidenced by a sense indicator that is no longer flashing

    g. Ensure that the pace indicator flashes as the pacemaker fires asynchronously

    h. Then increase the sensitivity slowly (i.e., decrease the millivolts) until flashing of the sense indicator is noted with each intrinsic beat

    i. The resultant setting is indicative of the sensing threshold

    j. Adjust the sensitivity to a setting that is less than half of the sensing threshold, or to the lowest number (most sensitive)

    k. Ensure that the rate is set back at the original position

    l. Repeat this process to determine the atrial sensing threshold by changing the atrial sensitivity; sensing of the P-wave should be noted on the monitor.

VII. Major complications and treatment

  A. Failure to capture—evidenced by appearance of pacemaker artifact without the appropriate complex following the spike (Figure 15.6)

    1. Position the patient on the left side

    2. Assess the chest x-ray for displacement

    3. Reprogram to increase the pacemaker amplitude

    4. Increase the milliampere output to maximum

    5. Change the battery (temporary) or the generator (permanent)

  B. Failure to pace—evidenced by absence of pacemaker artifact when firing of the pacemaker should have occurred (Figure 15.7)

    1. Position the patient on the left side

    2. Assess the chest x-ray for displacement

    3. Distance the patient from possible sources of electromagnetic interference such as MRI scanners and radio towers

    4. Warm the patient if the failure to pace is related to patient shivering

    5. Decrease the sensitivity by increasing the millivolts

    6. Change the battery (temporary) or the generator (permanent)

  C. Failure to sense—evidenced by random pacemaker spikes/artifacts throughout the patient's cardiac cycle that occur in competition with the patient's intrinsic cardiac rhythm (Figure 15.8)

    1. Position the patient on the left side

    2. Assess the chest x-ray for displacement

    3. Enhance sensitivity by decreasing the millivolts

    4. Use a magnet for a minimum length of time to check pacemaker function

    5. To prevent further competition and potentially life-threatening arrhythmias such as ventricular tachycardia, ventricular fibrillation, and asystole, turn off the pacemaker if the patient's cardiac output is stable

    6. Change the battery (temporary) or the generator (permanent)

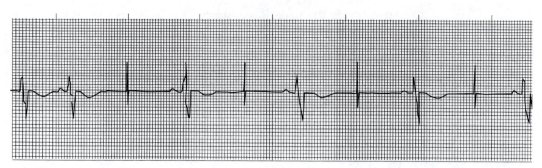

Figure 15.6. VVI mode. Rate = 71; V-V interval = 840 ms. Spikes occur at the appropriate time (the end of the V-V interval), but are not follwed by a QRS complex. The pacemaker is firing appropriately but is failing to capture. Adapted with permission from *Critical Care Skills: A Clinical Handbook* (2nd ed.), by B. C. Mims, M. K. Roberts, K. H. Toto, J. D. Brock, L. E. Leuke, and T. E. Tyner. Copyright 2004 by Saunders Elsevier.

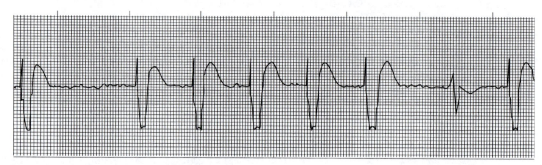

Figure 15.7. Ventricular pacemaker shows two long pauses where the pacemaker failed to pace as soon as it should have.

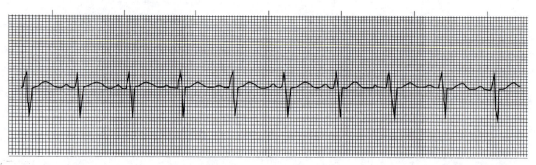

Figure 15.8. Pacing spikes falling at random: failure to sense. From Critical Care Skills: A Clinical Handbook (2nd ed.), by B. C. Mims, K. H. Toto, L. E. Leuke, et al., 2004, St. Louis: WB Saunders. Adapted with permission.

Table 15.3	NASPE/BPEG defibrillator (NBO) code		
Antitachycardia	**Tachycardia**	**Antibradycardia Shock Chamber**	**Pacing Chamber**
O = None	O = None	E = Electrogram	O = None
A = Atrium	A = Atrium	H = Hemodynamic	A = Atrium
V = Ventricle	V = Ventricle		V = Ventricle
D = Dual (A + V)	D = Dual (A + V)		D = Dual (A + V)

Note. NASPE = North American Society of Pacing and Electrophysiology; BPEG = British Pacing and Electrophysiology Group. From Andreoli's Comprehensive Cardiac Care (8th ed.), by M. Kinney, D. Packa, K. Andreoli, et al., 1995, St. Louis: Mosby; and "The NASPE/BPEG Defibrillator Code," by A. Bernstein, A. J. Camm, J. D. Fisher, et al., 1993, *PACE, 16*, p. 1776. Adapted with permission.

AUTOMATIC INTERNAL CARDIOVERTER/DEFIBRILLATOR (AICD)

I. **Definition**
  A. Electronic device implanted subcutaneously to automatically treat life-threatening arrhythmias
II. **Indications/general comments**
  A. Survival of sudden cardiac arrest unrelated to myocardial infarction
  B. Primary prevention for sudden cardiac death was approved by the Centers for Medicare and Medicaid Services in 2005 to include patients with coronary artery disease and an EF less than 35%, known dilated and other cardiomyopathies with EF less than 35%
  C. Patients with life-threatening ventricular arrhythmias that are refractory to pharmacological therapy
  D. It is estimated over 120,000 people worldwide have AICDs.
III. **Equipment**
  A. The AICD consists of a pulse generator and a lead system, similar to those of a pacemaker.
  B. The pulse generator, designed to last longer than 5 years, is usually implanted subcutaneously in the patient's subclavian area. Older AICDs were placed in the abdomen.
  C. The transvenous lead system is inserted through the left subclavian vein into the right ventricle and then is tunneled and connected to the pulse generator. One ventricular patch is also connected to the pulse generator. Some models have two transvenous leads (that use the right and the left subclavian veins) and two ventricular patches.
IV. **Programmability**
  A. Defibrillation
  B. Cardioversion
  C. Antitachycardia pacing
  D. Antibradycardia pacing

Table 15.4	NASPE/BPEG defribillator (NBD) code, short form
ICD-S	ICD with schock capability only
ICD-B	ICD with bradycardia pacing, as well as shock
ICD-T	ICD with tachycardia (and bradycardia) pacing, as well as shock

Note. NASPE = North American Society of Pacing and Electrophysiology; BPEG = British Pacing and Electrophysiology Group; ICD = internal cardioverter-defibrillator. From Andreoli's Comprehensive Cardiac Care (8th ed.), by M. Kinney, D. Packa, K. Andreoli, et al., 1995, St. Louis: Mosby; and "The NASPE/BPEG Defibrillator Code," by A. Bernstein, A. J. Camm, J. D. Fisher, et al., 1993, PACE, 16, p. 1776. Adapted with permission.

V.   Codes—two types depict the functions of the AICD (Tables 15.3 and 15.4)

VI.   Patient teaching

   A. Document device-related events

   B. Maintain MedicAlert identification

   C. Families and significant others should be trained in cardiopulmonary resuscitation

   D. Magnets may activate or deactivate the device. Monitor for tones emitted from the device that signal deactivation after exposure to external magnets

BIBLIOGRAPHY

Birnie, D. H., Healey, J. S., Wells, G. A., Verma, A., Tang, A. S., Krahn, A. D., . . . Essebag, V. (2013). Pacemaker or defibrillator surgery without interruption of anticoagulation. *New England Journal of Medicine, 368*(22), 2084–2093. doi:10.1056/NEJMoa1302946

Braunschweig, F., Boriani, G., Bauer, A., Hatala, R., Herrmann-Lingen, C., Kautzner, J., . . . Schalij, M. J. (2010). Management of patients receiving implantable cardiac defibrillator shocks: Recommendations for acute and long-term patient management. *Europace, 12*(12), 1673–1690. doi:10.1093/europace/euq316

Centers for Medicare and Medicaid Services. (2005). *NCD for Implantable Automatic Defibrillator. CMS Manual System.* Retrieved from http://www.cms.gov/medicare-coverage-database/details/ncd-details.aspx?NCDId=110&ncdver=3&IsPopup=y&NCAId=102&NcaName=Implantable+Defibrillators+-+Clinical+Trials&bc=AAAAAAAAIAAA&

Epstein, A. E., DiMarco, J. P., Ellenbogen, K. A., Estes, N. A. M., III, Freedman, R. A., Gettes, L. S., . . . Varosy, M.D. (2013). 2012 ACCF/AHA/HRS focused update incorporated into the ACCF/AHA/HRS 2008 guidelines for device-based therapy of cardiac rhythm abnormalities. *Journal of the American College of Cardiology, 61*(3), e6–75.

Goldberger, J. J., Buxton, A. E., Cain, M., Costantini, O., Exner, D. V., Knight, B. P., . . . Zipes, D. P. (2011). Risk stratification for arrhythmic sudden cardiac death: Identifying the roadblocks. *Circulation*, *123*(21), 2423–2430.

Healey, J. S., Connolly, S. J., Gold, M. R., Israel, C. W., Van Gelder, I. C., Capucci, A., . . . ASSERT Investigators. (2012). Subclinical atrial fibrillation and risk of stroke. *New England Journal of Medicine, 366*(2), 120–129. doi:10.1056/nejmoa1105575

Hillis, L. D., Smth, P. K., Anderson, J. L., Bittl, J. A., Bridges, C. R., Byrne, J. G., … Winniford, M. D. (2011). 2011 ACCF/AHA guideline for coronary artery bypass graft surgery. A report of the American College of Cardiology Foundation/American Heart Association Task Force on Practice Guidelines. Developed in collaboration with the American Association for Thoracic Surgery, Society of Cardiovascular Anesthesiologists, and Society of Thoracic Surgeons. *Journal of the American College of Cardiology*, *58*(24), 123–210.

Kushner, F. G., Hand, M., Smith, S. C., Jr., King, S. B., III, Anderson, J. L., Antman, E. M., . . . American College of Cardiology Foundation/American Heart Association Task Force on Practice Guidelines. (2009). 2009 focused updates: ACC/AHA guidelines for the management of patients with ST-elevation myocardial infarction (updating the 2004 guideline and 2007 focused update) and ACC/AHA/SCAI guidelines on percutaneous coronary intervention (updating the 2005 guideline and 2007 focused update) a report of the American College of Cardiology Foundation/American Heart Association Task Force on Practice Guidelines. *Circulation, 120*(22), 2271–2306. doi:10.1161/circulationaha.109.192663

Krishna, M., & Zacharowski, K. (2009). Principles of intra-aortic balloon pump counterpulsation. *Continuing Education in Anaesthesia, Critical Care and Pain, 9*(1), 24–28. doi:10.1093/bjaceaccp/mkn051

Perera, D., Stables, R., Thomas, M., Booth, J., Pitt, M., Blackman, D., . . . BCIS-1 Investigators. (2010). Elective intra-aortic balloon counterpulsation during high-risk percutaneous coronary intervention: A randomized controlled trial. *JAMA, 304*(8), 867. doi:10.1001/jama.2010.1190

Perera, D., Stables, R., Clayton, T., De Silva, K., Lumley, M., Clack, L., . . . BCIS-1 Investigators. (2013). Long-term mortality data from the balloon pump-assisted coronary intervention study (BCIS-1): A randomized, controlled trial of elective balloon counterpulsation during high-risk percutaneous coronary intervention. *Circulation, 127*(2), 207. doi:10.1161/circulationaha.112.132209

Rassin, M., Zilcha, L., & Gross, D. (2009). 'A pacemaker in my heart' - classification of questions asked by pacemaker patients as a basis for intervention. *Journal of Clinical nursing, 18*(1), 56–62.

Theologou, T., Bashir, M., Rengarajan, A., Khan, O., Spyt, T., Richens, D., & Field, M. (2011). Preoperative intra aortic balloon pumps in patients undergoing coronary artery bypass grafting. *Cochrane Database of Systematic Reviews, 19*(1). doi:10.1002/14651858.cd004472.pub3

Zipes, D. P., Camm, A. J., Borggrefe, M., Buxton, A. E., Chaitman, B., Fromer, M., . . . Tracy, C. (2006). ACC/AHA/ESC 2006 guidelines for management of patients with ventricular arrhythmias and the prevention of sudden cardiac death: A report of the American College of Cardiology/American Heart Association Task Force and the European Society of Cardiology Committee for Practice Guidelines (writing committee to develop guidelines for management of patients with ventricular arrhythmias and the prevention of sudden cardiac death). *Circulation*, 114, e385–e484. doi:10.1161/circulationaha.106.178233

CHAPTER 16

Peripheral Vascular Disease

THERESA M. WADAS • THOMAS W. BARKLEY, JR.

PERIPHERAL VASCULAR DISEASE: OVERVIEW

I. **Definition/incidence/prevalence**
   A. Definition: disorders of the peripheral arteries and veins
   B. Affects approximately 1:5 adults
      1. Prevalence increases with age; increases 15% to 20% among individuals older than 70 years
      2. Often coexists with other atherosclerotic disorders
   C. Includes two categories of disease:
      1. Peripheral arterial disease (PAD) or peripheral arterial occlusive disease (PAOD)
      2. Chronic venous insufficiency (CVI)

II. **Etiology/predisposing factors**
   A. Same as for coronary artery disease (see Coronary Artery Disease and Hyperlipidemia chapter)
   B. Strongest associations demonstrated with diabetes mellitus and smoking
   C. More common in the lower extremities than in the upper extremities because of the higher incidence of obstructive lesions in this region

III. **Peripheral arterial disease**
   A. Subjective/physical exam findings
      1. Only half of men and a quarter of women have symptoms or recognize their symptoms
      2. The six P's:
         a. Pain-intermittent claudication (i.e., pain to calf, thigh, or buttock)
         b. Pallor
         c. Pulse absent or diminished distal to the obstruction

      d. Paresthesias

      e. Paralysis

      f. Poikilothermia

  3. Presence of bruits over the narrowed artery

  4. Loss of hair on toes or lower legs

  5. "Glossy," thin, cool, dry skin

  6. Reduced skin temperature

  7. Peripheral edema if extremity is kept in dependent position

  8. Atypical leg pain is often seen in the elderly.

      a. Limb heaviness, numbness, or soreness

B. Classification

  1. The two most widely used clinical classifications are the following:

      a. Fontaine's (stages of PAD), used in Europe

      b. Rutherford's (categories of PAD), used in the United States

         i. Stage 0—Asymptomatic

         ii. Stage 1—Mild claudication

         iii. Stage 2—Moderate claudication: The distance that delineates mild, moderate and severe claudication is not specified in the Rutherford classification, but is mentioned in the Fontaine classification as 200 meters.

         iv. Stage 3—Severe claudication

         v. Stage 4—Rest pain

         vi. Stage 5—Ischemic ulceration not exceeding ulcer of the digits of the foot

         vii. Stage 6—Severe ischemic ulcers or frank gangrene

C. Diagnostic testing

  1. Ankle-brachial index (ABI): 1.0 or higher in normal individuals and less than 1.0 in patients with PAD; individuals with long-standing diabetes, chronic renal failure, and/or the very elderly often have dense calcified vessels that are poorly compressible, which may result in high ankle pressures and ABI values

  2. Doppler ultrasonography: does not provide visualization of arterial anatomy

  3. Duplex ultrasonography: accuracy diminished in certain individuals such as obesity

  4. Treadmill testing: assesses functional limitations; decline in ABI after exercise supports the diagnosis of PAD

  5. Magnetic resonance angiography (MRA): contraindicated in patients with certain devices, such as implantable cardiac devices, intracranial metallic stents, clips, coils, and other devices

  6. Computed tomographic angiography (CTA): useful for individuals where magnetic resonance angiography (MRA) is contraindicated, such as elderly with implantable cardiac devices; disadvantages include image interference from calcified arteries, radiation exposure, and use of contrast dye.

7. Contrast angiography: useful in defining anatomy and determining hemodynamic significance of arterial lesions to assist in planning revascularization procedures; associated with risk of bleeding, infection, vascular access complications, contrast allergy, and contrast nephropathy

D. Management
   1. Supportive measures
      a. Meticulous care of feet, which must be kept clean and protected against excessive drying with moisturizing creams
      b. Protective shoes that fit well to reduce trauma
      c. Patient should avoid the use of elastic support hose because it reduces blood flow
      d. Supervised exercise program
   2. Medications
      a. Cilostazol (Pletal), 100 mg PO BID to treat claudication by inhibiting platelet aggregation and inducing vasodilation; contraindicated in elderly with heart failure
      b. Pentoxifylline (Trental), 400 mg PO TID; considered second-line therapy as an alternative therapy to cilostazol (Pletal) to improve walking distance; decreases viscosity and increases red blood cell flexibility
      c. Aspirin (acetylsalicylic acid, 81–325 mg daily) or clopidogrel (Plavix, 75 mg daily) to reduce risk of myocardial infarction, stroke, or thrombotic complications; dual therapy can be considered for individuals with increased cardiovascular risk, but not for individuals with increased bleeding risk.
   3. Revascularization interventions: indicated for patients with disabling, progressive, or severe symptoms despite medical therapy, for those with critical limb ischemia, and a very favorable risk-benefit ratio
      a. Percutaneous transluminal angiography, stent placement, atherectomy, cutting balloons, thermal devices, and lasers are particularly useful for elderly and frail patients.
      b. Bypass surgery depends on the location and extent of obstruction as well as overall medical condition of the patient; not suitable for those with diffuse arterial occlusions, veins that are not suitable for grafting, and multiple comorbidities
   4. Risk factor modification
      a. Diabetes
      b. Smoking cessation
      c. Hypertension
      d. Hyperlipidemia
   5. Refer to vascular specialist for patients with progressive reduction of walking distance despite risk factor modification and consistent walking programs for those with limitations that interfere with their activities of daily living

IV.   **Chronic venous insufficiency**

    A.   Results from venous outflow disturbance of the limbs; may or may not be associated with venous valvular insufficiency and involves the superficial and/or deep venous system of the lower extremities

    B.   Subjective/physical exam findings

      1.   Dull ache in the leg that worsens with prolonged standing and resolves with leg elevation

      2.   Tingling, burning, muscle cramps, sensation of throbbing, or heaviness in affected leg

      3.   Restless legs

      4.   Fatigue

      5.   Dependent edema to the feet

      6.   Leg swelling or "tightness"

      7.   Increased leg circumference

      8.   Shiny, taut, hyperpigmented skin

      9.   Brown blotches

     10.   Ulcerations or varicosities on legs or feet

    C.   Classification and scoring

      1.   Clinical, etiologic, anatomic, and pathophysiologic (CEAP) classification schema: characterizes severity based on range of symptoms and signs; includes seven categories that indicate presence or absence of symptoms

      2.   Venous severity score: provides a numeric score based on three components:

        a.   Venous clinical severity score

        b.   Anatomic segment disease score

        c.   Disability score

    D.   Diagnostic testing

      1.   Venous duplex imaging: confirms the diagnosis of CVI and assesses its etiology and severity

      2.   Photoplethysmography: assesses the overall physiological function of the venous system; venous refill time less than 18–20 seconds depending on patient's position, indicative of CVI

      3.   Air plethysmography: measures the components of the pathophysiological mechanisms of CVI; includes the components of reflux, obstruction, and muscle pump dysfunction

      4.   Phlebography or venography: performed if venous reconstruction is planned or if duplex scan results are inconclusive

        a.   Ascending: injection of contrast in the dorsum of the foot with the visualization of contrast traveling up the lower extremity in the deep venous system; determines patency of veins

        b.   Descending: proximal injection of contrast in a semivertical posture on a tilt table with the use of the Valsalva maneuver; useful to identify reflux in the common femoral vein and at the saphenofemoral junction

5. Computed tomography and magnetic resonance venography: used to identify pelvic venous obstruction or iliac venous stenosis in patients with lower limb varicosity when a proximal obstruction or iliac vein compression is suspected

6. Intravascular ultrasound: used to evaluate iliac vein compression or obstruction and to monitor patient after venous stenting

E. Management

1. The specific treatment is based on disease severity.
   a. CEAP Classes 4–6 often require reconstructive treatment.
   b. CEAP Classes 4–6 and Class 3 with edema indicate referral to vascular specialist.

2. Supportive measures
   a. Elevate legs to minimize edema and decrease intra-abdominal pressure
   b. Compressive stockings
      i. Prescription for elastic compression stockings; tension is based on clinical severity
         (a) CEAP Classes 2–3: 20–30 mmHg
         (b) CEAP Classes 4–6: 30–40 mmHg
         (c) Recurrent ulcers: 40–50 mmHg
      ii. Length: most common is knee length
   c. Meticulous wound and skin care
   d. Weight reduction as appropriate
   e. Review medications for agents that may potentially cause edema (e.g., calcium channel blockers).
   f. Graded exercise program

3. Reconstructive interventions
   a. Sclerotherapy: used for obliterating telangiectases, varicose veins, and venous segments with reflux; may be used as primary intervention or in conjunction with other interventions
   b. Ablative therapy with radiofrequency and/or laser
      i. Radiofrequency
         (a) Frequently used for great saphenous vein reflux as an alternative to stripping
   c. Complications
      i. Saphenous vein nerve injury
      ii. Deep vein thrombosis (DVT): requires the use of duplex ultrasound surveillance
   d. Endovascular or stent therapy
      i. Indicated to restore outflow of venous system and obstruction relief
      ii. Commonly used with iliac vein stenosis and obstruction
      iii. Close follow-up is required to ensure stent patency

      iv. Surgical treatment indicated for individuals who are refractory to medical therapy; also considered for individuals who are unable to comply with medical therapy

    e. Ligation and stripping, and venous phlebectomy

      i. Used with CEAP Classes 2–6 with superficial venous reflux

      ii. Commonly used with great saphenous vein

    f. Subfascial endoscopic perforation surgery

      i. Ligate incompetent perforator veins from a remote site on the leg that is away from ulcer area

    g. Valve reconstruction

      i. Performed for individuals with advanced CVI who have recurrent ulcerations with severe and disabling symptoms

    h. Valvoplasty: open and closed technique

    i. Refer to:

      i. Vascular specialist: patients with significant saphenous reflux for ablation

      ii. Wound care specialist: patients with ulcers

SPECIFIC DISORDERS

I.   **Occlusive arterial disease**

   A. Arteriosclerosis obliterans

     1. Definition/incidence/prevalence

      a. Definition: stenosis or occlusion of arterial lumen that results from atherosclerosis, may be acute or chronic

      b. Increased incidence in men (3:1 male-to-female ratio), commonly between 50 and 70 years of age

      c. Higher incidence among diabetic patients

      d. Prevalence increases with age

     2. Etiology/predisposing factors

      a. Same as for coronary artery disease (see Coronary Artery Disease and Hyperlipidemia)

      b. Strongest associations demonstrated with diabetes mellitus and smoking

      c. CAD is more common in the lower extremities than in the upper extremities (femoropopliteal, popliteal-tibial, and aortoiliac vessels); thus, the lower extremities are most commonly affected

     3. Subjective/physical examination findings

      a. Same as for PAD

      b. Acute limb ischemia

        i. Acute and sudden severe pain, paresthesia, numbness, and coldness of involved extremity

        ii. Paralysis with severe and persistent ischemia; sensory and motor function preserved if sufficient collateral circulation present

        iii. Loss of distal pulse to the occlusion

        iv. Cyanosis, pallor, or mottling of affected extremity

        v. Decreased skin temperature

        vi. Weakened or absent deep tendon reflexes

4. Diagnostic testing

    a. Same as for PAD

5. Management

    a. Chronic: same as for PAD

    b. Acute limb ischemia

        i. Initiate anticoagulation with heparin IV immediately

        ii. Revascularization interventions

            (a) Intra-arterial thrombolysis with recombinant tissue plasminogen activator (rt-PA) is often effective in management of occlusive arterial disease. This treatment is also indicated when a patient's overall condition contraindicates surgical intervention or when the patient's smaller distal vessels are occluded.

            (b) Endovascular clot removal techniques (e.g., percutaneous mechanical thrombectomy)

            (c) Surgery: thromboembolectomy

B. Thromboangiitis obliterans (Buerger's disease)

1. Definition/incidence/prevalence

    a. Definition: non-atherosclerotic-inflammatory vasculopathy involving small- and medium-sized arteries and veins in the distal upper and lower extremities caused by an inflammatory, highly cellular intraluminal thrombus

    b. More common in men (ages 20–40 years); rarely occurs in women

    c. Prevalence is higher in Asians and Eastern Europeans

    d. Strongly associated with smoking

2. Etiology/predisposing factors

    a. The etiology is unknown, but it is postulated that the immune system plays a central role in the etiology.

    b. Smoking plays a major role in initiation and progression of disease.

    c. Potential genetic disposition

3. Phases

    a. Acute phase: characterized by acute inflammation involving all layers of the vessel wall, especially the veins in association with occlusive thrombosis; microabscesses in the periphery of the thrombus

      b. Intermediate phase: progressive development of occlusive thrombus in the arteries and veins; prominent inflammatory cell infiltrates within the thrombus, less inflammation in the vessel wall

      c. Chronic phase: end-stage lesion characterized by occlusive thrombus with extensive recanalization, prominent vascularization of the media, and adventitial, perivascular fibrosis

4. Subjective/physical exam findings

      a. Intermittent claudication, particularly calf pain, which often begins in the arch of the foot

      b. Pain at rest

      c. Pain relieved by dependent positioning

      d. Coldness, numbness, or pallor of the extremity or extremities

      e. Absent or diminished pulse, especially distal pulses

      f. Ulcerations

5. Diagnostic testing

      a. Physical examination is the most accurate method for diagnosis

      b. Same as for PAD

      c. Laboratory tests to exclude autoimmune or connective tissue diseases and diabetes mellitus

      d. Transthoracic echocardiography and arteriography to exclude proximal source of emboli

6. Management

      a. Same as for PAD; smoking cessation is the only definitive treatment to prevent the disease's progression

      b. Vasodilators promote vasodilation and may improve blood flow.

            i. Vasodilators, such as α-blockers, calcium channel blockers, and sildenafil may be helpful but have not been studied in prospective clinical trials.

            ii. Prostaglandins, administered intravenously or intra-arterially; may be beneficial

      c. Surgical interventions

            i. Surgical revascularization: rarely possible because of the diffuse vascular damage and the distal nature of disease

            ii. Sympathectomy decreases arterial spasm, provides short-term pain relief, and promotes ulcer healing; it is usually performed laparoscopically

            iii. Ilizavor's technique induces neoangiogenesis.

            iv. Spinal cord stimulators are used to provide pain relief and promote peripheral microcirculation.

            v. Stem cell therapy induces angiogenesis.

      vi. Amputation occurs at a rate of 50% for individuals who continue to smoke.

VENOUS DISEASE

I.   **Definition**
- **A.** Condition in which alteration in the character of veins results in thrombosis or decreased venous return
- **B.** Manifests as superficial thrombophlebitis or DVT

II.   **Etiology/incidence**
- **A.** Stasis of blood (e.g., immobility)
- **B.** Hypercoagulability
- **C.** Other
- **D.** DVT is more common in women than in men.

III.   **Superficial thrombophlebitis**
- **A.** Etiology/incidence
  - **1.** Intravenous cannulation of veins—most common cause
  - **2.** Trauma to preexisting varices
  - **3.** Infection: Staphylococcus, most common cause
  - **4.** Accounts for 10% of all nosocomial infections
  - **5.** One in five cases associated with DVT
- **B.** Physical exam findings
  - **1.** Palpable, cordlike, and reddened vein (i.e., linear appearance of redness)
  - **2.** Involved area is tender and warm
  - **3.** Absence of significant swelling of the extremities
  - **4.** Fever in 70% of patients
- **C.** Management
  - **1.** Elevation of affected limb
  - **2.** Warm compresses
  - **3.** Nonsteroidal anti-inflammatory drugs (e.g., indomethacin [Indocin SR]) once or BID

IV.   **Deep vein thrombosis**
- **A.** Risk factors: internal and acquired
  - **1.** Internal: Virchow's triad
    - **a.** Stasis of blood flow
    - **b.** Endothelial injury
    - **c.** Hypercoagulability
  - **2.** Acquired factors
    - **a.** Increased age (greater than 40 years)
    - **b.** Major surgery
    - **c.** Trauma (especially to pelvis or lower extremities)
    - **d.** Malignancy
    - **e.** Lupus anticoagulant
    - **f.** Female hormones
    - **g.** Obesity

   h. Chronic heart failure
   i. The elderly are particularly susceptible because of limited or restricted mobility and comorbidities; furthermore, 60% of first time DVT occurs in nursing home residents.
B. Physical exam findings
   1. Aching/"throbbing" pain
   2. Tenderness to palpation
   3. Positive Homans' sign (pain upon dorsiflexion of the foot) occurs in approximately 40% of patients
   4. Increased body temperature
   5. Localized edema/swelling distal to the occlusion
   6. Other signs of inflammation (e.g., redness, swelling, fever, and extremity warm to touch) may be present.
C. Pretest probability/laboratory/diagnostic findings
   1. Assessment of pretest clinical probability
      a. Includes nine clinical parameters with scores of 0 points or higher
      b. If the d-dimer is elevated and the score is 3 or higher, duplex ultrasonography is indicated.
   2. Laboratory findings
      a. The d-dimer level may be normal or elevated; 90% of hospitalized elderly have elevated d-dimer levels secondary to infections and tissue damage.
      b. Clotting factor studies
   3. Duplex ultrasonography is used for suspected symptomatic proximal lower extremity DVT; accuracy may be lower for distal DVT, asymptomatic DVT, and upper extremity thrombosis.
   4. Venography is indicated if ultrasonography results are inconclusive, laboratory findings are unclear, and no other explanation for symptoms can be found.
D. Management
   1. Supportive measures
      a. Bed rest with elevation of involved extremity; mobilize as soon as clinically feasible
      b. Local heat to affect area
      c. Compression stocking for acute DVT in lower extremity, use below the knee compression stocking (30–40 mmHg at the ankle)
   2. Anticoagulation therapy may vary from institution to institution.
      a. Unfractionated heparin
         i. Weight-based nomogram: bolus of 80 units/kg ideal body weight, followed by continuous intravenous drip of 18 units/kg/hr
         ii. Fixed dose: 5000 units bolus followed by 1000 units/hr
         iii. The literature supports an activated partial thromboplastin time (aPTT) goal range of 1.5–2.5 x baseline aPTT.

      iv. Disadvantages: higher incidence of heparin-induced thrombocytopenia (HIT), variable bioavailability, bone demineralization, and the need for inpatient treatment

b. Low molecular weight heparin

    i. Enoxaparin (Lovenox), 1 mg/kg subcutaneous BID or 1.5 mg/kg subcutaneous once daily

      (a) Advantages: lower incidence of HIT; more predictable pharmacokinetics and bioavailability, does not require laboratory monitoring

      (b) Contraindicated in patients with severe renal dysfunction

    ii. Dalteparin (Fragmin), 200 units/kg SQ every 24 hr

    iii. Tinzaparin (Innohep), 175 units/kg SQ daily

      (a) May be contraindicated in morbidly obese patients or those with severe renal impairment

c. Factor Xa inhibitors

    i. Fondaparinux (Arixtra)

      (a) Weight based: general dose to 5 mg SQ once daily (if body weight less than 50 kg), 7.5 mg SQ once daily (if body weight 50–100 kg), 10 mg SQ daily (if body weight greater than 100 kg)

      (b) Advantages: 100% bioavailability, daily dosing, and does not cause HIT

    ii. Rivaroxaban (Xarelto), 15 mg PO BID for 21 days, followed by 20 mg PO once daily

d. Warfarin (Coumadin), initiate at time of diagnosis of VTE, typically first dose is 5–10 mg PO daily

    i. Continue heparin/LMWH/fondaparinux until therapeutic anticoagulant levels are achieved with warfarin. Or administer dabigatran (Pradaxa), 150 mg PO BID once warfarin has been administered for 5–10 days.

    ii. Monitor international normalized ratio (INR) after initial daily doses of warfarin

    iii. Adequate oral anticoagulant effect is achieved when INR is at least 2–2.5 (goal INR is 2–3)

e. Duration of therapy is usually 3–6 months for first time episode and indefinitely for recurrent DVT and/or individuals with the following: cancer, anticardiolipin antibodies, lupus anticoagulant, homozygous factor V, prothrombin (factor II) gene mutation, antithrombin deficiency, protein C or S deficiency, or combination of two or more thrombophilias

f. Catheter-directed thrombolytic therapy

    i. Regimens may vary depending on institution, size of thrombus, vessel occluded, etc.

    ii. Used for thrombosis less than 1 week, extends above the inguinal ligament or proximally in an upper limb, associated with severe symptoms and significant edema

    iii. Contraindicated if patient has an increased risk of bleeding

g. Inferior vena cava (IVC) filter: used in patients for whom anticoagulation is contraindicated for prevention of pulmonary embolus, especially elderly, who may be susceptible to frequent falls, or in patients with recurrent DVT despite adequate anticoagulation

BIBLIOGRAPHY

Anderson, J. L., Halperin, J. L., Albert, N., Bozkurt, B., Brindis, R. G., Curtis, L. H., . . . Shen, W. K. (2013). Management of patients with peripheral artery disease (compilation of 2005 and 2011 ACCF/AHA guideline recommendations). A report of the American College of Cardiology Foundation/American Heart Association Task Force on Practice Guidelines. *Journal of the American College of Cardiology, 61*(14), 1555–1570.

Chang, R. N., Wang, S., Kirsner, R. S., & Federman, D. G. (2011). The elderly and peripheral arterial disease. *Clinical Geriatrics, 19*(7). Retrieved from http://www.clinicalgeriatrics.com/articles/Elderly-and-Peripheral-Arterial-Disease

Creager, M. A., & Loscalzo, L. (2012). Vascular disease of the extremities. In D. L. Longo, A. S. Fauci, D. L. Kasper, J. Hauser, L. Jameson, and J. Loscalzo (Eds.), *Harrison's principles of internal medicine* (18th ed.). Retrieved from http://accessmedicine.mhmedical.com/content.aspx?bookid=331&sectionid=40727028

Gloviczki, P., Comerota, A. J., Dalsing, M. C., Eklof, B. G., Gillespie, D. L., Gloviczki, M. L., . . . American Venous Forum. (2011). The care of patients with varicose veins and associated chronic venous diseases: Clinical practice guidelines of the Society for Vascular Surgery and the American Venous Forum. *Journal of Vascular Surgery, 53*(5 Suppl), 2S–48S. doi:10.1016/j.jvs.2011.01.079

Jones, W. S., Schmit, K. M., Vemulapalli, S., Subherwal, S., Patel, M. R., Hasselblad, V., . . . Dolor, R. J. (2013). *Treatment strategies for patients with peripheral artery disease.* Comparative Effectiveness Reviews, No. 118. (Prepared by the Duke Evidence-based Practice Center under Contract No. 290-2007-10066-I.) . Rockville, MD: Agency for Healthcare Research and Quality (US). Retrieved from https://www.ncbi.nlm.nih.gov/books/NBK148574/

Kane, R. L., Ouslander, J. G., Abrass, I. B., & Resnick, B. (2013). Peripheral vascular disease. In R. L. Kane, J. G. Ouslander, I. B. Abrass, & B. Resnick (Eds.), *Essentials of clinical geriatrics* (7th ed.). New York, NY: McGraw-Hill Medical. Retrieved from http://accessmedicine.mhmedical.com.libdata.lib. ua.edu.aspx?bookid=678

Lambert, M. A., & Belch, J J. F. (2013). Medical management of critical limb ischemia: Where do we stand? *Journal of Internal Medicine, 274,* 295–307. doi:10.1111/joim.12102

Piazza, G., & Creager, M. A. (2010). Thromboangiitis obliterans. *Circulation, 121,* 1858–1861.

Rapp, J. H., Owens, C. D., & Johnson M. D. (2014). Blood vessel & lymphatic disorders. In M. A. Papadakis, S. J. McPhee, & M. W. Rabow (Eds.), *CURRENT medical diagnosis and treatment.* New York, NY: McGraw-Hill Medical.

Shanmugasundaram, M., Ram, V. K., Luft, U. C., Szerlip, J., & Alpert, J. S. (2011). Peripheral arterial disease—What do we need to know? *Clinical Cardiology, 34*(8), 478–482. doi:10.1002/clc.20925

Veli-Pekka, H. (2011). *Deep vein thrombosis.* Helsinki, Finland: Wiley Interscience.

Vijayakumar, A. K., Tiwari, R., & Prabhuswamy, V. K. (2013). Thromboangiitis obliterans (Buerger's disease): Current practices. *International Journal of Inflammation, 2013.* doi:10.1155/2-13/156905

Wennber, P. W., & Rooke, T. W. (2011). Diagnosis and management of diseases of the peripheral arteries and veins. In V. Fuster, R. A. Walsh, & R. A. Harrington (Eds.), *Hurst's the heart* (13th ed.). New York, NY: McGraw-Hill Medical.

CHAPTER 17

Inflammatory Cardiac Diseases

SHEILA MELANDER • THOMAS W. BARKLEY, JR.

PERICARDITIS

I. **Definition/general comments**
    A. Acute, painful inflammation of the pericardium
    B. May be mild or life-threatening
    C. May also be subacute, chronic, recurrent, or constrictive
    D. Accurate patient history is of paramount importance in making the diagnosis

II. **Etiology/predisposing factors/incidence**
    A. Viruses: most common cause, especially infections with coxsackieviruses and echoviruses, Epstein-Barr virus, influenza, hepatitis, HIV, varicella, and mumps
    B. MI: affects 10%–15% of patients within the first week after MI
    C. Higher incidence among males
    D. Cardiac surgery
    E. Rheumatic fever
    F. Neoplasia
    G. Radiation therapy
    H. Uremia
    I. Tuberculosis
    J. Idiopathic
    K. Trauma
    L. Other causes, such as drug allergy or autoimmune disease
    M. Acutely affects 2%–6% of the general population

III. **Subjective findings**
    A. Reports of precordial/retrosternal, localized, "pleuritic" chest pain; pain that usually lasts for only a few seconds; patient may report pain under the breast

214

    B. Pain reports as being intensified with coughing, swallowing, inspiration (patient may complain of shortness of breath), or recumbent positioning; relieved by sitting in a forward position

    C. Fever may or may not be present (underlying cause)

IV.   **Physical examination findings**

    A. Pericardial friction rub—classically heard best with the patient sitting up and leaning forward

    B. Pleural friction rub may or may not be present

    C. Dyspnea

V.   **Laboratory/diagnostic findings**

    A. ST segment elevation: concave ST segment elevation in multiple, if not all, leads mimicking "smiling face"—ST segment elevation is not specific enough for differentiation between AMI and pericarditis

        1. Needs to be noted in multiple leads with smiling face appearance

        2. Elevation will return to normal in a few days; this is followed by possible T-wave inversion

    B. Depressed PR interval: highly diagnostic of pericarditis

    C. Elevated erythrocyte sedimentation rate

    D. Leukocytosis

    E. Consider ordering the following:

        1. CBC (to rule out infection/leukemia)

        2. Electrolytes or basic metabolic profile

        3. BNP (can help differentiate if cardiac or pulmonary in etiology)

        4. Blood cultures (if bacteria/infection is suspected)

        5. Echocardiogram (to confirm pericardial fluid)

VI.   **Management**

    A. Depends on underlying cause (i.e., tuberculous pericarditis or other)

    B. Colchicine (Colcrys), 0.6 mg PO twice a day

    C. NSAIDs

        1. Ibuprofen (Motrin), 600 mg PO three times a day with meals

            a. Preferred regimen, better tolerated than aspirin or indomethacin, less expensive than naproxen and available OTCs

        2. Aspirin (acetylsalicylic acid [ASA]), 650 mg PO every 6–8 hr for 2 weeks

        3. Naproxen, 500 mg BID with meals

        4. Ketorolac (Toradol), 60 mg IV/IM for 1 dose, followed by 15–30 mg IV/IM every 6 hr PRN for pain (max 120 mg/day, not to exceed 5 days)

            a. In adults 65 or older, or those who weigh less than 50 kg, recommended dose is 15 mg IV single dose or 15 mg IV every 6 hr (max 60 mg/day)

        5. Indomethacin (Indocin), 25–50 mg every 8 hr with meals

        6. PPI therapy may be required due to the risk of gastrointestinal toxicity (i.e., pantoprazole 40 mg PO daily)

D. Corticosteroids—indicated only after contraindication to NSAID therapy or failure of high-dose NSAIDs of several weeks' duration because corticosteroids may enhance viral replication

    1. Prednisone (Deltasone), 60 mg daily

    2. Then, taper and discontinue; lack of taper may cause recurrent pericarditis

E. Antibiotics—as indicated for bacterial infections

F. Hydrocodone 5 mg/acetaminophen 325 mg (Norco) PO every 4 hr PRN for pain

G. Monitor patient closely for cardiac tamponade

ENDOCARDITIS

I.   **Definition**

    A. Inflammation/infection of the endothelial layer of the heart, usually involving the cardiac valves

    B. Endocarditis should be ruled out in any patient who presents with fever of unknown origin and development of a new heart murmur.

II.   **Etiology/incidence/predisposing factors**

    A. Most commonly caused by bacteria

        1. *Staphylococcus aureus*

        2. *Streptococcus pyogenes*

        3. *Pneumococcus*

        4. *Neisseria* organisms

    B. May also be caused by fungi and viruses, especially in immunocompromised patients

    C. Increased incidence associated with congenital heart disease and with valvular disease

    D. Predisposing factors include recent invasive procedures such as dental surgery, genitourinary surgery, the use of invasive catheters, hemodialysis, or burn treatment.

III.   **Subjective findings**

    A. Fever lasting for several weeks

    B. Headache

    C. Weight loss

    D. Fatigue

    E. Night sweats

    F. Exertional dyspnea

    G. Cough

    H. General malaise

IV.   **Physical examination findings**

    A. Fever—medium to high grade

    B. Murmur—may not be detectable in some patients, especially those with right-sided endocarditis

   C. Skin changes

     1. Pallor, purpura, petechiae

     2. Osler's nodes—painful, red nodules in distal phalanges

     3. Splinter hemorrhages—linear, subungual; resembling splinters

     4. Janeway's lesions—macules on palms and soles; rarely observed; smaller than Osler's nodes and not painful

     5. Roth's spots—small, white retinal infarcts, encircled by areas of hemorrhage

     6. Pallor

     7. Splenomegaly

V.   **Diagnostics/laboratory findings**

   A. Patient may have normochromic, normocytic anemia

   B. WBC count may be elevated; always a "left shift" in the differential with band formation

   C. Erythrocyte sedimentation rate is usually elevated.

   D. Microscopic hematuria and proteinuria may be present.

   E. Consider ordering the following:

     1. Blood cultures—most important diagnostic test; perform three cultures from three different sites

     2. Echocardiogram to assess valvular involvement

     3. Basic metabolic panel (BMP)

   F. Duke Criteria bases diagnosis on the following:

     1. Direct evidence based on histological findings, or

     2. Positive Gram stain or culture from surgery/autopsy, or

     3. Two major clinical criteria: positive blood culture of common causative organisms, vegetations/abscesses found on echocardiogram, endocardial damage, *Coxiella burnetii* infection, or

     4. Five minor clinical criteria: fever, predisposing valvular condition/IV drug abuse, vascular phenomenon, immunologic phenomenon, other positive blood cultures, or

     5. Combination of one major and three minor criteria

VI.   **Management**

   A. Infectious disease consultation

   B. Generally, while results are pending, empiric therapy may be necessary if the patient is critically ill.

   C. Empiric therapy

     1. Vancomycin dose adjusted to achieve vancomycin trough level of 15–20 mcg/ml (provides coverage for staphylococci [MSSA & MRSA] and enterococci) PLUS or MINUS

       a. Cefotaxime, 1–2 grams IV every 6 hr or ceftriaxone 1–2 grams IV every 12 hr (provides coverage for streptococci [PCN susceptible and PCN resistant], as well as the HACEK and non-HACEK Gram-negative bacilli)

2. When pathogens have been identified and susceptibility data is available, the antimicrobial regimen is adjusted accordingly.

a. Penicillin-susceptible viridans group Streptococci and *Streptococcus bovis*

  i. Penicillin G, 3 million units IV every 4 hr (12–18 million units per 24 hr), plus or minus gentamicin; dose adjusted to achieve peak of 3–4 mcg/ml and trough of 1–1.5 mcg/ml

b. Staphylococci (methicillin-susceptible strains: MSSA)

  i. Nafcillin or oxacillin, 12 grams every 24 hr IV in 4–6 equally divided doses, PLUS or MINUS

  ii. Gentamicin dose adjusted to achieve peak of 3–4 mcg/ml and trough of 1–1.5 mcg/ml

  iii. For penicillin-allergic patients:

    (a) Cefazolin (Ancef), 2 grams IV every 8 hr, or vancomycin (Vancocin), dose adjusted to achieve vancomycin trough level of 15–20 mcg/ml

c. Enterococci:

  i. Ampicillin, 2 grams IV every 4 hr, PLUS or MINUS

  ii. Gentamicin dose adjusted to achieve peak of 3–4 mcg/ml and trough of 1–1.5 mcg/ml

  iii. For penicillin-allergic patients:

    (a) Vancomycin, dose adjusted to achieve vancomycin trough level of 15–20 mcg/ml PLUS or MINUS

    (b) Gentamicin dose adjusted to achieve peak of 3–4 mcg/ml and trough of 1–1.5 mcg/ml

VII. Endocarditis prophylaxis

A. Endocarditis prophylaxis recommendations have been revised and are a major departure from previous AHA recommendations.

1. Infective endocarditis (IE) is much more likely to result from frequent exposure to random bacteremia associated with daily activities than from bacteremia caused by a dental, GI tract, or GU tract procedure.

2. The risk of antibiotic-associated adverse events exceeds the benefit, if any, from prophylactic antibiotic therapy. Maintenance of optimal oral health and hygiene may reduce the incidence of bacteremia from daily activities and is more important than prophylactic antibiotics for a dental procedure to reduce the risk of IE.

B. According the latest recommendations, there are no prospective, randomized, placebo-controlled studies that exist on the efficacy of antibiotic prophylaxis to prevent IE in patients who undergo a dental procedure.

1. Although the absolute risk for IE from a dental procedure is impossible to measure precisely, the best available estimates are that less than 1% of all cases result in streptococcal IE annually in the United States.
2. The overall risk in the general population is estimated to be as low as one case of IE per 14 million dental procedures.

C. Cardiac conditions associated with the highest risk of adverse outcomes from endocarditis for which prophylaxis with dental procedures is reasonable include:
   1. Prosthetic cardiac valve or prosthetic material used for cardiac valve repair
   2. Previous IE
   3. Congenital heart disease (CHD)
      a. Unrepaired cyanotic CHD, including palliative shunts and conduits
      b. Completely repaired congenital heart defect with prosthetic material or device, whether placed by surgery or by catheter intervention, during the first 6 months after the procedure
      c. Repaired CHD with residual defects at the site or adjacent to the site of a prosthetic patch or prosthetic device (which inhibits endothelialization)
   4. Cardiac transplantation recipients who develop cardiac valvulopathy
   5. Mitral valve prolapse (MVP) is the most common underlying condition for which antibiotics have previously been prescribed for in the Western world; however, the absolute incidence of endocarditis is extremely low for the entire population with MVP, and it is not usually associated with the grave outcome associated with the conditions identified above.

D. Procedures in which prophylaxis is recommended:
   1. Dental procedures for patients with underlying cardiac condition
      a. All dental procedures that require or involve manipulation of the gingival tissue
      b. All dental procedures that involve the periapical region of the teeth
      c. Any procedure that involves perforation of the oral mucosa
   2. Gastrointestinal tract procedures
      a. The administration of prophylactic antibiotics solely to prevent endocarditis is not recommended for those undergoing GU or GI procedures, including diagnostic esophagogastroduodenoscopies or colonoscopies.
      b. Latest recommendations suggest that due to increasing antibiotic-resistant strains, unless the above discussed cardiac situations exist in conjunction with a procedure, or if there is an established GI or GU tract infection, antibiotic prophylaxis does not decrease risk

Table 17.1	Indications for antibiotic use	
Situation	**Agent**	**Regimen—Single Dose 30–60 minutes before procedure**
Oral	Amoxicillin	2 grams
Unable to take oral medication	Ampicillin OR Cefazolin or ceftriaxone	2 grams IV/IM 1 gram IV/IM
Allergic to penicillins or ampicillin— Oral regimen	Cephalexin[a] OR Clindamycin OR Azithromycin or clarithromycin	2 grams 600 mg 500 mg
Allergic to penicillins or ampicillin and unable to take oral medication	Cefazolin or Ceftriaxone* OR Clindamycin	1 gram IV/IM 600 mg IV/IM

[a]Cephalosporins should not be used in an individual with a history of anaphylaxis, angioedema, or urticaria with penicillins or ampicillin.

3. Respiratory tract procedures
   a. Tonsillectomy and/or adenoidectomy
   b. Surgical procedures that include respiratory mucosa
   c. Bronchoscopy, only if incision of the respiratory mucosa is involved
4. See Table 17.1 for indications for antibiotic use

BIBLIOGRAPHY

Ballweg, R., Sullivan, E. M., Brown, D., & Vetrosky, D. (2012). *Physician assistant: A guide to clinical practice* (5th ed.). Philadelphia, PA: Elsevier Saunders.

Burton, M. A., & Ludwig, L. J. M. (2010). *Fundamentals of nursing care: Concepts, connections, & skills*. Philadelphia, PA: F.A. Davis.

Domino, F. J., Baldor, R. A., Grimes, J. A., & Golding, J. (2013). *The 5 minute clinical consult* (22nd ed.). Philadelphia, PA: Lippincott Williams & Wilkins.

Ferri, F. F. (2011). *Ferri's clinical advisor: Instant diagnosis and treatment* (1st ed.). Philadelphia, PA: Elsevier Mosby.

Fowler, V. G., Jr., Scheld, W. M., & Bayer, A. S. (2009). Endocarditis and intravascular infections. In G. L. Mandell, J. E. Bennett, & R. Dolin (Eds.), *Principles and practice of infectious diseases* (7th ed.). Philadelphia, PA: Elsevier Churchill Livingstone.

Imazio, M., Spodick, D. H., Brucato, A., Trinchero, R., & Adler, Y. (2010). Controversial issies in the management of pericardial diseases. *Circulation, 121*(7), 916–928. doi:10.1161/CIRCULATIONAHA.108.844.753

Karchmer, A. W. (2011). Infective endocarditis. In R. O. Bonow, D. L. Mann, D. P. Zipes, & P. Libby (Eds.), *Braunwald's heart disease: A textbook of cardiovascular medicine* (9th ed.). Philadelphia, PA: Saunders Elsevier.

Khandaker, M., Espinosa, R., Nishimura, R., Sinak, L., Hayes, S., Melduni, R., & Oh, J. (2010). Pericardial disease: Diagnosis and management. *Mayo Clinic Proceedings, 85*(6), 572–593. Retrieved from http://www.ncbi.nlm.nih.gov/pmc/articles/PMC2878263/

Nel, S. H., & Naidoo, D. P. (2014). An echocardiographic study of infective endocarditis, with special reference to patients with HIV. *Cardiovascular Journal of Africa, 25*(2), 50–57. doi: 10.5830/CVJA-2013-084

Palraj, R., Knoll, B. M., Baddour, L. M., & Wilson, W. R. (2014). Prosthetic valve endocarditis. In J. E. Bennett, R. Dolin, and M.J. Blaser (Eds.), *Mandell, Douglas, and Bennett's principles and practice of infectious diseases* (pp. 1029–1040). Philadelphia, PA: Elsevier Saunders.

Rajendram, R., Ehtisham, J., & Forfar, C. (2011). *Oxford case histories in cardiology.* Oxford: Oxford University Press.

Sexton, D. J. (2013). Infective endocarditis: Historical and Duke criteria. In S. B. Calderwood & E. L. Baron (Eds.), *UpToDate.* Waltham, MA: UpToDate. Retrieved from http://www.uptodate.com/contents/infective-endocarditis-historical-and-duke-criteria?source=search_&search=Infective+endocarditis%3A+Historical+and+Duke+criteria&selectedTitle=1~150

Sharif, N. & Dehghani, P. (2013). Acute pericarditis, myocarditis, and worse! *Canadian Family Physician, 59*(1), 39–41. Retrieved from http://www.cfp.ca/content/59/1/39.full?sid=59957acb-83a1-4a59-975b-731815481c6b

CHAPTER 18

Heart Failure

JOAN KING · ROBERT FELLIN · THOMAS W. BARKLEY, JR.

I.   Definition/general comments

    A. Heart failure (HF) is a clinical syndrome, rather than a disease, caused by a variety of pathophysiologic processes in which the heart is unable to pump an adequate amount of blood to meet the metabolic demands of tissues.

    B. HF may be defined as left-sided HF, right-sided HF, or combined failure, in which there is dysfunction of both ventricles. Characteristics include the following:

        1. Dilatation or hypertrophy of either the left or right ventricle or both

        2. Elevated cardiac filling pressure

        3. Inadequate oxygen delivery caused by cardiac dysfunction

        4. Most commonly, left-sided HF occurs first. After one side of the heart fails, the other may eventually fail because of increased strain and workload.

        5. Two classification systems exist:

            a. The New York Heart Association (NYHA) classification classifies HF into four groups that differ by symptoms (Table 18.1).

            b. The American Heart Association (AHA) has developed four stages with the focus of the first two stages on identifying patients who are at high risk for asymptomatic HF (Table 18.2).

    C. Current practice divides HF in terms of the type of ventricular dysfunction

        1. Systolic HF: defined as signs of failure (Table 18.1)

Table 18.1	New York Heart Association Heart Failure Functional Classification	
Functional Class	**Patient Description**	**Manifestations**
Class I	No limitation of activity	Suffer no symptoms from ordinary activities
Class II	Slight, mild limitation of activity	Comfortable at rest or with mild exertion
Class III	Marked limitation of activity	Comfortable only at rest
Class IV	Should be at complete rest, confined to bed or chair	Any activity brings discomfort, and symptoms occur at rest

Table 18.2	American Heart Association Stages of Heart Failure	
Stage of HF	**Definition**	**Manifestations**
Stage A	High risk for HF without structural heart disease	HTN, CAD, DM, obesity, metabolic syndrome
Stage B	Structural heart disease present and strongly associated with HF, but asymptomatic	Previous MI Left ventricular remodeling, including LVH and low EF; asymptomatic valvular disease
Stage C	Structural heart disease with current or prior symptoms	Structural heart disease and symptoms of HF
Stage D	Refractory heart failure	Marked symptoms of HF at rest Recurrent hospitalizations despite guided directed medical therapy

Note. HF = heart failure; HTN = hypertension; CAD = coronary artery disease; DM = diabetes mellitus; MI = myocardial infarction; LVH = left ventricular hypertrophy; EF = ejection fraction.

    a. With an ejection fraction (EF) less than 40%

    b. Impaired contractility that leads to reduced stroke volume and cardiac output

    c. Associated with eccentric hypertrophy

2. Diastolic HF: defined as signs of failure

    a. With an EF of greater than 50%

    b. A nondilated left ventricle (LV) but elevated LV filling pressures

    c. Normal contractility but impaired ventricular filling related to impairment of ventricular relaxation

    d. Associated with concentric hypertrophy but with a cardiothoracic ratio less than 55% on anteroposterior chest radiograph

      e. Also referred to as heart failure with preserved ejection fraction (HFpEF)

      f. HFpEF (borderline refers to individuals who have an EF between 41% and 49%, and they are treated with protocols similar to HFpEF)

      g. May be caused by valvular disease or other conditions

D. Other terms that may be used to describe HF include the following:

  1. Myocardial remodeling—pathologic myocardial hypertrophy or dilatation

  2. HF with a dilated LV

  3. Asymptomatic left ventricle dysfunction—EF less than 40% but no clinical signs or symptoms of HF

II. Incidence/etiology/predisposing factors

A. Affects more than 6 million persons in the United States

B. Estimated 550,000 new cases diagnosed each year

C. Most common inpatient diagnosis in patients older than 65 years

D. Single largest Medicare hospitalization expenditure; cost estimated at $32 billion per year

E. HF is more common in men than in women until age 75; at that time, incidence becomes approximately equal in both genders

F. Estimated death rate among African Americans is 50% higher than among Caucasians.

G. Predisposing factors

  1. Left ventricular dysfunction from coronary artery disease (CAD) is the most common cause; patients experiencing myocardial infarction (MI) with atherosclerotic cardiovascular disease have an 8–10 times increased risk for subsequent HF.

  2. Hypertension—risk is 3 times higher in patients with hypertension; leading risk factor for acute HF; CAD is the most common cause of chronic HF.

  3. Diabetes

  4. Physical inactivity

  5. Obesity

  6. Excessive alcohol intake

  7. Smoking

H. Other precipitating factors/disease states

  1. Infections such as pericarditis and viral or bacterial systemic infections

  2. Endocrine abnormalities such as hyperthyroidism, thyrotoxicosis, and pheochromocytoma

  3. Nutritional disorders such as beriberi (thiamine deficiency) and kwashiorkor (protein deficiency)

  4. Preeclampsia

     5. Cardiomyopathy including dilated cardiomyopathy, restrictive cardiomyopathy, and takotsubo cardiomyopathy (broken heart syndrome)

     6. Musculoskeletal disorders such as muscular dystrophy and myasthenia gravis

     7. Autoimmune disorders such as lupus erythematosus, sarcoidosis, and amyloidosis

     8. Genetic factors leading to hypertrophic cardiomyopathy

     9. Valvular heart disease

    10. Rheumatic or congenital heart disease

III. **Compensatory mechanisms common with heart failure**

  A. Hypertrophy

     1. Cardiac wall thickens with increased muscle mass over time because of increased strain and workload

     2. Wall thickening leads to higher myocardial oxygen demands.

  B. Dilatation

     1. Chambers enlarge to compensate for increased blood volume.

     2. Because of increased volume, muscle fibers become stretched and, up to a point, increase contractile force (Frank Starling law)

     3. However, overstretching of cardiac muscle fibers impairs appropriate actin-myosin interaction, and there is a decrease in contractile force.

  C. Sympathetic nervous system: Inadequate cardiac output activates the sympathetic nervous system to release epinephrine and norepinephrine. As a result, there is:

     1. An increase in heart rate

     2. An increase in systemic vascular resistance, which increases afterload, and

     3. An increase in myocardial oxygen demand

  D. Renal response (renin-angiotensin-aldosterone cascade)

     1. Blood filtration in the kidneys decreases when cardiac output decreases.

     2. The kidneys respond to a falsely decreased blood volume with an increased release of renin.

     3. Renin activates release of angiotensin I and angiotensin II.

     4. Angiotensin causes peripheral vasoconstriction (increase in systemic vascular resistance) and release of aldosterone.

     5. Aldosterone causes sodium retention.

     6. Sodium retention is detected by the posterior pituitary, and antidiuretic hormone is secreted.

     7. Antidiuretic hormone increases water absorption in the renal tubules, resulting in water retention.

IV. Right- versus left-sided HF: Physical examination findings

A. Right-sided HF: The right ventricle is impaired and blood backs up into the right ventricle, the right atrium, and the systemic venous circulation. Signs include the following:

1. Increased central venous pressure
2. Jugular venous distention
3. Peripheral edema
4. Hepatomegaly (liver enlargement) and presence of hepatojugular reflux
5. Ascites
6. S3 and/or S4 heart sounds

B. Left-sided heart failure: The LV is impaired, and blood backs up into the left ventricle, left atrium, pulmonary veins, and lungs. Signs include the following:

1. Increased pulmonary capillary wedge pressure
2. Crackles (rhonchi and/or rales)
3. Adventitious breath sounds (crackles)
4. Dyspnea
5. Atrial fibrillation related to atrial distention
6. Pulsus alternans (every other pulse beat is diminished)
7. S3 common and, rarely, S4 heart sounds
8. Bilateral infiltrates on chest radiograph
9. Evidence of pulmonary edema

V. Subjective/physical examination findings of HF

A. Fatigue—may be an early sign
B. Dyspnea—related to poor gas exchange associated with fluid retention
C. Orthopnea
D. Paroxysmal nocturnal dyspnea (PND) or nocturnal cough
E. Tachycardia—related to the sympathetic nervous system response to decreased cardiac output
F. Edema

1. Legs (peripheral)
2. Liver (hepatomegaly) along with hepatojugular reflux
3. Spleen (splenomegaly)
4. Abdominal cavity (ascites)
5. Lungs (pulmonary edema)

G. Nocturia—at night, when the body is in the supine position, fluid shifts from the interstitial spaces back into the intravascular space, resulting in increased renal blood flow and diuresis
H. Skin changes—related to increased tissue capillary oxygen extraction; skin may look dusky and may also be diaphoretic
I. Behavioral changes—related to impaired cerebral circulation, especially in the presence of atherosclerosis (e.g., unexplained fatigue, restlessness, confusion, delirium, decreased attention span, and decreased memory)

J. Chest pain—in the presence of atherosclerosis, chest pain is related to decrease of coronary perfusion

K. Weight gain with an increase in weight of 1 kg, representing 1 liter of fluid retention

VI.   **Laboratory/diagnostics**

A. History and physical examination are very important for diagnosis and follow-up treatment

B. Arterial blood gases (respiratory alkalosis due to compensatory hyperventilation is common; as the failure progresses, the patient may develop metabolic and respiratory acidosis)

C. B-type natriuretic peptide (BNP) indicates LV dysfunction, and elevated levels are correlated with myocardial ischemia/damage; may serve to predict severity of current/future cardiac complications, including HF and mortality

1. Normal BNP levels vary with age and sex, with women having slightly higher normal values.

2. Mean levels are as follows:
   a. Ages 55–64 years = 26 pg/ml
   b. Ages 65–74 years = 31 pg/ml
   c. 75 years and older = 63 pg/ml

3. Expected levels associated with concurrent MI = 100–400 pg/ml

4. With HF, monitoring of trends in elevation is appropriate.

5. When the diagnosis of HF is uncertain with patients in whom the condition is suspected, the N-terminal portion of the pro-BNP peptide nasotracheal (NT-proBNP) levels should be assessed. (The assessment is necessary because BNP is rapidly eliminated from the body.)
   a. Normal range for NT-proBNP for individuals younger than 75 years is less than 125 pg/ml
   b. Normal range for NT-proBNP for individuals 75 years or older is less than 450 pg/ml
   c. NT-proBNP levels will increase with both age and renal dysfunction.

6. BNP is not recommended for routine evaluation of structural heart disease in patients at risk for, but without signs of HF.

D. Erythrocyte sedimentation rate (decreased)

E. Electrolyte analyses via basic metabolic panel

F. BUN, creatinine levels, and glomerular filtration rate (GFR) to assess for renal insufficiency

G. Chest radiograph (may reveal cardiomegaly and/or congestion)

H. ECG to assess for the following:

1. Evidence of current or previous myocardial infarction

2. Dysrhythmias such as atrial fibrillation or atrial flutter

3. Ectopy such as premature ventricular contractions

4. Evidence of left or right bundle branch block or prolonged conduction time
5. Reduced ECG complex size

I. Echocardiogram to assess valvular function, wall motion abnormalities, and EF

J. Nuclear stress test to assess baseline tolerance and evidence of areas of reversible ischemia

VII. Management considerations (Figure 18.1)

A. The management of asymptomatic patients with reduced LVEF focuses on controlling cardiovascular risk factors and preventing/reducing ventricular modeling.

1. Regular exercise (American College of Cardiology Foundation/American Heart Association 2013 Guidelines)
2. Smoking cessation
3. Discouraging alcohol consumption
4. Aggressive blood pressure control
5. Angiotensin-converting enzyme (ACE) inhibitor therapy is recommended for all patients with reduced LVEF less than 40% who do not have renal insufficiency.
6. Angiotensin receptor blockers (ARBs) are recommended for asymptomatic patients with reduced LVEF who cannot take ACE inhibitors because of cough or angioedema.
7. β-blocker therapy is recommended for all patients with reduced LVEF regardless of DM status.
8. Diuretic therapy if patient begins to show evidence of fluid retention

B. Nonpharmacologic management for patients with chronic heart disease

1. Patients should receive carbohydrate and caloric restraint teaching.
2. Sodium restriction
   a. Two to 3 grams of sodium daily is recommended for patients with the clinical syndrome of HF and preserved or depressed LVEF
   b. Less than 2 grams of sodium daily should be considered in moderate to severe HF
3. Fluid restriction: less than 2 L is recommended for patients with severe hyponatremia (Na less than 130 mEq/L) and for all patients with fluid retention, regardless of diuretic therapy
4. Specifically monitor caloric intake, prealbumin, BUN for patients with unintentional weight loss/wasting
5. Daily multivitamin recommended, especially for those on restricted diets or diuretic therapy
6. Assess quality-of-life issues (e.g., depression, sexual dysfunction, and impact on daily activities of living) at regular intervals.
7. Pneumococcal vaccine and annual flu vaccine, as appropriate

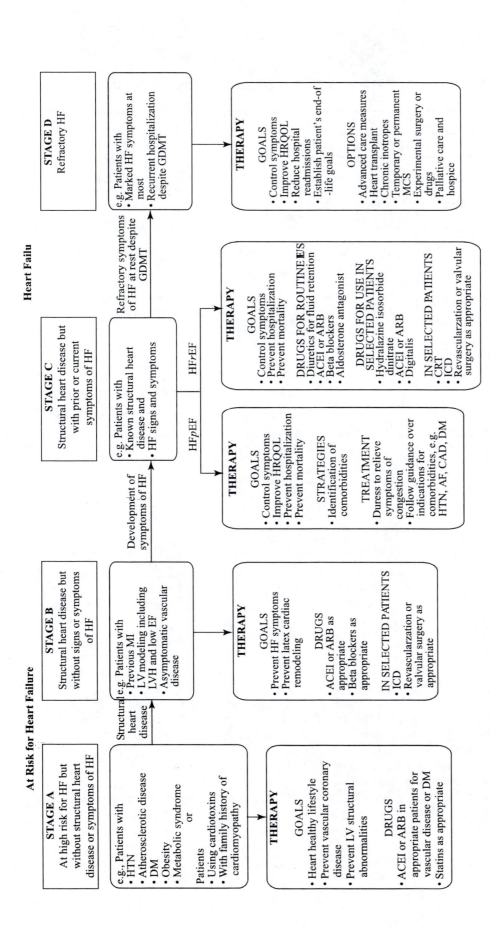

Figure 18.1. Stages in the development of HF and recommended therapy by stage. ACEI = angiotensin-converting enzyme inhibitor; AF = atrial fibrillation; ARB = angiotensin-receptor blocker; CAD = coronary artery disease; CRT = cardiac resynchronization therapy; DM = diabetes mellitus; EF = ejection fraction; GDMT = guideline-directed medical therapy; HF = heart failure; HFpEF = heart failure with preserved ejection fraction; HFrEF = heart failure with reduced ejection fraction; HRQOL = health-related quality of life; HTN = hypertension; ICD = implantable cardioverter-defibrillator; LV = left ventricular; LVH = left ventricular hypertrophy; MCS = mechanical circulatory support; and MI = myocardial infarction. Adapted from "2013 ACCF/AHA Guideline for the Management of Heart Failure. A Report of the American College of Cardiology Foundation/American Heart Association Task Force on Practice Guidelines," by C. W. Yancy, M. Jessup, B. Bozkurt, J. Butler, D. E. Casey Jr, M. H. Drazner, G. C. Fonarow, . . . B. L. Wilkoff, 2013, *Circulation, 128.*

Table 18.3	Cardiovascular Medications Useful for Treatment of Patients at Various Stages of Heart Failure		
Drug	**Stage A**	**Stage B**	**Stage C**
ACE inhibitors			
Benazepril	H	–	–
Captopril	H, DN	Post-MI	HF
Enalapril	H, DN	Asymptomatic LVSD	HF
Fosinopril	H	–	HF
Lisinopril	H, DN	Post-MI	HF
Moexipril	H	–	–
Perindopril	H, CV risk	–	–
Quinapril	H	–	HF
Ramipril	H, CV risk	Post-MI	Post-MI
Trandolapril	H	Post-MI	Post-MI
Angiotensin receptor blockers			
Candesartan	H	–	HF
Eprosartan	H	–	–
Irbesartan	H, DN	–	–
Losartan	H, DN	CV risk	–
Olmesartan	H	–	–
Telmisartan	H	–	–
Valsartan	H, DN	Post-MI	Post-MI, HF
Aldosterone blockers			
Eplerenone	H	Post-MI	Post-MI
Spironolactone	H	–	HF

Note. Stage A = patients at high risk for developing heart failure; Stage B = patients with cardiac structural abnormalities who have not developed HF symptoms; Stage C = patients with current of prior symptoms of HF; CV risk = cardiovascular risk; DN = diabetic neuropathy; H = hypertension; HF = heart failure; LVSD = left ventricular systolic dysfunction; Post-MI = reduction in heart failure or other cardiac events following myocardial infarction. Adapted from "2009 Focused Update Incorporated Into the ACC/AHA 2005 Guidelines for the Diagnosis and Management of Heart Failure in Adults: A Report of the American College of Cardiology Foundation/American Heart Association Task Force on Practice Guidelines Developed in Collaboration With the International Society for Heart and Lung Transplantation," by F. G. Kushner, M. Hand, S. C. Smith, et al., 2009, Journal of the American College of Cardiology, 53, p. e30. Copyright 2009 by the American College of Cardiology Foundation and the American Heart Association, Inc. Adapted with permission. β-blockers, along with ACE inhibitors, are established routine therapy in patients with LV systolic dysfunction. Further, this combination is recommended as routine therapy for asymptomatic patients with an LVEF 40% or less

Table 18.3	Cardiovascular Medications Useful for Treatment of Patients at Various Stages of Heart Failure		
Drug	**Stage A**	**Stage B**	**Stage C**
β-blockers			
Acebutolol	H	–	–
Atenolol	H	Post-MI	–
Betaxolol	H	–	–
Bisoprolol	H	–	HF
Carteolol	H	–	–
Carvedilol	H	Post-MI	HF, Post-MI
Labetalol	H	–	–
Metoprolol succinate	H	–	HF
Metoprolol tartrate	H	Post-MI	–
Nadolol	H	–	–
Penbutolol	H	–	–
Pindolol	H	–	–
Propranolol	H	Post-MI	–
Timolol	H	Post-MI	–
Digoxin	–	–	HF

C. Basic management considerations for patients with LV systolic dysfunction (Table 18.3)

1. ACE inhibitors are recommended for symptomatic and asymptomatic patients with LVEF 40% or less, with doses titrated as tolerated during concomitant; up titration of β-blockers

2. Substitute other therapies for ACE inhibitors in the following circumstances:

   a. If the patient cannot tolerate ACE inhibitors because of cough, ARBs are recommended. If the patient cannot tolerate ARBs, the combination of hydralazine plus oral nitrate may be considered.

   b. If the patient cannot tolerate ACE inhibitors because of hyperkalemia or renal insufficiency, a similar response is expected in terms of adverse effects as with ARBs. A combination of hydralazine plus an oral nitrate should be considered.

3. β-blockers, along with ACE inhibitors, are established routine therapy in patients with LV systolic dysfunction. Further, this combination is recommended as routine therapy for asymptomatic patients with an LVEF 40% or less.

   a. β-blockers are recommended for all patients with an LVEF 40% or less.

   b. β-blockers are recommended in most patients and in those with LV systolic dysfunction, even if diabetes, chronic obstructive pulmonary disease, or peripheral vascular disease is present.

   c. β-blockers should be used with caution in patients with diabetes who have recurrent hypoglycemia, asthma, or resting limb ischemia; considerable caution is warranted in those with bradycardia or hypotension.

   d. β-blockers are not recommended in patients who have asthma with active bronchospasms.

4. ARBs are recommended for routine therapy in asymptomatic and symptomatic patients with an LVEF 40% or less who are intolerant to ACE inhibitors for reasons other than hyperkalemia or renal insufficiency.

   a. Individual ARBs, rather than ACE inhibitors, are considered initial therapy for the following patients:

      i. HF after MI

      ii. Chronic HF and systolic dysfunction

   b. ARBs should be considered in patients with angioedema while on ACE inhibitors; the combination of hydralazine plus oral nitrates may be considered when patients do not tolerate ARB therapy.

   c. In patients with recent MI and LV dysfunction, routine administration of ARBs is not recommended when in addition to ACE inhibitors and β-blockers.

5. Aldosterone antagonists (or mineralocorticoid receptor antagonists) are recommended for patients with the NYHA Class II-IV (previously Class IV or Class III) HF with a LVEF of 35% or less, unless contraindicated, to reduce morbidity and mortality.

   a. Patients with NYHA class II HF should have a history of prior cardiovascular hospitalization or elevated plasma natriuretic peptide levels to be considered for aldosterone receptor antagonists.

   b. Creatinine should be 2.5 mg/dl or less in men or 2.0 mg/dl or less in women (or estimated glomerular filtration rate greater than 30 ml/min/1.73 m^2)

   c. Potassium should be less than 5.0 mEq/L

    d. Careful monitoring of potassium, renal function, and diuretic dosing should be performed at initiation and closely followed thereafter to minimize risk of hyper-kalemia and renal insufficiency.

6. For African Americans with LV systolic dysfunction, the combination of hydralazine plus oral nitrates is recommended as part of standard therapy (in addition to β-blockers and ACE inhibitors).

    a. NYHA Class II, III, or IV HF

    b. Hydralazine plus oral nitrates may be considered in others (i.e., non-African Americans) with LV systolic dysfunction, which remains symptomatic despite optimal standard therapy.

7. Polypharmacy in patients with LV systolic dysfunction—required for optimal management

    a. ACE inhibitor plus β-blocker = standard therapy

    b. An ARB can be substituted for an ACE inhibitor as indicated.

    c. An ARB can be added to an ACE inhibitor in patients for whom β-blockers are contraindicated or are not tolerated.

        i. Additional agents should be considered in patients with systolic dysfunction HF who have persistent symptoms or worsening of the disease despite optimal therapy with an ACE inhibitor and a β-blocker, as well as in those who are unable to tolerate a β-blocker.

        ii. The specific agent chosen should be selected on the basis of numerous entities, including clinical considerations, renal status, chronic K+ levels, blood pressure, and volume status, among others.

        iii. Triple combination therapy of an ACE inhibitor, an ARB, and an aldosterone agonist is not recommended because of the potential risks associated with hyperkalemia (Box 18.1).

        iv. Example regimens include the following:

            (a) Addition of an ARB

            (b) Addition of an aldosterone antagonist for moderate or severe HF

            (c) Addition of the combination of hydralazine plus isosorbide dinitrate for African Americans and perhaps others

8. Diuretic therapy: Loop and distal tubular agents are necessary adjuncts for HF when symptoms are due to sodium and water retention (Tables 18.4 and 18.5).

    a. Loop diuretics are considered the class of choice for HF treatment.

Box 18.1	Guidelines for minimizing the risk of hyperkalemia in patients treated with aldosterone antagonists

1. Impaired renal function is a risk factor for hyperkalemia during treatment with aldosterone antagonists. The risk of hyperkalemia increases progressively when serum creatinine exceeds 1.6 mg/dL. *In elderly patients and others with low muscle mass in whom serum creatinine does not accurately reflect glomerular filtration rate, the determination that glomerular filtration rate or creatinine clearance exceeds 30 ml/min is recommended.

2. Aldosterone antagonists should not be administered to patients with baseline serum potassium in excess of 5.0 mEq/L.

3. An initial dose of spironolactone 12.5 mg or eplerenone 25 mg is recommended, after which the dose may be increased to spironolactone 25 mg or eplerenone 50 mg, if appropriate.

4. The risk of hyperkalemia is increased with the concomitant use of higher doses of ACEIs (e.g., captopril, 75 mg or more daily; enalapril or lisinopril, 10 mg or more daily).

5. Nonsteroidal anti-inflammatory drugs and cyclooxygenase-2 inhibitors should be avoided.

6. Potassium supplements should be discontinued or reduced.

7. Close monitoring of serum potassium is required; potassium levels and renal function should be checked in 3 days and at 1 week after initiation of therapy and at least monthly for the first 3 months.

8. Diarrhea or other causes of dehydration should be addressed immediately.

Note. Although the entry criteria for the trials of aldosterone antagonists included creatinine greater than 2.5 mg/dl, the majority of patients had creatinine much lower; in one trial (335a), 95% of patients had creatinine less than or equal to 1.7 mg/dl. ACEI = angiotensin converting enzyme inhibitor. Adapted from "2009 Focused Update Incorporated Into the ACC/AHA 2005 Guidelines for the Diagnosis and Management of Heart Failure in Adults: A Report of the American College of Cardiology Foundation/American Heart Association Task Force on Practice Guidelines Developed in Collaboration With the International Society for Heart and Lung Transplantation," by F. G. Kushner, M. Hand, S. C. Smith, et al., 2009, Journal of the American College of Cardiology, 53, p. e30. Copyright 2009 by the American College of Cardiology Foundation and the American Heart Association, Inc. Adapted with permission.

Table 18.4	Oral diuretics Recommended for Use in the Treatment of Patients in Chronic Heart failure		
Drug	**Initial Daily Dose**	**Maximum Total Daily Dose**	**Duration of Action**
Loop diuretics			
Bumetanide	0.5–1.0 mg once or twice	10 mg	4–6 hr
Furosemide	20–40 mg once or twice	600 mg	6–8 hr
Torsemide	10–20 mg once	200 mg	12–16 hr
Thiazide diuretics			
Chlorothiazide	250–500 mg once or twice	1000 mg	6–12 hr
Chlorthalidone	12.5–25 mg once	100 mg	24–72 hr
Hydrochlorothiazide	25 mg once or twice	200 mg	6–12 hr
Indapamide	2.5 mg once	5 mg	36 hr
Metolazone	2.5 mg once	20 mg	12–24 hr
Potassium-sparing diuretics			
Amiloride	5 mg once	20 mg	24 hr
Spironolactone	12.5–25 mg once	50 mg	2–3 days
Triamterene	50–75 mg twice	200 mg	7–9 hr
Sequential nephron blockade			
Metolazone	2.5–10 mg once plus loop diuretic		
Hydrochlorothiazide	25–100 mg once or twice plus loop diuretic		
Chlorothiazide (IV)	500–1000 mg once plus loop diuretic		

Note. Higher doses may occasionally be used with close monitoring. IV = intravenous. Adapted from "2009 Focused Update Incorporated Into the ACC/AHA 2005 Guidelines for the Diagnosis and Management of Heart Failure in Adults: A Report of the American College of Cardiology Foundation/ American Heart Association Task Force on Practice Guidelines Developed in Collaboration With the International Society for Heart and Lung Transplantation," by F. G. Kushner, M. Hand, S. C. Smith, et al., 2009, Journal of the American College of Cardiology, 53, p. e21. Copyright 2009 by the American College of Cardiology Foundation and the American Heart Association, Inc. Adapted with permission.

Table 18.5	Intravenous Diuretic Medications Useful for the Treatment of Patients With Severe Heart Failure	
Drug	**Initial Dose**	**Maximum Single Dose**
Loop diuretics		
Bumetanide	1 mg	4–8 mg
Furosemide	40 mg	160–200 mg
Torsemide	10 mg	100–200 mg
Thiazide diuretics		
Chlorothiazide	500 mg	1000 mg
Sequential nephron blockade	Chlorothiazide, 500–1000 mg IV once or twice, plus loop diuretics once—multiple doses per day	
	Metolazone (as Zaroxolyn or Diulo), 2.5–5 mg PO, once or BID with loop diuretic	
IV infusions		
Bumetanide	1-mg IV load, then 0.5–2 mg/hr infusion	
Furosemide	40-mg IV load, then 10–100 mg/hr infusion	
Torsemide	20-mg IV load, then 5–20 mg/hr infusion	

Note. IV = intravenous; PO = per os (by mouth). Adapted from "2009 Focused Update Incorporated Into the ACC/AHA 2005 Guidelines for the Diagnosis and Management of Heart Failure in Adults: A Report of the American College of Cardiology Foundation/American Heart Association Task Force on Practice Guidelines Developed in Collaboration With the International Society for Heart and Lung Transplantation," by F. G. Kushner, M. Hand, S. C. Smith, et al., 2009, Journal of the American College of Cardiology, 53, p. e25. Copyright 2009 by the American College of Cardiology Foundation and the American Heart Association, Inc. Adapted with permission.

b. Diuretic therapy is recommended to restore and maintain normal volume status in patients with symptomatic HF; again, loop diuretics, rather than thiazide types, are typically necessary.

c. Initial doses are usually increased as necessary to relieve signs/symptoms; after initial therapy with short-acting loop diuretics; increasing administration frequency (e.g., twice or thrice daily) provides greater diuresis with fewer physiologic adverse effects than are produced by larger, single doses.

    d. For patients with poor absorption of oral medication or with erratic diuretic effects, oral toresmide may be considered, particularly in a patient who has right-sided HF and refractory fluid retention despite high doses of other loop diuretics.

    e. Once or BID addition of chlorothiazide or metolazone to loop diuretic regimens should be considered in patients with persistent fluid retention, despite high-dose loop therapy; long-term daily use, especially of metolazone, should be avoided because of potential electrolyte shifts and volume disturbances; rather, consider using these agents periodically (e.g., every other day or weekly).

    f. Because chlorothiazide diuretics delete potassium, electrolytes should be monitored frequently, especially when starting chlorothiazide diuretics or adjusting dosages

    g. Patients requiring diuretic therapy to treat fluid retention will generally require long-term treatment, yet at lower doses than those initially required to promote diuresis; monitor for electrolyte abnormalities, hypotension, and renal dysfunction.

9. Digoxin: Debate and lack of consensus are noted in the literature regarding the use of digoxin in patients with normal sinus rhythm; most agree to the benefits of use in patients with symptomatic LV systolic dysfunction who have atrial fibrillation or in patients who remain symptomatic and are in AHA Stage C or D of HF.

    a. Digoxin should be considered in patients with symptomatic LV systolic dysfunction (LVEF occurs in 40% or less) who are receiving standard therapy, including ACE inhibitors and β-blockers (i.e., NYHA Classes II-IV).

    b. On the basis of lean body mass, renal function, and other current medications, the dose of digoxin should be 0.125 mg daily in most patients, with maintenance of a digoxin level below 1 nanogram/ml.

    c. Maintained rate control of the ventricular response to atrial fibrillation is recommended, although high doses of digoxin (greater than 0.25 mg daily) are not recommended to achieve this result.

    d. Digoxin has a narrow therapeutic range. Digoxin levels and potassium levels should be monitored closely in patients assessed for signs of digoxin toxicity, especially in patients in with a history of hypokalemia.

10. Anticoagulants and antiplatelet agents: warfarin, aspirin, and clopidogrel all have potential benefits in treating patients with HF

a. Warfarin treatment to maintain a goal international normalized ratio (INR) of 2:3 is recommended for all patients with HF; the same treatment is also recommend for patients with chronic or documented atrial fibrillation with a CHADS2 score of 1 or greater, a history of pulmonary embolus, and stroke or transient ischemic attack, unless otherwise contraindicated. Also considered when patient's EF falls below 20%–25%

b. In some instances, dabigatran (Pradaxa) may be prescribed for anticoagulation in atrial fibrillation. However, extreme caution must be taken when used in a patient with renal or liver impairment.

c. Patients with asymptomatic or symptomatic cardiomyopathy and documented recent large anterior MI or recent MI with documented LV thrombus should also be treated with warfarin to maintain a goal INR of 2:3, or another oral anticoagulation agent, for the initial 3 months after MI, unless otherwise contraindicated.

d. In the absence of the indicators above, warfarin may be considered in those with cardiomyopathy and an LVEF 35% or less.

   i. Long-term treatment with an antithrombotic agent is recommended for patients with HF with ischemic cardiomyopathy, regardless of whether they are receiving ACE inhibitors.

   ii. Aspirin is recommended in most patients for whom anticoagulation therapy is not specifically indicated.

   iii. Warfarin (INR; goal, 2:3) and clopidogrel, 75 mg, may be considered as alternatives to aspirin.

   iv. Routine use of aspirin and an ACE inhibitor in combination may be considered for patients with HF when simultaneous indications for both drugs exist.

D. Electrophysiologic testing and use of devices in HF

  1. Electrophysiologic testing

    a. Immediate evaluation is recommended in patients with HF who present with syncope.

    b. Routine electrophysiologic testing is not recommended in patients with LV systolic dysfunction who have asymptomatic nonsustained ventricular tachycardia in the absence of prior infarction.

  2. Implantable cardioverter defibrillator (ICD) placement

a. In patients with or without CAD (including MI longer than 40 days postinfarction), prophylactic ICD placement should be considered (LVEF 30% or less) and may be considered (LVEF 31%–35%) for patients with mild to moderate HF (NYHA Classes II-III).

b. Concomitant ICD placement should be considered in patients undergoing implantation of a biventricular pacing device.

c. ICD placement is recommended for survivors of cardiac arrest from ventricular fibrillation or hemodynamically unstable ventricular tachycardia without evidence of MI. ICD placement is also recommended if cardiac arrest occurs longer than 48 hr after onset of infarction in the absence of a recurrent ischemic event.

d. ICD placement is not recommended in chronic, severe refractory HF when no reasonable expectation for improvement exists.

3. Biventricular resynchronization pacing improves hemodynamics in patients in which an echocardiogram reveals asynchronous contractions of the right and left ventricles.

a. For patients who have persistent, moderate to severe HF (NYHA Class II and Class III) despite optimal therapy, biventricular pacing therapy should be considered if the following signs are also present: sinus rhythm, left bundle branch block with a quantitative reference standard complex (120–150 or more milliseconds), and severe LV systolic dysfunction (LVEF 35% or less, with LV dilatation greater 5.5 cm).

b. Some ambulatory NYHA Class IV patients may be considered for biventricular pacing if ambulatory.

c. Biventricular pacing is not recommended in patients who are asymptomatic, have mild symptoms of HF, or have quantitative reference standard that is fewer than 120 ms.

4. Dual-chamber (atrioventricular) pacemakers

a. Routine use is not recommended for patients with HF in the absence of symptomatic bradycardia or high-grade atrioventricular block.

E. Basic management considerations for patients with HF and preserved left ventricular function, defined as having an LVEF greater than 41%–50%

1. Ischemic heart disease evaluation is recommended

2. Aggressive blood pressure control

3. Low-sodium diet/sodium restriction

4. Diuretic therapy: Treatment may begin with a low-thiazide or loop preparation; for patients with more severe fluid retention, loop therapy should be implemented. Avoid excessive diuresis.

5. ARBs or ACE inhibitors should be considered in patients with HF and preserved LVEF.
   a. ACE inhibitors should be considered in all patients with HF and preserved LVEF who have symptomatic atherosclerotic cardiovascular disease, diabetes, and one additional risk factor; for those intolerant to ACE inhibitors, ARBs should be considered.
6. β-blocker therapy is recommended in patients with HF and preserved LVEF who have had prior MI, hypertension, or atrial fibrillation requiring ventricular rate control.
7. Calcium channel blockers are contraindicated in patients with systolic HF; diltiazem or verapamil should be considered in patients with the following conditions:
   a. Symptom-limiting angina
   b. If hypertension is present, then consider amlodipine
8. Continuous positive airway pressure is recommended to address obstructive sleep apnea

F. Basic management considerations for patients with acute decompensated HF (ADHF)
   1. Diagnosis should be made primarily on the basis of signs and symptoms; when unsure, obtain BNP or NT-proBNP in patients who have dyspnea and comparable HF signs; BNP should not be interpreted in isolation but rather within the context clinical data.
   2. Hospitalization is recommended or should be considered for symptomatic patients with ADHF.
      a. Recommended hospitalization: hypotension, worsening renal function, altered mental status, dyspnea at rest (primarily reflected as tachypnea first, then falling oxygen saturation), hemodynamically significant arrhythmia (including new-onset atrial fibrillation), acute coronary syndromes, and so on
      b. Hospitalization considered: worsened congestion (even without dyspnea; typically reflected by 5 kg or more weight gain), signs or symptoms of pulmonary/systemic congestion (even in the absence of weight gain), PND, major electrolyte disturbances, associated comorbidities (e.g., pneumonia, pulmonary embolus, diabetic ketoacidosis, symptoms suggestive of transient ischemic attack, cerebrovascular accident, repeated ICD firings, previously undiagnosed HF with signs systemic or pulmonary congestion, and so on.
   3. Inpatient monitoring considerations
      a. Daily weight: determine after morning void, noting that a 1-kg increase in weight reflects a liter of fluid retained. Increase in weight needs to be correlated with other signs of fluid retention.
      b. Daily intake and output
      c. Vital signs, including orthostatic blood pressure measurements

    d. Daily electrolyte assessment, especially serum potassium, magnesium, and sodium

    e. Daily renal function assessment (BUN and serum creatinine)

    f. Monitor potential signs (e.g., edema, ascites, rales, hepatomegaly, jugular venous distention, hepatojugular reflux, liver tenderness, etc.)

    g. Monitor potential symptoms (e.g., orthopnea, PND, nocturnal cough, dyspnea, fatigue, etc.)

4. Recommended initial treatment of fluid overload with loop diuretics intravenously, then orally. Upon an inadequate response to diuretic therapy, consider sodium and fluid restriction, increased doses of loop diuretics, continuous loop diuretic infusion, or addition of a second type of oral (e.g., metolazone) or intravenous (e.g., chlorothiazide) diuretic; finally, ultrafiltration may be considered.

5. Fluid restriction (less than 2 L/day) is recommended for patients with moderate hyponatremia (Na less than 130 mEq/L) and should be considered in other patients to assist in treatment of fluid overload; more strict fluid restriction may be warranted for patients with Na less than 125 mEq/L.

6. In the absence of hypoxia, routine oxygen administration is not recommended.

7. For patients without hypotension, intravenous nitroglycerin, nitroprusside, or nesiritide may be considered because of their vasodilation properties, in addition to diuretic therapy, to rapidly improve congestive symptoms; intravenous vasodilator agents such as nitroglycerin or nitroprusside and diuretics are recommended for rapid improvement in patients with acute pulmonary edema or severe hypertension.

8. Continuous positive airway pressure, in an emergent or urgent situation, may decrease venous return to the heart and decrease preload while waiting for diuretics to relieve fluid overload.

9. Intravenous inotropes such as milrinone or dobutamine may be considered in patients with advanced HF characterized by LV dilatation, reduced LVEF, diminished peripheral perfusion, or end-organ dysfunction, particularly if these patients are hypotensive or have an inadequate response/intolerance to intravenous vasodilators.

    a. Administration of vasodilators instead of intravenous inotropes (e.g., milrinone, dobutamine) should be considered when adjunct therapy is needed in other patients with ADHF

    b. Agents such as milrinone and dobutamine are not recommended unless HF filling pressures are known to be elevated on the basis of direct measurement or clear clinical signs.

10. Routine invasive hemodynamic monitoring in patients with ADHF is not recommended. However, it should be considered for ADHF patients who are refractory to initial therapy, whose volume status and cardiac filling pressures are unclear, who present with significant hypotension or worsening renal function, and who need adequate documentation of hemodynamic response to inotropic agents.

11. Patients who are refractory to therapy placement of a left ventricular assist device (LVAD) may be considered as candidates for either destination therapy or bridge to transplantation.

G. Basic management considerations for patients with HF in the setting of ischemic heart disease:

1. CAD risk factor assessment is recommended in all patients with chronic HF, regardless of EF because CAD is the most common cause of chronic HF.

2. Cardiac catheterization is recommended for patients with HF and angina.

3. Patients with HF and no angina but with known CAD (and those at high risk for CAD) should undergo noninvasive stress imaging and/or coronary angiography.

4. Examples of imaging tests to be used include exercise or pharmacologic stress myocardial perfusion imaging, exercise or pharmacologic stress echocardiography, cardiac magnetic resonance imaging, and positron emission tomography scanning.

5. Management of risk factors (e.g., lipids, smoking, physical inactivity, weight, and hypertension) is of primary importance.

6. Specific therapies for patients with HF and CAD:

   a. Antiplatelet therapy is recommended in patients with HF and CAD, unless contraindicated.

   b. ACE inhibitors are recommended in all patients with systolic dysfunction or preserved systolic dysfunction after MI.

   c. β-blockers are recommended for management of all patients with reduced LVEF or post-MI.

   d. ACE inhibitors and β-blockers are recommended to be started within 48 hr during hospitalization in hemodynamically stable post-MI patients with LV dysfunction or HF.

   e. Nitrates should be considered in patients with HF when additional anti-anginal pain relief is needed.

   f. Amlopidine (calcium channel blocker) should be considered in HF patients with angina, despite the optimal use of β-blockers and nitrates, especially in patients with both angina and decreased systolic function.

Table 18.6	Inhibitors of the Renin-Angiotensin-Aldosterone System and β-Blockers Commonly Used for the Treatment of Patients With HF With Low Ejection Fraction	
Drug	**Initial Daily Dose(s)**	**Maximum Dose(s)**
ACE inhibitors		
Captopril	6.25 mg 3 times	50 mg 3 times
Enalapril	2.5 mg twice	10–20 mg twice
Fosinopril	5–10 mg once	40 mg once
Lisinopril	2.5–5 mg once	20–40 mg once
Perindopril	2 mg once	8–16 mg once
Quinapril	5 mg twice	20 mg twice
Ramipril	1.25–2.5 mg once	10 mg once
Trandolapril	1 mg once	4 mg once
Angiotensin receptor blockers		
Candesartan	4–8 mg once	32 mg once
Losartan	25–50 mg once	50–100 mg once
Valsartan	20–40 mg twice	160 mg twice
Aldosterone antagonists		
Spironolactone	12.5–25 mg once	25 mg once or twice
Eplerenone	25 mg once	50 mg once
β-blockers		
Bisoprolol	1.25 mg once	10 mg once
Carvedilol	3.125 mg twice	25 mg twice (50 mg twice for patients weighing more than 85 kg)
Carvedilol CR	10 mg once daily	80 mg once daily
Metoprolol succinate extended release (metoprolol CR/XL)	12.5–25 mg once	200 mg once

Note. ACE = angiotensin-converting enzyme; HF = heart failure. Adapted from "2009 Focused Update Incorporated Into the ACC/AHA 2005 Guidelines for the Diagnosis and Management of Heart Failure in Adults: A Report of the American College of Cardiology Foundation/American Heart Association Task Force on Practice Guidelines Developed in Collaboration With the International Society for Heart and Lung Transplantation," by F. G. Kushner, M. Hand, S. C. Smith, et al., 2009, Journal of the American College of Cardiology, 53, p. e29. Copyright 2009 by the American College of Cardiology Foundation and the American Heart Association, Inc. Adapted with permission.

> **g.** Drugs that should be avoided in HF patients, or withdrawn if possible, include most antiarrhythmic drugs, calcium channel blockers except for amlodipine, NSAIDs, and thiazolidinediones (ACCF/AHA guidelines).
>
> **h.** Coronary revascularization is recommended in patients with HF for relief of refractory angina or acute coronary syndromes, when possible.

H. The basic management considerations for patients with hypertension and HF are as follows:

1. Aggressive blood pressure control (less than 130/80 mmHg is preferred in clinical practice; however, current heart failure guidelines do not identify a goal blood pressure)

2. The use of several agents should be considered; usually, an ACE inhibitor or an ARB, a diuretic, and often, a β-blocker or amlodipine should be included.

3. For asymptomatic LV dysfunction with LV dilatation and low EF, the following treatments are suggested:

   a. An ACE inhibitor (20 mg enalapril daily) is recommended

   b. Addition of a β-blocker is recommended even if blood pressure is controlled.

   c. If BP remains elevated, the addition of a diuretic is recommended followed by another antihypertensive agent.

4. For symptomatic LV dysfunction with LV dilatation and low EF (Table 18.6), the following recommendations apply:

   a. Target doses of the following are recommended: ACE inhibitors, ARBs, β-blockers, aldosterone inhibitors, and isosorbide dinitrate/hydralazine in various combinations (with a diuretic if needed).

   b. If BP remains above 130/80 mmHg, a non-cardiac depressing calcium antagonist, such as amlodipine, may be considered, or consider increasing the doses of other antihypertensive medications.

I. Specific considerations for special populations experiencing HF include the following:

1. Elderly

   a. Cardiovascular changes with aging, including a decrease in peak contractility, responsiveness of heart rate to sympathetic nervous system stimulation, peripheral vasodilation, and decrease in renal function, all contribute to increase incidence of ADHF in the elderly.

   b. β-blocker and ACE inhibitor therapy is also standard in all patients with HF from LV systolic dysfunction; however, these medications need to be titrated slowly, and therapeutic goals should be adjusted appropriately.

   c. Monitor carefully for fluid overload, noting jugular venous distension, S3 gallop, and peripheral edema as the hallmark signs of ADHF in elderly

2. Women: β-blocker therapy and ACE inhibitor therapy are recommended for HF that results from symptomatic or asymptomatic LV systolic dysfunction.

3. African Americans with HF: β-blocker therapy and, to some extent, ACE inhibitor therapy are recommended as part of standard care for patients with HF due to symptomatic or asymptomatic LV systolic dysfunction.

   a. ARBs may be substituted for African Americans with HF who are intolerant to ACE inhibitors.

   b. A combination of hydralazine and isosorbide dinitrate is recommended as a standard therapy, in addition to β-blockers and ACE inhibitors, for African Americans with LV systolic dysfunction and NYHA Class III or IV HF (and may be considered for some with NYHA Class II HF).

BIBLIOGRAPHY

Chisholm-Burns, M. A., Wells, B. G., Schwinghammer, T. L., Malone, P. M., Kolesar, J. M., & Dipiro, J. T. (2013). *Pharmacotherapy: Principles and practice* (3rd ed.). New York, NY: McGraw Hill Medical.

Foreman, M. D., Milisen, K., & Fulmer, T. T. (2009). *Critical care nursing of older adults: Best practices* (3rd ed.). New York, NY: Springer Publishing Company.

Foster, J. G. W. & Prevost, S. S. (Eds.). (2012). *Advanced practice nursing of adults in acute care.* Philadelphia, PA: F.A. Davis Company.

Go, A. S., Mozaffarian, D., Roger, V. L., Benjamin, E. J., Berry, J. D., Borden, W. B., . . . Turner, M. B. (2013). Heart Disease and Stroke Statistics—2013 Update: A Report from the American Heart Association. *Circulation, 127*(1), e6-e245. doi: 10.1161/CIR.0b013e31828124ad

Godara, H., Hirbe, A., Nassif, M., Otepka, H., & Rosenstock, A. (Eds.). (2014). *The Washington manual of medical therapeutics* (34th ed.). Philadelphia, PA: Wolters Kluwer/Lippincott, Williams, & Wilkins.

Griffin, B. P., Callahan, T. D., & Menon, V. (Eds.). (2012). *Manual of cardiovascular medicine* (4th ed.). Philadelphia, PA: Wolters Kluwer/ Lippincott, Williams, & Wilkins.

Heidenreich, P. A., Trogdon, J. G., Khavjou, O. A., Butler, J., Dracup, K., Ezekowitz, M. D., . . . Woo, Y. J. (2011). Forecasting the future of cardiovascular disease in the United States: A policy statement from the American Heart Association. *Circulation, 123*(8), 933-944. doi: 10.1161/ CIR.0b013e31820a55f5

Management of patients with cardiovascular disorders. (2014.) In T. W. Barkley Jr. (Ed.), *Adult nurse practitioner certification review manual.* West Hollywood, CA: Barkley & Associates.

Marini, J. J., & Wheeler, A. P. (2009). *Critical care medicine: The essentials* (4th ed.). Philadelphia, PA: Wolters Kluwer/Lippincott, Williams, & Wilkins.

Marino, P. L. (2013). *The ICU book* (4th ed.). Philadelphia, PA: Wolters Kluwer Health/Lippincott, Williams, & Wilkins.

Parrillo, J. E., & Dellinger, R. P. (2013). *Critical care medicine: Principles of diagnosis and management in the adult* (4th ed.). Philadelphia, PA: Elsevier Saunders.

Yancy, C. W., Jessup, M., Bozkurt, B., Butler, J., Casey, D. E., Drazner, M. H., . . . Wilkoff, B. L. (2013). 2013 ACCF/AHA guideline for the management of heart failure: Executive summary: A report of the American College of Cardiology Foundation/American Heart Association Task Force on Practice Guidelines. *Circulation, 128*(16), 1810–1852. doi: 10.1161/CIR.0b013e31829e8807

Yancy, C. W., Jessup, M., Bozkurt, B., Butler, J., Casey, D. E., Drazner, M. H., . . . Wilkoff, B. L. (2013). 2013 ACCF/AHA guideline for the management of heart failure: A report of the American College of Cardiology Foundation/American Heart Association Task Force on Practice Guidelines. *Journal of the American College of Cardiology, 62*(16), e147–e239. doi:10.1016/j.jacc.2013.05.019.

CHAPTER 19

Valvular Disease

THERESA M. WADAS • ROBERT FELLIN • THOMAS W. BARKLEY, JR.

I. **Definition**
   A. Impairment of unidirectional flow that results from damaged cardiac valves
   B. Two types
      1. Stenosis ("narrowing: obstructed forward blood flow")
      2. Regurgitation ("insufficiency: backward blood across the valve")
   C. May occur with all cardiac valves
   D. Aortic stenosis and mitral regurgitation: most common valvular disease in the elderly

II. **Mitral stenosis**
   A. Definition: narrowing of the mitral valve that results in obstructed forward blood flow
   B. Etiology/incidence
      1. Rheumatic heart disease, including endocarditis from rheumatic fever, is most common
      2. Fibrosis and calcification of the valve with scarring
      3. Valve leaflets become immobilized and narrow the orifice
      4. Approximately two thirds of patients are female
   C. Subjective and physical examination findings
      1. Fatigue
      2. Dyspnea
      3. Orthopnea
      4. Hemoptysis—associated with pulmonary venous hypertension and elevated left atrial pressures
      5. Other findings consistent with left-sided heart failure
      6. Palpitations—associated with atrial fibrillation

7. Loud S1 heart sound with low-pitched, mid-diastolic murmur; does not radiate, heard best at the apex and in the left lateral position
8. Apical crescendo rumble
9. Mitral facies with malar flush

D. Diagnostic tests
1. Echocardiogram (two-dimensional)—confirms diagnosis; demonstrates restricted motion of the valve and quantifies severity
2. Doppler echocardiogram—prolonged pressure half-time across the valve; quantifies severity
3. Transesophageal echocardiogram (TEE)—check for valvular measurements, estimates of transvalvular peak and mean gradients, assessment of LV and RV function, chamber sizes estimate of pulmonary artery pressure, and presence of thrombus
4. ECG—check for atrial fibrillation; if in sinus rhythm, tall and peaked P waves in lead II and upright in V1 seen with severe pulmonary hypertension
5. Chest X-ray—check for the appearance of a straight left-sided heart border or large left atrium, prominence of main pulmonary arteries, dilation of the upper lobe pulmonary vein, and posterior displacement of the esophagus, and Kerley B lines
6. Cardiac catheterization to assess associated lesions and presence of coronary artery disease

E. Medical therapy
1. Anticoagulation: warfarin or heparin is indicated in patients with:
   a. Mitral stenosis (MS) and atrial fibrillation (AF) (paroxysmal, persistent, or permanent)
   b. MS and a prior embolic event
   c. MS and a left atrial thrombus
   d. Efficacy of oral anticoagulant agents in preventing embolic events has not been studied in patients with MS. It is controversial as to whether long-term anticoagulation should be given to patients with MS in normal sinus rhythm on the basis of left atrial enlargement or spontaneous contrast on TEE.
2. Heart rate control: can be beneficial in patients with MS and atrial fibrillation and fast ventricular response
3. Heart rhythm control: cardioversion may be necessary to improve hemodynamic instability in select patients
   a. In stable patients, the decision for rate versus rhythm, control depends on multiple factors (duration, left atrial size, etc.). It is much more difficult to achieve rhythm control in patients with MS because of the rheumatic process.

        4. Antibiotic prophylaxis for surgical or dental procedures (refer to Inflammatory Cardiac Disease chapter section on endocarditis prophylaxis for appropriate indications/criteria and definitive therapy)

   F. Intervention

        1. Percutaneous mitral balloon commissurotomy (PMBC) is recommended for symptomatic patients with severe MS. There is no role for percutaneous mitral balloon or surgical commissurotomy for patients with MS due to calcification.

        2. Mitral valve surgery (replacement or repair) is indicated in severely symptomatic patients who are not high risk for surgery and who are not candidates for or failed previous PMBC.

           a. Patients with calcification are often elderly and debilitated, have multiple comorbidities, and are at high risk for surgery; therefore, intervention should be delayed until symptoms are severely limiting and cannot be managed with medical therapy.

III. **Mitral regurgitation**

   A. Definition: backflow of blood into the left atrium as a result of deficient mitral valve closure

   B. Etiology

        1. Rheumatic disease

        2. "Floppy" mitral valve

        3. Papillary muscle dysfunction related to ischemic heart disease

        4. Infective endocarditis

        5. Ruptured chordae tendineae

        6. Hypertrophic obstructive and dilated cardiomyopathy

        7. Systemic lupus erythematosus

        8. Commonly associated with heart failure in the elderly

   C. Subjective and physical examination findings

        1. Fatigue

        2. Weakness

        3. Exertional dyspnea

        4. Palpitations—associated with atrial fibrillation

        5. S3 heart sound with holosystolic murmur at the fifth intercostal space/midclavicular line (apex)—may radiate to base or left axilla; blowing, musical, or high-pitched at times

        6. Apical thrill may be palpable (grade IV/VI).

   D. Diagnostic tests

        1. Echocardiogram (two-dimensional)—thickened valve with or without flailing leaflets or vegetation; indicated to assess the mechanism of the MR and its hemodynamic severity, also provides rapid assessment of clinical change

        2. Doppler echocardiogram—regurgitant flow into the left atrium

        3. Transesophageal echocardiogram

4. ECG—check for atrial fibrillation and left ventricular hypertrophy, if in sinus rhythm, tall and peaked P waves in lead II and upright in VI/VI seen with severe pulmonary hypertension
5. Chest X-ray—check for enlarged left atrium and/or ventricle.
6. Cardiac catheterization—same as for mitral stenosis

E. Management
  1. Acute MR
    a. Vasodilating agents (sodium nitroprusside or nicardipine): decreases MR while simultaneously increasing forward output
    b. Intra-aortic balloon counterpulsation: temporizing measure for achieving hemodynamic stability until definitive mitral surgery can be performed
    c. Mitral valve surgery (repair or replacement) is recommended for symptomatic patients with acute severe primary MR
  2. Chronic MR
    a. Primary MR
      i. Standard regimen for HF: β-blockers, ACE inhibitors, or ARBs
      ii. Vasodilator therapy not indicate for normotensive asymptomatic patients with chronic primary MR and normal systolic LV function
      iii. MV surgery (repair or replacement) recommended for symptomatic patients with chronic severe primary MR
      iv. Transcatheter MV repair may be considered for severely symptomatic patients with chronic severe primary MR who have a reasonable life expectancy, but a prohibitive surgical risk because of severe comorbidities
    b. Secondary MR
      i. Standard regimen for HF: β-blockers, ACE inhibitors, or ARBs
      ii. Cardiac resynchronization therapy with biventricular pacing is recommended for symptomatic patients with chronic severe secondary MR who meet the indications for device therapy.
      iii. MV surgery may be considered for severely symptomatic patients with chronic severe secondary MR. MV repair may be considered for patients with chronic moderate secondary MR who are undergoing other cardiac surgery.
  3. Antibiotic prophylaxis for surgical or dental procedures (refer to Inflammatory Cardiac Disease chapter section on endocarditis prophylaxis for appropriate indications/criteria and definitive therapy)

IV.   Mitral valve prolapse
  A. Definition/etiology/incidence
    1. Protrusion of the mitral valve into the left atrium during systole as the result of damaged leaflets of the valve
    2. Cause often unknown; appears to have genetic disposition to collagen disorders such as Marfan syndrome, osteogenesis imperfecta, and Ehlers-Danlos syndrome
    3. Usually benign
    4. Affects up to 2%–6% of the population
    5. More prevalent in women between the ages of 15 and 30 than in men; if observed in men, often older (older than 50 years of age)
    6. Familial incidence for some—suggesting autosomal dominant form of inheritance
  B. Physical examination findings
    1. Often asymptomatic
    2. Fatigue
    3. Dizziness or lightheadedness
    4. Dyspnea
    5. Chest pain or palpitations may occur
    6. Syncope
    7. Dysrhythmias—most commonly ventricular premature contractions, paroxysmal supraventricular and ventricular tachycardia, and atrial fibrillation
    8. Midsystolic click frequently followed by a late systolic crescendo-decrescendo murmur, medium to high pitched sound, heard best at the apex
      a. Increases during the straining phase of the Valsalva maneuver or any intervention that increases LV volume
      b. Decreases during squatting and isometric exercises
  C. Diagnostic tests
    1. Same as for other mitral disorders
  D. Management
    1. Antibiotic prophylaxis for procedures only for those with a prior history of endocarditis (refer to Inflammatory Cardiac Disease chapter section on Endocarditis prophylaxis for appropriate indications/criteria and definitive therapy)
    2. Avoid stimulants in patients with palpitations
    3. β blockers for patients with mild tachyarrhythmias
    4. Aspirin, 81–325 mg daily for patients with documented neurological focal events who are in sinus rhythm with no atrial thrombi
    5. Same additional treatment as for mitral stenosis and regurgitation
    6. Monitor patient for complications
      a. Mitral regurgitation—most common complication
      b. Bacterial endocarditis—risk is 2–3 times that of the general population
      c. Supraventricular arrhythmias

V. Aortic stenosis (AS)

A. Definition: narrowing of the aortic valve resulting in obstructed forward blood flow

B. Etiology/incidence
1. Rheumatic disease is the most common cause.
2. Degenerative or senile calcific disease most common cause in elderly
3. Idiopathic calcification of the aortic valve
4. Congenital
5. Most common valvular disorder in the U.S. and among the elderly

C. Subjective and physical examination findings
1. Dyspnea—may be marked
2. Angina—occurs in approximately 70% of patients
3. Syncope—occurs in approximately 20% of patients
4. Murmur—systolic, "blowing," rough, harsh at the second right intercostal space, usually radiating to the neck and apex; classic crescendo-decrescendo quality; may especially radiate to the apex in elderly patients
5. A thrill or anacrotic "shudder" may be palpable over carotid arteries—commonly found on left; may be normal due to concurrent atherosclerosis and increased vascular stiffness in elderly patients
6. Pulsus parvus et tardus—peripheral arterial pulse rises slowly to a delayed peak
7. Presence of S4—reflects LV hypertrophy and elevated LV end-diastolic pressure
8. LV impulse displaced laterally
9. Absence of A2 component of second heart sound (absence of aortic component); intensity of S2 is a reliable marker of AS severity (softer the S2 sound, the more severe the AS)
10. Because onset of symptoms may be subtle, elderly may not have any limitations or may unconsciously alter habits to avoid symptoms

D. Diagnostic tests
1. Echocardiogram—same as for mitral disorders
2. ECG—check for LV hypertrophy seen with severe AS
3. Chest X-ray—check for concentric hypertrophy of the left ventricle with a calcified valve, dilated proximal ascending aorta along the upper right heart border, enlargement of heart chambers, and pulmonary artery
4. Cardiac catheterization: same as for mitral disorders

E. Management
1. Surgery—mortality rate is dependent upon preoperative clinical and hemodynamic state; for elderly, pay particular attention to pulmonary, renal, and hepatic function

      a. 10-year survival rate is 60%

      b. 30% of bioprosthetic valves demonstrate valve failure in 10 years, requiring re-replacement

      c. Equal percentage of patients develop hemorrhagic complications secondary to anticoagulants, particularly among the elderly and frail elderly

2. Percutaneous balloon aortic valvuloplasty—preferred approach in young adults with congenital, noncalcific AS

3. Transcatheter Aortic Valve Implantation (TAVI)

      a. Implantation procedure involves accessing a femoral artery, performing balloon valvuloplasty, and then advancing the device across the native valve. During rapid right ventricular pacing, a balloon is inflated to deploy the valve and the frame.

4. Nitrates should be used with caution in patients with symptomatic coronary artery disease with AS due to their effect on coronary artery perfusion.

5. Medical therapy for hypertension should follow standard guidelines, starting at a low dose and gradually titrating upward PRN to achieve BP control. There are no studies addressing specific antihypertensive medications in patients with AS, but diuretics should be avoided if the LV chamber is small, because even smaller LV volumes may result in a fall in cardiac output.

6. Avoid strenuous physical activity and competitive sports; avoid dehydration and hypovolemia to safe guard against significant reduction in cardiac output

7. Antibiotic prophylaxis for procedures for patients with prior history of endocarditis (refer to Inflammatory Cardiac Disease chapter section on endocarditis prophylaxis for appropriate indications/criteria and definitive therapy)

VI. **Aortic regurgitation**

A. Definition: backflow of blood into the left ventricle as a result of deficiencies of the aortic valve leaflets or the aorta

B. Etiology

    1. Rheumatic fever

    2. Rheumatoid arthritis

    3. Infectious endocarditis is the most common cause of acute presentation.

    4. Idiopathic valve calcification

C. Subjective and physical examination findings

    1. Fatigue

    2. Dyspnea

    3. Syncope

    4. Sinus tachycardia during exertion or with emotion

    5. Feeling of head pounding or palpitations

    6. Chest pain even in the absence of coronary artery disease

7. Jarring of the entire body and the bobbing motion of the head with each systole and abrupt distention and collapse of the larger arteries
8. Corrigan's pulse—rapidly rising "water-hammer" pulse, which collapses suddenly as arterial pressure falls rapidly during late systole and diastole
9. Quincke's pulse—alternate flushing and paling of the skin at the root of the nail while pressure is applied to the nail tip
10. Widened pulse pressure—result of both systolic hypertension and a lowering of the diastolic pressure
11. S3 heart sound
12. LV impulse—heaving and laterally displaced
13. Murmur—high pitched, blowing, decrescendo diastolic, murmur at the third left intercostal space along the left sternal border; heard best with patient sitting up, leaning forward, and with the breath held in forced expiration
14. Signs of congestive heart failure

D. Diagnostic tests
  1. Same as for mitral disorders
  2. Chest X-ray—check for moderate to severe left ventricular enlargement

E. Management
  1. Surgical—guided by the stage of AR as well as clinical setting (i.e., aortic dissection or hemodynamic instability)
    a. Acute AR: in presence of hemodynamic instability, surgery is usually not delayed
      i. Intra-aortic balloon counterpulsation is contraindicated in patients with acute severe AR
      ii. AVR (repair or replacement) is indicated for symptomatic patients with severe AR regardless of LV systolic function
    b. Chronic AR: requires staging/surgical risk assessment
      i. AVR is indicated for asymptomatic patients with chronic severe AR and LV systolic dysfunction
  2. Pharmaceutical
    a. Acute AR:
      i. Vasodilating agents: sodium nitroprusside
      ii. β blockers, diltiazem and verapamil; unless treating aortic dissection, these agents should be used cautiously, if at all, because they will block the compensatory tachycardia and could precipitate a marked reduction in BP
      iii. Antibiotic prophylaxis against bacterial endocarditis for dental or other surgical procedures (refer to Inflammatory Cardiac Disease chapter section on endocarditis prophylaxis for appropriate indications/criteria and definitive therapy)

  b. Chronic AR:

   i. Treatment of hypertension (systolic BP greater than 140 mmHg) is recommended in patients with chronic AR, preferably with dihydropyridine calcium channel blockers or ACE inhibitors/ARBs

   ii. β blockers less effective because reduction in heart rate is associated with an even higher stroke volume, which contributes to elevated systolic pressure in patients with chronic severe AR

   iii. ACE inhibitors/ARBs and β blockers are reasonable in patients with severe AR who have symptoms and/or LV dysfunction when surgery is not performed because of comorbidities.

   iv. Vasodilating drugs are effective in reducing systolic BP in patients with chronic AR, however they are not routinely recommended in patients with chronic asymptomatic AR and normal LV systolic function.

BIBLIOGRAPHY

Adams, D. H., Carabello, B. A., & Castillo, J. G. (2011). Mitral valve regurgitation. In V. Fuster, R. A. Walsh, & R. A. Harrington (Eds.), *Hurst's the heart* (13th ed.). [E-reader version]. Retrieved from http://accessmedicine.mhmedical.com.libdata.lib.ua.edu/content.aspx?bookid=376&sectionid=40279811

Carbello, B. A. (2011). Mitral stenosis. In V. Fuster, R. A. Walsh, & R. A. Harrington (Eds.), *Hurst's the heart* (13th ed.). [E-reader version]. Retrieved from http://accessmedicine.mhmedical.com.libdata.lib.ua.edu/content.aspx?bookid=376&sectionid=40279812

Cawley, P. J., & Otto, C. M. (2011). Valvular heart disease in the elderly. *Current Cardiovascular Risk Reports, 5*(5), 413–421. doi:10.1007/s12170–011–0187–z

Chikwe, J., Filsoufi, F., & Carpentier, A. (2011). Prosthetic heart valves. In V. Fuster, R. A. Walsh, & R. A. Harrington (Eds.), *Hurst's the heart* (13th ed.). [E-reader version]. Retrieved from http://accessmedicine.mhmedical.com.libdata.lib.ua.edu/content.aspx?bookid=376&sectionid=40279814

Cupido, B. J., & Commerford, P. J. (2013). Rheumatic fever and valvular heart disease. In C. Rosendorff (Ed.), *Essential cardiology: Principles and practice*. New York, NY: Springer.

Freeman, R. V. & Otto, C. M. (2011). Aortic valve disease. In V. Fuster, R. A. Walsh, & R. A. Harrington (Eds.), *Hurst's the heart* (13th ed.). [E-reader version]. Retrieved from http://accessmedicine.mhmedical.com.libdata.lib.ua.edu/content.aspx?bookid=376&sectionid=40279810

Gongidi, V. R. & Hamaty, J. N. (2011). Aortic stenosis: A focused review in the elderly. *Clinical Geriatrics, 19*(3), 19–22.

Lazar, H. L. (2012). The year in review: The surgical treatment of valvular disease-2011. *Journal of Cardiac Surgery, 27*(4), 493–510. doi:10.1111/j.1540–8191.2012.01494.x

Nishimura, R. A., Otto, C. M., Bonow, R. O., Carabello, B. A., Erwin, J. P., Guyton, R. A. . . . Thomas, J. D. (2014). 2014 AHA/ACC guideline for the management of patients with valvular heart disease: A report of the American College of Cardiology/American Heart Association Task Force on Practice Guidelines. *Circulation.* doi:10.1161/CIR.0000000000000029

O'Gara, P. & Loscalzo, J. (2012). Valvular heart disease. In D. L. Longo, A. S. Fauci, D. L. Kasper, S. L. Hauser, J. L. Jameson, & J. Loscalzo (Eds.), *Harrison's principles of internal medicine* (18th ed.). [E-reader version]. Retrieved from ttp://accessmedicine.com/content/aspx?aID=9127003

Saikrishnan, N., Kumar, G., Sawaya, F. J., Lerakis, S. & Yoganathan, A. P. (2014). Accurate assessment of aortic stenosis: A review of diagnostic modalities and hemodynamics. *Circulation, 129*(2), 244–253. doi:10.1161/CIRCULATION AHA.113.002310

Vahanian, A., Alfierei, O., Andreotti, F., Antunes, M. J., Baron-Esquivias, G., Baumgartner, H., . . . Zembata, M. (2012). Guidelines on the management of valvular heart disease (version 2012). *European Heart Journal, 33*(19), 2451–2496. doi:10.1093/eurheartj/ehs109

Whitlock, R. P., Sun, J. C., Fremes, S. E., Rubens, F. D., & Teoh, K. H. (2012). Antithrombotic and thrombolytic therapy for valvular disease: Antithrombotic therapy and prevention of thrombosis, 9th ed: American College of Chest Physicians evidence-based clinical practice guidelines. *Chest, 141*(2 Suppl), 576S–600S. doi:10.1378/chest.11–2305

CHAPTER 20

Cardiomyopathy

SHEILA MELANDER • THOMAS W. BARKLEY, JR.

I. **Definition**
   A. Idiopathic disorder causing cardiac muscle dysfunction that may result in systolic or diastolic dysfunction not due to atherosclerosis, hypertension, or valvular disease

II. **Types**
   A. Dilated
      1. Abnormal systolic pump function
      2. Dilated ventricles without proportionate compensatory hypertrophy
      3. Systolic heart failure
   B. Hypertrophy
      1. Autosomal dominant disorder
      2. Stiff left ventricle during diastole that restricts ventricular filling
      3. Ventricular hypertrophy that occurs without dilatation or a thickening septum
      4. Diastolic heart failure
   C. Restrictive
      1. Inadequate diastolic filling
      2. Rigid ventricular walls
      3. Diastolic heart failure

III. **Etiology/incidence**
   A. Dilated
      1. Caused by ischemic heart disease, alcoholism, persistent tachycardia, that is, inappropriate sinus tachycardia or AFib with RVR, systemic lupus erythematosus, toxins, cocaine; also, idiopathic causes
      2. Most common type of cardiomyopathy

3. Approximately 1% of the general population is affected; 10% of these patients are older than 80 years of age.

B. Hypertrophic
   1. Cause is idiopathic
   2. Chronic hypertension has been associated with increased incidence.

C. Restrictive
   1. Related to a variety of conditions
      a. Sarcoidosis
      b. Endomyocardial fibrosis (after open heart surgery)
      c. Exposure
      d. Idiopathic causes
   2. Relatively uncommon

IV. Subjective/physical exam findings

A. Dilated cardiomyopathy is associated with left or biventricular congestive heart failure (CHF).
   1. Increased jugular venous distention
   2. Low pulse pressure
   3. S3 and/or S4 heart sounds
   4. Peripheral edema
   5. Rales
   6. Dyspnea
   7. Orthopnea
   8. Paroxysmal nocturnal dyspnea
   9. Mitral or tricuspid regurgitation
   10. Cardiomegaly

B. Hypertrophic
   1. Dyspnea
   2. Chest pain
   3. Syncope
   4. Murmur—harsh, "diamond-shaped" (crescendo-decrescendo) systolic, at the left sternal border; decreases with squatting and increases with the Valsalva maneuver
   5. S4 heart sound
   6. Maximized apical pulse (double or triple)

C. Restrictive—associated with right-sided heart failure
   1. Dyspnea
   2. Fatigue
   3. Weakness
   4. Edema
   5. Jugular venous distention
   6. Ascites
   7. Murmurs (regurgitant)
   8. Kussmaul breathing (possibly)

V. **Diagnostics**
   A. Dilated cardiomyopathy
      1. Chest x-ray
         a. Marked cardiac enlargement
         b. Pulmonary edema (interstitial)
      2. ECG
         a. ST segment/T-wave changes with left ventricular hypertrophy
         b. Right or left bundle branch block
         c. Arrhythmias common
            i. Atrial fibrillation
            ii. Premature atrial contractions
            iii. Premature ventricular contractions
            iv. Ventricular tachycardia
      3. Echocardiogram
         a. Left ventricular dilatation and dysfunction with low ejection fraction
      4. Routine blood and urine chemistries
   B. Hypertrophic
      1. Chest x-ray
         a. Mild cardiomegaly or normal heart size
      2. ECG
         a. Abnormal Q waves in anterolateral and inferior leads
         b. Left ventricular hypertrophy
      3. Echocardiogram (diagnosis confirmed by two-dimensional approach)
         a. Left ventricular hypertrophy
         b. Increased or at times normal ejection fraction
      4. Exercise stress testing and 24-hr Holter monitor screening
      5. Routine blood and urine chemistries
   C. Restrictive
      1. Chest x-ray
         a. Evidence of CHF, possibly including pleural effusion
         b. Cardiomegaly is usually mild to moderate.
      2. ECG
         a. ST segment/T-wave changes
         b. Atrial fibrillation, left axis deviation, and other arrhythmias are possible
      3. Echocardiogram
         a. Thickened cardiac valves
         b. Increased wall thickness
         c. Normal or small left ventricle size with mild to normal left ventricle function
      4. Routine blood and urine chemistries
      5. Cardiac catheterization/MRI to distinguish from constrictive pericarditis

      a. Impairment of the left ventricle is more evident than impairment of the right ventricle (e.g., pulmonary capillary wedge pressure is greater than central venous pressure) with restrictive cardiomyopathy.

      b. MRI reveals greater thickening of the pericardium with restrictive cardiomyopathy.

      c. With constrictive pericarditis, both ventricles are usually involved.

   6. Myocardial biopsy for definitive diagnosis

VI.   **Management**

   A. Dilated cardiomyopathy

     1. Treatment of the underlying condition (e.g., discontinuing use of alcohol, treating endocrine causes, and rapid heart rate arrhythmias)

     2. For heart failure (see Heart Failure chapter)

      a. Rest

      b. Daily weights

      c. Restricted sodium

      d. Diuretics

      e. ACE inhibitors

      f. Digitalis if needed to reduce heart rate and thus workload in associated tachyarrhythmias

     3. Vasodilators, especially combined with ACE inhibitors and nitrates

     4. Oral anticoagulation for emboli prophylaxis

     5. β-blockers such as Carvedilol or Coreg, or Metoprolol (Lopressor; Toprol XL)—low-dose β-blockade

     6. Diltiazem (Cardizem)—especially effective for idiopathic causes; however, not advocated for use in patients with left ventricular depression

     7. Antiarrhythmics PRN

   B. Hypertrophic

     1. β-blocking drugs are recommended for the treatment of symptoms (angina or dyspnea) in adult patients with obstructive or nonobstructive HCM, but should be used with caution in patients with sinus bradycardia or severe conduction disease.

     2. If low doses of β-blocking drugs are ineffective for controlling symptoms, titrate the dose to a resting heart rate of less than 60-65 bpm (up to generally accepted and recommended maximum doses of these drugs).

      a. Metoprolol, 25 mg PO every 12 hr (maximum 400 mg/day)

      b. Atenolol, 25 mg PO daily (maximum 200 mg/day)

      c. Verapamil (Calan), 120-480 mg daily to BID, for obstructive and nonobstructive disease in those for whom β-blockers are contraindicated/intolerable)

3. With acute heart failure, IV normal saline in addition to propranolol (Inderal) or verapamil (Calan)
4. Antibiotic prophylaxis for invasive procedures, may be indicated depending upon individual valvular diagnoses
5. Amiodarone (Cordarone) or other antiarrhythmics to prevent recurrence of atrial fibrillation
6. Avoidance of alcohol
7. Consider dual-chamber pacing to prevent progression of the disease, as indicated
   a. ACE inhibitors, nitrates, diuretics, and digoxin are contraindicated with hypertrophic obstructive disease
8. Consider implantation of internal cardioverter defibrillator for the prevention of sudden death

C. Restrictive
1. Control major cause(s) of death due to heart failure
   a. Restrict sodium intake
   b. Use diuretics PRN
   c. Administer antiarrhythmics as appropriate
2. Perform repeated phlebotomies to decrease iron deposition in the heart for patients with cardiomyopathy caused by hemochromatosis
3. Corticosteroids for sarcoidosis
4. Symptomatic treatment

BIBLIOGRAPHY

Bojar, R. M. (2011). *Manual of perioperative care in adult cardiac surgery* (5ᵗʰ ed.). Boston, MA: Wiley/Blackwell Publishing.

Carvalho, V. O., Bocchi, E. A., & Guimarães, G. V. (2009). Hydrotherapy in heart failure: A case report. *Clinics, 64*(8).

Dunphy, L. H. (2004). *Management guidelines for nurse practitioners working with adults* (2ⁿᵈ ed.). Philadelphia, PA: FA Davis.

England, B., Lee, A., Tran, T., Faw, H., Yang, P., Lin, A., . . . Ross, B. D. (2005). Magnetic resonance criteria for future trials of cardiac resynchronization. *Journal of Cardiovascular Magnetic Resonance, 7*(5), 827–834.

Ferri, F. F. (2011). *Ferri's clinical advisor 2011: Instant diagnosis and treatment.* Philadelphia, PA: Elsevier Health Sciences.

Gersh, B. J., Maron, B. J., Bonow, R. O., Dearani, J. A., Fifer, M. A., Link, M. S., . . . & Yancy, C. W. (2011). 2011 ACCF/AHA guideline of the diagnosis and treatment of hypertropic cardiomyopathy: Executive summary. *Circulation, 124*, 2761–2796.

Gheorghiade, M., Flaherty, J. D., Fonarow, G. C., Desai, R. V., Lee, R., McGiffin, D., . . . Ahmed, A. (2011). Coronary artery disease, coronary revascularization, and outcomes in chronic advanced systolic heart failure. *International Journal of Cardiology, 151*(1), 69–75.

Grimes, J. A. (2013). *The 5-minute clinical consult*. Philadelphia, PA: Lippincott Williams & Wilkins.

Hare, J. M. (2011). The dilated, restrictive, and infiltrative cardiomyopathies. In R. O. Bonow, D. L. Mann, D. P. Zipes, & P. Libby (Eds.). *Braunwald's heart disease: A textbook of cardiovascular medicine* (9th ed.). Philadelphia, PA: Saunders Elsevier.

Klabunde, R. E. (2004). *Cardiovascular physiology concepts*. Philadelphia, PA: Lippincott Williams & Wilkins.

Maron, B., & Maron, M. (2013). Hypertrophic cardiomyopathy. *Lancet, 381*(9862), 242-255. doi:10.1016/S0140-6736(12)60397-3

Schiros, C. G., Ahmed, M. I., Sanagala, T., Zha, W., McGiffin, D. C., Bamman, M. M., . . . Dell'Italia, L. J. (2013). Importance of 3-dimensional geometric analysis in the assessment of the athlete's heart. *American Journal of Cardiology, 111*(7), 1067–1072.

Wackett, A., & Fan, R. (2005). *Cardiomyopathy, restrictive*. Retrieved September 4, 2007, from www.emedicine.com/EMERG/topic81.htm

Wexler, R. K., Elton, T., Pleister, A., & Feldman, D. (2009). Cardiomyopathy: An overview. *American Family Physician, 79*(9), 778–784.

CHAPTER 21

Arrhythmias

FREDRICK CARLSTON • ROBERT FELLIN • THOMAS W. BARKLEY, JR

COMMON CARDIAC RHYTHMS/ARRHYTHMIAS AND TREATMENT

I. **Normal sinus rhythm (NSR) (Figure 21.1)**
   A. Characteristics
      1. Regular rate and rhythm
      2. PR interval and QRS complex normal
         a. PR interval 0.20 seconds or less
         b. QRS complex 0.12 seconds or less
   B. Rate is 60–100 beats/minute (bpm)
II. **Sinus bradycardia (SB) (Figure 21.2)**
   A. Characteristics
      1. Regular rate and rhythm
      2. PR interval and QRS complex normal
   B. Rate 60 bpm or less than expected relative to underlying condition or cause
   C. Etiology
      1. Increased vagal tone (e.g., in athletes)
      2. Medications: AV nodal blockers (e.g., digitalis, β blockers, calcium channel blockers)
      3. Recreational drug abuse
      4. Metabolic or electrolyte abnormalities
      5. Autonomic dysfunction or neurologic causes
      6. Ischemic or valvular heart disease
      7. Sinus node dysfunction; includes inappropriate sinus bradycardia and tachy-brady syndrome
   D. Clinical manifestations
      1. May be asymptomatic

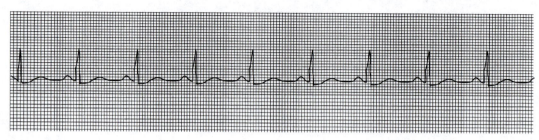

Figure 21.1. Normal sinus rhythm.

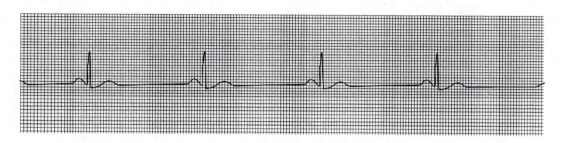

Figure 21.2. Sinus bradycardia.

2. Presyncope or syncope, dizziness, orthostatic, fatigue, or weakness
3. Signs of decreased perfusion, hypotension, or confusion

E. Treatment
1. Consult/refer to cardiologist or electrophysiologist
2. If asymptomatic, treatment may not be indicated
3. Diagnostic testing could include Holter monitor or rhythm patch, labs, and tilt-table test
4. If indicated, may require permanent pacemaker
5. For acute symptomatic bradycardia, initiate transcutaneous pacing Medication (e.g., atropine, dopamine, isoproterenol) can be used

III. Sinus arrhythmia (Figure 21.3)
A. Characteristics
1. Rate is variable (i.e., variable R-R interval)
2. Normal PR interval and QRS complex
3. Rate varies with respirations

B. Etiology: common in children and the elderly
C. Clinical manifestations: none known
D. Treatment: none indicated

IV. Junctional rhythm (Figure 21.4)
A. Characteristics
1. Because the beat originates in the atrioventricular (AV) node, usually no P waves precede QRS complexes
2. Occasionally, P waves are retrograde conducted, resulting in a downward deflection before or after the QRS complex.
3. Rate is usually 40–60 bpm (i.e., the intrinsic AV node rate)

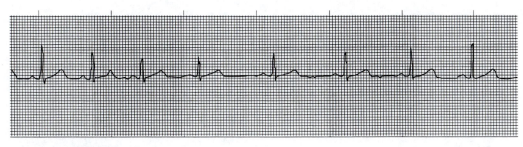

Figure 21.3. Sinus arrythmia

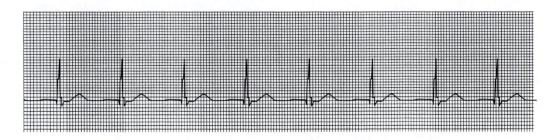

Figure 21.4. Accelerated junctional rhythm (strip is approximately 80 bpm)

     4. Accelerated junctional rhythms have the same criteria, but rates range from 60–100 bpm.

     5. Rarely seen in adult patients

  B. Etiology (common causes)

     1. Digitalis toxicity

     2. Theophylline

     3. Dopamine

  C. Treatment

     1. Consult/refer to cardiologist or electrophysiologist

     2. Atropine, 0.5 mg intravenous push (IVP), to a maximum of 3 mg (for unstable patient)

     3. Consider pacing if patient is severely bradycardic (for unstable patient)

V.   **Sinus tachycardia (ST) (Figure 21.5)**

  A. Characteristics

     1. Regular rate and rhythm

     2. PR interval and QRS complex normal

  B. Rate 100 bpm or more and typically less than 150–160 bpm

  C. Etiology

     1. Usually reflects an underlying process, metabolic state, or medication use (e.g., fever, shock, CHF, pain, cocaine or other illicit drug use, hypovolemia)

     2. Inappropriate sinus tachycardia

  D. Clinical manifestations

     1. May be asymptomatic

     2. Chest tightness, SOB, palpitations, fatigue, facial flushing

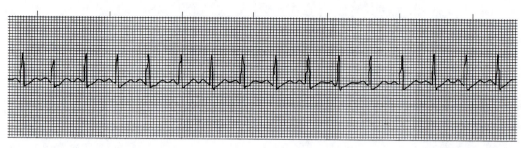

Figure 21.5. Sinus tachycardia.

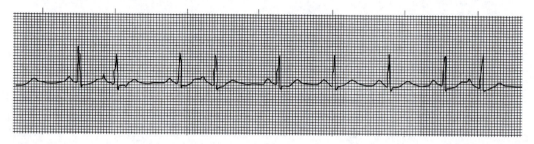

Figure 21.6. Premature atrial contractions

        3. Hypertension

        4. If poor perfusion: hypotension, loss of consciousness (LOC)

    E. Treatment

        1. Treat the underlying problem or cause

        2. If all causes of sinus tachycardia have been excluded, consult/refer to cardiologist or electrophysiologist for evaluation of inappropriate sinus tachycardia

            a. β-blockers or non-dihydropyridine calcium channel blockers (i.e., diltiazem or verapamil) may be indicated

            b. Can lead to tachycardia-induced cardiomyopathy

            c. Refractory cases may require SA node ablation

VI. **Premature atrial contractions (PACs) (Figure 21.6)**

    A. Characteristics

        1. Occur when an ectopic focus in the atria fires before the next sinus node impulse; P waves usually look different (i.e., either smaller or peaked)

        2. Rate usually "resets" itself, resulting in one premature beat followed by a normal series of beats in sinus rhythm

    B. Etiology: not considered an abnormal finding

    C. Clinical manifestations: usually asymptomatic; rarely can cause symptoms of palpitations and SOB

    D. Treatment: in general, none; in patients who are symptomatic, β-blockers or non-dihydropyridine calcium channel blockers (i.e., diltiazem or verapamil) are usually effective

VII. **Atrial tachycardia**

    A. Characteristics

1. Often sudden onset and sudden stop, sustained atrial tachycardia is relatively rare
2. Rate of 140–220 bpm
3. Ventricle is a "slave" to the atrium
4. P wave morphology usually different; QRS remains unchanged
5. Pacemaker is coming from a single ectopic focus that is outside the SA node

B. Etiology
1. Usually occurs in patients with abnormal automaticity or pulmonary problems
2. Can be caused by medications including Digoxin excess
3. Can be caused by increased catecholamine state or volume overload (atrial stretch)

C. Clinical manifestations
1. Patients can be asymptomatic
2. Patients can report chest pressure, palpitations, syncope or presyncope, SOB, or fatigue
3. Patients with poor perfusion may have hypotension, LOC, shock

D. Treatment
1. Consult/refer to cardiologist or electrophysiologist.
2. Treat underlying cause
3. Can try vagal maneuvers by asking the patient to cough, strain as though having a bowel movement, or elicit the patient's gag reflex
4. AV nodal blockers (β-blockers, non-dihydropyridine calcium channel blockers [i.e., diltiazem or verapamil])
5. Antiarrhythmics may be required if AV nodal blockers are not effective (see Table 21.1)
6. Cardiac ablation of ectopic focus may be indicated and has a 95% success rate
7. For unstable patient, follow ACLS guidelines

VIII. Multifocal atrial tachycardia

A. Characteristics
1. P waves of three or more different morphologies
2. P-P, P-R, and R-R intervals vary
3. Rates usually 100–180 bpm
4. Irregular and is often mistaken for atrial fibrillation
5. Can degenerate into atrial fibrillation

B. Etiology
1. Occurs in the elderly or acutely ill patients
2. Common in patients with pulmonary disorders and associated with hypoxia
3. Occasionally seen with sepsis, volume overload, and theophylline toxicity

C. Treatment
1. Rhythm itself is rarely associated with instability

Table 21.1	Antiarrhythmic Agents	
Agent	**Indication**	**Adverse Effects**
Class IA: Sodium Channel Blockers **All may cause new or worsen dysrhythmias** **Effective for atrial and ventricular arrhythmias, however infrequently used due to their significant toxicity**		
Disopyramide phosphate (Norpace)	AF, PSVT, PVC, VT, WPW	constipation, nausea, muscle weakness, blurred vision, fatigue, heart failure
Procainamide HCl (Pronestyl)	AF, PVC, VT, WPW	agranulocytosis, SLE, hypotension, hepatotoxicity, ventricular arrhythmia,
Quinidine gluconate (Quinaglute)	AF, PVC, VT, WPW	nausea, abdominal pain, diarrhea, hemolytic anemia, thrombocytopenia, hepatitis, ventricular tachycardia (torsade de pointe)
Class IB: Sodium Channel Blockers **Cannot be used to treat atrial arrhythmias**		
Lidocaine	PVC, VT, VF	hypotension, nausea, blurred vision, methemoglobinemia, paresthesias, confusion, seizure, tremors
Mexiletine (Mexitil)	PVC, VT, VF	nausea, vomiting, dizziness, lightheadedness, tremor, blurred vision, visual disturbance, agranulocytosis, hepatotoxicity
Class IC: Sodium Channel Blockers **Do not use in patients with structural heart disease**		
Flecainide (Tambocor)	AF, PSVT, ventricular arrhythmias	palpitations, nausea, dizziness, headache, blurred vision, fatigue
Propafenone (Rythmol)	AF, ventricular arrhythmias, WPW	chest pain, edema, palpitations, constipation, altered sense of taste, vomiting, dizziness, anxiety, fatigue, agranulocytosis, heart failure
Class II: β-Adrenergic Blockers **Primarily used for rate control**		
Acebutolol (Sectral)	Atrial tachyarrhythmias AF (rate control; control ventricular rate)	hypotension, dizziness, bradycardia, 2nd or 3rd degree heart block, fatigue, insomnia, nausea
Atenolol (Tenormin)		
Esmolol (Brevibloc)		
Metoprolol (Lopressor)		
Propranolol (Inderal)		

Table 21.1	Antiarrhythmic Agents	
Agent	**Indication**	**Adverse Effects**
Class III: Potassium Channel Blockers **All may cause new or worsen dysrhythmias** **Effective for atrial and ventricular arrhythmias**		
Amiodarone (Cordarone, Pacerone)	AF, PSVT, VF, ventricular arrhythmias	bradyarrhythmia, hypotension, photodermatitis, photosensitivity, thyroid dysfunction, nausea, vomiting, increased liver enzymes, dizziness, paresthesia, visual disturbance, optic neuritis, fatigue, toxic epidermal necrolysis, pulmonary fibrosis
Dofetilide (Tikosyn)	AF/atrial flutter	chest pain, dizziness, headache, heart block, ventricular arrhythmia
Ibutilide (Corvert)	AF/atrial flutter	bradyarrhythmia, heart block, ventricular arrhythmia, headache, hypotension
Sotalol (βpace)	AF, PSVT, ventricular arrhythmias	dizziness, weakness, fatigue, nausea, vomiting, diarrhea, bradycardia, heart block, heart failure, bronchospasm
Dronedarone (Multaq)	AF	abdominal pain, diarrhea, indigestion, nausea, vomiting, heart failure, CVA, liver failure Doubles the risk of death in patients with symptomatic heart failure
Class IV: Calcium Channel Blockers **Primarily used for rate control**		
Diltiazem (Cardizem)	Atrial tachyarrhythmias, AF (rate control; control ventricular rate)	peripheral edema, hypotension, dizziness, bradycardia, 2nd or 3rd degree heart block, fatigue, insomnia, constipation
Verapamil (Calan)	Supraventricular tachycardia, PSVT	
Miscellaneous Agents **May produce new dysrhythmias or worsen existing ones**		
Adenosine (Adenocard)	PSVT	chest discomfort, flushing, abdominal discomfort, dizziness, headache, dyspnea
Digoxin (Lanoxin)	AF (rate control; control ventricular rate)	nausea, vomiting, headache, visual disturbances Monitor drug levels

Note. AF = atrial fibrillation; PAC = premature atrial complex; PSVT = paroxysmal supraventricular tachycardia; PVC = premature ventricular complex; VF = ventricular fibrillation; VT = ventricular tachycardia; WPW = Wolff-Parkinson-White syndrome

2. Treat the underlying disorder
3. Magnesium, one dose of 2 grams followed by infusion of 1–2 grams per hr over 5 hr, may reduce atrial ectopy. Mg levels may rise to 2.5–3 mg/dl
4. Verapamil or β-blockers for rate control; caution recommended when using β-blockers in patients with pulmonary disease
5. No need for anticoagulation; no increased stroke risk

IX. **Atrial fibrillation (A-fib) (Figure 21.7; also see Figure 21.20 at the end of this chapter)**
  A. Characteristics
    1. No discernible P waves; fibrillatory waves are noted instead
    2. PR interval is not measurable (wavy baseline).
    3. QRS complex is regularly irregular.
    4. Atrial rate is commonly 400–700 bpm.
    5. Ventricular rate is usually 100–160 bpm or greater
    6. Most common sustained arrhythmia; estimated 2.2 million people in the U.S. have atrial fibrillation
  B. Classifications
    1. Lone atrial fibrillation
    2. Paroxysmal atrial fibrillation
    3. Post-operative atrial fibrillation
    4. Persistent (longer than 7 days)
    5. Permanent or chronic atrial fibrillation
    6. Associated with increased morbidity, mortality, and preventable stroke
  C. Etiology
    1. Can be caused by various factors (e.g., catecholamine surges, volume overload causing atrial stretch, medications, hyperthyroidism, and autonomic tone)
    2. Etiology is unknown; irregular electrical signals from pulmonary veins entering the left atrium as a trigger source are becoming increasingly appreciated
    3. Prevalence increases with age with 0.4%–1% in the general population and as high as 8% in patients 80 years or older.
    4. Because the atrium is not contracting normally, blood clots could form in left atrium (left atrial appendage) and the patient is at higher risk of embolic stroke

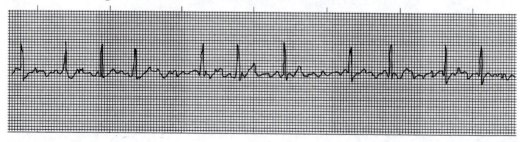

Figure 21.7. Atrial fibrillation.

5. The HAS-BLED Bleeding Risk Score can be used to assess the risk of bleeding for atrial fibrillation management; comprised of evaluating the following clinical characteristics: hypertension, abnormal renal and liver function, stroke, bleeding tendency/predisposition, labile INRs for patients taking warfarin, elderly, and drugs/alcohol

6. Use the CHADS2 score to assess the risk of atrial fibrillation by attributing and adding the specified number of points (see table 21.2)

7. The CHADSVASC scoring is becoming the standard.

X. Clinical manifestations

1. Patient may be asymptomatic
2. Patient may report palpitations, SOB, presyncope, diaphoresis, fatigue, weakness, chest pressure or tightness
3. Patient with decreased perfusion may have hypotension and LOC

A. Treatment

1. Referral to cardiologist or electrophysiologist
2. Treatment is immediate direct-current cardioversion (DCC) for an unstable patient in rapid atrial fibrillation
3. Treatment strategy of the stable patient is individualized, decision is made to pursue rate control strategy vs rhythm control strategy; both strategies include stroke risk reduction (see Tables 21.4 & 21.5).
   a. AV nodal blockers for rate control (see Table 21.1)
   b. Antiarrhythmics (see Table 21.1) and/or planned TEE and cardioversion (see Tables 21.4 & 21.5) for rhythm control
   c. Anticoagulation for stroke risk reduction
      i. Aspirin vs Coumadin based on individual stroke risk
      ii. Newer direct thrombin inhibitors are becoming more prevalent in part because INR testing is not required (e.g., dabigatran).

Table 21.2	CHADS2 Score: Stroke risk assessment in atrial fibrillation
Score	**CHADS2 Risk Criteria**
1 point	Heart failure
1 point	Hypertension
1 point	Age greater than 75 years
1 point	Diabetes mellitus
2 points	Stroke/transient ischemic attack

4. Catheter ablation with pulmonary vein isolation is available to patients who are symptomatic and not responsive to AV nodal blockers or antiarrhythmics (has 75% success rate and often requires more than one ablation).

5. Treatment recommendations when using the CHADS2 Risk Assessment scoring guidelines (see table 21.3)

Table 21.3	CHADS2 Risk Assessment scoring guidelines	
CHADS2 Score	**Risk**	**Recommendation**
0	Low	Aspirin (81–325 mg) daily
1	Intermediate	Aspirin (81–324 mg) daily or warfarin (INR 2.0–3.0)
2 or more	High	Warfarin (INR 2.0–3.0) unless contraindicated

Table 21.4	Therapeutic interventions for cardioversion of atrial fibrillation
Intervention	**Comments**
Direct-Current Cardioversion	• Recommended for patients with AF or atrial flutter as a method to restore sinus rhythm. If cardioversion is unsuccessful, repeated direct-current cardioversion attempts may be made after adjusting the location of the electrodes or applying pressure over the electrodes, or following administration of an antiarrhythmic medication • Recommended when a rapid ventricular response to AF or atrial flutter does not respond promptly to pharmacological therapies and contributes to ongoing myocardial ischemia, hypotension or HF • Recommended for patients with AF or atrial flutter and pre-excitation when tachycardia is associated with hemodynamic instability
Amiodarone	• Maintains efficacy in patients with atrial fibrillation present for more than 7 days • Many drug-drug interactions and adverse effects
Dofetilide	• Dofetilide therapy should not be initiated out of hospital due to the risk of excessive QT prolongation that can cause Torsades de pointes. • MD must be registered by manufacturer to prescribe • Dofetilide is prescribed and dispensed only by healthcare providers, hospitals, and pharmacies that are certified to have received appropriate dofetilide dosing and treatment initiation education.
Flecainide	Avoid in patients with structural heart disease; increased risk of arrhythmia
Ibutilide (IV form only)	Avoid in patients with structural heart disease; increased risk of arrhythmia
Propafenone	Avoid in patients with structural heart disease; increased risk of arrhythmia

Table 21.5	Recommended antiarrhythmic drug therapy for maintenance of sinus rhythm in patients with recurrent paroxysmal or recurrent persistent atrial fibrillation
Condition	**Recommendation**
No structural heart disease	First line: flecainide, propafenone or sotalol Second line: amiodarone or dofetilide or catheter ablation
Heart Failure	First line: amiodarone or dofetilide Second line: catheter ablation
Coronary artery disease	First line: sotalol (should be used only if patients have normal left ventricular systolic function) Second line: amiodarone or dofetilide or catheter ablation
Hypertension without significant LVH	First line: flecainide, propafenone or sotalol Second line: amiodarone or dofetilide or catheter ablation
Hypertension with significant LVH	First line: amiodarone Second line: catheter ablation

Note. LVH = left ventricular hypertrophy

XI.   Atrial flutter (A-flutter) (Figure 21.8; also see Figure 21.20)
   A. Characteristics
      1. Sawtooth appearance of flutter waves (F waves), especially if the rhythm strip is turned upside down
      2. PR interval is not measurable
      3. Atrial rate ranges from 240–340 bpm
      4. QRS complex is usually normal
      5. Incidence varies from 0.4%–1.2%
      6. Considered to have the same stroke risk as atrial fibrillation

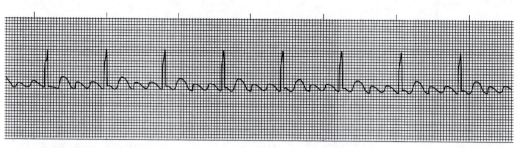

Figure 21.8. Atrial flutter.

B. Etiology
  1. Same causative factors as atrial fibrillation; catecholamine surge, volume overload causing atrial stretch, medications, hyperthyroidism, or autonomic tone
  2. Manifested by reentrant electrical circuit that travels within the right atrium in a counter-clockwise rotation (typical atrial flutter); clockwise may also be seen (atypical atrial flutter)
C. Clinical manifestations
  1. May be asymptomatic
  2. Symptoms include palpitations, SOB, diaphoresis, fatigue, weakness, presyncope, chest pressure or tightness
  3. Patients with decreased perfusion may have hypotension and LOC
D. Treatment
  1. Similar to atrial fibrillation; atrial flutter does not often respond as well to rate control strategy
  2. Ablation of reentrant circuit has 95% success rate
XII. **AV nodal re-entry tachycardia (AVNRT)**
  A. Characteristics
    1. Most common SVT (excluding A-fib and A-flutter)
    2. An AV nodal dependent arrhythmia
    3. Rates 150–190 but can exceed 200
    4. Involves the slow and fast pathway within the AV node
    5. P waves are hidden within the QRS
    6. Usually found in patients without underlying heart disease; more common in women
  B. Etiology
    1. Caused by a PAC that travels down a slow pathway within the AV node, causing the conduction to create a re-entrant pathway within the AV node
  C. Clinical manifestations
    1. Patients may experience palpitations, SOB, presyncope, fatigue, or diaphoresis
    2. Patients with poor perfusion may experience hypotension, LOC, or shock
  D. Treatment
    1. Vagal maneuvers to attempt termination

2. Adenosine, 6 mg rapid IV push; if not successful, increase to 12 mg
3. Referral to cardiologist or electrophysiologist
4. β-blockers and non-dihydropyridine calcium channel blockers (i.e., diltiazem, verapamil) help to prevent recurrence
5. Ablation is the curative therapy with a 95% success rate (Heart block is the major complication risk with 0.8% of patients requiring permanent pacemaker due to the proximity of the AV node)
6. Antiarrhythmics are used for patients not wanting ablation and not responding to AV nodal blockers (see Table 21.1)

XIII. AV reentrant tachycardia (AVRT)

A. Characteristics
1. Type of SVT that is AV node dependent
2. Rates similar to AVNRT, however, more often greater than 200 bpm
3. Relies on the presence of an accessory pathway; this abnormal conduction pathway between the atrium and the ventricle can be on the left or right sides of the heart, the free wall or septum
4. P waves are usually within the ST segment or T wave

B. Etiology
1. Conduction through a reentry circuit that travels through the accessory pathway and back through the AV node

C. Clinical manifestations
1. Patients may experience palpitations, SOB, presyncope, fatigue, or diaphoresis.
2. Patients with poor perfusion may experience hypotension, LOC, or shock.

D. Treatment
1. Vagal maneuvers to attempt termination
2. Adenosine, 6 mg rapid IV push; if not successful, increase to 12 mg; can repeat once
3. For unstable AVNRT, proceed to direct-current cardioversion.
4. Referral to cardiologist or electrophysiologist
5. β-blockers and non-dihydropyridine calcium channel blockers (i.e., diltiazem or verapamil) help to prevent recurrence
6. Ablation of accessory pathway is the curative therapy with a 95% success rate. Heart block is a complication risk if the accessory pathway is close to septum.
7. Antiarrhythmics used for patients not wanting ablation and not responding to AV nodal blockers (see Table 21.1)

XIV. Wolff-Parkinson White syndrome (WPW)

A. Characteristics
1. Defined as the presence of short PR and Delta wave on EKG along with evidence of SVT

2. Delta wave: short PR and "slurring" of initial portion of the QRS
3. 0.2% of general population, about 70% asymptomatic
4. 60%–70% men
5. Predisposition to tachyarrhythmias
6. In asymptomatic patients, a Delta wave does not confirm WPW syndrome but rather a "WPW pattern" (WPW pattern should not be treated, but can be monitored; these patients should be referred to a cardiologist)

B. Etiology
1. Conduction through an accessory pathway that can conduct both antegrade and retrograde; the antegrade conduction produces a Delta wave, due to "pre-excitation" of the ventricle.
2. Can present as SVT and Delta waves after conversion back to NSR

C. Clinical manifestations
1. Patients may experience the same symptoms as SVT: palpitations, SOB, presyncope, fatigue, or diaphoresis.
2. Patients who present with atrial fibrillation present with wide and bizarre QRS's d/t pre-excitation; ventricular rates can be as high as 200–300 and can degenerate to ventricular fibrillation; these patients can be very symptomatic.

D. Treatment
1. Referral to cardiologist or electrophysiologist
2. WPW pattern on EKG: monitor, refer for expert consultation
3. WPW that presents in SVT, treat the same as you would SVT; vagal maneuvers, adenosine
4. WPW that presents in atrial fibrillation: avoid AV nodal blockers which can cause 1:1 conduction through the accessory pathway (e.g., HR's could be greater than 300 bpm).
5. In stable patients with atrial fibrillation, use drugs that prolong the refractory period of the bypass tract (procainamide or amiodarone) or consider transesophageal echocardiogram (TEE) and direct-current cardioversion (DCCV); in the unstable patient, move directly toward DCCV.
6. EP study and ablation of accessory pathway is the curative therapy and preferred choice.
7. Can also use antiarrhythmics (see Table 21.1)

XV. **Premature ventricular contractions (PVCs) (Figure 21.9)**
A. Etiology
1. Irritability of the myocardium due to the following:
   a. Electrolyte imbalance
   b. Hypoxia
   c. Acidosis
   d. Myocardial infarction
   e. Other

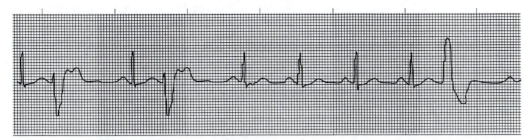

Figure 21.9. Premature ventricular contractions.

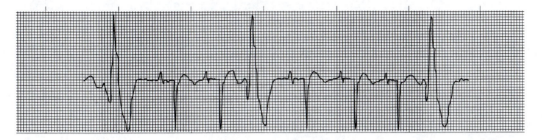

Figure 21.10A. Onifocal premature ventricular contractions

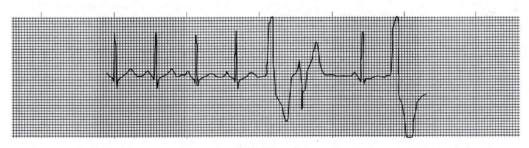

Figure 21.10B. Multifocal premature ventricular contractions

      2. A stimulus from the ventricle replaces the sinoatrial (SA) node as the pacemaker for one or more beats, and contraction occurs without the usual transmission from the atrium.

B. Clinical manifestations

      1. Patients may or may not be aware of PVCs

      2. Symptoms are usually related to the number and frequency of abnormal beats

      3. Patients may complain of "fluttering" or "palpitations" of the heart

      4. On the monitor, PVCs exhibit a wide QRS configuration that differs from that of the normal beat

C. Implications

      1. Unifocal PVCs that occur infrequently or have the same focus (i.e., have the same shape [Figure 21.10, A]), have limited significance, and may occur in the absence of heart disease

      2. An increase in the frequency of these beats is more significant, especially if the PVCs occur more often than 6 times per minute, or if the patient has had a very recent myocardial infarction.

3. PVCs that are the result of more than one focus (i.e., multifocal [Figure 21.10, B]) are more serious and may precede ventricular tachycardia or ventricular fibrillation.
   a. The risk is minimal if the beats are isolated.
   b. The danger increases if beats do the following:
      i. Are frequent (i.e., more than six per minute)
      ii. Are multifocal (have different shapes) (Figure 21.11)
      iii. Occur with every other beat (bigeminal) (Figure 21.12)
      iv. Occur with every third beat (trigeminal) (Figure 21.13)
      v. Occur repetitively (pairs)
      vi. Appear on the downslope of the T wave (when the heart is relatively refractory and electrically unstable)
   c. If a PVC lands on the downslope of the T wave, the patient may experience ventricular tachycardia and/or ventricular fibrillation.

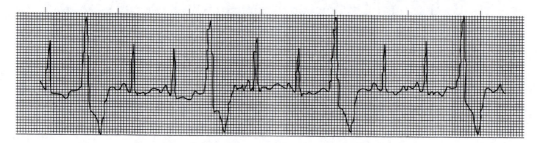

Figure 21.11. Multifocal premature ventricular contractions.

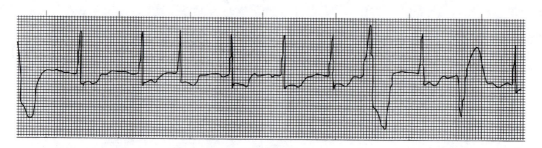

Figure 21.12. Regular sinus rhythm with bigeminal premature ventricular contractions.

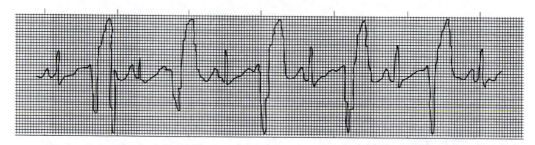

Figure 21.13. Regular sinus rhythm with trigeminal premature ventricular contractions.

D. Treatment
  1. None if asymptomatic
  2. Check electrolytes and replace PRN
  3. First line treatment for symptomatic PVCs is β-blockers which help to decrease sympathetic tone
  4. For symptomatic treatment of PVCs, consult cardiologist or electrophysiologist for consideration of antiarrhythmics or VT ablation.

XVI. Ventricular tachycardia (VT) (Figure 21.14)
  A. Etiology
    1. 3 or more wide complex QRS (greater than 120ms) that are ventricular in origin with a rate greater than 100 bpm
    2. Can originate anywhere below the AV node
    3. Monomorphic is the most common; uniform QRS and regular
    4. Non-sustained is defined as less than 30 seconds
    5. Can be caused by ischemia, scar tissue, electrolyte disturbances, QT prolongation, cardiomyopathy, or be idiopathic
  B. Clinical manifestations
    1. Patient can be asymptomatic
    2. Patients may feel palpitations, SOB, chest pain, or presyncope
    3. Patients could have VT arrest or sudden cardiac death
  C. Implications
    1. If untreated, VT produces rapid hemodynamic decompensation caused by inadequate filling and emptying of the ventricles
    2. If untreated, VT leads to VF, asystole, and death
  D. Treatment of VT
    1. Consult cardiologist or electrophysiologist—causes should be ruled out and treatment guided by experts; for stable VT and nonsustained VT, β-blockers are the mainstay
      a. Blocks the sympathetic response
      b. Slows sinus rate
    2. Treatment with amiodarone, sotalol, and mexiletine is used frequently to reduce the number and frequency of shocks.
      a. May be controversial due to a high side effect profile

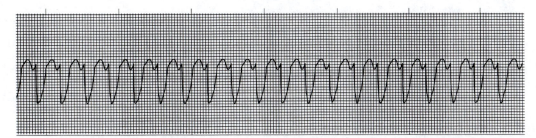

Figure 21.14. Ventricular tachycardia.

      b. Blocks potassium repolarization which increases wavelength for reentry

  3. Consider magnesium, 1–2 grams IV if torsades de pointes with prolonged QT interval is present

  4. Be prepared for cardioversion

  5. Treat underlying cause

      a. If ischemia is the cause, may need to go to cath lab or OR for revascularization

      b. Monitor and replace electrolytes

      c. Monitor QT for prolongation; if prolonged (general rule greater than 500), look for QT medication offenders

      d. Patients with cardiomyopathy may require ICD placement (e.g., primary prevention of sudden cardiac death in patients with an ejection fraction less than 35%)

  6. Consult electrophysiologist for consideration of EP study, ablation, and/or AICD placement

      a. AICD placement has supplanted the use of antiarrhythmics for the chronic management of ventricular arrhythmias. Concomitant antiarrhythmic therapy can be used in patients who often receive shocks to reduce the incidence of appropriate shocks from VT or VF, reduce the VT rate so that it can be terminated with antitachycardia pacing, reduce the incidence of inappropriate shocks triggered by the AF or atrial flutter and prolong the device's battery life.

E. Treatment of unstable VT. Follow ACLS guidelines:

  1. Begin high quality CPR with interruptions kept to a minimum; early defibrillation; CPR resumed for 5 cycles between shocks

  2. Epinephrine 1 mg every 3–5 minutes; vasopressin 40 units can replace 1st or 2nd dose of epinephrine; consider amiodarone 300 mg IVP after 3rd shock, 2nd dose of amiodarone 150 mg IVP.

  3. Lidocaine, 1–1.5 mg/kg with a 2nd dose of 0.5–0.75 mg/kg for refractory VT that does not respond to amiodarone

  4. Consider magnesium, 1–2 grams IV if torsades de pointes with prolonged QT interval is present

  5. For airway management, consider capnography

XVII. Ventricular fibrillation (V-fib) (Figure 21.15)

A. Etiology

  1. Often precipitated by VT

  2. No organized electrical activity

  3. Chaotic "wavy" baseline

  4. Characterized as course vs fine

  5. Same causes as VT

B. Clinical manifestations

  1. Sudden loss of consciousness and/or seizure-like activity

  2. Absence of pulse or respirations

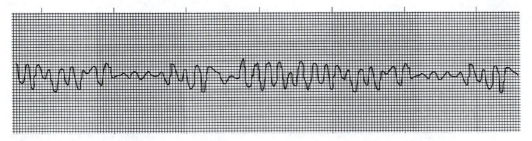

Figure 21.15. Ventricular fibrillation.

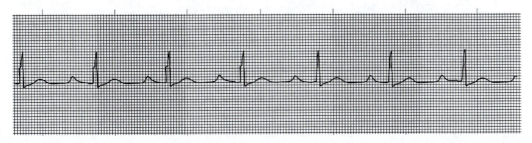

Figure 21.16. First-degree AV block

3. Cyanosis
4. Dilated pupils
C. Implications
   1. V-fib results in sudden death unless the arrhythmia is immediately terminated.
   2. Although V-fib may be reversed, irreversible brain damage may result from lack of perfusion.
D. Treatment of unstable V-fib. Follow ACLS guidelines:
   1. Begin high quality CPR with interruptions kept to a minimum; early defibrillation; CPR resumed for 5 cycles between shocks
   2. Epinephrine 1 mg every 3–5 minutes; vasopressin 40 units can replace 1st or 2nd dose of epinephrine; consider amiodarone 300 mg IVP after 3rd shock, 2nd dose of amiodarone 150 mg IVP
   3. Lidocaine, 1–1.5 mg/kg with a 2nd dose of 0.5–0.75 mg/kg for refractory VT that does not respond to amiodarone
   4. Consider magnesium, 1–2 grams IV if torsades de pointes with prolonged QT interval is present
   5. Airway management, consider capnography

XVIII. First-degree AV block (Figure 21.16)
A. Characteristics
   1. Delay in the impulse from the atria to the ventricles characterized by a PR interval of longer than 0.20 seconds
   2. Rhythm is regular, and the QRS complex is not affected
B. Etiology
   1. Occurs in all ages in both normal and diseased hearts
   2. Drugs
      a. Digoxin

        b. β-blockers

        c. Calcium channel blockers

        d. Damage to the junction

C. Clinical manifestations: usually asymptomatic

D. Treatment

    1. Rarely, if ever, needs treatment; untreated if asymptomatic

    2. If PR interval prolonged greater than 0.4 seconds and/or the patient is symptomatic, consult a cardiologist or electrophysiologist for consideration of permanent pacemaker.

XIX. Second-degree block (Mobitz type I) (Wenckebach) (Figure 21.17)

A. Characteristics

    1. Usually transient and occurs at the AV node

    2. Progressive prolongation of the PR interval until an impulse is completely blocked (dropped)

    3. Then, the pattern usually repeats

    4. R-R interval decreases prior to the blocked beat

    5. Atrial rhythm is usually regular, and the ventricular rhythm is usually irregular, with progressive shortening of the R-R interval before the blocked impulse.

    6. QRS complex is not affected

B. Etiology

    1. Usually from drug effects (e.g., digitalis, verapamil, propranolol)

    2. Myocardial infarction

    3. Sometimes seen in young athletes

C. Clinical manifestations

    1. Often asymptomatic

    2. If symptomatic, may see the following:

        a. Decreased cardiac output

        b. Hypotension

        c. LOC

D. Treatment

    1. Rarely an unstable arrhythmia, often no treatment needed

    2. If symptomatic consult expert

    3. Can progress to complete heart block; patients should be monitored for worsening conduction disease. This can be done as outpatient at regular intervals

    4. Evaluation of all medications, electrolytes, and thyroid function may be indicated. Echocardiogram to rule out structural heart disease

XX. Second-degree block (Mobitz type II) (Figure 21.18)

A. Characteristics

    1. Usually occurs below the level of the AV node

    2. Commonly associated with an organic lesion in the conduction pathway

    3. Associated with poorer prognosis than Mobitz type I

    4. PR interval does not lengthen prior to a dropped beat

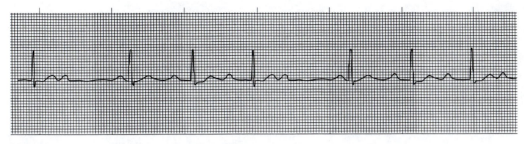

Figure 21.17. Second-degree block, Mobitz type I.

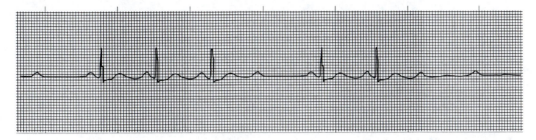

Figure 21.18. Second-degree block, Mobitz type II.

      5. More than one dropped beat may occur in succession

      6. Sometimes associated with widened QRS complex

      7. Overall, the atrial rate is unaffected, but the ventricular rate is less than the atrial rate.

  B. Etiology

      1. Failure of conduction below the AV node; generally secondary to structural damage to the conduction system (e.g., infarction, fibrosis, necrosis).

  C. Clinical manifestations: same as second-degree type 1

  D. Treatment

      1. Urgent cardiologist or electrophysiologist consultation for permanent pacemaker

      2. While waiting for cardiologist or electrophysiologist, patient should be hospitalized, on telemetry with transcutaneous pacemaker and closely monitored

      3. Work up of alternative causes (e.g., Lyme's disease, medications, metabolic abnormalities); echocardiogram to rule out structural heart disease

      4. IV atropine, 0.5 mg given every 3–5 minutes with a maximum of 3 mg, should be administered to patients with signs or symptoms of poor perfusion (altered mental status, chest pain, hypotension, shock).

      5. For treatment of symptomatic bradycardia, dopamine, epinephrine, and isoproterenol are alternatives when patient unresponsive to atropine, or as a temporizing measure while waiting for an available pacemaker.

XXI. **Third-degree AV block (complete heart block) (Figure 21.19)**

  A. Characteristics

      1. Complete absence of conduction between the atria and the ventricles

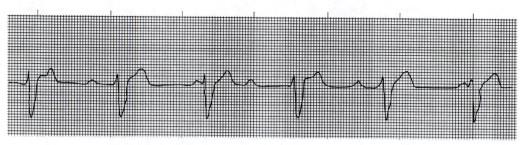

Figure 21.19 Third-degree AV block (complete heart block)

    2. Atrial rate is unaffected, and the ventricular rate is slower than the atrial rate

    3. Ventricular rate is usually 40–60 bpm

    4. PR interval will vary because the atria and the ventricles are depolarized from different pacemakers.

B. Etiology

    1. Myocardial ischemia or scar is the most common cause

    2. May also be caused by medications (e.g., digitalis), metabolic abnormalities, or any other degeneration of the conduction system

C. Clinical manifestations

    1. Asymptomatic if the ventricular rate is adequate

    2. Otherwise, progressive decrease in cardiac output leads to LOC

D. Treatment

    1. Urgent cardiologist or electrophysiologist consultation for permanent pacemaker

    2. While waiting for expert, patient should be hospitalized, on telemetry, with transcutaneous pacemaker and close monitoring.

    3. Work up for alternative causes (e.g., Lyme's disease, medications, metabolic abnormalities); echocardiogram to rule out structural heart

    4. IV atropine, 0.5 mg given every 3–5 minutes with a maximum of 3 mg, should be administered to patients with signs or symptoms of poor perfusion (altered mental status, chest pain, hypotension, shock)

    5. For treatment of symptomatic bradycardia, dopamine, epinephrine, and isoproterenol are alternatives when patient is unresponsive to atropine, or as a temporizing measure while waiting for an available pacemaker

Adult Tachycardia
(With Pulse)

1

Asses appropriateness for clinical condition.
Heart rate typically ≥ 150/min if tachyarrhythmia

2

Identify and treat underlying cause

- Maintain patent airway; assist breathing as necessary
- Oxygen (if hypoxemic)
- Cardiac monitor to identify rhythm; monitor blood pressure and oximetry

3

Persistent tachyarrhythmia
Causing:

- Hypotension?
- Acutely altered mental status?
- Signs of shock?
- Ischemic chest discomfort?
- Acute heart failure?

Yes →

4

Synchronized cardioversion
- Consider sedation
- If regular narrow complex, consider adenosine

No

5

Wide QRS?
≥ 0.12 second

Yes →

6

- IV access and 12-lead ECG if available
- Consider adenosine only if regular and monomorphic
- Consider antiarrhythmic infusion
- Consider expert consultation.

No

7

- IV access and 12-lead ECG if available
- Vagal maneuvers
- Adenosine (if regular)
- ß-blocker or calcium channel blocker
- Consider expert consultation

Doses/Details

Synchronized Cardioversion
Initial recommended doses:
- Narrow regular: 50-100 J
- Narrow irregular: 120-200 J biphasic or 200 J monophasic
- Wide regular: 100 J
- Wide irregular: defibrillation dose (Not synchronized)

Adenosine IV Dose:
First dose: 6 mg rapid IV push; follow with NS flush.
Second dose: 12 mg if required.

Antiarrhythmic Infusions for Stable Wide-QRS Tachycardia

Procainamide IV Dose:
20-50 mg/min until arrhythmia suppressed, hypotension ensues, QRS duration increases > 50%, or maximum dose 17 mg/kg given. Maintenance infusion: 1-4 mg/min. Avoid if prolonged QT or CHF.

Amiodarone IV Dose:
First dose: 150 mg over 10 minutes.
Repeat as needed if VT recurs.
Follow by maintenance infusion of 1 mg/min for first 6 hours.

Sotalol IV Dose:
100 mg (1.5 mg/kg) over 5 minutes.
Avoid if prolonged QT.

Figure 21.20. Tachycardia Algorithm. QRS = ventricular complex; IV = intravenous; ECG = electrocardiogram. Adapted from "2010 American Heart Association Guidelines for Cardiopulmonary Resuscitation and Emergency Cardiovascular Care Science," by R. W. Neumar, C. W. Otto, M. S. Link, S. L. Kronick, C. W. Callaway, P .J. Krudenchuck . . . L. J. Morrison, 2010, *Circulation, 122.*

BIBLIOGRAPHY

Anderson, J. L., Halperin, J. L., Albert, N. M., Bozkurt, B., Brindis, R. G., Curtis, L. H., . . . Shen, W. (2013). Management of patients with atrial fibrillation (compilation of 2006 ACCF/AHA/ESC and 2011 ACCF/AHA/HRS recommendations). *Journal of the American College of Cardiology, 61*(18), 1935–1944.

Cohn, E. G. (2012). *Flip and see ECG* (4th ed.). Philadelphia, PA: Elsevier Health Sciences.

Hazinski, M. F., Samson, R., & Schexnayder, S. (2010). *2010 Handbook of Emergency Cardiovascular Care for Healthcare Providers*. Dallas, TX: American Heart Association.

Sinz, E. (2013). *ACLS for experienced providers: Manual and resource text*. Dallas, TX: American Heart Association.

January, C. T., Wann, S., Alpert, J. S., Calkins, H., Cleveland, J. C., Cigarroa, J. E., . . . Yancy, C. W. (2014). 2014 AHA/ACC/HRS guideline for the management of patients with atrial fibrillation: Executive summary. *Journal of the American College of Cardiology*. doi:10.1016/j.jacc.2014.03.021

Karch, A. M. (2013). *2014 Lippincott's nursing drug guide*. Riverwoods, IL: Lippincott Williams & Wilkins.

Kee, J. L., Hayes, E. R., & McCuistion, L. E. (2012). *Pharmacology: A nursing process approach* (7th ed.). St. Louis, MO: Elsevier Saunders.

Levine, E. (2014). *CHADS2 score for stroke risk assessment in atrial fibrillation*. Retrieved from http://emedicine.medscape.com/article/2172597-overview

Lip, G. Y. (2014). Anticoagulation in older adults. In L. Leung, K. E. Schmader, & J. S. Tirnauer (Eds), *Uptodate*. Waltham, MA: UpToDate.

Peberdy, M. A., Callaway, C. W., Neumar, R. W., Geocadin, R. G., Zimmerman, J. L., Donnino, M., . . . Kronick, S. L. (2010). American Heart Association guidelines for cardiopulmonary resuscitation and emergency cardiovascular care. *Circulation, 122*, 5640–5933.

Poldermans, D., Bax, J. J., Boersma, E., Hert, S. D., Eeckhout, E., Fowkes, G., . . . Vermassen, F. (2009). Guidelines for pre-operative cardiac risk assessment and perioperative cardiac management in non-cardiac surgery. The task force for preoperative cardiac risk assessment and perioperative cardiac management in non-cardiac sugery of the European Society of Cardiology (ESC) and endorsed by the European Society of Anaesthesiology (ESA). *European Heart Journal, 30*(22), 2769–2812.

Tracy, C. M., Epstein, A. E., Darbar, D., DiMarco, J. P., Dunbar, S. B., Estes, M., . . . Varosy, P. D. (2012). 2012 ACCF/AHA/HRS focused update of the 2008 guidelines for device-based therapy for cardiac rhythm abnormalities: A report of the American College of Cardiology Foundation/American Heart Association Task Force on Practice Guidelines and the Heart Rhythm Society. *Circulation, 126*, 1784–1800.

Urden, L. D., Stacy, K. M., & Lough, M. E. (2010). *Critical care nursing: Diagnosis and management* (6th ed.). St. Louis, Mo.: Mosby/Elsevier.

Management of Pulmonary Disorders

Diagnostic Concepts of Oxygenation and Ventilation

AMITA AVADHANI • CHARLENE M. MYERS

PULMONARY PERFUSION

I. **Definition**
   A. Movement of mixed venous blood through the pulmonary capillary bed for the purpose of gas exchange between the blood and the alveolar air

II. **The pulmonary vascular system is a high-volume system with low capillary resistance.**
   A. Pulmonary blood flow is about 6 L/minute.
   B. Mean pulmonary arterial pressure is 15 mmHg.

III. **Regional differences in blood flow in the lungs**
   A. Lung bases receive a greater percentage of blood flow than do the apices.
   B. Factors that affect the distribution of pulmonary blood flow:
      1. Gravity and hydrostatic pressure differences within the blood vessels: a patient's blood must flow against gravity to the apices when the person is in the upright position.
      2. Effect of alveolar pressure: alveolar pressure may be greater than pulmonary capillary pressure in the apical and middle regions of lungs because of the following:
         a. Positive pressure ventilation
         b. Decreased right ventricular preload (decreased hydrostatic pressure), dehydration, and hemorrhage
         c. Air trapping in chronic obstructive pulmonary disease
      3. Effect of decreased PaO_2 (partial pressure of oxygen in arterial blood) (alveolar gas): local reflex that causes vasoconstriction of pulmonary arterioles supplying hypoxic alveoli

VENTILATION

I. **Definition**
   A. Mechanical movement of air into and out of the alveoli for the purpose of gas exchange between the atmosphere and capillary blood
   B. Gas flows from higher atmospheric to lower intrapulmonary pressure during inhalation.

II. **Regulation of ventilation**
   A. Central nervous system control
      1. Brain stem centers (medulla and pons): cells fire automatically to trigger inhalation, others fire to halt inhalation, and exhalation occurs passively.
      2. Cerebral cortex: allows voluntary control to override brain stem centers in response to chemical stimuli and lung inflation changes
   B. Chemical regulation
      1. Central chemoreceptors in medulla respond to increased partial pressure of carbon dioxide in arterial blood ($PaCO_2$) (hypercapnia) and decreased pH (acidosis) through medullary stimuli by increasing ventilatory depth and rate; hypercapnia is the major stimulus to alter ventilation.
      2. Peripheral chemoreceptors in aortic and carotid bodies respond to decreased PaO_2 (hypoxemia) by stimulating medullary centers to enhance ventilation.
      3. Patients with chronically high $PaCO_2$: hypercapnic ventilatory drive is lost; these patients respond only to changes in PaO_2 by stimulation of peripheral receptors to adjust ventilation (hypoxemic respiratory drive)
         a. Supplemental O_2: Administer low liter flows very carefully to prevent apnea (e.g., begin with 1–2 L/minute and assess).
         b. Do not withhold O_2 if needed; be prepared to assist with mechanical ventilation if respiratory drive is depressed.

III. **Work of breathing (WOB)**
   A. Definition: amount of effort required to overcome the elastic and resistive properties of the lungs and chest wall
   B. Elasticity (elastic recoil): tendency of the lungs to return to their original shape
      1. Lungs try to collapse because of tension between the interstitial elastic fibers and the surface of the alveoli
      2. Chest wall attempts to resist inward-moving recoil
   C. Compliance: measure of distensibility, or how easily the lungs and thorax can be stretched; describes resistance as a result of elastic properties. Increased compliance means less pressure is needed to stretch the lungs and/or thorax
      1. High compliance: easier to expand lung tissue (e.g., chronic obstructive pulmonary disease)

      2. Low compliance: stiff lungs; chest wall less distensible (e.g., pneumonia and acute respiratory distress syndrome)

  D. Resistance is determined by the radius of the airway through which air is flowing. Increased resistance means increased effort for ventilation and increased WOB.

IV. **Alveolar ventilation: amount of air that reaches alveoli and participates in gas exchange**

  A. $PaCO_2$: best indicator of alveolar ventilation

  B. Normal: $PaCO_2$ is 35–45 mmHg

ALVEOLAR DIFFUSION

I. **Definition**

  A. Exchange of O_2 and CO_2 across the alveolocapillary membrane

  B. Oxygen diffuses down the concentration gradient from higher alveolar pressure (PAO_2) to lower pulmonary capillary pressure (PaO_2).

  C. CO_2 diffuses at a rate 20 times greater than that of O_2 from capillary to alveolus

II. **A-a gradient: alveolar-to-arterial oxygen gradient; $AaDO_2$: alveolar-to-arterial oxygen difference**

  A. A calculation to aid in diagnosing the degree of a patient's hypoxemia

  B. Formula: difference between partial pressure of O_2 in the alveoli (PAO_2) and partial pressure of O_2 in arterial blood (PaO_2)

    1. PAO_2: calculated

    2. PaO_2: from arterial blood gases

    3. Note: A-a gradient OR $AaDO_2 = PAO_2 - PaO_2$

    4. Formula to calculate PAO_2

$$PaO_2 = \frac{PIO_2 - PaCO_2}{0.8 \text{ (respiratory quotient)}}$$

$$PIO_2 = \text{Partial pressure of inspired oxygen: } 21\%–100\%$$

$$Pb = \text{Barometric pressure: } 760 \text{ mmHg (at sea level)}$$

$$PH_2O = \text{Water vapor pressure: } 47 \text{ mmHg}$$

$$PaO_2 = \frac{[0.21 \times (760 - 47)] - 40}{0.8}$$

$$PaO_2 = 0.21 \times 713 - 50$$

$$PaO_2 = 100 \text{ mmHg}$$

$$\text{Normal } PaO_2 = 60–100 \text{ mmHg}$$

  C. Normal values: difference between alveolar and arterial oxygen

    1. Young adult breathing room air ($FIO_2 = 21\%$): less than 10 mmHg difference

    2. Adult older than age 60 on room air: less than 20 mmHg difference

    3. Breathing FIO_2 100% = less than 50 mmHg difference

OXYGEN TRANSPORT IN THE CIRCULATION

I.   **O_2 Carried in the blood**
   A. O_2 dissolved in plasma (3% of total) = PaO_2 (normal is 80–100 mmHg)
   B. O_2 bound to hemoglobin (Hgb) (97% of total) = SaO_2 (oxygen saturation) (normal is 95%–100%)
   C. Note: reserve for times of increased demand
   D. Note: assess Hgb level for oxygen-carrying capacity. If Hgb level is decreased yet adequately saturated, the patient is not adequately oxygenated

II.   **PaO_2 and SaO_2: indirect measurement of O_2 available to tissues**

III.   **O_2 that stays bound to Hgb is useless to body cells.**
   A. Affinity: ability of Hgb to release O_2
      1. Weak affinity: easily releases O_2 to tissues
      2. Strong affinity: easily accepts and retains O_2

IV.   **Oxyhemoglobin dissociation curve: demonstrates affinity of Hgb for O_2**
   A. Flat part of curve: binding portion in lungs
      1. Increased affinity; binds easily: PaO_2 is 60–100 mmHg, with SaO_2 greater than 90%
   B. Steep part of curve: dissociation portion at the tissue level
      1. Weaker affinity: Hgb readily dissociates O_2 when PaO_2 falls to below 60 mmHg.

V.   **Shifts in oxyhemoglobin dissociation curve: other patient variables affect affinity of Hgb for O_2**
   A. Shift to the left: greater affinity
      1. Binds easily in the lung; less unloading to tissues
      2. Increased affinity leads to possible tissue hypoxia due to strong bond between Hgb and O_2; need for O_2 may have decreased
      3. Causes:
         a. Alkalosis
         b. Hypothermia
         c. Decreased 2,3-diphosphoglycerate
   B. Shift to the right: decreased affinity
      1. Hgb unloads more O_2 to tissues
      2. Delivery of O_2 to tissues improves as long as loading of O_2 in lungs is adequate
      3. Causes:
         a. Acidosis
         b. Increased tissue metabolism, anaerobic metabolism, and hyperthermia
         c. Increased 2,3-diphosphoglycerate

VI. **Continuous SvO_2 (mixed venous oxygen saturation) monitoring: monitoring O_2 transport and extraction**

    A. Measure of mixed venous O_2 saturation by the pulmonary artery catheter

        1. Continuous measure and display of mixed venous oxygen saturation

        2. Hgb reflects light, which can be measured according to its saturation.

    B. Normal SvO_2: 75%; Hgb unloads 25% of its O_2 before returning to the heart.

        1. Normal ratio of supply of O_2 to demand: 4:1

        2. Acceptable SvO_2 range: 60%–80%

Venous blood gases	Arterial blood gases
pH = 7.36	pH = 7.4
$PvCO_2$ = 47 mmHg	$PaCO_2$ = 40 mmHg
HCO_2 = 24 mEq/L	HCO_3 = 24 mEq/L
PvO_2 = 40 mmHg	PaO_2 = 100 mmHg
SvO_2 = 75%	SaO_2 = 99%
Hgb = 15 g	Hgb = 15 g

    C. Trends in changes in SvO_2: assesses the effectiveness of peripheral oxygen delivery; may signal need to assess cardiac profile

        1. SvO_2 less than 60% or trend downward: patient has tapped the venous reserve of O_2

            a. Implies increased tissue extraction of O_2

                i. Note: greater risk for anaerobic metabolism

            b. Causes

                i. Decreased O_2 supply (e.g., decreased FIO_2, anemia, and decreased CO)

                ii. Increased O_2 demand (e.g., fever, increased WOB, shivering, pain, and agitation)

            c. SvO_2 less than 40% = anaerobic metabolism leading to organ dysfunction

        2. SvO_2 greater than 80%: implies decreased tissue extraction of oxygen

            a. High return of O_2 is often an earlier indicator of change in patient status than change in hemodynamic parameters

            b. Causes:

                i. Increased O_2 supply (e.g., FIO_2 greater than need and polycythemia)

                ii. Decreased O_2 demand (e.g., sleep and hypothermia)

                iii. Decreased effective O_2 delivery and uptake by cells (e.g., sepsis, cyanide toxicity, and shift of O_2/Hgb curve to left)

VII. Oxygen supply/demand balance: calculations

ROI_2 = venous O_2 return to heart

$= CI \times$ (venous O_2 content) $\times 10$

$= CI \times (1.34 \times Hgb \times Svo_2) \times 10$

$= 3 \times (1.34 \times 15 \times .75) \times 10$

$= 3 \times (15) \times 10$

$= 450$ mL/min/m²

DOI_2 = arterial O_2 delivery to tissues

$= CI \times$ (arterial O_2 content) $\times 10$

$= CI \times (1.34 \times Hgb \times SaO_2) \times 10$

$= 3 \times (1.34 \times 15 \times 0.98) \times 10$

$= 3 \times (20) \times 10$

$= 600$ mL/min/m²

VO_2 = tissue O_2 demand

$DOI_2 - ROI_2 = VO_2$

600 mL $- 450$ mL $= 150$ mL/min/m²

Note. CI = cardiac index; Prolonged Svo_2 and/or prolonged Vo_2 are poor prognosis.

VENTILATOR ADJUSTMENTS

I. Respiratory acidosis
A. The goal is to increase PCO_2
B. Make the following ventilator adjustments:
  1. Increase the respiratory rate; watch for auto-PEEP with high respiratory rate (beware of hypotension from reduced preload)
  2. Increase the tidal volume:
     a. In assist control mode, directly increase the tidal volume.
     b. In pressure control or pressure support modes, increase the inspiratory pressure to increase tidal volume.
  3. In acute lung injury, some extent of hypercapnia/respiratory acidosis should be generally tolerated, rather than raising the tidal volume greater than 8 ml/kg.

II. Respiratory alkalosis
A. The goal is to decrease the PCO_2
B. Make the following ventilator adjustments:
  1. Decrease the respiratory rate
  2. Decrease the tidal volume
  3. If the patient is breathing faster than the set rate, these strategies will not work.
C. Determine the cause of respiratory alkalosis and correct the cause, for example, sepsis, pulmonary embolism, pain, and so forth.

III. Hypoxemia
A. The goal is to improve tissue oxygenation by improving SaO_2, PO_2, and PaO_2.
B. Increase FiO_2; increase PEEP. (Watch out for the drop in cardiac output from decreased preload associated with increase in PEEP. Preload can be augmented with IV fluids.)

IV.   Difficult ventilation may first manifest itself as increase in peak inspiratory pressure, resulting from the following:

    A. Bronchospasm

    B. Secretions in the airways, endotracheal tube, and ventilator tubing

    C. Pulmonary edema

    D. Pneumothorax

    E. Intubation in the right mainstem

    F. Mucus plug

    G. Worsening airspace disease (adult respiratory distress syndrome, pneumonia, and pulmonary edema)

    H. Agitated patient with ventilator dyssynchrony

    I. Therefore, it would be important to address the cause to correct the ventilatory issue.

BIBLIOGRAPHY

Andreoli, T. E., & Cecil, R. L. (2010). *Andreoli and Carpenter's Cecil essentials of medicine* (8th ed.). Philadelphia, PA: Saunders/Elsevier.

Criner, G. J., Barnette, R. E., & Alonzo, G. E. (2010). *Critical care study guide text and review* (2nd ed.). New York, NY: Springer.

Cyna, A. M. (2011). *Handbook of communication in anaesthesia and critical care: A practical guide to exploring the art.* Oxford: Oxford University Press.

Galvagno, S. M. (2014). *Emergency pathophysiology clinical applications for prehospital care.* Hoboken: Teton NewMedia, Inc.

George, R. B. (2005). *Chest medicine: Essentials of pulmonary and critical care medicine.* Philadelphia, PA: Lippincott Williams & Wilkins.

Goroll, A. H., & Mulley, A. G. (2009). *Primary care medicine: Office evaluation and management of the adult patient* (6th ed.). Philadelphia: Wolters Kluwer Health/Lippincott Williams & Wilkins.

Marino, P. L. (2013). *Marino's the ICU book* (4th ed.). Philadelphia, PA: Lippincott Williams & Wilkins.

Respiratory Therapy Cave: Oxyhemoglobin Dissociation Curve. (2010, July 7). *Respiratory Therapy Cave: Oxyhemoglobin Dissociation Curve.* Retrieved September 23, 2014, from http://respiratorytherapycave.blogspot.com/2010/07/oxyhemoglobin-dissociation-curve.html

Scanlon, C. L., Wilkins, R. L., & Stoller, J. K. (2012). *Egan's fundamentals of respiratory care* (10th ed.). St. Louis, MO: Mosby.

Wiegand, D. J. (2013). *AACN Procedure Manual for Critical Care* (6th ed.). London: Elsevier Health Sciences.

Wilkins, R. L., Dexter, J. R., & Heuer, A. J. (2010). *Clinical assessment in respiratory care* (6th ed.). St. Louis, MO: Mosby.

CHAPTER **23**

Measures of Oxygenation and Ventilation

BIMBOLA AKINTADE • CHARLENE M. MYERS

OXYGENATION AND VENTILATION

I. **Definition**
   A. Closely interrelated terms that collectively refer to the processes by which oxygen (O_2) and carbon dioxide (CO_2) are transported between atmosphere and tissue via concentration gradients, perfusion, and affinity of hemoglobin for oxygen
   B. Oxygenation refers to movement of oxygen into the blood and its transport and delivery to tissue.
      1. Diffusion pressures, determined by gradients between the respective partial pressures of alveolar, plasma, and tissue oxygen, allow for movement of oxygen from alveoli to blood to tissue.
      2. Hemoglobin and its affinity for oxygen allows for blood transport of far more oxygen than could be dissolved in plasma alone.
      3. Perfusion, determined by cardiac output and vascular tone, affects oxygen delivery to tissue capillaries.
   C. Ventilation refers to the exchange of extrapulmonary and intra-alveolar gas mixtures.
      1. Resupply of oxygen diffused into blood and removal of CO_2 diffused from blood allow for maintenance of their respective alveolar-capillary pressure gradients
      2. Patent airway(s), neuromuscular function, and structural integrity of chest wall allow for inspiratory and expiratory air flow.
II. **Clinical measurements**
   A. Exercise tolerance: Ability to perform a normal exercise load (e.g., climb a flight of stairs without stopping) suggests adequate oxygenation and ventilation.
   B. Dyspnea, air hunger, work of breathing

      1. Does the patient report distress?

      2. Does the patient appear distressed?

C. Cyanosis

      1. Dusky bluish tint from excessive amounts of unsaturated hemoglobin

      2. The more central the cyanosis, the greater its severity. For example, cyanosis evident on the face and chest is more severe than cyanosis limited to the fingertips.

D. Arterial blood gases (ABGs)

      1. Partial pressures of oxygen and carbon dioxide

      2. Oxygen saturation of arterial hemoglobin

      3. pH

      4. Presence or absence of metabolic imbalance

      5. Normal values for arterial blood gas

         a. pH = 7.35–7.45

         b. Partial pressure of oxygen in arterial blood (PaO_2) = 80–97 mmHg

         c. Partial pressure of carbon dioxide in arterial blood ($PaCO_2$) = 35–45 mmHg

         d. Bicarbonate (HCO3) = 22–26 mEq/L

         e. Base excess, -3 to +3 mEq/L

         f. Saturation of arterial oxygen (SaO_2) greater than 98%

      6. Partial pressures of arterial oxygen and carbon dioxide and arterial oxygen saturation decline as altitude above sea level increases.

      7. Oxygenation

         a. Interpret PaO_2 in light of fraction of inspired oxygen (FIO_2). As a general rule, PaO_2 should be 4–5 times the percentage of O_2 (e.g., the FIO_2 of room air is 21%, and a normal PaO_2 is 80–97 mmHg).

         b. PaO_2/FiO_2 ratio describes the degree of impairment in pulmonary gas exchange. Normal ratios are 300–500 mmHg. Low ratios indicate impaired oxygen exchange, while ratios less than 200 mmHg indicated severe hypoxemia.

      8. Ventilation

         a. Ventilation is reciprocally reflected by $PaCO_2$. For example, a rising $PaCO_2$ means that a decrease in ventilation has occurred (and vice versa).

         b. Every 10 mmHg shift in $PaCO_2$ should produce a reciprocal 0.08 shift in pH. A $PaCO_2$ of 50 mm would thus predict a pH of 7.32. Any difference from that predicted shift must be attributed to a concurrent metabolic imbalance or compensation.

III. Limitations

    A. Invasiveness

        1. Drawing blood for an ABG measurement is often painful for the patient and involves significant risk of injury and compromise of perfusion distal to the site.

        2. If frequent measurements are required, as in a critically ill or mechanically ventilated patient, an indwelling arterial catheter should be placed.

    B. An ABG is not a continuous measurement, and its accuracy is specific only to the time it was drawn.

        1. A more continuous measurement would be peripheral oxygen saturation, measured by a pulse oximeter or an end-tidal CO_2 measurement device.

    C. The ABG sample must be handled with care.

        1. The sample must not be allowed to clot and must be heparinized.

        2. Excessive amounts of heparin in a small blood sample will alter the pH.

        3. Any air bubbles must be expelled from the syringe because oxygen and carbon dioxide in the sample will equilibrate with the air bubble.

        4. If more than a few minutes may pass before the sample is measured, it must be chilled to limit the ongoing metabolism of cellular components.

    D. Sample may inadvertently be taken from a vein in close proximity to the intended arterial site.

        1. The clinician must make an astute analysis for results inconsistent with an arterial sample.

PULSE OXIMETRY

I. Definition

    A. Pulse oximetry is a noninvasive, continuous, and relatively inexpensive method for transcutaneous measurement of the degree to which hemoglobin in arterial blood is saturated with oxygen (SaO_2).

II. Mechanism

    A. Pulse oximetry (SpO_2) uses a light-emitting diode to transmit light in the trans-red and near-infrared wavelengths through perfused tissue to a receiving sensor.

    B. The device compares light emitted versus light received by the sensor to calculate light absorbed by oxyhemoglobin and thus, the saturation of hemoglobin with oxygen.

    C. The device can detect a pulsatile fluctuation in saturation and can selectively display the highest measurement as the SpO_2 (presumed to reflect the SaO_2).

    D. The pulse oximetry probe may be applied for intermittent or continuous measurements. It is typically placed on a digit but can be placed on an earlobe, cheek, nose, or toe.

    E. The accuracy of the displayed reading may be affected by several factors.

        1. Abnormal hemoglobins

        2. Movement of the probe may create artifact, causing the measurement to be rejected. Alternative placement or stabilization with tape may be required.

        3. It is recommended but not always necessary that nail polish be removed so an accurate reading is obtained.

III. **Normal values are variable and must be interpreted in light of altitude, the patient's age, and cardiopulmonary function.**

    A. Remember that the relationship between oxygen saturation and partial pressure of oxygen is nonlinear. It is prudent to commit to memory the following:

        1. SpO_2 of 90% represents a PaO_2 of 60 mmHg

        2. SpO_2 of 75% is a PaO_2 of 40 mmHg

        3. SpO_2 of 50% is a PaO_2 of 27 mmHg

    B. Factors that can distort the normal relationship between oxygen saturation and partial pressure of oxygen must be considered.

        1. With alkalosis or hypothermia, the PaO_2 may be lower than predicted by the SpO_2.

        2. With acidosis or hyperthermia, the PaO_2 may be higher than predicted by the SpO_2.

IV. **Limitations of pulse oximetry**

    A. Pulse oximetry is only a presumptive reflection of SaO_2 and does not provide information regarding pH, $PaCO_2$, or respiratory rate.

    B. Pulse oximetry is confounded by the presence of carbon monoxide.

        1. The device will misinterpret carboxyhemoglobin as oxyhemoglobin and thereby provide a false elevation.

        2. When carbon monoxide poisoning is suspected, an ABG analysis is a more reliable measurement of oxygenation.

    C. Methylene blue dye and, similarly, methemoglobinemia will be misinterpreted by the oximeter as deoxygenated hemoglobin, thus falsely indicating a lowered oxygen saturation.

    D. Pulse oximetry is most valuable as a reading of central oxygenation.

        1. In some circumstances (e.g., shock, hypothermia, severe peripheral vascular disease, use of high-dose vasopressors), a peripherally placed oximeter will not accurately reflect central oxygenation.

        2. Remember that pulse oximetry measures oxygen saturation, not oxygen content. For example, an anemic patient may have high oxygen saturation, but low oxygen content. (100% of half is still half!)

MEASUREMENT OF CLINICAL PERFUSION

I. **Definition**

    A. Technique of using blood flow to direct a balloon-tipped catheter from the central venous circulation through the right side of the heart into the pulmonary artery (PA) for the purpose of hemodynamic monitoring

II. **General description**

    A. The most basic PA catheter consists of three lumina, each accessed by its separate respective port.

        1. A distal lumen opens at the tip of the catheter.

        2. A proximal lumen opens approximately 30 cm from the distal tip.

        3. A lumen opens into a balloon immediately proximal to the distal tip.

    B. The catheter is approximately 100–110 cm long and has markings every 10 cm to allow measurement of how far the catheter has been inserted.

    C. Most PA catheters have a temperature sensor at the tip that provides an accurate core temperature and permits calculation of cardiac output via a thermodilution technique.

        1. A known temperature change is induced in the blood flow upstream from the probe.

            a. Rapid manual injection of 10 ml of room temperature saline via the proximal port for intermittent measurements

            b. Frequent sequential heating via a heating coil located 10–20 cm from the distal tip for "continuous" measurements

        2. As ongoing blood flow dilutes the temperature change (thermodilution), cardiac output is calculated on the basis of rate of return to baseline blood temperature.

            a. A faster return to baseline will result in a higher cardiac output calculation (and vice versa).

    D. Common versions of the catheter may incorporate additional ports and functions.

        1. A venous infusion port is usually located within a centimeter of the proximal port and may be used interchangeably.

        2. An oximetry sensor on the distal tip can allow measurement of mixed venous oxygen saturation (SvO_2).

        3. SvO_2 is an important value in guiding resuscitation, and supplies information about both respiratory and circulatory systems.

        4. It is a valuable measure of systemic oxygenation. It reflects the relationship between supply and demand, and tissue oxygenation.

        5. Measure of less than 70% indicates systemic delivery is impaired.

        6. Pacing capabilities may be provided via integrated pacing electrodes or a dedicated port through which a pacing wire may be inserted.

III. **Catheter placement**
   A. Central venous access, most commonly at an internal jugular, subclavian, or femoral site, is first attained with a large-bore (6–8.5 French) introducer catheter.
   B. The PA catheter is advanced through the introducer and is positioned by flow-directed balloon flotation.
   C. The catheter is positioned with the distal tip in a branch of the pulmonary artery.
      1. The most common placement leaves the distal tip in the right branch.
      2. With normal anatomy, the proximal port will be positioned in the right atrium.
      3. Ongoing assessment of catheter placement is essential.
         a. Proper placement will most commonly occur with the catheter inserted approximately 50–60 cm
         b. Astute analysis of chest X-ray and pressure waveforms measured at distal and proximal ports can confirm placement.

IV. **Indications for placement**
   A. PA catheterization is indicated only in the following circumstances:
      1. Specific hemodynamic parameters cannot be adequately inferred by less invasive clinical assessment
         a. Differentiation between cardiogenic (high pulmonary capillary wedge pressure [PCWP], normal pulmonary artery pressure [PAP]) and pulmogenic (normal PCWP, high PAP) pulmonary edema
         b. Cardiac output/cardiac index (CO/CI), systemic vascular resistance (SVR), pulmonary vascular resistance (PVR), SvO_2
      2. Accurate, direct measurements are required to guide titration of therapy.

V. **Contraindications to placement of a PA catheter**
   A. No absolute contraindications
   B. Relative contraindications include the following:
      1. Coagulopathies (for fear of uncontrolled bleeding at deep central vascular puncture site)
      2. Left bundle branch blocks (for fear of complete heart block resulting from interruption of right bundle branch function during catheter placement)
      3. Presence of temporary pacing catheter (for fear of disruption of pacing)

VI. **Information provided by the pulmonary catheter is extensive; however, the quality of this information is highly dependent on the integrity of the monitoring system (monitor, transducers, tubing) and the ability of the clinician to assess the reliability of the information and the system that generates it.**

A. Pressure in the central venous space (CVP) is measured though the proximal port.
   1. Reflects right ventricular (RV) end-diastolic filling pressure (RV preload)
   2. Most often used to infer general systemic volume status
   3. Used in calculation of SVR
B. Pressure measured at the distal port is dependent on whether the balloon is inflated
   1. When the balloon is not inflated, the pressure measured is the PAP.
   2. When the balloon is inflated (and properly positioned), it occludes ("wedges") the branch of the PA in which it is positioned.
   3. Pressure measured is the PCWP
   4. Reflects left ventricular (LV) end-diastolic filling pressure (LV preload)
   5. Most often used to infer left ventricular function
   6. Used in calculation of PVR
C. The temperature probe accurately measures core temperature.
D. Directly measured pressures and temperature are used as variables included in calculation of hemodynamic parameters, most prominently CO/CI, SVR, and PVR

VII. Complications
A. Sepsis
   1. Limit risk by scrupulous site care/protection
   2. Limit duration at site to 7–10 days
B. Pulmonary hemorrhage
   1. Use minimal inflation of balloon that achieves wedge
   2. Inflate only as long as required to get the measurement
   3. Do not inflate against resistance.
   4. Avoid unnecessary inflations.
   5. Pulmonary hemorrhage is usually heralded by hematemesis.
C. Cardiac rhythm disturbances—associated with ventricular stimulation by catheter tip
   1. Usually occurs during placement as catheter passes through RV
   2. May herald displacement of catheter from PA into RV
D. Thrombocytopenia—may be associated with prolonged catheter placement

FLUID RESUSCITATION

I. Definition
A. Process by which optimal cardiac output, and thus adequate perfusion to vital organs, is restored by increasing intravascular volume from exogenous or endogenous sources

II. Indicators of inadequate intravascular volume
A. No reason to suspect cardiogenic or neurogenic shock
B. Evidence of inadequate ventricular filling pressures (preload)

1. Hypotension, tachycardia, low CVP, low PCWP
2. Flat neck veins in the Trendelenburg position

C. Decreased urine output—less than 0.5 ml/kg/hour

D. Obvious history of significant volume wasting disease
   1. Hemorrhage
   2. Prolonged emesis or diarrhea
   3. Prolonged diaphoresis
   4. Excess diuresis
   5. Sepsis

E. Poor response to early goal-directed therapy

III. **Fluid resuscitation in a seriously ill patient should be managed in a critical care setting.**

A. Consideration should be given to the placement of adequate monitoring devices, including the following:
   1. Arterial catheter for monitoring and sampling purposes
   2. CVP which is a hemodynamic parameter to measure and monitor fluid status
   3. Urinary bladder catheter to provide an accurate measurement of urine production

B. Body temperature should be monitored during large-volume resuscitations
   1. Substantial amounts of room temperature fluids or chilled blood products can rapidly chill a patient.
   2. Fluids should be warmed before administration, if hypothermia is evident.
   3. In actively bleeding patients or patients with hemorrhagic shock, administration of cool/cold blood products may lead to coagulopathy.

C. At least two large-bore (at least 16-gauge) intravenous catheters may be lifesaving.
   1. Catheter should be placed in as large a vessel as can be accessed readily
   2. Peripheral access should be no more distal than the anticubital veins

IV. **Choices for Fluid Resuscitation**

A. Crystalloid solutions
   1. Normal saline (0.9% NS) is a good choice for routine fluid resuscitation.
      a. When administering 1 L, only approximately 250 ml remain intravascular; the rest remains in the interstitial space.
   2. Lactated Ringer's solution has a wider variety of elemental constituents than normal saline and is commonly employed in the operating suite.
      a. When infused in large volumes, can lead to hyperchloremic acidosis due to high concentration of chloride

3. Dextrose-containing solutions come in a wide variety of concentrations.
   a. These should be used only after the patient's need for dextrose is considered.
   b. Dextrose-containing solutions are not first-line agents for volume expansion.
B. Packed RBCs
   1. Fluid of choice for major hemorrhage after PRBCs
   2. Each unit of red cells typically increases the hematocrit of a 70-kg person by 3%.
C. Colloid solutions, such as albumin, may be thought of as intravascular sponges that, through oncotic attraction, absorb volume from the extravascular space and hold it within the intravascular space.
   1. Use with caution because this effect is transient and does little to correct the primary problem of decreased intravascular volume.
   2. Colloid solutions should be reserved for specific indications, such as refractory hypovolemia, among others.
D. Fresh frozen plasma, platelets, and cryoprecipitate are not useful in fluid resuscitation, except as these relate to correction of underlying hemorrhagic conditions.

V. **Adequacy of fluid resuscitation may be judged by clinical indicators such as the following:**
A. Normalization of blood pressure and heart rate
B. Increasing urinary output
C. Normalization of hemodynamic parameters such as CVP, PCWP, CO/CI, and SVR

BIBLIOGRAPHY

Dries, D. J. (2013). Traumatic shock and tissue hypoperfusion: Nonsurgical management. In J. E. Parrillo & R. P. Dellinger (Eds.), *Critical care medicine: Principles of diagnosis and management in the adult* (4th ed., pp. 409–431). Philadelphia, PA: Elsevier Saunders.

Eskaros, S. M., Papadakos, P. J., & Lachmann, B. (2009). Respiratory monitoring. In R. D. Miller, L. I. Eriksson, L. A. Fleisher, J. P. Weiner-Kronish, & W. L. Young (Eds.), *Miller's anesthesia* (7th ed., pp. 1411–1442). Philadelphia, PA: Churchill Livingstone Elsevier.

Fontes, M. L., Skubas, N., & Osorio, J. (2011). Cardiac tamponade. In F. F. Yao, M. L. Fontes, & V. Malhotra (Eds.), *Yao and Artusio's anesthesiology: Problem-oriented patient management* (7th ed.). Philadelphia, PA: Wolters Kluwer/Lippincott, Williams & Wilkins.

Gadepalli, S. K., & Hirschl, R. B. (2014). Mechanical ventilation in pediatric surgical disease. In G. W. Holcomb, P. J. Murphy, & D. J. Ostlie (Eds.), *Ashcraft's pediatric surgery* (6th ed.). Philadelphia, PA: Elsevier Saunders.

Galvagno, S. M. (2013). *Emergency pathophysiology: Clinical applications for prehospital care.* Jackson, WY: Teton NewMedia.

Green, D., & Paklet, L. (2010). Latest developments in peri-operative monitoring of the high-risk major surgery patient. *International Journal of Surgery, 8*(2), 90–99. doi:10.1016/j.ijsu.2009.12.004

Kieninger, A. N., & Lipsett, P. A. (2009). Hospital-acquired pneumonia: Pathophysiology, diagnosis, and treatment. *Surgical Clinics of North America, 89*(2), 439–461.

Kraft, M. (2011). Approach to the patient with respiratory disease. In L. Goldman & A. I. Schafer (Eds.), *Goldman's Cecil medicine* (24th ed.). Philadelphia, PA: Elsevier Saunders.

Leppikangas, H., Järvelä, K., Sisto, T., Maaranen, P., Virtanen, M., Lehto, P., . . . Lindgren, L. (2011). Preoperative levosimendan infusion in combined aortic valve and coronary bypass surgery. *British Journal of Anaesthesia.* doi:10.1093/bja/aeq402

Mishra, N., & Pothal, S. (2013). Pulmonary manifestations of liver diseases. *World Clinics: Pulmonary and Critical Care Medicine, 2*(2), 424–443.

Murphey, E. D., Sherwood, E. R., & Toliver-Kinsky, T. (2012). The immunological response and strategies for intervention. In D. N. Herndon (Ed.), *Total Burn Care* (4th ed., pp. 265–276). Philadelphia, PA: Elsevier Saunders.

Ohye, R. G., & Hirsch, J. C. (2012). Congenital heart disease and anomalies of the great vessels. In A. G. Coran, N. S. Adzick, T. M. Krummel, J. M. Laberge, R. C. Shamberger, & A. A. Caldamone (Eds.), *Pediatric Surgery* (7th ed., pp. 1647–1672). Philadelphia, PA: Elsevier Saunders Mosby.

Schroeder, R. A., Barbeito, A., Bar-Yosef, S., & Mark, J. B. (2009). Cardiovascular monitoring. In R. D. Miller, L. I. Eriksson, L. A. Fleisher, J. P. Weiner-Kronish, & W. L. Young (Eds.), *Miller's Anesthesia* (7th ed., pp. 1267–1328). Philadelphia, PA: Churchill Livingstone Elsevier.

Tamura, T. (2014). Sensing technologies for biomedical telemetry. In K. S. Nikita (Ed.), *Handbook of Biomedical Telemetry* (pp. 76–107). Hoboken, NJ: John Wiley and Sons.

Villar, J., Blanco, J., Añón, J. M., Santos-Bouza, A., Blanch, L., Ambrós, A., . . . Kacmarek, R. M. (2011). The ALIEN study: Incidence and outcome of acute respiratory distress syndrome in the era of lung protective ventilation. *Intensive Care Medicine, 37*(12), 1932–1941. Retrieved from http://icmjournal.esicm.org/Journals/abstract.html?doi=10.1007/s00134–011–2380–4

Weinberger, S. E., Cockrill, B. A., & Mandel, J. (2013). *Principles of pulmonary medicine* (6th ed.). Philadelphia, PA: Elsevier Saunders.

West, J. B. (2012). *Pulmonary pathophysiology: The essentials* (8th ed.). Philadelphia, PA: Wolters Kluwer Health/Lippincott, Williams, & Wilkins.

CHAPTER 24

The Chest X-ray

VICTORIA F. KU • THOMAS W. BARKLEY, JR.

GENERAL PRINCIPLES

I. **Most common views as an inpatient**
   A. Anteroposterior (AP) films with back against the film plate
      1. Usually obtained with a portable x-ray machine
         a. Indicated when patient's condition precludes prudent travel
         b. Most often done supine unless specified as upright
      2. May limit attainment of optimal image
         a. Increase magnification and decrease sharpness of the image
         b. Supine position
            i. May limit inspiration and lead to misinterpretation
            ii. Unable to accurately assess free pleural fluid level due to distribution of fluid throughout the whole lung
            iii. Flattening of posterior surface of heart, causing heart to be falsely widened up to 15%
   B. Posteroanterior (PA) films with chest against film plate
      1. Usually obtained in the x-ray suite
      2. Allows for optimal image
         a. Less magnification, with sharper image
         b. Done in the upright position
            i. Deeper inspiration shows more of the lung
            ii. Dependent free pleural fluid level more evident
            iii. Less distortion (widening) of cardiac silhouette
   C. Lateral films
      1. Most often done with film against left side
      2. Particularly useful in evaluating structures in the posterior mediastinal and retrocardiac spaces
      3. Also useful in evaluating the thoracic vertebrae
      4. May reveal free pleural fluid level not evident in supine AP

II. **Adequacy of the film**

A. Some portion of the x-ray beam is absorbed by the material(s) it passes through before reaching the film plate

   1. Air, fat, soft tissue (water), and bone (metal) absorb progressively more radiation

B. Only the portion of the beam that penetrates the material and is not absorbed will create a darker image on the film

   1. A high degree of penetration (low absorption) will create a black or radiolucent area on the film.

   2. A low degree of penetration (high absorption) will create a white or radiopaque area on the film.

C. Sufficient detail in the image is largely determined by the intensity of the x-ray beam

   1. Optimal penetration is generally judged by the clarity of the vertebral bodies on the image

   a. Overpenetration: beam too intense, resulting in an overly dark image with subtle details rendered invisible

   b. Underpenetration: beam insufficiently intense, producing an overly white image; all details are lost in the glare

D. The x-ray beam should be perpendicular to the film and/or anatomic plane, so as to avoid distortion of structural relationships and sizes. The x-ray should also be taken a minimal of six feet away to decrease magnification and increase sharpness.

   1. In the PA/AP view, clavicular symmetry is a general indicator of chest rotation from the perpendicular plane

   a. Clavicles should be approximately equal in length

   b. Clavicular heads should be equal distances from the spinal process

E. The film should be exposed during a deep inspiration to produce good alveolar inflation and avoid diaphragmatic displacement of the heart.

   1. A general indicator of adequate inspiration is the seventh rib visible at or above the diaphragm

   2. Inadequate inspiration flattens the inferior border of the heart, causing the lateral borders to falsely widen

READING A CHEST X-RAY

I. **Keys to consistent accuracy**

A. Understanding of normal anatomic relationships in three dimensions

B. Understanding the impact of pathologic changes on image

C. Organized search pattern and persistent repetition of this ordered approach film after film

D. Always compare with previous films, when available

II. **Basic impact of disease on image**

A. Silhouette sign

1. A loss of the normal border between different densities, such as when lungs with normal air density become filled with fluid and, therefore, become water dense
2. Useful in localizing infiltrate or fluid; for example, if an area of increased density in the right lower lung field obscures the border of the hemidiaphragm, the infiltrate is in the right lower lung; if only the border of the right heart is lost, the infiltrate is in the right middle lung

B. Interstitial pattern
1. As the pulmonary interstitium or tissues in the lungs outside of the alveoli, the bronchial tree, and vasculature acquire more water (more density), such become more distinct.
2. Appears as aerated lung with distinct linear or nodular markings
3. Diseases with interstitial pattern include idiopathic pulmonary fibrosis, radiation pneumonitis, and scleroderma.

C. Alveolar pattern
1. As alveoli fill, consolidate, or collapse, interstitial markings become less distinct (similar to silhouette sign).
2. Remaining air-filled bronchi may show up in contrast against otherwise non-aerated lung (air bronchogram)
3. Alveolar patterns are likely acute whether focal, multifocal, or diffuse.
4. Diseases with alveolar pattern may include pulmonary edema, bronchopneumonia, hemorrhage, and atelectasis, among others.

III. **Reviewing the x-ray with an organized approach**
A. Ensure that you are looking at the proper film
1. Identify the patient
2. Verify the date and time of the film

B. Examine the film for orientation, rotation, and image quality
1. PA/AP views should be hung as if facing the patient's front
2. Clavicles should be of equal length with heads astride chest midline
3. Outline of separate vertebral bodies should be evident
4. Compare side by side with prior x-rays
5. Check the film for adequate inspiration

C. Use systematic ways to examine the x-ray, by using the ABCDEHI pneumonic
1. Airway
   a. The trachea should be midline
      i. A displaced trachea can indicate thyroid enlargement
   b. The carina should be between T4 and T6 and should be examined when the patient is intubated to ensure inflation of both lungs.
   c. The right main bronchus is straighter than the left main bronchus.

    i. Aspiration pneumonia is suspected when the consolidation occurs in the right lower lobe.

2. Bones
- **a.** Include spine, clavicle, ribs, and scapula
- **b.** Anterior ribs appear more flat versus the posterior ribs, which have a sharper downward angle
- **c.** Each rib should be examined for fracture
- **d.** Intercostal spaces should be noted for widening or asymmetry, which can indicate diseases that cause hyperinflation of the lungs or chest wall tumors

3. Circulation or cardiac
- **a.** Examine the mediastinum
  - **i.** A widened mediastinum can indicate heart failure or aortic aneurysm
- **b.** Calcification is indicative of atherosclerosis
- **c.** The normal cardiac to thoracic ratio should be less than 50%
- **d.** The left mediastinal border consists of the brachiocephalic vein, the aortic arch, the pulmonary artery, the atrial appendage, and the left ventricle
- **e.** The right mediastinal border consists of the brachiocephalic vein, the superior vena cava, the ascending aorta, the right pulmonary artery, the right atrium, and the inferior vena cava

4. Diaphragm
- **a.** The right diaphragm is normally 1–3 cm higher than the left diaphragm due to the liver elevating the left diaphragm.
- **b.** The costophrenic angles should be sharp
- **c.** Air under the diaphragm can be indicative of a perforated portion of the bowels, and such is a medical emergency

5. Edges
- **a.** Examine the edges of the lung and chest wall. Disease processes to keep in mind include the following:
  - **i.** Subcutaneous emphysema
  - **ii.** Pneumothorax
  - **iii.** Hemothorax
  - **iv.** Pleural effusions, and others
    - **(a)** Pleural effusions require 175–250 ml of fluid to blunt at least one of the costophrenic angles

6. Fields
- **a.** Lung parenchyma is examined for density changes or consolidations that are incongruent with the rest of the lung fields.

7. Gastric bubble
- **a.** Loss of the gastric air bubble can indicate a hiatal hernia
- **b.** A large gastric bubble can be correlated with bloating

Table 24.1 Invasive devices and positioning on chest X-ray	
Devices	Proper Location on the CXR
Endotracheal tube	2–4 cm above the carina, not deviating to one bronchus
Chest tubes	All opening of the chest tube are inside the chest wall, tube travels up to drain air, down to drain fluids
Nasogastric tube	Below the diaphragm with tip and side holes 10 cm into the antrum of the stomach, without looping back to the fundus
Small-bore feeding tube	Tip should be into the duodenum, pass the pylorus, confirmed with abdominal film
Central venous catheter	Tip should be in the superior vena cava, above the right atrium
Dialysis catheters	Tip ends in the superior vena cava
Pulmonary artery catheter	Travels around the heart into the left or more commonly, the right pulmonary artery, 2–4 cm from midline, not in the periphery of the lung
Peripherally inserted center catheter	Tip should be within the superior vena cava above the right atrium
Intra-aortic balloon pump	Tip should be in the aorta, 2 cm below the aortic arch
Pacemakers	Lead touching the right atrium and right ventricle. Pacemaker catheters should lie along lower right cardiac (right ventricular) border
Automatic internal cardiac defibrillator	Lead in the superior vena cava or brachial cephalic vein, and apex of the right ventricle.

      c. Air density outside of the gastric bubble and gastrointestinal tract can indicate pneumoperitoneum

   8. Hilum

      a. The hilar is the overlapping of pulmonary arteries and veins, and the left hilum is usually 1–2 cm above the right.

      b. Widening of the hilum can be indicative of pulmonary hypertension

   9. Invasive lines

      a. Assess tubes, lines, drains, catheters, and wires

      b. Please refer to table 24.1 for correct positioning of invasive devices

SPECIFIC DISEASE ENTITIES

I.   **Congestive heart failure**

    A. It often manifests as an enlarged cardiac shadow, along with increased pulmonary vascular markings

B. Cardiogenic pulmonary edema can be seen on the chest x-ray as Kerley B lines, which are horizontal lines that are less than 2 cm long, found near the costophrenic angle of the lungs.

C. Pleural effusions often occur along with the diagnosis of congestive heart failure.

II. **Pericardial effusion**

A. The chest x-ray is not sensitive enough to detect pericardial effusion.

1. Changes in the size and/or hazy borders of the cardiac silhouette seen in serial films may, however, be suggestive of an effusion

2. Previous films should be reviewed for recognition and documentation of subtle changes

B. Cardiac echocardiography is more reliable than chest x-ray for detection of pericardial effusions

III. **Emphysema**

A. Pulmonary parenchyma tends to be more lucent than normal, reflecting the loss of tissue and hyperinflation.

B. The cardiac silhouette is often narrow

C. Diaphragmatic domes are often flattened

D. Lung volumes appear larger

IV. **Pneumonia**

A. A chest x-ray is an essential part of the initial workup of a suspected diagnosis of pneumonia.

B. Pneumonia is suspected when an infiltrate is seen in a specific segment of the lung. The diagnosis of pneumonia requires clinical and laboratory findings as well.

C. Improvement in the appearance of a chest film often lags behind clinical improvement by a factor of weeks

V. **Pulmonary nodules (also called coin lesions)**

A. A nodule is defined as "a lesion smaller than 3 cm in size." Larger lesions are referred to as "masses."

B. Solitary nodules should always be evaluated

C. The most valuable method for evaluation of a pulmonary nodule involves comparison with earlier films.

1. Nodules should be followed by serial chest x-rays and yearly computed tomography scans

2. Benign nodules are often found in nonsmokers younger than 35 years

3. Benign nodules tend to be calcified

4. Calcifications in benign nodules are typically described as central, laminar, diffuse, or popcorn

5. Nodules described as eccentric or stippled may be benign or malignant

6. Benign nodules tend to remain unchanged over time

D. Computerized tomography and positron emission tomography are useful in evaluating questionable nodules.

E. Persons ages 55–74 years old, are current smokers or have quit smoking within the past 15 years, and/or have a smoking history of 30 pack-years should receive lung cancer screening

1. A pack-year is calculated by the number of packs smoked per day multiplied by the years smoked.
2. Screening should be performed with low dose computed tomography scan and has been shown to decrease mortality by 20%.

BIBLIOGRAPHY

Antin-Ozerkis, D., Rubinowitz, A., Evans, J., Homer, R. J., & Matthay, R. A. (2012). Interstitial lung disease in the connective tissue diseases. *Clinics in Chest Medicine, 33*(1), 123–149.

Bejan, C. A., Xia, F., Vanderwende, L., Wurfel, M.W., Yetisgen-Yildiz, M. (2012). Pneumonia identification using statistical feature selection. *Journal of the American Medical Informatics Association.* Advance online publication. doi:10.1136/amianjnl-2011–000752

Castañer, E., Gallardo, X., Ballesteros, E., Andreu, M., Pallardó, Y., Mata, M. M., & Riera, L. (2009). CT diagnosis of chronic pulmonary thromboembolism 1. *Radiographics, 29*(1), 31–50. doi:10.1148/rg.291085061.

Daffner, R. H., & Hartman, M. S. (2014). *Clinical radiology: The essentials* (4th ed.). Philadelphia, PA: Lippincott, Williams & Wilkins.

Erkonen, W. E., & Smith, W. L. (2010). *Radiology 101: The basics and fundamentals of imaging* (3rd ed.). Philadelphia, PA: Lippincott Williams & Wilkins.

Gorgan, M., Bockorny, B., Lawlor, M., Volpe, J., & Fiel-Gan, M. (2013). Pulmonary hemorrhage with capillaritis secondary to mycophenolate mofetil in a heart-transplant patient. *Archives of Pathology and Laboratory Medicine, 137*(11), 1684–1687.

Hasegawa, N., Nishimura, T., Ohtani, S., Takeshita, K., Fukunaga, K., Tasaka, S., . . . & Ishizaka, A. (2009). Therapeutic effects of various initial combinations of chemotherapy including clarithromycin against mycobacterium avium complex pulmonary disease. *Chest Journal, 136*(6), 1569–1575.

Herrmann, C. (2009). *As easy as black and white: CXR interpretation.* Retrieved from http://www.aacn.org/wd/nti2009/nti_cd/data/papers/main/30978.pdf

Jiang, M., Chen, Y., Liu, M., Rosenbloom, S. T., Mani, S., Denny, J. C., Xu, H. (2011). *Journal of the American Medical Informatics Association, 18*, 601–606. doi:10.1136/amiajnl-2011–000163

Joarder, R., & Crundwell, N. (Eds.). (2009). *Chest x-ray in clinical practice.* New York, NY: Springer.

Li, F., Hara, T., Shiraishi, J., Engelmann, R., MacMahon, H., & Doi, K. (2011). Improved detection of subtle lung nodules by use of chest radiographs with bone suppression imaging: Receiver operating characteristic analysis with and without localization. *American Journal of Roentgenology, 196*(5), W535-W541.

Light, R. W. (2007). *Pleural diseases*. Philadelphia, PA: Lippincott Williams & Wilkins.

Napolitano, L. M., (2010). Use of severity scoring and stratification factors in clinical trials of hospital-acquired and ventilator-associated pnemonia [Supplemental material]. *Clinical Infectious Diseases, 51*(S1), S67-S80. doi:10.1086/653052

National Cancer Institute. (2010). *National lung screening trials*. Retrieved from: http://www.cancer.gov/clinicaltrials/noteworthy-trials/nlst/updates

Ozawa, Y., Hara, M., Kato, M., Shimizu, S., & Shibamoto, Y. (2014). Contrast enhancement of posterior mediastinal ganglioneuromas—Correlation between the level of enhancement and histopathological features. *Open Journal of Radiology, 4*(1), 123–129. doi:10.4236/ojrad.2014.41016

Pezzotti, W. (2014). Chest x-ray interpretation: Not just Black & White. *Nursing2014, 44*(1), 40–47.

del Portillo, I. P., Vázquez, S. T., Mendoza, J. B., & Moreno, R. V. (2014). Oxygen therapy in critical care: A double-edged sword. *Health, 6*(15), 2035–2046. doi:10.4236/health.2014.615238

Sussmann, A. R., & Ko, J. P. (2009). Understanding chest radiographic anatomy with MDCT reformations. *Clinical Radiology, 65*(2), 155–166.

Test, M., Shah, S. S., Monuteaux, M., Ambroggio, L., Lee, E. Y., Markowitz, R. I., . . . & Neuman, M. I. (2013). Impact of clinical history on chest radiograph interpretation. *Journal of Hospital Medicine, 8*(7), 359–364. doi:10.1002/jhm.1991

Tozzetti, C., Adembri, C., & Modesti, P. A. (2009). Pulse oximeter, the fifth vital sign: A safety belt, or a prison of the mind? *Internal and emergency medicine, 4*(4), 331–332.

West, J. B. (2012). *Pulmonary pathophysiology. The essentials* (7th ed.). Philadelphia, PA: Lippincott Williams & Wilkins.

CHAPTER 25

Pulmonary Function Testing

HALEY M. HOY • THOMAS W. BARKLEY, JR. • CHARLENE M. MYERS

I. **Purpose of a pulmonary function test (PFT)**
   A. To determine the existence of pulmonary function that may then be used to do the following:
      1. Assign a potential diagnosis to explain a patient's symptoms
      2. Differentiate between obstructions of airways and decreased pulmonary parenchymal compliance as the source of a patient's symptoms
      3. Evaluate the response to treatment of a pulmonary disease process
   B. Indications for a PFT
      1. Evaluate unexplained dyspnea and cough
      2. Assess severity of pulmonary dysfunction
      3. Determine potential reversibility of airway obstruction
   C. Limitations of the PFT
      1. The patient must be able to cooperate with the testing (inadequate cooperation negates the value of the testing), the person administering the test must be skilled, and the person interpreting the test must be knowledgeable in PFT interpretation.
      2. The patient should be relatively stable with respect to symptoms. Temporary worsening of symptoms may invalidate the severity of the dysfunction assessed.

II. **Types of PFTs**
   A. Spirometry continues to be recommended as the objective measurement of pulmonary function and for the diagnosis and management of respiratory dysfunction.
      1. Determines forced vital capacity (FVC) and forced expiratory flow rates

  a. Forced expiratory volume in one second (FEV_1) is considered the gold standard by which obstructive airway disease is measured. More specifically, the ratio of FEV_1/FVC is diagnostic for obstructive lung disease.

  b. Values are compared with predicted values derived from population-based reference groups

  c. Decreased FEV_1/FVC (less than 70% of normal) indicates the presence of airflow obstruction or an obstructive disorder

 2. If expiratory airflow obstruction is defined, the response to an aerosolized bronchodilator should be measured

  a. An increase of 12% or 200 ml or greater is often accepted as a reason to use a bronchodilator

  b. However, although controversial, a smaller improvement in flow rate in the presence of more severe obstruction is often a reason to consider using a bronchodilator.

 3. Graphic display of inspiration and exhalation (flow volume loops) provides a comprehensive view of respiratory mechanics, allows the identification of subtle changes, can identify the location of airflow obstruction, and aids in differentiating between obstructive and restrictive disease.

 4. Results correlate with morbidity and life expectancy

 5. Safe, inexpensive, and fast

 6. Spirometry, however, is effort dependent, and some patients have difficulty performing the process because of advanced age or acute illness.

B. Spirometry with bronchodilator therapy (evaluation for bronchospasm)

 1. Determines the vital capacity and expiratory flow rates before and after aerosolized bronchodilator therapy

 2. Degree of responsiveness may be useful in determining the need for bronchodilator therapy

C. Body plethysmography (volume displacement techniques)

 1. Useful in determining all lung volumes, including the following:

  a. Vital capacity (measured during spirometry)

  b. Residual volume in the chest after expiration

  c. Total lung capacity (TLC)

 2. More completely differentiates between a restrictive ventilatory defect (lowered lung volumes) and an obstructive ventilatory defect (increased total lung volume and residual volume)

  a. TLC is decreased with restrictive disorders

  b. TLC is normal or increased with obstructive disorders

  c. Interpret cautiously in patients with neuromuscular weakness because this can sometimes decrease TLC and may prevent differentiation between restrictive and obstructive disorders

D. Measurement of exhaled nitrous oxide

 1. Noninvasive marker of airway inflammation

      a. Appears to reflect lower airway inflammation—a hallmark of the asthma disease process

      b. Useful in recognizing inflammation in symptom-free asthmatic patients who have normal lung function

      c. Helps with the titration of inhaled steroid therapy, in that inhaled steroids quickly reduce exhaled nitrous oxide levels, indicating a reduction in airway inflammation

E. Diffusing capacity of the lung for carbon monoxide (CO) (single-breath technique)

  1. Uses CO as a substitute for O_2 to assess the gas transfer function of the lungs

      a. Decreased diffusion capacity of carbon monoxide in the lung (DLCO) may indicate disorders of pulmonary parenchyma, vascular problems, or decreases in alveolar function (such as occur with lung resection or emphysema)

      b. Increased DLCO may indicate asthma, obesity, polycythemia, or cardiac left-to-right shunting

  2. Modified techniques to measure DLCO must be used for patients with end-stage heart disease and after heart transplant

F. Maximal (inspiratory) respiratory pressures

  1. Helps in the diagnosis of neuromuscular causes of respiratory dysfunction

      a. Decreased inspiratory and expiratory pressures indicate generalized neuromuscular diseases such as amyotrophic lateral sclerosis

      b. Decreased inspiratory pressures suggest dysfunction of the diaphragm

      c. Decreased expiratory pressures are often seen with spinal cord injuries

  2. Important in the prognosis of neuromuscular dysfunction

      a. Helps in the evaluation of airway protective capacity (adequate cough)

      b. Helps predict successful weaning from mechanical ventilators

      c. Helps assess severity and progression of neuromuscular weakness

G. Bronchial provocation testing (challenge)

  1. Aids in the identification of suspected asthma

      a. Useful test when spirometry is normal and cough is unexplained

  2. Involves the inhalation of methacholine, histamine, or other chemical stimulants to induce bronchial smooth muscle constriction

      a. Bronchial smooth muscle constriction occurs in asthmatic patients at much lower doses than that in nonasthmatic patients.

        b. Positive results for asthma are indicated by an FEV_1 that has decreased by 20% or more at a dose of 16 mg/ml or less.

        c. The test is 95% sensitive for the diagnosis of asthma; negative results make a diagnosis of asthma unlikely.

    H. High-resolution computed tomography

        1. Useful in examining specific individual airways and structural alterations associated with pathologic change

            a. Provides a way to view airways during expansion and contraction and to assess changes in airway size with changes in lung volume

        2. May show lesions missed on plain radiography

III. **Understanding "normal" values or "predicted" values**

    A. Pulmonary function testing laboratories compare the patient being studied versus a larger population of persons of similar age, race, gender, height, and weight.

    B. The nomograms used vary among laboratories and may prevent absolute comparison when testing is done in different locations.

IV. **Lung volume measurements and the meaning of lung "capacities" (See table 25.1 and 25.2)**

    A. Lung volume is reported as a single value

    B. Lung capacity refers to the combination of lung volumes

Table 25.1	Lung Volumes and Lung Capacities	
Lung volume	**Lung capacity**	
Inspiratory reserve volume (IRV) The amount of air that can be inhaled after a full inspiration	Vital capacity (forced) (FVC)	Total lung capacity (TLC)
Tidal volume (VT) The amount of air that is inhaled or exhaled during a normal breath		
Expiratory reserve volume (ERV) The amount of air that can be forced out of the lungs after a full expiration		
Residual volume (from plethysmography) RV The amount of air remaining in the lungs after a forced expiration		

Table 25.2	Expiratory Flow Rates
Flow rate measurement	
FEV$_1$ **Forced expiratory volume in one second**	Parameter assessed, comment on effort dependency Central and smaller airways
FEV$_1$% (FEV$_1$/FVC) **FEV$_1$ as a percentage of forced vital capacity**	How much of the vital capacity can be exhaled forcibly in one second? Effort dependent
FEF$_{25-75}$ **Forced expiratory flow rate over the midportion of exhalation**	Small airways Relatively effort independent

V. Determination of the presence of obstructive and restrictive ventilatory defects

   A. Obstructive ventilatory defects

      1. Flow rates are reduced when compared with normal values for similar persons

      2. Lung volumes generally are within the normal range or are larger than the normal range because of air trapping and hyperinflation (with increased reserve volume and TLC).

   B. Restrictive ventilatory defects

      1. Flow rates are normal or increased

      2. Lung volumes are proportionately reduced

VI. Determining severity of defects (lung volumes and flow rates)

   A. Values greater than 70% of predicted volumes/flow rates are considered within normal limits

   B. Values 60%–70% of predicted volumes/flow rates are mildly reduced

   C. Values 50%–60% of predicted volumes/flow rates are moderately reduced

   D. Values lower than 50% of predicted volumes/flow rates are severely reduced

   E. When values for residual volume and TLC exceed 120% of predicted, air trapping and hyperinflation are present

   F. When airflow obstruction is present, bronchodilator responsiveness is considered significant if expiratory airflow measurements improve by at least 15% over baseline values

      1. The absence of such a response is, by itself, not justification for withholding these medications

      2. Bronchodilators may improve other parameters of lung function, including secretion clearance.

VII. **Peak expiratory flowmeter and asthma**
  A. Simple and inexpensive device (indeed, usually provided by
    pharmaceutical companies that manufacture bronchodilators) intended
    for home use by asthmatic patients and those with other forms of
    potentially reversible airway obstruction
    1. Still recommended for daily monitoring
  B. Ideally, the patient will measure his or her peak expiratory flow rate
    (PEFR) at least once daily initially, at the same time each day, to
    provide a measure of functional airflow limitation over time.
    1. Values are recorded in a diary provided with the device
      a. Patients may demonstrate low compliance in terms of
        accurately and consistently recording results
    2. The patient's "best" flow rate, typical flow rates, and altered
      flow rates may then be used to determine the need for additional
      medication.
      a. PEFR 80%–100% of baseline
        i. The "green" zone
        ii. No change in therapy is needed
      b. PEFR 50%–80% of baseline
        i. The "yellow" zone
        ii. Temporary increase in intensity of therapy, or additional
          therapy, should be considered
      c. PEFR below 50% of baseline
        i. The "red" zone
        ii. Urgent/emergency care is advised
VIII. **Implications for geriatric patients**
  A. Many older adults experience changes in elastic recoil and
    musculoskeletal changes of the chest wall
    1. TLC usually remains constant but vital capacity decreases because
      residual volume increases
    2. Tidal volume may be decreased
    3. Alveoli collapse more easily
    4. Number of cilia diminish
    5. Decreased cough reflex
  B. It is important to allow extra time when performing lung function
    testing on older adults.

BIBLIOGRAPHY

Chang, J. E., White. A. A., & Simon, R. A. (2014). Non-steroidal anti-inflammatory drug hypersensitivity and sinus disease. In C. C. Chang, G. A. Incaudo, & M. E. Gershwin (Eds.), *Diseases of the sinuses: A comprehensive textbook of diagnosis and treatment* (2nd ed., pp. 195–208). New York, NY: Springer.

Goldman, L., & Schafer, A. (2011). *Goldman's Cecil Medicine* (24th ed.). Philadelphia, PA: Elsevier Saunders.

King, G. G. (2011). Cutting edge technologies in respiratory research: Lung function testing. *Respirology, 16*(6), 883–890. doi:10.1111/j.1440–1843.2011.02013.x

Liang, B. M., Lam, D. C., & Feng, Y. L. (2012). Clinical applictions of lung function tests: A revisit. *Respirology, 17*(4), 611–619. doi:10.1111/j.1440–1843.2012.02149.x

MacIntyre, N. R. (2012). The future of pulmonary function testing. *Respiratory Care, 57*(1), 154–161. doi:10.4187/respcare.01422

Meiner, S. E. (2010). *Gerontologic nursing* (4th ed.). St. Louis, MO: Elsevier Mosby.

Pretto, J. J., Brazzale, D. J., Guy, P. A., Goudge, R. J., & Hensley, M. J. (2013). Reasons for referral for pulmonary function testing: An audit of 4 adult lung function laboratories. *Respiratory Care, 58*(3), 507–510. Retrieved from http://rc.rcjournal.com/content/58/3/507.full.pdf

Ruppel, G. L., & Enright, P. L. (2012). Pulmonary function testing. *Respiratory Care, 57*(1), 165–175. doi:10.4187/respcare.01640

West, J. B. (2012). *Pulmonary pathophysiology* (8th ed.). Philadelphia, PA: Wolters Kluwer Health/Lippincott, Williams, & Wilkins.

Wheaton, A. G., Ford, E. S., Thompson, W. W., Greenlund, K. J., Presley-Cantrell, L. R., & Croft, J. B. (2013). Pulmonary function, chronic respiratory symptoms, and health-related quality of life among adults in the United States—National Health and Nutrition Examination Survey 2007–2010. *BMC Public Health, 13*(854). Retrieved from http://www.biomedcentral.com/1471–2458/13/854

CHAPTER 26

Obstructive (Ventilatory) Lung Diseases

THOMAS W. BARKLEY, JR. • ROBERT FELLIN • TOBIAS P. REBMANN

CHRONIC OBSTRUCTIVE PULMONARY DISEASE (COPD)

I. **Definition**
   A. COPD is a mixture of diseases, including emphysema, chronic bronchitis, and bronchospastic airway disease, all of which are characterized by limitation of expiratory airflow
   B. Acute exacerbations are superimposed upon chronic symptoms

II. **Etiologies/incidence**
   A. Tobacco smoking (cigarettes, cigars, and pipes) is the most common cause
      1. Most persons who smoke a pack of cigarettes per day for longer than 40 years will have manifestations of COPD.
      2. Note: One pack of cigarettes per day multiplied by the number of years smoked equals the number of pack-years of cigarettes smoked
   B. Inhalation of environmental pollutants (e.g., oxides of sulfur and nitrogen)
      1. Incidence depends on duration and concentration of exposure in heavily polluted areas
   C. Occupational exposure to inorganic chemicals (chlorine and fluorine) and organic chemicals (e.g., toluene) may result in obstructive airway disease.

III. **Subjective findings**
   A. Cough, dry and occasionally productive, especially in the early morning
   B. Sputum production
      1. Usually clear in color but may be discolored (e.g., yellow, purulent, and green)

2. A change in the amount produced or the color of the sputum is important in management decisions
   a. Exertional dyspnea
C. Weight loss with progressive disease due to early satiety and difficulty breathing after food is consumed, especially in the elderly
D. Fatigue
E. Complaints of chest tightness, owing to one of the following:
   1. Alterations that are slowly occurring in the chest wall (e.g., increase in anteroposterior chest diameter)
   2. Acute air retention within the thorax

IV. **Physical exam findings**
A. General
   1. Respiratory rate is normal or increased
   2. Mental status should be alert and oriented
   3. Note sitting position for the presence of classic "emphysema stance"
      a. The patient sits with the chest forward and the arms straightened
      b. The upper body is lifted to allow for greater expansion of the chest, as gravity pulls the abdominal contents downward and away from the diaphragm
   4. Inspect for clubbing of the nail beds and for pursed-lip breathing
B. Chest inspection
   1. Increase in the anteroposterior diameter of the chest
      a. Gives rise to a "barrel" configuration
      b. Normally, the diameter of the chest from axilla to axilla is about twice the anteroposterior diameter
      c. Loss of muscle strength in elderly may accelerate this
   2. Use of accessory muscles of respiration
      a. Sternocleidomastoids
      b. Intercostals
C. Chest percussion
   1. Hyperresonance
   2. Low diaphragm
D. Chest auscultation
   1. Diminished breath sounds throughout the chest
   2. Prolonged forced expiratory time (auscultation while the patient forcibly exhales shows that the effort needed to exhale the air requires longer than 3 seconds)
   3. Rhonchi on inspiration and/or expiration, especially when secretions are increased
   4. Occasional wheezing on expiration
      a. Asthma
      b. Chronic bronchitis

V. **Laboratory/diagnostics**
- **A.** Pulmonary function testing
  1. Expiratory flow rates are reduced
     - **a.** Early disease: reduction in small airway flow rates
     - **b.** Late disease: reduction in FEV_1 (forced expiratory volume in 1 second, a measure of the potential for severe complications of COPD)
  2. Lung volume changes
     - **a.** Air trapping indicated by increased residual volume
     - **b.** Hyperinflation indicated by increased total lung capacity
     - **c.** Forced vital capacity (FVC) may be reduced by air trapping.
     - **d.** The reduction in FVC is, on a percentage of a normal basis, less than the percentage reduction in predicted expiratory airflow.
- **B.** Arterial blood gases (ABGs) and pulse oximetry
  1. Earlier in the course of disease, and often during the later stages, both studies show normal oxygenation, and ABGs show no evidence of chronic respiratory acidosis
  2. Seen more frequently later in the course of disease, or during exacerbations of moderately severe disease
     - **a.** Hypoxemia (partial pressure of oxygen in arterial blood [PaO_2] less than 55 mmHg)
     - **b.** Hypercarbia (chronic respiratory acidosis)
  3. During acute exacerbations of COPD, hypoxemia and acute hypercarbia may be seen.
     - **a.** Assessment requires at least one ABG analysis
     - **b.** Increasing respiratory distress and changes in mental status (confusion, stupor) require more frequent checks of ABGs
  4. Pulse oximetry
     - **a.** Used frequently to assess for adequacy of oxygen transport within the blood at rest and during exertion
     - **b.** Adequate oxygenation is implied when SaO_2 (oxygen saturation) is greater than 88% when the hemoglobin level is above 10 grams/dl
- **C.** Other laboratory values
  1. Hemoglobin and hematocrit
     - **a.** Hemoglobin less than 10 grams/dl may be suboptimal for oxygen transport
     - **b.** Hematocrit greater than 55 ml/dl indicates secondary polycythemia is due to chronic hypoxemia
  2. Serum bicarbonate is often elevated with chronic hypercarbia
- **D.** Chest x-ray
  1. Air trapping

2. Blebs and bullae (dilated air spaces within the pulmonary parenchyma) may be seen, although usually require CT imaging to be recognized
3. Flattened diaphragm
4. Hyperinflation is noted by the following:
    a. Hyperlucency in upper lung zones
    b. Widening of intercostal spaces
    c. Ten or more ribs identified above diaphragm
5. Retrosternal air noted on lateral view

VI. **Nonpharmacological management**
   A. Smoking cessation (perhaps most difficult to achieve)
      1. Behavioral modification
      2. Nicotine replacement therapy (gum, lozenges, and transdermal) are all available over the counter. Decisions regarding the initial dosing should rely on the product chosen and the daily nicotine exposure. The provider should discuss this with the patient.
      3. Pharmacological
          a. Bupropion (Zyban), 150 mg daily for 3 days, then BID for 7–12 weeks
          b. Varenicline (Chantix) available in a starter month pack, then 1 mg BID for 8–16 additional weeks
   B. Nonpharmacological therapy provided with heated or cooled aerosols of water in combination with chest physiotherapy may help thin airway secretions.
   C. The value of chest physiotherapy (percussion and postural drainage) in COPD is controversial, but it may be worthwhile when patients perceive a benefit from it.

VII. **Pharmacological management**
   A. All pharmacotherapy must take into consideration comorbid conditions, concomitant use of other medications, and dose adjustments for age, renal and hepatic function, and body mass where indicated
   B. Symptom assessment in patients with COPD can be made using a standard assessment tool such as the COPD Assessment Tool (CAT, 2012) with its User Guide for Healthcare Professionals (CAT User Guide, 2012). The test evaluates cough, phlegm production, perceived chest tightness, dyspnea, impact on ADLs and IADLs, sleep, and energy; it is at least semiquantitative over time.
      1. Classifying the degree of severity of COPD by severity of airflow obstruction (GOLD, 2014)
          a. Four categories
              i. GOLD 1: Mild—FEV_1 80% or greater of predicted
              ii. GOLD 2: Moderate—50% or less FEV_1 less than 80% predicted

        iii. GOLD 3: Severe—30% or less FEV$_1$ less than 50% predicted

        iv. GOLD 4: Very severe—FEV$_1$ less than 30% predicted

    b. Exacerbation of COPD (GOLD, 2014)

        i. Worsening of symptoms that leads to a change in therapy

        ii. Two or more exacerbations per year is suggestive of deteriorating lung function (a higher GOLD category)

    c. Evaluate for possible worsening or co-existing conditions (comorbidities)

        i. Cardiovascular, depression/anxiety, muscle weakness, metabolic syndrome, co-existing lung disease

        ii. Treat these as indicated.

C. Drug management, stable COPD (GOLD, 2014)

  1. Anticholinergic agents

    a. Decrease airway secretions and airway smooth muscle tone

    b. Anticholinergic agents of choice in COPD

        i. Ipratropium bromide (Atrovent), two puffs 4 times a day; also premixed in saline for use in handheld nebulizer, or

        ii. Tiotropium bromide (Spiriva) 18 mcg, once daily by HandiHaler

        iii. Aclidinium (Tudorza) 400 mcg inhaled BID

        iv. Umeclidinium (Incruse Ellipta) 62.5 mcg inhaled daily

    c. Mainstay of therapy for COPD

    d. Adverse effects: dry mouth and dry, hacking cough, oral candidiasis (teach patient to rinse mouth after use), and urinary retention (especially elderly males with concomitant prostate hypertrophy)

  2. Bronchodilators

    a. Beta$_2$-adrenergic receptor agonists

        i. Relax smooth muscle tone and improve airflow

        ii. Stimulate ciliary motion to promote secretion mobilization

    b. Short-acting inhaled β_2 agonists: used for episodic symptom exacerbations

        i. Albuterol (Proventil, Ventolin), also premixed in saline for handheld nebulizer use

        ii. Levalbuterol (Xopenex); metered dose inhalers and nebulizer solutions, possibly less tachycardia and tremor effect than albuterol

    c. Other agents available (caution urged if severe coronary artery disease, history of rapid supraventricular or ventricular arrhythmias, or cardiomyopathy). These are maintenance drugs in the therapy of COPD.

    i.   Long-acting inhaled β_2 agonists (LABA): used for maintenance therapy only; bronchodilation for up to 12 hr, currently not recommended without concomitant use of inhaled corticosteroid (GOLD, 2014)

        (a)   Salmeterol (Serevent Diskus): prolonged receptor binding requires patient education about proper use to avoid induction of cardiac arrhythmias. (Advair: contains salmeterol 50 mcg, and fluticasone, 100, 250, or 500 mcg; dosage, 1 puff BID)

        (b)   Formoterol (Foradil inhaler): similar prolonged receptor binding (Symbicort: contains formoterol 4.5 mcg and budesonide, 80 or 160 mcg; dosage, 2 puffs BID maximum. Dulera contains formoterol 5 mcg and mometasone 100 mcg; dosage, 2 puffs BID)

        (c)   Vilanterol/fluticasone (Breo Ellipta): similar prolonged receptor binding; contains vilanterol (25 mcg) and fluticasone (100 mcg); dosage, 1 puff daily; NOT for patients with asthma

        (d)   Vilanterol/umeclidinium (Anoro Ellipta): combination of long-acting β agonist and an anticholinergic agent; vilanterol (25 mcg) and umeclidinium (62.5 mcg), 1 inhalation daily; NOT for patients with asthma

3. Combination corticosteroid and LABA inhalation is recommended and should be administered at a standard dose of LABA with various doses of corticosteroid. This regimen is primarily indicated for asthma, although it does cross over to COPD with bronchospastic component (bronchitis).

    a.   The 2014 GOLD report reiterates that when the FEV_1 less than 60% of predicted, inhaled corticosteroids improve symptoms, lung function, and quality of life, and reduce frequency of exacerbations.

4. Anti-inflammatory corticosteroids (can be used alone when stable after using with long-acting β agonist bronchodilators)

    a.   Reduce acute and chronic effects of inflammation

    b.   Can improve lung function

    c.   Provide symptomatic relief of emphysema but do not improve lung function (FEV_1)

    d.   Patients taking systemic doses of corticosteroids need to be warned of adverse effects that may result from the abrupt withdrawal of these agents, such as Addisonian crises (e.g., weakness, headache, fever, tachycardia, hypotension, tachypnea, and others).

   e. Oral (enteral) and parenteral doses should generally be rapidly tapered over several days until it is clear such agents have contributed to improving the patient's general condition.
   - **i.** Oral tablets
     - **(a)** Prednisone (Deltasone), 60 mg/day, tapered quickly to less than 20 mg/day
     - **(b)** Methylprednisolone (Medrol), 64 mg/day, tapered to less than 16 mg/day
   - **ii.** Intravenous preparations
     - **(a)** Methylprednisolone sodium succinate (Solu-Medrol), 20–40 mg IV every 6–8 hr for severe exacerbations of COPD; tapered as patient condition allows
   - **iii.** Intramuscular preparations (evidence of effectiveness above oral dosing is questionable)
     - **(a)** Methylprednisolone (Depo-Medrol), 80–240 mg IM in divided doses to decrease discomfort
   f. Caution use of systemic corticosteroids in elderly due to immunosuppressive, hyperglycemic, and bone demineralization effects, even in short-term use if repeated frequently due to exacerbations.
5. Phosphodiesterase 4 inhibitors
   a. Used in later stages of disease
   b. Increases intracellular cAMP in lung tissue
   c. Reduces neutrophil and eosinophil counts in the lung
   d. Roflumilast (Daliresp), 500 mcg daily
D. COPD Stepwise treatment plans
1. GOLD 0: at risk
   a. Normal lung function
   b. Cough and sputum production
   c. Remove toxins
2. GOLD I: mild
   a. FEV_1 greater than 80% (see Pulmonary Function Testing chapter)
   b. Asymptomatic or may have chronic cough and sputum
   c. Short-acting beta agonist
3. GOLD II: moderate
   a. FEV_1 50%–80%
   b. Asymptomatic or may have chronic cough and sputum
   c. Add long-acting β_2 agonist
4. GOLD III: severe
   a. FEV_1 30%–50%
   b. Some symptoms daily
   c. Add inhaled corticosteroid
5. GOLD IV: very severe

      a. FEV_1 less than 30% or less than 50% with severe respiratory failure

      b. Multiple symptoms

      c. Long-term oxygen for severe hypoxia

      d. Consider surgical treatment

E. Exacerbations: most common cause is bronchial infection

    1. Systemic corticosteroids and antibiotics

    2. Positive pressure noninvasive ventilation (BiPAP) helps decrease CO_2 retention and prevent intubation

    3. Mechanical ventilation

F. Palliative care and end-of-life issues should be discussed and offered to patients with patients who have COPD, especially those who have severe disease, significant symptoms and are of advanced age.

G. Periodic review of proper use of metered dose inhalers is strongly recommended

H. Drugs for respiratory muscles (i.e., diaphragm and intercostals) and bronchodilator activity

    1. Theophylline

      a. Theo-Dur, 300 mg BID

      b. Uni-Dur, 400–600 mg in the evening

      c. Theophylline timed-release (Uniphyl), 400–600 mg in the evening

    2. Therapeutic drug levels are recommended to be lower than 20 mg/L

      a. Note: Evening doses acknowledge the circadian increase in airway smooth muscle tone.

      b. Monitor for side effects, especially in elderly. Systemic adverse effects can occur even with serum levels within therapeutic range

I. Comments

    1. Maintenance therapy for COPD may incorporate as many different classes of pharmacological agents PRN to maintain the patient's usual performance status. From a step-wise point of view, short-acting bronchodilators are used for mild disease, and then adding regular doses of anticholinergics, long-acting bronchodilators with inhaled corticosteroids, and then considering theophylline, 4-phosphodiesterase inhibitors, and other medications for more severe disease.

    2. During exacerbations, inhaled bronchodilators may be needed more frequently than every 4 hr

    3. Parenteral steroids should be added and rapidly tapered over several days until it is clear whether or not these preparations have contributed to improving the patient's general condition.

J. Antimicrobial agents

    1. Indications

    a. Changes in sputum quantity and color are considered important
      i. Gram's stain may be helpful
      ii. Sputum culture is not indicated for initiation of treatment
      iii. In most instances, sputum and blood cultures should be obtained prior to initiation of antimicrobial therapy if pneumonia is suspected.
    b. Recent upper respiratory infection (Note: upper respiratory infection is the most common cause of COPD exacerbation)
    c. Radiographic evidence compatible with pneumonia is present
    d. Bacteremia is suspected

  2. Agents chosen should cover usually expected respiratory pathogens (see Lower Respiratory Tract Pathogens chapter), without being unnecessarily broader in spectrum than is required.

K. Agents to thin the sputum:

  1. Guaifenesin (Mucinex, Robitussin) may be of help to thin respiratory secretions, although total body hydration is clearly more important. Thus, these agents should be combined with adequate hydration.

  2. Acetylcysteine (Mucomyst 10% or 20%)
    a. Reduces sputum viscosity
    b. 1–10 ml of solution is inhaled every 6–8 hr, generally after a β_2 agonist is inhaled (see Bronchodilator section under pharmacological management of COPD)
    c. Can provoke bronchospasm
    d. "Tastes like rotten eggs" because of sulfur content

L. Supplemental oxygen (see Oxygen Supplementation chapter)

M. Antitussives are generally contraindicated for long term or chronic use in stable COPD

N. Risk prevention
  1. Flu vaccine
  2. Pneumonia vaccine

O. Surgical treatment: referral to a pulmonologist experienced with lung transplantation in COPD is recommended
  1. Lung transplantation
  2. Lung volume reduction surgery may help to relieve dyspnea and improve exercise tolerance
  3. Surgical intervention may be associated with significant adverse effects in elderly

P. Therapy: realities
  1. No treatment will restore lung function
  2. Removing toxins, including tobacco, occupational chemicals, and pollutants, is the only method of preventing continued deterioration of lung function

3. Exercise training may help to improve respiratory function but does show improvement in exercise tolerance and symptoms

4. Treatment will not change decline in lung function; treatment is based on preventing symptoms

Q. Special considerations in pharmacological management of COPD in the elderly

1. Increased risk of adverse drug events (reduced hepatic metabolism and renal excretion)

   a. Short-acting β_2 agonist bronchodilators can induce tremor and tachycardia. Consider using an anticholinergic (ipratropium) with the β_2 adrenergic agent

   b. Inhaled corticosteroids: increased risk of cataracts

   c. Theophylline toxicity risk increases after age 75, especially due to drug interactions (e.g., with cimetidine)

   d. Systemic corticosteroids increase the risk of confusion, agitation, poor glycemic control, and osteoporosis (especially with less mobility due to breathing problems

2. Increased risk for non-adherence due to difficulty with using hand-activated metered dose inhalers (arthritis) or forgetfulness (dementia)

3. Polypharmacy increases the risk for non-adherence and for overuse of inhaled medications, requiring medication reconciliation at every encounter

4. Those with comorbid conditions

   a. Gastroesophageal reflux

   b. Overweight or obese status

   c. Diabetes mellitus

   d. Obstructive sleep apnea

   e. Allergic rhinitis or sinusitis

   f. Cardiovascular disease

ASTHMA

I. **Definition**

A. Clinical disorder characterized by periodic cough often with episodic wheezing, although wheezing less commonly heard among the elderly

B. Sputum is usually described as "plugs" of sputum

C. When the disorder is exacerbated, the patient may report "tightness" in the chest and dyspnea

1. Symptoms may worsen with certain "triggers" (exercise; viral infection; strong emotions; weather changes)

2. Symptoms may persist with exposure to animal dander, house dust, mold (home or external environment), smoke, pollen, airborne chemicals

D. Patient often has a family history of asthma

E. Inflammatory reaction

    1. Hypertrophy of bronchial smooth muscle and mucous glands

    2. Hyperactive airway and inflammation

    3. Causes bronchospasm and mucous production with airway edema

  F. Usually begins in childhood, with or without genetic predisposition

  G. Increased incidence in areas with environmental pollutants

II. **Physical exam findings**

  A. Reduced air entry sounds

  B. Prolonged expiration with expiratory wheezing

  C. Associated symptoms of hay fever or allergic rhinitis

III. **Differential diagnosis in older adults**

  A. COPD

  B. Heart failure

  C. Pulmonary embolism

  D. Endobronchial obstruction (tumor)

  E. Cough related to co-administration of certain medications (e.g., angiotensin converting enzyme inhibitors and β adrenergic blockers)

  F. Vocal cord dysfunction

IV. **Diagnostics**

  A. Diagnosis is based upon symptoms (due to episodic airflow obstruction), at least partially reversible airflow obstruction (based on spirometry), and exclusion of other diagnoses (especially important among elderly patients)

  B. Chest x-ray can be entirely normal or may show hyperinflation; among the elderly it may show evidence of comorbid cardiopulmonary conditions

  C. Spirometry to demonstrate the severity airflow obstruction and reversibility after inhalation of a short-acting bronchodilator

    1. Peak expiratory flow meters are used in monitoring asthma, not in diagnosing asthma

    2. Spirometry should be measured using American Thoracic Society standards.

V. **Management (see tables 26.1 & 26.2)**

  A. Engage the elderly patient as a partner in self-management

    1. Understanding which medications are for quick relief (See SABAs, step 1; systemic corticosteroids, steps 5 and 6) and which are for long-term control (see ICS, leukotriene modifiers, LABAs)

    2. Report changes in symptom patterns/exacerbations (nighttime awakenings; more frequent short-acting β adrenergic inhaler use; work absence; alteration in daily activities; worsening quality of life)

    3. Report significant changes, following the patient's asthma action plan, if used

    4. Report visits to the emergency room or hospitalizations for asthma

Step UP if needed (first check inhaler technique, adherence, environmental control, and comorbid conditions)
ASSESS CONTROL
Step DOWN if possible (and asthma is well controlled for at least 3 months)

	Step 1	Step 2	Step 3	Step 4	Step 5	Step 6
	Intermittent Asthma	Persistent Asthma: Daily Medication				
		Consult with asthma specialist if step 4 care or higher is required. Consider consultation at step 3.				
Preferred	SABA as needed	Low-dose ICS	Low-dose ICS + LABA or Medium-dose ICS	Medium-dose ICS + LABA	High-dose ICS + LABA	High-dose ICS + LABA + Oral Corticosteroid
Alternative		Cromolyn, LTRA, nedrocromil, or theophylline	Low-dose ICS + LTRA, theophylline, or zileuton	Medium-dose ICS + LTRA, theophylline, or zileuton	Consider omalizumab for patients who have allergic asthma	Consider omalizumab for patients who have allergic asthma

Patient education and environmental control, and management of comorbidities at each step.
Step 2–4: Consider subcutaneous allergen immunotherapy for patients who have allergic asthma

Rescue Medication	• SABA as needed for symptoms—up to 3 treatments at 20-minute intervals intiially. Treatment intensity depends on symptom severity. • Short course of corticosteroids may be needed. • Use of SABA > 2 days a week for symptom relief (not prevention of EIB) generally indicates inadequate control and the need to step treatment.

Figure 26.1. Stepwise approach for managing asthma in those ≥ 12 years of age. SABA = short-acting beta$_2$-agonist; ICS = inhaled corticosteroids; LTRA = leukotreine recepter antagonist; LABA = long-acting inhaled beta$_2$-agonist. Adapted from "Expert Panel Report 3: Guidelines for the Diagnosis and Management of Asthma" by the National Institutes of Health, National Heart, Lung, and Blood Institute, 2007.

Table 26.1   Classifying asthma severity and initiating treatment in youths ≥ 12 and adults

Components of Severity		Classification of Asthma Severity ≥ 12 years of age			
		Intermittent	Persistent		
			Mild	Moderate	Severe
Impairment **Normal FEV$_1$/FVC:** **8-19 yr 85%** **20-39 yr 80%** **40-59 yr 75%** **60-80 yr 70%**	Symptoms	≤ 2 days/week	> 2 days/week but not daily	Daily	Throughout the day
	Nighttime awakenings	≤ 2x/month	3-4x/month	1x/week but not nightly	Often 7x/week
	Short-acting beta$_2$ agonist use for symptom control (not prevention of EIB)	≤ 2 days/week	>2 days/week but not daily, and not more than 1x on any day	Daily	Several times per day
	Interference with normal activity	None	Minor limitation	Some limitation	Extremely limited
	Lung function	-Normal FEV$_1$ between exacerbations -FEV$_1$ > 80% predicted -FEV$_1$/FVC normal	-FEV$_1$ > 80% predicted -FEV$_1$/FVC normal	-FEV$_1$ > 60% but < 80% predicted -FEV$_1$/FVC reduced 5%	-FEV$_1$ < 60% predicted -FEV$_1$/FVC reduced > 5%
Risk	Exacerbations requiring oral systemic corticosteroids	0-1/year (see notes)	≥2/year (see notes)		
		Consider severity and interval since last exacerbation. Frequency and severity may fluctuate over time for patients in any severity category. Relative annual risk of exacerbations may be related to FEV1.			
Recommended Step for Initiating Treatment **See figure 26.1 for treatment steps**		Step 1	Step 2	Step 3	Step 4
			And consider short course of oral systemic corticosteroids		
		In 2-6 weeks, evaluate level of asthma control that is achieved and adjust therapy accordingly.			

Notes: FEV$_1$ forced expiratory volume in 1 second; FVC: forced vital capacity

From the National Heart, Lung, and Blood Institute, Department of Health and Human Services, National Institutes of Health: Guidelines for the diagnosis and management of asthma (EPR-3), Section 4, Managing asthma long term: youth ≥ 12 years and adults, 2007: http://www.nhlbi.nih.gov/guidelines/asthma/09_sec4_lt_12.pdf, Tables 4.5, 4.6, 4.7. Accessed December 3, 2014.

Table 26.2	Assessing asthma control in those ≥ 12 years of age			
Components of Control		**Well Controlled**	**Not Well Controlled**	**Very Poorly Controlled**
Impairment	Symptoms	≤ 2 days/week	> 2 days/week	Throughout the day
	Nighttime awakenings	≤ 2x/month	1–3x/week	≥ 4x/week
	Interference with normal activity	None	Some limitation	Extremely limited
	SABA use for symptom control (not prevention of EIB)	≤ 2 days/week	> 2 days/week	Several times per day
	FEV$_1$ or peak flow	> 80% predicted/personal best	60%–80% predicted/personal best	< 60% predicted/personal best
	Validated questionnaires			
	ATAQ	0	1–2	3–4
	ACQ	≤ 0.75[a]	≥ 1.5	n/a
	ACT	≥ 20	16–19	≤ 15

Note. SABA = short-acting beta$_2$ agonist; EIB = exercised-induced bronchospasm; FEV$_1$ = forced expiratory volume in 1 second; ATAQ = asthma therapy assessment questionnaire; ACQ = asthma control questionnaire; ACT = asthma control test. Adapted from "Expert Panel Report 3: Guidelines for the Diagnosis and Management of Asthma" by the National Institutes of Health, National Heart, Lung, and Blood Institute, 2007.

[a]ACQ values of 0.76–1.4 are indeterminate regarding well-controlled asthma.

[b]The level of control is based on the most severe impairment or risk category. Assess impairment domain by patient's recall of previo us 2–4 weeks and by spirometry/ or peak flow measures. Symptom assessment for longer periods should reflect a global assessment, such as inquiring whether the patient's asthma is better or worse since the last visit. At present, there are inadequate data to correspond frequencies of exacerbations with different levels of asthma control. In general, more frequent and intense exacerbations (e.g., requiring urgent, unscheduled care, hospitalization, or ICU admission) indicate poorer disease control. For treatment purposes, patients who had ≥ 2 exacerbations requiring oral systemic corticosteroids in the past year may be considered the same as patients who have not-well-controlled asthma, even in the absence of impairment levels consistent with not-well-controlled asthma

Table 26.2	Assessing asthma control in those ≥ 12 years of age		
Components of Control	**Well Controlled**	**Not Well Controlled**	**Very Poorly Controlled**
Risk			
Exacerbations requiring oral corticosteroids	0–1/year	≥ 2/year[b]	
	Consider severity and interval since last exacerbation		
Progressive loss of lung function	Evaluation requires long-term followup care		
Treatment-related adverse effects	Medication side effects can vary in intensity from none to very troublesome and worrisome. The level of intensity does not correlate to specific levels of control but should be considered in the overall assessment of risk.		
Recommended Action for Treatment (see figure 26.1 for treatment steps)	Maintain current steps Regular followups every 1–6 months to maintain control. Consider step down if well controlled for at least 3 months	Step up 1 step and Reevaluate in 2–6 weeks. For side effects consider alternative treatment options	Consider short course of oral systemic corticosteroids Step up 1–2 steps, and Reevaluate in 2 weeks. For side effects, consider alternative treatment options

B. Stepwise Management of Asthma (assessment for hypoxemia should be done if health assessment and/or co-morbidities warrant this during any step in asthma management of elderly patients.) See figure 26.1.

C. Step 1—Intermittent: symptoms less than or equal to 2 days/week, less than or equal to 2 nighttime awakenings/month, less than or equal to 2 days/week use of SABA for symptom relief, no interference with normal activity, normal FEV_1 between exacerbations, FEV_1 greater than 80% predicted, and normal FEV_1/FVC

  1. Management

    a. SABA PRN. Examples include

      i. Albuterol HFA inhaler; 2 inhalations every 4 hr PRN

      ii. Albuterol 2.5 mg via nebulizer every 4 hr PRN

      iii. Levalbuterol inhaler; 2 inhalations every 4–6 hr PRN

      iv. Levalbuterol 0.63–1.25 mg every 4–6 hr PRN

      v. Pirbuterol inhaler; 2 inhalations every 4–6 hr PRN

    b. Patient education (including about proper use of inhaler or nebulizer), environment control, and management of comorbidities

    c. Reevaluate level of asthma control and adjust therapy in 2–6 weeks

D. Step 2—Mild persistent: symptoms greater than 2 days/week but not daily, 3–4 nighttime awakenings/month, greater than 2 days/week but not daily and not more than one time per day use of an SABA for symptom relief, minor limitation with normal activity, FEV_1 greater than 80% predicted, and normal FEV_1/FVC

  1. Management

      i. Preferred: low-dose inhaled corticosteroid (ICS). Examples include:

        (a) Budnesonide (Pulmicort Flexhaler), 180–360 mcg BID

        (b) Ciclesonide (Avlesco), 80 mcg BID

        (c) Fluticasone (Flovent HFA), 88 mcg BID

        (d) Mometasone (Asmanex), 220 mcg daily or BID

      ii. Alternative: leukotriene modifier (less effective than inhaled corticosteroids)

        (a) Leukotriene modifiers. Examples include:

          1. Montelukast (Singulair), 10 mg orally daily

          2. Zafirlukast (Accolate), 20 mg orally BID

    a. Consider subcutaneous allergen immunotherapy for patients with possible allergic asthma (based upon history)

    b. Assess for medication and treatment adherence

    c. Patient education (including about proper use of inhalers), environment control, and management of comorbidities

    d. Reevaluate level of asthma control and adjust therapy in 2–6 weeks

E. Step 3—Moderate persistent: daily symptoms, more than 1 time/week that the patient experiences nighttime awakening but not nightly awakening; daily use of an SABA for symptom relief, some limitation with normal activity, FEV_1 greater than 60% but less than 80% predicted, FEV_1/FVC reduced 5%

1. Management
    i. Preferred: low-dose ICS plus LABA or medium-dose ICS (prolonged receptor binding requires patient education about proper use and frequency to avoid induction of cardiac arrhythmias)
        (a) Advair (100 mcg), one inhalation BID
        (b) Symbicort (80 mcg), two inhalations BID
        (c) Dulera, 2 inhalations BID
    ii. Consider a short course of oral systemic corticosteroids
    iii. Consider consulting asthma specialist
    a. Consider subcutaneous allergen immunotherapy for patients with allergic asthma
    b. Assess for medication and treatment adherence
    c. Patient education (including for all inhalers used), environment control, and management of comorbidities
    d. Reevaluate level of asthma control and adjust therapy in 2–6 weeks

F. Steps 4, 5, and 6—severe persistent: symptoms throughout the day, often to seven nighttime awakenings per week, several times per day use of an SABA for symptom relief, extremely limited normal activity, FEV_1 less than 60% predicted, FEV_1/FVC reduced by more than 5%. Assessment for hypoxemia should be done for steps 4, 5, and 6

1. Management
    a. Steps 4
        i. Preferred: medium-dose ICS plus LABA
            (a) Advair 250 mcg, 1 inhalation BID
            (b) Symbicort 160 mcg, 2 inhalations BID
        ii. Consider a short course of oral systemic corticosteroids
        iii. Assess for medication and treatment adherence
        iv. Consider asthma specialist (allergist; pulmonologist) consultation
        v. Consider subcutaneous allergen immunotherapy for patients with allergic asthma
        vi. Patient education, environment control, and management of comorbidities
        vii. Reevaluate level of asthma control and adjust therapy in 2–6 weeks or sooner

      b. Step 5:
         i. Preferred: high-dose ICS plus LABA (Advair 500)
         ii. Consider omalizumab (Xolair)
         iii. Strongly consider a short course of oral, systemic corticosteroids
         iv. Assess for medication and treatment adherence
         v. Consult an asthma specialist
         vi. Patient education (including for all inhalers), environment control, and management of comorbidities
         vii. Reevaluate the patient's level of asthma control and adjust therapy in 2–6 weeks or sooner

      c. Step 6:
         i. Preferred: high-dose ICS plus LABA (Advair 500) plus higher dose oral corticosteroid
         ii. Consideration for omalizumab (Xolair) for patients who have allergies and frequent exacerbations
         iii. Consideration for hospitalization should be made
         iv. Assess for medication and treatment adherence
         v. Consult an asthma specialist

G. Step down therapy if possible and if asthma has been well controlled for at least 3 months

H. Special considerations in the pharmacological management of asthma in the elderly (See special considerations in pharmacological management in the elderly in Pharmacological Management section of COPD, above)

    1. If the older patient has not been evaluated for reversible airway obstruction, consideration of three weeks of oral corticosteroids (20 mg. prednisone daily) and repeat spirometry to assess for reversible component.

    2. Periodic review of proper use of metered dose inhalers is strongly recommended

COPD AND ASTHMA DUAL DIAGNOSIS

I. **Special consideration for the elderly patient**

    A. Over 40% of COPD patients self-report a history of asthma, and the prevalence of the dual diagnosis increases with age.

        1. The dual diagnosis patients tend to progress more rapidly than either diagnosis alone.

        2. Dual diagnosis patients have increased comorbid diagnoses and rates of healthcare utilization.

    B. Current understanding of those at most risk for dual diagnosis of COPD and asthma

        1. Occurrence earlier in life

        2. African-Americans

        3. Female gender

    4. Less inhaled tobacco use that those with just COPD

    5. Higher rates of exacerbation

II. Need greater attention to preventing exacerbations (see COPD and Asthma sections on management)

BRONCHIECTASIS

I. Definition

    A. Clinical disorder characterized by periodic cough with production of copious sputum

    B. Copious sputum means one or more cups per day and occasionally bloody

    C. Often postinflammatory

        1. After severe pneumonia or obstruction of a bronchus by a foreign body

        2. After healing of tuberculosis

II. Physical exam findings

    A. Inspiratory rhonchi during acute exacerbations

    B. Noisy expiration

III. Diagnostics

    A. Chest x-ray may show fibrotic changes

    B. Chest CT scan will usually document dilatation of airways and thickening of bronchial walls.

IV. Management

    A. See Pharmacological Management section of COPD (above)

    B. Strong role for percussive therapy and postural drainage (airway clearance and pulmonary toilet)

        1. Flutter valve

        2. Percussive nebulizers

        3. Percussive garment (VEST)

        4. Positive expiratory pressure devices

    C. Generous use of mucolytics

    D. Emphasis is placed on use of antibiotics (even prophylactically)

OBSTRUCTIVE AIRWAY LESIONS

I. Endobronchial lesions (e.g., tumors and foreign bodies)—seen on chest x-ray or suspected because of atelectasis

    A. Subjective findings

        1. Cough

        2. Dyspnea

        3. Hemoptysis

        4. Weight loss

        5. May include findings outside the chest in other regions of the body when metastatic from another organ

   B. Diagnostics
- **1.** Computed tomographic scan showing a solid mass or irregularly shaped cavity within one lung
- **2.** Chest x-ray demonstrating a mass
- **3.** Fiberoptic bronchoscopy with biopsy
- **4.** Positron emission tomography scan to assist in identifying areas of metastasis

   C. Treatment: based on discovered pathology; may include the following:
- **1.** Surgical removal
- **2.** Chemotherapy
- **3.** Radiation therapy
- **4.** Combination of the preceding

BIBLIOGRAPHY

GlaxoSmithKline. (2012). *COPD Assessment Test (CAT) Health Professional User Guide.* Retrieved June 1, 2014, from http://www.catestonline.org/images/ UserGuides/ CATHCPUser%20guideEn.pdf

GlaxoSmithKline. (2012). *COPD Assessment Test (CAT).* Retrieved June 1, 2014, from http://www.catestonline.org/images/pdfs/CATest.pdf

Global Institute for Chronic Obstructive Lung Disease (GOLD). (2014). *Global strategies for the diagnosis, management, and prevention of COPD, updated May, 2014.* Retrieved June 1, 2014, from http://www.goldcopd.org/Guidelines/ guidelines-resources.html

Hanania, N. A., Sharma, G., & Sharafkhaneh, A. (2010). COPD in the elderly patient. *Seminars in Respiratory and Critical Care Medicine, 31*(5), 596–606.

Hardin, M., Silverman, E. K., Barr, R. G., Hansel, N. N., Schroeder, J. D., Make, B. J., . . . D., & Hersh, C. P. (2011). The clinical features of the overlap between COPD and asthma. *Respiratory Research, 12*, 127. doi:10.1186/1465–9921–12–127

U.S. Department of Health and Human Services. National Institutes of Health: National Heart, Lung, and Blood Institute. (2007). *Expert panel report 3: Guidelines for the diagnosis and management of asthma.* Retrieved from http://www.nhlbi.nih.gov/files/docs/guidelines/asthgdln.pdf

Wechsler, M. E. (2009). Managing asthma in primary care: Putting new guideline recommendations into context. *Mayo Clinic Proceedings, 84*(8), 707–717.

CHAPTER 27

Restrictive (Inflammatory) Lung Diseases

THOMAS W. BARKLEY, JR. • TOBIAS P. REBMANN • DAVID A. MILLER

PNEUMONIA

I. **Definition of pneumonia**
   A. Acute febrile inflammatory disorder of the lung(s), associated with cough and exertional dyspnea
   B. Infiltrate is present on chest x-ray; the appearance of the infiltrate may lag behind the appearance of symptoms by 24–48 hr, justifying a repeat chest x-ray at that time
   C. Leukocytosis may be present

II. **Incidence/etiology**
   A. Pneumonia is one of the most common of all serious lung conditions and a frequent cause of acute care hospitalization and mortality.
   B. Elderly are especially at risk due to poor immune systems, debilitation, and weakness preventing adequate airway clearance
   C. Organisms that are potential causes of community-acquired pneumonia:
      1. Bacteria
         a. *Streptococcus pneumoniae* (most common bacterial cause in adults)
         b. *Haemophilus influenza*
         c. *Klebsiella pneumoniae*
         d. Gram-negative organisms
      2. "Atypical" pathogens
         a. *Chlamydia pneumoniae*
         b. *Mycoplasma pneumoniae*
         c. *Mycobacterium tuberculosis*
      3. Viruses
         a. Respiratory syncytial virus

   b. Adenovirus

   c. Rhinovirus

D. Overzealous treatment of mild respiratory infection in the past has contributed to the development of antimicrobial drug resistance, especially to *S. pneumoniae*

E. Comorbidity from the following conditions contributes to high mortality from pneumonia:

   1. Chronic obstructive pulmonary disease (COPD)

   2. Heart failure

   3. Diabetes mellitus

   4. Chronic liver and renal disease

F. The very young and the very old are at increased risk of death from pneumonia, despite the remarkable array of antimicrobial agents available to treat this disorder.

III. **Classification of pneumonia**

A. "Typical" pneumonias manifest with "classic" findings

   1. Fever

   2. Chills

   3. Leukocytosis

   4. Cough

   5. Sputum production

   6. Increased fremitus

B. "Atypical" pneumonias vary in their presentation

   1. Fever may be high

   2. Leukocytosis

      a. May be absent

      b. May be associated with a "left shift" in the differential white blood cell count (WBC) to include a high number of "band" forms

   3. Cough is often dry

   4. Headache

   5. Sore throat

   6. Excessive sweating

   7. Soreness in the chest

C. Both forms demonstrate an infiltrate on chest x-ray

   1. Atypical pneumonias are more often diffuse

   2. Atypical pneumonias may particularly involve more than one lung segment or both lungs

D. Occurrence information may assist in defining the type of pneumonia present

   1. Time of year

   2. Known epidemic disease

   3. Presence of comorbid conditions

E. Community-acquired pneumonias (CAPs) are those acquired within the community setting

F. Nosocomial pneumonias result from exposure to infection during a stay in a health care facility

1. Hospital-acquired pneumonia (HAP)

   a. Pneumonia that occurs 48 hr or more after admission, which was not incubating at the time of admission (includes VAP and HCAP). *Staphylococcus aureus*, *Streptococcus pneumoniae*, and *Haemophilus influenzae* are the most common causative organisms.

2. Ventilator-acquired pneumonia (VAP)

   a. Pneumonia that arises more than 48–72 hr after endotracheal intubation

   b. *Pseudomonas* is the most common causative organism

3. Healthcare-associated pneumonia (HCAP)

   a. Includes any patient who was hospitalized in an acute care hospital for two or more days within 90 days of the infection; resided in a nursing home or long-term care facility; received recent intravenous antibiotic therapy, chemotherapy, or wound care within the past 30 days of the current infection; or attended a hospital or hemodialysis clinic

   b. Organisms in HCAP are more similar to those of HAP than CAP (e.g., higher rates of *Staphylococcus aureus* and *Pseudomonas aeruginosa*, and less *Streptococcus pneumoniae*, *Haemophilus influenzae*, and MRSA)

G. Pneumonias are often categorized by risk factors present that predispose the patient to pneumonia

1. Aspiration pneumonias (related to altered mental status or dysphagia from stroke or neuromuscular disease, i.e., Parkinson's disease)

2. Obstructive lesions of the airway

   a. Tumor

   b. Retained bronchopulmonary secretions

3. Inhalation injury-related pneumonia

   a. Hypersensitivity pneumonia

   b. Near drowning

H. Pneumonia Index Severity Index may be helpful; grades severity based on age, sex, comorbid diseases, physical exam, and labs

IV.   Evaluation for possible pneumonia

A. Historical information

B. Physical examination

1. Tachypnea

2. Tachycardia

3. Fever

4. Discomfort

5. Rales (or "crackles") on auscultation over the affected area(s)

6. Mental status changes and confusion

C. Chest x-ray, in a search for new pulmonary infiltrates

D. Laboratory/diagnostics

1. Complete blood count (CBC), including differential WBC count
2. Blood cultures
3. Gram stain and culture of sputum
4. Arterial blood gases (ABGs) and/or pulse oximetry
5. Procalcitonin levels, when available, may aid in diagnosis of bacterial pneumonia and guide duration of antimicrobial therapy

V. **Treatment**

A. Antimicrobial therapy with cultures pending (for specific treatment guidelines, see Lower Respiratory Tract Pathogens chapter)

B. Antimicrobial therapy should be revised as culture information becomes available and as improvement occurs. In general, the narrowest spectrum antimicrobial to which known organisms are expected to respond should be used.

C. Need to cover anaerobic organisms in cases of known or suspected aspiration

D. Simultaneous treatment of coexisting illnesses is needed

1. COPD
2. Heart failure
3. Diabetes
4. Dehydration

E. Not all patients, especially young adults, need hospitalization for pneumonia

1. The decision to hospitalize a patient with pneumonia should be guided by the following:
   a. The possibility of rapidly progressive disease
   b. The overall status of the patient (coexisting problems)
   c. The patient's ability to reliably self-administer medication for this illness
2. If in doubt, it is reasonable to observe the patient in hospital during initial therapy and to reassess early response to treatment

VI. **Prevention of pneumonia**

A. Vaccination against influenza: Influenza virus vaccine

1. Repeated annually
2. Some revaccinate within a season if the patient:
   i. Is immunocompromised
   ii. Has severe underlying COPD or heart disease

B. Vaccination against *S. pneumoniae*: pneumococcal vaccine polyvalent (Pneumovax)

1. PCV13: pneumococcal conjugate vaccine for infants, children, and adults older than 19 years at high risk for disease
2. PPSV23: pneumococcal polysaccharide vaccine for adults older than 65 years and those older than 2 years at high risk for disease

3. If giving both vaccines, start with PCV 13 and give PPSV23 at least 8 weeks later
4. Guidelines change frequently; refer to the Centers for Disease Control and Prevention for the latest recommendations

TUBERCULOSIS (TB)

I.   **Etiology:** *Mycobacterium tuberculosis*
II. **Incidence**
   A. The rates of new infection by *M. tuberculosis* are increasing, especially among the homeless and among those living in crowded conditions, such as nursing homes and prisons in larger metropolitan areas.
   B. Alarmingly, the incidence of multidrug-resistant TB (defined as resistant to isoniazid and rifampin) also appears to be rising, especially along the East and West Coasts of the United States.
   C. This rise has coincided with increased numbers of patients with HIV and AIDS
III. **Clinical findings**
   A. Symptoms
      1. Most patients are asymptomatic
      2. Fever
      3. Cough, generally productive of purulent sputum that may contain blood
      4. Weight loss
      5. Night sweats that may require changing of bed linen
   B. Physical exam findings
      1. Body temperature elevation
      2. Cachexia may be noted.
      3. Rales over the affected areas: apical posttussive rales for apical disease
   C. Laboratory/diagnostics
      1. Normal CBC
      2. Low serum cortisol level if disseminated disease to the adrenal glands has destroyed the adrenal cortices
      3. Sputum
         a. Acid-fast smears are often positive, but therapy may have to be started empirically if other findings are suggestive of TB in the absence of positive smears
         b. Cultures for *M. tuberculosis* are usually positive within 6 weeks
      4. TB skin testing (intradermal purified protein derivative [PPD])
         a. Indicates only exposure, not necessarily active infection
         b. PPD (0.1 ml) injected intradermally; read 48 hr later
         c. Interpretation based on measurement of the largest diameter of the indurated area (not including flat but erythematous area):
            i. Less than 5 mm: negative test

      ii. 5 mm or more: positive test in an HIV-infected patient, recent TB exposure, immunocompromised, or patient with chest film typical for TB

      iii. 10 mm or more: positive test in health care workers, HIV-negative injection drug users, residents of nursing homes/homeless shelters, recent immigrants, etc.

      iv. 15 mm or more: positive test in any person

  5. QuantiFERON TB Gold test

    a. Serum test used for diagnosis of TB, either latent or active, instead of PPD

    b. Not affected by prior exposure to bacille Calmette-Guérin (BCG) vaccination

D. Chest x-ray

  1. Infiltrate

    a. Especially present in the upper lobes of the lungs or in the superior segments of the lower lobes

    b. Can be present in any portion of the lungs

  2. Cavity within the lungs

IV. Treatment

A. Patient isolation during initial evaluation and treatment, according to the Occupational Safety and Health Administration standards, is mandatory

B. Suspected disease, or smear-positive disease, pending the return of sputum cultures

  1. Four-drug therapy

    a. Isoniazid, 300 mg PO daily (or 5 mg/kg; maximum, 300 mg daily), with pyridoxine, 50 mg PO, to prevent INH-induced peripheral neuropathy

    b. Rifampin (Rifadin/Rimactane) 600 mg PO each day (or 10 mg/kg daily; maximum, 600 mg/dose)

    c. Ethambutol (Myambutol), 15–25 mg/kg PO each day (maximum, 2.5 grams/dose), preceded by screening of color vision

      i. Note: Ethambutol (Myambutol) may cause red/green color blindness as an adverse effect, as well as changes in visual acuity.

    d. Pyrazinamide, 15–30 mg/kg in three divided doses daily (maximum, 2 grams/dose)

  2. Modification of regimen may be necessary if drug susceptibility studies demonstrate resistance to first-line drugs

    a. If isolate proves to be fully susceptible to INH and RIF, then ethambutol may be dropped

  3. Therapy is continued usually for 6–9 months (6 months for most patients, 9 months for HIV-positive and/or immunocompromised patients)

    4. Intermittent directly observed therapy may follow one of three regimens:

        a. INH + rifampin + pyrazinamide + ethambutol daily for 2 months, followed by INH + rifampin 2–3 times weekly for an additional 4 months, especially if susceptibility to INH/rifampin is noted

        b. INH + rifampin + pyrazinamide + ethambutol daily for 2 weeks, followed by the same agents 2 times weekly for 6 weeks, then INH + rifampin 2 times weekly for 4 months, if susceptibility to INH/rifampin is noted

        c. Thrice-weekly dosing of INH + rifampin + pyrazinamide + ethambutol for 24 doses (8 weeks); followed by thrice-weekly dosing of INH + rifampin for 54 doses (18 weeks)

        d. Patients with advanced HIV (CD4 counts less than 100/µl) should be treated with daily or three-times-weekly therapy in both the initial and the continuation phases.

    5. For nonadherent patients, directly observed treatment may be initiated at 3 times per week, usually after 2 weeks of observed therapy, often in hospital

C. Prophylaxis

    1. Consider for the following patients:

        a. Asymptomatic, with a positive PPD and a normal chest x-ray

        b. Exposed to active TB who have a negative PPD

        c. Undergoing immunosuppressive therapy for other reasons

        d. HIV infected

    2. Treatment

        a. INH, 300 mg PO daily, although controversy exists as to whether 6 months or up to 1 year of therapy should be given; the standard regimen consists of a duration of 9 months, which is also the preferred duration for HIV-positive patients

        b. Pyridoxine, 50 mg PO daily, may be also chosen during INH therapy to prevent neuropathy

ACUTE RESPIRATORY DISTRESS SYNDROME (ARDS)/ ACUTE LUNG INJURY (ALI)

I. **Etiologies: any of the numerous causes of acute systemic inflammation**

    A. Bacteremia or other severe systemic infections

    B. Massive trauma or injury, including burns and smoke inhalation

    C. Pancreatitis

    D. Shock (any cause)

    E. Cardiopulmonary bypass

    F. Increased intracranial pressure, especially after trauma or intracranial bleeding

G. Aspiration of fluid, including gastrointestinal contents and near drowning

II. **Incidence**

    A. Annual incidence is unknown, largely owing to lack of required reporting and misunderstanding about when and how the diagnosis is made

    B. Overall incidence in any locale will be proportionate to the incidence of known causes of the syndrome itself

III. **Clinical findings**

    A. Severe respiratory distress occurring during the course of one of the inciting events

    B. Respiratory distress often requires the early institution of mechanical ventilatory assistance; refractory hypoxemia is a classic finding

    C. Symptoms:

        1. Breathlessness

        2. Agitation

        3. Confusion

        4. Obtundation as oxygen delivery and uptake by tissues falls

    D. Other manifestations include failure of other organ systems

        1. Kidneys

        2. Liver

        3. Bone marrow (reduced platelet count)

        4. Multisystem organ failure

    E. Physical findings depend on the presentation of the condition, placing the patient at risk for ARDS. Lungs often sound clearer than the chest x-ray would suggest.

    F. Laboratory/diagnostics

        1. Arterial blood gas (ABG): PaO_2/FiO_2 ratio. If less than 300, then acute lung injury; if less than 200, then acute respiratory distress syndrome (ARDS)

        2. Complete blood count with differential white count and platelet count

        3. Coagulation studies

            a. Prothrombin time

            b. Partial thromboplastin time

            c. Fibrinogen level

            d. Fibrin degradation products

        4. Renal and liver function

        5. Urinalysis

        6. Blood and urine cultures

        7. Sputum culture and Gram stain

    G. X-rays

        1. Chest x-ray—often shows evolving bilateral infiltrates (e.g., "whited out")

      2. Other x-rays—as indicated by the patient's presenting problems (e.g., trauma)

IV. **Treatment**

  A. Airway

     1. Assess the adequacy of ventilation and the degree of work used during spontaneous ventilation

     2. Intubate if ventilation is significantly compromised, especially if altered mentation is noted

  B. Breathing: institute mechanical ventilation

     1. If work of breathing is not being met, as evidenced by the following:

       a. Patient fatigue

       b. Elevated $PaCO_2$ (partial pressure of carbon dioxide in arterial blood)

     2. If measured, hypoxemia is not correctable with an FIO_2 (fraction of inspired oxygen) of 0.5

  C. Circulation: vigorous fluid resuscitation should be started if hypotension is present

     1. Regulated by hemodynamic parameters, especially left ventricular ejection fraction

  D. Correct the underlying etiology of the ARDS

  E. Support needed

     1. Mechanical ventilatory assistance often requires the institution of positive end-expiratory pressure

     2. Ventilatory pressures over 45 cm H_2O may require the use of:

       a. Reduced tidal volumes

       b. Pressure-cycled ventilation

       c. High-frequency oscillatory ventilation

       d. Permissive hypercapnia, with bicarbonate repletion to avoid excessive acidosis

     3. The patient should be sedated for comfort

     4. Nutritional support should be started early

       a. Use enteral route (total parenteral nutrition may be used with caution when enteral route is unavailable)

       b. Most patients require nearly twice their usual daily caloric requirements to counteract the tremendous energy expenditure used in combating ARDS

V. **Despite refinements in the provision of care for patients with ARDS, overall mortality remains at nearly 40%**

VI. **Special considerations**

  A. The risk of pulmonary barotrauma, including pneumothorax or pneumomediastinum, is high with this disorder.

  B. Sudden increases in ventilating pressure with desaturation in arterial oxygen tension indicate the need for an immediate repeat chest x-ray and for possible chest tube insertion

C. Repeated physical and radiographic assessments of the lungs may be needed to rule out barotrauma in the mechanically ventilated patient with ARDS

IDIOPATHIC PULMONARY FIBROSIS (IPF)

I. **Etiology/general concepts**
 A. Etiology is unknown; strongly linked to cigarette smoking
 B. Prior to treatment, rule out the following:
  1. Inhalation exposure
  2. Autoimmune disorders
  3. Chronic lung infection
   a. Tuberculosis
   b. Deep fungal infection
    i. Histoplasmosis
    ii. Coccidioidomycosis
 C. In patients with prior malignancy, the lymphangitic spread of tumor to the lungs should be excluded.

II. **Incidence**
 A. Unknown; IPF is the most common cause of interstitial lung disease among elderly patients
 B. More common in men than in women

III. **Clinical findings**
 A. Symptoms
  1. Progressive (slow or rapid) dyspnea
  2. Cough (nonproductive)
  3. Specific questioning of the patient about prior exposure to the following:
   a. Inorganic dusts
    i. Silica
    ii. Asbestos
   b. Organic dusts (e.g., in silos, where hypersensitivity pneumonia may be acquired)
   c. Fumes
    i. Chlorine
    ii. Sulfur dioxide
   d. Drugs
    i. Chemotherapeutic agents (e.g., bleomycin)
    ii. Antibiotics (e.g., nitrofurantoin and sulfa)
    iii. Gold salts (during the course of therapy for rheumatoid arthritis)
    iv. Amiodarone (for cardiac arrhythmias)
   e. Radiation to lung parenchyma
   f. Risk factors for *Pneumocystis carinii* pneumonia
    i. Immunosuppression from HIV infection

       ii. Chemotherapy for lymphoma or lymphocytic leukemia and other malignancies

       iii. Immunosuppression for organ transplantation

    g. Known chronic heart failure

B. Physical exam findings

    1. Rales ("Velcro crackles") may be heard on auscultation

C. Laboratory/diagnostics

    1. Changes within the lung parenchyma, especially in the lower lobes, demonstrated by chest x-ray and high-resolution CT scanning

       a. Interstitial infiltrates

       b. Nodules

       c. Cystic (or "honeycombing") changes

    2. Pulmonary function testing typically demonstrates a restrictive ventilatory defect.

       a. Some patients may show a coexisting bronchoconstriction in small airways

       b. The diffusing capacity of lung for carbon monoxide is commonly reduced—a manifestation of altered ventilation and perfusion relationships within the lungs.

    3. ABG analysis and pulse oximetry

       a. May demonstrate hypoxemia, typically as the disease progresses

       b. Carbon dioxide retention indicates severe disease

    4. Laboratory findings generally are not helpful

       a. PPD testing should be done

       b. Prior exposure to deep fungi, including *Histoplasma capsulatum* (chicken coops in the Midwest) and *Coccidioides immitis* (dust in the Southwest desert and Central Valleys of California), may be assessed with complement fixation serologic studies for deep fungi, although prior exposure does not necessarily equate with active disease

          i. Histoplasmosis

          ii. Coccidioidomycosis

          iii. Blastomycosis

    5. Obtaining tissue for diagnosis

       a. Fiber-optic bronchoscopy with transbronchial biopsy of the lung parenchyma is safe and should be done first

       b. Bronchoalveolar lavage to assess for inflammation and to obtain secretions for culture (e.g., acid-fast bacilli, fungi, and *Nocardia*) may be performed at the same time

      c. Because biopsies obtained at bronchoscopy may be inadequate for diagnosis and are subject to sampling error, patients deemed healthy enough to undergo open lung biopsy should be considered for thoracoscopic lung biopsy. If further assurance is required, then the diagnosis of IPF is correct.

        i. Obtain preoperative pulmonary function tests

D. Vaccination: influenza and pneumococcal polysaccharide vaccine should be offered to patients with IPF, as these infections are poorly tolerated in patients with interstitial lung disease

E. Therapy

    1. Corticosteroids (prednisone 1 mg/kg/day for 12 weeks)

      a. Used for acute exacerbation, although scientific evidence/support for benefit is lacking

      b. Many patients report subjective improvement

      c. Far fewer demonstrate objective improvement radiographically or on pulmonary function testing

      d. Use caution with elderly because of its significant side effects (bone demineralization, immunosuppression, and hyperglycemia)

    2. Alternative treatments that may be considered in selected patients include cyclophosphamide (Cytoxan), 1 mg/kg/day, or azathioprine (Imuran), 3 mg/kg/day, although data to support immunosuppressive therapy in this setting is limited.

    3. Noninvasive use of positive airway pressure (by mask) may be beneficial in selected patients

F. Prognosis: IPF is usually a progressive illness, and the prognosis is often poor over time

G. Patients with rapidly progressive or end-stage disease should be counseled on palliative care and end-of-life issues.

SARCOIDOSIS

I. **Definition**

A. Characterized pathologically by the presence of non caseating granulomas and interstitial lung disease

B. Systemic manifestations:

    1. Lymphadenopathy

    2. Cardiac involvement

    3. Iritis

    4. Cutaneous lesions

    5. Arthritis

    6. Gastrointestinal involvement

    7. Other organs may be involved

II.   Incidence

   A. Unknown

   B. More common among females, North Americans, African Americans, and northern European Caucasians

   C. May be seen in all races

   D. Typically, the onset of symptoms is between the ages of 20 and 40 years

III.   Clinical findings

   A. Symptoms

      1. Progressive dyspnea (slow or rapid)

      2. Nonproductive cough

   B. Physical exam findings

      1. Depends on specific organ involvement

      2. Lung examination may be normal.

      3. Rales ("Velcro crackles") may be heard on auscultation when interstitial disease (for example, fibrosis) is present

   C. Laboratory/diagnostics

      1. Chest x-ray may demonstrate the following: (The stages shown are useful in staging pulmonary involvement by sarcoidosis.)

         a. Stage 0: normal chest x-ray

         b. Stage I: bilateral hilar lymphadenopathy (BHL)

         c. Stage II: BHL plus pulmonary infiltrates

         d. Stage III: pulmonary infiltrates without BHL

         e. Stage IV: pulmonary fibrosis

      2. Pulmonary function testing typically demonstrates a restrictive ventilatory defect

         a. Some patients may show a coexisting bronchoconstriction in small airways

         b. The diffusing capacity of lung for carbon monoxide is commonly reduced—a manifestation of altered ventilation and perfusion relationships within the lungs

      3. ABG analysis and pulse oximetry

         a. May demonstrate hypoxemia, typically as the disease progresses

         b. Carbon dioxide retention indicates severe disease

      4. Laboratory findings generally are not helpful

         a. PPD testing should be done

         b. Prior exposure to deep fungi may be assessed with complement fixation serologic studies for deep fungi, although prior exposure does not necessarily equate active disease.

            i. Histoplasmosis

            ii. Coccidioidomycosis

            iii. Blastomycosis

5. Obtaining tissue for diagnosis of pulmonary sarcoidosis
   a. Fiberoptic bronchoscopy with transbronchial biopsy of the lung parenchyma is safe and should be done first.
   b. Bronchoalveolar lavage to assess for inflammation and to obtain secretions for culture (e.g., acid-fast bacilli, fungi, and *Nocardia*) may be performed at the same time.
   c. Because biopsies obtained at bronchoscopy may be inadequate for diagnosis and are subject to sampling error, patients deemed healthy enough to undergo open lung biopsy should be considered for thoracoscopic lung biopsy if further assurance is required that the diagnosis of sarcoidosis is correct
   d. If other organs are involved, biopsy of one of those sites may be beneficial in establishing the diagnosis.
   e. If BHL is present, cervical mediastinal exploration with biopsy of a node is reasonable.
6. Blood tests
   a. CBC
   b. Calcium (sarcoidosis is associated with hypercalcemia)
   c. Liver function tests
   d. BUN
   e. Creatinine
7. ECG
8. Urinalysis
9. PPD
10. Ophthalmologic examination
D. Therapy
   1. Corticosteroids
      a. Initial dose of prednisone includes 0.3–0.6 mg/kg ideal body weight (usually 20–40 mg/day) x 6 weeks. No formal data is available to guide maintenance dosing of oral glucocorticoids.
      b. Maintenance dose of prednisone is 0.25–0.5 mg/kg (usually 10–20 mg) per day dose. Maintenance dose is continued for at least 6–8 months, with a total treatment time of about 1 year.
      c. Many patients report subjective improvement. Proper length of therapy in patients who respond to treatment is unknown.
      d. Far fewer demonstrate objective improvement radiographically or by pulmonary function testing
      e. Use is cautioned with elderly due to significant side effects (bone demineralization, immunosuppression, and hyperglycemia)
   2. Alternative treatments that may be considered in selected patients; a variety of immunosuppressive agents have been used to treat refractory pulmonary sarcoidosis include:

        a. Cyclophosphamide (Cytoxan), 25–50 mg/day (not to exceed 150 mg/day), or

        b. Azathioprine (Imuran), 2 mg/kg or 50 mg PO daily. Due to the toxicity of cyclophosphamide, it is reserved as a "third-line" drug

    3. Methotrexate, 7.5 mg PO daily (which can be increased by 2.5 mg every two weeks with a maximum dose of 10–15 mg per week) and chloroquine (250–750 mg PO daily or every other day) also have been used alternatively in sarcoidosis.

HEART FAILURE/CARDIOGENIC PULMONARY EDEMA

I. **Etiology: numerous causes are known**
- **A.** Coronary artery disease with myocardial ischemia and infarction, aggravated by the following:
  - **1.** Obesity
  - **2.** Limited exercise
  - **3.** Dyslipidemia
  - **4.** Cigarette smoking
- **B.** Cardiac arrhythmias
  - **1.** Tachycardia (especially)
  - **2.** Bradycardia
- **C.** Hypertension
- **D.** Valvular dysfunction of the heart
- **E.** Thyroid dysfunction, including the following:
  - **1.** Hyperthyroidism
  - **2.** Hypothyroidism
- **F.** Diabetes mellitus
- **G.** Viral myocarditis
- **H.** Idiopathic cardiomyopathy
- **I.** Renal failure
- **J.** Drug therapy, especially certain chemotherapeutic agents

II. **Incidence**
- **A.** Heart failure is a common disorder that leads to frequent outpatient visits and inpatient hospitalizations, despite the availability of modern therapeutic interventions
- **B.** In general, heart failure can be described in the following ways:
  - **1.** Is progressive
  - **2.** Eventuates in frequent hospitalizations
  - **3.** Carries a guarded prognosis over time

III. **Clinical manifestations are related to the development of restrictive ventilatory defects within the lung parenchyma that are initially mild and later severe.**
- **A.** Symptoms
  - **1.** Progression from exertional dyspnea to orthopnea and paroxysmal nocturnal dyspnea

2. Frank respiratory failure may be noted
3. Dry cough is commonly seen
4. The time course of this progression may be slow or abrupt

B. Classification is based on New York Heart Association (NYHA) functional scale
   1. NYHA 1: no limitations from ordinary activities
   2. NYHA 2: slight limitations with moderate exertion
   3. NYHA 3: marked limitation with activity and comfortable only at rest
   4. NYHA 4: patients who should be on complete rest; symptoms with any activity and occasionally at rest

C. Physical exam findings: secondary responses lead to detectable signs of fluid retention
   1. Edema and jugular venous distention
   2. Rales
   3. Tachycardia or bradycardia
   4. Inability to tolerate lying flat in the supine position (orthopnea)
   5. Tachypnea
   6. Pleural effusions
   7. Ascites (when heart failure is advanced)

D. Diagnosis
   1. ECG
      a. Assess for ischemia or infarction
      b. Determine cardiac rhythm
   2. Chest x-ray, looking for the following:
      a. Vascular redistribution to upper lung fields
      b. Presence of the following:
         i. Interstitial edema
         ii. Kerley B lines
      c. Pleural effusions (usually bilateral or on the right)
      d. Cardiomegaly
   3. Assessment of oxygenation to ensure adequate oxygenation of blood and to assess for carbon dioxide retention
      a. ABG analysis
      b. Pulse oximetry
   4. CBC to rule out anemia
   5. Chemistries
      a. Thyroid function: thyroid-stimulating hormone
         i. If thyroid-stimulating hormone is abnormal, perform free triiodothyronine (Free T3) and free thyroxine (Free T4) to determine true disease versus euthyroid sick state, especially in acutely ill
      b. Renal function
         i. BUN
         ii. Creatinine

      c. Liver function

      d. Electrolytes (including magnesium levels)

  6. Cardiac enzyme evaluation, especially if recent myocardial infarction or unstable angina pectoris is suspected

  7. Echocardiography to assess the following:

      a. Systolic function of the heart; rate of demise is more significant than the actual ejection fraction

      b. Valvular function

      c. Dyskinesia

          i. Global

          ii. Segmental

      d. Diastology

      e. Right heart pressures and function (right ventricular systolic pressure) to determine presence of pulmonary hypertension, either acute or chronic

  8. Pulmonary function studies are not useful during acute pulmonary edema, but when the patient is stable, they have the following purposes:

      a. May help to demonstrate the presence of a restrictive ventilatory defect in early heart failure (reduced vital capacity)

      b. May help to evaluate for coexisting COPD, especially among smokers

  9. Occasionally, patients with heart failure will require pulmonary artery catheterization to document the severity of the problem, especially when hypotension is present.

      a. Aggressive fluid therapy could further aggravate heart failure

      b. If needed, determination can be made of the following:

          i. Cardiac output

          ii. Cardiac index

          iii. Systemic vascular resistance

          iv. Pulmonary capillary wedge pressure

  10. In general, insertion of a pulmonary artery catheter is not necessary in treating patients with heart failure.

E. Treatment

  1. Correct the cause of the heart failure, if known (especially ischemia). Nitrates may be indicated clinically; however, these may or may not be appropriate, depending on the underlying cause (arrhythmia, valvular heart disease, etc.)

      a. Sublingual nitroglycerin

      b. Nitroglycerin patches, such as Nitro-Dur 0.4 mg, applied daily

      c. Oral, long-acting nitrates, such as isosorbide

  2. Emphasize long-term priorities of improved diet (sodium restriction), weight control, and exercise

  3. Control dyslipidemia with diet, exercise, and pharmacologic therapy

4. Supplement oxygen, usually via nasal cannula at low flow rates (e.g., 2 L/min).
   a. In frank pulmonary edema, oxygen should be supplied in higher amounts
   b. Use mask delivery PRN to adequately oxygenate the blood
5. If the patient is unable to sustain the work of breathing during an acute episode of heart failure, attempt should be made at noninvasive positive pressure ventilation via continuous positive airway pressure (CPAP) followed by intubation and mechanical ventilatory assistance, if necessary. This will help to redistribute edema out of the lungs and back into the vascular space, as well as to offload the work of breathing and save energy.
6. Improve contractility of the myocardium
   a. Eliminate cardiac depressants
      i. Calcium channel blockers
      ii. β-blockers (in acute decompensation)
   b. Supply additional inotropic force in acute decompensation (dobutamine and milrinone)
   c. Decrease afterload with an ACE inhibitor as blood pressure tolerates
   d. Decrease preload with morphine and diuresis
   e. Use β-adrenergic antagonists to help regulate catecholamines if blood pressure and heart rate will tolerate
   f. These measures will reduce interstitial edema and ventilatory restriction, thereby improving respiratory symptoms.
   g. Aggressiveness of these measures must be proportionate to the severity of interstitial edema and the degree of respiratory distress present

BIBLIOGRAPHY

Bartlett, J. G. (2010). *Workshop on issues in the design of clinical trials for antibacterial drugs for hospital acquired pneumonia and ventilator associated pneumonia*. Chicago, IL: Univ. of Chicago Press.

Cecil, R. L., Goldman, L., & Schafer, A. I. (2012). *Goldman's Cecil medicine* (24th ed.). Philadelphia, PA: Elsevier/Saunders.

Centers for Disease Control and Prevention. (2005). Guidelines for the investigation of contacts of persons with infectious tuberculosis: Recommendations from the National Tuberculosis Controllers Association and CDC. *Morbidity and Mortality Weekly Report, 54*(RR-15), 1–37.

Emanuel, L. L. (2011). *Palliative care: Core skills and clinical competencies* (2nd ed.). Philadelphia, PA: Saunders.

Guidelines for the prevention of ventilator-associated pneumonia in adults in Ireland. (2011). Dublin: Health Protection Surveillance Centre.

Hawkins, N. M. (2010). *Heart failure and chronic obstructive pulmonary disease common partners, common problems*. Glasgow: University of Glasgow.

Kamangar, N., Royani, P., & Shorr, A. F. (2013). In S. P. Peters (Ed.), *Sarcoidosis*. Retrieved November 30, 2013, from http://www.emedicine.medscape.com/article/301914-overview

Longo, D. L., Fauci, A., Hauser, S., Jameson, J., & Loscalzo, J. (2012). *Harrison's principles of internal medicine* (18th ed.). New York, NY: McGraw-Hill.

Mall, M. A. (2014). *Cystic fibrosis*. Sheffield: European Respiratory Society.

McPhee, S. J., Papadakis, M. A., & Rabow, M. W. (Eds.). (2013). *CURRENT medical diagnosis and treatment 2013* (52nd ed.). New York, NY: McGraw Hill/Appleton & Lange.

Murali, S. (2012). *Pulmonary hypertension*. Philadelphia, PA: Saunders/Elsevier.

Nathanson, N. (2007). *Viral pathogenesis and immunity* (2nd ed.). Amsterdam: Elsevier Academic Press.

Pneumonia Severity Index Calculator. (2003). Agency for Healthcare Research and Quality. Rockville, MD. http://pda.ahrq.gov/psicalc.as

Pokorski, M. (2013). *Neurobiology of respiration*. Dordrecht: Springer.

Weinstock, M. B., Neides, D. M., Chan, M., Schumick, D. R. (2009). *Resident's guide to ambulatory* care (6th ed.). Colombus, OH: Anadem Publishing Inc.

Yancy, C. W., Jessup, M., Bozkurt, B., Butler, J., Casey, D. E., Drazner, M. H., . . . Wilkoff, B. L. (2013). 2013 ACCF/AHA guidelines for the management of heart failure: Executive summary: A report of the American College of Cardiology Foundation/American Heart Association Task Force on practice guidelines. *Journal of the American College of Cardiology*, *62*(16), 1495–1539.

CHAPTER **28**

Pulmonary Hypertension and Pulmonary Vascular Disorders

HALEY M. HOY • IVAN ROBBINS • THOMAS W. BARKLEY, JR.

PULMONARY HYPERTENSION

I. **Etiology**
   A. Increased pulmonary vascular resistance
      1. Vasoconstriction (e.g., due to hypoxemia and acidosis)
      2. Loss of vasculature (e.g., due to emphysema and lung resection)
      3. Occlusion of the pulmonary vasculature (e.g., due to pulmonary embolism [PE])
      4. Relative stenosis of the pulmonary vasculature (e.g., vasculitis)
   B. Increased pulmonary venous pressure
      1. Left ventricular failure or hypertrophy
      2. Valvular heart disease (e.g., mitral valve stenosis and aortic valve stenosis)
      3. Constrictive pericarditis
   C. Increased pulmonary blood flow (left-to-right shunt)
   D. Polycythemia (primary or secondary; e.g., from hypoxemia)
   E. Idiopathic pulmonary arterial hypertension, seen most often in young women
      1. World Health Organization (WHO) classification:
         a. WHO group I: pulmonary arterial hypertension
            i. Idiopathic pulmonary arterial hypertension
            ii. Familial pulmonary arterial hypertension

   iii. Associated pulmonary arterial hypertension: collagen vascular disease (e.g., scleroderma), congenital shunts between systemic and pulmonary circulation, portal hypertension, HIV infection, drugs, toxins, or other diseases or disorders

   iv. Associated with venous or capillary disease

  b. WHO group II: pulmonary hypertension associated with left heart disease

   i. Atrial or ventricular disease

   ii. Valvular disease (e.g., mitral stenosis)

  c. WHO group III: pulmonary hypertension associated with lung diseases and/or hypoxemia

   i. Chronic obstructive pulmonary disease (COPD), interstitial lung disease

   ii. Sleep-disordered breathing, alveolar hypoventilation

   iii. Chronic exposure to high altitude

   iv. Developmental lung abnormalities

  d. WHO group IV: pulmonary hypertension due to chronic thrombotic and/or embolic disease

   i. PE in the proximal or distal pulmonary arteries

   ii. Embolization of other matter, such as tumor cells or parasites

  e. WHO group V: miscellaneous, hematologic, and systemic disorders

   i. Myeloproliferative disorders

   ii. Sarcoidosis

   iii. Sickle cell disease

II. **Incidence**

 A. Note: The incidence of secondary pulmonary hypertension is related to the incidence of the cause of pulmonary hypertension.

III. **Signs/symptoms**

 A. Dyspnea with exertion

 B. Those related to the cause of the pulmonary hypertension

 C. Substernal discomfort

 D. Fatigue

 E. Syncope

 F. Palpitations

IV. **Subjective/physical examination findings**

 A. Splitting of the second cardiac sound; pulmonic valve component of the second heart sound (P2) is increased in intensity

 B. Peripheral edema related to right ventricular (RV) failure

 C. Ascites

 D. RV heave

 E. Loud pulmonic valve

V. Laboratory/diagnostics
  A. Lab:
    1. Complete blood count: increase in hemoglobin and hematocrit if hypoxemia present
  B. Radiographs:
    1. Chest x-ray: increased size of the proximal pulmonary arteries; visible narrowing of the pulmonary arteries in the medial third of the lung (typically seen in emphysema)
  C. Cardiac: electrocardiogram, echocardiogram, and right heart catheterization
    1. Two-dimensional echocardiography is used to diagnose pulmonary hypertension
    2. Cardiac catheterization is used to confirm the diagnosis
      a. Elevated mean pulmonary artery pressure with normal pulmonary capillary wedge pressure, elevated pulmonary artery systolic pressure, and tricuspid regurgitation velocity
  D. Pulmonary function testing: to assess for obstructive and restrictive ventilatory defects
  E. Consider tests to rule out thromboembolic disorders
    1. Lower-extremity Doppler
    2. Ventilation/perfusion lung scan
    3. Computed tomography (CT)

VI. Treatment
  A. Treatment of underlying disorders that may contribute to hypoxemia, including the following:
    1. COPD
    2. Congestive heart failure
    3. Obstructive sleep apnea
  B. Supplemental oxygen during the night
  C. Consider anticoagulation due to increased risk for intrapulmonary thrombosis and thromboembolism.
  D. If polycythemia is severe, with hematocrit above 60%, therapeutic phlebotomy should be considered to yield a hematocrit of approximately 55%. Consider adding diuretics for fluid retention
  E. Pharmacologic therapy—usually started for symptomatic patients in WHO functional classes II, III, or IV if patients showed no acute vasoreactivity or did not respond well to calcium channel blockers
    1. Prostanoids
      a. Calcium channel blockers
        i. Nifedipine, 90–240 mg PO daily
        ii. Diltiazem, 240–720 mg daily
        iii. Limited role in therapy; should not be use empirically to treat pulmonary arterial hypertension in the absence of demonstrated acute vasoreactivity
        iv. May be used in WHO functional classes I-IV

        v.   If improvement in functional class to class I or II is not seen, additional or alternative therapy should be instituted.

    b. Prostacyclins

        i.   Epoprostenol (Flolan, Veletri)

           (a) Initiated in controlled setting/hospital

           (b) Initial: 2 ng/kg/min IV; titrate upward in increments of 2 ng/kg/min every 15 min or longer until dose-limiting effects or intolerance develops

        ii. Treprostinil (Remodulin, Tyvaso)

           (a) Initiated in controlled setting/hospital

           (b) Injection: 1.25 ng/kg/min continuous SQ or central line IV infusion; decrease to 0.625 ng/kg/min if initial dose cannot be tolerated

           (c) Oral: 3 breaths (18 mcg) via oral inhalation per treatment session, QID during waking hours approximately 4 hr apart; reduce to 1 or 2 breaths if 3 breaths is not tolerated

        iii. Iloprost (Ventavis)

           (a) Oral: 2.5 mcg inhaled; if tolerated, increase dose to 5 mcg inhaled six to nine times per day (no more than every 2 hr) during waking ts; maximum daily dose of 45 mcg

  2. Endothelin receptor antagonists

    a. Ambrisentan (Letairis)

        i.   Must enroll in Letairis education and access program

        ii. 5 mg PO once daily; may increase to 10 mg once daily if 5-mg dose is tolerated

    b. Bosentan (Tracleer)

        i.   Must enroll in Tracleer access program

        ii. Initial: 62.5 mg PO BID for 4 weeks

        iii. Maintenance: up to 125 mg PO BID

  3. PDE5 inhibitors

    a. Sildenafil (Revatio), 5–20 mg PO TID

    b. Tadalafil (Cialis), 40 mg PO once daily

F. Consider referral for transplantation

PULMONARY VASCULAR DISORDERS

I.   **Pulmonary embolism**

  A. Definition

    1. Clot (thromboembolus) or other undissolved solid, liquid, or gaseous material that has traveled to the lung via the venous system and become lodged in the pulmonary arterial circulation, interrupting blood flow

2. Extent of lung tissue injury is determined by the size of the embolus, which is considered massive if more than 50% of flow is obstructed
3. Accurate diagnosis is the key to reducing associated mortality
4. Death occurs as a result of RV failure

B. Etiology/incidence/predisposing factors
1. Predisposing factors for thrombotic emboli (Virchow triad) include the following:
   a. Venous stasis: deep venous thrombosis in lower extremities and pelvis leads to 70% of pulmonary emboli
      i. Prolonged immobility or surgery involving general anesthesia longer than 30 min
      ii. Congestive heart failure
      iii. Dehydration
      iv. Obesity
      v. Advanced age
   b. Vessel wall injury (e.g., surgery, fractured hip and/or pelvis)
   c. Hypercoagulability (e.g., increased owing to estrogen supplies, malignancy)
   d. Genetic predisposition
2. Other etiologies
   a. Fat embolism: orthopedic trauma (especially through marrow-containing bone) and surgery
   b. Air embolism (e.g., from a central line)
   c. Tumor fragments
   d. Amniotic fluid embolism
   e. Septic debris (e.g., indwelling venous access device)

C. Signs/symptoms
1. Dyspnea, insidious or sudden in onset, is the most common symptom
2. Apprehension, anxiety, and perception of "impending doom"
3. Substernal discomfort
4. Pleuritic pain with PE with infarction
5. Hemoptysis with pulmonary infarction
6. Syncope

D. Subjective/physical examination findings (may range from none to frank cardiovascular collapse)
1. Tachycardia
2. Tachypnea and dyspnea
3. Initially elevated blood pressure
4. Diaphoresis
5. Chest pain (dull, central, and pleuritic with pulmonary infarction)
6. Decreased cardiac output
7. Hypotension and shock
8. Signs of RV overload

        a. Jugular venous distention

        b. Increased intensity, second heart sound

  9. Peripheral phlebitis

 10. Signs of fat embolization

        a. Sudden, marked dyspnea in a susceptible patient

        b. Altered consciousness

        c. Body temperature elevation higher than 102°F

        d. Petechiae over the thorax, shoulders, and axillae

E. Laboratory/diagnostics

  1. Arterial blood gas analysis

        a. Acute respiratory alkalosis

        b. Variable degrees of hypoxemia

  2. ECG: nonspecific changes

        a. Most common is sinus tachycardia; atrial fibrillation is common as well

  3. Chest x-ray: normal, or with small infiltrates and/or effusion

  4. Ventilation/perfusion lung scan

        a. If read as high probability for PE, treat with anticoagulants

        b. If read as indeterminate or low probability for PE, consider pulmonary angiography if clinical suspicion remains high

        c. If the chest x-ray is abnormal, or if COPD is present, lung scanning may lead to an erroneous interpretation. Consider CT angiogram

  5. Pulmonary angiography remains the accepted gold standard for detecting the presence of pulmonary emboli

  6. Venous Doppler studies of the lower extremities may reveal the presence of deep venous thrombosis, which requires anticoagulation, in part obviating the need for evaluation of PE.

  7. Some authorities believe that spiral-cut, high-resolution CT scan of the chest reliably shows central PE

F. Management

  1. These agents have the FDA labeling for pulmonary embolism:

        a. Fondaparinux (Arixtra)

            i. 5 mg SQ once daily for patients whose weight is less than 50 kg

            ii. 7.5 mg SQ once daily for patients whose weight ranges from 50–100 kg

            iii. 10 mg SQ once daily for patients whose weight exceeds 100 kg

        b. Argatroban

            i. Use weight-based dosing to achieve a partial thromboplastin time of 1.5–3 times the baseline

        c. Dabigatran (Pradaxa), 150 mg PO BID

  2. Anticoagulation for venous thromboembolism

    a. Heparin may be started while confirmatory tests are being conducted

        i. Weight-based dosing

            (a) Initial bolus of 80 units/kg followed by a continuous infusion of 18 units/kg/hr

        ii. Dosage sufficient to maintain the partial thromboplastin time (PTT) at 2–2.5 times control

        iii. Some hospitals use a heparin protocol, with PTT checks every 6 hr, to guide heparin therapy.

    b. Low-molecular weight heparin (e.g., enoxaparin [Lovenox]), 1 mg/kg subcutaneously every 12 hr, is an acceptable alternative to heparin

        i. It also carries a lower risk of bleeding and of heparin-induced thrombocytopenia.

        ii. No extensive monitoring of coagulation parameters is needed

    c. Warfarin (Coumadin)

        i. Begun at the time diagnosis of PE is confirmed; usual first dose is 5–10 mg PO

        ii. Heparin is continued until therapeutic anticoagulant levels are achieved with warfarin.

        iii. Monitor the international normalized ratio (INR) after initial daily doses of Coumadin

            (a) Adequate oral anticoagulant effect is achieved when the INR is 2–2.5 for at least 2–3 days

        iv. Length of treatment: 3–6 months for the initial episode of PE; for recurrent episodes, treat for 6–12 months or longer, or consider placement of an indwelling vena cava filter to protect against massive embolization in patients with ongoing risk factors

    d. Rivaroxaban (Xarelto), 15 mg PO BID with food for 21 days, followed by 20 mg PO once daily with food

        i. Is an oral Xa inhibitor in the anticoagulant family

        ii. Approved in patients with deep vein thrombosis/PE

        iii. No monitoring required (no INRs to be checked)

        iv. Must be renally dosed

        v. May cause irreversible bleeding, which is treatable only with fresh frozen plasma

3. Fibrinolytic treatment: note contraindications before instituting this therapy (see fibrinolytic therapy for myocardial infarction in Angina and Myocardial Infarction)

4. May be appropriate for massive proximal PE associated with persistent systemic hypotension and signs of right heart strain, as well as in patients with very little cardiopulmonary reserve

5. Recombinant tissue plasminogen activator (Alteplase): 100 mg as a continuous infusion over 2 hr
6. Streptokinase: 250,000 units over 30 min; then 100,000 units/hr for 24 hr
   a. Rarely used; streptokinase has been associated with increased bleeding risk (compared to alteplase), increased incidence of allergic response (compared to alteplase), and resistance to affect due to antibody formation
7. Fibrinolytic therapy: after completed, begin heparin or enoxaparin when the PTT is less than 2 times control
8. Hemodynamic support may be needed for massive emboli with hypotension
9. Surgical embolectomy: reserved for those patients with massive emboli in central pulmonary arteries in whom the clot is creating hypotension and shock
10. Inferior vena cava interruption ("umbrella" device; Greenfield filter)
    a. Indicated when the risk of further emboli is perceived to be high
    b. Indicated with an absolute risk to anticoagulation
11. Supplemental oxygen is indicated to keep oxygen saturation above 90%

II. **Pulmonary vasculitis**
   A. Wegener granulomatosis
      1. Necrotizing granulomas of the respiratory tract (upper and lower), pulmonary microangiitis, and glomerulonephritis
      2. Associated with the following:
         a. Hemoptysis
         b. Dyspnea
         c. Cough
         d. Pulmonary infiltrates
      3. Antineutrophilic cytoplasmic antibodies are often positive.
      4. Treatment includes prednisone, 1 mg/kg per day, or cyclophosphamide (Cytoxan), 2 mg/kg/day, with reasonable chance of remission within 1 year
      5. Treatment has two components:
         a. Induction of remission with initial immunosuppressive therapy
         b. Maintenance immunosuppressive therapy for a variable period to prevent relapse
      6. Treatment is based on disease severity (mild, moderate, to severe disease)
         a. Glucocorticoids in combination with methotrexate, cyclophosphamide, or rituximab
      7. Prophylaxis against opportunistic infections (i.e., PCP/PJP) during induction therapy may be necessary

8. When initiating glucocorticoid therapy, there is disagreement among experts as to whether therapy should begin with pulse methylprednisolone (7–15 mg/kg to a maximum dose of 500–1,000 mg/day for 3 days) in all patients or only in those with necrotizing or crescentic glomerulonephritis or more severe respiratory disease.

   a. Induction:
      i. Prednisone, 1 mg/kg/day (maximum of 60–80 mg per day)
      ii. Oral cyclophosphamide, 1.5–2 mg/kg per day
      iii. IV cyclophosphamide, 0.5g/m^2 every 2 weeks for 3–6 months
      iv. Rituximab, 375 mg/m^2 per week for 4 weeks
      v. Methotrexate—not FDA labeled for this indication; trial data suggests 20–25 mg PO per week

   b. Maintenance
      i. Methotrexate, 0.3 mg/kg per week (maximum dose of 15 mg); if tolerated, the dose increases in 2.5 mg increments each week to a dose of 20–25 mg per week
      ii. Azathioprine, 2 mg/kg per day

B. Lymphomatoid granulomatosis
   1. Systemic granulomatous angiitis involving the following:
      a. Lung
      b. Brain
      c. Skin (especially)
      d. Upper respiratory tract (rarely)
      e. Kidneys (rarely)
   2. Associated with the eventual development of lymphoma in many cases
   3. In general, treatment options for pulmonary lymphomatoid granulomatosis follow those for diffuse large B-cell lymphoma.
   4. The choice of treatment should be based upon the presence of symptoms, history of using an inciting medication, extent of extrapulmonary involvement, and careful assessment of the histopathologic grade of the lesion. When a medication is implicated, it should be stopped and the patient observed for changes in the extent of the disease.
   5. Refer to hematology oncology specialist for consultation and/or treatment

III. **Implications for geriatric patients**
   A. Heart failure with preserved ejection fraction is a commonly under-recognized cause of pulmonary hypertension in the elderly

B. Very unlikely to be pulmonary artery hypertension; more likely to be pulmonary venous hypertension due to left ventricular systolic or diastolic failure, aortic or mitral valve disease, or left atrial non-compliance in the elderly

BIBLIOGRAPHY

Benza, R. L., Miller, D. P., Barst, R. J., Badesch, D. B., Frost, A. E., & McGoon, M. D. (2012). An evaluation of long-term survival from time of diagnosis in pulmonary arterial hypertension from the REVEAL Registry. *Chest, 142*(2), 448–456.

Bishop, B. M., Mauro, V. F., & Khouri, S. J. (2012). Practical considerations for the pharmacotherapy of pulmonary arterial hypertension. *Pharmacotherapy, 32*(9), 838–855. doi:10.1002/j.1875–9114.2012.01114.x

Boilson, B. A., Schirger, J. A., & Borlaug, B. A. (2010). Caveat medicus! Pulmonary hypertension in the elderly: A word of caution. *European Journal of Heart Failure, 12*, 89–93.

Bonderman, D., Wexberg, P., Heinzl, H., & Lang, I. M. (2012). Non-invasive algorithms for the diagnosis of pulmonary hypertension. *Thrombosis and Haemostasis, 108*(6), 1037–1041. doi:10.1160/th12–04–0239

Bossone, E., D'Andrea, A., D'Alto, M., Citro, R., Argiento, P., Ferrara, F., . . . Naeije, R. (2013). Echocardiography in pulmonary arterial hypertension: From diagnosis to prognosis. *Journal of the American Society of Echocardiography, 26*(1), 1–14. doi:10.1016/j.echo.2012.10.009

Chan, L., Kennedy, M., Woolstenhulme, J. G., Nathan, S. D., Weinstein, A. A., Connors, G., . . . Keyser, R. E. (2013). Benefits of intensive treadmill exercise training on cardiorespiratory function and quality of life in patients with pulmonary hypertension. *Chest, 143*(2), 333–343.

Charalampopoulos, A., Raphael, C., Gin-Sing, W., & Gibbs, J. S. (2012). Diagnosing and managing pulmonary hypertension. *Practitioner, 256*(1756), 21–25.

Cracowski, J. L., & Leuchte, H. H. (2012). The potential of biomarkers in pulmonary arterial hypertension. *American Journal of Cardiology, 110*(6 Suppl), 32s-38s. doi:10.1016/j.amjcard.2012.06.014

de Man, F. S., Tu, L., Handoko, M. L., Rain, S., Ruiter, G., François, C., . . . Guignabert, C. (2012). Dysregulated renin-angiotensin-aldosterone system contributes to pulmonary arterial hypertension. *American Journal of Respiratory and Critical Care Medicine, 186*(8), 780–789. doi:10.1164/rccm.201203–0411OC

Foris, V., Kovacs, G., Tscherner, M., Olschewski, A., & Olschewski, H. (2013). Biomarkers in pulmonary hypertension: What do we know? *Chest, 144*(1), 274–283. doi:10.1378/chest.12–1246

Frazier, A. A., & Burke, A. P. (2012). The imaging of pulmonary hypertension. *Seminars in Ultrasound, CT, and MR, 33*(6), 535–551. doi:10.1053/j.sult.2012.06.002

Gabler, N. B., French, B., Strom, B. L., Liu, Z., Palevsky, H. I., Taichman, D. B., . . . Halpern, S. D. (2012). Race and sex differences in response to endothelin receptor antagonists for pulmonary arterial hypertension. *Chest, 141*(1), 20–26.

Georgiopoulou, V. V., Kalogeropoulos, A. P., Borlaug, B. A., Gheorghiade, M., & Butler, J. (2013). Left ventricular dysfunction with pulmonary hypertension: Part 1: Epidemiology, pathophysiology, and definitions. *Circulation. Heart Failure, 6*(2), 344–354. doi:10.1161/circheartfailure.112.000095

Gologanu, D., Stanescu, C., & Bogdan, M. A. (2012). Pulmonary hypertension secondary to chronic obstructive pulmonary disease. *Romanian Journal of Internal Medicine, 50*(4), 259–268.

Guazzi, M., Castelvecchio, S., Bandera, F., & Menicanti, L. (2012). Right ventricular pulmonary hypertension. *Current Heart Failure Reports, 9*(4), 303–308. doi:10.1007/s11897–012–0106–8

Humbert, M., Gerry Coghlan, J., & Khanna, D. (2012). Early detection and management of pulmonary arterial hypertension. *European Respiratory Review, 21*(126), 306–312. doi:10.1183/09059180.00005112

Iwasawa, T. (2013). Diagnosis and management of pulmonary arterial hypertension using MR imaging. *Magnetic Resonance in Medical Sciences, 12*(1), 1–9.

Judge, E. P., & Gaine, S. P. (2013). Management of pulmonary arterial hypertension. *Current Opinion in Critical Care, 19*(1), 44–50. doi:10.1097/MCC.0b013e32835c5137

Lewczuk, J., Romaszkiewicz, R., Lenartowska, L., Piszko, P., Jagas, J., Nowak, M., . . . Wrabec, K. (2013). The natural history of thromboembolic pulmonary hypertension. Since when is it chronic? A proposal of an algorithm for the diagnosis and treatment. *Kardiologia Polska, 71*(5), 522–526. doi:10.5603/kp.2013.0102

Ling, Y., Johnson, M. K., Kiely, D. G., Condliffe, R., Elliot, C. A., Gibbs, J. S., . . . Peacock, A. J. (2012). Changing demographics, epidemiology, and survival of incident pulmonary arterial hypertension: Results from the pulmonary hypertension registry of the United Kingdom and Ireland. *American Journal of Respiratory and Critical Care Medicine, 186*(8), 790–796. doi:10.1164/rccm.201203–0383OC

Liu, C., Chen, J., Gao, Y., Deng, B., & Liu, K. (2013). Endothelin receptor antagonists for pulmonary arterial hypertension. *Cochrane Database of Systematic Reviews, 2*. doi:10.1002/14651858.CD004434.pub5

Malenfant, S., Margaillan, G., Loehr, J. E., Bonnet, S., & Provencher, S. (2013). The emergence of new therapeutic targets in pulmonary arterial hypertension: From now to the near future. *Expert Review of Respiratory Medicine, 7*(1), 43–55. doi:10.1586/ers.12.83

Mandel, J., & Poch, D. (2013). In the clinic. Pulmonary hypertension. *Annals of Internal Medicine, 158*(9). doi:10.7326/0003–4819–158–9-201305070–01005

Mauritz, G. J., Kind, T., Marcus, J. T., Bogaard, H. J., Postmus, P. E., Boonstra, A., . . . Vonk-Noordegraaf, A. (2012). Progressive changes in right ventricular geometric shortening and long-term survival in pulmonary arterial hypertension. *Chest, 141*(4), 935–943.

McLaughlin, V. V., Langer, A., Tan, M., Clements, P. J., Oudiz, R. J., Tapson, V. F., . . . Rubin, L. J. (2013). Contemporary trends in the diagnosis and management of pulmonary arterial hypertension: An initiative to close the care gap. *Chest, 143*(2), 324–332.

Ng, C., & Jenkins, D. P. (2013). Surgical management of chronic thromboembolic pulmonary hypertension. *British Journal of Hospital Medicine (London), 74*(1), 31–35.

Nider, V. (2013). Pulmonary arterial hypertension. Recognition is the first essential step. *Advance for NPs and PAs, 4*(5), 33–37.

O'Callaghan, D. S., & Humbert, M. (2012). A critical analysis of survival in pulmonary arterial hypertension. *European Respiratory Review, 21*(125), 218–222. doi:10.1183/09059180.00003512

Peacock, A. (2013). Pulmonary hypertension. *European Respiratory Review, 22*(127), 20–25. doi:10.1183/09059180.00006912

Poor, H. D., & Ventetuolo, C. E. (2012). Pulmonary hypertension in the intensive care unit. *Progress in Cardiovascular Diseases, 55*(2), 187–198. doi:10.1016/j.pcad.2012.07.001

Rabinovitch, M. (2012). Molecular pathogenesis of pulmonary arterial hypertension. *Journal of Clinical Investigation, 122*(12), 4306–4313. doi:10.1172/jci60658

Rajdev, A., Garan, H., & Biviano, A. (2012). Arrhythmias in pulmonary arterial hypertension. *Progress in Cardiovascular Diseases, 55*(2), 180–186. doi:10.1016/j.pcad.2012.06.002

Rubin, L. J., Simonneau, G., Badesch, D., Galie, N., Humbert, M., Keogh, A., . . . Kymes, S. (2012). The study of risk in pulmonary arterial hypertension. *European Respiratory Review, 21*(125), 234–238. doi:10.1183/09059180.00003712

Singh, G. K., Levy, P. T., Holland, M. R., & Hamvas, A. (2012). Novel methods for assessment of right heart structure and function in pulmonary hypertension. *Clinics in Perinatology, 39*(3), 685–701. doi:10.1016/j.clp.2012.06.002

Skoro-Sajer, N. (2012). Optimal use of treprostinil in pulmonary arterial hypertension: A guide to the correct use of different formulations. *Drugs, 72*(18), 2351–2363. doi:10.2165/11638260–000000000–00000

Sood, N. (2013). Managing an acutely ill patient with pulmonary arterial hypertension. *Expert Review of Respiratory Medicine, 7*(1), 77–83. doi:10.1586/ers.12.73

Stacher, E., Graham, B. B., Hunt, J. M., Gandjeva, A., Groshong, S. D., McLaughlin, V. V., . . . Tuder, R. M. (2012). Modern age pathology of pulmonary arterial hypertension. *American Journal of Respiratory and Critical Care Medicine, 186*(3), 261–272. doi:10.1164/rccm.201201–0164OC

Tackett, K. L., & Stajich, G. V. (2013). Combination pharmacotherapy in the treatment of pulmonary arterial hypertension: Continuing education article. *Journal of Pharmacy Practice, 26*(1), 18–28. doi:10.1177/0897190012466046

Thomas, M., Ciuclan, L., Hussey, M. J., & Press, N. J. (2013). Targeting the serotonin pathway for the treatment of pulmonary arterial hypertension. *Pharmacology and Therapeutics, 138*(3), 409–417. doi:10.1016/j.pharmthera.2013.02.002

Tonelli, A. R., Arelli, V., Minai, O. A., Newman, J., Bair, N., Heresi, G. A., & Dweik, R. A. (2013). Causes and circumstances of death in pulmonary arterial hypertension. *American Journal of Respiratory and Critical Care Medicine, 188*(3), 365–369. doi:10.1164/rccm.201209–1640OC

Vachiery, J. L., & Gaine, S. (2012). Challenges in the diagnosis and treatment of pulmonary arterial hypertension. *European Respiratory Review, 21*(126), 313–320. doi:10.1183/09059180.00005412

Ventetuolo, C. E., & Klinger, J. R. (2012). WHO Group 1 pulmonary arterial hypertension: Current and investigative therapies. *Progress in Cardiovascular Diseases, 55*(2), 89–103. doi:10.1016/j.pcad.2012.07.002

Voelkel, N. F., Mizuno, S., & Bogaard, H. J. (2013). The role of hypoxia in pulmonary vascular diseases: A perspective. *American Journal of Physiology. Lung Cellular and Molecular Physiology, 304*(7), L457–465. doi:10.1152/ajplung.00335.2012

Waxman, A. B. (2012). Exercise physiology and pulmonary arterial hypertension. *Progress in Cardiovascular Diseases, 55*(2), 172–179. doi:10.1016/j.pcad.2012.07.003

Waxman, A. B., & Zamanian, R. T. (2013). Pulmonary arterial hypertension: New insights into the optimal role of current and emerging prostacyclin therapies. *American Journal of Cardiology, 111*(5 Suppl), 1A-16A; quiz 17A-19A. doi:10.1016/j.amjcard.2012.12.002

Wilkins, M. R., Wharton, J., & Gladwin, M. T. (2013). Update in pulmonary vascular diseases 2012. *American Journal of Respiratory and Critical Care Medicine, 188*(1), 23–28. doi:10.1164/rccm.201303–0470UP

Wilson, S. R., Ghio, S., Scelsi, L., & Horn, E. M. (2012). Pulmonary hypertension and right ventricular dysfunction in left heart disease (Group 2 pulmonary hypertension). *Progress in Cardiovascular Diseases, 55*(2), 104–118. doi:10.1016/j.pcad.2012.07.007

Wu, W. H., Yang, L., Peng, F. H., Yao, J., Zou, L. L., Liu, D., . . . Jing, Z. C. (2013). Lower socioeconomic status is associated with worse outcomes in pulmonary arterial hypertension. *American Journal of Respiratory and Critical Care Medicine, 187*(3), 303–310. doi:10.1164/rccm.201207–1290OC

Yao, A. (2012). Recent advances and future perspectives in therapeutic strategies for pulmonary arterial hypertension. *Journal of Cardiology, 60*(5), 344–349. doi:10.1016/j.jjcc.2012.08.009

Zimner-Rapuch, S., Amet, S., Janus, N., Deray, G., & Launay-Vacher, V. (2013). Pulmonary hypertension: Use of oral drugs in patients with renal insufficiency. *Clinical Drug Investigation, 33*(1), 65–69. doi:10.1007/s40261–012–0045-x

CHAPTER 29

Chest Wall and Secondary Pleural Disorders

JENNIFER COATES • THOMAS W. BARKLEY, JR. • CHARLENE M. MYERS

DISORDERS OF THE CHEST WALL

I. **Components of the chest that may contribute to respiratory dysfunction**
   A. Spine
   B. Rib cage
   C. Costosternal margins
   D. Pleura
   E. Respiratory muscles

II. **Disorders of the spine**
   A. Congenital scoliosis
      1. The spine assumes an S-shaped curvature
      2. May induce a restrictive ventilatory defect
      3. Most often, scoliosis remains an insignificant variable, unless one of the following occurs:
         a. The curvature is severe
         b. Superimposed chest disease makes the work of breathing difficult
      4. In these instances, the risk of respiratory failure may increase.
   B. Kyphosis of the spine
      1. The spine has an accentuated dorsal curve
      2. May induce a restrictive ventilatory defect
      3. May coexist with scoliosis
      4. Can increase the risk of breathing problems in the presence of other chest diseases
      5. Acquired kyphosis
         a. Results from osteoporosis

  b. Common clinical problem resulting from vertebral collapse with pain

  c. Treatment of the pain may introduce the additional risk of ventilatory compromise

 C. Ankylosing spondylitis

  1. Chronic inflammatory disease of the joints of the axial skeleton

  2. Patient will have pain and progressive stiffening of the spine

  3. Chest expansion becomes limited as the disease progresses

III. **Rib and sternal fracture and sternal dehiscence after cardiac surgery**

 A. Fracture of the ribs, or even of the sternum, can occur spontaneously or as the result of trauma or surgery

 B. The instability of the chest wall, with flailing of the wall outward during inspiration and associated chest pain resulting from fractures, limits chest wall movement, especially if multiple fractures are present.

 C. Abnormal movement of the chest wall can result in hypoventilation and in poor secretion clearance

 D. Pain medication may facilitate breathing, but it can also lead to hypoventilation and ventilatory failure

 E. Milder problems theoretically can be helped with chest wall binders; however, with significant impairment of ventilation, positive pressure ventilation to stabilize the chest wall may be necessary.

 F. Sternal dehiscence following open heart surgery or surgical procedures involving the mediastinum similarly can result in respiratory compromise.

IV. **Costochondral junctions**

 A. Costosternal junctions may become inflamed owing to the following:

  1. Arthritis (autoimmune in origin)

   a. Rheumatoid disease

   b. Systemic lupus erythematosus

  2. Costochondritis (Tietze syndrome)

   a. Inflammation of the cartilage that connects rib to the sternum; causes pain and tenderness at costosternal joint, when taking deep breath, or upon coughing

 B. Although typically not serious, costochondritis may be confused with other more serious conditions within the chest.

 C. Costochondritis is more common in young women

 D. Tenderness over the affected area is common

 E. NSAIDs and heat are helpful in relieving the pain

PLEURAL DISORDERS

I. **Pleuritis**
   A. Also called pleurisy
   B. Defined as pain due to acute pleural inflammation
   C. Pain is typically localized, sharp, and fleeting and made worse by coughing, sneezing, and deep breathing.
   D. Multiple different possible etiologies, treatment depends on cause

II. **Pleural effusion**
   A. Increased amounts of fluid within the pleural space
      1. Transudative: due to increased hydrostatic or decreased oncotic pressure
         a. Causes include congestive heart failure, cirrhosis, and hypoalbuminemia
      2. Exudative: due to increased production of fluid due to abnormal capillary permeability or decreased lymphatic clearance from pleural space
         a. Causes include malignancy, rheumatoid arthritis, vasculitis, and lupus
      3. Empyema: infection and pus accumulation in the pleural space
      4. Hemothorax: blood in the pleural space
      5. Chylothorax: due to ruptured thoracic ducts and accumulation of chyle in the pleural space
      6. Parapneumonic effusion: exudate that accompanies an infection accumulating in the pleural space
   B. Symptoms
      1. Dyspnea
      2. Pleuritic chest pain
   C. Physical examination findings
      1. Tachypnea
      2. Dullness on percussion, with diminished or absent breath sounds over the affected area
      3. Pleural friction rub
      4. Fever, especially if the fluid is infected
   D. Chest x-ray
      1. Increased amount of fluid between the visceral and the parietal pleura
      2. Layering out of the fluid on decubitus chest x-rays
      3. Loculation of fluid along the lateral chest wall (may be confirmed by ultrasonography over the affected area)
      4. Blunting of the costophrenic angles: appears as a linear shadow ascending vertically and clinging to the ribs in a meniscus pattern
         a. Lateral check x-ray: at least 75 ml of pleural fluid needed
         b. Posteroanterior chest x-ray: at least 175 ml of pleural fluid needed

    c. Lateral decubitus x-ray: amounts as small as 5 ml may blunt the costophrenic angle

E. Management

  1. Observation with or without diuresis: If risk of infection is small, and if it is likely that the effusion is due to heart failure, then the response may be assessed by doing the following:

    a. Following the effusion by serial chest x-rays

    b. Looking for a decrease in the amount of fluid over time during diuresis

  2. Thoracentesis is indicated in the following circumstances:

    a. The cause of the effusion must be evaluated for the following:

      i. Risk of infection

      ii. Malignancy

    b. The patient is dyspneic

      i. Procedure is therapeutic

      ii. Procedure can be used diagnostically when fluid is sent for laboratory evaluation

  3. Laboratory evaluation of pleural fluid

    a. Cell count and differential white blood cell count

    b. Chemistries—collect serum and pleural fluid levels of the following studies:

      i. Total protein

      ii. Glucose

      iii. Lactate dehydrogenase (LDH) levels

      iv. Amylase level

      v. A pleural exudate is an effusion that has one or more of the following:

        (a) Ratio of pleural fluid protein to serum protein greater than 0.5

        (b) Ratio of pleural fluid LDH to serum LDH greater than 0.6

        (c) Pleural fluid LDH more than two-thirds the upper limit of normal serum LDH

      vi. A transudative effusion typically has a serum glucose equal to pleural fluid glucose, and a pH between 7.40 and 7.55.

    c. Gram's stain and fluid cultures, as indicated by the patient's clinical status

      i. Bacteria (aerobic and anaerobic)

      ii. Acid-fast bacilli

      iii. Fungi

    d. Special serologic tests may be considered.

      i. Carcinoembryonic antigen in a patient with known colon cancer

      ii. CA125 in a woman with known ovarian cancer

      e. Determination of fluid pH, which tends to be low in the following situations:

         i. Empyema due to tuberculosis or anaerobic bacterial pathogens

         ii. Rheumatoid involvement of the pleura

      f. Pleural fluid cytologic examination to assess for metastatic cancer to the pleura

    4. Further management issues:

      a. If the fluid is bloody, insertion of a chest tube is often required.

      b. Empyema requires chest tube insertion and probable surgical intervention.

         i. Antimicrobials alone are not curative when empyema is present.

         ii. All antimicrobials used should be selected on the basis of pleural fluid culture results, including antimicrobial sensitivity data.

      c. Repeated thoracentesis is an acceptable method of draining reaccumulations of malignant effusions, especially when the procedure is needed infrequently.

      d. Malignant effusions treated with chest tube drainage may also be sclerosed (creating scar tissue, in hopes of preventing recurrence).

         i. A sclerosing agent is introduced through the chest tube after drainage of the effusion is completed.

         ii. This sclerosing process is called pleurodesis.

F. Gerontologic considerations

    1. The chest wall muscle compliance decreases with age because the ribs become ossified (less flexible) and joints become stiffer.

    2. Respiratory muscle strength and endurance decrease with aging

    3. Antibiotic doses may need to be reduced in the elderly patient due to alterations in renal function or predisposition to medication side effects.

    4. The incidence of lung cancer increases with age; therefore, malignancy needs to be included in the list of pleural effusion differential diagnoses in the elderly patient.

BIBLIOGRAPHY

Girdhar, A., Shujaat, A., & Bajwa, A. (2012). Management of infectious processes of the pleural space: A review. *Pulmonary Medicine.* doi:10.1155/2012/816502

Goldman, L., & Ausiello, D. (Eds.). (2011). *Cecil textbook of medicine* (24th ed.). Philadelphia, PA: WB Saunders.

Halter, J., Ouslander, J., Tinetti, M., Studenski, S., High, K., & Asthana, S. (2009). *Hazzard's geriatric medicine and gerontology* (6th ed.). New York, NY: McGraw-Hill.

Light, R. W. (2007). *Pleural diseases*. Philadelphia, PA: Lippincott Williams & Wilkins.

Longo, D., Fauci, A. S., Kasper, D. L., Hauser, S. L., Jameson, L. J., & Loscalzo, J. (2012). *Harrison's principles of internal medicine* (18th ed.). New York, NY: McGraw-Hill.

McCance, K. L., & Huether, S. E. (Eds.). (2013). *Pathophysiology: The biologic basis for disease in adults and children.* Philadelphia, PA: Elsevier Health Sciences.

McGrath, E. E., & Anderson, P. B. (2011). Diagnosis of pleural effusion: A systematic approach. *American Journal of Critical Care, 20*(2), 119–128.

Papadakis, M. A. (2014). *Current medical diagnosis & treatment 2013.* S. J. McPhee (Ed.). New York, NY: McGraw-Hill Education Medical.

Rubenstein, W., & Talbot, Y. (2013). *Medical teaching in ambulatory care.* Toronto, ON: University of Toronto Press.

CHAPTER 30

Respiratory Failure

DAVID A. MILLER • THOMAS W. BARKLEY, JR.

DEFINITIONS AND CONCEPTS

I. **Breathing**
   A. Breathing is understood as the movement of air into and out of the lungs.
   B. Physiologically, breathing is controlled by the metabolic needs of the body (i.e., oxygen and carbon dioxide levels in the blood) as perceived by the central nervous system (chemoreceptor input).
   C. Breathing is also under voluntary control in conscious, alert individuals.

II. **Ventilation**
   A. Ventilation is the aspect of breathing that refers to the actual movement of air into and out of the lungs.
   B. Ventilation is determined by the volume of air moved (tidal volume) and by the ventilatory rate.
   C. Individuals who are alert and spontaneously breathing vary the amount of air inhaled and exhaled with each breath, as well as the respiratory rate, responding to the control of the central nervous system over the ventilatory act.
   D. Yawning and sighing are normal variations seen during the act of ventilation.

III. **Respiration**
   A. Respiration refers to the following:
      1. Actual use of oxygen at the cellular level
      2. Removal from the cellular environment of the following products:
         a. Carbon dioxide
         b. Metabolic wastes, especially metabolic acids
            i. Lactic acid
            ii. Ketoacids

    B. Cellular respiration is dependent on two variables:
        1. Perfusion of capillaries with oxygen and nutrient-laden blood in adequate amounts
            a. Cellular uptake and use of oxygen normally are independent of oxygen delivery.
        2. Venous blood flow that removes cellular metabolic wastes to the heart, lungs, and kidney
            a. For distribution to other cells, especially the following:
                i. Alveoli
                ii. Liver
                iii. Kidneys
            b. For further metabolism PRN and eventual removal from the body via these routes:
                i. Expiration
                ii. Stool
                iii. Urine

THE EFFECTS OF AGING ON THE NEED FOR RESPIRATORY ASSISTANCE, INCLUDING INTUBATION

I.   **Physiological changes**
    A. Reduced lung elasticity and increased ventilation–perfusion mismatching
    B. Reduced chest wall compliance and diaphragmatic and intercostal muscle strength
    C. Reduced clearance of airway secretions
    D. Altered responsiveness to hypoxemia and hypercarbia
II.   **Effects of comorbidities**
    A. Increase the risk of respiratory failure
        1. Heart failure
        2. Chronic obstructive pulmonary disorder (COPD)
        3. Dementia
        4. Chronic inactivity
        5. Chronic kidney disease
III. **Ethical issues**
    A. Assessing for prior autonomous choices in the use of life-prolonging interventions among the elderly is essential, if possible. Family members are crucial in this regard.
    B. Patient age is not an indication to withhold ventilator assistance

VENTILATORY FAILURE

I. **Ventilatory failure refers to absent or inadequate movement of oxygen into the lungs and/or of carbon dioxide out of the lungs.**
  A. Apnea—absence of movement of respiratory gases
  B. Hypopnea—inadequate movement of respiratory gases

II. **Ventilatory failure is best assessed by measurement of the partial pressure of carbon dioxide in arterial blood ($PaCO_2$) and/or end-tidal CO_2 levels.**

III. **Causes of ventilatory failure**
  A. Ventilatory failure may be induced by overdose of medications (e.g., sedatives, hypnotics, and opioids) relative to the body's ability to continue to respond to metabolic and cellular respiratory needs while influenced by these drugs. Elderly persons are particularly susceptible to the respiratory depression associated with the use of these drugs.
    1. Unintentional overdose (e.g., iatrogenic oversedation in the presence of COPD)
    2. Intentional overdose
      a. Iatrogenic sedation with the intent to control ventilation
      b. Drug overdose with suicidal intent
  B. The ability to get oxygen into and carbon dioxide out of the lungs is impaired by acquired acute pathology related to the following:
    1. Infections of the lungs (e.g., in patients with COPD)
    2. Neuromuscular disease
      a. Myasthenia gravis in crisis
      b. Guillain-Barré syndrome
      c. Traumatic head or spinal cord injury
    3. Pulmonary edema of cardiogenic or noncardiogenic origin

RESPIRATORY FAILURE

I. **Definition**
  A. Failure of adequate oxygen delivery to cells (e.g., during hypotension)
  B. Failure of the cell's ability to use oxygen (e.g., cyanide poisoning, carbon monoxide poisoning)

II. **The term "shock" is best reserved for situations in which respiratory failure is generalized throughout the body.**
  A. The sepsis syndrome with hypotension poses risk not only to the lungs but also to critically important organs, including the kidneys, heart, liver, gut, and central nervous system.
  B. In sepsis syndrome, oxygen delivery to cells becomes pathophysiologically supply dependent. Hence,
    1. Ventilation must ensure an adequate supply of oxygen to the body.
    2. Circulation requires adequate volume support and systemic vascular resistance to ensure delivery of oxygen and nutrients to cells without overloading the ability of the heart to pump blood into the circulation.

3. Pulmonary artery catheter monitoring may become necessary on a temporary basis for determining cardiac status and systemic vascular resistance.

4. The amount of oxygen returning to the heart reflects the overall distribution of oxygen and nutrients to cells (mixed venous oxygen saturation [SvO_2] monitoring).

III.   **The goal of treating respiratory failure is prevention of cellular ischemia and death while the cause of respiratory failure is corrected.**

A. Control of ventilation, and oxygen and nutrient supplies, is critical

1. Control of the airway is essential

B. Also critical is the prevention of problems associated with mechanical ventilation.

1. Pneumothorax
2. Nosocomial pneumonia
3. Indwelling catheter-related sepsis
4. Malnutrition during the course of respiratory failure

TREATMENT

I.   **Various modalities are potentially indicated**

A. For hypoxemia when ventilation appears unlabored and sustainable

1. Supplemental oxygen by mask

B. For hypoxemia and hypercapnia and the patient is fully alert

1. Supplemental oxygen via nasal prongs
2. Consideration for bilevel positive airway pressure to keep ventilation near normal for patient

C. For hypoxemia when ventilation is labored and/or hypercapnia is worsening

1. Bilevel positive airway pressure
2. Intubation and mechanical ventilation

II.   **Support measures for comorbid illnesses need to be continued as indicated.**

III.   **Nutritional support should be started as soon as possible to avert caloric restriction during a time of higher caloric need.**

BIBLIOGRAPHY

Brown, C. A. (2013). The decision to intubate. In D. S. Basow (Ed.), *UpToDate.* Waltham, MA: UpToDate.

Brown, C. A., & Arbelaez, C. (2013). Emergency airway management in the geriatric patient. In D. S. Basow (Ed.), *UpToDate.* Waltham, MA: UpToDate.

Centers for Medicare & Medicaid Services (CMS). (2013). *2014 ICD-10 PCS and GEMs.* Retrieved November 25, 2013, from http:///www.cms.gov/Medicare/ Coding/ICD10/2014-ICD-10-PCS.html

Dirkes, S. (2011). Acute kidney injury: Not just acute renal failure anymore? *Critical Care Nurse, 3*(1), 37–49.

Goldman, L., & Shafer, A. I. (Eds.) (2012). *Goldman's Cecil medicine* (24th ed.). Philadelphia, PA: Saunders.

Longo, D. L., Kasper, D. L., Jameson, J. L., Fauci, A. S., Hauser, S. L., & Loscalzo, J. (Eds.) (2011). *Harrison's principles of internal medicine* (18th ed.). New York, NY: McGraw Hill.

Slutsky, A. S., & Ranieri, V. M. (2013). Ventilatory-induced lung injury. *New England Journal of Medicine, 369*, 2126–2136. doi:10.1056/NEJMra1208707

University of Miami Geriatric and Ethics Programs. (2013). *Geriatrics: Decision-making, autonomy, valid consent and guardianship.* Retrieved November 27, 2013, from http://www.miami.edu/index.php/ethics/projects/geriatrics_and_ ethics/decision-making_autonomy_valid_consent_and_guardianship/

University of Miami Geriatric and Ethics Programs. (2013). *Geriatrics: End-of-life issues.* Retrieved November 27, 2013, from http://www.miami.edu/index. php/ethics/projects/geriatrics_and_ethics/end-of-life_issues/

CHAPTER 31

Pneumothorax

BIMBOLA AKINTADE • THOMAS W. BARKLEY, JR.

I. Definition

A. The presence of air in the pleural space, resulting from perforation of the chest wall or pleura, causes the lung to collapse

B. Types

   1. Spontaneous: disruption of the visceral pleura

      a. Air enters the pleural space from the lung

      b. Occurs in individuals with or without underlying lung disease

   2. Traumatic

      a. Open: penetrating chest trauma

         i. Parietal pleura is disrupted

         ii. Air enters the pleural space from the atmosphere

      b. Closed: blunt chest trauma

         i. The visceral pleura is disrupted

         ii. Air enters the pleural space from the lung

      c. Iatrogenic

         i. Disruption of the visceral pleura as a complication of an invasive thoracic procedure

         ii. May also occur after procedures involving the neck or the abdomen

   3. Tension

      a. As a result of a spontaneous or traumatic pneumothorax, air enters the pleural space but is unable to exit.

      b. As pressure rises in the pleural space, the lung collapses, the mediastinum shifts to the other side, and venous return to the right heart is impaired.

      c. Tension pneumothorax is a medical emergency

II. **Etiology/incidence/predisposing factors**
  - **A.** Penetrating or blunt chest trauma
  - **B.** Rupture of a subpleural bleb or invasion of visceral pleura by disease (e.g., necrotizing pneumonia)
  - **C.** Intrinsic lung disease
    1. Chronic obstructive pulmonary disease
    2. Tuberculosis
    3. Sarcoidosis
    4. Pulmonary fibrosis
    5. Bronchogenic carcinoma
  - **D.** Barotrauma resulting from mechanical ventilation with increased positive end-expiratory pressure.
  - **E.** Complication of invasive thoracic, neck, or abdominal diagnostic of therapeutic procedures
    1. Insertion of intravenous access devices
    2. Needle biopsy of liver or lung
    3. Thoracentesis

III. **Subjective/physical exam findings: depend on degree of lung collapse and mechanism involved**
  - **A.** Possible sudden onset of dyspnea and shortness of breath
  - **B.** Pleuritic chest pain, may be sharp and severe
  - **C.** Apprehension and agitation

IV. **Physical examination findings: depend on degree of lung collapse and mechanism involved**
  - **A.** Splinting and decreased inspiratory expansion of involved hemithorax
  - **B.** Bulging of the intercostal spaces on the affected side during exhalation
  - **C.** Decreased breath sounds and fremitus, along with a hyperresonant percussion note over the affected area
  - **D.** Tracheal deviation toward the unaffected side
  - **E.** Subcutaneous emphysema
  - **F.** Possible Hamman sign (mediastinal crepitus on auscultation)
  - **G.** In the mechanically ventilated patient with positive end-expiratory pressure, development of high peak inspiratory pressure with decreased compliance may occur.
  - **H.** In patients with tension pneumothorax, signs of decreased cardiac output resulting from impaired venous return

V. **Laboratory/diagnostics**
  - **A.** Arterial blood gases: mild to moderate hypoxemia and hypercapnia
  - **B.** Chest x-ray
    1. Increased translucency confirms the degree of lung collapse
    2. Recognition of small pneumothoraces, particularly in mechanically ventilated patients, crucial to prevention of tension pneumothorax

VI. **Management**
  - **A.** Tension pneumothorax

1. Immediate decompression with 14- to 16-gauge needle into the second intercostal space, midclavicular line
2. Insertion of chest tube at the fourth or fifth intercostal space midaxillary line to closed water-seal drainage
   B. Spontaneous pneumothorax: depends on size
   1. If small, give supplemental oxygen with 100% non-rebreather mask and observe
   2. If collapse is greater than 20%, insert a chest tube and connect it to a water-seal drainage
   C. Traumatic pneumothorax
   1. Prompt chest tube insertion, fourth or fifth intercostal space midaxillary line with closed chest drainage
   D. Negative pressure (application of suction to chest drainage apparatus)
   1. Use when water seal fails to re-expand the lung after 24–48 hr
   2. Use when persistent pneumothorax perpetuates hypoxemia and/or hypercapnia

BIBLIOGRAPHY

Baird, M. S., & Bethel, S. (2010). *Manual of critical care nursing: nursing interventions and collaborative management* (6th ed.). St. Louis, MO: Mosby.

Corbridge, T. C., & Singer, B. D. (2009). Basic invasive mechanical ventilation. *Southern Medical Journal, 102,* 1238–1245.

Dellinger, R. P., & Parrillo, J. E. (2013). *Critical care medicine: principles of diagnosis and management in the adult* (4th ed.). St. Louis, MO: Mosby.

Feller-Kopman, D., & Yarmus, L., (2012). Pneumothorax in the critically ill patient. *Chest, 141,* 1098–1105.

Fix, B., & Jones, J. (2009). *Critical care notes: Clinical pocket guide.* Philadelphia, PA: F.A. Davis.

Goldman, G., & Ausicello D. (2012). *Cecil textbook of medicine* (24nd ed.). Philadelphia, PA: WB Saunders.

Rakel, R. E., & Bope, E. T. (2013). *Conn's current therapy.* Philadelphia, PA: WB Saunders.

Ureden, L. D., Stacey, K. M., & Lough, M. E. (2013). *Thelan's critical care nursing: Diagnosis and management* (7th ed.). St. Louis, MO: Mosby.

Ureden, L. D., Stacey, K. M., & Lough, M. E. (2011). *Priorities in critical care nursing* (6th ed.). St. Louis, MO: Mosby.

CHAPTER 32

Lower Respiratory Tract Pathogens

DAVID A. MILLER • THOMAS W. BARKLEY, JR.

I. **Defined as pathogens found below the larynx**
   A. Note that pathogens in all parts of the lower respiratory tract are the same
   B. Recommended pharmacological treatment may require revision after the results of sputum and blood cultures are obtained (see Table 32.1)
   C. Considerations in older adults
      1. Comorbid conditions (heart failure, chronic obstructive pulmonary disease [COPD], diabetes, altered mental status, dementia, dysphagia, and cancer)
      2. Altered immunological status with aging
      3. Aspiration and residence in long-term care facilities may require broader-spectrum antibiotic coverage.
      4. More than 50% of all cases of pneumonia occur in adults older than 65 years. Comorbidity is a strong predictor of mortality from community-acquired pneumonia in the elderly, as is low body temperature, hypotension, elevation of creatinine above 1.5 mg/dl, debility, and being older than 85 years.
      5. Microbiology
         a. *Streptococcus pneumoniae* still predominates
         b. May be polymicrobial, including other bacteria and respiratory viruses
         c. Causative organisms are not identified in 60% of cases among the elderly.
         d. Antimicrobial resistance patterns in the local community and in long-term care facilities need to be reviewed, if available.

      e. Antimicrobial choices need to be addressed by these resistance patterns due to the prevalence of resistance among all bacteria responsible for pneumonia in elderly patients. This resistance is a global problem.

    D. Immunization against the pneumococcus and annual influenza vaccines is important. Pneumococcal vaccination does not guarantee pneumococcal pneumonia will be prevented by the vaccine.

II. **Milder disease requires only narrow-spectrum antimicrobials, if any.**

III. **Severe disease requires a combination of antimicrobials while cultures are pending.**

IV. **The suggestions in Table 32.1 apply to therapy that is chosen empirically while sputum and blood cultures are pending.**

    A. When culture data are available, antimicrobials used should be reviewed and changed if necessary.

    B. The narrowest-spectrum antimicrobial that is reasonably expected to effectively treat the patient's lower respiratory tract infection should be used.

V. **Recall that antimicrobial therapy is intended to help clear pulmonary infection.**

    A. Other pharmacological and nonpharmacological therapies should be considered as well.

    B. Examples:

        1. Supplemental oxygen

        2. Treatment of underlying COPD

        3. Hydration and nutritional support

VI. **The most common causes of community-acquired pneumonia are shown in Table 32.2.**

VII. **Organism and treatment considerations for various pneumonias are depicted in Tables 32.4 through 32.8.**

VIII. **Table 32.10 lists pharmacological treatment options selected on the basis of suspected/known organisms for lower respiratory tract infection.**

Table 32.1	Lower Respiratory Tract Pathogens and Treatment Considerations (Modified From Karmanger, 2013)	
Lower respiratory tract infection	**Organism**	**Recommended pharmacological treatment**
Acute tracheo-bronchitis	Viral	No therapy indicated
	Mycoplasma pneumoniae	Doxycycline, macrolides (note the risk of QT segment prolongation and torsade de points, including azithromycin)
	Chlamydia pneumoniae	Doxycycline, macrolides (note the risk of QT segment prolongation and torsade de points, including azithromycin)
	Bordetella pertussis	Macrolides (note the risk of QT segment prolongation and torsade de points, including azithromycin)
Acute bacterial exacerbation of COPD	Viral, with secondary bacterial infection	Therapy may be unnecessary
	Streptococcus pneumoniae	Consider amoxicillin, trimethoprim-sulfamethoxazole, doxycycline, second-generation cephalosporin
	Haemophilus pneumoniae	Amoxicillin preferred if susceptible Consider fluoroquinolones, azithromycin (risk as noted above), and tetracyclines
	Moraxella catarrhalis	For severe cases, consider amoxicillin-clavulanate, clarithromycin or azithromycin (risk as noted above), oral cephalosporin, telithromycin, fluoroquinolone (with resistant *S. pneumoniae* coverage)
Influenza	Influenza H and B (winter months)	Zanamivir (Relenza), 10 mg (two inhalations BID), or Oseltamivir (Tamiflu), 75 mg BID
	Other viral	Supportive therapy; may check for respiratory syncytial virus in elderly or immunocompromised patients, although ribavirin (Virazole) effectiveness in this setting is unknown
Pneumonia	Community-acquired	See Tables 32.4 and 32.5

Table 32.2	Pathogens in Community-Acquired Pneumonia
Typical bacterial pathogens (approx. 85%)	*Streptococcus pneumoniae* Penicillin-sensitive *S. pneumoniae* Penicillin-resistant *S. pneumoniae* *Haemophilus influenzae* Ampicillin-sensitive *H. influenzae* Ampicillin-resistant *H. influenzae* *Moraxella catarrhalis* (all strains penicillin resistant)
Atypical respiratory pathogens (approx. 15%)	*Legionella* species *Mycoplasma* species *Chlamydia pneumoniae*
Less common bacterial pathogens	*Klebsiella pneumoniae* (only in those with chronic alcoholism) *Staphylococcus aureus* (postviral, influenza setting) *Pseudomonas aeruginosa* (especially in patients with bronchiectasis)

Table 32.3	Outpatient Bacterial Pneumonia With Comorbidity in Patients 60 years or Older (Modified From Karmanger, 2013)

Organisms	*Streptococcus pneumoniae*
	Haemophilus influenzae
	Aerobic Gram-negative bacilli
	Staphylococcus aureus
	Miscellaneous:
	     Moraxella catarrhalis
	     Legionella species
	     Mycoplasma species

Therapy for Specific Comorbidity:	COPD (no recent antibiotics or oral corticosteroids, past 3 months): First choice: newer macrolides (warning regarding prolonged QT and torsade de pointes, including azithromycin) Second choice: doxycycline
	COPD (recent antibiotics or oral corticosteroids in past 3 months): First choice: respiratory fluoroquinolone Second choice: amoxicillin/clavulanate plus macrolide (warning, as above), or second-generation cephalosporin plus macrolide
	Suspected microaspiration, oral anaerobes: First choice: amoxicillin/clavulanate and/or macrolide or fourth-generation fluoroquinolone (e.g., moxifloxacin) Second choice: third-generation fluoroquinolone (e.g., levofloxacin) plus clindamycin or metronidazole

Table 32.4	**Patients With Community-Acquired Bacterial Pneumonia Admitted to a Hospital (Modified From Karmanger, 2013)**

Organisms:	*Streptococcus pneumoniae*
	Haemophilus influenzae
	Polymicrobial (including aerobic bacteria)
	Aerobic Gram-negative bacilli
	Legionella species
	Staphylococcus aureus
	Chlamydia pneumoniae
	Miscellaneous
	       Mycoplasma pneumoniae
	       Moraxella catarrhalis

Therapy:	First choice: respiratory fluoroquinolone Second choice: second- or third-generation cephalosporin plus macrolide

Table 32.5	**Patients With Severe Community-Acquired Bacterial Pneumonia Admitted to an ICU**
Organisms:	*Streptococcus pneumoniae* *Legionella* species Aerobic Gram-negative bacilli *Mycoplasma pneumoniae* Miscellaneous *Haemophilus influenzae*
Therapy:	First choice: antipseudomonal fluoroquinolone (e.g., ciprofloxacin) plus antipseudomonal β-lactam (e.g., ceftazidime, piperacillin-tazobactam, carbapenem) or aminoglycoside (e.g., gentamicin, tobramycin, amikacin) Second choice: triple therapy with antipseudomonal β-lactam plus aminoglycoside plus macrolide

Table 32.6	Patients With Mild to Moderate Hospital-Acquired Bacterial Pneumonia, No Unusual Risk Factors, and Onset at Any Time; or Patients With Severe Hospital-Acquired Pneumonia With Early Onset (Excludes Immunosuppressed Elderly Patients) (Modified From Karmanger, 2013)
Core organisms:	Enteric Gram-negative bacilli (Nonpseudomonal) *Enterobacter* species *Escherichia coli* *Klebsiella* species *Proteus* species *Serratia marcescens* *Haemophilus influenzae* Methicillin-sensitive *Staphylococcus aureus* *Streptococcus pneumoniae*
Core antibiotics:	Cephalosporin Second-generation or antipseudomonal third-generation β-lactam/β-lactamase inhibitor combination If allergic to penicillin, fluoroquinolone or clindamycin plus aztreonam

Table 32.7	Patients With Mild to Moderate Hospital-Acquired Bacterial Pneumonia With Risk Factors, Onset at Any Time (Modified From Karmanger, 2013)
Organisms:	Core organisms, plus one of the following: -Anaerobes (recent abdominal surgery, witnessed following aspiration) -*Staphylococcus aureus* (coma, head trauma, diabetes mellitus, and renal failure) -*Legionella* (high-dose steroids) -*Pseudomonas aeruginosa* (prolonged ICU stay, steroids, antibiotics, and structural lung disease)
Therapy:	Core antibiotics plus: -Clindamycin or β-lactam/β-lactamase inhibitor alone or with vancomycin (until methicillin-resistant *Staphylococcus aureus* is excluded) -Erythromycin, possibly with rifampin -Linezolid -Treat as severe hospital-acquired pneumonia (see Table 32.8)

Table 32.8	Patients With Severe Hospital-Acquired Bacterial Pneumonia With Risk Factors and Early Onset or Patients With Severe Hospital-Acquired Pneumonia and Late Onset.
Core organisms, plus the following:	*Pseudomonas aeruginosa* *Acinetobacter* species Consider methicillin-resistant *Staphylococcus aureus*
Therapy:	Aminoglycoside or ciprofloxacin plus one of the following: -Antipseudomonal penicillin -β-lactam/β-lactamase inhibitor -Ceftazidime or cefoperazone -Imipenem, possibly with vancomycin -Linezolid

Table 32.9	Select Pharmacological Treatment Options Based on Suspected/Known Organism	
Organism	**Drug**	**Recommended pharmacological treatment options**
***Haemophilus influenzae* (β-lactamase positive)**	Amoxicillin/clavulanate (Augmentin)	500 mg/125 mg PO every 8 hr or 875 mg/125 mg every 12 hr
	Cefuroxime (Ceftin)	500 mg PO BID
	Erythromycin (EES, Erythrocin, E-mycin) (significant resistance but active against most strains)	250–500 mg PO BID
	Clarithromycin (Biaxin) (significant resistance but active against most strains) (macrolide risks as noted above)	250–500 mg PO every 12 hr or extended-release 1000 mg BID for 7 days
	Azithromycin (Zithromax) (significant resistance but active against most strains) (macrolide risks as noted above)	Day 1: 500 mg PO Days 2–5: 250 mg/day PO
	Moxifloxacin (Avelox)	400 mg PO daily for 7–14 days
	Telithromycin (Ketek)	800 mg PO daily for 7–10 days

Table 32.9	Select Pharmacological Treatment Options Based on Suspected/Known Organism	
Organism	**Drug**	**Recommended pharmacological treatment options**
***Haemophilus influenzae* (β-lactamase negative)**	Amoxicillin	500 mg–1 gram PO every 8 hr
	Amoxicillin/clavulanate (Augmentin)	500 mg/125 mg PO every 8 hr or 875 mg/125 mg every 12 hr
	Cefuroxime (Ceftin)	500 mg PO BID
	Erythromycin (EES, Erythrocin, E-mycin) (significant resistance but active against most strains)	250–500 mg PO BID
	Clarithromycin (Biaxin) (significant resistance but active against most strains)	250–500 mg PO every 12 hr or extended-release 1000 mg BID for 7 days
	Azithromycin (Zithromax) (significant resistance but active against most strains) (risks as noted previously)	Day 1: 500 mg PO Days 2–5: 250 mg/day PO
	Moxifloxacin (Avelox)	400 mg PO daily for 7–14 days
	Telithromycin (Ketek)	800 mg PO daily for 7–10 days
***Streptococcus pneumoniae* (resistant)**	Amoxicillin (significant resistance, but active against most strains)	500 mg–1 g PO every 8 hr (Note: Doses of 80 mg/kg/day may be effective against nonmeningeal, penicillin-resistant *Streptococcus pneumoniae*.)
	Moxifloxacin (Avelox)	400 mg PO daily for 7–14 days
	Telithromycin (Ketek)	800 mg PO daily for 7–10 days
Chlamydia pneumoniae	Azithromycin (Zithromax) (macrolide risks as noted above)	Day 1: 500 mg PO Days 2–5: 250 mg PO daily Community-acquired pneumonia: 500 mg PO/IV daily for 7–10 days
	Telithromycin (Ketek)	800 mg PO daily for 7–10 days
	Levofloxacin (Levaquin)	500 mg PO/IV daily for 7–14 days or 750 mg PO/IV daily for 5 days
	Moxifloxacin (Avelox)	400 mg PO daily

Table 32.9	Select Pharmacological Treatment Options Based on Suspected/Known Organism	
Organism	**Drug**	**Recommended pharmacological treatment options**
Legionella/ legionellosis	Erythromycin (EES, E-Mycin, Ery-Tab) (macrolide risks as noted above)	250 mg erythromycin stearate/ base (or 400 mg ethylsuccinate) every 6 hr PO 1 hr before meals, or 500 mg every 12 hr or 333 mg PO every 8 hr; increase to 4 g/day, depending on severity of infection; 15–20 mg/kg/day IV every 6 hr in divided doses; not to exceed 4 g daily
	Levofloxacin (Levaquin)	500 mg PO/IV daily; adjust dose in renal disease
	Trovafloxacin (Trovan)	100–200 mg PO daily; 200 mg IV daily
	Azithromycin (Zithromax) (macrolide risks as noted above)	Day 1: 500 mg PO Days 2–5: 250 mg PO daily or 500 mg IV daily
	Clarithromycin (Biaxin) (macrolide risks as noted above)	250 mg PO BID; may increase to 500 mg PO 3 times a day or500 mg PO every 12 hr
	Ciprofloxacin (Cipro)	250–750 mg PO every 12 hr; 200–400 mg IV every 12 hr
	Ofloxacin (Floxin)	400 mg PO/IV every 12 hr
	Sparfloxacin (Zagam)	200 mg PO daily
	Doxycycline (Vibramycin)	100 mg PO/IV every 12 hr
	Moxifloxacin (Avelox)	400 mg PO daily for 10 days

Table 32.9	Select Pharmacological Treatment Options Based on Suspected/Known Organism	
Organism	**Drug**	**Recommended pharmacological treatment options**
Streptococcus pneumoniae	Amoxicillin	500 mg–1 g PO every 8 hr
	Amoxicillin/Clavulanate	500 mg/125 mg every 8 hr or 875 mg/125 mg every 12 hr
	Cefuroxime (Ceftin)	500 mg PO BID
	Erythromycin (EES, Erythrocin, E-mycin)	250–500 mg PO BID
	Clarithromycin (Biaxin)	250–500 mg PO every 12 hr or extended-release 1000 mg BID for 7 days
	Azithromycin (Zithromax)	Day 1: 500 mg PO Days 2–5: 250 mg/day PO
	Moxifloxacin (Avelox)	400 mg PO daily for 7–14 days
	Telithromycin (Ketek)	800 mg PO daily for 7–10 days
Mycoplasma pneumoniae	Tetracycline (Sumycin)	500 mg PO BID for 1–4 weeks
	Erythromycin (EES, Erythrocin, E-mycin) (macrolide risks as noted above)	500 mg PO 4 times a day for 7–10 days
	Azithromycin (Zithromax) (macrolide risks as noted above)	Day 1: 500 mg PO Days 2–5: 250 mg/day PO
	Clarithromycin (Biaxin) (macrolide risks as noted above)	250–500 mg PO BID for 7–14 days
	Moxifloxacin (Avelox)	400 mg PO daily for 7–14 days
	Telithromycin (Ketek)	800 mg PO daily for 7–10 days
	Tetracycline (Sumycin)	500 mg PO 4 times a day
	Doxycycline (Vibramycin)	100 mg PO BID
	Erythromycin (EES) (macrolide risks as noted above)	500 mg PO/IV every 6 hr
	Clarithromycin (Biaxin) (macrolide risks as noted above)	500 mg PO BID or 1 g PO every day 7–14 days

BIBLIOGRAPHY

Centers for Medicare & Medicaid Services. (2013). *2014 ICD-10 PCS and GEMs.* Retrieved November 25, 2013, from http:///www.cms.gov/Medicare/Coding/ICD10/2014-ICD-10-PCS.html

Food and Drug Administration. (2013). *FDA drug safety communication: Azithromycin (Zithromax or Zmax) and the risk of potentially fatal heart rhythms.* Retrieved November 25, 2013, from http://www.fda.gov/downloads/Drugs/DrugSafety/UCM343347.pdf

Garlington, W., & High, K. (2013). Evaluation of infection in the older adult. In D. S. Basow (Ed.), *UpToDate.* Waltham, MA: UpToDate.

Gilbert, D. N., Moellering, R. C., & Eliopoulos, G. M. (Eds.). (2013). *The Sanford guide to antimicrobial therapy 2013.* Sperryville, VA: Antimicrobial Therapy.

Goldman, L, & Shafer, A. I. (Eds.) (2012). *Goldman's Cecil medicine* (24th ed.). Philadelphia, PA: Saunders.

Kamanger, N. (2013). *Bacterial pneumonia. Practice essentials update.* Retrieved November 26, 2013, from http://emedicine.medscape.com/article/300157-overview

Longo, D. L., Kasper, D. L., Jameson, J. L., Fauci, A. S., Hauser, S. L., & Loscalzo, J. (Eds.). (2011). *Harrison's principles of internal medicine* (18th ed.). New York, NY: McGraw Hill.

Mandell, G. L., Bennett, J. E., & Dolin, R. (2010). *Principles and practice of infectious disease.* (7th ed.). Philadelphia, PA: Churchill Livingston.

Marrie, T. J. (2013). Epidemiology, pathogenesis, and microbiology of community-acquired pneumonia in adults. In D. S. Basow (Ed.), *UpToDate.* Waltham, MA: UpToDate.

CHAPTER 33

Obstructive Sleep Apnea

JENNIFER COATES • THOMAS W. BARKLEY, JR.

CHARACTERISTICS OF BREATHING AND SLEEP

A. Tidal volume and respiratory rate decline as a person becomes more deeply asleep. Skeletal muscle tone decreases progressively in deeper stages of sleep, with frank atony occurring during rapid eye movement sleep.

B. Peak airway resistance tends to be highest from 2:00 a.m. to 6:00 a.m. and lowest from 2:00 p.m. to 6:00 p.m.

C. Cough and shortness of breath may be aggravated during the normal sleeping period at night

D. Normal pauses in respiration are infrequent and brief, lasting 5–10 seconds. These pauses are central in origin and are not associated with physical obstruction of the oropharynx or hypopharynx.

OBSTRUCTIVE SLEEP APNEA (OSA)

I. **Etiology**

A. Obstruction of the upper airway caused by loss of normal pharyngeal muscle tone during sleep

B. Obstruction causes arousals and awakenings from sleep, and effective sleep time is reduced

II. **Incidence**

A. The incidence is unknown. However, OSA and hypopnea are often under recognized in clinical practice.

B. OSA is more commonly noted among obese individuals, but the absence of obesity does not rule out the possible existence of OSA.

C. OSA is more common among males

III. Clinical manifestations
  A. The classic manifestation of significant OSA is excessive daytime sleepiness
  B. Snoring is commonly heard, although severe sleep apnea may be accompanied by quiet snoring
  C. Severe daytime sleepiness interferes with normal daytime functioning
    1. Additional attempts to "catch up" on sleep fail
    2. Driving a vehicle or operating heavy machinery may become dangerous
  D. Hypoxemia during the apneic and hypopneic episodes may lead to adverse health consequences, including the following:
    1. Myocardial ischemia, infarction, arrhythmias, and heart failure
    2. Cerebral ischemia and stroke
    3. Sudden death
    4. Cardiorespiratory arrest after surgery or administration of sedatives, hypnotics, and opioids

IV. Physical findings
  A. Mental status reflects less than optimal alertness
  B. Obesity with fatty infiltration of the soft palate and pharyngeal wall can be found as well as a decrease in the posterior pharyngeal space; tonsillar enlargement, if present, aggravates the obstruction, as it does enlargement of the adenoids
  C. Right-sided heart failure, with peripheral edema, may be seen

V. Diagnosis
  A. Polysomnography (PSG), an overnight sleep study that measures airflow, muscle tone, and brain wave activity, is required
  B. The finding of more than 10 obstructive apneas/hypopneas (respiratory effort in the absence of, or significant reduction in, airflow during sleep) per hour is abnormal and justifies treatment, especially when oxygen desaturation values below 88% are documented.
  C. Oxygen desaturation measurements below 88% during sleep may require supplemental oxygen if therapy produces no improvement.

VI. Treatment
  A. General
    1. Avoidance of alcohol, sedatives, hypnotics, and opioids until effective therapy is begun
    2. Weight loss and maintenance, if indicated
    3. Avoidance of driving and operating heavy machinery until effective treated is provided and a significant reduction in daytime sleepiness is noted
  B. Specific
    1. Institution of nasal continuous positive airway pressure (nCPAP) or nasal bilevel positive airway pressure (nBIPAP) to stent the posterior pharynx

        a. Pressure is delivered by a mechanically driven device and is applied through a mask that is snugly and appropriately fitted over the nose or a pair of fitted nasal "pillows."

        b. A chin strap may be required to avoid pressure leaks through the mouth

        c. Humidification added to the mechanical circuitry may help prevent mucosal dryness

    2. Pressure needed to treat patients with OSA is usually between 5 and 15 cm H_2O and may be empirically chosen; however, optimal therapy is best determined by repeat PSG and titration of pressure to the level that fully alleviates obstructive events and oxygen desaturation.

    3. Follow-up to determine adherence to recommended therapies is crucial. The patient should use nCPAP during all sleeping periods.

  C. Other therapies

    1. Surgical removal of excessive tissue in the posterior pharynx if nCPAP or nBIPAP fails to alleviate excessive daytime sleepiness and to reduce the frequency of apnea and hypopnea and oxygen desaturation, as determined by follow-up PSG

        a. Uvulopalatopharyngoplasty (UPPP)

        b. Tonsillectomy and/or adenoidectomy

    2. Mandibular advancement to pull the tongue forward to create additional posterior pharyngeal space

    3. Oral devices to enhance the posterior pharyngeal space tend to be uncomfortable and, therefore, are ineffective in treating patients with OSA.

    4. Tracheostomy relieves OSA promptly and was the definitive therapy before nCPAP became available. It is now reserved for those individuals with severe disease who are unable to use nCPAP or nBIPAP, or who are not candidates for surgical resection of redundant tissue.

VII. **Gerontologic considerations**

  A. The prevalence of OSA increases with age. Untreated OSA may increase the risk of metabolic syndrome or early mortality.

  B. Cognitive changes may be present in elderly patients with OSA; experts are unsure if these effects are due to hypoxia, hypersomnolence, or both. These changes may include the following:

    1. Impairments in attention

    2. Impairments in concentration

    3. Difficulty with executive functioning

    4. Working memory less

  C. Treatment with nCPAP or nBIPAP may improve cognitive functioning

BIBLIOGRAPHY

Downey, R., Gold, P. M., Rowley, J. A., & Wickramasinghe, H. (2014). Obstructive sleep apnea. *Medscape*. Retrieved from http://emedicine.medscape.com/article/295807-overview#showall

Epstein, L. J., Kristo, D., Strollo, P. J., Friedman, N., Malhotra, A., Patil, S. P., . . . Weinstein, M. D. (2009). Adult Obstructive Sleep Apnea Task Force of the American Academy of Sleep Medicine. Clinical guideline for the evaluation, management and long term care of obstructive sleep apnea in adults. *Journal of Clinical Sleep Medicine, 5,* 263–276.

Halter, J., Ouslander, J., Tinetti, M., Studenski, S., High, K., & Asthana, S. (2009, March 9). *Hazzard's geriatric medicine and gerontology* (6th ed.). New York, NY: McGraw-Hill Professional.

Kryger, M., Roth, T., & Dement, W. (2010). *Principles and practice of sleep medicine* (5th ed.). Philadelphia, PA: Elsevier.

Longo, D., Fauci, A., Kasper, D., Hauser S., Jameson, J., & Loscalzo, J. (2012). *Harrison's principles of internal medicine* (18th ed.). New York, NY: McGraw-Hill.

McPhee, S. J., & Papadakis, M. A. (2014). *Current medical diagnosis and treatment* (53rd ed.). New York, NY: McGraw Hill Lange.

Olaithe, M., & Bucks, R. S. (2013). Executive dysfunction in OSA before and after treatment. *Sleep, 36,* 1297.

Vasu, T. S., Grewal, R., Doghramji, K. (2012) Obstructive sleep apnea syndrome and perioperative complications: A systematic review of the literature. *Journal of Clinical Sleep Medicine, 8,* 199–207.

CHAPTER **34**

Oxygen Supplementation

CAROL THOMPSON • THOMAS W. BARKLEY, JR. • CHARLENE M. MYERS

BASIC PRINCIPLES OF OXYGEN SUPPLEMENTATION

I. **The goal of oxygen supplementation is to increase the fraction of inspired oxygen (FIO$_2$).**
   A. The diffusion gradient is increased, thereby facilitating an increased partial pressure of oxygen in arterial blood (PaO$_2$)

II. **Supplemental oxygen supply is accessed through a wall source or a portable oxygen cylinder.**
   A. Wall oxygen is sourced from outlets fed from a large bulk tank outside the facility
      1. Supplied at a constant pressure of 50 lb per square inch (PSI)
      2. Requires only a flowmeter (Thorpe tube) for delivery
      3. Duration of flow is generally not an issue for the clinician
   B. Cylinder oxygen is sourced from portable metal cylinders of various sizes
      1. Cylinder sizes are identified in descending order by letter designations H, E, D, B, A, AA, and DD
         a. The most common cylinder for providing portable oxygen in the hospital is the E cylinder
      2. All cylinders have a pressure of 2200 PSI when full
         a. Pressure will fall as oxygen in the cylinder is used
         b. Oxygen supply should be considered unreliable at less than 500 PSI
      3. Cylinders require a regulator for reduction of pressure and control of flow
         a. Pressure is maintained at constant 50 PSI despite changing pressure within the cylinder
         b. Flow is metered by a Bourdon gauge

4. When portable oxygen is needed, duration of flow is an important consideration (i.e., "How long will this tank last?")
   a. Duration of flow in minutes is calculated by multiplying the PSI (subtract 500 for safety buffer) by the "cylinder factor" (0.28 for an E cylinder), then dividing by liters per minute of flow. The D cylinder factor is 0.16 and M cylinder factor is 1.56.
   b. Example: $[(2200 - 500) \times 0.28] \div 4 = 119$ minutes
   c. A full E cylinder that delivers 4 L per minute should safely last about 2 hr

C. Oxygen outlets, meters, gauges, and tanks are color coded (green) to distinguish them from other gases (various colors) or suction sources (white).
   1. Caution is required because neighboring Canadian standards color code oxygen as white
   2. Always read label on the cylinder

III. **Oxygen supplementation is indicated when an actual or potential deficit of global or specific tissue oxygenation is present.**

A. Deficit may result from decreased supply of oxygen or increased demand for oxygen (or combination)
   1. Decreased supply may be due to ventilation, diffusion, or perfusion defects (or combination)
      a. Ventilation defect examples
         i. Overdose
         ii. Sedation
         iii. Flail chest
         iv. Asthma
      b. Diffusion defect examples
         i. Pneumonia
         ii. Acute respiratory distress syndrome (ARDS)
         iii. CHF
         iv. Chronic obstructive pulmonary disease (COPD)
      c. Perfusion defect examples
         i. Shock
         ii. Anemia
         iii. Hypovolemia
         iv. Stroke
         v. Angina/MI
         vi. Sickle cell crisis
   2. Increased demand may be due to exertion or hypermetabolic states.
      a. Examples of exertion
         i. Fatigue
         ii. Seizures

        b. Examples of hypermetabolism

           i. Hyperthermia

           ii. Hyperthyroidism

B. Supplemental oxygen should be provided at the lowest FIO_2 that will abolish significant threats of real or potential tissue oxygenation deficits.

    1. Avoid FIO_2 that exceeds 0.50 for longer than 24 hr

        a. Risk for effects of oxygen toxicity

           i. Alveolar damage

           ii. Loss of surfactant

           iii. Atelectasis

    2. Anticipate risk of ventilatory suppression in patients with history of carbon dioxide retention (e.g., COPD)

        a. Avoid overcorrection of mild hypoxemia (may depress primary ventilatory stimulus), especially if unable to closely monitor

        b. Severe hypoxemia (may result in tissue damage) should be corrected with anticipation of risk for ventilatory suppression (prepare for ventilatory assistance)

C. Assess frequently (at least daily) for need to continue supplementation

    1. Wean or discontinue supplemental oxygen as indicated by confidence for the following:

        a. PaO_2 greater than 60

        b. Oxygen saturation (SaO_2) greater than 90%

        c. Potential threat ruled out or abolished

        d. No overt distress

FACILITATION OF VENTILATION

I. **Occasionally, patients are unable to maintain spontaneous ventilation.**

    A. Examples:

        1. Impaired structure

           a. Trauma (flail chest, pneumothorax)

           b. Decreased compliance (ARDS)

           c. COPD

        2. Impaired function

           a. CNS depression (drugs, spinal cord injury [SCI])

    B. Patients require both oxygen supplementation and ventilatory assistance

II. **Airway maintenance and bag-valve-mask ventilation are the first lines of ventilatory assistance in the clinical setting.**

    A. Airway maintenance focuses on upper airway patency

        1. Primary actions to ensure patency such as proper head position and jaw thrust maneuver are well covered in basic and advanced life support courses

      a. Proper head position includes positioning to avoid aspiration of emesis

  2. Secondary actions to ensure patency consist of effective upper airway suction efforts (using Yankauer suction handle)

  3. Tertiary actions to ensure patency may include insertion of oropharyngeal airway

      a. May not be tolerated by conscious patient

      b. Proper insertion technique is needed to avoid trauma and airway compromise

      c. Insert by sliding lateral to the tongue and then rotating the tip to the posterior part of the tongue

      d. Secure and monitor closely to avoid or detect displacement and airway compromise

B. Bag-valve-mask ventilation focuses on delivery of adequate tidal volume and FIO_2.

  1. Self-inflating bag provides reservoir for oxygen and means of delivering volume

      a. High-flow oxygen (12–15 L/minute) produces FIO_2 of near 1 (100%) in the reservoir

      b. Manual compression of the bag displaces reservoir volume into the airway through positive pressure

      c. Degree to which the bag is compressed determines volume delivered

  2. Valve prevents aspiration of expired air into the bag-reservoir during bag reinflation

  3. Sealing of the upper airway with a mask is required for positive-pressure ventilation

      a. Improper seal will result in failure to deliver volume and FIO_2

      b. Efforts to produce a seal must include maintenance of head and jaw position to avoid compromise of airway patency

      c. The "C-E grip" with thumb and forefinger (forming C) around the bag/mask junction and the third, fourth, and fifth fingers (forming E) hooked under the end of the jaw can be effective in producing a seal.

      d. Assistance provided by a second person is preferred but may be required if teeth/dentures are absent.

  4. Mouth-to-mouth ventilation should be considered "last resort" in clinical settings.

      a. Ventilation with exhaled air via mouth-to-mouth delivers decreased FIO_2 (0.16 vs 0.21) and increased carbon dioxide (CO_2) (0.05 vs greater than 0.01).

      b. Oral shielding device such as a pocket mask should be used to prevent body fluid exposure of both victim and rescuer

C. Even well-administered mouth-to-mouth breathing delivers an FIO_2 of only 16% to 17%, compared with 21% oxygen in room air.

III. **A pocket mask device allows mouth-to-mouth ventilation without personal contact.**

   A. Some pocket masks have a port that allows administration of supplemental oxygen

   B. Pocket mask devices are eminently portable

IV. **Bag-valve-mask devices**

   A. Bag-valve-mask devices allow administration of supplemental oxygen via a face mask and a reservoir bag

   B. Depending on oxygen flow and operator skill, high concentrations of oxygen may be administered

   C. Self-inflating bags are as follows:

   1. Versatile

   2. Can be used with or without supplemental oxygen

   3. Available in various sizes appropriate for infants, children, and adults

   D. The major complication of a bag-valve-mask device involves inflation of the stomach resulting from poor airway maintenance or high ventilation pressures.

   1. Be alert for the development of gastric distention

   2. Relieve distention through placement of a nasogastric tube

   3. Do not compress the distended stomach manually; emesis may result

   E. The mask is an essential component of the device and should be sized to the patient.

   1. A well-fitting mask with a seal that encompasses the nose and the mouth is important in ensuring adequate ventilation.

   2. The mask should be clear to allow visualization of emesis.

   F. The airway in an unconscious patient is more easily maintained with an oropharyngeal airway.

   1. The device will lift the tongue from the posterior pharynx.

   2. Oropharyngeal airways are not tolerated by patients with intact gag reflexes.

   3. A small degree of skill is required for placement of the oropharyngeal airway.

   a. Inept placement may traumatize the soft tissues of the oropharynx or may occlude the airway

   b. To safely place the airway, the following steps must be taken:

   i. Open the patient's mouth

   ii. Move the tongue aside with a tongue blade

   iii. Insert the oropharyngeal airway with the tip pointing laterally, then rotate once posterior to the tongue

   G. A nasopharyngeal airway is a soft plastic device placed through the nares that provides a passage through the posterior pharynx

   1. Lubrication with lidocaine jelly facilitates placement and enhances patient tolerance

2. A nasopharyngeal airway is usually tolerated by a conscious patient.
3. Nasopharyngeal airways are especially useful in the following patients:
   a. Those with orofacial trauma
   b. Those in whom the oropharynx is not accessible

V. **Suction devices are an important adjunct to ventilation.**
   A. Sudden cessation of ventilation may be due to airway occlusion caused by emesis or a mucous plug
   B. Accumulation of saliva and airway secretions can also cause occlusion
   C. A rigid suction device (e.g., Yankauer suction) is generally more useful than a flexible catheter for airway maintenance in the posterior pharynx.

DEVICES FOR OXYGEN SUPPLEMENTATION

I. **Nasal prongs are the simplest means of delivering supplemental oxygen.**
   A. Inspired room air is mixed with oxygen that has been stored in the reservoir (nasal cavity).
      1. Prongs deliver oxygen into the nasal cavity, which acts as a reservoir.
      2. Inspiratory air flow through the oropharynx creates lower pressure at the posterior nasopharynx (Bernoulli's principle), and oxygen stored in nasal cavity is drawn in via the nasopharynx.
   B. FIO_2 is generally determined by liter flow of oxygen per minute (L/minute) into the reservoir (nasal cavity).
      1. Generally ordered in terms of L/minute up to maximum of 6 L/minute
      2. As a general rule, each L/minute of oxygen flow increases FIO_2 by approximately 0.04 (4%).
         a. For 2 L/minute, FIO_2 is approximately 0.28–0.32
         b. For 4 L/minute, FIO_2 is approximately 0.35–0.38
         c. For 6 L/minute, FIO_2 is approximately 0.42–0.45
      3. Oral breathing is assumed; only a patent nasal airway is required
   C. Advantages
      1. Well tolerated during eating, speaking, or activity
      2. Relatively inexpensive, simple to use
   D. Disadvantages
      1. Effectiveness can be sensitive to placement
         a. Prongs must be within nares to be effective
      2. May require humidification to prevent drying of nasal mucosa
         a. Always use humidification at flows greater than 3 L/minute
      3. Caution is required to prevent pressure injury at contact points over ears, cheeks, and nares

II. **Face masks can provide a higher FIO$_2$ than is attained with nasal prongs.**

   A. A properly functioning face mask can provide an FIO$_2$ level of 0.40 to almost 1 (100%).

   B. Supplemental oxygen masks do not require a tight seal to the face.

      1. Mask design assumes or prevents entrainment of room air under edge of mask

   C. Simple face masks use relatively low flow rates (5–8 L/minute).

      1. Low flow allows room air to be entrained under edge of mask on inspiration.

         a. FIO$_2$ is imprecise and is limited to less than 0.6 because of variable mixing with room air.

      2. Lower cost and less drying than with nasal cannula

      3. Patients may feel claustrophobic, which may interfere with eating or speaking.

   D. Venturi masks use velocity to create pressure gradient for more precise control of FIO$_2$ up to 0.6

      1. Oxygen is funneled through Venturi nozzle past "window" entraining room air (Bernoulli's principle) precisely to desired FIO$_2$

         a. Size of Venturi or window may be adjusted to produce desired FIO$_2$

      2. High-velocity flow into confined space of mask produces pressure greater than room air

         a. Inhaled air comes from precise FIO$_2$ in mask

         b. No room air pulled under edge of mask to dilute FIO$_2$

      3. More expensive but produces more reliable FIO$_2$; otherwise, same advantages and disadvantages as simple mask

   E. Non-rebreather masks use high flow rates (11–15 L/minute), reservoir bags, and valves to deliver FIO$_2$ near 100%

      1. High rate of flow fills large-volume reservoir bag with 100% oxygen with greater pressure than room air.

         a. Reservoir bag must be fully distended for proper function

         b. Inhaled volume comes from high-pressure reservoir bag with FIO$_2$ near 1

         c. High-pressure source prevents entrainment or room air under edge of mask

      2. Exhalation into mask closes one-way valve, preventing mixing with inhaled air source

         a. Exhaled air is blown out under edge of mask and is, thus, not "re-breathed."

      3. Can deliver maximal oxygen supplementation short of assisted ventilation device

      4. Expensive and bulky; otherwise, similar advantages and disadvantages as other masks

BIBLIOGRAPHY

Boyer, A., Vargas, F., Delacre, M., Saint-Léger, M., Clouzeau, B., Hilbert, G., & Gruson, D. (2011). Prognostic impact of high-flow nasal cannula oxygen supply in an ICU patient with pulmonary fibrosis complicated by acute respiratory failure. *Intensive Care Medicine, 37,* 558–559. doi: 10.1007/s00134–010–2036–9

Considine, J., Botti, M., & Thomas, S. (2012). Descriptive analysis of emergency department oxygen use in acute exacerbation of chronic obstructive pulmonary disease. *Internal Medicine Journal, 42*, e38-e47. doi:10.1111/j.1445–5994.2010.02220.x

Gerstein, N. S., Carey, M. C., Braude, D. A., Tawil, I., Persen, T. R., Deriy, L., & Anderson, M. S. (2013). Efficacy of facemask ventilation techniques in novice providers. *Journal of Clinical Anesthesia, 25,* 193–197. Retrieved from http://dx.doi.org/10.1016/j.jclinane.2012.10.009

Ehrenwerth, J., Elsenkraft, J. B., & Berry, F. M. (2013). *Anesthesia equipment: Principles and applications*. Philadelphia, PA: Saunders.

Hegde, S. & Prodhan, P. (2013). Serious air leak syndrome complicating high-flow nasal cannula therapy: A report of 3 cases. *Pediatrics, 131,* e939–944. doi:10.1542/peds.2011–3767

Hemmings, H. C., & Egan, T. D. (2013). *Pharmacology and physiology for anesthesia: Foundations and clinical applications*. Philadelphia, PA: Elsevier/Saunders.

Lee, J. H., Rehder, K. J., Williford, L., Cheifetz, I. M., & Turner, D. A. (2013). Use of high flow nasal cannula in critically ill infants, children, and adults: A critical review of the literature. *Intensive Care Medicine, 39*, 247–257. doi:10.1007/s00134–012–2743–5

Martí, S., Pajares, V., Morante, F., Ramón, M., Lara, J., Ferrer, J. & Güell, M. (2013). Are oxygen-conserving devices effective for correcting exercise hypoxemia? *Respiratory Care, 58,* 1606–1613. doi:10.4187/respcare.02260

Peel, D., Neighbour, R., & Eltringham, R. J. (2013). Evaluation of oxygen concentrators for use in countries with limited resources. *Anaesthesia, 68*, 706–712. doi:10.1111/anae.12260

Restrepo, R., D., Hirst, K. R., Wittnebel, L., & Wettstein, R. (2012). AARC clinical practice guidelines: Transcutaneous monitoring of carbon dioxide and oxygen: 2012. *Respiratory Care, 57,* 1955–1962. doi:10.4187/respcare.02011

Rice, K. L., Schmidt, M. F., Buan, J. S., Lebahn, F., & Schwarzock, T. K. (2011). Accu[Osub2] oximetry-driven oxygen-conserving device versus fixed-dose oxygen devices in stable COPD patients. *Respiratory Care, 56,* 1901–1905. doi:10.4187/respcare.01059

Ritchie, J. E., Williams, A. B., Gerard, C., & Hockey, H. (2011). Evaluation of a humidified nasal high-glow oxygen system, using oxygraph, capnography and measurement of upper airway pressures. *Anaesthesia Intensive Care, 39*(6), 1103–1110.

Schibler, A., Pham, T. M., Dunster, K. R., Foster, K., Barlow, A., Gibbons, K., & Hough, J. L. (2011). Reduced intubation rates for infants after introduction of high-flow nasal prong oxygen delivery. *Intensive Care Medicine, 37*, 847–853. doi:10.1007/s00134–011–2177–5

Urbano, J., Castillo, J., López-Herce, J., Gallardo, J. A., Solana, M. J., & Carrillo, Á. (2012). High-flow oxygen therapy: Pressure analysis in a pediatric airway model. *Respiratory Care, 57*, 721–726. doi:10.4187/respcare.01386

CHAPTER 35

Mechanical Ventilatory Support

AMITA AVADHANI • THOMAS W. BARKLEY, JR. • CHARLENE M. MYERS

INDICATIONS FOR MECHANICAL VENTILATION

I. **Inadequate intrinsic respiratory capacity to prevent or compensate for severe hypoxia and/or hypercarbia due to the following:**

   A. Neuromuscular (NM) depression or failure

      1. Drugs

         a. Opioids

         b. Sedatives

         c. NM blockers

      2. Trauma

         a. Spinal cord injury

         b. Phrenic nerve injury

      3. Disease

         a. Guillain-Barré syndrome

         b. Amyotrophic lateral sclerosis

         c. Myasthenia gravis

         d. Shock

      4. Exhaustion

         a. Status asthmaticus

         b. Sustained severe work of breathing

      5. Sustained apnea of any cause

   B. Persistent hypoxia (partial pressure of oxygen in arterial blood [PaO_2] less than 60 mmHg) and/or hypercarbia (partial pressure of carbon dioxide in arterial blood [$PaCO_2$] greater than 50 mmHg) refractory to noninvasive supplemental oxygen and/or airway maintenance (suction and position)

      1. Diffusion defects

      a. Aspiration

      b. Pulmonary edema

      c. Acute respiratory distress syndrome

      d. Chronic obstructive pulmonary disease

      e. Pneumonia

  2. Ventilation defects

      a. Chronic obstructive pulmonary disease

      b. Pickwickian syndrome

      c. Flail chest

      d. Pneumothorax

      e. Atelectasis

  3. Perfusion defects

      a. Shock

      b. Pulmonary embolus

      c. Malignant arrhythmias

GENERAL PRINCIPLES OF VENTILATION

I. **Inspiratory airflow occurs as the result of a pressure gradient in which extrapulmonary pressure is greater than intrapulmonary pressure.**

  A. This can result from lowering intrapulmonary pressure to below extrapulmonary pressure or by raising extrapulmonary pressure to above intrapulmonary pressure.

    1. Normal human inspiration occurs when chest volume is expanded by contraction of the diaphragm and elevation of the ribs, creating a negative intrapulmonary pressure and drawing air into the lungs. ("People suck to breathe.")

    2. Mechanical ventilation creates positive extrapulmonary pressure generated by a device that forces air into the lungs. ("Ventilators blow to breathe.")

      a. Positive-pressure ventilation requires a sealed airway, most commonly attained by an endotracheal tube (ETT) with an inflatable cuff.

II. **Expiratory airflow occurs as the result of a pressure gradient in which intrapulmonary pressure is raised to above extrapulmonary pressure.**

  A. Normal expiration, whether inspiration is spontaneous or mechanical, relies on passive elastic recoil of lung tissue and of chest wall muscles

    1. Chest wall and abdominal musculature can actively augment passive elastic recoil

    2. Mechanical positive-pressure ventilators cannot create an expiratory pressure gradient

VARIABLES FOR MECHANICAL VENTILATORS

I. **Tidal volume refers to the volume of air entering (inhaled) or leaving (exhaled) the lungs with each breath.**

A. When a ventilator mode uses a target tidal volume in adults, the settings should be in the range of 6–8 ml/kg ideal body weight in adults. (The goal is not to exceed the plateau pressure of 30 cm of H_2O to prevent barotrauma.)

1. The most common practice is to approximate tidal volume within 50 ml (400, 450, 500, 550, etc.) and then to adjust the effect

2. To avoid barotrauma, minimal effective tidal volume should be used

B. When the target is airway pressure, tidal volume may vary with compliance

II. **Rate is the number of mechanical breaths delivered each minute**

A. A mechanical breath cycle may be defined by a tidal volume target or by a pressure target

B. Set ventilator rates will be adjusted to achieve pH and $PaCO_2$ goals

III. **Fraction of inspired oxygen (FIO$_2$) is the decimal value produced by dividing partial pressure of oxygen (PO$_2$) by total pressure of the mixture.**

A. FIO_2 is most correctly expressed by a decimal value rather than a percentage

1. FIO_2 of room air is approximately 0.21

2. FIO_2 of 100% oxygen is 1

B. FIO_2 settings on ventilators typically range from 0.35–1, depending on patient requirements

1. FIO_2 that exceeds 0.5 for longer than 24 hr may result in oxygen toxicity

IV. **Inspiratory cycles vary as follows**

A. Volume cycled: pressure limited (volume targeted)

1. A preset tidal volume is delivered unless a set pressure limit is reached, terminating the cycle.

a. Ensures that tidal volume is not determined by compliance but has higher risk of barotrauma

B. Pressure cycled: volume limited (pressure targeted)

1. A preset pressure is delivered unless a volume limit is reached, terminating the cycle

a. Allows more natural tidal volume with less risk of barotrauma

b. Rate may have to be adjusted to compensate for variable tidal volumes

V. **Positive end-expiratory pressure (PEEP) prevents the return of intrapulmonary pressure to equal extrapulmonary pressure at the end of expiration.**

  A. Effect is that of an incomplete expiration: increased functional residual volume (FRV) remains

    1. The result of increased FRV is twofold

      a. A greater number of alveoli opened for gas exchange throughout ventilatory cycle

      b. Additional alveoli opened at peak inspiration because of tidal volume "stacked" on increased functional residual volume

  B. Effect of increased alveolar ventilation is twofold

    1. Increased PaO_2 without increase in FIO_2

    2. Reduced atelectasis

  C. Risks

    1. Barotrauma due to hyperdistention and high intrapulmonary pressures

    2. Impedance of central venous return, resulting in lower cardiac output

      a. Most significant with low central venous pressure or right ventricular diastolic dysfunction

      b. Increased intracranial pressure

  D. Typical PEEP settings range from 5–10 cm H_2O

    1. "Higher" PEEP up to 10–20 cm H_2O may be used with low-compliance conditions such as acute respiratory distress syndrome

VI. **Continuous positive airway pressure (CPAP) is functionally equivalent to PEEP**

  A. CPAP is effectively PEEP without mechanically delivered inspirations (rate = 0)

  B. Patient must have independent inspiratory capability

  C. Has the same risks and benefits as PEEP

VII. **Pressure support reflects an augmentation of flow rate during spontaneous inspiration**

  A. The result is to overcome resistance to flow through ventilator circuit (valves, corrugated tubing, and narrow lumina), thus reducing spontaneous inspiratory effort or work of breathing.

  B. At higher levels of pressure, it can provide full ventilatory support

VIII. **Alarms alert the clinician to unacceptable deviations from various critical ventilator variables**

  A. High-pressure alarms when proximal airway pressures exceed set limits

    1. Secretion accumulation

    2. Patient coughing

    3. Spontaneous dyssynchrony

    4. Decreasing compliance

5. Pneumothorax
6. Airway occlusion

B. Low-pressure alarms when proximal airway pressure does not reflect current ventilator function
   1. Disconnected tubing
   2. ETT cuff leak

C. Low-volume alarms when volume returned to the ventilator is less than the set limit
   1. May result from disconnecting tubing, from ETT cuff leak
   2. May result from decreased patient tidal volumes (shallow breaths)

D. Low FIO_2 alarms if below set FIO_2
   1. Interruption in oxygen supply

E. Apnea alarms if no spontaneous or mechanical breath detected within set time frame
   1. Patient apnea
   2. Mechanical failure

MODES OF MECHANICAL VENTILATION

I. **Controlled mandatory ventilation**
   A. Patient receives only set tidal volume at a set rate
      1. Patient cannot add spontaneous breaths
         a. Sedation and/or NM blockade will be required to reduce anxiety and prevent interference with ventilator function
      2. Minute volume will be equal to set rate x set tidal volume

II. **Assist control ventilation**
   A. Patient will receive set tidal volume at set rate
      1. Patient can add spontaneous breaths but will receive set tidal volume with the initiation of each spontaneous breath
         a. The delivery of ventilator breaths will not be synchronized with spontaneous breaths.
         b. Sedation may be required to prevent hyperventilation (hypocarbia) and ventilator dyssynchrony.
      2. Minute volume will be equal to (set rate + spontaneous rate) x set tidal volume

III. **Intermittent mandatory ventilation (IMV)**
   A. Patient will receive set tidal volume at set rate
      1. Patient can add spontaneous breaths at own tidal volume
         a. The delivery of ventilator breaths may not be synchronized with spontaneous breaths (IMV)
         b. The delivery of ventilator breaths can be synchronized with spontaneous breaths (synchronized IMV)
      2. Minute volume will be equal to (set rate x set tidal volume) + (spontaneous rate x own tidal volume)
      3. Typically used with pressure support ventilation, which augments spontaneous breaths and minute volume

IV.   Pressure control ventilation
  A. The patient will receive a set rate delivered up to a set pressure.
  B. The tidal volume will vary with each breath according to compliance, and minute volume may be adversely affected with poor compliance if the tidal volumes are very low.
  C. May be used with inverse ratio ventilation
     1. Inspiratory time is lengthened, and expiratory time is shortened
     2. Barotrauma risk is reduced
     3. Oxygenation may be improved

SPECIAL ASPECTS OF VENTILATOR MANAGEMENT

I.   Ventilator settings: mode, rate, tidal volume, PEEP, and FiO$_2$ written as: mode/FiO$_2$/tidal volume/rate/PEEP/PS
  A. Example: assist control (AC) / 1 (100%) / 14 / 450 / +5 / +5
II.   Assessment
  A. Complete physical assessment of all organ systems is warranted
  B. Particular attention to respiratory assessment is required
     1. Observe for distress, cyanosis, symmetry, spontaneous/mechanical ratio, location, and placement (centimeter mark at lips) of ETT
     2. Palpate for fremitus, crepitus, and subcutaneous emphysema
     3. Auscultate for the following:
        a. Bilateral and equal distribution of normal breath sounds
        b. Adventitious sounds
        c. Evidence of ETT cuff leak
     4. Percuss for hyperresonance
III.   Airway management
  A. Humidification is essential to avoid extreme drying of respiratory mucosa
     1. A heat-moisture exchanger is an "artificial nose" that traps expired moisture to humidify inspired air.
        a. Placed in ventilator tubing near ETT
     2. Cascade acts as "bubbler" to humidify oxygen before it enters the inspiratory circuit
  B. ETT cuff pressure should be adequate to seal the airway but not exceed the capillary filling pressure of the tracheal mucosa.
     1. Optimal pressure can be approximated with the minimal leak technique.
        a. Use syringe to add or remove air in the cuff until very minimal air leak is auscultated
     2. More precisely, optimal cuff pressure can be obtained with the use of a bulb manometer to adjust pressure to 2–4 mmHg below average capillary filling pressure of 25–28 mmHg
        a. Be aware of conditions in which capillary filling pressures are below average

C. ETT position should not extend the distal tip beyond the level of the carina
1. ETT 22-cm mark even with lips is a good approximation for most adults
2. On chest x-ray, tip of ETT should be 2–4 cm above the carina
3. Breath sounds should be audible bilaterally

IV. **Suctioning**
A. Suction only as necessary
B. Use small catheter with only moderate suction
C. Oxygenate pre-peri-post to maximize oxygen saturation (SaO_2)
D. Minimize or avoid the use of saline lavage to prevent iatrogenic pneumonia
E. Make no more than a three 10-second suction passes before allowing the patient to rest
F. Monitor vitals, pulse oximetry, and SpO_2
G. Perform subglottal suction to reduce risks of aspiration and ventilator-related pneumonia
H. In-line suction systems reduce risks of hypoxemia and ventilator-related pneumonia.

V. **Nutrition**
A. Feed early and adequately
B. Consider placement of a small-bore feeding tube beyond the pylorus to reduce risks of reflux and aspiration pneumonia

VI. **Weaning from mechanical ventilation**
A. The basic requirement is that the initial indication for ventilation has been improved or eliminated
B. Other factors will affect readiness to wean:
1. Time on ventilator
2. Psychological readiness
3. Nutritional status
4. Ability to clear airway (cough)
5. Hemodynamic stability
C. Assessing readiness to wean
1. Conduct a spontaneous breathing trial daily when the following conditions are met:
a. FiO_2 of 0.40 or less and PEEP of 8 or less
b. PEEP and FiO_2 less than or equal the values of previous day
c. Patient has acceptable spontaneous breathing efforts (may decrease vent rate by 50% for 5 minutes to detect effort)
d. Systolic BP of 90 mmHg or more without vasopressor support
e. No NM blocking agents or blockade (acute respiratory distress syndrome network protocol)
2. Additional factors to consider before attempting weaning:
a. Physical ability
i. Respiratory rate less than 30 breaths per minute

        ii. Minute ventilation less than 12 L/minute
- **b.** Mechanical efficiency
  - **i.** Vital capacity 10–15 ml/kg
  - **ii.** Negative inspiratory force greater than 20 cm H_2O
- **c.** Oxygenation and ventilation
  - **i.** PaO_2 greater than 60 on FIO_2 less than 0.50
  - **ii.** $PaCO_2$ less than 50 with pH 7.35–7.45
  - **iii.** PEEP +5 or less with SaO_2 greater than 92%
- **d.** Hemodynamics
  - **i.** Cardiac index greater than 2.3 L/min/m², mean arterial pressure less than 60 mmHg, heart rate less than 120 beats per minute and more than 60 beats per minute, and pulmonary capillary wedge pressure less than 18 mmHg
- **e.** Secretions
  - **i.** Not copious, easily coughed to tip of ETT for suction

D. Techniques
- **1.** Spontaneous breathing trial for 30–120 minutes
  - **a.** If trial is successful, patient usually will tolerate extubation
  - **b.** If trial is not tolerated, weaning should be delayed until the next day
  - **c.** Trials should take place daily until patient is ready to be extubated, or a different method is determined to be more effective.
- **2.** Alternate periods on ventilator and CPAP to condition respiratory muscles
- **3.** Use pressure support to minimize ventilator-induced work of breathing

E. Extubation

F. Criteria for termination of wean
- **1.** Opposite of readiness to wean
- **2.** Do early in day
- **3.** Patient should be rested, aware, and cooperative
- **4.** Have suction, O_2 device, and reintubation equipment close at hand
- **5.** Elevate head of bed (HOB)
- **6.** Suction well
- **7.** Extubate
- **8.** Monitor closely

BIBLIOGRAPHY

Bagga, S., Paluzzi, D. E., Chen, C. Y., Riggio, J. M., Nagaraja, M., Marik, P. E., & Baram, M. (2014). Improved compliance with lower tidal volumes for initial ventilation setting—using a Computerized Clinical Decision Support System. *Respiratory Care, 59*(8), 1172–1177. doi:10.4187/respcare.02223

Beaudin, A. E., Walsh, M. L., & White, M. D. (2012). Central chemoreflex ventilatory responses in humans following passive heat acclimation. *Respiratory Physiology & Neurobiology, 180*(1), 97–104. doi:10.1016/j. resp.2011.10.014

Burkhart, C. S., Dell-Kuster, S., Gamberini, M., Moeckli, A., Grapow, M., Filipovic, M., . . . Steiner, L. A. (2010). Modifiable and non-modifiable risk factors for postoperative delirium after cardiac bypass surgery with cardiopulmonary bypass. *Journal of Cardiothoracic and Vascular Anesthesia, 24*(4), 555–559. doi:10.1053/j.jvca.2010.01.003

Cairo, J. M. (2012). *Pilbeam's Mechanical Ventilation: Physiological and clinical applications* (5th ed.). St Louis, MO: Elsevier Mosby.

Carpene, N., Vagheggini, G., Panait, E., Gabbrielli, L., & Ambrosino, N. (2010). A proposal of a new model of long-term weaning: Respiratory intensive care unit and weaning center. *Respiratory Medicine, 104*(10), 1505–1511. doi:10.1016/j. rmed.2010.05.012

Carter, A., Fletcher, S. J., & Tuffin, R. (2013). The effect of inner tube placement on resistance and work of breathing through tracheostomy tubes: A bench test. *Anesthesia, 68*(3), 276–282. doi:10.1111/anae.12094

Chui, K. K., & Lusardi, M. M. (2012). Aging and activity tolerance: Implications for orthotic and prosthetic rehabilitation. In M. M. Lusardi, M. Jorge, & C. C. Nielsen (Eds.), *Orthotics and prosthetics in rehabilitation* (3rd ed., pp. 14–37). Philadelphia, PA: Elsevier Saunders.

Finucane, B. T., Tsui, B. C. H., & Santora, A. H. (2010). *Principles of airway management* (4th ed.). New York, NY: Springer.

Güldner, A., Carvalho, N. C., Pelosi, P., & Gama de Abreu, M. (2012). Biphasic PAP/airway pressure release ventilation in ALI. In M. Ferrer and P. Pelosi (Eds.), *European Respiratory Monograph 55: New developments in mechanical ventilation* (pp. 81–96). Sheffield, UK: European Respiratory Society.

Haas, C. F., & Loik, P. S. (2012). Ventilator discontinuation protocols. *Respiratory Care, 57*(10), 1649–1662. doi:10.4187/respcare.01895

Hasan, A. (2010). *Understanding mechanical ventilation: A practical handbook.* London, UK: Springer-Verlag.

Hess, D. R. (2011). Patient-ventilator interaction during noninvasive ventilation. *Respiratory Care, 56*(2), 153–167. doi:10.4187/respcare.01049

Hraiech, S., Brégeon, F., Brunel, J.-M., Rolain, J.-M., Lepidi, H., Andrieu, V., ... Roch, A. (2012). Antibacterial efficacy of inhaled squalamine in a rat model of chronic *Pseudomonas aeruginosa* pneumonia. *Journal of Antimicrobial Chemotherapy, 67*(10), 2452–2458. doi:10.1093/jac/dks230

Kahn, A., Gnanapandithan, K., & Agarwal, R. (2011). Weaning from mechanical ventilation. In P. S. Shankar, S. Raoof, & D. Gupta (Eds.), *Textbook of pulmonary and critical care medicine, Vols. 1 and 2* (pp. 1974–1982). New Delhi: Jaypee Brothers Medical Publishers Ltd.

Krüger, W., & Ludman, A. J. (2014). *Core knowledge of critical care medicine.* New York, NY: Springer.

Marchese, S., Corrado, A., Scala, R., Corrao, S., & Ambrosino, N. (2010). Tracheostomy in patients with long-term mechanical ventilation: A survey. *Respiratory Medicine, 104*(5), 749–753. doi:10.1016/j.rmed.2010.01.003

Mittal, M. K., & Wijdicks, E. F. M. (2013). Muscular paralysis: Myasthenia gravis and Guillain-Barré syndrome. In J. E. Parrillo and R. P. Dellinger (Eds.), *Critical care medicine: Principles of diagnosis and management in the adult* (4th ed., pp. 1121–1129). Philadelphia, PA: Elsevier Saunders.

Papaioannou, V., Dragoumanis, C., & Pneumatikos, I. (2010). Biosignal analysis techniques for weaning outcome assessment. *Journal of Critical Care, 25*(1), 39–46. doi:10.1016/j.jcrc.2009.04.006

Patel, V. P., & Shapiro, J. M. (2012). Mechanical ventilation in the cardiac care unit. In E. Herzog (Ed.), *The cardiac care unit survival guide* (pp. 279–293). Philadelphia, PA: Wolters Kluwer Health/Lippincott, Williams, & Wilkins.

Petrucci, N., & De Feo, C. (2013). Lung protective ventilation strategy for the acute respiratory distress syndrome. *Cochrane Database of Systematic Reviews, 2*, CD003844. doi:10.1002/14651858.CD003844.pub4

Porteus, C., Hedrick, M. S., Hicks, J. W., Wang, T., & Milsom, W. K. (2011). Time domains of the hypoxic ventilatory response in ectothermic vertebrates. *Journal of Comparative Physiology B, 181*(3), 311–333. doi:10.1007/s00360–011–0554–6

Sessler, C. N., & Murevich, K. M. (2013). Use of sedatives, analgesics, and neuromuscular blockers. In J. E. Parrillo & R. P. Dellinger (Eds.), *Critical care medicine: Principles of diagnosis and management in the adult* (4th ed., pp. 255–271). Philadelphia, PA: Elsevier Saunders.

Skaar, D. J., & Weinert, C. G. (2011). Sedatives and hypnotics. In J.-L. Vincent, E. Abraham, F. A. Moore, P. M. Kochanek, & M. P. Fink (Eds.), *Textbook of critical care* (6th ed., pp. 1366–1373). Philadelphia, PA: Elsevier Saunders.

Stevens, J. P., & Howell, M. D. (2012). Preventing harm and improving quality in the intensive care unit. *Hospital Medicine Clinics, 1*(1), e12-e35. doi:10.1016/j.ehmc.2011.11.008

Von Dossow-Hanfstingl, V., Deja, M., Zwissler, B., & Spies, C. (2011). Postoperative management: Extracorporeal ventilatory therapy. In P. Slinger, R. S. Blank, J. Campos, E. Cohen, & K. McRae (Eds.), *Principles and practice of anesthesia for thoracic surgery* (pp. 635–648). New York, NY: Springer.

Widjicks, E. F. M. (2010). *The practice of emergency and critical care neurology.* New York, NY: Oxford University Press.

Management of Patients with Gastrointestinal Disorders

CHAPTER 36

Peptic Ulcer Disease

ALICIA HUCKSTADT · CHARLENE M. MYERS

PEPTIC ULCER DISEASE

I. **Definition**
    A. A gastrointestinal (GI) ulcer is a loss of enteric surface epithelium that extends deep enough to penetrate the muscularis mucosae, and is usually over 5 mm in diameter.
    B. Peptic ulcer disease (PUD) refers to a chronic disorder in which the patient has a lifelong underlying tendency to develop mucosal ulcers at sites that are exposed to peptic juice (i.e., acid and pepsin).
        1. The most common locations are the duodenum and the stomach.
        2. Ulcers may also occur in the esophagus, jejunum, and ileum and at the gastroenteric anastomoses.

II. **Etiology**
    A. PUD is a common disorder with approximately 500,000 new cases diagnosed each year in the United States and 4 million causes of ulcer recurrence.
    B. *Helicobacter pylori* is present in more than 75%–90% of duodenal ulcers; it occurs at a lower rate with gastric ulcers but is found in most gastric ulcers in which nonsteroidal anti-inflammatory drugs (NSAIDs) cannot be implicated.
    C. An imbalance exists between mucosal defense mechanisms (protective factors) and mucosal damaging mechanisms (aggressive factors).
        1. Protective factors
            a. Mucosal barrier (bicarbonate and gastric mucus)
            b. Sufficient blood supply to gastric mucosa and submucosa
            c. Competent sphincters (pyloric and lower esophageal sphincter [LES]), which prevent bile salt reflux into the stomach and the esophagus

    d. Certain medications
        i. H2 blockers
        ii. Antacids
        iii. Sucralfate (Carafate)
        iv. Colloidal bismuth suspension
        v. Anticholinergics
        vi. Misoprostol (Cytotec)
        vii. Omeprazole (Prilosec)

  2. Aggressive factors
    a. *H. pylori* infection
    b. Gastric acid
    c. Pepsin
    d. Bile acids
    e. Decreased blood flow to gastric mucosa
    f. Incompetent sphincters
    g. Various medications
        i. Aspirin
        ii. NSAIDs
        iii. Glucocorticoids
        iv. Cigarette smoking
        v. Gastrinoma
        vi. Stress (especially posttraumatic)
        vii. Alcohol
        viii. Impaired proximal duodenal bicarbonate secretion

III.   **Risk factors**
  A. Highly associated
    1. Smoking more than one half pack of cigarettes per day
    2. Drugs (NSAIDs)
    3. Genetics
    4. Acid hypersecretory states such as the Zollinger-Ellison syndrome (condition caused by non-insulin-secreting tumors of the pancreas, which secrete excess amounts of gastrin)
    5. Cytomegalovirus
    6. Crohn's disease
    7. Lymphoma
  B. Possibly associated with:
    1. Alcohol
    2. Corticosteroids
    3. Stress
    4. Decreased prostaglandin levels associated with aging
  C. Low association or no association with:
    1. Spices
    2. Alcohol
    3. Caffeine
    4. Acetaminophen

IV. **Types of peptic ulcers**
   A. Duodenal ulcers
      1. Ulcers occur five times more in the duodenum
      2. In all, 90%–95% occur in the first portion of the duodenum.
      3. Duodenal ulcers are four times more common than gastric ulcers.
      4. Duodenal ulcers have 10% lifetime prevalence for men and 5% for women.
      5. New cases have declined over the last 30 years
      6. The most common age range is 30–55 years
   B. Gastric ulcers
      1. They are most commonly seen in the lesser curvature of the stomach near the incisura angularis.
      2. New cases are increasingly likely because of widespread NSAIDs and aspirin use
      3. Gastric ulcers are three to four times more prevalent than duodenal ulcers in NSAID users.
      4. The peak age of incidence is 55–70 years (rare before age 40)

V. **Subjective/physical exam findings**
   A. Duodenal ulcers
      1. Epigastric pain ("gnawing," "aching," and "hunger-like") occurs 1–3 hr after eating. The pain is rhythmic and periodic.
      2. Nocturnal pain that awakens a patient from sleep
      3. Usually relieved by antacid or food ingestion
      4. Heartburn (suggests reflux disease)
      5. Epigastric tenderness: usually midline or right of midline
   B. Gastric ulcers
      1. Epigastric pain similar to that associated with duodenal ulcers and also rhythmic and periodic
      2. Pain is not usually relieved by food
      3. Food may precipitate symptoms
      4. Nausea and anorexia
   C. Often unremarkable
   D. The most common exam finding is epigastric tenderness to palpation.
      1. At or to the left of the midline with gastric ulcer
      2. Located 1 inch or farther to the right of midline with duodenal ulcer
   E. Signs and symptoms of shock from acute or chronic blood loss
   F. Nausea and vomiting if the pyloric channel is obstructed
   G. Boardlike abdomen and rebound tenderness in the event of perforation
   H. Hematemesis or melena if the ulcer is bleeding

VI. **Laboratory/diagnostics**
   A. Laboratory findings do not play a major role in diagnosing PUD but may assist the clinician in defining an underlying disorder or complication
   B. Laboratory studies are typically normal in uncomplicated disease

C. For detection of *H. pylori*, the following tests are performed:
  1. Histopathology (endoscopic biopsy)—gold standard
  2. Urea breath test
    a. Positive test implies active infection
    b. More expensive than serum and fecal tests
    c. Proton pump inhibitors (PPIs) may cause false-negative results and should be withheld for at least 7–14 days before testing is done.
  3. Serum *H. pylori* antibody test
    a. Positive test does not necessarily imply an active infection; it may reflect previous infection
    b. Lower sensitivity (85%) and specificity (79%) than fecal antigen or urea breath (both have 95% sensitivity and specificity)
  4. Fecal antigen for *H. pylori*
    a. Detects active infection by measuring fecal excretion of *H. pylori* antigens
    b. Good test to use to assess whether treatment has been successful
    c. PPIs may cause false-negative results and should be withheld for at least 7–14 days before testing is done
D. Complete blood count may indicate anemia due to acute or possibly chronic blood loss
E. Leukocytosis suggests ulcer penetration or perforation
F. Elevated serum amylase level with severe epigastric pain suggests possible ulcer penetration into the pancreas
G. Fasting serum gastrin levels to identify the Zollinger-Ellison syndrome
H. Upper GI barium studies
  1. For uncomplicated dyspepsia
  2. Those diagnosed with gastric ulcers should undergo endoscopy after 8–12 weeks of treatment to distinguish benign from malignant ulcers.
I. Endoscopy
  1. Procedure of choice for diagnosis of duodenal and gastric ulcers
  2. Identifies superficial and very small ulcers
  3. Biopsy may be performed
  4. Electrocautery of any bleeding ulcers can be carried out
  5. Gastric pH can be measured in suspected gastrinoma
  6. Esophagitis, gastritis, or duodenitis can be diagnosed
  7. *H. pylori* can be detected
  8. Higher cost than barium studies
VII. **Complications of PUD**
  A. GI bleeding (20% of cases)
    1. Clinical manifestations
      a. Hematemesis

        b. Melena

        c. Hematochezia

        d. "Coffee ground" emesis

2. Physical examination
   - **a.** Pallor
   - **b.** Tachycardia
   - **c.** Hypotension
   - **d.** Diaphoresis

3. Laboratory findings
   - **a.** Decreased hematocrit due to bleeding or hemodilution from IV fluids
   - **b.** Blood urea nitrogen may rise owing to absorption of blood nitrogen from the small intestine and as a result of prerenal azotemia.

4. Diagnostics: endoscopy after the patient has stabilized

5. Management
   - **a.** In approximately 80% of cases, bleeding stops spontaneously within a few hours after admission to the hospital.
   - **b.** IV hydration with normal saline
   - **c.** Blood transfusion as required
   - **d.** Continuous IV infusion of H_2 blockers at a dose adequate to maintain gastric pH greater than 4
   - **e.** Vasopressin (Pitressin) and IV octreotide (Sandostatin) should not be used for bleeding ulcers
   - **f.** Surgery if bleeding persists

B. Perforation (5%–10% of cases)

1. Subjective data
   - **a.** Severe abdominal pain
   - **b.** Epigastric pain that radiates to back or right upper quadrant

2. Physical examination
   - **a.** Ill appearance
   - **b.** Boardlike abdomen
   - **c.** Severe epigastric tenderness
   - **d.** Absent bowel sounds
   - **e.** Knee-to-chest position
   - **f.** Patient may have symptoms of hypovolemia, fever

3. Laboratory findings
   - **a.** Leukocytosis is almost always present
   - **b.** Amylase levels may be mildly elevated

4. Diagnostics
   - **a.** Abdominal x-rays may reveal free air in the peritoneal cavity
   - **b.** Upper GI radiography with water-soluble contrast may be useful
   - **c.** Barium studies are contraindicated

5. Therapy

      a. Surgery

      b. Patients who are considered poor candidates for surgery or who present more than 24 hr after perforation and are stable, may be followed closely while on IV fluids, nasogastric suction, and broad-spectrum antibiotics

      c. If their condition deteriorates, they should be taken to surgery

C. Gastric outlet obstruction (2% of cases)

    1. Caused by edema or narrowing of the pylorus or duodenal bulb

    2. Subjective findings:

      a. Early satiety

      b. Nausea

      c. Vomiting of undigested food

      d. Epigastric pain unrelieved by food or antacids

      e. Weight loss

    3. Physical examination findings:

      a. "Succussion splash" may be audible on physical examination and is caused by large amounts of air and fluid in the stomach

      b. Nasogastric aspiration may return a large amount (more than 200 ml) of foul-smelling fluid

    4. Diagnostics

      a. Upper GI endoscopy should be performed after 24–72 hr to determine the source of obstruction

      b. At 72 hr, all patients should be given the saline load test, accomplished by instilling 750 ml of normal saline into the stomach and checking the residual in 30 minutes.

      c. Residual volume greater than 400 ml is considered positive

      d. Patient should remain on nasogastric suction for 5–7 additional days

    5. Laboratory: metabolic alkalosis and hypokalemia may be present

    6. Therapy:

      a. Normal saline IV infusion with potassium chloride, if patient has an electrolyte imbalance due to vomiting and poor digestion (i.e., 1 liter normal saline with 40 mEq potassium chloride per liter at 100 ml/hour, titrated up or down according to the patient's condition)

        i. For example, someone who is dehydrated with an increased heart rate, decreased urinary output, and decreased central venous pressure/pulmonary capillary wedge pressure may require more fluids.

        ii. By comparison, those with a history of heart failure or who have signs and symptoms of cardiac overload (e.g., crackles, jugular venous distention, or edema) may require less fluid.

      b. IV H_2 blockers

        i. Ranitidine (Zantac), 50 mg every 6–8 hr up to 150 mg/day
        ii. Famotidine (Pepcid), 20 mg at bedtime or BID
        iii. Cimetidine (Tagamet), 400 mg at bedtime or BID
        iv. Nizatidine (Axid), 300 mg at bedtime
    c. Nasogastric decompression
    d. Total parenteral nutrition for the severely malnourished
  7. Surgery: traditional
  8. Upper GI endoscopy with dilatation of the obstruction has proven successful

VIII. Medical therapy for PUD

  A. Acid-antisecretory agents
    1. Acid-antisecretory agents (H_2-receptor antagonists): Although these drugs are effective, proton pump inhibitors (PPIs) are now preferred for those with known PUD because of their ease of use and superior efficacy.
      a. Decrease gastric acid secretion by blocking histamine H_2 receptors on parietal cells
      b. Effectively inhibit nocturnal acid output but not as effective at inhibiting meal-stimulated acid secretion
      c. Agents:
        i. Ranitidine (Zantac)
        ii. Famotidine (Pepcid)
        iii. Nizatidine (Axid)
        iv. Cimetidine (Tagamet): rarely used today because it inhibits hepatic cytochrome P-450 metabolism, which raises serum concentrations of theophylline, warfarin, lidocaine, and phenytoin and may cause gynecomastia or impotence, among other interactions
      d. Dosages:
        i. Ranitidine, 150 mg PO BID or 300 mg at bedtime
        ii. Nizatidine, 150 mg PO BID or 300 mg at bedtime
        iii. Famotidine, 20 mg PO BID or 40 mg at bedtime
        iv. Cimetidine, 300 mg PO QID or 800 mg at bedtime
      e. Symptom relief usually occurs within 2 weeks
      f. Healing of duodenal ulcers is usually attained within 6 weeks of initiation of therapy
      g. Gastric ulcer healing is delayed by 2–4 weeks compared with duodenal ulcers, but the duration of therapy of 8 weeks is sufficient.

2. PPIs
   a. Suppress gastric acid secretion by inhibition of the hydrogen/potassium adenosine triphosphate (H+K+-ATPase) enzyme system at the secretory surface of the gastric parietal cell
   b. Indications for treatment of the following:
      i. Duodenal ulcers
      ii. Severe erosive esophagitis
      iii. Poorly responsive gastroesophageal reflux disease
   c. Agents: each of the following PPIs, when given once daily, results in healing of greater than 90% of duodenal ulcers after 4 weeks and 90% of gastric ulcers after 8 weeks
      i. Omeprazole (Prilosec), 20 mg PO daily (duodenal ulcer) or 40 mg PO daily (gastric ulcer)
      ii. Lansoprazole (Prevacid), 15 mg PO daily (duodenal ulcer) or 30 mg PO daily (gastric ulcer)
      iii. Rabeprazole (Aciphex), 20 mg PO daily (duodenal ulcer)
      iv. Pantoprazole (Protonix), 40–80 mg PO daily (duodenal/gastric ulcer)
      v. Esomeprazole (Nexium), 20 mg PO daily (duodenal ulcer) or 20–40 mg PO daily (gastric ulcer)
      vi. Dexlansoprazole (Dexilant), 30 mg PO daily (duodenal ulcer) or 3060 mg PO daily (gastric ulcer)
   d. Should be administered 30 minutes before meals
   e. PPIs are remarkably safe in short-term therapy. Serum gastrin levels may rise by more than 500 pg/ml in 10% of patients given long-term therapy; therefore, serum gastrin levels should be checked after 6 months of therapy, and treatment should be terminated or decreased if levels rise to above 500 pg/ml.
      i. Long-term use may decrease vitamin B12, iron, and calcium absorption, and may cause enteric infections (including *Clostridium difficile*), hip fracture, or pneumonia.
B. Agents that enhance mucosal defenses:
   1. Sucralfate
      a. Forms a protective barrier against acid, bile, and pepsin
      b. May cause constipation
      c. May bind some medications; therefore, doses should be separated by at least 2 hr. Requires dosage adjustment in renal impairment, as it may cause aluminum toxicity.
      d. Associated with decreased incidence of nosocomial pneumonia in some studies
      e. Requires an acidic environment; therefore, antacids, PPIs, and H2 blockers should be avoided

   f. One gram four times a day has the same efficacy as H2 blockers in the treatment of duodenal ulcers (6–8 weeks' duration)

   g. Efficacy against gastric ulcers is less firmly established

   h. Maintenance dose: 1 gram BID

  2. Prostaglandin analog (misoprostol [Cytotec])

   a. Promotes ulcer healing by stimulating mucous and bicarbonate secretion and by modestly inhibiting acid secretion

   b. Used solely as a prophylactic agent in the prevention of NSAID-induced ulcers rather than for treatment of active ulcers

    i. With the advent of PPIs and cyclooxygenase-2-selective NSAIDs, misoprostol is now used less for this indication

   c. High incidence of diarrhea

   d. May stimulate contractions in pregnant patients and may induce abortion

   e. Initial dose: 100 mcg four times a day with food; increased to 200 mcg four times a day if well tolerated

  3. Antacids

   a. No longer used as first-line agents; commonly used, as required, to supplement other antiulcer therapies owing to rapid relief of symptoms

   b. Low-dose aluminum- and magnesium-containing antacids promote ulcer healing by stimulating gastric mucosal defenses, rather than neutralizing gastric acidity.

   c. Dosage: 30 ml 1–3 hr after meals and at bedtime

   d. High dosages are associated with diarrhea, hypermagnesemia, and hypophosphatemia

 C. *H. pylori* eradication therapy

  1. Combination drug therapy is necessary to achieve adequate rates of eradication and to decrease failures due to antibiotic resistance

  2. Combination therapy consists of two antibiotics, plus a PPI with or without bismuth.

  3. Regimens using PPIs include the following:

   a. Omeprazole, 20 mg

   b. Rabeprazole, 20 mg

   c. Lansoprazole, 30 mg

   d. Pantoprazole, 40 mg

   e. Esomeprazole, 40 mg

   f. All PPIs are given BID, except for esomeprazole, which is given once daily

    g. Examples:

        i. Metronidazole + omeprazole + clarithromycin (MOC)

            (a) Metronidazole (Flagyl) (if allergic to penicillin), 500 mg BID with meals

            (b) Omeprazole, 20 mg BID before meals (may use PPI of choice)

            (c) Clarithromycin (Biaxin), 500 mg BID with meals for 7 days

            (d) Instruct patient that Flagyl should not be taken with alcohol or vinegar

        ii. Amoxicillin + omeprazole + clarithromycin (AOC)

            (a) Amoxicillin (Amoxil), 1 gram BID with meals

            (b) Omeprazole, 20 mg BID before meals (may use PPI of choice)

            (c) Clarithromycin (Biaxin), 500 mg BID with meals for 7 days

            (d) Preferred for those whose disease is resistant to metronidazole

        iii. Metronidazole + omeprazole + amoxicillin (MOA)

            (a) Metronidazole 500 mg BID with meals

            (b) Omeprazole, 20 mg BID before meals (may use PPI of choice)

            (c) Amoxicillin, 1 gram BID with meals for 7–14 days

4. Regimens that use bismuth compounds:

    a. Require four times a day dosing and have a greater number of adverse effects than PPI regimens

    b. BMT:

        i. Bismuth subsalicylate, 2 tablets four times a day

        ii. Metronidazole, 250 mg four times a day

        iii. Tetracycline (Tetracyn), 500 mg four times a day

        iv. All pills are taken with meals and at bedtime

    c. BMT + Omeprazole (above regimen with the following):

        i. Omeprazole, 20 mg BID before meals for 7 days

5. A 5-day treatment regimen with three antibiotics (amoxicillin, 1 gram BID; clarithromycin, 250 mg BID; and metronidazole, 400 mg BID), plus either lansoprazole, 30 mg BID; or ranitidine, 300 mg BID is an effective, cost-saving option for patients older than 55 years who have no history of PUD. This regimen may be cost-effective; however, efficacy needs to be further evaluated.

6. Antiulcer therapy is recommended for 3–7 weeks after the treatment regimens described previously to ensure symptom relief and ulcer healing.

    a. Duodenal ulcers: omeprazole, 40 mg daily, or lansoprazole, 30 mg daily, should be continued for 7 additional weeks.

    b. H2 blockers or sucralfate can be given for 6–8 weeks

    c. Testing for confirmation of eradication; typically recommended for:

      i. Any patient with an *H. pylori* associated ulcer

      ii. Patients with persistent dyspeptic symptoms, despite test-and-treat strategy

      iii. Patients with *H. pylori* associated MALT lymphoma

      iv. Patients who have undergone resection of early gastric cancer

D. Surgery for refractory ulcers is rarely performed today. If needed, methods include selective vagotomy for duodenal ulcer or ulcer removal with antrectomy, or hemigastrectomy without vagotomy for gastric ulcers.

IX. **Suggested follow-up**

A. Duodenal ulcer: no further evaluation is necessary if the patient is symptom-free after 8 weeks of therapy

B. Gastric ulcer: repeat endoscopy should be performed 4–6 weeks after therapy is completed

    1. Completely healed ulcers require no follow-up

    2. Partially healed ulcers

      a. If greater than 50% healing occurs and findings are negative for carcinoma, 6 weeks of additional therapy is required, followed by reevaluation.

      b. If healing is greater than 59% but findings are positive for carcinoma, surgical intervention is required.

      c. Less than 50% healing requires surgery

GASTROESOPHAGEAL REFLUX DISEASE (GERD)

I. **Definition**

A. Chronic condition in which gastric contents enter into and remain within the lower esophagus because of impaired esophageal function

B. GERD is a symptomatic clinical condition or histologic alteration that results from episodes of gastroesophageal reflux that may produce inflammation of the esophagus (reflux esophagitis).

II. **Etiology**

A. Anatomic factors

    1. Hypotensive LES pressures

    2. Hiatal hernia

      a. Decreased esophageal clearance of gastric contents: severity depends on length of contact time between the gastric contents and the esophagus

      b. Composition and volume of refluxate: the combination of acid, pepsin, and bile produces a potent refluxate that may cause damage to the esophagus; acidic gastric fluid (pH less than 4.0) is extremely caustic to the mucosa

    c. Delayed gastric emptying (due to gastroparesis or partial gastric outlet obstruction) may contribute to gastroesophageal reflux by producing an increase in gastric volume that may increase the frequency and amount of fluid that is refluxed.

III. **Incidence**

    A. Affects 20% of U.S. adults with at least weekly episodes, 10% have daily symptoms

    B. Contributing factors

        1. Dietary

            a. Caffeinated food and/or drinks

                i. Coffee

                ii. Tea

                iii. Cola

                iv. Chocolate

            b. Esophageal irritants

                i. Citrus fruits

                ii. Vinegar

                iii. Spicy foods

                iv. Tomatoes

            c. Excessive fluids with meals

            d. Large meals

            e. Fatty meals

            f. Meals within 2–3 hr of bedtime

            g. Lower esophageal sphincter relaxants

                i. Onions

                ii. Garlic

                iii. Mint

                iv. Alcoholic beverages

            h. Lying down immediately after eating

        2. Non-dietary

            a. Anxiety

            b. Obesity

            c. Pregnancy

            d. Tight-fitting clothing

            e. Smoking

        3. Pharmacologic agents

            a. α-adrenergic antagonists

            b. Anticholinergics

            c. Antihistamines

            d. Aspirin

            e. Benzodiazepines

            f. Calcium channel blockers

            g. β-adrenergic agonists

            h. Cholecystokinin

            i. Levodopa

      j. Nitrates

      k. NSAIDs

      l. Opioids

      m. Progestins

      n. Prostaglandins

      o. Secretin

      p. Somatostatin

      q. Theophylline

      r. Tricyclic antidepressants

      s. Transdermal nicotine

IV.   **Signs/symptoms**

    A. Hallmark symptom: heartburn (pyrosis)

      1. Described as substernal sensation of warmth or burning that may radiate to the neck, throat, and/or back

      2. Generally associated with large meals; occurs 30–60 minutes after eating

      3. Often aggravated by the supine position and bending over

    B. Regurgitation

    C. Water brash (hypersalivation)

    D. Dysphagia (difficulty swallowing)

    E. Odynophagia (pain on swallowing)

    F. Hemorrhage

    G. Belching

    H. Early satiety

    I. Atypical symptoms

      1. Pulmonary symptoms

        a. Recurrent pneumonia

        b. Bronchospasm

      2. Chest pain

      3. Cough

      4. Hoarseness

      5. Hiccups

      6. Sore throat

      7. Nighttime choking

      8. Halitosis

V.   **Laboratory/diagnostics**

    A. Clinical history, including presenting symptoms and associated risk factors, is the most useful tool in the diagnosis of GERD.

    B. Barium swallow is the simplest, least expensive test but is also the least sensitive. Useful as a screening tool to accomplish the following:

      1. To rule out the following complications:

        a. Inflammation

        b. Ulcers

        c. Strictures

      2. To evaluate the following:

    a. Dysphagia
    b. Odynophagia
    c. Significant weight loss
    d. Occult blood loss

C. Endoscopy is an excellent study for the diagnosis and evaluation of reflux esophagitis and other complications of GERD (strictures and Barrett esophagus). During endoscopy:

    1. Biopsy specimens can be obtained
    2. Strictures can be dilated

D. The Bernstein test is an intraesophageal acid perfusion study that can be used to confirm that the patient's symptoms are acid related.

    1. The test requires an alternating infusion of 0.1 N hydrochloric acid and normal saline into the esophagus.
    2. With reflux esophagitis, symptoms of heartburn occur with infusion of acid but not with infusion of saline.

E. The most specific and sensitive diagnostic test used to detect the presence of abnormal acid reflux is 24-hour ambulatory pH monitoring.

    1. This test remains the gold standard for many practitioners.
    2. It is performed by passing a small electrode pH probe intranasally and placing it approximately 5 cm above the LES.
    3. The frequency and severity of reflux can be determined with this study.

F. Esophageal manometry measures esophageal pressure

    1. Identifies abnormalities of the LES
    2. Identifies esophageal muscle contraction abnormalities

VI. **Management**

A. Phase 1 treatment modalities

    1. Elevate head of the bed 4–6 inches (increases esophageal clearance)
    2. Avoid vigorous exercise 2–3 hr before bedtime
    3. Avoid large, high-fat meals and eating 2–3 hr before bedtime (decreases gastric volume)
    4. Avoid foods that may decrease LES pressure
        a. Fats
        b. Chocolate
        c. Alcohol
        d. Peppermint
        e. Spearmint
    5. Avoid foods that have an irritant effect directly on the esophageal mucosa
        a. Spicy foods
        b. Citrus juice
        c. Tomato juice
        d. Coffee

6. Add protein-rich meals to the diet (to augment LES pressure)
7. Reduce weight (to reduce symptoms)
8. Eliminate smoking, if applicable (to decrease spontaneous esophageal sphincter relaxation)
9. Avoid alcohol (to increase amplitude of the LES and peristaltic waves and the frequency of contractions)
10. Avoid tight-fitting clothes
11. Eliminate exacerbating medications (see Contributing Factors of GERD, above)
12. Use antacids and alginic acid PRN
    a. After meals and at bedtime, 80–100 mEq of neutralizing activity (usually 30 ml/8–10 tablets)
        i. Chooz
        ii. Gaviscon
        iii. Gelusil
        iv. Gelusil II
        v. Maalox Plus
        vi. Maalox TC
        vii. Mylanta
        viii. Mylanta II
        ix. Riopan
        x. Tums
    b. Liquid and tablet form are preferred.
13. Try over-the-counter H_2 blockers
    a. Famotidine, 10 mg up to BID
    b. Ranitidine, 50–100 mg up to BID
    c. Cimetidine, 200 mg up to BID

B. Phase 2 treatment modalities
    1. Continue the nonpharmacologic therapies. Weight loss is recommended for GERD patients who are overweight or have had recent weight gain. Head of bed elevation and avoidance of meals 2–3 hrs before bedtime recommended for patients with nocturnal GERD.

C. Phase 3 treatment modalities
    1. Inadequate response after 2–4 weeks of phase 2 management necessitates progression to phase 3
    2. Increase the dose of the initial drug
    3. The initial course of therapy is usually 8–12 weeks. Long-term therapy may be necessary to maintain remission in some patients who relapse.
        a. Omeprazole (Prilosec), 20 mg PO daily
        b. Lansoprazole (Prevacid), 15–30 mg PO daily
        c. Rabeprazole (Aciphex), 20 mg PO daily
        d. Pantoprazole (Protonix), 40 mg PO daily
        e. Esomeprazole (Nexium), 20 mg PO daily

   f. Dexlansoprazole (Dexilant), 30 mg PO daily
      i. PPI therapy should be initiated at once a day dosing
      ii. For patients with partial response to once daily therapy, BID dosing should be considered.
      iii. Non-responders to PPI should be referred for evaluation.
 D. Step-up versus step-down theory in management
   1. Step up: begins with lifestyle modifications and use of over-the-counter medications. Medication may be stepped up to other drugs if symptoms are not resolved.
   2. Step down: begins with a PPI, the most effective treatment, and then is reduced to a lower dosage or a less effective drug (this does not work in patients with severe esophagitis)
 E. Phase 4 treatment modalities
   1. Surgical intervention
      a. Reserved for those in whom medical management has failed or complications have developed
      b. Indications include the following:
         i. Reflux-related pulmonary disease
         ii. Persistent ulcerative esophagitis
         iii. Recurrent esophageal strictures
         iv. Large hiatal hernia
      c. The Nissen fundoplication procedure has a cure rate of approximately 90%.
      d. Stretta procedure
         i. Involves application of radiofrequency energy into the LES in an outpatient setting
         ii. Indicated by a prolonged history of GERD with stable or worsening symptoms after use of PPIs

BIBLIOGRAPHY

Bredenoord, A. J., Pandolfino, J. E., & Smout, P. M. (2013). Gastro-esophageal reflux disease. *Lancet, 381*, 1933–1942.

DiMarino, M. C. (2014). Drug treatment of gastric acidity. *Merck Manuals.* Retrieved from http://www.merckmanuals.com/professional/gastrointestinal_ disorders/gastritis_and_peptic_ulcer_disease/drug_treatment_of_gastric_ acidity.html

Dunphy, L. M., Winland-Brown, J. E., Porter, B. O., & Thomas, D. J. (2011). Abdominal problems. *Primary care: The art and science of advanced practice care nursing* (3rd ed.). Philadelphia, PA: FA Davis.

Laine, L., & Jensen, D. M. (2012). Management of patients with ulcer bleeding. *American Journal of Gastroenterology, 107*, 345–360. doi:10.1038/ ajg.2011.480

Lanza, F. L., Chan, F. K., Quigley, E. M., & Practice Parameters Committee of the American College of Gastroenterology. (2009). Guidelines for prevention of NSAID-related ulcer complications. *American Journal of Gastroenterology, 104*, 728–738. doi:10.1038/ajg.2009.115

McQuaid, K. R. (2013). Gastrointestinal disorders. In M. A. Papadakis & S. J. McPhee (Eds.), *Current medical diagnosis & treatment*. New York, NY: McGraw Hill.

National Institutes of Health, National Institute of Diabetes and Digestive and Kidney Diseases, National Digestive Diseases Informative Clearinghouse. *What I need to know about peptic ulcers*. Retrieved on May 8, 2014, from http://digestive.niddk.nih.gov/ ddiseases/pubs/pepticulers_ez/

Tang, R. S, & Chan, F. K. (2012). Therapeutic management of recurrent peptic ulcer disease. *Drugs, 72*(12), 1605–1616.

Woo, T. M., & Wynne, A. L. (2011). *Pharmacotherapeutics for nurse practitioner prescribers* (3rd ed.). Philadelphia, PA: FA Davis.

CHAPTER 37

Liver Disease

MICHALYN D. PELPHREY • CHARLENE M. MYERS

MAJOR LIVER DISEASES

I. **Hepatitis**
   A. Definition: Hepatitis refers to an inflammation of the liver that can be caused by many drugs and toxic agents, as well as viruses. Hepatitis A, C, D, E, and G are all RNA viruses. Hepatitis B is the only DNA virus. All types of hepatitis produce similar illnesses.
   B. Viral hepatitis
      1. Hepatitis A virus (HAV)
         a. Etiology
            i. Usually, it is spread by fecal–oral route, including contaminated food sources, water, and shellfish; spread by parenteral route is rare
            ii. Spread is enhanced by crowding and by poor sanitation.
            iii. Maximum infectivity occurs 2 weeks before clinical illness.
            iv. Blood and stool are infectious during a 2- to 6-week incubation period.
            v. Mortality rate is low, and fulminant hepatitis A is uncommon
         b. Laboratory/diagnostics
            i. Immunoglobulin IgM anti-HAV: excellent diagnostic test
            ii. First laboratory test ordered with acute illness with increased alanine transaminase (ALT) and aspartate transaminase (AST)
            iii. IgM occurs during the first week of clinical disease
            iv. IgM disappears after 3–6 months

           (a) Positive interpretation: HAV infection within the preceding 6 months

           (b) Negative interpretation: no HAV infection within the preceding 12 months

      v. IgG anti-HAV—presence of IgG

           (a) Indicates previous exposure and noninfectivity

           (b) Confers lifelong immunity

      vi. Negative interpretation: no previous HAV infection

   c. Medical management

      i. Supportive

           (a) Consists of bed rest until jaundice resolves

           (b) No heavy lifting, straining, or activity

      ii. High-calorie diet

           (a) Small, frequent meals with supplements

           (b) High carbohydrates

           (c) Low proteins

           (d) No fatty foods

      iii. Potentially hepatotoxic medications should be avoided

      iv. Restriction of alcohol

      v. Most patients do not require hospitalization

      vi. If patients show signs of encephalopathy or severe coagulopathy, fulminant hepatic failure should be suspected, and hospitalization is necessary.

      vii. Administer antiemetics to decrease nausea and vomiting

   d. Vaccinations

      i. Hepatitis A: In the United States, two vaccines are available: Havrix and VAQTA. Both consist of inactivated HAV.

      ii. Hepatitis A vaccination is recommended for all children aged 1 year, for persons who are at increased risk for infection, for persons who are at increased risk for complications from hepatitis A, and for any person wishing to obtain immunity.

2. Hepatitis B virus (HBV)

   a. Etiology

      i. HBV: blood-borne virus that is present in saliva, semen, and vaginal secretions

      ii. Transmission

           (a) Sex

           (b) Contaminated blood and blood products

           (c) Parenteral drug abuse

           (d) Perinatal

           (e) Body piercing

           (f) Tattooing

           (g) Recreational cocaine

      iii. Approximately 350 million people are chronically infected worldwide

      iv. 15%–40% of carriers of HBV are likely to develop serious hepatic sequela in their lifetime

      v. Coinfection, superinfection, or chronic infection with hepatitis D virus markedly increases mortality and morbidity.

b. Diagnosis

      i. Hepatitis B surface antigen or hepatitis B core antigen (HBsAg or anti-HBc IgM [IgM antibody to hepatitis B core antigen]). HBsAg is often detected in patients with acute HBV infection and is detectable in the serum of patients with active viral replication. Anti-HBc IgM can facilitate differentiation of acute from chronic HBV.

      ii. Total hepatitis B core antibody (anti-HBc) is very useful as a serologic marker of acute hepatitis during a gap when patients have cleared HBsAg, but anti-HBs (antibody to hepatitis B surface antigen) cannot be detected. It also indicates past exposure or infection with hepatitis B.

      iii. Hepatitis B surface antibody (anti-HBs) appears after clearance of HBsAg and/or after successful hepatitis vaccination.

      iv. The appearance of anti-HBs and disappearance of HBsAg indicate the following:

        (a) Recovery from HBV

        (b) Noninfectivity

        (c) Protection from recurrent infection

      v. Hepatitis B e-antigen (HBeAg) found during acute or chronic infection. Presence indicates viral replication with high level of HBV.

      vi. Hepatitis B e-antibody (HBeAb) produced by immune system temporarily during acute HBV infection or during or after a burst in replication. Conversion from e-antigen to e-antibody is a predictor of long-term clearance of HBV in patients being treated with antiviral therapy and indicates lower viral HBV.

c. Medical management

      i. The treatment of chronic hepatitis B is indicated if the risk of liver-related morbidity and mortality in 5–10 years and the likelihood of achieving viral suppression are high.

      ii. Treatment not indicated if the risk of liver-related morbidity or mortality in the next 20 years and the likelihood of achieving viral suppression are low

    iii. Many considerations such as safety and efficacy of treatment, risks of resistance, and cost should be given when picking antiviral therapy agent for chronic HBV treatment. The following are approved agents:

       (a) Peginterferon α: 180 mcg SQ once a week for 48 weeks; has many side effects; efficacy is limited to a small percentage of selected patients

       (b) Lamivudine: 100 mg PO daily; not preferred due to resistance; adjust dose for renal impairment

       (c) Adefovir: 10 mg PO daily; adjust dose for renal impairment; less potent than other agents and linked to increasing rate of antiviral resistance; best used as a second-line drug following the first year of therapy

       (d) Entecavir: 0.5–1 mg PO daily; adjust dose for renal impairment

       (e) Telbivudine: 600 mg PO daily; adjust dose for renal impairment; not preferred due to resistance

       (f) Tenofovir: 300 mg PO daily

       (g) Peginterferon, entecavir, or tenofovir are the first-line drugs recommended for treatment of hepatitis B.

    iv. Can be complicated by cirrhosis or hepatocellular carcinoma leading for need for liver transplant

  d. Vaccination

    i. Hepatitis B vaccine (Hep B) contains HBsAg, the primary antigenic protein in the viral envelope.

    ii. Promotes synthesis of specific antibodies directed against HBV

    iii. Marketed under the trade names Recombivax HB and Engerix B

       (a) These vaccines are made from a viral component rather than from a live virus; therefore, they cannot cause disease.

       (b) All vaccines should be administered in three doses. Once the first dose has been given, the second dose is given 1 month (or longer) later; the third dose is given in 6 months.

    iv. In 2001, the FDA approved a new vaccine directed against both hepatitis A and hepatitis B. This agent, marketed as Twinrix, is approved for use in adults, adolescents, and children between the ages of 1 and 18 years.

      v. Postexposure prophylaxis with immune globulin can be used to prevent HBV infection and subsequent development of liver disease

3. Hepatitis C virus (HCV/non-A non-B virus)

    a. Etiology

      i. HCV: blood-borne virus

      ii. Most common chronic blood-borne infection in the United States

      iii. Approximately 3.2 million people are chronically infected

      iv. Risk of sexual and perinatal transmission is small

      v. Of those infected, 70%–85% develop chronic HCV infection

      vi. Approximately 70%–90% of HCV infection from former or current IVDU

      vii. Majority of people infected may not be aware of infection because most people are asymptomatic

      viii. Six genotypes with several subtypes have been identified. Genotypes 2 and 3 are more sensitive to antiviral treatment. Genotype 1, which is the most common in the United States, is more difficult to treat.

    b. Diagnosis

      i. Anti-HCV (anti-HCV antibody)

        (a) First-line test when diagnosis is suspected

        (b) Highly sensitive—if negative, infection is unlikely

        (c) Specificity depends on the situation—if positive in a person with risk factors and elevated liver enzymes, specificity is high

        (d) Positive anti-HCV—hepatitis C infection is present until it is proven otherwise

      ii. Most recombinant immunoblot assay—positive patients are infectious, and a polymerase chain reaction can be used to confirm HCV infection

        (a) Gold standard for confirmation of infection

        (b) Detects actual virus, not antibodies

        (c) Differentiates prior exposure from current viremia

    c. Medical management

i. In patients with chronic hepatitis C, standard of care therapy has been the use of peginterferon and ribavirin. It is administered for 48 weeks for HCV genotypes 1, 4, 5, and 6 and for 24 weeks for HCV genotypes 2 and 3. Sustained viral response is achieved when HCV polymerase chain reaction is negative at 6 months after the completion of treatment. This is considered a virological cure for HCV. Sustained virological response (SVR) is achieved in 40%–50% of genotype 1 patients. SVR is achieved in 80%–90% of genotype 2 and 3 patients. Depending on the patient's weight, dosing varies as follows:

   (a) 66–80 kg: peginterferon alfa-2b 1.5 mcg/kg/week SQ with ribavirin 400 mg PO BID for 48 weeks for genotype 1 or 24 weeks for genotypes 2 and 3

   (b) 81–105 kg: peginterferon alfa-2b 1.5 mcg/kg/week SQ with ribavirin 600 mg PO BID for 48 weeks for genotype 1 or 24 weeks for genotypes 2 and 3

   (c) Over 105 kg: peginterferon alfa-2b 1.5 mcg/kg/week SQ with ribavirin 600 mg PO in the morning and 800 mg PO in the evening for 48 weeks for genotype 1 or 24 weeks for genotypes 2 and 3

ii. The American Association for the Study of Liver Diseases recommends the addition of protease inhibitors Boceprevir or Telaprevir to markedly improve SVR rates in genotype 1 patients.

   (a) Boceprevir 800 mg PO with food three times a day OR telaprevir 750 mg PO with food (not low-fat) three times per day (every 7–9 hr) in combination with peginterferon alfa and ribavirin

   (b) At this time, boceprevir and telaprevir should not be used to treat patients with genotype 2 or 3 HCV infections.

iii. Newly approved medications are due to be released. These medications have had such promising results during study that it is believed that it will now be possible to cure most people of hepatitis C infection in the very near future.

iv. It is estimated that between 15% and 20% of patients with chronic HCV develop cirrhosis within 20 years of disease onset, which may lead to need for liver transplant

v. HCV cirrhosis patients have 2%–8% annual risk of developing hepatocellular carcinoma

d. Vaccination/screening

          i. Hepatitis C: no vaccination for active or passive immunity available

          ii. New CDC recommendation for an age-based screening strategy consisting of one-time testing for HCV for those at highest risk, including everyone born between 1945 and 1965

4. Hepatitis D virus (delta agent)

    a. An uncommon incomplete RNA virus that causes hepatitis only when accompanied by HBV infection

    b. Combined infection has a worse prognosis than HBV alone, along with an increased incidence of fulminant hepatitis

    c. There is no vaccination or specific treatment for the hepatitis D virus, but it can be prevented with HBV vaccination.

5. Hepatitis E virus (enterically transmitted or epidemic non-A non-B virus)

    a. An acute infection, does not lead to chronic infection, and rare in the United States

    b. Ingestion of fecal matter, even in microscopic amounts; usually associated with contaminated water supply in countries with poor sanitation

    c. Incubation period is 2–9 weeks (the mean is 6 weeks)

    d. Clinical disease is similar to HAV, except it is more severe

    e. Mortality rate is 1%–2% in general population and 10%–20% in pregnant women—significantly higher than HAV

    f. No current approved vaccination

6. Hepatitis G virus (HGV)

    a. Uncertain what role, if any, it plays in etiology of liver disease

    b. A recently identified virus that is transmitted percutaneously and may cause mild acute hepatitis and chronic viremia lasting as long as 9 years

    c. Detected in 50% of intravenous drug abusers and in 20% of hemophiliac patients

    d. Diagnostic tests are not currently available

7. Viral hepatitis risk factors

    a. Health care providers/other occupational risks; positive needlestick

    b. Hemodialysis patients

    c. Recipients of blood and/or blood products

    d. Intravenous drug users

    e. Sexually active men who have sex with men or those with multiple heterosexual partners

    f. Household exposure

    g. Intimate exposure

    h. Persons in underdeveloped countries

    i. Body piercing

      j. Tattooing
- **8.** Viral hepatitis subjective findings (extremely variable)
  - **a.** Prodromal phase
    - **i.** Malaise, myalgia, arthralgia, and easy fatigue
    - **ii.** Upper respiratory symptoms (nasal discharge and pharyngitis)
    - **iii.** Anorexia, nausea, and vomiting are common.
    - **iv.** Diarrhea or constipation may occur.
    - **v.** Aversion to smoking (HBV)
    - **vi.** Skin rashes, arthritis, or serum sickness may be seen early in HBV.
    - **vii.** Fever usually less than 103.1°F (39.5°C) (more common in HAV)
    - **viii.** Mild, constant abdominal pain in the right upper quadrant or epigastrium that is often aggravated by exertion
  - **b.** Icteric phase
    - **i.** Clinical jaundice occurs after 5–10 days but may occur at the same time as the initial symptoms
    - **ii.** Most patients never develop clinical icterus
    - **iii.** Intensification of prodromal symptoms usually occurs with the onset of jaundice; this is generally followed by progressive improvement
    - **iv.** Dark urine/clay-colored stools
    - **v.** Patient may be asymptomatic
- **9.** Viral hepatitis physical findings
  - **a.** Jaundice
  - **b.** Tender hepatomegaly
  - **c.** Splenomegaly
  - **d.** Posterior cervical lymphadenopathy (rare)
  - **e.** Rash (HBV)
  - **f.** Arthritis (rare)
  - **g.** Examination findings may be normal
- **10.** Laboratory/diagnostics
  - **a.** WBC count is normal or may be low
  - **b.** Urinalysis—proteinuria is common; bilirubinuria may occur before jaundice
  - **c.** Greatly increased ALT and AST levels (greater than 500 IU/L; normal, 0–35 IU/L)
  - **d.** Increased bilirubin and alkaline phosphatase levels; may remain elevated after ALT and AST have normalized
  - **e.** Prothrombin time (PT) and glucose level are usually normal; increased PT or decreased glucose level indicates severe liver damage
- **C.** Autoimmune hepatitis (AIH)
  - **1.** Etiology

        a. Generally unresolving inflammation of liver of unknown cause

        b. Working model for pathogenesis postulates environmental triggers, failure of immune tolerance mechanisms and a genetic predisposition together lead to a t cell-mediated immune attack of the liver

        c. Symptoms range from asymptomatic or similar to viral hepatitis symptoms

    2. Laboratory/diagnostics

        a. Based on histologic abnormalities, abnormal levels of serum globulins and presence of one or more autoantibodies

        b. Women are more frequently affected than men

        c. Abnormal serum aminotransferases, especially with lower or normal alkaline phosphatase

        d. Serum globulin or IGG greater than one and a half times normal

        e. Positive ANA, SMA, or LKM 1 antibodies at titers greater than 1:80

        f. In patients with negative conventional autoantibodies in whom AIH is suspected, other serological markers including at least anti-SLA and atypical p-ANCA should be tested.

        g. Diagnosis of AIH should be considered in all patients with acute or chronic hepatitis of undetermined cause

    3. Medical treatment

        a. Prednisone monotherapy

            i. Induction therapy: 50–60 mg PO daily

            ii. Maintenance therapy: 5–20 mg PO daily

        b. Prednisone and azathioprine

            i. Induction therapy:

                (a) Prednisone 30 mg PO daily

                (b) Azathioprine 50 mg PO daily

            ii. Maintenance therapy:

                (a) Prednisone 5–10 mg PO daily

                (b) Azathioprine 50 mg PO daily

        c. Conventional therapy is continued until remission, treatment failure, incomplete response, or drug toxicity.

        d. May lead to liver transplant in both the acute and chronic settings

D. Nonalcoholic steatohepatitis

    1. Etiology

    a. Nonalcoholic fatty liver disease (NAFLD) occurs where there is evidence of hepatic steatosis by either imaging or histology and there are no other causes for secondary hepatic fat such as significant alcohol consumption, medication, or hereditary disorders that could be cause. There is a presence of steatosis with no evidence of hepatocellular injury in the form of ballooning of hepatocytes.

    b. Nonalcoholic steatohepatitis (NASH) is steatosis with inflammation, with hepatocyte injury or ballooning without fibrosis.

    c. Obesity, diabetes, and dyslipidemia are associated risk factors

2. Laboratory/diagnostics

    a. When evaluating those with suspected NAFLD, it is important to exclude competing etiologies for steatosis or other common liver diseases.

    b. Serum aminotransferase levels and imaging such as ultrasound, CT scan, or MRI can be used as initial screening but are not reliable in determining steatohepatitis or fibrosis.

    c. Liver biopsy may need to be performed to determine if hepatic inflammation or fibrosis is present.

    d. A validated scoring system called the "NAFLD fibrosis score" is now being used to predict advanced fibrosis.

        i. A score less than negative 1.455: 90% sensitivity and 60% specificity of excluding advanced fibrosis

        ii. A score greater than 0.676 has a 67% sensitivity and 97% specificity of identifying the presence of advanced fibrosis

3. Treatment

    a. Lifestyle intervention

        i. Weight loss

        ii. Exercises

    b. Medications

        i. Vitamin E, 800 IU/day, has been shown to improve liver histology in nondiabetic adults with biopsy proven NASH.

        ii. There have been some studies that pioglitazone and rosiglitazone have shown improvement in liver histology for NASH patients; however, these have not been established as a recommendation.

    c. Bariatric surgery

        i. Premature to consider as an established option for specific treatment of NASH but is not contraindicated if otherwise eligible for the surgery

    d. May lead to cirrhosis and need for liver transplantation

II. **Primary biliary cirrhosis**
  A. Etiology
    1. Primary biliary cirrhosis (PBC) is often considered a model autoimmune disease because of its hallmark serologic signature or antimitochondrial antibody and specific bile duct pathology.
      a. Antimitochondrial antibody positive in 90%–95% of patients
      b. A unique feature of PBC is the high degree of involvement of the small intrahepatic bile ducts
    2. Thought to be a combination of environmental triggers and genetic predisposition
    3. Cholestatic disease with progressive course, which can extend over many decades
  B. Laboratory/diagnostics
    1. Abnormal liver tests, including alkaline phosphatase, mild elevation of ALT and AST, and present and increased immunoglobulins
    2. In patients without cirrhosis, the degree of elevation of alkaline phosphatase is strongly related to the severity of ductopenia and inflammation.
    3. Hyperbilirubinemia also reflects the severity of ductopenia and biliary necrosis.
    4. Histologic evidence of nonsuppurative destructive cholangitis and destruction of interlobular bile ducts
  C. Treatment
    1. The only approved drug to treat PBC is ursodiol (ursodeoxycholic acid [UDCA]), 13–15 mg/kg/day
    2. May lead to need for liver transplantation
III. **Primary sclerosing cholangitis**
  A. Etiology
    1. Chronic cholestatic liver disease characterized by inflammation and fibrosis of both intrahepatic and extrahepatic bile ducts leading to multifocal bile duct strictures
    2. Likely immune-mediated and progressive disorder usually leading to cirrhosis
  B. Diagnosis
    1. Made with patients that have cholestatic biochemical profile (elevated alkaline phosphatase and AST/ALT) and cholangiography by either magnetic resonance cholangiopancreatography or endoscopic retrograde cholangiopancreatography showing characteristic bile duct changes with multifocal strictures and segmental dilations
    2. Patients often asymptomatic and diagnosis is made incidentally
    3. Episodes of cholangitis are very uncommon at presentation.

4. Approximately 60%–80% of patients with primary sclerosing cholangitis (PSC) also have either Crohn disease or ulcerative colitis as well
5. Endoscopic retrograde cholangiopancreatography is the gold standard for diagnosing PSC, but magnetic resonance cholangiopancreatography can also be used.
6. Patients with PSC are at increased risk for developing cholangiocarcinoma. The estimated ten-year cumulative risk of developing cholangiocarcinoma is approximately 7%–9%.

C. Treatment
1. The endoscopic management of strictures to relieve biliary obstruction is the major treatment for PSC.
2. Patients with symptoms from dominant stricture such as cholangitis, jaundice, pruritus, and worsening liver function are appropriate for endoscopic management.
3. The only long-term effective treatment for PSC is liver transplantation.

IV. **Hereditary hemochromatosis**
A. Etiology
1. Most common genetic disorder in Caucasians; most prevalent in northern European origin, particularly Nordic or Celtic ancestry
2. Genetic predisposition increases the inappropriate absorption of dietary iron that can lead to cirrhosis, hepatocellular carcinoma, diabetes, and heart disease

B. Diagnosis
1. Diagnosis is based on increased iron stores demonstrated by elevated ferritin levels and increased hepatic iron content. Hemochromatosis gene detection can further define the diagnosis. C282y homozygotes account for 80%–85% of typical patients with hereditary hemochromatosis.
2. Phenotypic expression does not always lead to severe iron overload and the accompanied organ damage and clinical manifestations of hemochromatosis. Three stages of progression of hemochromatosis have been identified.
    a. Stage 1—patients with the genetic disorder, with no increase in iron stores
    b. Stage 2—patients with the genetic disorder, with evidence of iron overload, with no evidence of tissue or organ damage
    c. Stage 3—those who have the genetic disorder with iron overload and deposition to the degree that tissue and organ damage occurs

C. Treatment/screening
1. Those with iron overload should undergo therapeutic phlebotomy weekly as tolerated. Goal is target ferritin level of 50–100 µg/L.
2. Vitamin C and iron supplements should be avoided

3. Dietary restrictions are unnecessary

4. Those with cirrhosis should be screened for hepatocellular carcinoma. There is an annual incidence of 3%–4% risk of developing hepatocellular carcinoma with hemochromatosis cirrhosis

5. Family screening is recommended for patients with hereditary hemochromatosis for all first-degree relatives with iron studies, ferritin, and hemochromatosis gene mutation analysis.

V. Alcoholic liver disease

A. Etiology

1. It is the most common cause of cirrhosis and accounts for 40% of deaths from cirrhosis in the United States.

2. It is estimated that more than 7.4% of Americans meet the Diagnostic and Statistical Manual of Mental Disorders, Fourth Edition criteria for the diagnosis of alcohol abuse and or dependence in 1994.

3. The amount of alcohol is the most important risk factor; however, amount consumed and liver disease are not clearly linear

   a. Compared with men, women have been shown to be twice as sensitive to alcohol-mediated hepatotoxicity and may require less alcohol intake to lead to severe liver disease.

   b. Drinking outside meal times has been reported to increase the risk of alcoholic liver disease (ALD).

   c. Binge drinking (drinking five drinks for men and four drinks for women) in one sitting also increases the risk of ALD.

4. Obesity has been associated with the increased risk of ALD.

5. Genetic factors also predispose people to alcoholism and ALD.

B. Diagnosis

1. Diagnosis is based on history of significant alcohol intake, clinical evidence of liver disease, and supporting laboratory abnormalities

2. Denial and underreporting of alcohol intake make it a difficult diagnosis

3. Various questionnaires have been developed—CAGE, MAST, and AUDIT

4. No single laboratory definitely establishes ALD

5. In approximately 70% of patients, the AST/ALT ratio is higher than 2—suggestive of ALD

6. Alcoholic hepatitis has high mortality rate. Maddrey's discriminant function (MDF) is a prognostic score to stratify the severity of illness.

   a. MDF = 4.6 × patients PT − control PT plus total bilirubin

   b. Patients that score greater than or equal to 32 have 1 month mortality as high as 30%–50%

C. Treatment

1. Abstinence is the most important treatment for ALD

2. Alcoholic hepatitis treatment
    a. Assess and treat for nutritional deficiencies
    b. Severe MDF score greater than 32 should be considered for a 4-week course of prednisone 40 mg/day for 28 days
    c. Prednisolone may be preferred over prednisone because prednisone requires a conversion to the active prednisolone in the liver, a process that may be impaired in alcoholic hepatitis.
    d. If steroids are contraindicated, pentoxifylline, 400 mg TID for 4 weeks, can be used in patients with severe alcoholic hepatitis.
3. ALD is the second most common indication for liver transplant for chronic liver disease in the Western World.

VI. Wilson disease

A. Etiology
    1. A familial autosomal recessive disease that, if not treated, may be lethal. It may manifest with neurologic symptoms accompanied by chronic liver disease leading to cirrhosis.
    2. It is caused by the absence of a gene, which is expressed mainly in hepatocytes and functions with the transmembrane transport of copper within hepatocytes, which leads to the decreased excretion of copper into bile. Decreased excretion results in copper accumulation and injury.
    3. Eventually, the copper is released in the bloodstream and deposited in the brain, kidneys, and cornea.
    4. Wilson disease should be considered in any individual between the ages of 3 and 55 years with liver abnormalities of uncertain cause.

B. Diagnosis
    1. Abnormal aminotransferase generally abnormal
    2. Ceruloplasmin that is significantly low, less than 50 mg/L, should be taken as a strong evidence of Wilson disease
    3. A 24-hr urinary copper should be obtained on all patients with suspicion of Wilson disease. Findings greater than 40 μg may indicate Wilson disease.
    4. Liver biopsy for the measurement of hepatic copper content remains the best evidence of Wilson disease. Content greater than 250 μg/gram dry weight is indicative of Wilson disease.
    5. Wilson disease should be suspected in any patient presenting with acute hepatic failure with Coombs-negative intravascular hemolysis, modest elevation in AST and ALT or low alkaline phosphatase, and a ratio of alkaline phosphatase to bilirubin of less than 2.

C. Treatment
    1. Pharmacological therapy available
        a. D-Penicillamine general chelator

        i. Initial therapy: 750–1500 mg PO daily resulting in an initial 24 hr cupriuresis of over 2 mg/day; optimal dose is based on urinary copper excretion and free copper serum

        ii. Maintenance therapy: up to 2000 mg/day; dosing based on urinary copper excretion and free copper in serum

    b. Pyridoxine 25 mg PO daily may be given to prevent pyridoxal phosphate deficiency

    c. Trientine-general chelator 750–1250 mg/day PO in 2–4 divided doses, may be increased to a maximum of 2 grams/day

    d. Zinc, 50 mg PO 3 times a day; blocks intestinal absorption of copper

  2. Patients should avoid intake of food and water high in copper

  3. Liver transplant is the only option for those with decompensated cirrhosis or those who present with acute liver failure (ALF) unresponsive to medical therapy.

  4. Treatment is lifelong, unless liver transplant is performed

  5. All first-degree relatives of patients diagnosed with Wilson disease should be screened.

VII. Fulminant liver failure/acute liver failure (ALF)

  A. Definition

    1. ALF is a rare but catastrophic illness that results from sudden, marked impairment of liver cell function. Acute onset of liver disease occurs with coagulopathy, and with no previous history of liver disease. Hepatic encephalopathy develops within 8 weeks of onset of illness. It is referred to as "fulminant hepatic failure."

  B. Etiology

    1. Viral hepatitis (A, B, C, D, or E)

    2. Hepatitis caused by other viruses (cytomegalovirus; herpes viruses 1, 2, and 6; and Epstein-Barr virus)

    3. Drug-induced injury (e.g., acetaminophen)

    4. Toxins (e.g., Amanita phalloides mushrooms and organic solvents)

    5. Metabolic disorders

    6. Vascular events (e.g., heatstroke)

    7. Miscellaneous disorders (e.g., Wilson disease, AIH, and liver tumor)

    8. Estimated 2,000 cases in United States per year

    9. High morbidity and mortality

  C. Clinical manifestations/diagnosis

    1. Initial signs are vague and include the following:

      a. Weakness

      b. Fatigue

      c. Loss of appetite

      d. Weight loss

      e. Abdominal discomfort

    f. Nausea and vomiting

    g. Change in bowel pattern

  2. Patients with ALF should be hospitalized and monitored frequently in ICU.

  3. Transplant center should be contacted and plans for transfer should be initiated early in the evaluation process. Early transfer is important as the patient's condition may deteriorate very rapidly.

  4. Initial lab evaluation should be extensive to try to determine the etiology

    a. Chemistries, ABG, lactate, toxicology screen, acetaminophen level, viral hepatitis serologies, ceruloplasmin, autoimmune markers, HIV, amylase, lipase, and PT/international normalized ratio (INR)

D. Specific etiology management

  1. Acetaminophen toxicity

    a. If ingestion is within 4 hr, give activated charcoal (1 gm/kg orally)

    b. Begin N-acetylcysteine in any suspected or possible acetaminophen toxicity (140 mg/kg PO or nasogastrically, diluted in 5% solution, followed by 70 mg/kg every 4 hr × 17 doses or intravenous dose of 150 mg/kg in 5% dextrose over 15 min with 50 mg/kg given over 4 hr, followed by 100 mg/kg over 16 hr)

  2. Viral hepatitis

    a. Supportive care for viral hepatitis A and E; no virus-specific treatment is available

    b. Acute hepatitis B should be treated with one of the hepatitis B antiviral agents

  3. Wilson disease

    a. Should obtain ceruloplasmin, urinary copper level, and slit lamp exam for Kayser–Fleischer rings

    b. A high bilirubin-to-alkaline phosphatase ratio greater than 2.0 is a reliable indicator for Wilson disease.

  4. Acute fatty liver of pregnancy/HELLP syndrome

    a. Triad of jaundice, coagulopathy, and low platelets along with features of preeclampsia are indicators of HELLP.

    b. Steatosis on imaging

    c. Can have intrahepatic hemorrhage or hepatic rupture requiring emergent intervention

    d. Prompt delivery of baby critical in good outcome

  5. If etiology remains unclear, liver biopsy may be appropriate, but the risk/benefit ratio has to be weighed due to likely coagulopathy.

E. ICU management

1. Cerebral edema and intracranial hypertension are the most critical complications to monitor. If cerebral edema is identified, measures to decrease ICP must be done.
   a. Hyperventilation
   b. Hypertonic sodium chloride
   c. Mannitol
   d. Barbiturates if other measures fail
2. In cases of grade III or IV encephalopathy
   a. Intubate for airway protection
   b. CT scan of the head to evaluate for cerebral edema
   c. ICP monitoring recommended
3. Hemodynamics and renal failure
   a. Fluid resuscitation with normal saline for hypotension
   b. Dialysis if needed for renal failure
   c. Vasopressor such as norepinephrine for volume refractory hypotension
   d. Goal to keep MAP greater than 75 and CPP 60–80 mmHg
   e. Monitor closely for acidosis and hypoglycemia
F. Clinical predictors for poor prognosis in ALF
   1. King's College criteria—prognostic model for poor prognosis —only an indicator not absolute
      a. Acetaminophen-induced ALF is considered for liver transplant in case of the following:
         i. pH less than 7.3 or lactate greater than 3 after fluid resuscitation
         ii. Presence of grade 3 or 4 encephalopathy
         iii. INR greater than 6.5
         iv. Creatinine greater than 3.4
      b. Nonacetaminophen ALF—consider liver transplant if the following criteria are met:
         i. INR greater than 6.5 and encephalopathy present at all or any three of following:
            (a) Age less than 10 or greater than 40 years
            (b) Jaundice for greater than 7 days before encephalopathy
            (c) Bilirubin greater than 17 mg/dl
            (d) Unfavorable etiology such as Wilson disease, idiosyncratic drug reaction, and seronegative hepatitis
   2. Model for End-stage Liver Disease (MELD)—prognostic model used to determine severity of liver disease by using patient's laboratory values and the following formula:

$$MELD = 3.8 \text{ x } \log_e(\text{serum bilirubin [mg/dl]})$$
$$+ 11.2 \text{ x } \log_e(\text{INR})$$
$$+ 9.6 \text{ x } \log_e (\text{serum creatinine [mg/dl]})$$
$$+ 6.4$$

  a. Primarily used to prioritize patients on waitlist for liver transplantation based on liver disease severity and short-term mortality risk; can potentially be used to predict mortality rate for patients with acute alcoholic hepatitis and variceal hemorrhage

VIII. Chronic liver disease sequela and management
  A. Can lead to multiorgan failure
  B. Reduced liver metabolic processes
  C. Impaired bile formation and flow
  D. Increased incidence of infection
  E. Cardiac
     1. Hyperdynamic circulation
     2. Portal hypertension
     3. Arrhythmias
     4. Edema
     5. Activity intolerance
  F. Dermatologic
     1. Jaundice
     2. Spider angiomas
     3. Pruritus
  G. Fluid and electrolytes
     1. Ascites
     2. Water retention
     3. Decreased vascular volume
     4. Hypokalemia
     5. Hyponatremia (hemodilution)
     6. Hypernatremia
     7. Hypoglycemia
     8. Hypoalbuminemia
  H. Gastrointestinal
     1. Abdominal discomfort
     2. Decreased appetite
     3. Diarrhea
     4. GI bleeding
     5. Varices
     6. Malnutrition
     7. Nausea and vomiting
  I. Hematologic
     1. Anemia
     2. Impaired coagulation
     3. Disseminated intravascular coagulopathy

J.   Immune system
   1. Increased risk for infection, which may lead to sepsis

K. Neurologic
   1. Hepatic encephalopathy

L.   Respiratory
   1. Dyspnea
   2. Hyperventilation
   3. Hypoxemia

M. Renal
   1. Renal failure (hepatorenal syndrome)—patients in end-stage liver disease may develop any of the following:
      a. Azotemia
      b. Oliguria
      c. Hyponatremia
      d. Low urinary sodium levels
      e. Hypotension

N. Laboratory findings/diagnostics
   1. Bilirubin—elevated (normal, 1 mg/dl)
   2. Albumin—decreased (normal, 3.5–5.5 grams/dl)
   3. PT—prolonged; high prognostic value in acute liver injury (normal, 10–12 seconds)
   4. Partial thromboplastin time—prolonged (normal, 25–41 seconds)
   5. Liver enzyme level assessment is not the same as a liver function test; liver enzyme levels assess the presence of dysfunction but do not actually determine how well the liver is working
   6. Liver enzymes can be classified into two major types:
      a. Aminotransaminases
         i. AST (formerly SGOT)—elevated (normal, 0–40 U/L)
         ii. ALT (formerly SGPT)—greater specificity for liver disease
         iii. In most liver diseases, AST increase is less than that of ALT
            (a) AST/ALT ratio, less than 1
            (b) Normal ALT, 0–35 U/L
      b. Phosphatases
         i. Alkaline phosphatase—normal, 30–120 U/L
         ii. Gamma-glutamyltranspeptidase—normal, 0–30 U/L
            (a) These liver enzymes are released during cellular injury and are no longer released when hepatocytes begin to heal.
            (b) If injury is severe enough to cause necrosis, these enzymes are initially very high and then decline because no additional enzymes are available for release.
   7. Ammonia—elevated (normal, 10–80 µg/dl)

O. Management
  1. Hepatic encephalopathy
     a. Administer lactulose (Cephulac), 15–30 ml every 3–4 hr (orally or nasogastrically) until the patient produces three to four loose stools daily
     b. Gut cleansing with enemas might also be used
     c. Limit protein to lean proteins
     d. Rifaximin, 550 mg BID, recommended for those not controlled or tolerating lactulose therapy
  2. Monitor for hypoglycemia.
     a. Intravenous infusion of 10% glucose
     b. Rate depends on blood glucose level
     c. May start at 50–100 ml/hr and is titrated depending on glucose levels
     d. Glucose intravenous push 50% if needed
  3. Coagulopathy
     a. Vitamin K, 10 mg subcutaneously daily for 3 days, if PT is greater than 14 seconds and INR is greater than 2
     b. Fresh frozen plasma
  4. Hyponatremia
     a. Free water restriction
     b. Less than 1000–1500 ml of water per day for those with a serum sodium level lower than 125 mEq/L
     c. Hold diuretics
  5. Hypokalemia: potassium chloride replacement
  6. Variceal bleeding: Refer to Gastrointestinal Bleeding chapter
  7. Ascites
     a. Low-sodium diet—2 grams daily
     b. Fluid restriction—1000–1500 ml daily for those with a serum sodium level less than 125 mEq/L
     c. Diuretic therapy
        i. Spironolactone, 100 mg/day in divided doses to 400 mg maximum
        ii. Furosemide (Lasix), 20–40 mg/day
        iii. Goal is to reduce weight 1 lb/day in those with ascites and 2 lb/day in those with ascites and edema
        iv. Dose may have to be increased for this weight loss to be achieved
     d. For those with tense ascites, paracentesis may be necessary to drain 3–6 L for comfort and to decrease the risk for respiratory complications.
        i. Administer albumin 6–8 grams for each liter removed, to protect intravascular volume

ii. The need for colloid replacement to prevent effective hypovolemia after LVP remains controversial; it is likely unnecessary for paracentesis of 5 L or less.

iii. Dextran may be rarely used as well

8. Intravenous bicarbonate may be necessary for severe acidosis in which there is too much acid in the body fluids. Bicarbonate prevents the pH of blood from becoming too acidic.

9. Monitor BUN/serum creatinine (Cr) for elevation. Dialysis may be necessary

10. Closely monitor respiratory and hemodynamic status. Vasopressors and intubation may be necessary

11. Avoid hepatotoxic substances

12. Cholestyramine for pruritis management
    a. Initial therapy: 4 grams PO once or BID
    b. Maintenance therapy: 8–16 grams PO daily in 2 or more divided doses; max dose should not exceed 24 grams daily

13. Colestipol, 2 grams PO every day or every 12 hr (tablets) OR 5 grams PO every day (granules) in water or juice, may be helpful for those with pruritus as well

14. When symptoms become unmanageable, transplantation should be considered.

BIBLIOGRAPHY

Ahmed, F. (2013). What about us? Recent advances in the treatment of chronic hepatitis C threaten to leave some parts of the world behind. *Journal of Viral Hepatitis, 20*(5), 367–368.

Bacon, B. R., Adams, P. C., Kowdley, K. V., Powell, L. W., & Tavill, A. S. (2011). *Diagnosis and management of hemochromatosis: 2011 practice guideline by the American Association for the Study of Liver Disease.* Retrieved from http://www.aasld.org/practiceguidelines/Documents/Bookmarked%20Practice%20Guidelines/Hemochromatosis%202011.pdf

Bride, G. M. (2013). *Clinical guidelines for advanced practice nursing: an interdisciplinary approach* (2nd ed.). Burlington, MA: Jones & Bartlett Learning.

Centers for Disease Control and Prevention. (2009). *Viral hepatitis A fact sheet.* Retrieved May 15, 2007, from www.cdc.gov/ncidod/diseases/hepatitis/a/fact.htm

Centers for Disease Control and Prevention. (2009). *Viral hepatitis B fact sheet.* Retrieved May 15, 2007, from www.cdc.gov/ncidod/diseases/hepatitis/b/fact.htm

Centers for Disease Control and Prevention. (2012). *Hepatitis B FAQs for health professionals.* Retrieved December 1, 2013, from http://www.cdc.gov/hepatitis/HBV/HBVfaq.htm

Centers for Disease Control and Prevention. (2012). *Hepatitis E FAQs for health professionals.* Retrieved December 1, 2013, from http://www.cdc.gov/hepatitis/HEV/HEVfaq.htm

Centers for Disease Control and Prevention. (2013). *Hepatitis A FAQs for health professionals.* Retrieved December 1, 2013, from http://www.cdc.gov/hepatitis/HAV/HAVfaq.htm

Centers for Disease Control and Prevention. (2013). *Hepatitis C FAQs for health professionals.* Retrieved December 1, 2013, from http://www.cdc.gov/hepatitis/HCV/HCVfaq.htm

Centers for Disease Control and Prevention. (2013). *Hepatitis D.* Retrieved December 1, 2013, from http://www.cdc.gov/hepatitis/HDV/index.htm

Centers for Disease Control and Prevention. (2013, July 16). *Vaccine recommendations of the ACIP.* Retrieved September 29, 2014, from http://www.cdc.gov/vaccines/hcp/acip-recs/vacc-specific/hepb.html

Chalasani, N., Younossi, Z., Lavine, J. E., Diehl, A. M., Brunt, E. M., Cusi, K., . . . Sanyal, A. J. (2012). *The diagnosis and management of the non-alcoholic fatty liver disease: Practice guideline by the American Association for the Study of Liver Disease, American College of Gastroenterology, and the American Gastroenterological Association.* Retrieved from http://www.aasld.org/practiceguidelines/Documents/NonalcoholicFattyLiverDisease2012_25762_ftp.pdf

Chapman, R., Fevery, J., Kalloo, A., Nagorney, D. M., Boberg, K. M., Shneider, B., & Gores, G. J. (2010). Diagnosis and management of primary sclerosing cholangitis. *AASLD practice guidelines.* Retrieved from http://www.aasld.org/practiceguidelines/Documents/Practice%20Guidelines/PSC_2-2010.pdf

Desai, M. C. (2013). *Successful strategies for the discovery of antiviral drugs.* Cambridge: Royal Society of Chemistry.

DiPiro, J. T. (2014). *Pharmacotherapy: A pathophysiologic approach* (9th ed.). New York, NY: McGraw-Hill.

Friedman, L. S. (2012). *Handbook of liver disease* (3rd ed.). Philadelphia, PA: Elsevier/Saunders.

Ghany, M. G., Nelson, D. R., Strader, D. B., Thomas, D. L., & Seeff, L. B. (2011). An update on treatment of genotype I chronic hepatitis C virus infection: *Practice guideline by the American Association for the Study of Liver Disease.* Retrieved from http://www.aasld.org/practiceguidelines/Documents/AASLDUpdateTreatmentGenotype1HCV11113.pdf

Greenberger, N. J. (2012). Current diagnosis & treatment gastroenterology, hepatology, & endoscopy (2nd ed.). New York: McGraw-Hill Medical.

Lange, C. (2013). O144: Vitamin D deficiency and hepatitis C. *Journal of Viral Hepatitis, 20,* 8–9.

Lee, M. (2012). Adherence with use of oral agents in the treatment of chronic hepatitis B. *Current Hepatitis Reports, 11*(2), 70–74.

Lee, W. M., Larson, A. M., & Stravitz, R. T. (2011). *AASLD position paper: The management of acute liver failure* (update 2011). Retrieved from http://www. aasld.org/practiceguidelines/Documents/AcuteLiverFailureUpdate2011.pdf

Lehne, R. A. (2010). *Study guide, pharmacology for nursing care* (7th ed.). St. Louis, MO: Saunders/Elsevier.

Lindor, K. D., Gershwin, M. E., Poupon, R., Kaplan, M., Bergasa, N. V., & Heathcote, E. J. (2009). Primary biliary cirrhosis. *AASLD practice guidelines.* Retrieved from http://www.aasld.org/practiceguidelines/Documents/ Bookmarked%20Practice%20Guidelines/PrimaryBillaryCirrhosis7–2009.pdf

Lok, A. S., & McMahon, B. J. (2009). Chronic hepatitis B: Update 2009. *AASLD practice guidelines.* Retrieved from http://www.aasld.org/practiceguidelines/ Documents/Bookmarked%20Practice%20Guidelines/Chronic_Hep_B_ Update_2009%208_24_2009.pdf

Manns, M. P., Czaja, A. J., Gorham, J. D., Krawitt, E. L., Vergani, G. M., Vergani, D., & Vierling, J. M. (2010). Diagnosis and management of autoimmune hepatitis. *AASLD practice guidelines.* Retrieved from http://www.aasld.org/ practiceguidelines/Documents/AIH2010.pdf

Mann, S. J. (2012). *Hypertension and you: Old drugs, new drugs, and the right drugs for your high blood pressure.* Lanham, Md.: Rowman & Littlefield Publishers.

McCaughan, G. W. (2012). *Advanced therapy for hepatitis C.* Chichester, West Sussex: Blackwell.

McPhee, S. J., & Papadakis, M. A. (2011). *Current medical diagnosis & treatment 2011* (50th ed.). New York, NY: McGraw-Hill Medical.

O'Shea, R. S., Dasarathy, S., & McCullough, A. J. (2010). Alcoholic liver disease. *AASLD practice guidelines.* Retrieved from http://www.aasld.org/ practiceguidelines/Documents/Bookmarked%20Practice%20Guidelines/ AlcoholicLiverDisease1–2010.pdf

Pagana, K. D., & Pagana, T. J. (2010). *Mosby's manual of diagnostic and laboratory tests* (4th ed.). St. Louis, MO: Mosby/Elsevier.

Roberts, E. A., & Schilsky, M. I. (2008). Diagnosis and treatment of Wilson disease: An update. *AASLD practice guidelines.* Retrieved from http://www. aasld.org/practiceguidelines/Documents/Bookmarked%20Practice%20 Guidelines/Diagnosis%20and%20Treatment%20of%20Wilson%20Disease.pdf

Runyon, B. A. (2013). Management of adult patients with ascites due to cirrhosis: Update 2012. *AASLD practice guideline.* Retrieved from http://www.aasld.org/ practiceguidelines/Documents/ascitesupdate2013.pdf

Schiff, E. R. (2012). *Schiff's diseases of the liver* (11th ed.). Chichester, West Sussex, UK: John Wiley & Sons.

Symposium, C. F. (2009). *Interferon.* Hoboken: John Wiley & Sons.

Wells, B. G. (2009). *Pharmacotherapy handbook* (7th ed.). New York, NY: McGraw-Hill Medical Pub. Division.

CHAPTER 38

Biliary Dysfunction

MICHALYN PELPHREY • CHARLENE M. MYERS

CHOLECYSTITIS

I.   **Definition**

   A. Inflammation of the gallbladder, acute or chronic, associated with gallstones (cholelithiasis) in more than 90% of cases

II.   **Etiology/contributing factors/risk factors**

   A. Gallstones
   1. Gallstones become impacted within the cystic duct
   2. Inflammation occurs behind the obstruction
   3. Gallstones are the most common form of gallbladder disease
   4. Most stones are formed from cholesterol

   B. Acalculous cholecystitis
   1. 5% of cases
   2. Should be considered with unexplained fever 2–4 weeks after surgery or any stressful situation
      a. Multiple trauma
      b. Critical illness with a prolonged period of poor oral intake

   C. Bacteria/infectious agents, especially in patients with AIDS (cytomegalovirus, *Cryptosporidium*)

   D. Neoplasms (primary or metastatic)

   E. Strictures of the common bile duct

   F. Ischemia

   G. Torsion (twisting of cystic duct)

   H. Possible contributing factors:
   1. Obesity
   2. Pregnancy
   3. Sedentary lifestyle
   4. Low-fiber diets

     I. Risk factors:
        1. Female
        2. Advanced age
        3. Rapid weight loss
        4. Fad diets
        5. High levels of cholesterol

III. **Signs/symptoms**
    A. Can be present for years without causing symptoms
        1. When symptoms do develop, they often present similarly to indigestion (i.e., bloating, gassiness, and abdominal discomfort).
    B. A stone may become lodged, causing biliary colic
        1. Sudden onset
        2. Intense epigastric or right upper quadrant pain that may radiate to the shoulder or back (infrascapular region)
        3. Often associated with a full or fatty meal
    C. Nausea and vomiting
        1. Occurs in approximately 70% of cases
        2. Vomiting offers some relief for many patients
    D. Feeling of abdominal fullness
    E. Anorexia (inability to finish an average-sized meal)
    F. Dyspepsia
    G. Recurrent episodes of biliary colic lasting longer than 12 hr

IV. **Subjective/physical exam findings**
    A. Elevated body temperature
    B. Local tenderness that is almost always accompanied by muscle guarding and rebound pain
    C. Positive Murphy's sign (deep pain on inspiration while fingers are placed under the right rib cage)
    D. Palpable gallbladder in 5% of cases
    E. Jaundice in 20% of cases
    F. Right upper quadrant pain, tenderness, guarding, fever, and leukocytosis that continues or progresses after 2–3 days indicates severe inflammation and possible gangrene, empyema, or perforation

V. **Laboratory/diagnostics**
    A. Mild leukocytosis: white blood cell (WBC) count, 12,000–20,000/mcl
    B. Serum bilirubin mildly increased (greater than 4 mg/dl)
    C. Increased levels of the following:
        1. Alanine transaminase (normal, 1–35 units/L)
        2. Aspartate transaminase (normal, 0–35 units/L)
        3. Lactate dehydrogenase (LDH) (normal, 50–150 units/L)
        4. Alkaline phosphatase (normal, 30–120 units/L)
    D. Amylase level (normal, 0–130 units/L)
        1. Elevated
        2. If greater than 500 units, concomitant pancreatitis should be suspected

E. Electrocardiogram
1. Normal
2. Electrocardiogram is important to rule out myocardial infarction as the cause of symptoms
F. Chest x-ray to rule out pneumonia
G. Flat plate of the abdomen may show radiopaque gallstones (20% of cases)
H. Hepato-iminodiacetic acid scan to visualize cystic duct obstruction
1. A positive test consists of nonvisualization of the gallbladder after 4 hr
2. This test is reliable if bilirubin is less than 5 mg/dl
I. Ultrasound: best study for diagnosing gallstones; dilated gallbladder with a thickened gallbladder wall, pericholecystic fluid, and sonographic Murphy's sign are seen in patients with acute cholecystitis
J. Endoscopic retrograde cholangiopancreatography (ERCP)
1. Can be used to diagnose stones in the gallbladder if noninvasive studies have been found negative
2. Gives information on the status of biliary and pancreatic ducts
K. Tokyo Guidelines for diagnostic criteria and severity assessment
1. Diagnostic criteria for acute cholecystitis
   a. Local signs of inflammation—Murphy's sign, right upper quadrant mass/pain/tenderness
   b. Systemic signs of inflammation—fever, elevated CRP, elevated WBC
   c. Imaging findings characteristics of acute cholecystitis
      i. Definite diagnosis—one item in a and one in b are positive
      ii. Item c confirms the diagnosis when acute cholecystitis is suspected clinically
2. Severity assessment
   a. Mild (grade I) acute cholecystitis—no findings of organ dysfunction and mild disease in the gallbladder
   b. Moderate (grade II) acute cholecystitis—accompanied by any one of the following:
      i. Elevated WBC greater than 18,000
      ii. Palpable tender mass in right upper quadrant
      iii. Duration of complaints greater than 72 hr
      iv. Marked local inflammation (gangrenous cholecystitis, emphysematous cholecystitis, abcess)
   c. Severe (grade III) acute cholecystitis
      i. Accompanied by dysfunctions of organ systems (hypotension, decreased level of consciousness, renal dysfunction, PaO_2/FiO_2 ration less than 300, hepatic dysfunction, hematological dysfunction)

VI.   Treatment
  A. Nothing by mouth (NPO) or low-fat, low-volume meals
  B. If NPO, nasogastric tube to low wall suction
  C. IV fluids
  1. To maintain intravascular volume and electrolytes, 5% dextrose in 0.45 normal saline (NS), 125 ml/hr
  2. Note signs of dehydration, and increase fluids PRN
     a. Tachycardia
     b. Hypotension
     c. Decreased urinary output
  D. Pain can be controlled with antispasmodics, NSAIDs, and if necessary, some opiate analgesics (morphine, hydromorphone [Dilaudid])
  E. IV antibiotics
  1. Typically, a third-generation cephalosporin (e.g., cefazolin, cefuroxime, ceftriaxone) with the addition of metronidazole (1 gram IV loading dose, followed by 500 mg IV every 6 hr) in mild-to-moderate cases of community-acquired acute cholecystitis
  2. Piperacillin/tazobactam (3.375 grams IV every 6 hr or 4.5 grams IV every 8 hr)
  3. Ampicillin/sulbactam (3 grams IV every 6 hr)
  4. Meropenem (1 gram IV every 8 hr)
  5. For more severe cases, use imipenem/cilastatin (500 mg IV every 6 hr)
  F. Antispasmodics and antiemetics
  G. Surgery consultation: Early laparoscopic cholecystectomy is considered the treatment of choice for most patients. In randomized trials and meta-analysis, early treatment has been associated with shorter hospitalization. When laparoscopic cholecystectomy is performed in patients with moderate to severe cholecystitis, it should be performed by a highly experienced surgeon. If anatomical identification is difficult, the surgery should be converted to open cholecystectomy.
  1. In those with severe cholecystitis, initial conservative management with antibiotics is recommended with the use of cholecystostomy, PRN.
  H. ERCP with sphincterotomy and extraction of stones can be performed along with cholecystectomy for patients with a stone in the common bile duct (choledocholithiasis).
  I. Gallstones that are primarily composed of cholesterol and are smaller than 2 cm in diameter can be treated by pharmacologic dissolution, which should not be used as a primary treatment in acute cholecystitis but can be used as a measure in chronic cholecystitis
  1. Ursodiol/ursodeoxycholic acid (10–15 mg/kg/day) for 12–24 months

   a. Monitor every 6 months with an ultrasound scan of the gallbladder
   b. Recurrence rate has been found to be high after discontinuation of the medication
   2. Non-overweight patients who have stones that are radiolucent, small, lacking in calcification, few in number, and floating may benefit from chenodeoxycholic acid/chenodiol, which blocks hepatic synthesis of cholesterol, and ursodeoxycholic acid/ursodiol, which blocks intestinal uptake.
   a. Chenodeoxycholic acid/chenodiol 250 mg PO, BID for the first 2 weeks; increase the dose by 250 mg/day each week until a range of 13–16 mg/kg/day in 2 divided doses or until the maximum tolerated dose is reached
   3. Contact dissolution by instillation of methyl tert-butyl ether percutaneously into the gallbladder

ACUTE PANCREATITIS

I. **Definition**
   A. Acute, inflammatory autodigestive process of the pancreas
II. **Etiology**
   A. Acute biliary tract disease (e.g., gallstones)
   B. Alcoholism and acute intoxication
   C. Smoking
   D. Hypertriglyceridemia
   E. Hypercalcemia
   F. Autoimmune pancreatitis
   G. Hereditary pancreatitis
   H. Sphincter of Oddi dysfunction
   I. Pancreatic divisum
   J. Traumatic pancreatitis
   K. Infectious causes (e.g., mumps, cytomegalovirus, *Mycobacterium avium-intracellulare complex*)
   L. Idiopathic pancreatitis
   M. Hypoperfusion induced pancreatitis
   N. ERCP
   O. Medications
      1. Azathioprine (Imuran)
      2. Sulfonamides
      3. Thiazide diuretics
      4. Estrogen
      5. Furosemide (Lasix)
      6. Corticosteroids
      7. Tetracycline
      8. Valproic acid
      9. Metronidazole

10. L-asparaginase
11. Methyldopa
12. Pentamidine
13. Ethacrynic acid
14. Procainamide
15. Sulindac
16. Nitrofurantoin
17. Angiotensin-converting-enzyme (ACE) inhibitors
18. Danazol
19. Cimetidine
20. Diphenoxylate
21. Piroxicam
22. Gold
23. Ranitidine
24. Sulfasalazine
25. Isoniazid
26. Acetaminophen
27. Cisplatin
28. Opiates
29. Erythromycin

III. **Signs/symptoms**
   A. Epigastric abdominal pain
      1. May radiate to the back or to the right or the left
      2. Usually
         a. Has an abrupt onset
         b. Is steady and severe
         c. Is worsened by walking or lying supine
      3. May be alleviated by
         a. Knee-to-chest position
         b. Leaning forward
         c. Sitting
   B. Nausea and vomiting
   C. In severe attacks
      1. Weakness
      2. Sweating
      3. Anxiety
   D. Epigastric tenderness and guarding
   E. Absent or hypoactive bowel sounds, distention (resulting from ileus)
   F. Fever
   G. Tachycardia, hypotension, cool/pale skin (due to decreased intravascular volume)
   H. Tachypnea, decreased breath sounds (caused by pleural effusion)
   I. Jaundice
   J. Steatorrhea
   K. If hypocalcemic

      1. Chvostek sign and/or

      2. Trousseau sign

  L. Ascites

  M. Crackles if pleural effusion is present

  N. Right upper quadrant mass may be palpated

  O. If intra-abdominal bleeding is present (hemorrhagic pancreatitis)

      1. Flank discoloration (Grey Turner's sign) and/or

      2. Umbilical discoloration (Cullen's sign)

IV. **Laboratory/diagnostics**

  A. Elevated serum amylase and lipase levels

      1. Serum lipase remains elevated longer than serum amylase and is more specific

      2. Isoamylase is preferred by some clinicians as the initial test for reducing the risk of erroneously diagnosing pancreatitis by excluding occasional cases of salivary hyperamylasemia.

      3. The recommended cutoff for diagnosis is amylase three times above normal range or less than three times with abdominal pain typical of pancreatitis with CT scan to confirm diagnosis.

      4. Normal amylase does not rule out pancreatitis

  B. Elevated urine amylase level

  C. Elevated serum trypsin levels, which are diagnostic of pancreatitis in the absence of renal failure, are the most accurate indicators of the disease. Measurements are obtained by radioimmunoassay; however, this test is not readily available in most laboratories.

  D. For those patients who present to the emergency department with acute abdominal pain and a high degree of suspicion for pancreatitis, a negative dipstick for urinary trypsinogen-2 is useful to rule out acute pancreatitis.

  E. Leukocytosis (10,000–30,000/μl)

  F. Hematocrit may be elevated initially owing to hemoconcentration; decreased hematocrit may suggest hemorrhage or disseminated intravascular coagulopathy

  G. Hyperglycemia (in severe disease) with islet cell damage

  H. Elevated BUN concentration (usually resulting from dehydration)

  I. AST and LDH levels may be elevated as the result of tissue necrosis

  J. Bilirubin and alkaline phosphatase levels may be increased as a result of common bile duct obstruction.

  K. Hypocalcemia (less than 7 mg/dl) in severe disease (due to saponification of fat)

  L. Hypokalemia may be present because of associated vomiting; hyperkalemia may occur as the result of acidosis or renal insufficiency

  M. Low albumin

  N. Elevated C-reactive protein concentration after 48 hr suggests the development of pancreatic necrosis

O. Monitor arterial blood gases for hypoxemia (due to acute respiratory distress syndrome, atelectasis, or pleural effusion) and acidosis (due to lactic acidosis, respiratory acidosis, or renal insufficiency)

P. Abdominal plain film may show the following:
1. A sentinel loop (ileus)
2. Pancreatic calcifications
3. Gallstones

Q. Abdominal ultrasonography for detecting gallstones and pancreatic pseudocysts

R. Contrast-enhanced CT scan is superior to ultrasound in defining the extent of pancreatitis and in diagnosing pseudocysts, necrosis, and fistulas

S. ERCP may be indicated for some patients but should not be performed during acute stages of the disease

T. Magnetic resonance imaging/cholangiopancreatography (MRI/MRCP) has several advantages over CT scan, including the evaluation of biliary tract and the pancreatic duct, and is free of radiation risk. MRI can assess the severity of acute pancreatitis by detecting the extent of necrosis and fluid collections like a CT scan but better allows definition of solid debris within collections. There is a magnetic resonance severity index that corresponds well with the Ranson score.

V.   Management

A. IV hydration to maintain intravascular volume
1. Fluid therapy is the cornerstone of management of acute pancreatitis
2. Note: remember that hypovolemia and shock are major causes of death early in the disease process. Patients may have sequestered up to 12 L of fluid on presentation of symptoms. It is imperative that the practitioner closely monitor fluid status and make fluid replacement a high priority when treating acute pancreatitis.
3. Lactated Ringer or NS solution with 20 mEq KCl/L at 75–100 ml/hr
4. Increase PRN to maintain adequate blood pressure (BP) (try to keep systolic blood pressure [SBP] higher than 100 mmHg and mean arterial pressure [MAP] higher than 60 mmHg), urinary output (try to keep more than 30 ml/hr), heart rate (try to keep less than 100 beats per minute), and pulmonary capillary wedge pressure (PCWP)/central venous pressure (try to keep PCWP between 11 and 14 mmHg). These are reasonable goals, but they should be individualized for each patient.
5. Fresh frozen plasma and albumin may also be infused
6. Patients with acute hemorrhagic pancreatitis may need red blood cells in addition to fluid therapy to restore vascular volume.
7. Those patients who fail to respond to fluid therapy alone may need vasoactive agents (e.g., dopamine and dobutamine) to support BP.

B. Pain control

    1. Morphine (Morphine sulfate, 2–10 mg IV every 4 hr, PRN), hydromorphone (Dilaudid, 0.5–1.5 mg IV or SQ, every 4 hr, PRN), and fentanyl (25–75 mcg IV/SQ, every 2 hr, PRN) are reasonable alternatives to meperidine and are more desirable due to adverse effects associated with meperidine

C. Antibiotics—not used prophylactically

    1. For patients who have evidence of the following:

        a. Septicemia

        b. Pancreatic abscess

        c. Inflammation caused by biliary stones

    2. Should be broad-spectrum agents (e.g., imipenem-cilastatin [Primaxin], 250–500 mg every 6–8 hr)

    3. Prophylactic antibiotics not recommended, regardless of type or severity

    4. Infected necrosis should be suspected in patients with pancreatic or extrapancreatic necrosis who deteriorate (clinical instability, sepsis, increased WBC, fevers) or fail to improve after 7–10 days of hospitalization.

    5. If empiric antibiotics initiated, antibiotics that penetrate pancreatic necrosis should be used.

        a. Carbapenems or quinolones plus metronidazole (500 mg IV every 8 hr)

D. NPO until clinical improvement, then the following:

    1. Supplements

    2. Small, frequent meals

        a. Low cholesterol

        b. High protein

        c. Low fat

        d. Bland

E. Nasogastric tube for ileus or vomiting

F. Monitor calcium levels and replace PRN

G. Monitor pulmonary function

H. Enteral nutrition may be necessary

    1. Has shown significant reduction in mortality and multiorgan failure, operative interventions and systemic infections compared to parenteral nutrition

    2. Pancreatic stimulation is overcome by feeding via nasojejunal tube delivering tube feeds beyond the ligament of Tritz into jejunum

I. Insulin may be needed in cases of hyperglycemia

J. Surgery in selected cases

    1. Gallstones

    2. Perforated peptic ulcer

    3. Need for excision or drainage

K. If pancreatitis is caused by biliary obstruction, stent placement via ERCP may be used to decrease the likelihood of recurrent episodes.

VI. Prognosis

A. The Ranson criteria have identified criteria for predicting the prognosis of patients with acute pancreatitis. The number of prognostic signs present within the first 48 hr after admission helps to determine the patient's chances of morbidity and mortality.

1. Fewer than three risk factors: approximately 1% mortality rate
2. Three to four risk factors: 16% mortality
3. Five to six risk factors: 40% mortality
4. More than seven risk factors: close to 100% mortality
5. Prognostic signs at admission or diagnosis
   a. Older than age 55 (older than age 70 for gallstones)
   b. WBC count greater than 16,000/mcl
   c. Blood glucose higher than 200 mg/dl
   d. LDH greater than 350 international units/L
   e. AST greater than 250 international units/L
6. Prognostic signs during initial 48 hr
   a. Hematocrit drops by more than 10 ml/dl
   b. BUN increases by more than 5 mg/dl
   c. Calcium level declines by 8 mg/dl
   d. Arterial oxygen pressure declines by 60 mmHg
   e. Base deficit exceeds 4 mEq/L
   f. Estimated fluid sequestration exceeds 6,000 ml

B. APACHE II predicts the severity of acute pancreatitis

1. Twelve physiological parameters and additional points for age and underlying medical conditions (rectal temperature, MAP, heart rate, respiration rate, FIO_2, arterial pH, serum sodium, serum potassium, serum creatinine, hematocrit, and WBC)
2. It can be applied at time of admission and daily to assess progression on disease.
3. A score of 8 or more points predicts 11%–18% mortality

C. BISAP score

1. The variables are as follows:
   a. Blood urea nitrogen level greater than 25 mg/dl
   b. Impaired mental status
   c. Systemic inflammatory response syndrome
   d. Age older than 60 years
   e. Pleural effusion
2. Each score is worth 1 point. There is a steady increase in the risk of mortality with the increasing number of points.
   a. 0 points: mortality rate of 0.1%
   b. 1 point: mortality rate of 0.4%
   c. 2 points: mortality rate of 1.6%
   d. 3 points: mortality rate of 3.6%
   e. 4 points: mortality rate of 7.4%
   f. 5 points: mortality rate of 9.5%

BIBLIOGRAPHY

Banks, P. A., Bollen, T. L., Dervenis, C., . . . Vege, S. S. (2012) Classification of Acute Pancreatitis. *Gut, 62*, 101–111. Retrieved from http://gut.bmj.com/content/62/1/102.short

Chauhan, S., & Forsmark, C. E. (2010). Pain management in chronic pancreatitis: A treatment algorithm. *Best Practice and Research Clinical Gastroenterology, 24*, 323–335.

Ferri, F. F. (2011). *Practical guide to the care of the medical patient* (8th ed.). St. Louis, MO: Mosby.

Fujikawa, T., Tada, S., Abe, T., Yoshimoto, Y., Maekawa, H., Shimoike, N., & Tanaka, A. (2012). Is early laparoscopic cholecystectomy feasible for acute cholecystitis for the elderly? *Journal of Gastroenterology and Hepatology Research, 1*(10).

Greenberger, N. J., & Sharma, P. (2014) Update in gastroenterology and hepatology. *Annals of Internal Medicine, 161*, 205–209.

Greenberger, N. J., & Paumgartner, G. (2011). Diseases of the gallbladder and bile ducts. In D. L. Kasper, E. Braunwald, A. S. Fauci, S. Hauser, D. Longo, & J. L. Jameson (Eds.), *Harrison's principles of internal medicine* (18th ed.). New York, NY: McGraw-Hill.

Greenberger, N., Blumberg, R., & Burakoff, R. (2011). *Current diagnosis and treatment, gastroenterology, hepatology & endoscopy* (2nd ed.). New York, NY: McGraw Hill.

Gurusamy, K., Samraj, K., Gluud, C., Wilson, E., & Davidson, B. R. (2010). Meta-analysis of randomized controlled trials on the safety and effectiveness of early versus delayed laparoscopic cholecystectomy for acute cholecystitis. *British Journal of Surgery, 97*, 141–150.

Hawkins, J., & Roberto-Nichols, D. M. (2011). *Guidelines for nurse practitioners in gynecologic settings* (10th ed.). New York, NY: Springer .

Imrey, P. B., & Law, R. (2012). Antibiotic prophylaxis for severe acute pancreatitis. *American Journal of Surgery, 203*, 556–557.

Krumberger, J. M., & Hammer, B. (2012). Gastrointestinal alterations. In M. L. Sole, D. Klein, & M. Moseley (Eds.), *Introduction to critical care nursing* (6th ed.). Philadelphia, PA: WB Saunders.

McPhee, S. J., Papadakis, M. A., & Tierney, L. M. (Eds.). (2014). *Current medical diagnosis and treatment* (46th ed.). New York, NY: McGraw Hill/Appleton & Lange.

Muniraj, T., Gajendran, M., Thiruvengadam, S., Raghuram, K., Rao, S., & Devaraj, P. (2012). Acute pancreatitis. *Disease-a-Month, 58*, 98–144. Retrieved from http://dx.doi.org/10.1016/j.disamonth.2012.01.005

Nikfarjam, M., Niumsawatt, V., & Christophi, C. (2011). Outcomes of contemporary management of gangrenous and non-gangrenous acute cholecystitis. *HPB (Oxford)*, *13*, 551–558.

Sitaramin, S., & Friedman, L. S. (2012). *Essentials of gastroenterology*. Hoboken, NJ: Wiley-Blackwell.

Stefanidis, D., Richardson, W. S., Chang, L., Earle, D. B., & Fanelli, R. D. (2009). The role of diagnostic laparoscopy for acute abdominal conditions: An evidence based review. *Surgical Endoscopy, 23,* 16–23.

Tenner, S., Baillie, J., DeWitt, J., & Vege, S. S. (2013). American College of Gastroenterology Guideline: Management of acute pancreatitis. *American Journal of Gastroenterology*, *108*, 1400–1415.

Wiseman, J. T., Sharuk, M. N., Singla, A., Cahan, M., Litwin, D. E., . . . Shah, S. A. (2010). Surgical management of acute cholecystitis at a tertiary care center in the modern era. *Archives of Surgery*, *145*, 439–444.

Wittau, M., Mayer, B., Scheele, J., Henne-Bruns, D., Dellinger, E. P., & Isenmann, R. (2011). Systematic review and meta-analysis of antibiotic prophylaxis in severe acute pancreatitis. *Scandinavian Journal of Gastroenterology, 46*, 261–270.

CHAPTER 39

Inflammatory Gastrointestinal Disorders

LISA A. JOHNSON • CHARLENE M. MYERS

DIVERTICULITIS

I. **Definition**
   A. Perforation of a colonic diverticulum; can either be a localized microperforation (most common) or a macroperforation with abscess formation or generalized peritonitis
   B. Fifty percent of people older than 50 years have diverticulosis; 10%–25% of those with diverticulosis develop diverticulitis

II. **Etiology**
   A. Not clearly proven
   B. Low-fiber diet believed to be the leading cause in Western societies
   C. Weakness and defects in the colon wall

III. **Subjective/physical examination findings**
   A. Lower left quadrant pain (mild to moderate) and fever are the main clinical features
   B. Patients with free perforation present with more generalized pain and peritoneal signs
   C. Constipation is common and may alternate with diarrhea
   D. Fever and abdominal tenderness, guarding, palpable mass, spasms, and rebound tenderness indicate inflammation due to abscess
   E. Nausea and vomiting
   F. Bowel sounds are usually hypoactive
   G. Dysuria and frequency may be present

IV. **Laboratory/diagnostics**
   A. Leukocytosis is common, although those with mild diverticulitis may have a normal white blood cell count
   B. Elevated procalcitonin level, erythrocyte sedimentation rate, and C-reactive protein are caused by inflammation

C. CT scan of the abdomen is obtained to look for evidence of diverticulitis, to determine its severity, and to exclude abscess or fistula formation

D. Presence of colonic diverticula with colonic wall thickening, pericolic fat inflammation (streaking), abscess formation, or extraluminal air, all suggest varying levels of diverticulitis

E. Barium enema may reveal strictures, obstruction, masses, or fistulas, but it should not be used in acute stages because it may cause free perforation

F. Flexible sigmoidoscopy may show inflamed mucosa but should be avoided during the acute phase. Patients should wait 4–6 weeks before having invasive examination of colon.

V.   **Management**

A. Outpatient:
   1. Patients with mild symptoms and no peritoneal signs can be managed as an outpatient.
   2. Oral antibiotics, clear liquids to 48- to 72-hour advancement to low-fiber (residue) diet as tolerated. Avoid laxatives. Most patients improve in 2–3 days.
   3. In patients with acute uncomplicated diverticulitis, antibiotic treatment duration is 7–10 days, depending upon resolution of symptoms.
      a. Ciprofloxacin (Cipro), 500 mg PO two times a day; or levofloxacin (Levaquin), 500 mg PO daily plus metronidazole (Flagyl), 500 mg PO every 8 hr
      b. Amoxicillin (Amoxil) and clavulanate, 500 mg PO three times a day; or 875 mg PO two times a day

B. Inpatient:
   1. IV antibiotics, bowel rest, +/–TPN, and nasogastric tube (NGT) if ileus is present
   2. Antibiotic options (duration 7–10days; switch to oral after 5 days if patient improved):
      a. Fluoroquinolone (ciprofloxacin 400 mg IV every 12 hr or levofloxacin 500 mg IV QD) + metronidazole 500 mg IV every 8 hr
      b. Third or fourth generation cephalosporin (i.e. cefotaxime, ceftriaxone, or cefepime) + metronidazole 500 mg IV every 8 hr
      c. Piperacillin-tazobactam (Zosyn), 3.375 grams IV every 6 hr; or 4.5 grams IV every 8 hr
      d. Ticarcillin-clavulanate (Timentin), 3.1 grams IV every 6 hr
      e. Immunocompromised patients: imipenem 500 mg IV every 6 hr

C. Surgical considerations:

1. Severe disease or failure to respond to treatment within 72 hr requires surgical consultation
2. Emergency surgical consultation is necessary for those patients who have an abscess, an obstruction, free air, or peritonitis; these conditions require surgery

INFLAMMATORY BOWEL DISEASE

I. **Ulcerative colitis**
   A. Definition
      1. Idiopathic inflammatory condition involving the mucosal surface of the colon; characterized by erosions with bleeding and friability
   B. Subjective/physical examination findings
      1. Bloody diarrhea is the cardinal sign
      2. Fecal urgency, tenesmus, and abdominal cramping
      3. Weight loss, malnutrition, anemia, and fever can occur
      4. Assessment of disease activity (Table 39.1)
   C. Laboratory/diagnostics
      1. See Table 39.1
      2. Leukocytosis during inflammation
      3. Anemia
      4. Electrolyte abnormalities (hypokalemia)
      5. Causes elevated values on liver function tests (if hepatobiliary disease is present)
      6. Stool cultures to rule out infectious colitis

Table 39.1	Assessment of disease activity in ulcerative colitis		
	Mild	**Moderate**	**Severe**
Albumin	Normal	3–3.5 grams/dl	Less than 3.0 grams/dl
Erythrocyte sedimentation rate	Less than 20 mm/hr or normal	20–30 mm/hr	More than 30 mm/hr
Heart rate (beats/minute)	Less than 90	90–100	Higher than 100
Hematocrit	Normal	30–40 mg/dl	Less than 30 mg/dl
Stool, #/day	Fewer than four	Four to six	More than six (bloody)
Temperature	Normal	99°F to 100°F	Above 100°F
Weight loss	None	1% to 10%	Greater than 10%

7. Sigmoidoscopy/colonoscopy with biopsy determines the extent of disease and provides histologic confirmation. Crohn's disease that only affects the colon can be difficult to determine as it may appear as ulcerative colitis.

8. Plain abdominal x-rays exclude dilatation and are helpful in the determination of disease state

9. Colonoscopy and barium enema should not be performed in an acute attack due to risk of perforation

D. Management

1. See table 39.2

2. Mild/moderate active distal disease

   a. First-line therapy: oral or topical (enema/suppository) aminosalicylates or topical corticosteroids. Derivatives of 5-acetylsalicylic acid (5-ASA; sulfasalazine, mesalamine, balsalazide, and olsalazine) are currently available and result in symptomatic improvement in 50%–75% of patients

   b. Patients refractory to oral aminosalicylates or topical steroids may respond to mesalamine enemas

   c. Patients refractory to all of the above agents in maximal doses or who are systemically ill, may require treatment with oral prednisone in doses up to 40–60 mg per day or infliximab with an induction regimen of 5 mg/kg at weeks 0, 2, and 6

3. Mild/moderate active extensive disease

   a. Sulfasalazine (Azulfidine) is the cornerstone of drug therapy for mild to moderate cases of ulcerative colitis, although it is associated with a greater number of adverse effects.

   b. First-line therapy: oral sulfasalazine or an alternate aminosalicylate at dose equivalent to 4.8 grams/day of mesalamine

   c. For active disease, dosage should be 4 grams/day, 2 grams daily for maintaining remission

   d. It should be initiated at 500 mg/day and increased every few days up to 4–6 grams/day for the therapeutic dose

   e. Because sulfasalazine inhibits folate absorption, folate supplementation is recommended

   f. Patients with sulfa allergies should avoid this drug

   g. Consider combined oral and topical therapy for patients with distal disease

   h. Patients with mild to moderate disease who do not improve in 2–3 weeks with 5-ASA therapy should be given additional corticosteroid therapy.

      i. Topical hydrocortisone foam or enemas (80–100 mg once or BID) or 5-ASA enemas (4 grams once daily) may be tried first.

      ii. If therapy fails after 2 weeks, systemic steroid therapy should be initiated. Prednisone (40 mg QD) and methylprednisolone (Medrol) are the most commonly used. The patient should be tapered off steroids slowly after 2 weeks at a rate of decrease of no more than 5 mg/week.

    i. Patients refractory to oral corticosteroids can be treated with azathioprine (2–2.5 mg/kg/day) or 6-mercaptopurine (1–1.5 mg/kg/day); can be used in combination with aminosalicylates

    j. Infliximab is an effective treatment for patients who are steroid refractory or steroid dependent despite adequate doses of a thiopurine, or who are intolerant of these medications

4. Severe disease

    a. Patients with severe symptoms refractory to oral/topical aminosalicylates or corticosteroids should be treated with a 7–10 day course of IV corticosteroids (300 mg hydrocortisone or 48 mg methylprednisolone equivalent/day).

    b. Patients refractory to IV corticosteroids are candidates for IV cyclosporine (4 mg/kg/day)

    c. Infliximab may also be effective in avoiding colectomy in patients failing intravenous steroids but its long-term efficacy is unknown in this setting

    d. Patients refractory to above are candidates for colectomy

    e. Patients with toxic megacolon should undergo bowel decompression, treatment with broad-spectrum antibiotics, and possibly colectomy

5. Problems of hypersensitivity and intolerance have been reported with sulfasalazine. New forms have been developed (e.g., mesalamine [Asacol], 1.2–1.6 grams; mesalamine [Pentasa], 1 gram four times a day; balsalazide [Colazal], 2.25 grams three times a day for active disease [three 750-mg capsules three times a day]).

6. Mesalamine suppositories, 500 mg BID for 3–12 weeks, are beneficial for patients with ulcerative proctitis

7. Patients with disease beyond the rectum but not beyond the descending colon may benefit from mesalamine enemas (4 grams daily)

8. Immunomodulators

    a. Maintenance of remission; acute flares unresponsive to steroids

    b. Agents: 6-mercaptopurine (Purinethol), azathioprine (Imuran), cyclosporine (Neoral), methotrexate (Trexall)

Table. 39.2	Agents Used in the Treatment of IBD			
Drug Class	Agent	MOA	Adverse Effects	Comments
Aminosalicylates (5-ASA)	Sulfasalazine (Azulfidine®) **Non-sulfa containing:** Mesalamine (Asacol®) Mesalamine (Pentasa®) Olsalazine (Dipentum®) Balsalazide (Colazal®)	Sulfasalazine is cleaved by gut bacteria in the colon to sulfapyridine and mesalamine (5-ASA). The active moiety (5-ASA) imparts a topical anti-inflammatory effect on the diseased bowel.	Sulfasalazine: nausea, vomiting, diarrhea, anorexia, and hypersensitivity reactions **Non-sulfa 5-ASA:** Generally better tolerated than sulfasalazine. Nausea, vomiting, HA, alopecia, anorexia, and folate malabsorption	Used for both induction and maintenance of remission Efficacy (less active in CD affecting small intestine due to colonic activation of drug) and toxicity are dose related Dosage adjustment required for renal dysfunction Mesalamine available as enema & suppository
Corticosteroids	Prednisone (Deltasone®) Budesonide (Entocort EC®) Hydrocortisone (Solu-Cortef®) Methylprednisolone (Solu-Medrol®)	Anti-inflammatory	Nausea, vomiting, weight gain, water retention, gastritis, psychosis, adrenal suppression, glucose intolerance, osteoporosis (with long-term use)	Work quickly to suppress acute flares **NO role for maintenance therapy** **Avoid chronic use** Budesonide approximately 15 times more potent than prednisone Available as IV, oral & enema

Table. 39.2	Agents Used in the Treatment of IBD			
Drug Class	**Agent**	**MOA**	**Adverse Effects**	**Comments**
Immunomodulators	6-mercaptopurine (Purinethol®) Azathioprine (Imuran®) Methotrexate Cyclosporine (Sandimmune®) Tacrolimus (Prograf®)	Inhibits immune response	Pancreatitis, bone marrow suppression, nausea, diarrhea, rash, hepatotoxicity	May provide steroid sparing effect Indicated only for maintenance Drug interactions: cyclosporine, methotrexate, tacrolimus Limited data available for tacrolimus dosage
Anti-TNF Monoclonal Antibodies	infliximab (Remicade), adalimumab (Humira), certolizumab (Cimzia)	Neutralizes tumor necrosis factor (TNF) and alters immune response	Most common adverse effects are infusion-related reactions: fever, chills, pruritus, urticaria, chest pain, hypotension, hypertension, dyspnea	Serious infections including sepsis and disseminated tuberculosis have been reported. A tuberculin skin test is recommended prior to initiating therapy Indicated only for Crohn's disease Very expensive

      c. Azathioprine (Imuran) has been shown to be effective in preventing relapse of ulcerative colitis for periods of up to 2 years

9. For severe cases of ulcerative colitis, hospitalization is required because the patient's condition may deteriorate rapidly.
   a. Nothing by mouth (NPO)—total parenteral nutrition may be necessary for those with poor nutritional status
   b. Avoid opioids and anticholinergics
   c. Administer IV resuscitation and blood products PRN (hematocrit less than 25%–28%)
   d. Monitor and correct electrolyte imbalances
   e. Plain abdominal x-ray (to detect toxic megacolon)
   f. Stool samples (to detect infectious disease)
   g. Surgery consultation
   h. Methylprednisolone (Solu-Medrol), 40–60 mg IV daily

10. Surgical indications include the following (25% of patients will require surgery):
    a. Toxic megacolon
    b. Fulminant colitis
    c. Perforation
    d. Hemorrhage
    e. High-grade dysplasia
    f. Carcinoma
    g. Refractory disease requiring high-dose steroids

11. Toxic megacolon
    a. Develops in less than 2% of patients; rapid disease progression with fever, dehydration, and transfusions for anemia
    b. Antibiotics (cover for gram-negative bacteria and anaerobes), NGT, and serial plain abdominal films to monitor for perforation
    c. Surgery within 72 hr if failure to respond to medical management

II.   Crohn's disease

A. Definition
   1. Transmural process that can result in mucosal inflammation and ulceration, stricturing, fistula development, and abscess formation
   2. Patients may present with a combination of the following: chronic inflammation, intestinal obstruction, fistula formation, and abscess formation
   3. Patients with colonic disease are at risk for developing colon cancer, lymphoma, and small bowel adenocarcinoma

B. Management
   1. Drug therapy

    a. Initial management with 5-aminosalicylic acid agents (mesalamine, 2.4–4.8 grams/day, or Pentasa, 4 grams/day orally)

    b. Corticosteroids for active disease with prednisone or methylprednisolone with long course and slow taper; flares common during tapering of steroids

    c. Immunomodulating drugs: azathioprine, mercaptopurine, or methotrexate used in two-thirds of patients who with Crohn's disease who have not responded to corticosteroids

    d. Anti–tumor necrosis factor therapies: infliximab, adalimumab, and certolizumab injections/infusions for refractory disease

2. Mild/moderate active distal disease

    a. First-line therapy for ileal, ileocolonic or colonic disease: oral aminosalicylate

    b. Metronidazole (Flagyl®) 10–20 mg/kg/day may be used in patients not responding to oral aminosalicylates

    c. Ciprofloxacin (Cipro®) 1 gram/day is considered as effective as mesalamine (generally second-line)

    d. Oral budesonide may be considered as first-line treatment.

3. Moderate-severe disease

    a. Corticosteroids (prednisone 40–60 mg/day or budesonide 9 mg/day) until resolution of symptoms

    b. Anti TNF monoclonal antibodies (infliximab, adalimumab, and certolizumab pegol) are effective in the treatment of moderate to severely active CD in patients who have not responded despite complete and adequate therapy with a corticosteroid or an immunosuppressive agent

4. Severe/fulminant disease

    a. Severe symptoms despite oral corticosteroid or anti-TNF monoclonal antibodies therapy

    b. Assess need for surgical intervention (mass, obstruction, abscess)

    c. Administer IV corticosteroids (40–60 mg prednisone equivalent)

    d. Possibly use IV cyclosporine (5–7.5 mg/kg/day) or methotrexate (25 mg SQ/IM weekly) if IV steroids fail

5. Maintenance

    a. No role for long-term corticosteroid use

    b. Azathioprine (2–3 mg/kg/day)/6-mercaptopurine (1.5 mg/kg/day) or infliximab 5 mg/kg at 0, 2, and 6 weeks, then every 8 weeks thereafter are appropriate as first-line therapies

    c. Diet: well-balanced; may need supplemental enteral therapy or TPN for short-term management in active disease with significant weight loss

PERITONITIS

I.   Definition

    A. Acute inflammation of the visceral and parietal peritoneum

II.   Etiology

    A. Primary—spontaneous bacterial peritonitis (SBP) of ascitic fluid as a complication of cirrhotic ascites

        1. For SBP prophylaxis in patients with cirrhosis and ascites, norfloxacin 400 mg oral daily is recommended. Oral ciprofloxacin has been associated with a higher rate of quinolone-resistant organisms, and should be avoided. Although trimethoprim-sulfamethoxazole may also be indicated for prophylaxis, studies are conflicted as to its effectiveness in comparison to norfloxacin.

        2. Most cases of SBP are caused by transmigration of bacteria through the bowel wall; enteric Gram-negative bacilli are common pathogens (70%).

        3. *Klebsiella*, *Pneumococcus*, and *Enterococcus* are common as well

    B. Secondary peritonitis; peritonitis with a surgically amenable source

        1. Often polymicrobial infection

        2. Abdominal trauma/penetrating wounds

        3. Perforation resulting from appendicitis, colitis, peptic ulcer disease, diverticulitis, pancreatitis, and cholecystitis

III. Subjective/physical examination findings

    A. SBP: fever and abdominal pain with often a change in mental status due to hepatic encephalopathy

    B. Secondary peritonitis

        1. Acute abdominal pain, exacerbated by motion, variable location of abdominal pain

        2. High fever

        3. Nausea and vomiting

        4. Constipation

        5. Abdominal examination:

            a. Distention

            b. Rebound tenderness

            c. Generalized rigidity

            d. Decreased bowel sounds

            e. Hyperresonance to percussion

        6. Ascites

        7. Dyspnea, tachypnea

        8. Dehydration (hypotension, tachycardia)

IV.   Laboratory/diagnostics

    A. For SBP, ascitic fluid analysis will reveal the following:

        1. Protein concentration less than 1 gram/dl

    2. Polymorphonuclear cell count greater than 250/mm; this is the most sensitive and specific test for SBP if the count is higher than 500/mm

    3. Bacteria present on Gram's stain

    4. Lactic acid level greater than 32 mg/dl

    5. Glucose concentration higher than 50 mg/dl

    6. Lactate dehydrogenase level less than 225 mU/ml

B. The secondary peritonitis ascitic fluid analysis will reveal the following:

    1. Leukocyte count greater than 10,000/mm

    2. Lactate dehydrogenase greater than 225 mU/ml

    3. Protein levels greater than 1 gram/dl

    4. Glucose less than 50 mg/dl

    5. Presence of multiorganisms on Gram's stain or culture

C. Blood cultures—positive in 25% of patients

D. Leukocytosis—more pronounced in secondary peritonitis

E. Elevated BUN levels

F. Hemoconcentration (increased hematocrit)

G. Metabolic and respiratory acidosis

H. Elevated amylase levels

I. Abdominal x-ray

    1. Free air in peritoneal cavity

    2. Dilatation of large or small bowel

J. Chest x-ray—elevated diaphragm

K. CT scan and ultrasound

    1. Ascites

    2. Intra-abdominal mass

V. **Management**

A. See table 39.2

B. SBP: antibiotic therapy—third-generation cephalosporin

    1. Cefotaxime (Claforan), 2 grams IV every 8 hr

    2. Ceftriaxone (Rocephin), 2 grams IV every 24 hr

    3. Ampicillin 1–2 grams every 6 hr plus gentamicin dosed to achieve peak of 8–10, and trough of less than 1.5

    4. Levofloxacin 750 mg IV every 24 hr can be used for patients with penicillin allergy.

    5. Fluoroquinolones should not be used in a patient who had been receiving a fluoroquinolone for SBP prophylaxis because the infecting organism may be resistant to fluoroquinolones

    6. Traditionally, 10 days of therapy is recommended, although recent studies suggest that 5 days is sufficient.

C. Secondary peritonitis

    1. Operative management is indicated to eliminate the source of contamination, to reduce bacterial load, and to prevent recurrence.

2. Empiric antimicrobial coverage to include gram-negative aerobes, enteric streptococci, and anaerobes
   a. Cefotaxime 2 grams IV every 8 hr + metronidazole 500 mg IV every 8 hr
   b. Duration of antibiotics, 7+ days
3. Monitor blood and bacterial cultures for antibiotic management
4. IV fluid resuscitation; NPO and possible NGT placement
5. Monitor vital signs, urinary output, and consider need for respiratory support

APPENDICITIS

I. **Definition**
   A. Acute inflammation of the vermiform appendix caused by obstruction of the appendiceal lumen by
      1. Fecaliths (most common)
      2. Inflammation
      3. Foreign body
      4. Intestinal worms
      5. Strictures
      6. Tumors
   B. Gangrene and perforation can develop if appendicitis is not treated within 36 hr
   C. Appendicitis is the most common intra-abdominal infection treated by surgeons, 250,000 appendectomies per year.

II. **Clinical manifestations**
   A. Abdominal pain
      1. Periumbilical pain initially, then right lower quadrant pain (McBurney's point)
      2. Rovsing's sign: referral of pain to the right quadrant with palpation of the lower left quadrant
      3. Psoas sign: pain with active extension of the right hip
      4. Obturator sign: pain with internal rotation of the right hip
   B. Anorexia
   C. Nausea with or without vomiting
   D. Constipation—urge to defecate, although some report diarrhea
   E. Low-grade fever (high fever suggests possible perforation or another diagnosis)
   F. Motionless, with right thigh drawn up
   G. Guarding of the right lower quadrant

III. **Laboratory/diagnostics**
   A. Moderate leukocytosis—10,000–20,000 in 75% of cases
   B. Urinalysis
      1. Elevated specific gravity
      2. Hematuria
      3. Pyuria

    4. Albuminuria

  C. Ultrasound is 98% accurate in diagnosing appendicitis, provided that the appendix can be visualized

  D. CT scan to detect the following:

    1. Perforation

    2. Periappendiceal abscess

  E. History and clinical findings are the cornerstones of diagnosis

IV.   **Management**

  A. See table 39.2

  B. Prompt surgical intervention with appendectomy is the mainstay of treatment

  C. IV fluids: correct fluid and electrolyte imbalances as indicated

  D. Cefoxitin [Mefoxin], 1–2 grams, every 6–8 hr IV, cefotetan [Cefotan]

  E. Gangrenous or perforated appendicitis

    1. Mild-to-moderate severity (perforated or abscessed appendicitis and other infections of mild-to-moderate severity)

      a. Single agent:

        i. Cefoxitin, 2 grams IV every 6 hr

        ii. Ertapenem, 1 gram IV every 24 hr

        iii. Moxifloxacin, 400 mg IV every 24 hr

        iv. Ticarcillin-clavulanic acid, 3.1 grams IV every 6 hr

      b. Combination therapy: one of the following drugs in combination with metronidazole, 500 mg IV every 8 hr

        i. Cefazolin, 1–2 grams IV every 8 hr

        ii. Cefuroxime, 1.5 grams every 8 hr

        iii. Ceftriaxone, 1–2 grams IV every 12–24 hr

        iv. Cefotaxime, 1–2 grams IV every 6–8 hr

        v. Ciprofloxacin, 400 mg every 12 hr

        vi. Levofloxacin, 750 mg every 24 hr

    2. High risk or severity (severe physiologic disturbance, advanced age, or immunocompromised state)

      a. Single agent:

        i. Imipenem-cilastatin, 500 mg every 6 hr

        ii. Meropenem, 1 gram every 8 hr

        iii. Doripenem, 500 mg every 8 hr

        iv. Piperacillin-tazobactam, 3.375 grams every 6 hr

      b. Combination therapy: one of the following drugs in combinations with metronidazole, 500 mg IV every 8 hr

        i. Cefepime, 2 grams IV every 12 hr

        ii. Ceftazidime, 2 grams IV every 8 hr

        iii. Ciprofloxacin, 400 mg every 12 hr

        iv. Levofloxacin, 750 mg every 24 hr

    3. Regardless of the initial empiric regimen, the therapeutic regimen should be narrowed/adjusted once culture and susceptibility results are available.

    4. Continue antibiotics for 7 days after surgery

F. Pain management after diagnosis is made, and surgery is scheduled

    1. Hydromorphone (Dilaudid), 1 mg IV/SQ, every 4 hr PRN for pain, or

    2. Morphine sulfate, 1–2 mg IV every 4 hr PRN for pain

BIBLIOGRAPHY

Longo, D., Fauci, A., Kasper, D., Hauser, S., Jameson, J., & Loscalzo, J. (2012). *Harrison's principles of internal medicine* (18th ed.). New York, NY: McGraw-Hill.

Halter, J. B., Ouslander, J. G., Tinetti, M. E., Studenski, S., High, K. P., & Asthana, S. (2009). *Hazzard's geriatric medicine and gerontology* (6th ed.). New York, NY: McGraw-Hill.

McPhee, S. J., & Papadakis, M. A. (2014). In M. W. Rabow (Eds.), *Gastrointestinal disorders: Medical diagnosis and treatment.* New York, NY: McGraw-Hill.

Auwaerter, P. G., Barltett, J. G., Pham, P., & Hsu, A. J. (Eds.). (2014). *The Johns Hopkins POC-IT ABX Guide.* Baltimore, MD: John Hopkins University.

U.S. Department of Health and Human Services, National Institues of Health: National Institutes of Diabetes and Digestive and Kidney Diseases. (2011). *Ulcerative colitis.* NIH Publication No. 12–1597. Retrieved November 13, 2013, from http://digestive.niddk.nih.gov/ddiseases/pubs/colitis/

CHAPTER 40

Anatomic Intestinal Disorders

CATHERINE FUNG • CHARLENE M. MYERS

SMALL BOWEL OBSTRUCTION

I. **Definition**
   A. Blockage of the lumen of the intestine that prevents normal functioning and results in distention and tremendous losses of fluid into the gut
   B. Necrosis with toxicity and possible perforation may occur with strangulation

II. **Etiology**
   A. Adhesions—most common
   B. Hernias—external and internal
   C. Volvulus—twisting of the bowel on itself, causing obstruction
   D. Strictures—due to:
      1. Crohn's disease—intestinal fibrosis occurs as a result of chronic transmural inflammation causing stricture that usually leads to obstruction.
      2. Radiation
      3. Ischemia
   E. Hematomas—related to:
      1. Trauma
      2. Anticoagulants
   F. Intussusception—slipping of one part of an intestine into another part just below it
   G. Feces (impaction)
   H. Tumors
   I. Foreign bodies

III.   Pathophysiology

  A. The intestine proximal to the obstruction fills up with gas and fluid. This fluid is not absorbed by the intestines, causing the bowels to distend.

  B. Intestinal distention causes vomiting, which leads to more loss of fluid and electrolytes.

  C. The obstruction causes the intestine to reverse its mechanism of absorbing fluids in the gut to secreting more fluid from the intravascular space to the obstructed lumen, causing further bowel distention.

  D. Dehydration commences as more fluids and electrolytes are lost into the obstructed intestinal lumen. Metabolic alkalosis, hypokalemia, and hypochloremia may result from dehydration due to fluid loss and vomiting.

  E. Low intestinal blood flow occurs as the intestinal luminal pressure increases. Strangulated bowel obstruction can occur, which is a condition of intestinal ischemia, necrosis, and perforation.

  F. Stasis of intestinal contents leads to overgrowth of aerobic and anaerobic bacteria proximal to the site of bowel obstruction

IV.   Clinical manifestations

  A. Cramping periumbilical pain initially occurs sporadically, lasting seconds to minutes

  B. The pain becomes constant and diffuses as distention develops.

  C. High or proximal bowel obstruction
    1. Variable upper abdominal pain
    2. Profuse vomiting

  D. Middle or distal small bowel obstruction (SBO)
    1. Cramping, colicky, periumbilical, or diffuse pain
    2. Distention
    3. Episodic vomiting

  E. The more distal the obstruction, the greater the distention
    1. More vomiting of feculent contents
    2. Increase in nasogastric output

  F. Obstipation (extreme constipation) develops in complete obstruction.

  G. Partial obstruction—watery, possibly mucous, diarrhea

  H. Mild tenderness

  I. High-pitched "tinkling" bowel sounds and peristaltic rushes are noted early on auscultation; these sounds may be absent later

  J. Visible peristalsis may be present

  K. Signs and symptoms of dehydration
    1. Orthostatic hypotension
    2. Oliguria
    3. Elevated temperature
    4. Tachycardia

V. **Diagnostics/laboratory findings**
   A. Leukocytosis may be present
   B. Hemoconcentration—elevated hemoglobin and hematocrit
   C. Electrolyte imbalances—metabolic alkalosis due to vomiting and lack of oral intake, metabolic acidosis due to gastrointestinal bicarbonate loss, and tissue hypoperfusion due to hypovolemia
   D. Hypokalemia—the most common electrolyte imbalance
   E. Blood urea nitrogen/creatinine may be elevated due to renal hypoperfusion

VI. **Imaging**
   A. Supine and upright abdominal x-rays
      1. Ladder-like pattern of dilated bowel with air-fluid levels
      2. Little or no air in the colon or rectum with complete obstruction
      3. Thickening or "thumbprinting" of the intestinal wall with strangulation
      4. Pneumatosis in the wall of the intestines, or portal venous gas, are ominous signs and suggest urgent surgical intervention
   B. Transabdominal ultrasonography
      1. Noninvasive, radiation-free method
      2. Well tolerated by patients with acute abdominal symptoms
      3. Accurate and highly specific in the diagnosis of SBO
      4. Dilated loops of bowel filled with fluids with or without peristalsis are readily seen.
      5. Not commonly the first choice in the initial workup
   C. Barium radiography confirms the diagnosis if there is uncertainty.
      1. Oral administration of about 100 ml of Gastrografin or barium followed by plain abdominal x-ray. If the contrast reaches the cecum within 24 hr, it is 95% likely there is a partial SBO. Otherwise, it should be considered a complete obstruction, and surgical intervention must be considered.
   D. Small bowel follow-through using barium can evaluate an SBO caused by Crohn's disease by identifying a tight stricture in the terminal ileum.
   E. CT scan is superior in identifying the cause of the SBO (such as internal hernia, Crohn's disease, mass, and ischemia) or signs of intestinal compromise such as ischemia, necrosis, pneumatosis, or pneumoperitoneum.
      1. Shows abdomen in cross section to uniquely diagnose
      2. Used to decide the level and cause of obstruction when undetermined by x-ray
      3. Superior to ultrasound and x-ray, with 94% accuracy in diagnosing SBO
      4. Reveals dilated loops of bowel proximal to the obstruction and decompressed or collapsed bowel distally

F. Multidetector CT scan assists in diagnosing SBO due to matted adhesions or single adhesive band; more sensitive than the standard CT

G. Small bowel feces sign
1. Found in CT scan of 50% of patients and common in high-grade obstruction. It is not a useful finding in SBO by itself.
2. Solid material containing gas bubbles found in a segment of dilated bowel
3. Be careful not to mistake feces in the cecum for SBO at the ileocecal valve

H. Whirl sign
1. Found in CT scan of SBO
2. A "swirl" of mesenteric fat and soft tissue attenuation with loops of intestine adjacent to the surrounding intestinal vessels

I. A key diagnostic sign is finding a discrete transition point between dilated SBO and collapsed, nondistended SBO; this localizes the point of obstruction.

VII. **Management**

A. Nil per os (NPO; nothing by mouth) — bowel rest

B. Rapid intravenous fluids and electrolyte replacement with isotonic solution with potassium provided there is adequate kidney function. Total parenteral nutrition (TPN) and nutritional support/dietary consult may be considered to provide adequate nutrition for partial bowel obstruction and recuperation after complete bowel obstruction.

C. Nasogastric tube (NGT) to low wall suction—for nasogastric bowel decompression and to prevent aspiration from vomiting

D. Foley catheter to accurately monitor intake and output

E. Obtain blood cultures, complete blood count (CBC), comprehensive metabolic panel (CMP), arterial blood gas (ABG) test, serum lactate, and amylase/lipase, in addition to diagnostic imaging

F. Initiate antibiotics for patients with suspected perforation or small bowel obstruction in setting of diverticulitis (e.g., cefoxitin [Mefoxin] piggyback, 2 grams IV every 6 hr , cefotetan [Cefotan], 2 grams IV every 12 hr). There is no role for antimicrobial therapy in uncomplicated small bowel obstruction.

G. Partial obstructions usually resolve spontaneously within a few days

H. Surgical consultation is indicated for complete obstruction or for partial obstruction that fails to improve with traditional treatment

I. Laparoscopic adhesiolysis for SBO due to adhesions

LARGE BOWEL OBSTRUCTION

I. Definition

    A. Large bowel (intestinal) obstruction occurs when there is a blockage in the large bowel that prevents food from passing through. The blockage cuts off blood supply to the bowel and a part of it dies. When this happens, the pressure causes a leak that spreads bacteria into the body or blood (translocation).

II. Etiology/Predisposing Factors

    A. Cancers of the:

        1. Colon (primary cause)

        2. Stomach

        3. Ovary

        4. Lung

        5. Breast

    B. Abdominal surgery

    C. Abdominal radiation

III. Signs and symptoms

    A. A history of bowel movements, flatus, obstipation, and associated symptoms should be obtained. Complaints in patients with LBO may include the following:

        1. Abdominal distention

        2. Nausea and vomiting

        3. Crampy abdominal pain

    B. Other symptoms that may be diagnostically significant include the following:

        1. Abrupt onset of symptoms (suggestive of an acute obstructive event)

        2. Chronic constipation, long-term cathartic use, and straining at stools (suggestive of diverticulitis or carcinoma)

        3. Changes in stool caliber (strongly suggestive of carcinoma)

        4. Recurrent left lower quadrant abdominal pain over several years (suggestive of diverticulitis, a diverticular stricture, or similar problems)

IV. Physical Exam Findings

    A. Although a complete physical examination is necessary, the examination should place special emphasis on the following key areas:

        1. Abdomen (inspection, auscultation, percussion, and palpation —evaluate bowel sounds, tenderness, rigidity, guarding, and any mass or fullness

        2. Inguinal and femoral regions—in particular, look for a possible incarcerated hernia

        3. Rectum—assess anal patency (in a neonate), contents of anal vault, and stool consistency; perform fecal occult blood testing as appropriate

V. **Laboratory/Diagnostics**

   A. The following laboratory studies may be helpful:

   1. Complete blood count (CBC)
   2. Hematocrit
   3. Prothrombin time (PT)
   4. Type and crossmatch
   5. Serum chemistries
   6. Serum lactate (if bowel ischemia is a consideration)
   7. Urinalysis
   8. Stool guaiac test

   B. Imaging modalities that may be considered are as follows:

   1. Plain radiography (flat and upright)

      a. Upright chest: useful screen for free air which would suggest perforation and ileus rather than obstruction. The absence of free air does not exclude perforation (this finding may be absent in half of all perforations).

      b. Flat and upright abdominal film: can help distinguish severe constipation from bowel obstruction. Plain films may also help localize the site of obstruction (large vs. small bowel).

      c. Sigmoid or cecal volvulus may have a kidney-bean appearance on the abdominal films

      d. Intramural air is an ominous sign that suggests colonic ischemia

   2. Contrast radiography with enema
   3. Computed tomography (CT)—this is the imaging modality of choice if a colonic obstruction is clinically suspected; contrast-enhanced CT can help distinguish between partial and complete obstruction, ileus, and small-bowel obstruction

VI. **Management**

   A. Initial therapy in patients with suspected large-bowel obstruction (LBO) includes volume resuscitation, appropriate preoperative broad-spectrum antibiotics, and timely surgical consultation

   B. A nasogastric tube should be considered for patients with severe colonic distention and vomiting. The patient's intravascular volume is usually depleted, and early intravenous fluid (IVF) resuscitation with isotonic saline or Ringer lactate solution is necessary.

   C. Surgical intervention is frequently indicated, depending on the cause of the obstruction. Closed loop obstructions, bowel ischemia, and volvulus are surgical emergencies.

MESENTERIC ISCHEMIA

I. **Definition**

   A. Mesenteric ischemia results when the bloodstream fails to carry sufficient amounts of oxygen and other nutrients to meet intestinal needs.

B. Ischemia may be related to an artery occluded by an embolus or thrombus, or no physical occlusion may be present.

II. Etiology

A. Acute arterial occlusion—occurs on patients who are older than 60 years of age; 3:1 male to female ratio

    1. Embolism—cardiac embolization causes 40%–50% of the cases

        a. Atrial fibrillation/flutter

        b. Valvular disease

        c. Atrial thrombus

    2. Thrombus—thrombus formation; a link has been found between prothrombin gene 20210G/A mutation and thrombosis of digestive vessels

        a. Arterial thrombus—may occur on atheromatous plaque

        b. Spontaneously (in women on oral contraceptives)

        c. Surgical accidents

        d. Abdominal trauma

        e. Tumors

B. Mesenteric venous thrombosis—patients tend to be younger (50s–60s)

    1. Primary coagulopathies (anti-thrombin III deficiency, protein C, protein S deficiencies)

    2. Hematologic prothrombotic conditions (polycythemia vera, hyperfibrinogenemia)

    3. Disseminated intravascular coagulopathy

    4. Liver cirrhosis with portal hypertension

    5. Congestive heart failure

    6. Low-flow states (abdominal trauma, intra-abdominal infections, systemic hypotension)

    7. Pancreatitis

C. Nonocclusive mesenteric vascular disease or nonocclusive mesenteric ischemia is more common than the preceding conditions and is related to low-flow conditions and mesenteric vasoconstrictive states. The mesenteric flow is slowed down, not by an obstructive mechanism, but by arterial spasm due to pharmacotherapy or physiologic response to shock, sepsis, or cardiac dysfunction.

    1. Congestive heart failure

    2. Aortic stenosis

    3. Shock

    4. Cardiac arrhythmias

    5. Vasoconstrictor drugs

III. Clinical manifestations

A. Severe cramping and generalized or periumbilical abdominal pain that is out of proportion to the clinical exam presentation

B. Early in the course of the disorder, no abnormalities are found on examination. Diagnosis requires a high index of suspicion.

C. Possible rectal bleeding with colonic ischemia

  D. Hypotension and abdominal distention suggest infarction

IV. **Laboratory/diagnostic findings**

  A. Leukocytosis

  B. Lactic acidosis—in the late stages, suggests infarction

  C. Creatine kinase

  D. Duplex ultrasound—shows bowel spasm and vessel occlusion in the early stages; reveals fluid-filled intestinal lumen and decreased or absent peristalsis in the late stages.

  E. CT angiography—reveals an emboli, thrombi, or stenosis in the lumen of the vessel in the early stage; reveals site of infarct, ileus, and bowel thinning in the late stage.

  F. Mesenteric arteriography (digital subtraction angiography [DSA]) —useful in locating vascular occlusion

  G. Barium contrast radiography—"thumbprinting" or thickening of the intestinal wall in late stages

  H. Contrast-enhanced magnetic resonance angiography has sensitivity and specificity approaching those of DSA in the detection of mesenteric ischemia

  I. CT scan imaging has evolved over several years; findings include focal or segmental bowel wall thickening, submucosal edema or hemorrhage, pneumatosis, and portal venous gas

  J. Contrast-enhanced CT detects acute mesenteric ischemia

  K. Helical CT has improved image quality and scanning times and can be used to detect nonvascular visceral abnormalities

  L. Biphasic mesenteric multidetector CT angiography (similar to CT arteriography)—efficient diagnostic tool for accurate and timely discovery of mesenteric ischemic changes

V. **Management**

  A. Occlusive disease

   1. NPO

   2. Transcatheter administration of papaverine infusion, 30–60 mg/hr within 24–48 hr

   3. Embolectomy or bypass of the occluded vessel to prevent infarction. Abdominal exploration and open surgical revascularization.

   4. If infarction has occurred, resection of that part of the bowel should be performed.

   5. Fluids and supportive care

   6. TPN may be needed and may be continued indefinitely if a large portion of the bowel is resected.

  B. Nonocclusive disease

   1. Correct hypovolemia

   2. Supportive care for heart failure, pancreatitis, or other underlying conditions

   3. Remove vasoconstricting agents and digoxin

C. The goals are to restore intestinal perfusion, reverse ischemia, and prevent infarction.

D. If vasopressors are required, β-adrenergic agonists, such as low-dopamine and dobutamine, are preferred.

E. NGT for decompression

F. Foley catheter for accurate intake and output measurement

G. Begin antibiotic coverage before surgery if peritonitis is suspected (broad spectrum for Gram-negative bacteria and anaerobes).
1. Imipenem-cilastatin, 500 mg IV every 6 hr
2. Meropenem, 1 gram IV every 8 hr
3. Doripenem, 500 mg IV every 8 hr
4. Piperacillin-tazobactam, 3.375 grams IV every 6 hr
5. Cefepime, 2 grams IV every 8 hr plus metronidazole, 500 mg IV every 8 hr
6. Ceftazidime, 2 grams IV every 8 hr plus metronidazole, 500 mg IV every 8 hr

H. Vasodilator drugs can also be administered via an intra-arterial catheter placed during angiography.
1. Papaverine (Paverine, Pavabid) infusion, 30–60 mg/hr
2. Vasodilator prostaglandins

I. Pain control with opioids such as morphine or hydromorphone (Dilaudid)

J. Stent placement for stenosis or occlusions have been effective as an adjunct therapy

K. Angioplasty or surgical revascularization is the primary method of treatment for chronic mesenteric ischemia.

L. Systemic anticoagulation is warranted in venous thrombotic event of the bowels that are inoperable; heparin therapy is the common choice of treatment.

BIBLIOGRAPHY

Adler, G., Parczewski, M., Czerska, E., Loniewska, B., Kaczmarczyk, M., Gumprecht, J., . . . Ciechanowicz, A. (2010). An age-related decrease in factor V Leiden frequency among Polish subjects. *Journal of Applied Genetics, 51*(3), 337–341.

Aschoff, A. J., Stuber, G., Becker, B. W., Hoffman, M. H. K., Schmitz, B. L., Schelzig, H., . . . Jaeckle, T. (2009). Evaluation of acute mesenteric ischemia: Accuracy of biphasic mesenteric multidetector CT angiography. *Abdominal Imaging, 34*, 345–357. doi:10.1007/s00261–008–9392–8

Baumgart, D. (2012). *Crohn's disease and ulcerative colitis from epidemiology and immunobiology to a rational diagnostic and therapeutic approach.* New York, NY: Springer.

Brott, T. G., Hobson, R. W., Howard, G., Roubin, G. S., Clark, W. M., Brooks, W., . . . Meschia, J. F. (2010). Stenting versus endarterectomy for treatment of carotid-artery stenosis. *The New England Journal of Medicine, 363*, 11–23.

Carr, J. C. (2012). *Magnetic resonance angiography principles and applications.* New York, NY: Springer.

Dayton, M. T., Dempsey, D. T., Larson, G. M., & Posner, A. R. (2012). New paradigms in the treatment of small bowel obstruction. *Current Problems in Surgery, 49*(11), 642–717. doi:1067/j.cpsurg.2012.06.005

Ferri, F. (2014). *Ferri's practical guide* (9th ed.). London, UK: Elsevier Health Sciences.

Harrison, T. R. (2012). *Harrison's manual of medicine* (18th ed.). New York, NY: McGraw-Hill Medical.

Krupp, M. A. (2011). *Current medical diagnosis & treatment.* New York, NY: McGraw-Hill.

Mason, V. (2014). *Nurse practitioner's guide on how to start an independent practice.* Quanah, TX: Quanah Publishing.

Ravipati, M., Katragadda, S., Go, B., & Zarling, E. J. (2011, August). Acute mesenteric ischemia: Diagnostic challenge in clinical practice. *Practical Gastroenterology*, 35–43. Retrieved from http://www.practicalgastro.com/ pdf/ August11/RavipatiArticle.pdf

Reginelli, A., Gebovese, E. A., Cappabianca, S., Iacobellis, F., Beritto, D., Fonio, P., . . . Grassi, R. (2013). Intestinal ischemia: US-CT findings correlations [Supplement 1]. *Critical Ultrasound Journal, 3*, 1–11. Retrieved from http:// www.criticalultrasoundjournal.com/content/pdf/2036–7902–5-S1-S7.pdf

Rubin, G. D., & Rofsky, N. M. (2009). *CT and MR angiography: Comprehensive vascular assessment.* Philadelphia, PA: Wolters Kluwer Health/Lippincott Williams & Wilkins.

Sarac, T. P., Altinel, O., Kashyap, V., Bena, J., Lyden, S., Sruvastava, S., . . . Clair, D. (2008). Endovascular treatment of stenotic and occluded visceral arteries for chronic mesenteric ischemia. *Journal of Vascular Surgery, 47*, 485–491. doi:10.1016/j.jvs.2007.11.046

Silva, A. C., Pimenta, M., & Guimaraes, L. S. (2009). Small bowel obstruction: What to look for. *Radiographics, 29*, 423–439. doi:10.1148/rg.292085514

Sise, M. J. (2014). Acute mesenteric ischemia. *Surgical Clinics of North America, 94*(1), 165–181.

Skinner, H. B. (2014). *Current diagnosis & treatment in orthopedics* (5th ed.). New York, NY: McGraw-Hill Medical.

Solomkin, J. S., Mazuski, J. E., Bradley, J. S., Rodvold, K. A., Goldstein, E. J., Baron, E. J., . . . Bartlett, J. G. (2010). Diagnosis and management of complicated intra-abdominal infection in adults and children: Guidelines by the Surgical Infection Society and the Infectious Diseases Society of America. *Clinical Infectious Diseases, 50,* 133–164.

Stanley, A., & Schneider, J. G. (2013). Mesenteric ischemia. In C. J. Yeo, J. B. Matthews, D. W. Mcfadden, J. H. Pemberton, & J. H. Peters (Eds.), *Shakelford's surgery of the alimentary tract* (pp. 1075–1093). Philadelphia, PA: Elsevier.

Winkel, N. V. D., Cheragwandi, A., Nieboer, K., Van Tussenbroek, F., De Vogelaere, K., & Delvaux, G. (2014). Superior mesenteric arterial branch occlusion causing partial jejunal ischemia: A case report. *Journal of Medical Case Reports, 6*(48).

Wyers, M. C. (2010). Acute mesenteric ischemia: Diagnostic approach and surgical treatment. *Seminars in Vascular Surgery*, *23*, 9–20. doi:10.1053/j.semvascsurg.2009.12.002

CHAPTER 41

Gastrointestinal Bleeding

NICOLE A. PEREZ • CHARLENE M. MYERS

ESOPHAGEAL VARICES

I.   Definition

    A. Dilated submucosal veins that may develop in patients with underlying portal hypertension that can result in severe GI bleeding

    B. Varices can rupture at any moment and become a medical emergency.

    C. Three of ten patients will die from the initial hemorrhage

    D. Overall mortality reaches nearly 60% because rebleeding claims the lives of another 3 of 10 patients

II.   Etiology

    A. Cirrhosis—most common

    B. Portal venous pressure of at least 12 mmHg is needed for varices to bleed (normal pressure, 2–6 mmHg)

    C. Bleeding from esophageal varices usually occurs in the distal 5 cm of the esophagus and in the upper portion of the stomach.

    D. Aspirin, used alone or in combination with other nonsteroidal anti-inflammatory drugs, has been associated with a first variceal bleeding episode in patients with cirrhosis.

III.   Clinical manifestations

    A. Hematemesis

    B. Melena

    C. Hematochezia (indicates massive bleed, more than 1,000 ml)

    D. Abdominal discomfort

    E. Signs and symptoms of hypovolemia or shock

IV.   Laboratory/diagnostics

    A. Esophagogastroduodenoscopy (EGD) is the gold standard for the diagnosis of esophageal varices

    B. Complete blood count (CBC)

1. Hemoglobin/hematocrit is normal, then decreases because of volume resuscitation
2. WBC count elevates as a result of the body's attempt to restore homeostasis
3. Platelet count increases then decreases because of attempts to restore homeostasis and finally reflects true blood loss

C. Coagulation panel
   1. Prolonged prothrombin time (PT) and partial thromboplastin time (PTT) as well as increased INR due to decreased synthetic activity of liver

D. Electrolyte panel, liver function test, and arterial blood gas
   1. K+: decreases as a result of emesis, then may increase due to acute kidney injury from hypovolemia
   2. Na++: decreases, then increases as a result of hemoconcentration/fluid resuscitation ·
   3. Ca++: normal or decreased
   4. Hyperglycemia: stress response
   5. BUN/Creatinine ratio: elevated because of poor perfusion to the kidneys
   6. Lactate levels: elevated (lactic acidosis related to anaerobic metabolism)
   7. Aspartate aminotransferase (AST)/alanine aminotransferase (ALT) ratio and bilirubin level are usually abnormal in patients with underlying chronic liver disease
   8. Albumin: usually low due to several reasons such as poor synthetic function of liver and poor nutrition in such patients
   9. Arterial blood gases: respiratory alkalosis/metabolic acidosis

E. Barium studies: can be performed to define the presence of peptic ulcers, bleeding sites, tumors, and inflammation

V. **Management**

A. Emergency resuscitation
   1. Insert two large-bore (16-gauge) intravenous lines, and establish central venous pressure (CVP) line access
   2. Laboratory/diagnostics: blood type and cross match, PT/PTT/INR, complete blood count (CBC), electrolyte panel, lactate, renal, and liver function tests
   3. Infuse crystalloids/colloid/blood products (lactated Ringer solution or normal saline) for treatment of hypotension until blood products can be administered. (Note: Overzealous hydration increases portal pressure and can exacerbate or cause rebleeding of varices.)
      a. Maintain
         i. Systolic blood pressure higher than 110 mmHg,
         ii. CVP 10 mmHg or less, and
         iii. Pulmonary capillary wedge pressure 8 mmHg or less (if pulmonary artery catheter is in place)

    b. Administer fresh frozen plasma for elevated international normalized ratio (INR)

    c. Administer platelets or cryoprecipitate depending on platelets or fibrinogen levels, respectively

  4. Administer oxygen at 5–10 L/min

  5. Insert a Foley catheter

  6. Nothing by mouth (NPO)—insert nasogastric tube (NGT)

    a. However, NGT insertion is contraindicated during active hematemesis.

  7. Consult a surgeon and a gastroenterologist

B. 60%–80% of patients stop bleeding spontaneously; however, without therapy, more than half rebleed within 1 week

C. Emergency endoscopy

  1. Endoscopic band ligation—most effective

  2. Sclerotherapy with the use of agents such as ethanolamine or tetradecyl sulfate or band ligation

D. Octreotide (Sandostatin), 50 mcg IV bolus, followed by 3–5 days of continuous infusion of 50 mcg/hr, works similarly to vasopressin, has better adverse effect profile, and is better at controlling variceal hemorrhage

E. Vasopressin—vasoconstrictor that decreases portal pressures by reducing splanchnic flow (successful in only 50% of cases)

  1. Dose: 0.2–0.4 units/min to a maximum of 0.8 units/min

  2. Taper down over 24 hr after the bleeding is controlled

  3. Monitor for vasopressin-induced adverse effects

    a. Chest pain

    b. Sweating

    c. Skin pallor

  4. Rarely used in U.S. for acute variceal hemorrhage management, due to adverse effect profile and greater benefit of octreotide

  5. Requires addition of nitroglycerin 40–400 mcg/min, titrated to maintain SBP over 90. Vasopressin should never be used without a nitrate

F. May replete with vitamin K, IM or IV, due low liver stores in cirrhosis (important for clotting factors II, VII, IX, and X; and proteins C and S)

G. Lactulose, 30 mL PO/NG BID for patients with severe liver disease, to prevent encephalopathy (titrate to 2–3 stools/day)

H. Balloon tamponade may be necessary to control bleeding

  1. Sengstaken-Blakemore tube (three ports) or

  2. Minnesota tube (four ports)

    a. Normal inflation pressure is 20–45 mmHg

    b. Inflation pressures must be continually monitored

    c. Balloons should be deflated every 8–12 hr

3. The esophageal balloon must be deflated before the gastric tube is removed to prevent tube displacement upward and occlusion of the airway
   a. Keep scissors at the bedside
   b. Possible complications:
      i. Gastric balloon rupture—occlusion of airway
      ii. Esophageal rupture—characterized by severe back pain
      iii. Ulcerations of the esophageal or gastric mucosa

VI. **Prevention of rebleeding**
   A. Routine follow-up with endoscopy
   B. β-blockers
      1. Propanolol (Inderal), 20 mg PO BID or nadolol (Corgard), 40 mg PO daily
      2. Adjusted to the maximal tolerated dose
         a. Increased gradually until heart rate falls by 25% or reaches 55 beats per minute
      3. Used frequently in combination with sclerotherapy
   C. Transjugular intrahepatic portosystemic stent (TIPS)—for patients with recurrent bleeds despite the therapies listed previously
   D. Portosystemic shunt—usually reserved for patients for whom β-blockers have failed or for those who are noncompliant (TIPS is used more commonly than portosystemic shunt)
   E. Liver transplantation

VII. **Prevention of first episode of variceal bleeding**
   A. A high mortality rate is associated with variceal hemorrhage
   B. All patients with cirrhosis should undergo diagnostic endoscopy to locate any varices that may be present.
   C. Banding prophylactically has been noted to decrease the incidence of first-time bleeding
   D. Nonselective β-blockers (i.e., propanolol)
   E. Sclerotherapy in patients who have never had a bleed results in increased mortality compared with those treated with a placebo or with β-blockers and, therefore, is not recommended.

UPPER GASTROINTESTINAL BLEEDING

I. **Definition**
   A. Acute upper gastrointestinal bleeding refers to loss of blood within the intraluminal gastrointestinal tract from any location between the upper esophagus and the duodenum at the ligament of Treitz.
   B. Patient history is very important in determination of the time of onset of bleeding, severity, and possible causes

II. **Etiology**
   A. Peptic ulcer disease (PUD)
   B. Esophageal and gastric varices as a result of portal hypertension
   C. Mallory-Weiss tear

D. Vascular abnormalities

E. Neoplasm

F. Gastric or duodenal erosion

G. Aortoenteric fistula

H. Dieulafoy vascular malformation—submucosal artery usually located in the proximal stomach abnormally close to the mucosa that causes erosion of the epithelium and may result in massive upper tract bleeding

I. Hematobilia—blood in the bile or bile ducts

J. Ménétrier disease

   1. Gastritis of unknown cause

   2. Marked by excessive proliferation of stomach mucosal folds

III. **Clinical manifestations**

A. Abdominal discomfort

B. Hematemesis presenting as bright red vomitus or "coffee grounds" emesis

C. Melena, in most cases evidenced by 50–100 mL of blood in the upper gastrointestinal (UGI) tract; hematochezia in massive UGI bleeds (more than 1,000 ml)

D. Signs and symptoms of hypovolemic shock, such as hypotension and tachycardia, are present in severe cases or with acute loss (e.g., more than 40% blood volume).

E. Orthostatic changes are noted in patients with a loss of 20% or more of blood volume.

F. Skin pallor

G. Spider angiomas, palmar erythema, caput medusae, and icterus suggest chronic liver disease

H. NGT aspirate—bright red blood indicates active bleeding and is associated with a higher mortality than melena

IV. **Laboratory/diagnostics**

A. Blood type and cross match for at least 4 units of packed red blood cells

B. Hemoglobin and hematocrit poorly reflect degree and severity of blood loss

C. PT/PTT/INR, platelet count, electrolytes, BUN/creatinine, and liver enzymes

D. ECG in the elderly and in patients with coronary artery disease (CAD) may indicate ischemia related to severe anemia

E. Barium studies are of little value

F. Endoscopy is both diagnostic and therapeutic. Endoscopic evaluation of the UGI tract should be considered in asymptomatic patients who present with a high suspicion for liver cirrhosis and esophageal varices who have a positive fecal occult blood test.

G. Capsule endoscopy: small camera ingested to examine entire length of small bowel. Provides direct visualization of the mucosa and sends images to the computer to be reviewed. Intervention cannot be provided by this method.

H. Nuclear bleeding scan and angiography

V.   Management

A. Rapid clinical evaluation and assessment of hemodynamic status (i.e., airway, breathing, and circulation [ABCs])

B. Endotracheal intubation may be indicated

C. Consult with a gastroenterologist and a surgeon

D. Patients with significant blood loss

1. Insert two large-bore intravenous lines (16-gauge) or a central line for fluid resuscitation

2. Blood transfusions for high-risk patients are made on a case-by-case basis with the goal to adequately oxygenate end organs and tissues

   a. Keep hematocrit above 30%

   b. Young/healthy patients: maintain hematocrit above 20%

3. Patients with coagulopathies (elevated INR): 1–2 units fresh frozen plasma and 2.5–10 mg vitamin K IM or IV

4. Low platelet counts: transfuse platelets

E. NGT placement—tap water gastric lavage

1. If aspirate does not clear after 2–3 L, continued active bleeding is assumed

2. More urgent resuscitation and endoscopic interventions are indicated

F. Endoscopy—should be considered in all patients with UGI bleeding

1. Should be performed as an emergency procedure in a patient with active hemorrhage after stabilization

2. Active, self-limiting bleeds: perform within 24 hr, unless one of the following occurs:

   a. Portal hypertension or aortoenteric fistula is suspected

   b. Bleeding recurs after initial stabilization

3. Patients with chronic blood loss may undergo elective endoscopy.

4. Treatment options include the following:

   a. Thermal coagulation (i.e., cauterization)

   b. Injection therapy with epinephrine or sclerosant

   c. Band ligation

G. Acute pharmacologic therapies

1. IV proton pump inhibitors

   a. Pantoprazole (Protonix) or esomeprazole (Nexium), 80 mg IV bolus, followed by continuous infusion of 8 mg/hr

H. Endoscopic therapy

   a. Band ligation

   b. Sclerotherapy

        c. Laser therapy

        d. Clips

I. Balloon tamponade

J. Surgery is indicated for the following:

    1. Severe bleeding or rebleeding in which two endoscopic treatments have failed;

    2. Massive exsanguinating hemorrhage in which resuscitative efforts have failed;

    3. When more than 6–8 units of blood were needed during the first 24-hr period;

    4. Slow, continuous bleeding that lasts longer than 48 hr; and

    5. Nonsurgical patients, consult an interventional radiologist for arteriography/embolization

K. Intra-arterial embolization or vasopressin (thermal ablation) —performed by interventional radiologists and rarely used; associated with severe adverse effects

L. TIPS

M. Supportive care

N. Antibiotic prophylaxis

    1. Significantly reduces bacterial infections and may reduce all-cause mortality, bacterial infection mortality, rebleeding events, and hospitalization length

    2. Short term (7 day maximum) antibiotic prophylaxis should be instituted in any patient with cirrhosis and GI hemorrhage.

        a. Norfloxacin (Noroxin), 400 mg PO twice a day or ciprofloxacin (Cipro) IV (in patients whom oral administration is not possible)

    3. Patients with advanced cirrhosis, particularly in areas with high resistance to quinolone organisms

        a. Ceftriaxone (Rocephin), 1 gram/day

LOWER GASTROINTESTINAL BLEEDING

I.   **Definition**

    A. Bleeding that originates below the ligament of Treitz, for example, in the small intestine or colon

    B. Up to 10% of patients who present with hematochezia have a UGI source of bleeding (e.g., PUD)

II.   **Etiology**

    A. Diverticulosis (40% of patients)

    B. Vascular ectasias

        1. Painless bleeding ranging from acute hematochezia to chronic occult blood loss

        2. Most common in patients older than 70 years or in patients with chronic renal failure

    C. Neoplasms

       1. Benign or malignant

       2. Usually manifest by chronic, occult blood loss

       3. Sometimes evidenced by periodic hematochezia

       4. Occasionally manifests by massive lower tract bleeding

   D. Inflammatory bowel disease (i.e., ulcerative colitis)

       1. Abdominal pain

       2. Tenesmus

          a. Spasmodic contraction of the anal sphincter

          b. Pain

          c. Persistent desire to empty the bowel, with involuntary ineffectual straining efforts

       3. Urgency

   E. Anorectal disease

       1. Small amounts of bright red blood on the toilet tissue, streaking in the stool, or dripping into the toilet

       2. Rarely results in significant blood loss

       3. Painless bleeding is indicative of internal hemorrhoids

       4. Painful bleeding may indicate anal fissure

   F. Ischemic colitis

       1. Seen in the elderly who have a history of atherosclerosis

       2. Results in hematochezia or bloody diarrhea

       3. Usually associated with pain and cramps

   G. Others

       1. Radiation-induced colitis

       2. Infectious colitis

          a. *Shigella* spp.

          b. *Campylobacter* spp.

          c. *Escherichia coli*

       3. Other systemic conditions (rare)

III. **Clinical manifestations**

   A. Most patients with lower gastrointestinal bleeding present with hematochezia; although occasionally, melena will be present in bleeding from the upper small intestine.

   B. Chronic blood loss

       1. Skin pallor

       2. Tachycardia

       3. Postural hypotension

   C. Acute blood loss

       1. Altered mental status

       2. Hypotension

       3. Shock

       4. Gross evidence of rectal blood loss

   D. Rule out vaginal and urethral bleeding in females

IV. **Laboratory/diagnostics**

   A. Rule out UGI source by placing an NGT

    B. CBC

        1. Anemia—when blood loss has been subacute or chronic

        2. CBC may be normal in acute and massive bleeds because of hemoconcentration.

    C. Serum iron, total iron-binding capacity, and ferritin help to confirm iron deficiency when the patient is anemic and GI blood loss is suspected.

    D. Fecal occult blood test in stable patients whose GI blood loss is questionable

    E. Anoscopy and sigmoidoscopy

    F. Colonoscopy should be performed in all patients with significant lower gastrointestinal bleeding within 6–24 hr after admission to the hospital after the colon has been cleansed.

    G. Arteriography or technetium-99m (^{99m}Tc)–labeled red blood cell scintigraphy

    H. Small intestine push enteroscopy is used in recurrent bleeding of unknown origin; consists of a long, small-diameter endoscope that may reach to the distal jejunum

    I. Capsule imaging may help in the identification of distal small intestinal bleeds.

V. **Management**

    A. Resuscitate hemodynamically compromised patients

        1. Place two large-bore (16-gauge) intravenous lines and/or pulmonary artery catheter

        2. Administer lactated Ringer solution or normal saline and/or blood products

        3. Monitor heart rate, blood pressure, mean arterial pressure, and pulmonary capillary wedge pressure/CVP

        4. Titrate infusion rate to maintain perfusion

    B. Discontinue aspirin and all nonsteroidal anti-inflammatory drugs; treat the cause of the bleeding

    C. IV proton pump inhibitor (treatment of choice)

        1. Pantoprazole (Protonix) or esomeprazole (Nexium), 80 mg IV bolus, followed by continuous infusion of 8 mg/hr

    D. Blood type and cross match for 4 units of packed red blood cells

    E. Colonoscopic therapies—Electrocoagulation is useful in the treatment of patients with vascular ectasia of the colon.

    F. Angiographic techniques

        1. Intra-arterial vasopressin

        2. Embolization

    G. Endoscopic hemostatic therapy

    H. Surgery

        1. Depends on the nature and location of the bleeding

        2. Usually a segmental or subtotal colectomy is indicated

BIBLIOGRAPHY

Alford, K. F. (2012). Gastrointestinal alterations. In M. L. Sole, D. Klein, & M. Moseley (Eds.), *Introduction to critical care nursing* (6th ed., pp. 312–315). Philadelphia, PA: WB Saunders.

Barkun, A. N., Bardou, M., Kuipers, E. J., Sung, J., Hunt, R. H., Martel, M., . . . Sinclair, P. (2010). International consensus recommendations on the management of patients with nonvariceal upper gastrointestinal bleeding. *Annals of Internal Medicine, 152*(2), 101–113.

Chavez-Tapia, N. C., Barrientos-Gutierrez, T., Tellez-Avila, F. I., Soares-Weiser, K., & Uribe, M. (2010). Antibiotic prophylaxis for cirrhotic patients with upper gastrointestinal bleeding. *Cochrane Database of Systematic Reviews, 9*, CD002907. doi:10.1002/14651858.CD002907.pub2

Chen, Y.-I., & Peter, G. (2012). Prevention and management of gastroesophageal varices in cirrhosis. *International Journal of Hepatology*, 1–6.

Ferri, F. F. (2010). *Practical guide to the care of the medical patient* (8th ed.). Philadelphia, PA: Mosby Elsevier.

Ferlitsch, A., Schoefl, R., Puespoek, A., Miehsler, M., Schoeniger-Hekele, M., Hofer, H., Gangl, A., & Homoncik, M. (2010). Effect of virtual endoscopy simulator training on performance of upper gastrointestinal endoscopy in patients: A randomized controlled trial. *Endoscopy, 42*(12), 1049–1056.

Garcia-Tsao, G., & Bosch, J. (2010). Management of varices and variceal hemorrhage in cirrhosis. *The New England Journal of Medicine, 362*, 823–832.

Inadomi, J. M., Bhattacharya, R., Dominitz, J. A., & Hwang, Ho J. (2013). In T. Yamada (Ed.), *Yamada's handbook of gastroenterology* (3rd ed.). Hoboken, NJ: Wiley-Blackwell.

Kappelman, M. D., Palmer, L., Boyle, B. M., & Rubin, D. T. (2010). Quality of care in inflammatory bowel disease: A review and discussion. *Inflammatory Bowel Diseases, 16*(1), 125–133.

Laine, L. (2013). Gastrointestinal bleeding. In D. L. Longo, A. S. Fauci, D. Kasper, S. Hauser, J. Jameson, & J. Loscalzo (Eds.), *Harrison's principles of internal medicine* (18th ed., pp. 320–324). New York, NY: McGraw-Hill.

McQuaid, K. R. (2014). Gastrointestinal bleeding. In S. McPhee, S. J. McPhee, M. A. Papadakis, N. Gleason, & G. Quinn (Eds.), *Current medical diagnosis and treatment.* (53rd ed., pp. 563–569). New York, NY: McGraw Hill.

Okten, R. S., Kacar, S., Kucukay, F., Sasmaz, N., & Cumhur, T. (2011). Gastric subthelial masses: Evaluation of multidetector CT (multiplanar reconstruction and virtual gastroscopy) versus endoscopic ultrasonography. *Abdominal Imaging, 37*(4), 519–530.

Sheasgreen, C., & Leontiadis, G. I. (2013). Recent advances on the management of patients with non-variceal upper gastrointestinal bleeding. *Annals of Gastroenterology, 26*(3), 191–197.

Singh, V., & Alexander, J. A. (2009). The evaluation and management of obscure and occult gastrointestinal bleeding. *Abdominal Imaging, 34*(3), 311–319.

Sonomura, T., Ono, W., Sato, M., Sahara, S., Nakata, K., Sanda, H., . . . Kishi, K. (2013). Emergency balloon-occluded retrograde transvenous obliteration for gastric varices. *World Journal of Gastroenterology, 19*(31), 5125–5130. doi:10.3748/wjg.v19.i31.5125

Tajiri, T., Yoshida, H., Obara, K., Onji, M., Kage, M., Kitano, S., . . . Idezuki, Y. (2010). General rules for recording endoscopic findings of esophagogastric varices (2nd ed.). *Digestive Endoscopy, 22*(1), 1–9.

SECTION FIVE

Management of Patients with Genitourinary Disorders

CHAPTER 42

Urinary Tract Infections

MICHELE H. TALLEY • CHARLENE M. MYERS

URINARY TRACT INFECTIONS

I. **Definition**
  A. Presence of a significant number of pathogenic organisms in the urine with the potential to invade tissues of the urinary tract and adjacent structures, including the bladder, urethra, prostate, renal parenchyma (kidneys), and collecting system
  B. Causes inflammation in the urinary epithelium
  C. Associated with a positive urine culture: more than 100,000 colonies in asymptomatic patients and between 100 and 10,000 colonies in symptomatic patients
  D. Classified as lower urinary tract (bladder and urethra) and upper urinary tract (kidney and ureters)
  E. Defined as uncomplicated (occurs in normal working urinary tract) versus complicated (occurs with defects in urinary tract or in individuals with other health problems)

II. **Etiology/incidence**
  A. Urinary tract infection (UTI) is more common in women than in men.
  B. UTIs are the most common bacterial infection in the elderly, and nursing home patients are more likely to have resistant pathogens compared with others of the same age.
  C. Common uropathogens
    1. *Escherichia coli* is the most common causative organism (64.5% of cases)
    2. *Staphylococcus aureus* (6% of cases)
    3. *Proteus mirabilis* (4.7% of cases)
    4. *Klebsiella saprophyticus* (4.3% of cases)
    5. *Enterococcus faecalis* (3.6% of cases)

6. *Proteus vulgaris* (2.7% of cases)
7. *Pseudomonas aeruginosa* (2.4% of cases)
8. *Enterobacter* spp. (1.9% of cases)
9. *Staphylococcus epidermidis* (1.8% of cases)
10. *Providencia* spp. (1.7% of cases)
11. High risk for those patients who are critically ill
12. Elderly patients have gender-associated differences in UTIs
    a. Elderly women most often have *E. coli*
    b. Elderly men are likely to have *P. mirabilis* but may also have *Enterococcus* spp. or coagulase-negative staphylococci
    c. The following organisms are also commonly found in the elderly: *Klebsiella pneumoniae, Serratia* spp., *Citrobacter* spp., *Enterobacter, Morganella morganii,* and *P. aeruginosa*
    d. *Providencia* spp. UTI is found in institutionalized patients
    e. Elderly patients with diabetes often have group B streptococcal UTIs
13. Catheter-associated UTI is caused by a biofilm (a layer of uropathogens living along the catheter); the best strategy to prevent these infections is to avoid catheterization when possible and remove urinary catheters as soon as possible once they are no longer medically necessary.
    a. *Candida* spp. are common fungal causes of UTIs
D. Risk factors for both genders:
   1. Diabetes mellitus
   2. Urinary instrumentation and catheterization
   3. Obstruction of normal flow of urine due to calculi, tumors, and urethral strictures
   4. Neurogenic bladder disease resulting from stroke, multiple sclerosis, and spinal cord injury
   5. Vesicoureteral reflux
E. Contributing factors in women:
   1. Short urethra
   2. Sexual intercourse
   3. Use of a spermicide
   4. Pregnancy
   5. Previous UTI
   6. New sexual partner (within the past year)
   7. History of UTI in first-degree female relative
F. Contributing factors in men:
   1. Prostatic enlargement, resulting in urine residual
   2. Prostatitis
   3. Lack of circumcision
   4. Homosexuality
   5. Having a sexual partner with vaginal colonization by uropathogens
   6. HIV infection

III. Signs/symptoms
  A. Lower urinary tract (cystitis/urethritis/prostatitis)
    1. Dysuria
    2. Urinary frequency
    3. Urgency
    4. Suprapubic pain
    5. Hematuria with bacteriuria
    6. Malodorous urine
    7. Incontinence
    8. Fever and chills are uncommon but may be present
    9. No flank or costovertebral pain
  B. Upper urinary tract (pyelonephritis, renal abscess)
    1. Flank pain or costovertebral-angle tenderness
    2. Fever (temperature higher than 38°F)
    3. Hematuria
    4. Nausea and vomiting
    5. Mental status changes (in elderly patients)
    6. Malaise
    7. Shaking chills (rigors)
    8. Tachypnea (related to fever)
    9. Tachycardia (related to fever)
    10. If symptoms last for longer than 3 days, abscess formation should be considered.

IV. Laboratory/diagnostics
  A. Urine culture and sensitivity testing: The detection of bacteria in the culture is considered the diagnostic gold standard. Culture results are not available until 24 hr after collection. Point-of-care testing aids in early detection.
  B. Point-of-care testing includes urinalysis and urine dipstick tests
    1. Clean-catch urinalysis (diagnose UTI with positive nitrite or leukocyte esterase positive test; may also diagnose UTI with blood in urine)
    2. Urine microscopy
      a. Pyuria: presence of more than 10 leukocytes/ml
      b. Bacteriuria: more than 100,000 bacteria/ml; indicates active infection
      c. Bacterial counts of 10,000–100,000/ml may also indicate infection, especially if accompanied by pyuria.
      d. In urine specimens obtained by suprapubic aspiration or in-and-out catheterization, bacterial colony counts of 100–10,000/ml indicate infection
      e. Occasional erythrocytes, white cell casts, and mild proteinuria may be present in acute pyelonephritis
      f. Elevated erythrocyte sedimentation rate in pyelonephritis

3. Leukocyte esterase dipstick test: positive (purple in 60 seconds) —signifies pyuria or white blood cells (WBCs) in the urine
    a. False positives may occur with kidney stones, tumors, urethritis, and poor collection techniques
    b. False negatives may occur with uncomplicated or early UTIs
4. Nitrate dipstick test: positive for protein, blood, nitrates (pink in 30 seconds)—may be false negative in uncomplicated UTI, with diuretics early in the course of UTI, with inadequate levels of dietary nitrates, or in the presence of bacteria that do not produce nitrate reductase, such as *Staphylococcus saprophyticus*, *Enterococcus*, and *Pseudomonas*

C. CBC: leukocytosis with a left shift in acute pyelonephritis
D. Blood culture may be indicated for suspected pyelonephritis or sepsis.
E. If sexually transmitted infections are suspected, order *Neisseria gonorrhoeae* (GC) culture and chlamydia test.
F. To rule out obstruction, calculi, and papillary necrosis in men with UTIs and in women with recurrent UTIs, consider the following:
   1. X-ray voiding cystourethrography
   2. Computed tomography (CT) scan of the abdomen and pelvis: with and without contrast
   3. Ultrasound: pelvis (urethra)
   4. Magnetic resonance imaging of the pelvis: with and/or without contrast

V. Management

A. Acute cystitis
   1. First-line therapy
      a. Single-dose regimen: fosfomycin trometamol (Monurol), 3-gram sachet in a single dose
      b. Three-day regimen (preferred over single-dose regimen due to high relapse rates related to single-dose regimen) to 7-day regimen
         i. Sulfonamides: trimethoprim-sulfamethoxazole (TMP-SMZ) (Bactrim DS), 160 mg/800 mg BID PO for 3 days (can be ineffective in many patients because of the emergence of resistant organisms)
         ii. Sulfonamides: trimethoprim, 100 mg BID PO for 3 days
            (a) Prescription should be informed by local antimicrobial resistance patterns
         iii. Urinary antiseptics: nitrofurantoin (Macrobid), 100 mg PO BID for 5 days with meals, use with caution in elderly patients
   2. Second-line therapy
      a. Quinolones: ciprofloxacin (Cipro), 250 mg BID PO for 3 days; levofloxacin, 250–500 mg once daily PO for 3 days

    b. β-lactams (e.g., amoxicillin-clavulanate, cefdinir, cefaclor, and cefpodoxime proxetil) for 3–7 days

        i. Appropriate choice for therapy when other recommended agents cannot be used due to inferior efficacy and more adverse effects, compared with other UTI antimicrobials

B. Uncomplicated upper UTI

  1. Outpatient therapy

    a. Quinolones: ciprofloxacin, 500 mg BID PO or 1 gram (extended release) once daily PO for 7 days (may consider giving an initial IV 400 mg dose with the oral dose); levofloxacin, 750 mg once daily PO for 5 days

        i. If fluoroquinolone resistance exceeds 10%, consider giving initial 1 gram ceftriaxone IV or a consolidated 24 hr dose of an aminoglycoside

    b. Sulfonamides: TMP-SMZ, 160 mg/800 mg BID PO for 14 days (if susceptibility is known; if susceptibility is unknown, consider giving initial IV 1 gram ceftriaxone or a consolidated 24-hr dose of an aminoglycoside)

    c. Oral β-lactams for 10–14 days (less effective than fluoroquinolones)

  2. Inpatient therapy

    a. Cefotaxime or ceftriaxone IV

    b. Fluoroquinolone IV (depending on local resistance prevalence for severe or anaphylactic PCN allergic patients)

    c. Aminoglycoside IV with or without ampicillin IV

C. Catheter-associated UTI

  1. If the microorganism is bacterial, treat with an antibiotic for 7–14 days

  2. If candiduria, treat with fluconazole, 200–400 mg/day for 14 days

D. Special considerations

  1. Patients with acute bacterial pyelonephritis

    a. Should be hospitalized

        i. Surgery may be necessary when a structural abnormality or a large stone is blocking the urinary tract.

    b. Inpatient therapy

        i. First-line therapy for complicated polynephritis and nosocomial/hospital-acquired UTI

           (a) Aminoglycosides: gentamicin or tobramycin

               1. Not to be used as monotherapy for pyelonephritis

               2. Doses are individualized and based on normal renal function with defined peak levels of 5–10 mg/L and trough levels less than 2

      3. Aminoglycosides are to be avoided in patients with pre-existing renal disease. Patients with normal renal functions may use a daily dose of 15 mg/kg (Hartford nomogram).

   (b) Penicillins: ampicillin, 1 gram every 4–6 hr IV (should cover *Enterococcus* if Gram-positive cocci present on culture or Gram stain)

   (c) Cephalosporins: cefazolin, 1–2 grams every 8 hr IV; not routinely used for empiric therapy

  ii. Others to consider (based on susceptibility and patient allergies)

   (a) Sulfonamides: TMP/SMX, 160/800 mg every 12 hr IV

   (b) Aminoglycosides: amikacin (reserved for highly resistant organisms), 15 mg/kg/day IV in patients whose renal function meets criteria, individualized to achieve peak of 20–30 mg/L and trough levels less than 10

   (c) Antipseudomonal penicillins: piperacillin, 3 grams every 4 hr IV

   (d) Penicillin-β-lactamase inhibitor combinations: piperacillin/tazobactam, 4 grams/500 mg every 8 hr IV

   (e) Cephalosporins: cefotaxime, 1–2 grams every 8 hr IV; ceftriaxone, 1–2 grams every 24 hr IV; cefepime, 2 grams every 12 hr IV; or ceftazidime, 0.5–2 grams every 8 hr IV. Doses are individualized and based on obesity and pre-existence of pulmonary infections.

   (f) Miscellaneous antibiotic class: aztreonam, 1–2 grams every 6 hr IV (although has limited use, active for Gram-negative bacteria including *P. aeruginosa*; good for those with nosocomial infection when aminoglycosides are contraindicated or when patient penicillin sensitive); imipenem/cilastatin, 500 mg every 6 hr IV (covers broad spectrum of bacteria: Gram-positive, Gram-negative, and anaerobic; active against *Enterococci* and *P. aeruginosa* and resistant organisms; can cause *Candida* superinfection); or vancomycin, 500 mg every 6 hr or 1 gram every 12 hr IV (evaluate renal function)

   (g) Quinolones: ciprofloxacin, 200–400 mg every 12 hr IV, or levofloxacin, 500 mg daily IV

2. Pregnant women

  a. Quinolones cannot be given during pregnancy

    b. Sulfonamides cannot be given near the time of delivery; cephalexin is a reasonable choice

E. Treatment for discomfort

    1. Phenazopyridine hydrochloride (Pyridium), 200 mg PO 3 times a day for 2 days, may be added for discomfort associated with irritation

F. Aseptic techniques are essential if indwelling catheters are required.

    1. Modification of catheter material to confer antimicrobial activity may play an important part in the prevention of catheter-related infection

    2. Silver-impregnated catheters have been shown to effectively reduce the number of catheter-related infections; silver has antimicrobial activity against both Gram-positive and Gram-negative bacteria

G. Behavioral modifications

    1. Recommend abstinence or reduction in sexual activity

    2. Discuss means of contraception other than the use of spermicides as they alter the normal flora of the vagina, thus promoting the colonization of uropathogens

    3. May suggest the following: increase water intake, decrease carbonated drink intake, not delaying urination, and wiping front to back after defecating

H. Consider prophylaxis in patients with recurrent lower UTI

    1. Prophylactic antibiotic selection made on basis of community-resistance patterns, side effects, and cost

    2. Postcoital antimicrobial prophylaxis: single dose of antimicrobial drug as soon as possible after intercourse

        a. Urinary antiseptics: nitrofurantoin, 50–100 mg PO

        b. Sulfonamides: TMP-SMX, 40 mg/200 mg PO or 80 mg/400 mg PO

        c. Sulfonamides: TMP, 100 mg PO

        d. Cephalosporins: cephalexin, 250 mg PO

    3. Continuous prophylaxis with antimicrobial

        a. Urinary antiseptics: nitrofurantoin, 50–100 mg PO at bedtime

        b. Sulfonamides: TMP-SMX, 40 mg/200 mg PO at bedtime

        c. Sulfonamides: TMP, 100 mg PO at bedtime

        d. Cephalosporins: cephalexin, 125–250 mg PO at bedtime

        e. No conclusive evidence supports selection of a particular drug, dosage, duration or schedule of treatment. However, 6 months of treatment, followed by observation for reinfection after discontinuing prophylaxis, has been recommended.

    4. Prophylactic antibiotic selection may reduce the risk of recurrent UTIs in female patients with two episodes of infection in the previous year.

     a. Antibiotic selection should be informed by community resistance patters, side effects, and local costs.

I. No need to repeat urinalysis with culture and sensitivity tests after therapy in uncomplicated cystitis and pyelonephritis; must repeat in pregnant women

J. Emphasize compliance with medication and follow-up

BIBLIOGRAPHY

Baron, E. J., Miller, J. M., Weinstein, M. P., Richter, S. S., Gilligan, P. H., Thompson, R. B., . . . Pritt, B. S. (2013). A guide to utilization of the microbiology laboratory for diagnosis of infectious diseases: 2013 recommendations by the Infectious Diseases Society of America (IDSA) and the American Society for Microbiology (ASM). *Clinical Infectious Diseases, 57*(4), e22-e121.

Giesen, L. G., Cousins, G., Dimitrov, B. D., van de Laar, F. A., & Fahey, T. (2010). Predicting acute uncomplicated urinary tract infection in women: A systematic review of the diagnostic accuracy of symptoms and signs. *BMC Family Practice, 11*, 78–92.

Glass, A. S., Kovshilovskaya, B., & Breyer, B. N. (2012). Sexually transmitted infection and long-term risk of lower urinary tract symptoms. *European Urological Review, 7*(1), 133–136.

Gupta, K., Hooten, T., Naber, K. G., Wullt, B., Colgan, R., Miller, L. G., . . . European Society for Microbiology and Infectious Diseases. (2011). International clinical practice guidelines for the treatment of acute uncomplicated cystitis and pyelonephritis in women: A 2010 update by the Infectious Diseases Society of America and the European Society for Microbiology and Infectious Diseases. *Clinical Infectious Diseases, 52*(5), e103-e120.

Halter, J. B., Ouslander, J. G., Tinetti, M. E., Studenski, S., High, K., & Asthana, S. (Eds.). (2009). *Hazzard's geriatric medicine and gerontology* (6th ed.). New York, NY: McGraw-Hill.

Hooten, T. M. (2012). Uncomplicated urinary tract infection. *NEJM, 366*(11), 1028–1037.

Hooten, T. M., Bradley, S. F., Cardenas, D. D., Colgan, R., Geerlings, S. E., Rice, J. C., . . . Infectious Diseases Society of America. (2010). Diagnosis, prevention, and treatment of catheter-associated urinary tract infection in adults: 2009 international clinical practice guidelines from the Infectious Diseases Society of America. *Clinical Infectious Disease, 50*(5), 625–663.

Kodner, C. M., & Gupton, E. K. (2010). Recurrent urinary tract infections in women: Diagnosis and management. *American Family Physician, 82*(6), 638–643. Retrieved from http://www.aafp.org/afp/2010/0915/p638.pdf.

Lazarus, E., Casalino, D. D., Remer, E. M., Arellano, R. S., Bishoff, J. T., Coursey, C. A., . . . Expert Panel on Urologic Imaging. (2011). *ACR appropriateness criteria recurrent lower urinary tract infection in women.* [online publication]. Reston, VA: American College of Radiology (ACR).

Linhares, I., Raposo, T., Rodrigues, A., & Almeida, A. (2013). Frequency and antimicrobial resistance patterns of bacteria implicated in community urinary tract infections: A ten-year surveillance study (2000–2009). *BMC Infectious Diseases, 13*(19), 1–14. doi:10.1186/1471–2334–13–19

Longo, D. L., Fauci, A. S., Kasper, D. L., Hauser, S., Jameson, J., & Loscalzo, J. (Eds.). (2012). *Harrison's principles of internal medicine* (18th ed.). New York, NY: McGraw-Hill.

Marinosci, F., Zizzo, A., Coppola, A., Rodano, L., Laudisio, R., & Antonelli Incalzi, R. (2013). Carbapenem resistance and mortality in institutionalized elderly with urinary tract infection. *JAMDA, 14*(7), 513–517.

McCance, K. L., Huether, S. E., Brashers, V. L., & Rote, N. S. (Eds.). (2010). *Pathophysiology: The biologic basis for disease in adults and children* (6th ed.). Philadelphia, PA: Mosby Elsevier.

Mishra, B., Srivastava, S., Singh, K, Pandey, A., & Agarwal, J. (2012). Symptom-based diagnosis of urinary tract infection in women: Are we over-prescribing antibiotics? *Interational Journal of Clinical Practice, 66*(5), 493–498.

Sheerin, N. S. (2011). Urinary tract infection. *Medicine, 39*(7), 384–389.

CHAPTER 43

Acute Kidney Injury and Chronic Kidney Disease

STEVEN W. BRANHAM • CHARLENE M. MYERS

PRIMARY KIDNEY REGULATION OF PHYSIOLOGIC FUNCTIONS:

I.   **Acid–base status**
II.   **Maintain water balance**
III.   **Electrolyte balance**
IV.   **Hormone production and metabolism**
V.   **Gluconeogenesis in fasting states**
VI.   **Various regulatory functions are lost at different states of disease progression. In early disease, the onset is often insidious.**

ACUTE KIDNEY INJURY

I.   **Acute kidney injury and chronic kidney disease in perspective**
    A. Acute kidney injury (AKI) is an abrupt loss of kidney function while chronic kidney disease (CKD) can develop over months to years. In both states, the degree of dysfunction is related to cause and comorbid factors.
    B. In AKI, recovery is often attained with medical management, while in CKD, progression is delayed by medical management.
    C. Both conditions may require dialysis based on the degree of dysfunction if conservative measures fail.
    D. AKI in the presence of CKD requires aggressive management to prevent permanent progression of CKD.
    E. Although recovery typically occurs in AKI, the condition is associated with a lifetime risk of developing CKD.

II.   **Definition**
    A. An acute loss of renal function typically occurring within 24–48 hr

Table 43.1	RIFLE Method for Acute Kidney Infection	
RIFLE class	**GFR rate reduction**	**Urine output reduction**
Risk	Increase serum creatine × 1.5 or decrease of GFR greater than 25% from baseline	UO less than 0.5 ml/kg/hr for 6 hr
Injury	Increase serum creatine × 2 or decrease of GFR greater than 50% from baseline	UO less than 0.5 ml/kg/hr for 12 hr
Failure	Increase serum creatine × 1.5 or decrease of GFR greater than 25% from baseline	UO less than 0.3 ml/kg/hr for 12 hr or anuria for 12 hr
Loss	Complete loss of renal function for greater than 4 weeks	
End-stage kidney disease	Need for RRT for greater than 3 months	

B. Overall incidence is 3/1,000 with approximately 5/100,000 requiring dialysis for short-term management

C. AKI accounts for 5%–7% of hospital admissions and 30% of intensive care unit admissions, which are associated with higher mortality

D. Increased cost, increased length of stay, and increased in/out-of-hospital mortality are associated with AKI

E. AKI progresses from the inability to excrete metabolic waste products, such as urea nitrogen and creatinine, to the inability to maintain proper fluid and electrolyte balance.

   1. Typically, acute increases in serum creatinine levels from baseline (i.e., an increase of at least 0.5 mg/dl) occur. AKI can progress to complete renal failure when serum creatinine level increases by at least 0.5 mg/dl/day and urine output is less than 400 ml/day (oliguria).

F. Generally, AKI resolves within three months of onset

G. There are age and comorbidity factors that are related to an increase in occurrence regardless of etiology of AKI. Even with full recovery from AKI, an episode increases the lifetime risk of development of CKD with the exact mechanisms and specific etiology yet unknown.

H. Two major methods are used to identify AKI

   1. The Acute Dialysis Quality Initiative group developed a stratification method based on abrupt onset of renal impairment, loss, and the need for renal replacement therapy (RRT) coupled with duration (see Table 43.1)

   2. A second widely accepted classification method is based on the global etiology of injury to the kidney consisting of prerenal, intrarenal, and postrenal causation.

III.   Risk, injury, failure, loss, end-stage kidney disease stratification method for AKI (RIFLE) (see table 43.1)

IV.   Etiology classification method prerenal, intrarenal, and postrenal (prerenal and postrenal have the greatest incidence of recovery and not progressing to end-stage kidney disease where RRT is required)

A. Prerenal (60%–70% of cases)
  1. Characterized by diminished renal perfusion resulting from a decrease in blood supply to the kidneys
     a. No nephron damage is present
  2. Causes
     a. Intravascular volume depletion (absolute decrease in blood volume)
        i. Hemorrhage
        ii. Gastrointestinal losses (e.g., diarrhea, vomiting, and large amount of nasogastric tube aspirate)
        iii. Urinary losses (e.g., diabetes insipidus and use of diuretics)
        iv. Skin losses (third spacing, large surface area burns, and/or wounds)
     b. Vasodilatory states (relative decrease in blood volume)
        i. Sepsis
        ii. Anaphylaxis
        iii. Drugs
           (a) Angiotensin-converting enzyme (ACE) inhibitors, which may inhibit intrinsic renal autoregulation
           (b) Nonsteroidal anti-inflammatory drugs (NSAIDs), which may decrease renal blood flow
     c. Decreased cardiac output (relative decrease in blood volume)
        i. Congestive heart failure
        ii. Myocardial infarction
        iii. Cardiogenic shock
     d. Arterial occlusion/vasoconstrictive states (catecholamines)
     e. Uncontrolled hypertension/atherosclerosis
     f. Liver disease (advanced hepatic disease that may cause hepatic renal syndrome due to vasoconstriction in the kidneys)
  3. Results in increased tubular sodium and water reabsorption (in an attempt at reexpansion of circulating blood volume)
     a. Oliguria
     b. Decreased urine sodium (less than 20 mEq/L)
     c. High urine osmolality (higher than 500 mOsm/L)
     d. Urine-specific gravity: increased (higher than 1.020)
  4. Decreased distal tubular flow may cause increased urea absorption and decreased potassium secretion with marginal effect on creatinine

5. BUN-to-creatinine ratio increased (20:1)
6. Ratio of urine-to-plasma (U/P) levels of creatinine greater than 40
7. Fraction excretion of sodium is a very sensitive test
   a. Formula:

$$\frac{U_{Na} \times P_{Cr}}{P_{Na} \times U_{Cr}} \times 100$$

   Note. U_{Na} = urine sodium; U_{Cr} = urine creatinine; P_{Na} = plasma sodium; P_{Cr} = plasma creatinine

   b. Less than 1% = prerenal
   c. Greater than 1% = intrinsic
   d. Greater than 2%–4% = postrenal
8. Increased renal "threshold" for plasma ions: increased bicarbonate (HCO_3^-) generation leads to contraction alkalosis
9. Increased uric acid reabsorption: hyperuricemia
10. Increased antidiuretic hormone secretion: increased water reabsorption; urinary osmolality greater than serum osmolality
11. Hyponatremia with free water loading until volume is restored
12. Urinary sediment: hyaline casts

B. Intrarenal (intrinsic) (25%–40% of cases)
   1. Abrupt decrease in glomerular filtration rate (GFR) due to tubular cell damage that results from renal ischemia or nephrotoxic injury
   2. Acute tubular necrosis—accounts for most hospital-associated cases of intrinsic acute renal failure (ARF) around 50%
      a. Ischemic
         i. Decreased cardiac output
         ii. Prolonged hypotension
         iii. Volume depletion
         iv. Catecholamines
         v. Volume shift
         vi. Liver disease ("hepatorenal syndrome")
      b. Nephrotoxic
         i. Endogenous (e.g., hemoglobinuria [hemolysis], myoglobinuria [rhabdomyolysis], hyperuricemia, and multiple myeloma)
         ii. Exogenous (e.g., aminoglycosides, contrast media, ethylene glycol, amphotericin B, cyclosporine, antineoplastics such as cisplatin, and heavy metals)
         iii. Drug-induced treatment principles
            (a) The ideal methods stop the offending agent
            (b) If discontinuing the drug is not an option, then the drug needs to be renally dosed based on creatinine clearance, which is based on specific drug recommendations and renal clearance rates.

iv. Treatment and prevention of contrast-related kidney injury
   (a) Fluid administration (high-level evidence)
      1. IV administration of fluids has not been proven superior over oral fluids in preventing contrast-related injury.
      2. Hydration is key to the likelihood of AKI prevention, but other factors such as concomitant heart failure must be considered when assessing volume status and adequacy of volume status
      3. Optimal prevention starts with oral or IV replacement prior to dye loading (1 L) and should continue for 24 hr
      4. Postcontrast fluids are administered to attain a urine output volume of 300 ml/hr (if no comorbid conditions and does not develop fluid overload symptoms)
      5. When IV methods are selected, 0.45% normal saline is frequently selected as the sodium content most closely approximates urine sodium output assisting in the prevention acute iatrogenic hypernatremia, which can occur when 0.9% normal saline is used at these rates.
   (b) Adjunctive prevention methods (limited or no proof of outcome difference)
      1. IV/oral administration of N-acetylcysteine, 600 mg every 12 hr for 48–72 hr (before and after contrast) has been used to prevent contrast-induced injury but has not been shown to be superior to fluid alone
         a. When N-acetylcysteine is used, it is typically given before and after contrast to decrease in the incidence of dye-induced nephrotoxicity.
   (c) The administration of sodium bicarbonate has also been used but has limited advantage over fluid administration and should be reserved in cases when acidosis is present.
   (d) In diabetic patients receiving metformin or combinations containing the drug should be withheld for 48 hr prior to the dye load (based on risk benefit of the need for the test in light of the potential for kidney damage).

       1. If at all possible, an alternate test should be used or noncontrast imaging if the drug has been dosed in the prior 24-hr period. In patients who present to the hospital and need to withhold nephrotoxic drugs, these medications should be considered.

3. Acute tubulointerstitial nephritis accounts for 10%–15% of cases of intrinsic renal failure. This is caused by the following:
   a. Bacterial pyelonephritis: infectious causes may include streptococcal infection, leptospirosis, cytomegalovirus, histoplasmosis, and Rocky Mountain spotted fever
   b. More than 70% of cases are related to drug-induced hypersensitivity to the following:
      i. Penicillins
      ii. Cephalosporins
      iii. Sulfonamides and sulfonamide-containing diuretics
      iv. NSAIDs
      v. Rifampin
      vi. Phenytoin
      vii. Allopurinol
   c. Immunologic disorders—more commonly associated with glomerulonephritis, but may also be associated with:
      i. Systemic lupus erythematosus (SLE)
      ii. Sjögren syndrome
      iii. Sarcoidosis
      iv. Cryoglobulinemia
   d. Idiopathic conditions
4. Urinalysis: urinary sediment, with the following:
   a. Renal tubular epithelial cells
   b. Cellular debris
   c. Pigmented granular casts
   d. Renal tubular cell casts
   e. "Muddy brown" coarse granular casts (Table 43.2)
5. Urine volume
   a. Anuria: less than 100 ml/24 hr
   b. Oliguria: 100–400 ml/24 hr
   c. Nonoliguria: greater than 400 ml/24 hr
   d. Polyuria: greater than 6 L/24 hr
6. Urine osmolality: isotonic (350 mOsm or less)
7. Urine-specific gravity: fixed (1.0008–1.012)
8. Urine Na greater than 20 mEq/L
9. FENA would be greater than 1%
10. BUN-to-creatinine ratio: less than 20:1
11. Low serum Na (less than 135 mEq)
12. Proteinuria may be seen, particularly in NSAID-induced interstitial nephritis, but is usually modest

Table 43.2	Urine abnormalities in renal failure			
	Prerenal	**Postrenal (acute)**	**Intrinsic renal (acute)**	**Intrinsic renal (chronic)**
Urine volume	Decreased	Absent-to-wide fluctuation	Oliguric or nonoliguric	1000 ml³ until end stage
Urine creatinine	Increased (U/P Cr ± 40)	Decreased (U/P Cr ± 20)	Decreased (U/P Cr less than 20)	Decreased (U/P Cr less than 20)
Osmolarity	Increased (±400 mOsm/kg)	Less than 350 mOsm/kg	Less than 350 mOsm/kg	Less than 350 mOsm/kg
Degree of proteinuria	Minimum	Absent	Varies with cause of renal failure: modest with ATN; nephrotic range common with acute glomerulopathies, usually less than 2 grams/24 hr with interstitial disease[a]	Varies with cause of renal disease (from 1–2 grams/day to nephrotic range)
Urinary sediment	Negative, or may have occasional hyaline cast	Negative, or hematuria with stones or papillary necrosis; pyuria with infectious prostate disease	ATN: muddy brown interstitial nephritis: lymphocytes, eosinophils (in stained preparations), and WBC casts; RPGN: RBC casts; nephrosis oval fat bodies	Broad casts with variable renal "residual" acute findings

Note: [a] Except NSAID-induced allergic interstitial nephritis with concomitant "nil disease." U/P = urine/plasma; Cr = creatinine; ATN = acute tubular necrosis; mOsm = milliosmole; RBC = red blood cells; WBC = white blood cells; RPGN = rapidly progressing glomerulonephritis; NSAID = non-steroidal anti-inflammatory drug. Adapted from F.F. Ferri's *Practical Guide to the Care of the Medical Patient Eighth Edition*, 2011. Copyright 2011 by Mosby Inc. Used with permission.

Table 43.3	Serum and radiographic abnormalities in renal failure			
	Prerenal	**Postrenal (acute)**	**Intrinsic renal (acute)**	**Intrinsic renal (chronic)**
BUN	Increased 10:1 greater than Cr	Increased by 20–40/day	Increased by 20–40/day	Stable; increase varies with protein intake
Serum creatinine	Normal/ moderate increase	Increased by 2–4/day	Increased by 2–4/day	Stable increase (production equals excretion)
Serum potassium	Normal/ moderate increase	Increase varies with urinary volume	Large increase (particularly when patient is oliguric); even larger increase with rhabdomyolysis	Normal until end stage, unless tubular dysfunction (type 4 RTA)
Serum phosphorus	Normal/ moderate increase	Moderate increase	Increased	Becomes significantly elevated when serum creatinine surpasses 3 mg/dl
Serum calcium	Normal	Normal/ decreased with PO_4^{3-}	Decreased (poor correlation with duration of renal failure)	Usually decreased
Renal size by ultrasound FENA	Normal/ increased by less than 1	Increased and with dilated calyces less than 1 to greater than 1	Normal/ increased greater than 1	Decreased and with ultrasound echogenicity greater than 1

Note: BUN = blood urea nitrogen; Cr = creatinine; RTA = renal tubular acidosis; PO_4^{3-} = phosphate; FENA = fractional excretion of sodium. Adapted from F.F. Ferri's *Practical Guide to the Care of the Medical Patient,* Eighth Edition, 2011. Copyright 2011 by Mosby Inc. Used with permission.

13. Other clinical findings may include fever (greater than 80%), rash (25%–50%), arthralgias, and peripheral blood eosinophilia

C. Postrenal (5%–10% of cases)

1. Associated with conditions that cause the obstruction of urinary flow and consequently a decrease in GFR

2. Mechanical

   a. Calculi

   b. Tumors (prostate cancer, cervical cancer)

   c. Urethral strictures

   d. Benign prostatic hyperplasia

      e. Blood clots

      f. Occluded Foley catheter

   3. Functional

      a. Neurogenic bladder

      b. Diabetic neuropathy

      c. Spinal cord disease

   4. Urine volume may fluctuate between anuria and polyuria.

   5. Urine osmolality: isotonic (less than 350 mOsm) (initially may be high)

   6. Urine-specific gravity: fixed (1.0008–1.012)

   7. Urine Na: greater than 40 mEq/L (initially may be low—variable)

   8. FENa: variable

   9. Urinary sediment

      a. Normal or red cells

      b. White cells

      c. Crystals

  10. BUN-to-creatinine ratio: greater than 20:1

  11. In-and-out catheter may reveal increased postvoid residual volume, and renal ultrasound may demonstrate hydronephrosis

  12. Plain film X-ray (kidney, ureter, and bladder) of the abdomen will document the presence of two kidneys and will provide a check for kidney stones (Table 43.3)

  13. Computed tomography scan or magnetic resonance imaging may also reveal obstruction

  14. Retrograde urography may be used to obtain information on the ureters and the lower urinary tract

  15. Renal biopsy with special immune stains and electron microscopy may assist in determining the cause of renal failure

  16. Therapy may include catheter drainage, urethral stents, and percutaneous nephrostomy

V. **Management**

  A. Therapy for ARF is aimed at:

   1. Treating the underlying cause

   2. Correcting fluid, electrolyte, and uremic abnormalities

   3. Preventing complications, including nutritional deficiencies (Figure 43.1)

  B. Adjust intake to output on the basis of fluid status. Take the use of diuretics into consideration because more often, patients are overloaded, especially if they are oliguric or anuric.

  C. The volume-depleted patient is usually resuscitated with saline.

  D. Furosemide (Lasix) is used to convert oliguric to nonoliguric ARF but has no outcome difference

   1. Furosemide, given IV every 6 hr, is the initial treatment for volume overload

Renal Insufficiency and Failure

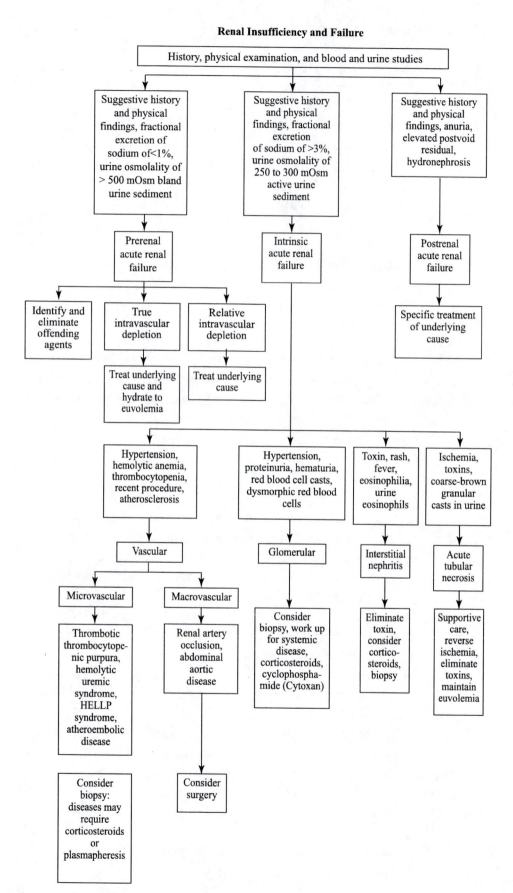

Figure 43.1. HELLP syndrome = abbreviation of symptoms associated with obstetric complication of pre-eclampsia: hemolysis, elevated liver enzymes, low platelet count; mOsm = milliosmole. Adapted from "Acute Renal Failure," by M. Agrawal and R. Swartz, 2000, Am Fam Physician, 61 (7), pp. 2077–2088. Copyright 2000 by the American Academy of Family Physicians. Used with permission.

      a. The initial dose can be 20–100 mg (this depends on whether the patient takes Lasix regularly)

  2. If the response is not adequate within 1 hr, the dose is doubled. This process is repeated until adequate urine output is achieved, but higher doses are associated with tinnitus and temporary deafness.

  3. A continuous Lasix drip may be used but has not proven superior over intermittent dosing in AKI. Diuretic use in AKI has not been shown to change the outcome, and should be used to manage physiologic needs, such as water balance.

E. Maximize cardiac function and maintain optimal blood pressure for renal perfusion

F. Discontinue offending drugs

G. If benign prostatic hyperplasia is known or suspected, avoid the use of sympathomimetic medications (often found in over the counter decongestants).

H. Use may precipitate acute outlet obstruction and lead to post renal obstruction

I. ARF is a catabolic state; therefore, patients can become nutritionally deficient. Total caloric intake should be 30–45 kcal/kg/day, most of which should come from a combination of carbohydrate and lipids. In patients who are not receiving dialysis, protein should be restricted to 0.6 grams/kg/day. In patients who are receiving dialysis, protein intake should be 1–1.5 grams/kg/day.

J. Monitor for complications

  1. Electrolyte imbalances

    a. Hyperkalemia

      i. Sodium polystyrene sulfonate (Kayexalate) adds 1 mEq Na+ for each 1 mEq K+ removed via the gastrointestinal tract

      ii. Administer 15–30 grams of sodium polystyrene sulfonate mixed with 100 ml of 20% sorbitol or as an enema (50 grams in 50 ml or 70% sorbitol and 150 ml of tap water)

      iii. IV administration of calcium (10 ml of a 10% solution of calcium gluconate) is cardioprotective and temporarily reverses the neuromuscular effects of hyperkalemia.

      iv. Potassium can also be temporarily shifted into the intracellular compartment with the use of IV insulin (10 units) and glucose (25 grams), inhaled β agonist, or IV sodium bicarbonate (150 mEq in 1 L of D5W)

      v. Dialysis is the definitive treatment in patients with significantly elevated potassium levels and renal failure

    b. Hypernatremia

    c. Hyponatremia

        d. Hypocalcemia

        e. Metabolic acidosis

            i. Acidosis is treated IV or orally with sodium bicarbonate when serum HCO_3 is less than 15 mEq/L, or pH is lower than 7.2

        f. Hypermagnesemia

        g. Hyperphosphatemia

    2. Volume overload: pulmonary edema

    3. Uremia: pericarditis

    4. Infection

    5. Gastrointestinal bleeding

K. Anticipate the need for dialysis. Between 20% and 60% of patients need short-term dialysis, particularly when BUN exceeds 100 mg/dl and serum creatinine exceeds 5–10 mg/dl.

    1. Intravascular volume overload: pulmonary edema

    2. Hyperkalemia

    3. Acidosis/alkalosis

    4. Uremia (symptomatic syndrome resulting from increase in nitrogenous wastes [azotemia])

        a. Central nervous system disturbances

        b. Gastrointestinal indications (nausea, vomiting, and anorexia)

        c. Level of azotemia (elevation of waste products): BUN 100–200 mg/dl

    5. Specific drug/toxin

L. Renally adjust dose all medications: assume that GFR is less than 10 ml/minute (normal, 80–120 ml/minute)

M. Adjust diet: low protein/Na/K

VI.   **RRT options in AKI and CKD**

A. Hemodialysis

    1. Intermittent (most common for chronic management)

        a. Requires specialized staff

        b. Useful in removing selected drugs in acute toxic states

        c. Typically requires adequate mean arterial pressure to attain flow rates for clearance (normally at least 60 mmHg)

    2. Continuous (similar creatine clearance to intermittent dialysis)

        a. Continuous arterial renal replacement therapy

            i. Requires arterial access and adequate mean blood pressure preferably at 60 mmHg

        b. Continuous veno venous hemodialysis

            i. Uses an external pump for flow rates so blood pressure requirements are lessened

            ii. Both can be performed by trained intensive care unit nurses

    iii. Benefits over intermittent dialysis have not been proven to reduce course, duration, outcome, or mortality in ARF even when the onset of treatment is started early

    iv. Use in ARF should be based on the need for fluid removal and correction of electrolyte imbalance when conventional medical management fails

    v. Choice should be made based on patient need, availability of services, and physiologic stability required by other replacement methods

    vi. Some form of dialysis is indicated if fluid uremic symptoms develop, such as encephalopathy or pericarditis

  B. Peritoneal dialysis

   1. Useful for long-term use

   2. Improved quality of life for patient over conventional dialysis methods

   3. Does not provide creatinine clearance rates at the level of other RRT methods, which may limit usefulness

   4. High risk for catheter site and intra-abdominal (peritoneal) infections

   5. Does not provide adequate creatinine clearance rates required in catabolic states such as major surgery, burns, or sepsis, which may require conversion to an alternate RRT method during the acute state until baseline physiological state is restored

  C. Renal transplantation

   1. Most cost-effective with the benefit realized at about 1½–2 years posttransplant

   2. Improved quality of life and functioning over chronic dialysis use

   3. Limited by organ availability

   4. Lifetime burden of immunosuppression use and the associated consequences

CHRONIC KIDNEY DISEASE

I. **Definition**

  A. Progressive azotemia over weeks, months, or years

   1. GFR 60 ml/minute or less for longer than 3 months, with or without kidney damage

  B. Isosthenuria is common

  C. Hypertension is common in most patients

  D. Ultrasound studies show evidence of bilateral small kidneys

  E. X-rays show evidence of renal osteodystrophy

II. **Etiology**

  A. Glomerular disease

  B. Polycystic kidney disease

  C. Hypertensive nephropathy

    D. Diabetic nephropathy

    E. Tubulointerstitial nephritis or necrosis

    F. Obstructive nephropathies

    G. Renal artery stenosis

III. **Stages based on the National Kidney Foundation Disease outcome quality initiative advisory board (recommended by the Center for Medicare Services to document renal damage–related complexity of care)**

    A. The progression of CKD occurs in five stages.

    B. Each stage reflects an increasing loss of nephrons

        1. Stage I

            a. GFR greater than 90 ml/minute

            b. Kidney damage with normal or increased GFR

        2. Stage II

            a. GFR 60–89 ml/minute

            b. Kidney damage with mild or decreased GFR

        3. Stage III

            a. GFR 30–59 ml/minute

            b. Moderate decrease in GFR with moderate complications

        4. Stage IV

            a. GFR 15–29 ml/minute

            b. Severe decrease in GFR with severe complications

        5. Stage V (kidney failure)

            a. End-stage renal disease

            b. GFR less than 15 ml/minute or dialysis

            c. Uremia and cardiovascular disease

            d. Monitor GFR. Normal is 80–120 ml/minute.

            e. Formula for calculation:

            f. Renal replacement is instituted when GFR falls to between 5 and 10 ml/minute.

            g. Creatinine clearance is used by many practitioners as a more accurate method of estimating GFR

                i. Age and gender dependent

                ii. Normal

                    (a) Males: 97–137 ml/minute/1.73 m^2

                    (b) Females: 88–128 ml/minute/1.73 m^2

            h. Cystatin C is a proteinase inhibitor that is not freely filtered by the glomerulus. It is felt to potentially be a better marker of renal function than creatine but is not widely available.

IV. **Signs/symptoms**

    A. General

        1. Fatigue

        2. Weakness

    B. Skin

        1. Pruritus

    2. Easy bruising

    3. Pallor, ecchymosis

    4. Excoriations

    5. Edema

    6. Xerosis

    7. Sallow complexion (ill, yellow appearing, jaundice if liver disease is present)

    8. Pale conjunctiva

    9. Reversible hair loss, nail changes

C. Ear, nose, and throat

    1. Metallic taste in the mouth

    2. Epistaxis

    3. Urinous breath

D. Pulmonary

    1. Shortness of breath

    2. Rales

    3. Pleural effusion

E. Cardiovascular

    1. Dyspnea on exertion

    2. Retrosternal pain on inspiration and pericardial friction rub caused by pericarditis related to uremia

    3. Hypertension caused by volume overload

    4. Cardiomegaly

F. Gastrointestinal

    1. Anorexia

    2. Nausea and vomiting

    3. Hiccups

G. Genitourinary

    1. Impotence

    2. Nocturia

    3. Iso-osmolar urine: Urine has an osmolarity similar to plasma osmolality despite variations in fluid intake; this indicates marked impairment in renal concentrating ability.

H. Neurologic

    1. Irritability

    2. Inability to concentrate

    3. Decreased libido

    4. Stupor

    5. Asterixis

    6. Myoclonus/hyperreflexia

    7. Peripheral neuropathy associated with diabetes, if present

    8. Restless leg syndrome/loss of vibratory sense

    9. Seizures (rare)

I. Anemia due to erythropoietin deficiency

V. **Management of common problems in CKD**

   A. Fluid overload

     1. Monitor weight, standing blood pressure, urine Na+ excretion, creatinine clearance (CrCl), and serum creatinine

     2. Decrease Na+ and fluid intake

     3. Diuretics

       a. Furosemide (Lasix), 20–80 mg/day initially

         i. Up to 600 mg/day; using too much of this drug may lead to side effects such as confusion, dehydration, and muscle cramps due to water and salt/mineral loss

         ii. Doses up to 1 gram/day have been used in congestive heart failure and renal failure

         iii. Continuous infusions of 100 mg/hr have been utilized

         iv. Remains effective when GFR is less than 25 ml/minute

       b. Other agents that may be used include the following but have not been proven to be more effective than furosemide:

         i. Metolazone (Zaroxolyn), 2.5–20 mg PO daily, in combination with loop diuretic only

         ii. Chlorothiazide (Diuril), 500 mg IV daily, in combination with loop diuretic only

         iii. Bumetanide (Bumex), 0.5–2 mg once daily (may repeat at 4- to 5-hour intervals, if needed, to a maximum of 10 mg/day). Continuous infusions of up to 2 mg/hr have been utilized.

         iv. Torsemide (Demadex), 10–20 mg once daily PO/IV (may increase up to 200 mg/day PRN)

   B. Hypertension

     1. Determine the patient's optimal Na+ and H_2O intact. Excess Na+/H_2O increases the level of hypertension

     2. Antihypertensive agents that maintain renal blood flow and reduce glomerular pressure and proteinuria are preferred

     3. If proteinuria is present, ACE inhibitors and calcium channel blockers may be superior to conventional treatment in decreasing proteinuria and reducing glomerular hypertension.

     4. Antihypertensives: Goal blood pressure for patients with chronic renal failure (CRF) is less than 140/80 mmHg; for those with proteinuria greater than 1–2 grams, it is less than 125/75 mmHg.

       a. ACE inhibitors

       b. Angiotensin II receptor blockers (if serum K+ and GFR permit)

       c. Calcium channel blockers

       d. Direct vasodilators

         i. Hydralazine (Apresoline)

         ii. Minoxidil (Loniten)

       e. Peripheral α blockers

         i.   Doxazosin mesylate (Cardura)

         ii.   Prazosin (Minipress)

    f.   β blockers

         i.   Propranolol (Inderal)

    g.   Central α blockers

         i.   Clonidine hydrochloride (Catapres)

C. Protein catabolism

  1. Limit protein intake (less than 8 grams/kg/day): The level of restriction may be increased to 0.6–0.8 grams/kg/day if restriction proves beneficial. Protein limitation is controversial as it has not shown to change the outcome of progress on CKD. It may lessen the need for dialysis times and frequency. Protein-related kidney disorders occur relatively late in CKD at GFRs of about 30. Protein restriction, if used, should be reserved for late Stage III, IV, and end-stage renal disease stage when protein abnormalities occur.

  2. Provide adequate calories

  3. Avoid stresses of trauma, infection, and immobilization, if possible

  4. Physical activity should be moderate

  5. Thyroid hormone, steroids, and tetracycline increase catabolism and must be avoided

  6. Anabolic agents may help some patients avoid a negative nitrogen balance (help stimulate erythropoiesis)

    a. Fluoxymesterone (Halotestin)

    b. Nandrolone decanoate (Deca-Durabolin)

D. Acidosis: alkalizing agents are indicated when plasma HCO_3 is less than 20 mEq/L

  1. $NaHCO_3$—1 gram + 13 mEq Na; generally used in emergencies because it may cause volume overload related to Na+

  2. Sodium citrate (Shohl solution, Bicitra): 1 mEq/ml of Na+

  3. Sodium and potassium citrate and citric acid (Polycitra): monitor K+ levels, and avoid in patients with hyperkalemia

E. Hyperkalemia

  1. Avoid foods and medications high in K+

  2. Avoid hypercatabolic states

  3. Medical emergency if K+ is greater than 7 mEq/L

    a. Administer hypertonic glucose, insulin, and HCO_3

    b. Calcium gluconate or calcium chloride IV to modify myocardial irritability

    c. Correct acidosis

    d. Administer K+ ion exchange resins to remove excess potassium ions

        i. Kayexalate, 30–60 grams/day (each gram of Kayexalate resin binds with 1 mEq of K+ and subsequently releases 1 mEq of Na+)

      e. Hemodialysis

      f. Monitor ECG for flat P waves, peaked T waves, PR interval greater than 0.20 seconds, QRS complex greater than 0.10 second, and bradycardia

F. Hyperphosphatemia (choose one or more from the following; the phosphorous level should be kept below 4.6 mg/dl):

  1. Restrict phosphorus to 800–1000 mg/day

      a. Limit foods such as colas, eggs, dairy products, and meat

  2. GFR less than 20–30 ml/minute usually requires phosphate-binding agents

  3. Calcium carbonate, 650 mg three times a day

      a. Phosphate-binding agent

      b. Prevents aluminum toxicity

  4. Sevelamer (Renvela), 800–3200 mg three times a day with meals

  5. Lanthanum (Fosrenol), 1500–3000 mg per day in divided doses with meals

  6. Calcium acetate, 667 mg (two to six tablets) three times a day, with meals

  7. Aluminium hydroxide is an effective phosphate binder that can be used in the acute setting for serum phosphorous levels greater than 7 mg/dl; however, long-term use should be avoided because it can cause osteomalacia and neurologic complications. Limit duration to 3 days to avoid aluminum toxicity.

  8. Hemodialysis

G. Hypocalcemia

  1. Maintain phosphorous level at less than 6 mg/dl

  2. Calcium carbonate supplements

  3. 1,25-OH$_2$ vitamin D in extreme cases

H. Hypermagnesemia: avoid Mg++ containing laxatives/antacids

I. Anemia

  1. Iron

  2. Vitamin supplements PRN

  3. Erythropoietin weekly injections; 50–100 units/kg IV/SQ three times a week; more dosing has a black box warning for increased cardiovascular disease risks

      a. Recommended for patients on hemodialysis

J. Neurologic problems

  1. Anticonvulsants

      a. Phenytoin

      b. Phenobarbital

  2. Sedatives

      a. Haloperidol

      b. Diphenhydramine

K. Renal osteodystrophy

1. Prevent acidosis, hypocalcemia, hyperphosphatemia; control hyperparathyroidism
2. Correct low Ca (less than 6.5 mg/dl)
   a. Administer calcium supplement, such as calcium carbonate and calcium gluconate, 1–2 grams/day
   b. Titrate as necessary to control serum phosphate and calcium levels
3. Correct high phosphorous levels (higher than 5 mg/dl). Administer phosphate binders.
4. Correct acidosis (HCO_3 less than 15 mEq/dl). Administer $NaHCO_3$, 2–5 mEq/kg, as a 4- to 8-hr infusion (for emergency situations), or 650 mg PO three times a day, and titrate PRN.
5. Administer vitamin D if Ca stays below 6 mg/dl (calcitrol, paricalcitol), bone pain is a problem, alkaline phosphatase levels increase, and X-rays reveal evidence of osteomalacia.
6. Identify and treat secondary hyperparathyroidism, which is triggered by low calcium levels
   a. Limit foods high in phosphorus
   b. Administer phosphate binders (Tums, Oscal) with meals
   c. Sevelamer hydrochloride (Renagel) is currently being used and is believed to have many advantages over calcium-based phosphate binders, although it is more expensive
   d. Calcitrol or paricalcitol

VI.   **RRT options**
   A. Hemodialysis
   B. Peritoneal dialysis
   C. Renal transplantation

MODIFICATION OF DRUG DOSAGES

I.   **Types of drugs**
   A. Type A: eliminated entirely by the kidney
   B. Type B: eliminated entirely by extrarenal mechanism
   C. Type C: eliminated by renal and extrarenal mechanisms
II.   **Decreased renal function results in the following:**
   A. Abnormal excretion rates
   B. Abnormal metabolism rates of certain drugs
   C. Abnormal sensitivity to certain drugs
III.   **Before administering any drug to a patient in renal failure, consider the following:**
   A. Does this drug depend on the kidney for excretion?
   B. Does an excess blood level affect the kidney or cause nephrotoxicity?
   C. Does the effect of the drug alter electrolyte imbalance?
   D. Is the patient susceptible to the drug because of kidney disease?

IV.   Modification of drug doses:

   A. Serum creatinine is greater than 10 mg/ml; renal function is 15% of normal: major modification is needed

   B. Serum creatinine is 3–10 mg/ml; renal function is 15%–20% of normal: modest changes are needed

BIBLIOGRAPHY

Acute kidney injury. (2013). *Nursing Standard, 28*(4), 21–21.

BET 3: RIFLE criteria versus acute kidney injury network (AKIN) criteria for prognosis of acute renal failure. (2011). *Emergency Medicine Journal, 28*(10), 900–901.

Bouchard, J., Soroko, S. B., Chertow, G. M., Himmelfarb, J., Ikizler, T. A., Paganini, E. P., & Mehta, R. L. (2009). Fluid accumulation, survival and recovery of kidney function in critically ill patients with acute kidney injury. *Kidney International, 76*(4), 422–427. doi:10.1038/ki.2009.159

Brar, S. S., Hiremath, S., Dangas, G., Mehran, R., Brar, S. K., & Leon, M. B. (2009). Sodium bicarbonate for the prevention of contrast induced-acute kidney injury: A systematic review and meta-analysis. *Clinical Journal of the American Society of Nephrology, 4*(10), 1584–1592. doi:10.2215/CJN.03120509; 10.2215/CJN.03120509

Cavalier, E., Delanaye, P., Vranken, L., Bekaert, A. C., Carlisi, A., Chapelle, J. P., & Souberbielle, J. C. (2012). Interpretation of serum PTH concentrations with different kits in dialysis patients according to the KDIGO guidelines: Importance of the reference (normal) values. *Nephrology, Dialysis, Transplantation, 27*(5), 1950–1956. doi:10.1093/ndt/gfr535; 10.1093/ndt/gfr535

Chao, C. T., Wu, V. C., Lai, C. F., Shiao, C. C., Huang, T. M., Wu, P. C., & Wu, K. D. (2012). Advanced age affects the outcome-predictive power of RIFLE classification in geriatric patients with acute kidney injury. *Kidney International, 82*(8), 920–927. doi:10.1038/ki.2012.237

Chawla, L. S., & Kimmel, P. L. (2012). Acute kidney injury and chronic kidney disease: An integrated clinical syndrome. *Kidney International, 82*(5), 516–524. doi:10.1038/ki.2012.208

Cheung, C. M., Ponnusamy, A., & Anderton, J. G. (2008). Management of acute renal failure in the elderly patient: A clinician's guide. *Drugs and Aging, 25*(6), 455–476.

Chronopoulos, A., Rosner, M. H., Cruz, D. N., & Ronco, C. (2010). Acute kidney injury in elderly intensive care patients: A review. *Intensive Care Medicine, 36*(9), 1454–1464. doi:10.1007/s00134–010–1957–7

Coyne, D. W. (2013). Anemia management in dialysis: Why the FDA and CMS have it right (and how KDIGO got it wrong). *Nephrology News and Issues, 27*(2), 16, 18, 20.

Faubel, S. (2013). Have we reached the limit of mortality benefit with our approach to renal replacement therapy in acute kidney injury? *American Journal of Kidney Diseases, 62*(6), 1030–033. doi:10.1053/j.ajkd.2013.09.004; 10.1053/j.ajkd.2013.09.004

Ferri, F. F. (2011). *Practical guide to the care of the medical patient* (8th ed.). Philadelphia, PA: Mosby Elsevier.

Fuchs, L., Lee, J., Novack, V., Baumfeld, Y., Scott, D., Celi, L., … Talmor, D. (2013). Severity of acute kidney injury and two-year outcomes in critically ill patients. *Chest, 144*(3), 866–875. doi:10.1378/chest.12–2967

Gocze, I., Wohlgemuth, W. A., Schlitt, H. J., & Jung, E. M. (2013). Contrast-enhanced ultrasonography for bedside imaging in subclinical acute kidney injury. *Intensive Care Medicine, 40*(3). doi:10.1007/s00134–013–3152–0

Hoste, E. A., Doom, S., De Waele, J., Delrue, L. J., Defreyne, L., Benoit, D. D., & Decruyenaere, J. (2011). Epidemiology of contrast-associated acute kidney injury in ICU patients: A retrospective cohort analysis. *Intensive Care Medicine, 37*(12), 1921–1931.

Joannidis, M., Metnitz, B., Bauer, P., Schusterschitz, N., Moreno, R., Druml, W., & Metnitz, P. G. (2009). Acute kidney injury in critically ill patients classified by AKIN versus RIFLE using the SAPS 3 database. *Intensive Care Medicine, 35*(10), 1692–1702. doi:10.1007/s00134–009–1530–4

Jorgensen, A., L. (2013). Contrast-induced nephropathy: Pathophysiology and preventive strategies. *Critical Care Nurse, 33*(1), 37–47. doi:10.4037/ccn2013680

Kellum, J. A., Lameire, N., & for the KDIGO AKI Guideline Work Group. (2013). Diagnosis, evaluation, and management of acute kidney injury: A KDIGO summary (Part 1). *Critical Care (London, England), 17*(1), 204. doi:10.1186/cc11454

Kovacevic, B., Ignjatovic, M., Zivaljevic, V., Cuk, V., Scepanovic, M., Petrovic, Z., & Paunovic, I. (2012). Parathyroidectomy for the attainment of NKF-K/DOQI and KDIGO recommended values for bone and mineral metabolism in dialysis patients with uncontrollable secondary hyperparathyroidism. *Langenbeck's Archives of Surgery, 397*(3), 413–420. doi:10.1007/s00423–011–0901–9; 10.1007/s00423–011–0901–9

Koyner, J. L. (2012). Assessment and diagnosis of renal dysfunction in the ICU. *Chest, 141*(6), 1584–1594. doi:10.1378/chest.11–1513

Lamb, E. J., Levey, A. S., & Stevens, P. E. (2013). The kidney disease improving global outcomes (KDIGO) guideline update for chronic kidney disease: Evolution not revolution. *Clinical Chemistry, 59*(3), 462–465. doi:10.1373/clinchem.2012.184259

London, G., Coyne, D., Hruska, K., Malluche, H. H., & Martin, K. J. (2010). The new kidney disease: Improving global outcomes (KDIGO) guidelines—Expert clinical focus on bone and vascular calcification. *Clinical Nephrology, 74*(6), 423–432.

Mårtensson, J., Martling, C. R., & Bell, M. (2012). Novel biomarkers of acute kidney injury and failure: Clinical applicability. *British Journal of Anaesthesia, 109*(6), 843–850. doi:10.1093/bja/aes357

Matzke, G. R., Aronoff, G. R., Atkinson, A. J., Jr., Bennett, W. M., Decker, B. S., Eckardt, K. U., & Murray, P. (2011). Drug dosing consideration in patients with acute and chronic kidney disease-A clinical update from kidney disease: Improving global outcomes (KDIGO). *Kidney International, 80*(11), 1122–1137. doi:10.1038/ki.2011.322; 10.1038/ki.2011.322

Li, P. K. T., Burdmann, E. A., & Mehta, R., L. (2013). Acute kidney injury: Global health alert. *Internet Journal of Nephrology, 8*(1), 1–1.

Sankarasubbaiyan, S., Janardan, J., D., & Kaur, P. (2013). Outcomes and characteristics of intermittent hemodialysis for acute kidney injury in an intensive care unit. *Indian Journal of Nephrology, 23*(1), 30–33. doi:10.4103/0971–4065.107193

Scharman, E. J., & Troutman, W. G. (2013). Prevention of kidney injury following rhabdomyolysis: A systematic review. *Annals of Pharmacotherapy, 47*(1), 90–105. doi:10.1345/aph.1R215

Serpa Neto, A., Veelo, D. P., Peireira, V. G., de Assuncao, M. S., Manetta, J. A., Esposito, D. C., & Schultz, M. J. (2013). Fluid resuscitation with hydroxyethyl starches in patients with sepsis is associated with an increased incidence of acute kidney injury and use of renal replacement therapy: A systematic review and meta-analysis of the literature. *Journal of Critical Care, 29*(1). doi:10.1016/j.jcrc.2013.09.031

Shavit, L., Korenfeld, R., Lifschitz, M., Butnaru, A., & Slotki, I. (2009). Sodium bicarbonate versus sodium chloride and oral *N*-acetylcysteine for the prevention of contrast-induced nephropathy in advanced chronic kidney disease. *Journal of Interventional Cardiology, 22*(6), 556–563. doi:10.1111/j.1540–8183.2009.00500.x

Singbartl, K., & Kellum, J. A. (2012). AKI in the ICU: Definition, epidemiology, risk stratification, and outcomes. *Kidney International, 81*(9), 819–825. doi:10.1038/ki.2011.339

CHAPTER 44

Benign Prostatic Hyperplasia

JENNIFER J. ROBERG • CHARLENE M. MYERS

I. **Definition**
  A. Benign prostatic hyperplasia (BPH) is the enlargement of the prostate gland, a condition commonly seen in men older than 50 years of age.
  B. Progressive condition that can cause obstruction of the urethra with interference in urine flow
  C. Hyperplastic process that results from an increase in cell numbers
II. **Etiology/incidence**
  A. Incidence is age related
    1. Men ages 41–50 years: 20%
    2. Men ages 51–60 years: 50%
    3. Men older than 80 years of age: more than 90%
  B. Exact cause is unknown
  C. May be a response of the prostate gland to androgen hormones over time
  D. Dietary fat may play a role
III. **Clinical manifestations**
  A. Irritative symptoms—consequence of bladder dysfunction
    1. Frequency
    2. Dysuria
    3. Urgency
    4. Nocturia
    5. Incontinence
  B. Obstructive symptoms
    1. Hesitancy
    2. Straining
    3. Starting and stopping

    4. Dribbling

    5. Retention

    6. Decreased force and caliber of stream

    7. Sensation of incomplete bladder emptying

    8. Double voiding (urinating a second time within 2 hr)

 C. Focal or uniform enlargement

    1. On digital rectal examination, the prostate may be enlarged. Size does not correlate with severity of symptoms or with degree of obstruction.

    2. The prostate should feel smooth and rubbery

    3. Focal enlargement, nodularity, or extreme hardness may represent malignancy; further investigation is indicated

        a. Transrectal ultrasound

        b. Biopsy

 D. Palpable bladder consistent with urinary retention

IV. **Laboratory findings**

 A. Urinalysis

    1. Pyuria suggests infection

    2. Hematuria may be a sign of malignancy

 B. Urine culture to rule out urinary tract infection (UTI) if irritative symptoms are present

 C. BUN/creatinine to assess for renal insufficiency

 D. Prostate-specific antigen (PSA)

    1. Considered optional, yet most practitioners include it in the initial evaluation

    2. Levels suggestive of prostate cancer

        a. Between 4 ng/ml and 10 ng/ml suggest a risk of approximately 25%

        b. Above 10 ng/ml suggest a risk of more than 50%

        c. Below 4 ng/ml does not guarantee that the patient does not have cancer

    3. Because an overlap is seen between levels in BPH and in prostate cancer, its use is controversial

    4. Other causes of elevated PSA include:

        a. Prostate cancer

        b. Bacterial prostatitis

        c. UTI

 E. Transrectal ultrasound with a palpable nodule or elevated PSA

V. **Management**

 A. Mild symptoms

    1. Patient may recover spontaneously over time ("watchful waiting")

    2. Avoid medications that can worsen symptoms

        a. Decongestants, diuretics, and other sympathomimetics (act on α receptors to enhance prostate muscle tone, which increases dynamic obstruction)

     b. Anticholinergics (antihistamines), bowel antispasmodics, tricyclic antidepressants, opiates, and antipsychotics; these decrease bladder muscle contraction, thus increasing urine retention

B. Mild to moderate symptoms

  1. Alpha (α) blockers, the preferred agents for BPH, relax muscle fibers in the prostate gland and capsule and in the internal urethral sphincter, thereby facilitating emptying of the bladder. No effect on blood pressure for the following agents:

     a. Terazosin (Hytrin), 1 mg at bedtime, increasing up to 10 mg at bedtime as necessary or tolerated

     b. Prazosin (Minipress), 1–5 mg PO BID

     c. Doxazosin (Cardura), 1–8 mg daily

     d. Hypotension and dizziness are the most commonly reported adverse effects.

     e. Combination therapy: tamsulosin (Flomax) (α1a blockade), 0.4 or 0.8 mg daily; alfuzosin (Uroxatral) 10 mg once daily; silodosin (Rapaflo), 8 mg once daily with a meal

  2. Hormonal manipulation

     a. Finasteride (Proscar), 5 mg/day

        i. Blocks conversion of testosterone to dihydrotestosterone

        ii. Works on the epithelial component of the prostate, resulting in reduction in the size of the gland and improvement in symptoms

        iii. Six months of therapy is required for maximal effect

     b. Dutasteride (Avodart), 0.5 mg once a day

     c. Estrogens, antiandrogens, or gonadotropin-releasing hormone (GnRH) may be used, but only if finasteride is not tolerated because of adverse effects

  3. Combination of α blockers and hormonal manipulation

  4. Phytotherapy

     a. Use of plants or plant extracts for medicinal purposes

     b. Several plant extracts have become popular:

        i. Saw palmetto berry

        ii. Bark of *Pygeum africanum*

        iii. Roots of *Echinacea purpurea* and *Hypoxis rooperi*

        iv. Pollen extract

        v. Leaves of the trembling poplar

        vi. Rye

        vii. Common or stinging nettle

        viii. Pumpkin/squash

     c. Herbal remedies sold as "dietary supplements"

     d. Safety and efficacy have not been evaluated by the FDA or any regulatory agency

     e. No requirement for proof of efficacy/safety prior to marketing

5. Safety and efficacy has not been evaluated by the FDA or any regulatory agency. Avoid medications that increase obstructive symptoms (as noted previously)

C. Severe symptoms
   1. Surgery may be necessary if significant urinary symptoms exist
   2. Types of surgeries:
      a. Transurethral resection of the prostate (TURP)
         i. Low mortality (1%) but moderate morbidity (18%)
         ii. Should bring improvement in the signs and symptoms of BPH
         iii. Repeat resection is needed in less than 10% of cases
         iv. Retrograde ejaculation may occur after the procedure has been performed
         v. Uncommon complications
            (a) Bladder neck contracture
            (b) Urethral stricture disease
            (c) Incontinence
      b. Open simple prostatectomy
      c. Transurethral incision of the prostate (TUIP)
         i. No tissue is resected
         ii. Antegrade ejaculation is usually maintained
         iii. Can usually be performed as an outpatient procedure
         iv. May benefit patients with BPH associated with smaller glands, especially younger men

D. The following options offer promise but few long-term data on their effectiveness have been gathered.
   1. Laser therapy
      a. Two primary energy sources of lasers have been used: neodymium: yttrium-aluminum-garnet (Nd:YAG) and holmium:YAG.
      b. Transurethral laser-induced prostatectomy (TULIP) is performed under transrectal ultrasound guidance.
      c. Advantages
         i. Minimal blood loss
         ii. Rare occurrence of transurethral resection syndrome
         iii. Ability of clinicians to treat patients on anticoagulation therapy
         iv. Outpatient therapy
      d. Disadvantages
         i. Lack of tissue for pathologic evaluation
         ii. Longer postoperative catheterization time
         iii. More frequent irritative voiding complaints
         iv. Expense of laser fibers and generators
   2. Transurethral needle ablation of the prostate (TUNA)

      a. A special catheter is passed into the urethra, and then interstitial radiofrequency needles are deployed from the end of the catheter to pierce the mucosa of the prostatic urethra.

      b. Tissue is heated by radiofrequencies; this results in coagulative necrosis. Improvement in voiding has been reported

  3. Transurethral electrovaporization of the prostate

      a. High current densities result in heat vaporization of tissue, which creates a cavity in the prostatic urethra

      b. Long-term comparative data versus other procedures are needed

  4. Transurethral microwave therapy (TUMT) (hyperthermia)

      a. Microwave hyperthermia is commonly delivered via transurethral catheter

      b. Long-term follow-up with large randomized trials is needed

  5. Urethral stents may be used for patients who are not candidates for standard surgery

      a. Can be performed under local anesthesia

      b. Preferred to chronic catheterization or suprapubic cystostomy

VI. **Gerontological considerations**

  1. Physiologic changes

      a. Diminished kidney mass, blood flow, and glomerular filtration rate (10% per decade after the age of 30 years)

      b. Kidneys are the primary route of elimination of most drugs or their metabolites

      c. Assessment of the estimated glomerular filtration rate (eGFR) or creatinine clearance is often required to adjust drug therapy

      d. Determine renal function through glomerular filtration rate by calculating the creatinine clearance in the elderly, using the Cockcroft-Gault equation

        i. Males:

          (a) Creatinine clearance (ml/min) = [(140 minus age in years) × (body weight in kg)]/[72 × (serum creatinine in mg/dl)]

        ii. Females: multiply the calculated value by 85% (0.85)

        iii. Normal creatinine clearance values in adults:

          (a) Males less than 40 years = 107–139 ml/min, or 1.8–2.3 ml/second

          (b) Females less than 40 years = 87–107 ml/min, or 1.5–1.8 ml/second

          (c) Creatinine clearance values usually decrease as one ages (e.g., decrease by 6.5 ml/min for every 10 years after the age of 20)

      e. Reduced bladder elasticity, muscle tone, and capacity

      f. Increased postvoid residual and nocturnal urine production

    g. Male reproductive system changes
- **i.** Prostate enlargement with risk of BPH
- **ii.** Decreased testosterone level leads to increased estrogen-to-androgen ratio
- **iii.** Decreased sperm motility; fertility reduced but extant
- **iv.** Increased incidence of gynecomastia

    h. Sexual function
- **i.** Slowed arousal-increased time to achieve erection
- **ii.** Erection less firm, shorter lasting
- **iii.** Delayed ejaculation and decreased forcefulness at ejaculation
- **iv.** Longer interval to achieving subsequent erection

    i. Prostate
- **i.** By fourth decade of life, stromal fibrous elements and glandular tissue hypertrophy, stimulated by dihydrotestosterone (DHT, the active androgen within the prostate); hyperplastic nodules enlarge in size, ultimately leading to urethral obstruction

2. Clinical implications

    a. History
- **i.** Many men are overly sensitive about complaints of the male genitourinary system; men are often not inclined to initiate discussion and seek help; important to take active role in screening with an approach that is open, trustworthy, and nonjudgmental.
- **ii.** Sexual function remains important to many men, even at 80 years of age and older
- **iii.** Lack of an available partner, poor health, erectile dysfunction, medication adverse effects, and lack of desire are the main reasons men do not continue to have sex.
- **iv.** Acute and chronic alcohol use can lead to impotence in men
- **v.** Nocturia is reported in 66% of patients over 65 years of age due to impaired ability to concentrate urine, reduced in bladder capacity or BPH-frequent cause of insomnia

    b. Physical
- **i.** Digital rectal exam is almost universally dreaded by men; provide privacy, allow for dignity

    c. Assessment
- **i.** In men diagnosed with BPH, periodic evaluation for prostate cancer must continue.

    d. Treatment
- **i.** A man may not want treatment for BPH because of fear of erectile dysfunction

3. Possible findings/results
    a. Decreased drug clearance and increased risk of:
        i. Adverse drug reactions
        ii. Nephrotoxicity
        iii. Renal complications
        iv. Volume/fluid overload (especially in heart failure patients)
        v. Hyponatremia and dehydration (especially in patients taking thiazide diuretics)
        vi. Hypernatremia (especially in patients with fever)
        vii. Hyperkalemia (especially in patients taking potassium-sparing diuretics)
        viii. Metabolic acidosis
        ix. Urinary urgency
        x. Incontinence
        xi. UTIs
        xii. Polyuria at night
        xiii. Falls

BIBLIOGRAPHY

American Cancer Society. (2014). *Prostate cancer*. Retrieved from http://www.cancer.org/cancer/prostatecancer/

Barry, M. J. (2009). Decision support in the treatment of prostate conditions. In A. Edwards & G. Elwyn (Eds.), *Shared Decision-Making in Health Care: Achieving Evidence-Based Patient Choice* (2nd ed.). New York, NY: Oxford University Press.

Deters, L. A., Costabile, R. A., Leveillee, R. J., Moore, C. R., & Patel, V. R. (2014). *Benign prostatic hypertrophy*. Retrieved from http://emedicine.medscape.com/article/437359-overview

Dowling-Castronovo, A., & Bradway, C. (2012). Urinary incontinence. In M. Boltz, E. Capuezuti, T. Fulmer, & D. Zwicker (Eds.), *Evidence-based geriatric nursing protocols for best practice* (4th ed., pp. 363–387). New York, NY: Springer Publishing Company.

Emberton, M. (2010). Medical treatment of benign prostatic hyperplasia: Physician and patient preferences and satisfaction. *International Journal of Clinical Practice, 64*(10), 1425–1435.

Filson, C., Hollingsworth, J., Clemens, J., & Wei, J. (2013). The efficacy and safety of combined therapy with α-blockers and anticholinergics for men with benign prostatic hyperplasia: A meta-analysis. *Journal of Urology, 190*(6), 2153–2160.

Gardiner, S. (2005). Need to know BPH. *Pulse, 65*, 34–37.

Kennedy-Malone, L., Fletcher, K. R., Martin-Plank, L. (2014). *Advanced Practice Nursing in the Care of Older Adults*. Philadelphia, PA: FA Davis.

Kigure, T., Nakata, K., Yuri, Y., Harada, T., Miyagata, S., Fujieda, N., . . . Etori, K. (2012). Microwave thermal therapy in the treatment of benign prostatic hyperplasia and prostate cancer. *Journal of Microwave Surgery, 30,* 239–245.

Lourenco, T., Shaw, M., Fraser, C., MacLennan, G., N'Dow, J., & Pickard, R. (2010). The clinical effectiveness of transurethral incision of the prostate: A systematic review of randomised controlled trials. *World Journal of Urology, 28,* 23–32.

Lee, A. G., Choi, Y. H., Cho, S. Y., & Cho, I. R. (2012). A prospective study of reducing unnecessary prostate biopsy in patients with high serum prostate-specific antigen with consideration of prostatic inflammation. *Korean Journal of Urology, 53*(1), 50–53.

Lerma, E. V. (2009). Anatomic and physiologic changes of the aging kidney. *Clinics in Geriatric Medicine, 25*(3), 325–329.

McPhee, S. J., Papadakis, M. A., & Rabow, M. W. (Eds.). (2014). *Current medical diagnosis and treatment* 2014. New York, NY: McGraw-Hill.

McVary, K. T., Roerhborn, C. G., Alvins, A. L., Barry, M. J., Bruskewitz, R. C., Donnel, R. F., . . . Wei, J. T. (2011). Update on AUA guideline on the management of benign prostatic hyperplasia. *The Journal of Urology, 185*(5), 1793–1803.

Miller, M. (2009). Disorders of fluid balance. In S. Studenski, K. P. High, & S. Asthana (Eds.), *Hazzard's geriatric medicine and gerontology* (6th ed., pp. 1047–1058). New York, NY: McGraw-Hill.

Neelima, D., & Bhagwat, D. (2011). Benign prostatic hyperplasia: An overview of existing treatment. *Indian Journal of Pharmacology, 43*(1), 6–12.

Paolone, D. R. (2010). Benign prostatic hyperplasia. *Clinics in geriatric medicine, 26*(2), 223–239.

Parsons, J. K., & Im, R. (2009). Alcohol consumption is associated with a decreased risk of benign prostatic hyperplasia. *Journal of Urology, 182*(4), 1463–68.

Péquignot, R., Belmin, J., Chauvelier, S., Gaubert, J. Y., Konrat, C., Duron, E., & Hanon, O. (2009). Renal function in older hospital patients is more accurately estimated using the Cockcroft-Gault formula than the modification diet in renal disease formula. *Journal of the American Geriatrics Society, 57*(9), 1638–1643. doi:10.1111/j.1532–5415.2009.02385.x

Shrivastava, A., & Gupta, V. B. (2012). Various treatment options for benign prostatic hyperplasia: A current update. *Journal of Midlife Health, 3*(1), 10–19.

Uphold, C., & Graham, M. (2013). *Clinical guidelines in family practice* (5th ed.). Gainesville, FL: Barmarrae Books, Inc.

Zhang, N., & Zhang, X. (2013). Controversy of the prostate-specific antigen test era: Should prostate cancer be detected and treated in all patients? *Chinese Medical Journal, 126*(15), 2803–2804.

CHAPTER 45

Renal Artery Stenosis

MICHELE H. TALLEY • CHARLENE M. MYERS

I. Definition

A. Renal artery stenosis (RAS) is defined as a stenosis or narrowing in the lumen of the main renal artery or in its proximal branches.

B. RAS is a progressive disease in which vascular supply is interrupted and perfusion to the kidney may lead to gradual loss of renal function due to ischemia and eventual death of the organ.

C. RAS is sometimes referred to as ischemic nephropathy (defined as decreased glomerular filtration rate [GFR] due to hemodynamically significant RAS).

II. Pathophysiology

A. Reduced blood flow through the renal artery causes the kidney to release increased amounts of the hormone, renin

B. Renin, a powerful blood pressure regulator, initiates a series of chemical events that result in hypertension.

C. Renal vascular hypertension can be very severe and difficult to control.

D. The kidney with RAS suffers from decreased blood flow and often shrinks (atrophies). This process is called "ischemic nephropathy."

E. The other kidney is at risk for the development of damage caused by hypertension.

F. Hypertensive nephrosclerosis often develops

G. Persistently elevated blood pressures in this non-stenotic kidney may cause progressive scarring (sclerosis) leading to progressive loss of filtering function in this kidney as well.

H. Compensatory contralateral hypertrophy may temporarily maintain renal function

I. Unilateral RAS and bilateral RAS can ultimately lead to chronic kidney disease.

III. Etiology
A. Atherosclerosis
B. Fibromuscular dysplasia
C. Dissection
D. Vasculitis (e.g., Takayasu arteritis)
E. Thromboembolic disease
F. Renal artery coarctation
G. Extrinsic compression
H. Radiation injury
I. Renal artery aneurysm

IV. Types of RAS
A. Fibromuscular dysplasia
1. Accounts for less than 10% of RAS
2. Due to an abnormality in the muscular lining of the renal artery
3. Occurs in ages 25–50 years in mostly women, compared to men
4. Familial tendency
B. Atherosclerosis
1. Leads to more than 90% of all cases of RAS
2. Most RAS is caused by atherosclerosis, or "hardening of the arteries." Atherosclerosis is the buildup of cholesterol deposits, or plaque, in the lining of the arteries.
C. Renovascular disease

V. Signs/symptoms
A. Usually asymptomatic until stenosis is severe
B. Symptoms are as follows:
1. Increase or decrease in urination
2. Edema
3. Drowsiness
4. Generalized itching
5. Dry skin
6. Headaches
7. Weight loss
8. Appetite loss
9. Nausea
10. Vomiting
11. Sleep problems
12. Discolored skin
13. Muscle cramping
C. RAS should be considered in the following circumstances:
1. Onset of hypertension (usually sudden) at younger than 30 years or older than age 55

2. Hypertension that was well controlled has become difficult to treat (despite using three or more different blood pressure control medications)
3. Malignant, accelerated, or resistant hypertension
4. No family history of hypertension
5. Unexplained heart failure or "flash" pulmonary edema
6. Asymmetric (differently sized and shaped) kidneys on ultrasound
7. Epigastric or renal artery bruits (upon auscultation or ultrasound)
8. Atherosclerotic disease of the aorta or peripheral arteries
9. A decline in estimated GFR by greater than 30% from baseline renal function after initiation of angiotensin converting enzyme (ACE-I) inhibitors or angiotensin receptor blockers (ARBs)
10. Metabolic acidosis

VI. Laboratory/diagnostics

A. Noninvasive tests: ultrasonography (US), computed tomography (CT) angiography, magnetic resonance angiography (MRA), captopril renal scintigraphy, and captopril test
  1. Doppler US may be used for initial diagnostic screening; however, if the stenosis is critical (greater than 80%–90%) when using Doppler US or MRI, an invasive diagnostic test may be required.
  2. CT angiography of the renal arteries: noninvasive and allows for 3D viewing of vessels
    a. Less specific than MRA but may be used in patients in whom MRA is contraindicated
    b. Risk of contrast-induced nephropathy is present
  3. MRA can provide a functional assessment of blood flow to the kidney and kidney function.
    a. Does not require use of radiation or iodinated contrast; uses gadolinium-based contrast medium and must be avoided in those with moderate- to end-stage renal failure
    b. Cannot use MRI/A in those with implanted devices

B. Invasive renal angiography: the most direct measure of hemodynamic or functional significance of a stenosis is differential pressure across the stenosis.
  1. Intra-arterial digital subtraction angiography is the definitive diagnostic test—currently, it is the gold standard. Renal artery differential pressure (RADP) can be measured during catheterization before percutaneous transluminal angioplasty (PTA), and this measurement can be used to guide treatment.
    a. A mean RADP of at least 10 mmHg or a peak RADP of at least 20 mmHg is considered significant; proceeding to PTA with either of these measurements is beneficial.
    b. The risk of contrast-induced nephropathy is present but volume of contrast needed may be controlled.

C. Renal vein renin sampling, peripheral renin levels, and captopril renal scintigraphy are not generally recommended due to low specificity and sensitivity.

VII. **Management**

A. Treatment and control of blood pressure and renal perfusion
1. Lifestyle changes
    a. Exercise
    b. Healthy body weight
    c. Healthy diet (low fat, low protein, low sodium, and high fiber)
    d. Smoking cessation
2. Medical management
    a. Optimize medical therapy for glycemic, blood pressure, and cholesterol management, as defined by current evidence-based guidelines and recommended therapy

Table 45.1	ACE Inhibitors and Angiotensin Receptor Blockers for Renal Artery Stenosis	
	Agent	**Usual Dose/Frequency**
ACE Inhibitors	Benazepril (lotensin®)	10–40 mg PO DAILY
	Captopril (capoten®)	12.5–100 mg PO BID or TID
	Enalapril (vasotec®)	5–40 mg PO DAILY or BID
	Fosinopril (monopril®)	10–40 mg PO DAILY
	Lisinopril (zestril®)	5–40 mg PO DAILY
	Moexipril (univasc®)	7.5–30 mg PO DAILY
	Perindopril (aceon®)	4–8 mg PO DAILY
	Quinapril (accupril®)	10–80 mg PO DAILY
	Ramipril (altace®)	2.5–20 mg PO DAILY
	Trandolapril (mavik®)	1–4 mg PO DAILY
Angiotensin II Receptor Antagonists	Azilsartan (edarbi®)	40–80 mg PO DAILY
	Candesartan (atacand®)	8–32 mg PO DAILY
	Eprosartan mesylate (teveten®)	400–800 mg PO DAILY or BID
	Irbesartan (avapro®)	75–300 mg PO DAILY
	Losartan (cozaar®)	25–100 mg PO DAILY
	Olmesartan (benicar®)	20–40 PO DAILY
	Telmisartan (micardis®)	20–80 mg PO DAILY
	Valsartan (diovan®)	40–320 mg PO DAILY or BID
	Azilsartan (edarbi®)	40–80 mg PO DAILY

      b. Medications (ACE inhibitors and ARBs have been shown to slow the progression of kidney disease); caution is necessary, as when ACE inhibitors or ARBs are used, further decline in GFR may occur in patients with RAS. Renin-angiotensin-aldosterone system (RAAS) blockade, statins, and antiplatelet therapy (i.e., aspirin) are the cornerstone for clinical management of atherosclerotic disease, including RAS. An important feature in the treatment of patients with atherosclerotic RAS is the reduction of serum lipids and cholesterol that are contributing to atherosclerosis in the renal artery and in the kidney itself.

      c. Blood pressure lowering medications, ACE inhibitors, and ARBs have been effective in slowing the progression of kidney disease (see table 45.1 for ACE inhibitor/ARB regimens).

            i. ACE inhibitors and ARBs can cause acute renal failure; patients should have their kidney function checked within 2 weeks after starting medication.

            ii. Many individuals require two or more medications to lower BP to recommended goals. In addition to an ACE inhibitor or ARB, a diuretic, β blocker, or calcium channel blocker may be needed (See Hypertension chapter for regimens of BP-lowering agents).

      d. Management of glycemia: see Diabetes Mellitus chapter

      e. Management of atherosclerotic disease: see Coronary Artery Disease/Hyperlipidemia and Peripheral Vascular Disease chapters

3. All patients should be assessed for coronary artery disease

4. Minimally invasive procedures to restore blood flow to the kidneys via revascularization. Revascularization is recommended by the American Heart Association when the renal artery is reduced more than 60% of its diameter. Associated risks include hemorrhage and contrast-induced nephropathy.

      a. Percutaneous transluminal angioplasty (PTA)

            i. Risks include renal artery dissection, rupture, thrombosis, and embolism

      b. PTA with stent placement

      c. Thrombolysis (in the event of acute thrombosis)

      d. Radioablation of renal nerves

5. Surgical procedures

      a. Renal artery bypass/reconstruction

      b. Endarterectomy

    c. Other considerations: all patients with atherosclerotic RAS should be assessed for coronary artery disease; most patients should receive an ACE inhibitor or an ARB and a statin. The latter not only reduces cardiac risk but also may induce regression of RAS. An important feature in the treatment of patients with atherosclerotic RAS is the reduction of serum lipids and cholesterol that are contributing to atherosclerosis in the renal artery and in the kidney itself

6. Regular medical prophylaxis may effectively prevent stone recurrence in patients with a history of recurrence, calcium oxalate dihydrate stones, hypercalciuria, or hyperuricuria

    a. Dietary advice for all patients

    b. Renal leak hypercalciuria: 50 mg HCTZ PO daily and 5 grams potassium citrate powder PO 3 times a day after meals

    c. Absorptive stones

    d. Uric acid and calcium oxalate calculi with hyperuricuria or gouty diathesis: 100 mg allopurinol PO twice daily, as well as potassium citrate

    e. Infected stones: potassium citrate and appropriate antibiotics

    f. Cost effectiveness, patient compliance, and gastrointestinal upset may limit patient acceptability and clinical use of medical prophylaxis

BIBLIOGRAPHY

Academy of Nutrition and Dietetics. (2010). *Recommendations summary: CKD: Assessment of medical health/history 2010*. Evidence Analysis Library. Retrieved September 24, 2014, from http://www.andeal.org/template.cfm?template=guide_summary&key=2595

Anderson, J. L., Halperin, J. L., Albert, N., Bozkurt, B., Brindis, R. G., Curtis, L. H., . . . Shen, W.-K. (2013). Management of patients with peripheral artery disease (compilation of 2005 and 2011 ACCF/AHA guideline recommendations): A report of the American College of Cardiology Foundation/American Heart Association Task Force on Practice Guidelines. *Journal of the American College of Cardiology, 61*(14), 1555–1570. doi:10.1016/j.jacc.2013.01.004

Colyer, W. R., Eltahawy, E., & Cooper, C. J. (2011). Renal artery stenosis: Optimizing diagnosis and treatment. *Progress in Cardiovascular Diseases, 54*(1), 29–35. doi:10.1016/j.pcad.2011.02.007

Creager, M. A., Belkin, M., Bluth, E. I., Casey, D. E., Chaturvedi, S., Dake, M. D., . . . Ziffer, J. A. (2012). 2012 ACCF/AHA/ACR/SCAI/SIR/STS/SVM/SVN/ SVS key data elements and definitions for peripheral atherosclerotic vascular disease: A report of the American College of Cardiology Foundation/American Heart Association Task Force on clinical data standards (writing committee to develop clinical data standards for peripheral atherosclerotic vascular disease). *Circulation, 125*(2), 395–467. doi:10.1161/CIR.0b013e31823299a1

Lao, D., Parasher, P. S., Cho, K. C., & Yeghiazarians, Y. (2011). Atherosclerotic renal artery stenosis—diagnosis and treatment. *Mayo Clinic Proceedings, 86*(7), 649–657. doi:10.4065/mcp.2011.0181

Longo, D. L., Fauci, A. S., Kasper, D. L., Hauser, S., Jameson, J., & Loscalzo, J. (Eds.). (2012). *Harrison's principles of internal medicine* (18th ed.). New York, NY: McGraw-Hill.

Madder, R. D., Hickman, L., Crimmins, G. M., Puri, M., Marinescu, V., McCullough, P. A., . . . Safian, R. D. (2011). Validity of estimated glomerular filtration rates for assessment of baseline and serial renal function in patients with atherosclerotic renal artery stenosis: Implications for clinical trials of renal revascularization. *Circulation: Cardiovascular Interventions, 4*(3), 219–225. doi:10.1161/CIRCINTERVENTIONS.110.960971

National Institute of Diabetes and Digestive and Kidney Diseases. (2014). *Renal artery stenosis.* National Kidney and Urologic Diseases Information (NKUDIC). Retrieved December 2, 2013, from http://kidney.niddk.nih.gov/ kudiseases/pubs/renalarterystenosis/index.aspx

National Institute of Neurological Disorders and Stroke. (2011). *Fibromuscular dysplasia information page.* Retrieved December 2, 2013, from http://www. ninds.nih.gov/disorders/fibromuscular_dysplasia/fibromuscular_dysplasia.htm

Plouin, P. F., & Bax, L. (2010). Diagnosis and treatment of renal artery stenosis. *Nature Reviews Nephrology, 6*(3), 151–159. doi:10.1038/nrneph.2009.230

Rooke, T. W., Hirsch, A. T., Misra, S., Sidawy, A. N., Beckman, J. A., Findeiss, L. K., . . . Zierler, R. E. (2011). 2011 ACCF/AHA focused update on the guideline for the management of patients with peripheral artery disease (updating the 2005 guideline): A report of the American College of Cardiology Foundation/ American Heart Association Task Force on Practice Guidelines. *Journal of the American College of Cardiology, 58*(19), 2020–2045. doi:10.1016/j. jacc.2011.08.023

Vasbinder, G. B., Nelemans, P. J., Kessels, A. G., Kroon, A. A., de Leeuw, P. W., & van Engelshoven, J. M. (2001). Diagnosis of renal artery stenosis. *Annals of Internal Medicine, 135*(6), S38.

CHAPTER 46

Nephrolithiasis

MARLA COUTURE • CHARLENE M. MYERS

RENAL CALCULI–NEPHROLITHIASIS

I.   Definition

A. Condition in which one or more stones are present in the pelvis, in the calyces of the kidney, or in the ureter

B. Calculi may be composed of calcium oxalate or calcium phosphate (two most common). Can also be composed of uric acid, struvite, or cystine

II.   Etiology

A. Approximately 10% of the population will develop urinary calculi during their lifetime.

   1. More common in men

   2. Usual age of onset is in the 30s

   3. Approximately 35%–50% of patients will have a recurrence within 5 years

B. Dehydration: occurs more frequently in hot, arid environments

C. Life stress

D. Supersaturation of urine with stone-forming salts

E. Dietary factors

   1. Low fluid intake

   2. High sodium intake

   3. High animal protein intake

   4. High fructose intake

   5. Low dietary calcium intake

      a. Can cause oxalate levels to rise

   6. Overload of calcium supplement intake

F. Decreased or absent stone inhibitors in the urine (e.g., citrate, magnesium, and pyrophosphate)

III. **Risk factors**
   A. Gender/age
   B. Family history
   C. Geography
   D. Genetic predisposition
   E. Preexisting medical conditions
      1. Primary hyperparathyroidism
      2. Obesity
      3. Diabetes
      4. Intestinal malabsorption
      5. Inflammatory bowel disease
      6. Sarcoidosis
      7. Gout
   F. Postsurgical comorbidities
      1. Small bowel resection
      2. Gastric bypass
      3. Colectomy
   G. Sleeping position
      1. Correlation between sleep posture and unilateral renal stone formation
   H. Immobility
   I. Low citrate levels
   J. Urinary tract infections
   K. Oxidative stress
      1. Stone formation linked to production of reactive oxygen species
      2. Oxidative stress linked to idiopathic calcium oxalate nephrolithiasis
   L. Drugs associated with stone formation:
      1. Triamterene (Dyrenium)
      2. Steroids
      3. Vitamin D supplements
      4. Carbonic anhydrous inhibitors
      5. Indinavir (Crixivan): protease inhibitor
      6. Colchicine
      7. Chemotherapy agents
   M. Dietary influences
      1. Decreased renal acid excretion, a precursor of uric acid, leads to hyperuricosuria and decreases calcium oxalate solubility
      2. Sodium ingestion: increases Na excretion, which increases Ca excretion and Ca mobilization from bone
      3. Foods high in oxalate: increases urinary oxalate excretion (e.g., nuts, chocolate, dark green leafy vegetables, rhubarb, beets, and okra)
   N. High urine pH level is the main risk factor for calcium oxalate and calcium phosphate

IV. Types

    A. Calcium stones constitute 80% of renal calculi

    B. Hypercalciuric calcium nephrolithiasis

        1. Can be caused by absorptive, resorptive, and renal disorders

        2. Absorptive (types I, II, and III)

            a. Caused by increased absorption of calcium at the level of the small bowel (i.e., jejunum)

            b. Treatment is focused on decreasing bowel absorption of calcium

            c. Type I is independent of calcium intake. Urine calcium is increased on a regular or even a low-calcium diet.

            d. Type II is diet-dependent. Dramatically decreasing dietary calcium may decrease hypercalciuria.

            e. Type III results from a renal phosphate leak that causes increased vitamin D synthesis and increased small bowel absorption of calcium

                i. Inhibits vitamin D synthesis but not intestinal absorption

        3. Resorptive

            a. Because of hyperparathyroidism

            b. Hypercalcemia, hypophosphatemia, and elevated levels of parathyroid hormones are present

            c. Surgical resection of the adenoma, which leads to hyperparathyroidism, cures the disease and the stones

        4. Renal leak

            a. Renal tubules are unable to reabsorb filtered calcium efficiently, and hypercalciuria occurs

    C. Hyperuricosuric calcium nephrolithiasis

        1. Caused by dietary excess or uric acid metabolic defects

        2. In contrast to uric acid calculi, these patients will maintain a urinary pH level higher than 5.5

    D. Hyperoxaluric calcium nephrolithiasis

        1. Due to primary intestinal disorders

        2. Patients usually have a history of chronic diarrhea, often with inflammatory bowel disease or steatorrhea.

        3. Calcium is unavailable to bind to oxalate, which is then freely and rapidly absorbed; this significantly promotes stone formation.

        4. Increased fluid intake must be emphasized.

    E. Hypocitraturic calcium nephrolithiasis

        1. May result from chronic diarrhea, type I renal tubular acidosis, or chronic or aggressive thiazide diuretic treatment; may also be idiopathic

        2. Citrate appears to bind to calcium in solution, thereby decreasing available calcium for stone formation.

    F. Uric acid calculi

1. Frequently have urinary pH levels lower than 5.5 (average urinary pH level is 5.85)
2. Increasing the pH to levels higher than 6.5 can dramatically increase solubility and can dissolve large stones

G. Struvite calculi
1. Magnesium-ammonium-phosphate stones
2. Commonly seen in women with recurrent urinary tract infections; most stones are large and cause obstruction and bleeding
3. Radiodense
4. Urinary pH level is high (greater than 7–7.5) = alkalotic
5. Caused by urease-producing organisms (*Proteus* spp., *Haemophilus* spp., *Klebsiella* spp., and *Ureaplasma urealyticum*)
6. Stones are soft and amenable to percutaneous nephrolithotomy or extracorporeal shock wave lithotripsy.
7. Treatment requires eradicating the infection with antibiotics and the above interventional techniques

H. Cystine calculi
1. Result of abnormal excretion of cystine, ornithine, lysine, and arginine
2. Cystine is the only amino acid that becomes insoluble in urine
3. Difficult to manage

V. **Clinical manifestations**
A. Acute flank pain (i.e., colic-like)
1. If flank pain increases in intensity and radiates downward to the groin, this indicates that the stone has passed to the lower third of the ureter.
B. Testicular pain
C. Pain not relieved by position
D. Nausea and vomiting
E. Costovertebral angle tenderness
F. Frequency, urgency, and dysuria suggest that the stone is located in the portion of the ureter within the bladder wall
G. Oliguria and acute renal failure may occur when both collecting systems are obstructed by stones
H. Hematuria

VI. **Radiologic studies/laboratory findings**
A. Noncontrast helical CT has proven to be the gold standard radiographic test for diagnosing nephrolithiasis.
B. Plain films of the abdomen will reveal opaque calculi
C. Renal ultrasound (involves no radiation, but less sensitive to detecting stones)
D. An excretory or retrograde pyelogram permits the exact definition of stones and reveals the presence or absence of obstruction.
E. Urinalysis reveals blood
F. Increased white blood cell count

G. Twenty-four-hour urine collection for calcium, uric acid, phosphate, oxalate, and citrate excretion is generally reserved for those with recurrent stones

H. Urine culture: positive for urease-producing organisms

I. Serum chemistries should include calcium, electrolytes, phosphate, and uric acid.

VII. **Management**

A. Relieve pain, nausea, and vomiting

   1. Randomized trials note parenteral nonsteroidal anti-inflammatory drugs are as effective as narcotics for treatment of renal colic (ketorolac). Avoid use in patients with renal dysfunction, as it may lower kidney blood flow and glomerular filtration.

   2. Opioids (hydromorphone) or combination analgesics (hydrocodone/acetaminophen) may be necessary when pain is unrelieved by nonsteroidal anti-inflammatory drugs.

   3. Antiemetics (ondansetron)

B. To hasten stone passage, induce high urine flow with oral intake of at least 2–3 L of fluids per 24 hr to ensure a urine output of at least 2 L per day

C. Urethral stones of up to 10 mm and eligible for observation may be offered medical expulsive therapy.

D. Medications

   1. Antispasmodics relax the smooth muscle of the ureters and have been shown to hasten stone passage by 5–7 days.

     a. α blockers

       i. Doxazosin (Cardura), 4 mg PO daily

       ii. Tamsulosin (Flomax), 0.4 mg PO daily

     b. Calcium channel blockers

       i. Nifedipine (Procardia XL), 30 mg PO daily

   2. Medications and supplements for specific type:

     a. Type I absorptive hypercalciuria: thiazide therapy

       i. Decreases renal excretion of calcium

       ii. Increases bone density by 1% per year

       iii. Has limited long-term use (less than 5 years)

     b. Type II absorptive hypercalciuria: no specific medical therapy is available

     c. Renal hypercalciuria: hydrochlorothiazides (HCTZs) are effective as long-term therapy

     d. Hyperuricemia: purine dietary restrictions or allopurinol, or both

     e. Hyperoxaluria: oral calcium supplements should be given with meals if diarrhea or steatorrhea cannot be effectively reduced

     f. Hypocitraturia: potassium citrate supplements (20 mEq 3 times a day) are usually effective

    g. Uric acid calculi: potassium citrate (liquid, crystals, or tablets—10 mEq), two tablets PO 3 or 4 times a day

      i. Fluid intake is less important; decrease protein intake

      ii. Many patients with uric acid calculi have gout

        (a) If hyperuricemia is present, allopurinol (Zyloprim) should be initiated at 300 mg/day

        (b) Doses greater than 300 mg should be divided and given BID

    h. Struvite calculi: acetohydroxamic acid is an effective urease inhibitor; however, it is poorly tolerated because of gastrointestinal adverse effects

    i. Cystine calculi:

      i. Increase fluid intake

      ii. Alkalinize the urine to pH greater than 7.5 and less than 8

      iii. Administer penicillamine (Cuprimine) or α-mercaptopropionylglycine (tiopronin) MPG

E. Shock wave lithotripsy and ureteroscopy

    1. Useful alternatives in treating the majority of stones

F. For larger, nonstandard stones greater than 10 mm

    1. Percutaneous antegrade ureteroscopy

    2. Laparoscopic techniques

    3. Open surgery

G. After removal, the goal is stone prevention. (see table 46.1)

    1. Recurrence rate is approximately 20%–50%

    2. Regular medical prophylaxis may effectively prevent stone recurrence in patients with a history of recurrence, calcium oxalate dihydrate stones, hypercalciuria, or hyperuricuria. (see Table 46.1)

      a. Cost effectiveness, patient compliance, and gastrointestinal upset may limit patient acceptability and clinical use of medical prophylaxis

Table 46.1	Prevention of Kidney Stones		
Type	**Dietary Modifications***	**Treatment**	**Rationale/ Comments**
ALL	Adequate fluid intake (make sure patient has more than 2 L of fluids/24 hr)	Promote low-glycemic diet Promote a healthy diet and exercise	
Hypercalciuria Calcium oxalate	Avoid foods high in salt (canned or processed foods, cheese, pickles, dried meats); do not add salt to food Reduce animal protein (meat, eggs) Calcium supplements if not getting enough calcium through diet Avoid foods high in oxalate (beans, spinach, rhubarb, chocolate, wheat, nuts, berries)	Thiazide diuretics: Hydrochlorothiazide 25–50 mg PO daily Potassium citrate 10–20 mEq PO TID with meals Calcium citrate 250–500 mg PO TID with meals	Increases the urinary excretion of calcium Raise the citrate and pH of urine Raise the citrate and pH of urine; bind urinary oxalate
Calcium phosphate	Avoid foods high in salt (canned or processed foods, cheese, pickles, dried meats); do not add salt to food reduce animal protein (meat, eggs) Calcium supplements if not getting enough calcium through diet Reduce phosphate intake Decrease intake of dairy products, legumes, chocolate and nuts by about one-third	Cranberry juice: at least 16 oz per day	Acidify urine
Uric acid stones	Decrease protein intake Limiting animal protein (red meat, fish, and shellfish) Reduce or eliminate alcohol intake	Allopurinol 300 mg PO daily (adjust dose for renal dysfunction) potassium citrate 10–20 mEq PO TID with meals	Decreases uric acid in the blood and urine Raise the citrate and pH of urine

Table 46.1	Prevention of Kidney Stones		
Type	**Dietary Modifications***	**Treatment**	**Rationale/ Comments**
Cystine stones	Decrease methionine (sulfur) intake Avoid dairy products, eggs, legumes, greens	**Tiopronin (Thiola)** 800 mg/day ORALLY in 3 divided doses Potassium citrate 10–20 mEq PO TID with meals Penicillamine (Cuprimine) 2 grams PO daily; range 1–4 grams/day	Decreases cystine in the urine Raise the citrate and pH of urine Lowers cystine concentrations and the prevents formation of cystine calculi in the urine
Struvite stones	Avoid supplemental magnesium	Antibiotics Acetohydroxamic acid (**Lithostat**) 15 mg/kg/day PO TID; MAX 1.5 grams/day	Eliminate infection Consider surgical intervention, especially for stones greater than 10 mm or if there is evidence of ongoing obstruction or infection

Note. More information can be found in the National Kidney and Urologic Diseases Information Clearinghouse fact sheet Diet for Kidney Stone Prevention at: http://kidney.niddk.nih.gov/kudiseases/pubs/kidneystonediet/index.aspx

BIBLIOGRAPHY

Asplin, J. R., Coe, F. L., & Favus, M. J. (2011). Nephrolithiasis. In D. L. Kasper, E. Braunwald, S. Hauser, D. Longo, J. L. Jameson, & A. S. Fauci (Eds.), *Harrison's principles of internal medicine* (18th ed.). New York, NY: McGraw-Hill.

Coe, F. L., Evan, A., & Worcester, E. (2008). Kidney stone disease. *Journal of Clinical Investigation, 115*(10), 2598–2608.

Fink, H. A., Wilt, T. J., Eidman, K. E., Garimella, P. S., MacDonald, R., Rutks, I. R., . . . Monga, M. (2013). Medical management to prevent recurrent nephrolithiasis in adults: A systematic review for an American College of Physicians clinical guideline. *Annals of Internal Medicine, 158*(7), 535–543.

Frassetto, L., & Kohlstadt, I. (2011). Treatment and prevention of kidney stones: An update. *American Family Physician, 84*(11), 1234–1242.

Hall, P. M. (2009). Nephrolithiasis: Treatment, causes, and prevention. *Cleveland Clinic Journal of Medicine, 76*(10), 583–591.

Khan, S. R. (2011). Is oxidative stress, a link between nephrolithiasis and obesity, hypertension, diabetes, chronic kidney disease, metabolic syndrome? *Urological Research, 40*(2), 95–112.

Marchini, G. S., Ortiz-Alvarado, O., Miyaoka, R., Kriedgberg, C., Moeding, A., Stessman, M., & Monga, M. (2013). Patient-centered medical therapy for nephrolithiasis. *Urology, 81*(3), 511–516.

McCance, K. L., Huether, S. E., Brashers, V. L., & Rote, N. S. (2013). *Pathophysiology: The biologic basis for disease in adults and children* (7th ed.). Maryland Heights, MD: Mosby.

National Kidney and Urologic Diseases Information Clearinghouse. (2013). *Kidney stones in adults*. In F. L. Coe (Ed.). Retrieved from http://kidney.niddk.nih.gov/kudiseases/pubs/stonesadults/#acknowledgments

Orson, W. M., Pearle, M. S., & Sakhaee, K. (2011). Pharmacotherapy of urolithiasis: Evidence from clinical trials. *Kidney International, 79*(4), 385–392.

Phillips, E., Kieley, S., Johnson, E. B., & Monga, M. (2009). Emergency room management of ureteral calculi: Current practices. *Journal of Endourology, 23*(6), 1021–1024.

Phipps, S., Tolley, D. A., Young, J. G., & Keeley, F. X., Jr. (2010). The management of ureteric stones. *Annals of the Royal College of Surgeons of England, 92*(5), 368–372.

Management of Patients with Endocrine Disorders

CHAPTER 47

Diabetes Mellitus

THOMAS W. BARKLEY, JR. • SUSAN J. APPEL

DIABETES MELLITUS: OVERVIEW OF PRINCIPLES

I. **Definition**
   A. A group of metabolic diseases resulting from a breakdown in the body's ability to produce and/or use insulin
   B. Characterized by hyperglycemia and associated with numerous acute and chronic complications
      1. Acute complications
         a. Diabetes ketoacidosis
         b. Hyperglycemic hyperosmolar nonketotic coma
      2. Chronic complications
         a. Neuropathy
         b. Nephropathy
         c. Retinopathy
         d. Gastroparesis
         e. Cardiovascular disease
         f. Peripheral vascular disease

II. **Incidence/predisposing factors**
   A. Approximately 14 million Americans have diabetes
   B. Diabetes affects approximately 8.3% of the U.S. population.
   C. Diabetes affects approximately 26.9% of individuals 65–74 years of age.
   D. In approximately 7 million of all individuals with diabetes mellitus, the condition is undiagnosed.
   E. Ethnic minorities, Native Americans in particular, are at highest risk
   F. A family history of diabetes mellitus indicates higher risk of development of diabetes.

III.   Classifications of diabetes mellitus and other forms of glucose intolerance
   A. Type 1 (previously, insulin-dependent or juvenile-onset diabetes)
   B. Type 2 (previously, non-insulin-dependent or adult-onset diabetes mellitus)
   C. Secondary diabetes related to the following:
      1. Hormonal excess
         a. Cushing's syndrome
         b. Acromegaly
         c. Hyperthyroidism
         d. Pheochromocytoma
      2. Medications
         a. Glucocorticoids
         b. Diuretics
         c. Phenytoin (Dilantin)
         d. Oral contraceptives
         e. Statins
      3. Pancreatic disease
         a. Pancreatitis
         b. Pancreatectomy
         c. Cystic fibrosis
      4. Other genetic factors
         a. β-cell defects
            i. Latent autoimmune diabetes of adulthood
            ii. Maturity-onset diabetes of the young
         b. Neoplasia
         c. Other genetic syndromes
            i. Down syndrome
            ii. Turner syndrome
            iii. Klinefelter syndrome
            iv. Wolfram syndrome
   D. Gestational diabetes
   E. Impaired glucose homeostasis
      1. Prediabetes
         a. Impaired fasting glucose (IFG)
         b. Impaired glucose tolerance (IGT)

IV.   Laboratory/diagnostic testing
   A. Symptoms of diabetes mellitus include:
      1. Polyuria
      2. Polydipsia
      3. Polyphagia
      4. Unexplained weight loss
   B. According to the American Diabetes Association, the diagnosis of diabetes mellitus and/or impaired glucose homeostasis may be made from positive findings from any of the following tests:

1. Random or casual (any time of day without regard to time since the last meal) plasma glucose concentration 200 mg/dl (11 mmol/L) or above
2. Two-hour post oral glucose tolerance test with 75 grams glucose load 200 mg/dl or above
3. Glycosylated hemoglobin (HbA1c) 6.5% or above
4. Fasting plasma glucose = 126 mg/dl (7.0 mmol/L) or above on two separate occasions
   a. Impaired glucose homeostasis: impaired fasting glucose/IGT/prediabetes

C. Diagnosis of prediabetes
   1. Fasting plasma glucose = 100–125 mg/dl
   2. 2 hr plasma glucose after a 75-gram glucose load = 140–199 mg/dl
   3. HbA1c = 5.7%–6.4%

D. Urinalysis: although this test is used less today because of the wide availability of glucose meters, it can be used to monitor for the following:
   1. Glycosuria—easily detected by Diastix or Clinistix paper strip testing
   2. Ketonuria—quantitatively evident in patients with type 1 diabetes via nitroprusside tests such as Acetest or Ketostix

E. Blood urea nitrogen and urinary creatinine
   1. Baseline
   2. To rule out dehydration (i.e., elevated)

F. Glycosylated hemoglobin (HbA1c)
   1. Elevated before diagnosis in approximately 85% of patients with diabetes
   2. Indicative of a patient's glycemic control over 2–3 months
   3. Now used for initial diagnosis of diabetes mellitus
   4. Appropriate for patients diagnosed with diabetes who have not reached stable glycemic control or are undergoing medication adjustments; the HbA1c should be measured quarterly
      a. Once optimal glycemic control has been reached, HbA1c should be measured every 6 months.
   5. Normal values are approximately 5.5%–6.4%; higher levels indicate higher blood glucose levels and thus, poorer glycemic control; most clinicians strive for less than 6% as the goal

V. **Management: diet, exercise, and eye and foot care for patients living with diabetes**
   A. Note: Treatment plans for all patients diagnosed with diabetes must be highly individualized. The following points provide general guidelines that may be tailored to the needs of each patient:
      1. Teach patients about the benefits of diet therapy:
         a. American Diabetes Association diets found at www.eatright. org or at www.ada.org

      b. Refer patient to a dietitian, as appropriate

      c. Total carbohydrate intake should be 55%–60% of total caloric intake

      d. Fiber intake should be 25 grams/1,000 calories

      e. Fats should account for 25%–35% of total calories (individualized according to serum lipid levels)

      f. Protein should make up 15%–20% of total calories

      g. Meal schedules for patients living with diabetes:

          i. Patients with type 1 diabetes should be encouraged to have three meals each day and three snacks on a schedule consistent with insulin regimen

          ii. Patients with type 2 diabetes should be taught to have meals about five hours apart with few or no snacks

          iii. Teach patients who are on insulin how to count carbohydrates

          iv. Low health-literacy patients can be taught the plate method, and all patients with diabetes should learn portion control.

      h. Artificial sweeteners instead of sugar may be encouraged

      i. Alcohol intake should be limited to modest use (e.g., two drinks or fewer per day); overuse of alcohol can lead to severe hypoglycemia

      j. Optimal glycemic control and weight reduction, PRN, are both important goals of therapy

2. Encourage exercise

      a. An essential component of care for all patients diagnosed with diabetes

      b. Encourage at least 30 min of exercise every day; allow for periods of warm-up (5–10 min) and cool down (5–10 min)

      c. Teach the patient to use silica gel or air midsoles and polyester or cotton blend socks to keep feet as dry as possible; wearing proper footwear and monitoring for blisters is of paramount importance.

      d. Monitor for dehydration; encourage intake of extra fluids

      e. Teach the patient to inject insulin at a body site far from that being exercised, if possible (e.g., abdomen instead of legs or arms)

      f. Additional carbohydrates should be ingested before exercise

      g. Teach that exercise diminishes the need for insulin

3. Foot care: Patients should be taught the importance of foot care in preventing infection, gangrene, and/or the need for amputation.

      a. The most important prevention strategy for foot complications is to examine the feet for injuries each day with a mirror, including the bottoms of the feet and between the toes.

    b. Report immediately any new problems such as broken skin, ulcers, or blisters (i.e., tell the patient not to wait until his or her next appointment)

    c. Have nails trimmed regularly by an experienced health care provider

    d. Wash feet daily with lukewarm water and a mild soap; pat feet dry with a soft cloth; apply lotion after washing but avoid lotion between toes

    e. Wear only shoes prescribed by a health care professional

    f. Always wear protective shoes and socks; do not wear socks alone

    g. Stop smoking

VI. **Complications**

    A. Diabetes-related retinopathy

      1. Occurs in approximately 15% of patients diagnosed with diabetes after 15 years; increases by 1% each year after diagnosis

      2. The most common cause of all blindness

      3. Annual ophthalmology examinations are indicated

    B. Cardiovascular disease

      1. Diabetes adds an independent risk factor to atherosclerotic development

      2. The prevalence of hypertension is 2 times greater in patients with type 2 diabetes than in the general population.

    C. Cataracts—increased incidence among patients diagnosed with diabetes

    D. Glaucoma—occurs among approximately 6% of patients living with diabetes

    E. Neuropathy (peripheral and autonomic)

      1. Most common complication

      2. Poorly understood

      3. May involve loss of sensation as well as pain along the autonomic and peripheral tracks

    F. Nephropathy: end-stage renal disease has a 40% incidence in patients with type 1 diabetes and a less than 20% incidence in patients with type 2 diabetes

    G. Infections

      1. Chronically common in patients diagnosed with diabetes

      2. Watch for necrobiosis lipoidica diabeticorum lesions over the anterior legs and dorsal surfaces of the ankles; these may predispose patients to infection

      3. Yeast infections are also common

    H. Gangrene of the feet: incidence is 20 times higher among patients diagnosed with diabetes

    I. Diabetes ketoacidosis (type 1 patients): see Diabetes-Related Emergencies

J. Hyperosmolar hyperglycemic nonketotic syndrome (HHNS) (type 2 patients): see Diabetes-Related Emergencies

TYPE 1 DIABETES MELLITUS

I. **Predisposing factors/general comments: type 1 diabetes**

A. Each year, 15 per 100,000 individuals with diabetes are diagnosed with type 1 diabetes.

B. Most commonly seen in Caucasians

C. African-Americans have the lowest incidence of this type in the United States.

D. Males and females are affected equally

E. Genetic predisposition

F. Approximately 70% acquire type 1 before age 20

G. Virtual absence of circulating insulin

H. Islet cell antibodies may be found in approximately 90% of patients within the first year of diagnosis.

I. Development of this type of diabetes is strongly associated with the presence of human leukocyte antigens HLA-DR3 and HLA-DR4

J. Absence of C-peptides

K. Ketone development usually occurs

L. Usually develops acutely over a period of days to weeks

II. **Signs/symptoms: type 1 diabetes**

A. Polyuria

B. Polydipsia

C. Polyphagia

D. Weight loss

E. Skin and genital infections

F. Nocturnal enuresis

G. Weakness/fatigue

H. Blurred vision

I. Changes in level of consciousness (irritability to coma)

J. Loss of subcutaneous fat and muscle wasting

III. **Laboratory/diagnostics: type 1 diabetes**

A. Essential criteria include the following:

1. Polyuria

2. Polydipsia

3. Polyphagia

4. Weight loss

5. Random serum glucose of 200 mg/dl or greater

6. Plasma glucose of 126 mg/dl or greater after an overnight fast for a recommended 9–12 hr

a. Performed on more than one occasion

7. Ketonemia, ketonuria, or both

IV. Management: type I diabetes

A. Note: Treatment plans for all patients living with diabetes must be highly individualized. The following points provide general guidelines that may be tailored to the needs of each patient:

1. Physician/endocrinologist referral—especially indicated for patients in whom condition is newly diagnosed and for those with comorbidities

2. Calculating insulin dosages

   a. As a general rule, the initiation of insulin commonly begins by prescribing 0.5 units/kg/day, with ⅔ of the dose given in the morning and the remaining ⅓ given in the evening.

      i. Note that dosages may be slightly lower for thinner patients and slightly higher for those who are obese.

   b. If serum glucose values remain above 140 mg/dl before the evening meal, dosages are generally changed by adding 2–5 units approximately every 3 days until the patient's levels are well regulated.

   c. Once afternoon postprandial glucose values are controlled (less than 140 mg/dl), fasting plasma levels are checked. If fasting levels are elevated, ⅔ of the insulin dose will be administered before breakfast, and the remaining ⅓ will be given before dinner until fasting glucose level reaches 120–140 mg/dl.

   d. After afternoon and pre-breakfast glucose levels have been regulated, late-morning glucose levels are assessed, and regular insulin may be added to the morning injection to keep glucose levels below 140 mg/dl.

      i. Note: regular insulin usually does not exceed 50% of the amount of insulin given at one time

3. For patients with type 1 diabetes, particularly those diagnosed by the findings of ketones and/or young age at onset, conventional use of insulin may be provided initially, especially during the early phases of the diagnosis.

   a. Physiologic regimens (preferred)

      i. Basal long-acting insulin (Lantus or Detemir) once daily at the same time (up to 50 units per site, as is poorly absorbed after that amount)

      ii. Bolus rapid-acting insulin (Lispro, Aspart, or Glulisine) before each meal

      iii. Therefore, a basal for a type 1 patient would be ⅓ daily insulin requirements

      iv. For a type 2 diabetes patient, kg × 0.2 = basal need or start in insulin-naive patients with 10 units SQ

   b. Non-physiologic regimens (conventional split-dose mixtures)

      i. The morning dose of insulin is ⅔ NPH and ⅓ regular

    ii. The evening dose is ½ NPH and ½ regular

    iii. Lispro (Humalog) dosage varies depending on patient, typically 0.5–1 unit/kg total, administered sq before breakfast and evening meals; insulin aspart (Novolog) 0.2–0.6 unit/kg total, administered SQ before breakfast and evening meals; insulin glulisine (Apidra) 0.5–1 unit/kg total, administered SQ 15 minutes before, or 20 minutes after, starting meal

    iv. Lispro (Humalog), insulin aspart (NovoLog), and insulin glulisine (Apidra) cause fewer episodes of severe hypoglycemia compared with regular insulin due to a more favorable kinetic profile (onset of action/lag time of regular insulin = 30 minutes vs. 5 minutes for lispro/aspart)

    v. Therefore, a 70-kg patient would receive 35 units of insulin each day: 10 units regular insulin and 15 units NPH every morning; and 5 units regular insulin and 5 units NPH every evening

4. Intensive therapy (used for patients who cannot maintain normal levels with conventional therapy without becoming hypoglycemic at night)

    a. Reducing/omitting the evening insulin dose and adding a portion at bedtime:

        i. 10 units regular insulin with 15 units NPH every morning,

        ii. 5 units of regular insulin before the evening meal, and

        iii. 5 units NPH insulin at bedtime

    b. Intensive therapy may be necessary several years after type 1 diabetes is diagnosed and may be the preferred method prescribed by some clinicians; however, this type of therapy is reserved for patients who are highly motivated and able to adhere to complex insulin regimens.

5. Home testing

    a. Blood glucose levels should be monitored 4 times a day (before breakfast, lunch, and dinner, and at bedtime)

6. Examples of insulin administration schedules—treatment plans must be highly individualized and based on the needs of the patient; however, the following examples may prove useful as a guide in practice:

    a. One-injection regimen: long-acting insulin glargine (Lantus) dosage depending on patient, administered SQ at same time every day

    b. Two-injection regimen: regular and NPH or insulin detemir (Levemir) in conventional split doses before breakfast and before dinner; usually ⅔ of total daily dose is administered in the morning

    c. Three-injection regimen: regular and NPH mixed in the morning before breakfast, regular insulin before dinner, and NPH at bedtime

        i. Used to prevent the dawn phenomenon and the Somogyi effect

    d. Four-injection regimen: lispro (Humalog), insulin aspart (Novolog), or insulin glulisine (Apidra) before meals (sometimes regular insulin instead) and NPH at bedtime

    e. Insulin pump regimen: with Humalog or regular insulin, administering 50% of total daily needs at a basal hourly rate, then boluses before meals and before bedtime snack

    f. Basal bolus as noted above

7. Types of insulin with most common examples (Table 47.1)

    a. Note: In addition to its use by patients with type 1 diabetes, insulin (usually beginning with NPH single-dose therapy, or long-acting single dose, or bid dosing for high insulin requirements) is indicated for patients with type 2 diabetes whose glucose levels fail to be adequately controlled by diet, exercise, and oral antidiabetic agents.

8. Sliding scales

    a. Used when around-the-clock therapy fails to maintain adequate glucose control

    b. When individual weight, height, and activity calculations are considered, a recommended initial example ordering regular insulin to be used on a sliding-scale basis might include the following:

Blood glucose level	Regular insulin dose	Lispro (Humalog)/ Insulin aspart (Novolog)/ Insulin glulisine (Apidra)
121–150 mg/dl	2 units	0 units
151–199 mg/dl	4 units	3 units
200–250 mg/dl	6 units	5 units
251–300 mg/dl	8 units	7 units
301–350 mg/dl	10 units	10 units
351–400 mg/dl	12 units, and call acute care nurse practitioner or physician	12 units, and call acute care nurse practitioner or physician

Table 47.1	Common Types of Insulin		
Insulin	**Onset**	**Peak**	**Duration**
Rapid-acting: covers insulin needs for meals eaten at the same time as the medication is administered; used in combination with longer-acting insulins			
Humalog (Lispro)	15–30 minutes	~30–90 minutes	3–5 hr
Novolog (Aspart)	10–20 minutes	~40–50 minutes	3–5 hr
Apidra (Glulisine)	20–30 minutes	~30–90 minutes	1–1.5 hr
<u>Short-acting</u>: **covers insulin needs for meals between 30 and 60 minutes after administration**			
Regular (Humulin R, Novolin R),	30–60 minutes	2–6 hr	5–8 hr
Humulin R U-500	30 minutes	1.7–4 hr	Up to 12 hr if given in high doses
<u>Intermediate-acting</u>: **covers insulin needs overnight or at least for half of the night; usually combined with rapid- or short-acting preparations**			
NPH (Humulin N, Novolin N)	2–4 hr	6–8 hr	12–15 hr
<u>Long-acting</u>: **covers insulin needs throughout an entire day/24-hour period; often combined with rapid- or short-acting preparations, but do not mix in same syringe. Do not exceed greater than 50 units long acting per injection site. Levemir and/or Lantus can be split in to b.i.d. dosing. Humulin R U-500 can be poteniated by oral hypoglycemics.**			
Levemir (Detemir)	1–2 hr	Maximal effect at 4–6 hr	Up to 24 hr
Lantus (glargine)	1–1.5 hr	Maximal effect at 4–6 hr	24+ hr
<u>Pre-mixed</u>: **combinations of intermediate- and short-acting preparations in a bottle or in an insulin pen; usually taken BID before meals**			
NPH/Regular 70/30 or 50/50	~30 minutes	Varies	18–24 hr
NPL/Humalog 75/25, 50/50	10–15 minutes	Varies	12–15 hr
Novolog 70/30	10–20 minutes	1–4 hr	Up to 24 hr

Note. B.I.D. = Bis in die (bid); NPH = neutral protamine hagedorn; NPL = neutral protamine lispro.

9. Monitoring control of glucose
    a. Patient testing
        i. Patients should be taught to document home glucose readings and bring their documentation to appointments with their clinician.
    b. Hemoglobin A1c
        i. Measurements are indicated every 3–4 months to assess glucose control over the past quarter
10. Management of poorly controlled early morning glucose
    a. Diagnosed by monitoring 3:00 a.m. blood glucose levels
        i. Somogyi effect
            (a) Nocturnal hypoglycemia develops, stimulating a surge of counter-regulatory hormones (Somogyi effect) that raise blood sugar, resulting in elevated early morning glucose levels.
            (b) The patient is hypoglycemic at 3:00 a.m. and rebounds with an elevated blood sugar at 7:00 a.m.
            (c) Treatment: Reduce or omit the bedtime dose of insulin. If using long-acting insulin, administer in the morning and not in the afternoon; actual peak occurs about five hours after administration
            (d) Levemir is shorter acting than Lantus and may help to avoid nocturnal hypoglycemic episodes
        ii. Dawn phenomenon
            (a) Decreased sensitivity to insulin occurs nocturnally, owing to the presence of growth hormone, which spikes at night.
            (b) Blood sugar becomes progressively elevated throughout the night, resulting in elevated glucose levels at 7:00 a.m.
            (c) Treatment: add or increase the bedtime dose of insulin
        iii. Waning of insulin levels: Insufficient dosage of intermediate-acting insulin may also cause elevated early morning glucose levels
            (a) Treatment: increase the amount of intermediate-acting insulin at bedtime
11. Major complications
    a. Diabetes ketoacidosis: see Diabetes-Related Emergencies
    b. Hypoglycemia

TYPE 2 DIABETES MELLITUS

I. **Predisposing factors/general comments: type 2 diabetes**
   A. Affects 3.5% of the general population

B. More than 90% of all patients diagnosed with diabetes have type 2 diabetes mellitus

C. Usually seen among adults, especially after age 45

D. Circulating insulin is sufficient to prevent ketoacidosis but is inadequate to meet the patient's insulin needs

E. Caused by tissue insensitivity to insulin, or by an insulin secretory defect that results in resistance and/or impaired production of insulin

F. Approximately 75%–80% of patients with type 2 diabetes in the United States are obese.

G. Ketone production does not usually occur in patients with type 2 diabetes

H. C-peptides are usually present

I. Associated with "metabolic syndrome," previously referred to as "syndrome X," a phenomenon characterized by three or more of the following:
1. Central obesity: waist circumference that is greater than or equal to 40 inches (101.6 cm) for men, greater than or equal to 35 inches (88.9 cm) for women, or a body mass index above 30 (due to Asians' small body habitus, more astringent waist cut points are used by the International Diabetes Foundation)
2. Hypertension: blood pressure of 130/85 mmHg or above
3. Abnormal high-density lipoprotein (HDL): less than 40 mg/dl in men and less than 50 mg/dl in women
4. Abnormal triglycerides: 150 mg/dl or greater
5. Fasting blood glucose of 100 mg/dl or greater (i.e., insulin resistance)

J. Usually develops insidiously

K. In addition to being hyperglycemic, the patient may be asymptomatic

II. Signs/symptoms: type 2 diabetes

A. Polyuria

B. Polydipsia

C. Polyphagia

D. Frequent infections, including vulvovaginitis and pruritus

E. Acute weight loss, yet the patient is often overweight

F. Fatigue

G. Blurred vision (recurrent)

H. Peripheral neuropathy

III. Laboratory/diagnostics: type 2 diabetes

A. Same as for type 1 diabetes mellitus, except that no ketone development (i.e., ketonemia or ketonuria) occurs

IV. Management: type 2 diabetes

A. Note: Treatment plans for all patients diagnosed with diabetes must be highly individualized. The following points provide general guidelines that may be tailored to the needs of each patient:

1. Physician/endocrinologist referral is especially indicated for patients with newly diagnosed diabetes and for those with comorbidities.
2. Diet and exercise
3. Oral pharmacologic agents should be initiated upon patients who fail to control glucose levels through diet and exercise
    a. Insulin therapy is reserved until oral therapy fails in patients with type 2 diabetes or their A1C is 8 or more; kg x 0.2 = basal need or start in insulin-naive patients with 10 units SQ
    b. Use of insulin therapy is common after 12–15 years of oral therapy
4. Oral hypoglycemic agent choices (Table 47.2)
    a. Biguanides
    b. Sulfonylureas
        i. Stimulate the pancreas to release more insulin
        ii. First-generation drugs are less commonly prescribed today because second-generation drugs are more effective and have less serious adverse effects.
        iii. Alcohol, chloramphenicol, methyldopa, miconazole, monoamine oxidase (MAO) inhibitors, salicylates, sulfonamides, warfarin, and phenylbutazone may potentiate hypoglycemic effects of sulfonylureas.
    c. α-glucosidase inhibitors
    d. Meglitinides
    e. Thiazolidinediones
    f. Incretin mimetics
    g. Dipeptidyl peptidase-4
    h. Glucagon-like peptide-1 receptor agonists
    i. Sodium-glucose cotransporter 2 inhibitors (SGLT-2 inhibitors)
5. Major complications
    a. HHNK (see Diabetes-Related Emergencies)

Table 47.2	Oral Hypoglycemic Agents			
Oral agent	**Duration**	**Starting dose**	**Daily dosage**	**Comment(s)**
Biguanides				
Metformin HCl (Glucophage) Oral Solution: Riomet 500 mg/5 ml	12–24 hr	500, 800, or1000 mg	500 mg–2.55 grams 1–3 times a day	"Insulin-sparing" agent that does not cause weight gain in patients with diabetes; therefore, extremely popular with obese patients and in combination with a sulfonylurea
Metformin, Extended Release (Glucophage XL)	Half-life: 6 hr	500 mg	500–2000 mg 1 time daily with evening meal	Dosage may be increased from starting dose by 500 mg weekly GI-related side effects are less severe with extended release
Sulfonylureas				
Glipizide (Glucotrol)	10–24 hr	5, 10 mg	5–40 mg per day single dose or in 2 divided doses	Should be taken on an empty stomach 30 minutes before meals
Glipizide Extended Release (Glucotrol XL)	Half-life, 2.5 hr	2.5, 5, 10 mg with meal	20 mg per day	
Glyburide (Diabeta, Micronase, Glynase)	24 hr	1.25, 2.5, or 5 mg	0.75–20 mg per day (Administered in single or 2 divided doses)	Use lower initial dose in the elderly, those with hepatic or renal impairment, and those at serious risk for hypoglycemia (may cause prolonged hypoglycemia); should not be taken on an empty stomach, or severe hypoglycemia may occur
Glimepiride (Amaryl)	24 hr	1, 2, or 4 mg	1–8 mg per day	Prescribed once each day as monotherapy or in combination with insulin

Table 47.2	Oral Hypoglycemic Agents			
Oral agent	Duration	Starting dose	Daily dosage	Comment(s)
α-Glucosidase Inhibitors				
Acarbose (Precose)	6–12 hr	25, 50, 100 mg once or TID	In patients weighing greater than 60 kg: 50 mg 3 times a day In patients weighing greater than 60 kg: 100 mg 3 times a day	May cause flatulence; dosage should be increased slowly to reduce GI adverse effects; take with first bite of meal. Do not use in patients with significant renal dysfunction (serum creatinine greater than 2 mg/dl)
Miglitol (Glyset)	2–4 hr	25, 50, 100 mg 3 times a day at the first bite of each meal; if severe GI adverse effects occur, may start at 25 mg each day	100 mg 3 times a day	Increases risk of hypoglycemia if taken with certain foods (e.g., garlic, celery, juniper berries, ginseng); contraindicated in type 1 diabetes. Do not use in patients with significant renal dysfunction (serum creatinine greater than 2 mg/dl). Take with first bite of meal.
Meglitinides				
Repaglinide (Prandin)	Half-life, 1 hr	0.5, 1, 2 mg 30 minutes or less before meals, 2–4 times a day	Maximum dose, 16 mg per day	Use cautiously in patients with hepatic or renal impairment; contraindicated in patients with type 1 diabetes; preferably taken less than 15 minutes prior to meal; omit if no meal eaten

Table 47.2	Oral Hypoglycemic Agents			
Oral agent	**Duration**	**Starting dose**	**Daily dosage**	**Comment(s)**
Meglitinides				
Nateglinide (Starlix)	Half-life, 1 hr	60, 100 mg 3 times a day	480 mg/day	Preferably taken less than 15 minutes prior to meal; omit if no meal eaten. Use cautiously in patients with hepatic or renal impairment.
Thiazolinediones				
Rosiglitazone maleate (Avandia)	Half-life, 3–4 hr	2, 4, 8 mg BID	8 mg, may take 4 mg BID or an 8-mg tablet once daily	Contraindicated in patients with established New York Heart Association Class III or IV heart failure. May be taken with or without food; after 12 weeks of therapy, may increase dosage to 8 mg; may be used with metformin and/or insulin
Pioglitazone hydrochloride (Actos)	Half-life, 3–7 hr	15, 30, 45 mg daily	45 mg once daily	Contraindicated in patients with established New York Heart Association Class III or IV heart failure. May be used as monotherapy or in combination with metformin and/or insulin; minor GI upset may occur; monitor liver enzymes. May increase risk of bladder cancer.

Table 47.2	Oral Hypoglycemic Agents			
Oral agent	Duration	Starting dose	Daily dosage	Comment(s)
Dipeptidyl Peptidase-4 Inhibitor (DPP-4)				
Linagliptin (Tradjenta)	8–14 hr	5 mg	5 mg once per day	
Saxagliptin (Onglyza)	8–14 hr	2.5, 5 mg	5 mg once per day	Contraindicated in end-stage renal disease; dose adjustment required for renal impairment
Sitagliptin (Januvia)	8–14 hr	25, 50, or 100 mg	100 mg once per day	Contraindicated in end-stage renal disease; dose adjustment required for renal impairment
Combination Preparations				
Actoplus met: pioglitazone (Actos) + metformin (Glucophage)		15 mg/500 mg, 15 mg/850 mg	Maximum dose is pioglitazone 45 mg or metformin 2550 mg daily	
Avandaryl: rosiglitazone (Avandia) 4 mg +glimepiride (Amaryl)		4 mg/1, 2, 4 mg once daily titrated carefully	Maximum dose is 8 mg rosiglitazone and 4 mg glimepiride	Given once daily with the first meal
Avandamet: metformin (Glucophage) + rosiglitazone (Avandia)		2 mg/500 mg once or BID	Maximum daily dose is 8 mg/2000 mg in divided doses	
Glucovance: glyburide (Diaβ) + metformin (Glucophage)		1.25, 2.5, 5 mg/250 or 500 mg once or BID with meals	Maximum dose is 20 mg/2000 mg daily in single or divided doses	Dosage may be increased every 2 weeks from initial dose to maximum dose

Table 47.2	Oral Hypoglycemic Agents			
Oral agent	**Duration**	**Starting dose**	**Daily dosage**	**Comment(s)**
Combination Preparations				
Metaglip: glipizide (Glucotrol) + metformin (Glucophage)		2.5, 5 mg/250 or 500 mg	20 mg glipizide/2000 mg metformin	May cause profound hypoglycemia; caution recommended if used in patients with cardiovascular heart disease risk
Linagliptin + metformin (Jentadueto)		2.5 mg/500, 850, or 1000 mg	2.5 mg/1000 mg twice a day	
Saxagliptin + Metformin (ext-rel) (Kombiglyze XR)		2.5, 5 mg/500 or 100 mg	5 mg/2 grams per day	
Sitagliptin + metformin (Janumet or Janumet XR)		50 mg/500 or 100 mg For XR: 50, 100 mg/500 or 1000 mg	100 mg/2 grams per day	

Combination Preparations

Pioglitazone + glimepride (Duetact)		30 mg/2 or 4 mg	30 mg/4 mg per day	
Rosiglitazone + glimepride (Avandaryl)		4 mg/1, 2, or 4 mg	8 mg/4 mg per day	

Table 47.2	Oral Hypoglycemic Agents			
Oral agent	Duration	Starting dose	Daily dosage	Comment(s)

Other Agents for Type 2 Diabetes

Amylin Receptor Agonist

Pramlintide (Symlin)	2–3 hr	Diabetes mellitus type 1: 15 mcg SQ immediately prior to major meals Diabetes mellitus type 2: 60 mcg SQ immediately prior to major meals	Diabetes mellitus type 1: titrate at 15 mcg increments to 30–60 mcg SQ as tolerated Diabetes mellitus type 2: 120 mcg SQ as tolerated	Adjunct therapy for type 1 and type 2 diabetes mellitus. Contraindicated in patients with hypoglycemic unawareness or gastroparesis. Black box warning for individuals while driving. Severe hypoglycemia with concurrent insulin or oral hypoglycemic agent. When initiating pramlintide, reduce dose of any secretagogues; reduce insulin dose by at least 50%

Glucagon-Like Peptide-1 Receptor Agonist

Liraglutide (Victoza)		6 mg/ml	Initially 0.6 mg/day x 1 week, then 1.2 mg/day and may increase to 1.8 mg/day	Several drug-drug interactions. Contraindicated in severe renal dysfunction, pancreatitis, or thyroid cancer

Table 47.2	Oral Hypoglycemic Agents			
Oral agent	**Duration**	**Starting dose**	**Daily dosage**	**Comment(s)**
Glucagon–Like Peptide-1 Receptor Agonist				
Exenatide (Byetta) for type 2 diabetes with oral agents such as metformin, a sulfonylurea, or both	9 hr	5-mcg and 10-mcg injection pen doses SQ	10 mcg twice a day SQ	Contraindicated in severe renal dysfunction, pancreatitis. Taken within 1 hr before meals. Administer as an SQ dose in the thigh, abdomen, or upper arm. Major side effects N/V/D. Warning: has been associated with acute pancreatitis
Exenatide Extended -Release (Bydureon		2 mg/vial	2 mg once every 7 days (weekly) SQ	Contraindicated in severe renal dysfunction, pancreatitis
Sodium-Glucose Co-Transporter 2 Inhibitors (SGLT-2 Inhibitor)				
Canaglifozin (Invokana)	10–13 hr	100, 300 mg	300 mg Take prior to first meal	Renal dosing advised Major side effect urinary infections

Note: HCl = hydrochloride; GI = gastrointestinal; XL, XR = extended release; SQ = subcutaneous; N/V/D = nausea, vomiting, diarrhea.

BIBLIOGRAPHY

Akhtar, N. (2013). Type 2 diabetes mellitus and invokana: An FDA approved drug. *Current Diabetes Reviews, 9*(6), 478–490. doi:10.2174/1573399811309 6660085

American Diabetes Association. (2013). *Diabetes care: Clinical practice recommendations, 36*(Supplement 1).

American Diabetes Association. (2013). Economic costs of diabetes in the United States in 2012. *Diabetes Care, 36*(6), 1033–1046. doi:10.2337/dc13-er06

Appel, S. J., & Jones, S. J. (2012). Latent autoimmune diabetes of adulthood: A case presentation. *Nurse Practitioner, 37*(10), 6–9. doi:10.1097/01. NPR.0000419302.54267.d8

Buttaro, T. M., Trybulski, J., Polgar-Bailey, P., & Sandberg-Cook, J. (2012). *Primary care: A collaborative practice* (4th ed.). St. Louis, MO: Elsevier Mosby.

Formosa, C., Gatt, A., & Chockalingam, N. (2012). The importance of diabetes foot care education in a primary care setting. *Journal of Diabetes Nursing, 16*(10), 410–414.

Jackson, B., & Grubbs, L. (2014). Basal-bolus insulin therapy and glycemic control in adult patients with type 2 diabetes mellitus: A review of the literature. *Journal of the American Association of Nurse Practitioners, 26*(6), 348–352. doi:10.1002/2327–6924.12033

Jameson, J. L. (2012). Principles of endocrinology. In D. L. Longo, A. S. Fauci, D. L. Kasper, S. L. Hauser, J. L. Jameson, & J. Loscalzo (Eds.), *Harrison's principles of internal medicine* (18th ed., pp. 2866–2875). New York, NY: McGraw-Hill.

Gastaldelli, A., Balas, B., Ratner, R., Rosenstock, J., Charbonnel, B., Bolli, G. B., . . . Balena, R. (2014). A direct comparison of long- and short-acting GLP-1 receptor agonists (taspoglutide once weekly and exenatide BID) on postprandial metabolism after 24 weeks of treatment. *Diabetes, Obesity and Metabolism, 16*(2), 170–178. doi:10.1111/dom.12192

Hill, A. N., & Appel, S. J. (2010). Diagnosing diabetes with A1C: Implications and considerations for measurement and surrogate markers. *Nurse Practitioner, 35*(10), 16–23. doi: 10.1097/01.NPR.0000388206.16357.02

Interactive Dosing Calculator. *Lantus Solostar*. Retrieved November 12, 2013, from http://www.lantus.com/hcp/dosing-titration/dosing-calculator.aspx

Mader, J. K., Neubauer, K. M., Schaupp, L., Augustin, T., Beck, P., Spat, S., . . . Plank, J. (2014). Efficacy, usability and sequence of operations of a workflow-integrated algorithm for basal-bolus insulin therapy in hospitalized type 2 diabetes patients. *Diabetes, Obesity and Metabolism, 16*(2), 137–146. doi:10.1111/dom.12186

Menke, A., Orchard, T. J., Imperatore, G., Bullard, K. M., Mayer-Davis, E., & Cowie, C. C. (2013). The prevalence of type 1 diabetes in the United States. *Epidemiology, 24*(5), 773–774. doi:10.1097/EDE.0b013e31829ef01a

Mompoint-Williams, D. F., Watts, P. I., & Appel, S. J. (2012). Detecting and treating hypoglycemia in patients with diabetes. *Nursing, 42*(8), 50–52. doi:10.1097/01.NURSE.0000414629.07884.7f

Novo Nordisk. (2013). *Using the Levemir FlexPen.* Retrieved November 12, 2013, from http://www.levemir.com/Levemir/UsingLevemir. aspx?campaign=000730601&WT.mc_id=Levemir_Patient- Brand&adgroup=Levemir_>_Dosing_(Exact)&WT.srch=1&utm_ source=Bing&utm_medium=cpc&utm_term=levemir%20dosage&utm_ content=Search&utm_campaign=Levemir%20Patient%20-%20Brand

Papadakis, M. A., McPhee, S. J., & Rabow, M. W. (Eds.). (2012). *Current medical diagnosis and treatment* (52nd ed.) New York, NY: McGraw-Hill/Appleton & Lange.

Powers, A. C. (2011). Diabetes mellitus. In D. Longo, A. Fauci, D. Kasper, S. Hauser, J. Jameson, & J. Loscalzo (Eds.), *Harrison's principles of internal medicine* (18th ed., pp. 2968–3002). New York, NY: McGraw-Hill.

Qaseem, A., Humphrey, L. L., Sweet, D. E., Starkey, M., & Shekelle, P. (2012). Oral pharmacologic treatment of type 2 diabetes mellitus: A clinical practice guideline from the American College of Physicians. *Annals of Internal Medicine, 156*(3), 218–231. doi:10.7326/0003–4819–156–3-201202070– 00011

Scheen, A. J. (2010). Pharmacokinetics of dipeptidylpeptidase-4 inhibitors. *Diabetes, Obesity and Metabolism, 12*(8), 648–658. doi:10.1111/j.1463– 1326.2010.01212.x

Smith, S. C., Jr., Benjamin, E. J., Bonow, R. O., Braun, L. T., Creager, M. A., Franklin, B. A, . . . Taubert, K. A. (2011). AHA/ACCF secondary prevention and risk reduction therapy for patients with coronary and other atherosclerotic vascular disease: 2011 update: A guideline from the American Heart Association and American College of Cardiology Foundation. *Circulation, 124*(22), 2458–2473. doi:10.1161/CIR.0b013e318235eb4d

Thomas, G., Shishehbor, M. H., Brill, D., & Nally, J. V. (2014). New hypertension guidelines: One size fits most? *Cleveland Clinic Journal of Medicine, 81*(3), 178–188. doi:10.3949/ccjm.81a.14003

U.S. Department of Health and Human Services, National Institutes of Health, National Heart, Lung, and Blood Institute. (2013). *Management of blood cholesterol in adults: Systematic evidence review from the Cholesterol Expert Panel.* Retrieved from http://www.nhlbi.nih.gov/health-pro/guidelines/in- develop/cholesterol-in-adults/

CHAPTER 48

Diabetes-Related Emergencies

THOMAS W. BARKLEY, JR. • SUSAN J. APPEL

DIABETIC KETOACIDOSIS

I. **Definition**
   A. A state of excessive intracellular dehydration that results from elevated blood glucose levels
   B. Hyperglycemia increases serum osmolality, causing a shift of intracellular water into the intravascular space.
   C. In addition to hyperglycemia, diabetic ketoacidosis (DKA) is characterized by hyperketonemia and an acidotic pH.

II. **Incidence/predisposing factors**
   A. Accounts for approximately 14% of all hospital admissions among patients living with diabetes mellitus (DM); although DKA usually occurs in patients with type 1 DM, it may occur in patients with type 2 DM who have lost 90% of β cell function
   B. Occurs in approximately 46 of 10,000 patients diagnosed with diabetes
   C. Increased incidence among patients with insulin pumps
   D. Mortality rate is approximately 5%
   E. Poor patient compliance—common causes include the following:
      1. Lack or omission of insulin: classically, the patient stops taking, or fails to appropriately take, insulin
      2. Too much food or insufficient exercise without an appropriate amount of insulin
      3. Failure to consume extra fluids and insulin during illness or acute stress
   F. Pancreatitis
   G. Sepsis/infection
   H. Surgery or trauma in the patient with DM

III.   Subjective/physical examination findings

  A. Polyuria (including nocturia)
  B. Polydipsia
  C. Polyphagia
  D. Nausea
  E. Vomiting
  F. Weight loss
  G. Sunken eyes and poor turgor
  H. Diminished vision
  I. Headache
  J. Abdominal pain related to bloating from gastric atony, leading to constipation
  K. Weakness/fatigue
  L. Altered level of consciousness ranging from drowsiness to coma
  M. Flushed, dry skin
  N. Fast, labored, and deep breathing (i.e., Kussmaul's respirations)
  O. Tachycardia with weak, rapid pulse
  P. Acetone (fruity) breath odor
  Q. Hyperkalemia
  R. Hypotension, especially orthostatic
  S. Usually, hypothermia is present if the patient is without infection. Patients with DKA and infection are usually normothermic or hyperthermic.

IV.   Laboratory/diagnostics

  A. Serum glucose levels greater than 250 mg/dl and frequently greater than 300 mg/dl
  B. Arterial pH is usually less than 7.3 mol/L and pCO_2 (partial pressure of CO_2) less than 40 mmHg, indicating metabolic acidosis; HCO_3 is less than 15 mEq/L
  C. Ketones present in serum and urine; serum ketones are acidic substances and further lower serum pH
  D. Hyperkalemia is related to shifting of hydrogen ions intracellularly in an attempt to buffer the acidosis; subsequently, hydrogen ions are exchanged for potassium ions.
  E. Increased blood/urea/nitrogen (BUN) level related to dehydration
  F. Glycosuria
  G. Increased hematocrit level related to dehydration
  H. Leukocytosis—white blood cell count may be 25,000/μL
  I. Serum hyperosmolality (greater than 280 mOsm/L) is common. Note: Osmolality greater than 320–330 mOsm/L usually results in coma. To effectively measure serum osmolality, use the following equation: mOsm/L = 2[Na(mEq/L) + K (mEq/L) Glucose/18]
  J. Note: Serum osmolality is approximately 2 times the Na value
  K. Expect an increased anion gap = $Na^+ - (HCO_3 + Cl)$
    1. Normal anion gap is 7–17 mEq/L

    2. Note that the higher the anion gap, the higher is the patient's acuity. Increasing fluids helps to close anion gap

L. Hypercholesterolemia may be present

M. Hypertriglyceridemia may be present

N. Hyperamylasemia may be present

V. **Management**

  A. Critical care monitoring is indicated. Consider invasive monitoring (e.g., central venous pressure/pulmonary arterial catheter) based on the patient's history of cardiovascular and/or pulmonary disease (e.g., heart failure, pulmonary edema).

  B. Parenteral fluid replacement should be initiated with 0.9% normal saline (NS) at 1,000 ml/hr for 1–2 hr; this should be followed by administration of 300–500 ml/hr for 4 hr to correct a usual fluid deficit of 4–8 L

    1. Once dehydration improves, 250 ml/hr is recommended

    2. Expect to order approximately 4–8 L of fluid to be administered during the first 24 hr of treatment

  C. Potassium values should be closely monitored during fluid resuscitation

  D. Isotonic fluids are generally used until the patient is hemodynamically stable

  E. Once the patient is hemodynamically stable, hypotonic solutions (e.g., 0.45 normal saline) are used to promote intracellular hydration

  F. As the patient's glucose levels fall to approximately 250 mg/dl, intravenous fluids are changed to dextrose-containing agents, such as D5 0.45 normal saline to prevent hypoglycemia and cerebral edema caused by lowering glucose too rapidly.

  G. Watch for potassium imbalance (i.e., hypokalemia post-treatment) and dysrhythmias. Potassium chloride, 20–30 mEq/L IV, should be added to intravenous fluids within the first 2–3 hr of therapy unless potassium levels exceed 5.0 mEq/L.

  H. Administer a loading dose of 0.1–0.15 units/kg of regular insulin intravenous followed by a continuous insulin drip (1:1) at 0.1 units/kg/hr

    1. If plasma levels of glucose do not fall by 10% within the first hr of therapy, a second loading dose is indicated

    2. Once the plasma glucose reaches 200 mg/dl, the insulin infusion can be decreased to 0.05 units/kg/hr

    3. The rate of insulin administration and the rate of infusion of D5W with 0.45% NaCl are adjusted to maintain the glucose value at around 200 mg/dl until the ketosis is resolved

    4. Once the metabolic acidosis has been corrected, subcutaneous insulin therapy may be initiated

   I. Sodium bicarbonate is rarely needed, but it may be administered via 50–100 mEq per liter of hypotonic saline if pH level is 7.0 mol/L or lower, or serum bicarbonate levels are lower than 9 mEq/L. Once pH reaches 7.1 mol/L and no signs of cardiac irritability are evident, bicarbonate should be discontinued to avoid overcompensation.

   J. Monitor for other electrolyte disturbances after treatment is completed (e.g., hypophosphatemia if diuresis and acidosis totally deplete levels of phosphorus)

HYPEROSMOLAR HYPERGLYCEMIC NONKETOSIS

I.   **Definition/general comments**
- **A.** A state of greatly elevated serum glucose, hyperosmolality, and severe dehydration without ketone production
- **B.** Usually occurs in patients who are able to produce enough insulin (those with type 2 DM) to prevent ketoacidosis but cannot produce enough insulin to prevent severe hyperglycemia, osmotic diuresis, and extracellular fluid depletion
- **C.** Because lipolysis from adipose tissue is inhibited, ketone production does not occur
  - **1.** Osmotic diuresis related to hyperglycemia leads to severe dehydration
  - **2.** Intracellular dehydration occurs, causing cerebral dehydration and neurologic signs and symptoms.
- **D.** The mortality rate may approach 30% to 50%

II.   **Incidence/predisposing factors**
- **A.** Recent onset of mild diabetes
- **B.** Patient receiving total parenteral nutrition or high-calorie feedings
- **C.** Neurologic changes that may be the most obvious presenting signs
- **D.** Illness, trauma, or stress
- **E.** Diet-controlled diabetes
- **F.** Pancreatitis
- **G.** Increased incidence among diabetes patients of advanced age (commonly missed among nursing home population)
- **H.** Nonadherence to diabetes treatment

III.   **Subjective/physical examination findings**
- **A.** Weakness
- **B.** Neurologic changes that may be the most obvious presenting signs include the following:
  - **1.** Disorientation
  - **2.** Lethargy
  - **3.** Seizures
  - **4.** Stupor
  - **5.** Coma
  - **6.** Flushed/dry skin, dry mucous membranes, and poor turgor (dehydration)

    C. Polyuria

    D. Hypotension

    E. Tachycardia

    F. Shallow breathing

IV. **Laboratory/diagnostics**

    A. Blood glucose levels 600 mg/dl or higher (commonly higher than 1,000 mg/dl)

    B. Elevated serum osmolarity (higher than 310 mOsm/L [normal serum osmolarity is 275–295 mOsm/L]) resulting in osmotic diuresis and severe dehydration

    C. Elevated BUN and creatinine

    D. Elevated serum sodium (to retain water, the kidneys try to conserve sodium)

    E. Relatively normal pH, higher than 7.3 mol/L; relatively normal sodium bicarbonate level, higher than 15 mEq/L (ketosis does not occur)

    F. Anion gap is normal

    G. When C-peptides are present, this is indicative of some level of insulin production

V. **Management**

    A. Critical care monitoring is indicated. Consider invasive monitoring (e.g., central venous pressure/pulmonary arterial catheter) based on the patient's history of cardiovascular and/or pulmonary disease (e.g., congestive heart failure, pulmonary edema).

    B. Massive fluid replacement; isotonic fluids are given until the patient becomes hemodynamically stable

    C. If the patient is not hypotensive, or once serum sodium level reaches 145 mEq/L, hypotonic solutions are used to hydrate the intracellular compartment (e.g., 0.45 normal saline).

    D. Expect to order approximately 4–6 L in the first 8–10 hr of therapy

    E. Overall fluid volume deficit may be 6–10 L

    F. Monitor for complications of too much fluid replacement

        1. Cardiac failure

        2. Cerebral edema

        3. Seizures

    G. Less insulin is required to control hyperosmolar hyperglycemic nonketotic syndrome than is required to control DKA

        1. Administer a loading dose of 0.1–0.15 units/kg of regular insulin intravenous followed by a continuous insulin drip (1:1) at 0.1 units/kg/hr

            a. If plasma levels of glucose do not fall by 10% within the first hr of therapy, a second loading dose is indicated.

            b. Once the plasma glucose reaches 200 mg/dl, the insulin infusion can be decreased to 0.05 units/kg/hr.

    c. The rate of insulin administration and the rate of infusion of D5W with 0.45% NaCl are adjusted to maintain the glucose value at around 200 mg/dl until the metabolic imbalances are resolved.

  2. Initial bolus of 0.1–0.15 units/kg IV, followed by 1–2 units/kg/hr titrated until blood glucose levels are acceptable (e.g., 60 mg/dl)

H. Continuous monitoring of electrolytes (Na, K, HCO3, Cl, and phosphorus) is necessary, with replacement PRN.

I. Cardiac monitoring for dysrhythmias—especially, monitor potassium levels as well as frequent blood glucose monitoring and clear documentation of glucose levels (e.g., bedside flow sheet)

HYPOGLYCEMIA

I. **Definition**
  A. A state of decreased serum glucose is produced by a variety of causes

II. **Incidence/predisposing factors**
  A. Frequently occurs in type 1 DM patients (i.e., patients on insulin therapy)
  B. Too much insulin
  C. Lack of food intake
  D. Excessive exercise, especially without adequate food intake
  E. Diarrhea and vomiting
  F. Alcohol consumption

III. **Subjective/physical examination findings**
  A. Dizziness
  B. Weakness
  C. Neurologic changes, including confusion, seizures, and coma
  D. Tremor, nervousness, and anxiety
  E. Sweating, pallor, and cold skin
  F. Tachycardia and palpitations
  G. Visual disturbances, including diplopia
  H. Paresthesia

IV. **Laboratory/diagnostics**
  A. Blood glucose level should be 70–60 mg/dl or lower.
    Note: Among patients with diabetes, symptoms of hypoglycemia may occur at higher glucose levels and may correlate with the speed of falling glucose values.
  B. Urine negative for glucose and/or acetone

V. **Management**
  A. In the acute care facility, a blood glucose level should first be obtained, and the hospital's protocol should be followed. Most protocols include several options, including:
  B. D50W, 25–50 ml
  C. Glucagon, 1 mg
  D. Glucose tablets, 16 grams

E. In the community setting, teach patient to take approximately 15 grams of carbohydrates, such as one of the following:

   1. Glucose tablets equaling 15–16 grams of carbohydrates (Note: Teach patients to stack tablets out in plain sight once they are aware of hypoglycemia so they can remember how many they have taken.)

   2. 4 oz. sweetened carbonated beverage or unsweetened fruit juice

   3. 1 tbsp. honey

   4. 5 pieces of hard candy with sugar

   5. 4 oz. regular soft drink

F. If the patient is unable to swallow:

   1. D50W per IV in the acute care facility, followed by an intravenous continuous infusion of D5W PRN to maintain glucose level higher than 100 mg/dl

   2. For patients with elevated serum creatinine, D10 may be indicated as an infusion because insulin will have prolonged action when there is renal impairment.

   3. Glucagon 1 mg intramuscularly (IM) in the deltoid if away from the acute care facility and intravenous access is not possible (this is most appropriate for type 1 DM patients who become hypoglycemic).

G. Give crackers and milk, or other protein and complex carbohydrate snack, after the event

H. Continue to monitor glucose levels as necessary. Patients taking oral anti-glycemic agents should be followed closely for 24–48 hr

BIBLIOGRAPHY

Arora, S., Probst, M. A., Andrews, L., Camilion, M., Grock, A., Hayward, G., & Menchine, M. (2012). A randomized, controlled trial of oral versus intravenous fluids for lowering blood glucose in emergency department patients with hyperglycemia. *Canadian Journal of Emergency Medicine, 15*, 1–6.

Chen, H. F., Wang, C. Y., Lee, H. Y., See, T. T., Chen, M. H., Jiang, J. Y., . . . Li, C. Y. (2010). Short-term case fatality rate and associated factors among inpatients with diabetic ketoacidosis and hyperglycemic hyperosmolar state: A hospital-based analysis over a 15-year period. *Internal Medicine, 49*(8), 729–737.

Cryer, P.E., & Davis, S. N. (2011). Hypoglycemia. In D. Longo, A. Fauci, D. Kasper, S. Hauser, J. Jameson, & J. Locscalzo (Eds.), *Harrison's principles of internal medicine* (18th ed.). New York, NY: McGraw-Hill.

Fadini, G. P., de Kreutzenberg, S. V., Rigato, M., Brocco, S., Marchesan, M., Tiengo, A., & Avogaro, A. (2011). Characteristics and outcomes of the hyperglycemic hyperosmolar non-ketotic syndrome in a cohort of 51 consecutive cases at a single center. *Diabetes Research and Clinical Practice, 94*(2), 172–179.

Fitzgerald, P. A. (2014). Endocrinology. In L. M. Tierney (Ed.), *Current medical diagnosis and treatment* (53rd ed.). New York, NY: McGraw Hill.

Kishore, P. (2014). Nonketotic hyperosmolar syndrome (NKHS). *Merck Manuals.* Retrieved from http://www.merckmanuals.com/professional/endocrine_and_ metabolic_disorders/diabetes_mellitus_and_disorders_of_carbohydrate_ metabolism/nonketotic_hyperosmolar_syndrome_nkhs.html

Mompoint-Williams, D. F., Watts, P. I., & Appel, S. J. (2012). Detecting and treating hypoglycemia in patients with diabetes. *Nursing, 42*(8), 50–51. doi:10.1097/01.NURSE.0000414629.07884.7f

Powers, A. C. (2011). Diabetes mellitus. In D. Longo, A. Fauci, D. Kasper, S. Hauser, J. Jameson, & J. Loscalzo (Eds.), *Harrison's principles of internal medicine* (18th ed.). New York, NY: McGraw-Hill.

Tzamaloukas, A. H., Sun, Y., Konstantinov, N. K., Ing, T. S., Dorin, R. I., Malhotra, D.D., . . . Shapiro, J. I. (2013). Principles of quantitative fluid and cation replacement in extreme hyperglycemia. *Cureus, 5*(3), e110. doi:10.7759/cureus.110

Tokuda, Y., Omata, F., Tsugawa, Y., Maesato, K., Momotura, K., Fujinuma, A., . . . Cook, E. F. (2010). Vital sign triage to rule out diabetic ketoacidosis and non-ketotic hyperosmolar syndrome in hyperglycemic patients. *Diabetes Research and Clinical Practice, 87*(3), 366–371.

CHAPTER 49

Thyroid Disease

RITA DELLO STRITTO • THOMAS W. BARKLEY, JR.

HYPERTHYROIDISM (THYROTOXICOSIS)

I. **Definition**
   A. A condition of excess secretion of thyroxine (T4) and triiodothyronine (T3) resulting from a variety of clinical disorders

II. **Etiology/predisposing factors/incidence**
   A. Graves' disease—the most common cause; associated with goiter and ocular changes
   B. Subacute thyroiditis
   C. Thyroid-stimulating hormone (TSH) pituitary tumor
   D. Toxic nodular goiter or thyroid carcinoma
   E. Other autoimmune causes:
      1. Pernicious anemia
      2. Diabetes mellitus
      3. Myasthenia gravis
   F. Most commonly seen between ages of 20 and 40
   G. Higher incidence among women; 8:1 female-to-male ratio
   H. May also occur in patients on high-dose amiodarone (Cordarone) therapy
      1. Note: high-dose amiodarone therapy may also cause signs of hypothyroidism

III. **Subjective/physical examination findings (thyrotoxic manifestations)**
   A. Hypermetabolism
   B. Heat intolerance
   C. Fatigue
   D. Anxiety
   E. Nervousness

      F. Manic behavior

      G. Confusion/restlessness

      H. Emotional lability

      I. Fine tremors

      J. Diaphoresis

      K. Hyperreflexia of deep tendon reflexes

      L. Resting tachycardia/palpitations/atrial fibrillation

      M. Exertional dyspnea

      N. Low-grade fever

      O. Increased appetite

      P. Weight loss

      Q. Frequent bowel movements

      R. Smooth, warm, moist, velvety skin with occasional pruritus

      S. Fine/thin hair

      T. Exophthalmos

      U. Eyelid lag

      V. Infrequent blinking

      W. Graves' ophthalmopathy: noted in 20%–40% of cases

IV. **Laboratory/diagnostic findings**

      A. TSH assay—most sensitive test; levels are low in most cases of hyperthyroidism

      B. Serum T3, T4, thyroid resin uptake, and free thyroxine index (FTI) values are elevated.

         1. Note: T4 may be normal, but T3 will be elevated

      C. Elevated erythrocyte sedimentation rate

      D. Serum antinuclear antibody (ANA) levels are usually elevated without evidence of systemic lupus erythematosus or other autoimmune disease.

      E. Hypercalcemia and anemia may be seen on complete blood cell count with decreased granulocytes.

      F. If unclear etiology for hyperthyroidism, radioactive iodine uptake tests may be performed:

         1. High iodine uptake is usually indicative of Graves' disease

         2. Low iodine uptake is usually indicative of subacute thyroiditis

      G. MRI of the orbits is used to assess Graves' ophthalmopathy, as indicated

V. **Management**

      A. Physician/endocrinologist consultation for newly diagnosed patients and those with comorbidities

      B. Symptomatic relief

         1. Propranolol (Inderal), 10 mg PO (may increase dosage to 80 mg) four times a day

         2. Metoprolol (Lopressor), 25 mg PO (may increase to 50 mg) every 6–8 hr

C. Antithyroid medications are used for mild cases of hyperthyroidism and in patients with small goiters who are afraid of using isotopes. However, a high rate of recurrence of the disease has been reported after 1 year.
   1. Methimazole (Tapazole)
      a. Initial dosing: 30–60 mg every day in three divided doses
      b. Maintenance dosing: 5–15 mg PO daily
   2. For patients intolerant of methimazole and/or in whom radioactive iodine or surgery is not appropriate:
      a. Propylthiouracil
         i. Initial dosing: 300–600 mg/day in four divided doses
         ii. Maintenance dosing: 100–150 mg/day in three divided doses

D. Radioactive iodine (131I)
   1. Used to destroy goiters
   2. Usually takes 3–4 months for the patient to become euthyroid
   3. May need to repeat in 6 months if persistent hyperthyroidism

E. Thyroid surgery to remove the gland
   1. Not a common modality
   2. Used in the following cases:
      a. Pregnant patients
      b. Patients suspected of having cancer
   3. Lugol's solution, 3–10 drops/day PO in 2–3 divided doses for 10 days, to reduce the vascularity of the thyroid preoperatively by blocking the release of hormones from the thyroid gland
   4. The patient must be euthyroid before the gland is removed.

F. Subacute thyroiditis—best treated with propranolol (symptomatically)

THYROID STORM (THYROTOXIC CRISIS)

I. **Definition**
   A. A deadly, hypermetabolic state caused by inadequately controlled hyperthyroidism
   B. This crisis manifests with exacerbated thyrotoxic symptoms.

II. **Predisposing factors/incidence/general comments for patients with existing diagnosed or undiagnosed hyperthyroidism**
   A. Trauma
   B. Major stress
   C. Infection
   D. Subtotal thyroidectomy or other thyroid surgery
   E. Uncontrolled diabetes
   F. Thyroid drug overdose
   G. Pregnancy
   H. Thyrotoxic crisis is a rare disorder.

III. **Subjective/physical examination findings**
   A. Fever (100°F–105.8°F [37.8°C–41°C])

B. Dilated vessels/flushing

C. Profuse diaphoresis (fluid loss may equal 4 L/24 hr)

D. Marked tachycardia (supraventricular tachycardia possible)/palpitations

E. Mental status changes

  1. Extreme agitation

  2. Delirium

  3. Psychosis

  4. Stupor/coma

F. Gastrointestinal disturbances: hyperdefecation may be an early sign of thyroid storm

G. Hyperglycemia

H. Others: see Subjective/physical examination findings (thyrotoxic manifestations) of hyperthyroidism

IV. Laboratory/diagnostic findings

A. See laboratory/diagnostic findings of hyperthyroidism

V. Management

A. Basic measures

  1. Supportive care, including decreasing environmental stimuli

  2. Hypothermic measures, antipyretics (e.g., acetaminophen)

  3. Avoid acetylsalicylic acid (aspirin) and NSAIDs because these potentially interfere with the binding of T4 and thyroid-binding globulin, possibly resulting in exacerbated hypermetabolism

B. Pharmacologic therapy (three classes)

  1. Agents that inhibit synthesis of thyroid hormone (antithyroid drugs)

    a. Propylthiouracil, 900–1,200 mg/day PO in divided doses, or

    b. Methimazole (Tapazole), 90–120 mg/day PO in divided doses

  2. Agents that inhibit the release of thyroid hormone (iodine preparations); administered an hour after administration of antithyroid drugs

    a. Lugol's solution, 10 drops PO three times a day, or

    b. Sodium iodine, 1 gram slowly IV with agents that block the effects of thyroid hormone

  3. Agents that block the effects of thyroid hormone (i.e., β blockers)

    a. Esmolol, 40–80 mg PO every 6 hr, with

    b. Hydrocortisone, 50 mg every 6 hr, followed by rapid tapering of the dosage as the patient improves

C. Surgery and treatment with radioactive iodine is delayed until the patient becomes euthyroid

HYPOTHYROIDISM (MYXEDEMA COMA)

I.   Definition

    A. A condition of greatly decreased metabolism resulting from a deficient amount of circulating thyroid hormone

II.   Incidence/predisposing factors/etiology

    A. Most common thyroid disease

    B. Affects all ages

    C. Women have a higher incidence, especially those with a history of thyroiditis or other autoimmune disorder (e.g., systemic lupus erythematosus, rheumatoid arthritis)

    D. Causes:

        1. Worldwide, hypothyroidism is most commonly related to iodine deficiency

        2. In the U.S., autoimmune thyroiditis processes (e.g., Hashimoto's) are the primary causal factor.

    E. Deficiency of pituitary TSH

        1. Pituitary tumor

        2. Hypophysectomy damage

    F. Hypothalamic deficiency of thyroid-releasing hormone (TRH)

    G. Thyroidectomy

    H. Failure to take thyroid medication

    I. High-dose amiodarone (Cordarone) therapy

        1. Note: high-dose amiodarone therapy may also cause signs of hyperthyroidism

III. Subjective/physical examination findings

    A. Extreme fatigue

    B. Changes in level of consciousness (i.e., confusion to depression to coma)

    C. Puffiness of face/eyes

    D. Hypoventilation

    E. Bradycardia

    F. Hypothermia

    G. Hypoglycemia

    H. Anorexia

    I. Decreased bowel sounds

    J. Weight gain

    K. Constipation

    L. Dry, cracked skin

    M. Coarse, brittle hair

    N. Brittle nails

    O. Cold intolerance

    P. Myxedema in extremities and periorbital edema

    Q. Decreased deep tendon reflexes

    R. Paresthesias

    S. Decreased sweating

    T. Enlarged tongue
    U. Ataxia
    V. Hair loss
    W. Hoarseness

IV. **Diagnostic/laboratory findings**
    A. Elevated TSH level
    B. Low or low normal T4 level
    C. Decreased resin T3 uptake; T3 is not a reliable test for hypothyroidism
    D. Hypoglycemia
    E. Hyponatremia
    F. Anemia (normochromic, normocytic)
    G. Elevated transaminases
    H. Hypercholesterolemia and elevated triglyceride levels

V. **Management**
    A. Hypothyroidism
       1. Levothyroxine (Synthroid) (T4)
          a. For patients younger than age 60 and without coronary artery disease: 50–100 mcg every day, with increase in dosage by 25 mcg every 1–2 weeks until symptoms stabilize and the patient becomes euthyroid
             i. TSH is rechecked 8 weeks after dose adjustment
          b. For patients older than age 60 with coronary artery disease: 25–50 mcg every day, with increase in dosage by 25 mcg every 1–2 weeks until symptoms stabilize and the patient becomes euthyroid
             i. TSH is rechecked 8 weeks after dose adjustment
    B. Myxedema coma
       1. Oxygen supplementation and mechanical ventilation for hypercapnia are almost always needed
       2. Consider fluid restriction and 3% normal saline for severe hyponatremia
       3. Consider D50W for severe hypoglycemia
       4. IV thyroid replacement:
          a. Levothyroxine (T4), one dose of 300–500 mcg IV; then, 50–100 mcg every day
          b. Alternative, use liothyronine sodium (Cytomel) (T3), 25–50 mcg IV every 4–6 hr
          c. Another alternative, levothyroxine (T4), 200 mcg and liothyronine sodium (T3), 25 mg, single dose
          d. If adrenal insufficiency is suspected, hydrocortisone (Solu-Cortef), 100 mg IV bolus, then 25–50 mg every 8 hr, to avoid excessive hyperadrenalism-like effects associated with rapid thyroid replacement
       5. Fluid replacement PRN (see Management of Fluid Disorders)
       6. Consider fluid restriction (see Management of Hyponatremia)

7. Consider D50W for severe hypoglycemia
8. Slow rewarming with blankets
   a. Note: hyperthermia blankets are contraindicated because rapid vasodilatation may further hypotension and lead to circulatory collapse
9. Patient teaching, including the need for levothyroxine replacement (usually 100–200 mcg/day) for life
10. Follow-up patient teaching to prevent future episodes

BIBLIOGRAPHY

Hershman, J. M., Hassani, S., & Samuels, M. H. (2009). Thyroid diseases. In J. B. Halter, J. G. Ouslander, M. E. Tinetti, S. Studenski, K. P. High, & S. Asthana (Eds.), *Hazzard's Geriatric Medicine and Gerontology* (6th ed.). New York, NY: McGraw-Hill.

Idrose, A. (2011). Thyroid disorders: Hyperthyroidism and thyroid storm. In J. E. Tintinalli, J. Stapczynski, O. Ma, D. M. Cline, R. K. Cydulka, & G. D. Meckler (Eds.), *Tintinalli's Emergency Medicine: A Comprehensive Study Guide* (7th ed.). New York, NY: McGraw-Hill.

Idrose, A. (2011). Thyroid disorders: Hypothyroidism and myxedema crisis. In J. E. Tintinalli, J. Stapczynski, O. Ma, D. M. Cline, R. K. Cydulka, & G. D. Meckler (Eds.), *Tintinalli's Emergency Medicine: A Comprehensive Study Guide* (7th ed.). New York, NY: McGraw-Hill.

Jameson, J., Weetman, A. P. (2012). Disorders of the thyroid gland. In D. L. Longo, A. S. Fauci, D. L. Kasper, S. L. Hauser, J. Jameson, & J. Loscalzo (Eds.), *Harrison's Principles of Internal Medicine* (18th ed.). New York, NY: McGraw-Hill.

Majeroni, A. (2009). Hypothyroidis, adult. In F. J. Domino (Ed.), *5-Minute Clinical Consult* (22nd ed.). Philadelphia, PA: Lippincott, Williams & Wilkins Health.

Paulson J. M., & Hollenberg A. N. (2012). Thyroid emergencies. In S. C. McKean, J. J. Ross, D. D. Dressler, D. J. Brotman, & J. S. Ginsberg (Eds.), *Principles and Practice of Hospital Medicine*. New York, NY: McGraw-Hill.

Sabharwal, A., & Kargi, D. (2009). Hyperthyroidism. In F. J. Domino (Ed.), *5-Minute Clinical Consult* (22nd ed.). Philadelphia, PA: Lippincott, Williams & Wilkins Health.

Weetman, A. P. (2010). The thyroid gland and disorder of thyroid functions. In D. A. Warrell, T. M. Cox, J. D. Firth, & G. S. Ogg (Eds.), *Oxford Textbook of Medicine* (5th ed.). New York, NY: Oxford University Press.

CHAPTER 50

Cushing's Syndrome

RITA DELLO STRITTO • THOMAS W. BARKLEY, JR.

I. **Definition/general comments**

  A. A group of symptoms resulting from hypercortisolism due to numerous causes

  B. Excess adrenocorticotropic hormone (ACTH) secretion by the pituitary accounts for 90% of Cushing's syndrome; therefore, it is referred to as Cushing's disease

II. **Incidence/predisposing factors**

  A. Ninety percent of Cushing's syndrome cases are non-iatrogenic.

  1. Excess ACTH production from the pituitary; approximately 70% of all cases of Cushing's syndrome are caused by benign pituitary adenomas.

  2. Adrenal neoplasms account for approximately 10% to 15% of cases; women are affected more often than men at a 3–5:1 ratio.

  3. Nonpituitary neoplasms, such as small cell lung cancer, account for approximately 15% of cases.

  B. Iatrogenic

  1. Excessive glucocorticoid administration, including prolonged use

III. **Subjective/physical examination findings**

  A. Obesity—central with muscle wasting

  B. Moon face

  C. Emotional lability

  1. Depression

  2. Anxiety

  3. Irritability

  D. Buffalo hump

  E. Acne

F. Purple striae

G. Protuberant abdomen

H. Hirsutism

I. Fragile ecchymotic skin on thin extremities

J. Hypertension

K. Weakness

L. Backache

M. Headache

N. Amenorrhea/impotence

O. Polyuria

P. Hyperglycemia

Q. Osteoporosis

IV. **Laboratory findings**

A. Hyperglycemia as evidenced by impaired glucose tolerance testing

B. Glycosuria

C. Hypokalemia

D. Hypernatremia

E. Leukocytosis

F. Elevated serum and free urinary cortisol

V. **Diagnosis**

A. Dexamethasone suppression test (DST)

1. Administer dexamethasone 1 mg at 11:00 p.m. and check serum cortisol at 8:00 a.m. the next day

   a. Cortisol levels greater than 1.8 mcg/dl (50 nmol/liter) is suggestive of CS

2. Administer dexamethasone, 2 mg/day for 48 hr DST (0.5 mg PO every 6 hr)

   a. On day two, urine is collected

   b. Cortisol levels greater than 1.8 mcg/dl (50 nmol/liter) is suggestive of CS

B. Urine Free Cortisol (UFC)

1. Measured by HPLC or LC/MS/MS in a 24-hour urine collection; highly accurate and specific

2. UFC is usually less than 50 mcg/24 hr (less than 135 nmol/24 hr) when measured by these methods

3. UFC greater than the normal range for the assay is considered diagnostic

C. Late Night Serum or Salivary Cortisol

1. Highly accurate in differentiating patients with CS from normal subjects/patients with pseudo-CS conditions

   a. Plasma cortisol level greater than 5.2–7 mcg/dl (140–190 nmol/L)

2. Salivary cortisol provides a simple, more convenient means of obtaining screening sample

   a. Salivary cortisol greater than 145 ng/dl (4 nmol/liter)

    D. Midnight cortisol level above 7.5 mcg/dl is diagnostic but requires the following:

      1. The patient must have been in the same time zone for 3 days

      2. The patient must have been without food for the previous 3 hr

      3. Indwelling arterial line is preferred for serum collection

VI. **Management**

    A. Depends on the cause; therefore, treat the underlying cause

      1. Transsphenoidal resection for pituitary adenomas

      2. Laparoscopic or more extensive surgery for adrenal neoplasms

      3. Resection of cortisol-secreting tumors

      4. Discontinuation, or at least reduction, of drugs that may cause the disease (i.e., glucocorticoids)

    B. Manage fluid and electrolyte imbalances

    C. Manage other complications, such as osteoporosis, as indicated

    D. Endocrinology referral

BIBLIOGRAPHY

Carroll, T. B., Aron, D. C., Findling, J. W., & Tyrrell, B. (2011). Glucocorticoids and adrenal androgens. In D. G. Garnder & D. Shoback (Eds.), *Greenspan's basic & clinical endocrinology* (9th ed.). New York, NY: McGraw Hill.

Loriaux, D. L. (2009). *Adrenal*. In E.G. Nabel (Ed.), *ACP Medicine* (section 3, chapter 4). Hamilton, ON: BC Decker.

Newell-Price, J. (2009). Diagnosis/differential diagnosis of Cushing's syndrome: A review of best practice. *Best Practice & Research Clinical Endocrinology & Metabolism, 23*(Suppl. 1), S5-S14.

Paniagua, L., & Gopalakrishnan, G. (2014). Cushing's disease and Cushing's syndrome. In F. J. Domino (Ed.), *The 5-minute clinical consult* (22nd ed.). Philadelphia, PA: Lippincott Williams & Wilkins.

Urden, L. D., Stacy, K. M., & Lough, M. E. (2010). *Thelan's critical care nursing diagnosis and management* (6th ed.). St. Louis, MO: Mosby Inc.

CHAPTER **51**

Primary Adrenocortical Insufficiency (Addison Disease) & Adrenal Crisis

RITA DELLO STRITTO · THOMAS W. BARKLEY, JR.

I. Definition
  A. A condition characterized by a deficiency of cortisol, androgens, and aldosterone as a result of destruction of the adrenal cortices

II. Incidence/predisposing factors
  A. Occurs in 40–60/1,000,000 individuals
  B. Female-to-male ratio is 2:1
  C. Sudden withdrawal of glucocorticoids (deficiency)
  D. Extreme stress
  E. Trauma
  F. Adrenal hemorrhage, post-adrenalectomy
  G. Sepsis
  H. Tuberculosis

III. Etiology
  A. Autoimmune destruction of the adrenal gland
  B. Bilateral adrenal hemorrhage (e.g., as a result of anticoagulant therapy)
  C. Metastatic cancer
  D. Pituitary failure resulting in decreased levels of adrenocorticotropic hormone (ACTH)

IV. Chronic subjective/physical examination findings
  A. Weakness/fatigue
  B. Headache
  C. Nausea
  D. Vomiting
  E. Abdominal pain with accompanying diarrhea

    F. Hyperpigmentation in the buccal mucosa and skin creases related to excess ACTH

        1. Apparent in knuckles, knees, posterior neck, elbows, and palmar creases

        2. Signifies a deficiency in cortisol, not in ACTH

    G. Sparse axillary hair

    H. Hypotension

    I. Arthralgias

    J. Weight loss

V. **Acute subjective/physical examination findings (adrenal crisis)**

    A. Marked and rapid worsening of the preceding chronic findings

    B. Fever

    C. Hypovolemia/hypotension

    D. Changes in mental status/level of consciousness

    E. Tachycardia

VI. **Laboratory/diagnostics**

    A. Hyponatremia

    B. Hyperkalemia

    C. Hypoglycemia

    D. Elevated erythrocyte sedimentation rate

    E. Neutropenia (approximately 5,000/μl)

    F. Eosinophil count above 300/μl

    G. Lymphocytosis in approximately 50% of patients

    H. Plasma cortisol less than 5 mg/dl at 8:00 a.m.

    I. Hypercalcemia may be present.

    J. Elevated blood/urea/nitrogen levels related to decrease in extracellular fluid volume caused by aldosterone deficiency

    K. Metabolic acidosis

        1. Related to hypotension, decreased renal function, and decreased hydrogen ion excretion; caused by lack of aldosterone

    L. If patient is exposed to bacteria, the patient may have positive cultures of blood, urine, and/or sputum

    M. Simplified cosyntropin (synthetic ACTH) test

        1. Cosyntropin, 0.25 mg IV, is administered. Note: For patients who are receiving glucocorticoid treatment, hydrocortisone must be discontinued at least 8 hr before the test.

        2. Plasma cortisol levels are checked 30–60 min after administration.

        3. Normally, cortisol levels rise 20 μg/dl or higher

        4. If the patient has primary adrenal disease, serum ACTH levels will not rise

    N. Chest and abdominal x-rays

    O. Abdominal CT scan, as indicated

VII. **Management**

    A. Outpatient management

        1. Consult with endocrinologist/specialist

2. Glucocorticoid and mineralocorticoid replacement therapy, PRN
   a. Hydrocortisone, 10–15 mg PO in the morning and 5–10 mg PO in the afternoon (4–5 p.m.) every day
   b. If additional therapy is needed, fludrocortisone acetate (Florinef Acetate) may be initiated at 0.05–0.2 mg orally in the a.m.
      i. Note: dosage should be increased if orthostatic hypotension, weight loss, or hyperkalemia occurs
      ii. Dosage should be decreased if hypertension, edema, or hypokalemia develops
      iii. About 10% of Addisonian patients can be managed with hydrocortisone and adequate dietary sodium intake alone and do not require fludrocortisones.
3. Teach the patient signs and symptoms of adrenal crisis and encourage the patient to wear a MedicAlert bracelet
B. Acute management
   1. Consult with endocrinologist/specialist
   2. Once the diagnosis of adrenal crisis is suspected, a cortisol level should be immediately obtained; hydrocortisone (Solu-Cortef) 100–300 mg should be administered intravenously with normal saline (NS) for pharmacologic and fluid replacement therapy.
   3. After initial administration, hydrocortisone phosphate (hydrocortisone sodium phosphate) or hydrocortisone sodium succinate 100 mg IV should be ordered.
      a. Hydrocortisone, via IV push or IVPB at 50–100 mg over 15–30 minutes, should be given every 6 hr during the first day of therapy
      b. Continue to give patient 100 mg via IV every 6 hr until the patient is stable; once stable, reduce to 50 mg every 6 hr
      c. By day 4 or 5, taper to maintenance therapy and add mineralocorticoid therapy PRN
   4. Volume may also be replaced with the use of D_5NS at 500 ml/hr for 4 hr, which is then tapered as indicated
   5. Initiate potassium replacement therapy. Even though the initial level may be high, a total body deficit usually occurs.
   6. Consider broad-spectrum antibiotics while cultures are pending because bacterial infections are frequently a causative factor in adrenal crises
   7. Once the patient's condition has stabilized, hydrocortisone 10–20 mg PO may be ordered every 6 hr, and the dose subsequently reduced to a satisfactory maintenance level
      a. May consider a twice-daily regimen: 10–20 mg PO in the morning and 5–10 mg PO in the evening
   8. Treat the underlying cause

BIBLIOGRAPHY

Brooke, A. M., & Monson, J. P. (2009). Addison's disease. *Medicine, 37*(8), 416–419.

Chrousos, G. P. (2012). Adrenocorticosteroids & adrenocortical antagonists. In B. G. Katzung, S. B. Masters, & A. J. Trevor (Eds.), *Basic and clinical pharmacology* (12th ed.). New York: NY: McGraw-Hill/Lange.

Clutter, W. E. (2014). Endocrine diseases. In H. Godara, A. Hirbe, M. Nassif, H. Otepka, & A. Rosenstock (Eds.). *The Washington manual of medical therapeutics* (34th ed.). Philadelphia, PA: Wolters Kluwer/Lippincott Williams & Wilkins.

Lin, Liew E. C, Sheehy, A. S., Wood, K. E., & Coursin, D. B. (2012). Adrenal insufficiency. In S. C. McKean, J. J. Ross, D. D. Dressler, D. J. Boyman, & J. S. Ginsberg (Eds.). *Principles and practice of hospital medicine.* New York, NY: McGraw-Hill Medical.

Stewart, P. M. (2010). Disorders of the adrenal cortex. In D. A. Warrell, T. M. Cox, & J. D. Firth (Eds.), *Oxford textbook of medicine* (5th ed.). New York, NY: Oxford University Press.

CHAPTER 52

Pheochromocytoma

MONIQUE LAMBERT • THOMAS W. BARKLEY, JR.

I. Definition/general comments

   A. A rare but serious condition often referred to as the "great masquerader" of medicine

      1. Results from excessive catecholamine release (norepinephrine and epinephrine), usually from an adrenal medullary tumor

      2. Characterized by paroxysmal or sustained hypertension

   B. Tumors may arise along the sympathetic nervous system chain, as well as in the thorax, bladder, and brain

II. Etiology/incidence/predisposing factors

   A. Patients may be diagnosed at any age but most commonly occur during the third, fourth, and fifth decade of life

   B. Occurs in both men and women in approximately equal frequency

   C. Rule of tens

      1. 10% familial

      2. 10% hereditary

      3. 10% malignant

      4. 10% occur without hypertension

      5. 10% extra-adrenal

      6. 10% bilateral

III. Subjective/physical examination findings

   A. The classic triad includes the following:

      1. Palpitations

      2. Severe headache

      3. Profuse diaphoresis

   B. Signs and symptoms may be intermittent or continuous.

      1. Hypertension sustained or paroxysmal

2. Tachycardia (may progress to a super ventricular tachycardia)
3. Flushing
4. Nausea
5. Weakness
6. Weight loss
7. Tremors
8. Anxiety and panic attacks
9. Chest pain mimicking a myocardial infarction
10. Dyspnea
11. Polyuria and polydipsia
12. Hyperglycemia
13. Hypercalcemia

IV. **Laboratory/diagnostics**
   A. Glycosuria may be present
   B. Hyperglycemia and leukocytosis are common
   C. Elevated erythrocyte sedimentation rate
   D. Thyroid-stimulating hormone, T4, free T4, and T3 levels are normal.
   E. Plasma metanephrine testing has the highest sensitivity (96%) for detecting a pheochromocytoma but a lower specificity (85%). High-risk patients (e.g., family history or genetic syndromes such as multiple endocrine neoplasia [MEN] 2A or 2B, von Hippel-Lindau disease, or neurofibromatosis) should be screened in this manner. In these scenarios, a higher-sensitivity test that lacks specificity is justified.
      1. A fractionated plasma-free metanephrine level may be obtained through simple venipuncture in a seated, ambulatory patient
   F. Assay of urinary catecholamines (total and fractionated), metanephrine, vanillylmandelic acid (VMA), and creatinine should suffice for all patients at lower risk for a pheochromocytoma (e.g., those with flushing spells, poorly controlled hypertension, or adrenal incidentalomas with an adrenocortical appearance), but these should be examined in all suspected patients.
      1. A 24-hr urine collection is preferred, but an overnight collection may be sufficient. Collecting urine during or immediately after a crisis is optimal.
      2. Results indicating pheochromocytoma include the following:
         a. Greater than 2.2 µg of metanephrine/mg of creatinine
         b. Greater than 135 µg total catecholamines/gram of creatinine
         c. Greater than 5.5 µg of VMA/mg of creatinine
      3. Metanephrine levels are considered the most sensitive and specific test for a pheochromocytoma.
      4. VMA is the least specific test; it has a false-positive rate greater than 15%
      5. To ensure adequacy of the collection, creatinine should be measured in all collections

6. The container should be dark, acidified, and kept cold to avoid degradation of catecholamines
7. Epinephrine and norepinephrine may be measured separately to confirm the total catecholamine level and to determine whether levels reflect the expected high norepinephrine-to-epinephrine ratio; for the same reason, normetanephrine may be examined separately.
8. Dopamine levels are not useful in this test (i.e., most of the dopamine is of renal origin)
9. Be aware that stress and numerous pharmacologic agents, such as foods, disorders, and chemicals, may affect tests for the disorder, including the following:
   a. Alcohol
   b. Sympathomimetics
   c. Vasodilators (e.g., labetalol)
   d. Levodopa
   e. Methyldopa
   f. Methylxanthines (e.g., aminophylline)
   g. Various disease states, such as
      i. Guillain-Barré syndrome
      ii. Hypoglycemia
      iii. Quadriplegia
      iv. Intracranial lesions
      v. Acute psychosis
   h. Isoproterenol
   i. Lithium
   j. Tricyclic antidepressants
   k. Chlorpromazine
   l. Sotalol
   m. Amphetamines
   n. Buspirone
   o. Benzodiazepines
10. Compounds that decrease 24-hr urine levels of metanephrines include methyltyrosine, methylglucamine (present in radiocontrast media), and reserpine
G. The clonidine suppression test may be useful in some patients: persistent elevations are indicative of pheochromocytoma
H. Multiple modalities may be utilized to localize pheochromocytoma, including the following:
   1. Computed tomography
   2. Magnetic resonance imaging
   3. Positron emission tomography
   4. Metaiodobenzylguanidine scintigraphy
I. If the mass is confirmed by metaiodobenzylguanidine, surgical resection is indicated

V. **Management**

    A. Treatment of hypertension in pheochromocytoma aims to bring out target blood pressure (BP) less than 120/80 mmHg (seated), with systolic BP greater than 90 mmHg (standing). Target BP readings may be modified in accordance with the patient's age and comorbid disease.

    B. Initial treatment is preoperative with α-blockers; once α-blockade has been established, β-blockers are added for heart rate control

        1. For acute treatment preoperatively, phentolamine (Regitine), 1–2 mg IV every 5 min until the patient becomes stabilized; then 1–5 mg IV every 12–24 hr

        2. Propranolol, 10 mg PO every 6 hr QID, titrate to goal BP

        3. For hypertensive crisis, nicardipine or nitroprusside intravenous may be used

            a. Nicardipine, 2.5–15 mg/hr by continuous infusion, titrate by 2.5 mg/hr every 5–15 min to maximum dose of 15 mg/hr; systolic BP is the clinical parameter for titration

            b. Nitroprusside, 0.1–5 mcg/kg/min to maximum dose of 10 mcg/kg/min; increase/decrease rate by minimum of 0.5 mcg/kg/min at intervals no longer than every 15 min; systolic BP is the parameter for titration

        4. For per os therapy, α-adrenergic blocking agents such as phenoxybenzamine (Dibenzyline), 10 mg PO every 12 hr, are indicated

            a. Increase the dose by 10–20 mg for 2–3 days until hypertension is controlled

            b. Maintenance doses range from 40–120 mg daily

            c. Avoid diuretics

            d. Phenoxybenzamine is the preferred drug for preoperative preparation to control blood pressure and arrhythmia in the U.S.

            e. When long-term pharmacologic treatment is indicated, selective α1-adrenergic blocking agents (e.g., prazosin, terazosin, doxazosin) are utilized due to a more favorable side-effect profile

    C. Do not restrict salt

    D. Achieve euvolemic state or infuse with intravenous normal saline before surgery

    E. Discontinue phenoxybenzamine 48 hr before surgery

    F. Consider autotransfusion of 1–2 units of packed red blood cells 12 hr preoperatively to reduce the risk of postoperative hypotension

    G. Post-operatively, monitor for the following:

        1. Hypotension from depleted catecholamines

        2. Adrenal insufficiency if a large part of the gland is removed

        3. Hemorrhage, as the adrenal gland is highly vascular

        4. Check urinary catecholamine levels at 1–2 weeks postoperatively in case metastatic tumors are present

BIBLIOGRAPHY

Blake, M. A. (2014). *Pheochromocytoma*. Retrieved from http://emedicine. medscape.com/article/124059-overview

Chen, H., Sippel, R., O'Dorisio, M. S., Vinik, A. I., Lloyd, R., & Pacak, K. (2010). The North American Neuroendocrine Tumor Society consensus guideline for the diagnosis and management of neuroendocrine tumors: pheochromocytoma, paraganglioma, and medullary thyroid cancer. *Pancreas, 39*(6), 775–83. doi:10.1097/mpa.0b013e3181ebb4f0

Därr, R., Lenders, J. W. M., Hofbauer, L. C., Naumann, B., Bornstein, S. R., & Eisenhofer, G. (2012). Pheochromocytoma: update on disease management. *Therapeutic Advances in Endocrinology and Metabolism, 3*(1), 11–26. doi:10.1177/2042018812437356

Fitzgerald, P. A. (2013). Endocrine Disorders. In M. A. Papadakis, S. J. McPhee, M. W. Rabow, & T. G. Berger (Eds.), *Current medical diagnosis & treatment 2014*. New York, NY: McGraw-Hill.

Goldman, L., & Schaefer, A. I. (2011). *Goldman's Cecil medicine: Expert consult premium edition* (24th ed.). Philadelphia, PA: WB Saunders.

McCance, K. L., Huether, S. E., Brashers, V. L., & Rote, N. S. (2010). *Pathophysiology: The Biologic basis for disease in adults and children* (6th ed.). St. Louis, MO: Mosby Elsevier.

Neumann, H. P. (2012). Pheochromocytoma. In D. L. Longo, A. S. Fauci, D. L. Kasper, S. L. Hauser, J. L. Jameson, & J. Loscalzo (Eds.), *Harrison's principles of internal medicine* (18th ed.). New York, NY: McGraw-Hill.

Yan, J., Min, J., & Zhou, B. (2013). Diagnosis of pheochromocytoma: A clinical practice guideline appraisal using AGREE II instrument. *Journal of Evaluation in Clinical Practice, 19*(4), 626–32. doi:10.1111/j.1365–2753.2012.01873.x

Syndrome of Inappropriate Antidiuretic Hormone

MONIQUE LAMBERT • THOMAS W. BARKLEY, JR.

I. **Definition/etiology**

A. A grouping of symptoms that results from secretion of antidiuretic hormone (ADH) independent of volume-dependent stimulation or osmolality

B. ADH is released from the posterior pituitary gland or from malignant tumors; this results in severe water retention despite a low serum osmolality.

II. **Incidence/predisposing factors/etiology**

A. Affects 1%–2% of patients with cancer

B. Central nervous system disorders
1. Brain tumors
2. Hemorrhages
3. Head trauma (including skull fractures)
4. Meningitis
5. Guillain-Barré syndrome
6. Systemic lupus erythematosus

C. Chronic lung diseases
1. Chronic obstructive pulmonary disease
2. Tuberculosis
3. Bacterial pneumonia
4. Aspergillosis
5. Bronchiectasis

D. Malignancies
1. Bronchogenic carcinoma
2. Pancreatic carcinoma
3. Prostatic carcinoma

4. Renal carcinoma
5. Leukemia
6. Malignant lymphoma
E. Pharmacologic agents that increase ADH production or potentiate ADH action
1. Antidepressants
2. Nonsteroidal anti-inflammatory drugs
3. Carbamazepine (Tegretol)
4. Morphine
5. Cyclophosphamide
6. Chlorpropamide
7. Vincristine
8. Nicotine
9. Alcohol
F. Other conditions that contribute to occurrence of syndrome of inappropriate diuretic hormone (SIADH) include the following:
1. AIDS
2. Physiologic stress
3. Pain

III. **Subjective/physical examination findings**
A. Neurologic changes from hyponatremia and usually if Na less than 120 mEq/L (mild headache to seizures, somnolence to respiratory failure)
B. Hypothermia may be present
C. Concentrated urine (ADH stimulates kidneys to reabsorb water)
D. Decreased urinary output
E. Decreased deep tendon reflexes
F. Weight gain and edema
G. Vomiting and abdominal cramping
H. Thyroid, cardiac, renal, adrenal, and liver function are not affected by the disease.

IV. **Laboratory/diagnostics**
A. Hyponatremia (less than 120 mEq/L), yet the patient is euvolemic
B. Decreased serum osmolality (less than 280 mOsm/kg)
C. Increased urine osmolality (more than 150 mOsm/kg)
D. Increased urine Na (usually less than 30 mEq/L)
E. Decreased blood urea nitrogen (BUN) (less than 10 mg/dl); may be normal in the absence of dehydration

V. **Management**
A. Treat the underlying cause
B. Symptomatic patients (usually with Na less than 120 mEq/L) should do the following:
1. Restrict water intake to approximately 500 ml/day

2. Increase serum Na by only 1–2 mEq/L/hr within the first day of therapy to avoid potential demyelination of nerves, cerebral edema, and seizures, but do not exceed 10–12 mEq/L in the first 24 hr
3. The rate of Na administration should be reduced to 0.5–1 mEq/L/hr once neurologic deficits improve.
4. The goal of therapy should be to reach a Na value of 125–130 mEq to avoid overcorrection.
5. Hypertonic 3% saline with or without furosemide (Lasix) 0.5–1 mg/kg IV over 1–2 min is indicated in symptomatic patients.
   a. If furosemide is not administered with hypertonic saline to the euvolemic patient, Na levels will temporarily increase, yet excess sodium will be excreted.
6. To determine the appropriate amount of 3% saline to be administered, the following steps should be followed:
   a. Check a random urinary Na after furosemide diuresis has begun
   b. Excreted Na is replaced with 3% saline at 1–2 ml/kg/hr; the infusion rate is then adjusted on the basis of urinary output and urinary sodium.
7. Seizure precautions should be followed for any patient with a markedly low serum Na level
8. Monitor serum Na levels at least every 2–4 hr
9. For hospitalized patients, vasopressin receptor antagonists may be used
   a. Should only be considered in the rare patients who have a persistent serum sodium below 120 mEq/L or persistent neurologic symptoms caused by hyponatremia
   b. May cause overly rapid correction of hyponatremia
   c. Intravenous parenteral conivaptan is an antagonist to the renal V-2 vasopressin receptor
      i. An initial loading dose of 20 mg over 30 min is recommended.
      ii. This is followed by a continuous infusion at a rate of 20–40 mg/day for an additional 1–3 days, up to 4 days in total
C. Asymptomatic patients
   1. Restrict water intake to 500–1,000 ml/day
   2. Increase serum Na by approximately 0.5 mEq/L/hr with normal saline (0.9%) given intravenous with furosemide 0.5–1 mg/kg to patients with Na values lower than 120 mEq/L. The electrolyte concentration of IV saline must be greater than the electrolyte concentration of the urine; this usually requires use of hypertonic saline
   3. Replace urinary sodium as described above

    4. Seizure precautions, as indicated

    5. Demeclocycline (Declomycin), 300–600 mg PO BID

        a. Rarely used due to cost and adverse effect profile

        b. May be used in patients who cannot follow fluid restriction and in those who require additional treatment for chronic SIADH

        c. Inhibits the effect of ADH in the kidneys

        d. May take 1–2 weeks for best effect to become apparent

        e. May increase risk of renal failure in patients with cirrhosis

  D. Medical emergencies

    1. Extracorporeal procedures such as continuous veno-venous hemofiltration and slow, low-efficiency daily dialysis

        a. More frequently seen in the cardiac patient who is hypervolemic with severe hyponatremia

BIBLIOGRAPHY

Blackburn, P. (2011). Emergency complications of malignancy. In J. E. Tintinalli, J. S. Stapczynski, O. J. Ma, D. M. Cline, R. K. Cydulka, & G. D. Meckler (Eds.), *Tintinalli's emergency medicine: a comprehensive study guide* (7th ed.). New York, NY: McGraw-Hill.

Chubb, S. A. P. (2010). Hyponatremia treatment guidelines 2007: Expert panel recommendations. *Clinical Biochemistry Review, 30*(1), 35–38.

Else, T., & Hammer G. D. (2010). Disorders of the hypothalamus & pituitary gland. In S. J. McPhee & G. D. Hammer (Eds.), *Pathophysiology of disease* (6th ed.). New York, NY: McGraw-Hill.

Fitzgerald, P. A. (2014). Endocrinology. In L. M. Tierney Jr., S. J. McPhee, & M. A. Papadakis (Eds.), *Current medical diagnosis & treatment* (45th ed.). Stamford, CT: Appleton & Lange.

Goldman, L., & Ausiello, D. (2011). *Cecil's textbook of medicine* (22nd ed.). Philadelphia, PA: W. B. Saunders.

Goroll, A. H., & Mulley A. G. (2009). *Primary care medicine* (5th ed.). St. Louis, MO: Mosby.

Gross, P. (2012). Management of SIADH. *Therapeutic Advances in Endocrinology and Metabolism, 3*(2), 62–73. doi:10.1177/2042018812437561

Huecker, M. R., & Danzl, D. F. (2011). Metabolic & endocrine emergencies. In R. L. Humphries & C. Stone (Eds.), *Current diagnosis & treatment emergency medicine* (7th ed.). New York, NY: McGraw-Hill.

Miller, M. (2009). Disorders of fluid balance. In J. B. Halter, J. G. Ouslander, M. E. Tinetti, S. Studenski, K. P. High, & S. Asthana (Eds.), *Hazzard's geriatric medicine and gerontology* (6th ed.). New York, NY: McGraw-Hill.

Papadakis, M. A., & McPhee, S. J. (2013). Syndrome of
inappropriate antidiuretic hormone (SIADH). *Access Medicine.*
Retrieved from http://accessmedicine.mhmedical.com/content.
aspx?bookid=548&sectionid=45863750&jumpsectionID=45884731

Reilly R. F., & Jackson E. K. (2011). Regulation of renal function and vascular
volume. In B. C. Knollmann (Ed.), *Goodman & Gilman's the pharmacological
basis of therapeutics* (12th ed.). New York, NY: McGraw-Hill.

Robinson, A. G. (2011). The posterior pituitary (neurohypophysis). In D. G.
Gardner & D. Shoback (Eds.), *Greenspan's basic & clinical endocrinology*
(9th ed.). New York, NY: McGraw-Hill.

Zietse, R., van der Lubbe, N., & Hoorn, E. J. (2009). Current and future treatment
options in SIADH. *Nephrology dialysis transplantation plus, 2*(3), iii12-iii19.
doi:10.1093/ndtplus/sfp154

CHAPTER 54

Diabetes Insipidus

RITA DELLO STRITTO • THOMAS W. BARKLEY, JR

I. Definition

   A. Polyuric syndrome that results from a deficiency of or insensitivity to antidiuretic hormone (ADH), causing volume depletion related to inability to concentrate urine

   B. Three types of diabetes insipidus (DI)

   1. Central (neurogenic)—deficiency of ADH production or release

   2. Nephrogenic—renal insensitivity to ADH

   3. Psychogenic

II. Incidence/predisposing factors

   A. Central—due to damage to the hypothalamus or the pituitary that results in a deficiency of ADH production or release

   1. Idiopathic

   2. Trauma

   3. More commonly seen with neurosurgical patients

   4. Brain tumors

   5. Intracranial hemorrhage

   6. Aneurysms

   7. Pituitary tumors

   8. Infections

   9. Meningitis

   10. Tuberculosis

   11. Syphilis

   12. Anoxic encephalopathy

   13. Vasopressinase induced

   14. Seen in the puerperium and during last trimester of pregnancy

   15. Associated with preeclampsia or liver dysfunction

    B. Nephrogenic—due to a defect in the renal tubules that results in renal insensitivity to ADH, thereby interfering with water reabsorption; unresponsive to vasopressin

        1. Familial X-linked trait (recessive)

        2. Renal disease (e.g., acquired via pyelonephritis or a defect in the renal tubules)

        3. Chronic hypokalemia or hypocalcemia

        4. Certain medications may induce nephrogenic DI, including the following:

            a. Lithium

            b. Methicillin

            c. Amphotericin B

        5. If psychogenic, then refer to a specialist

III. **Subjective/physical examination findings**

    A. May be physically asymptomatic (with central DI)

    B. Changes in level of consciousness

    C. Extreme thirst is present with cravings for ice water; the patient may report 5–20 L/day of fluid intake

    D. Hypotension

    E. Tachycardia

    F. Increased urinary output (2–20 L/24 hr)

    G. Nocturia may be present

    H. Low urine specific gravity (less than 1.006)

    I. Poor skin turgor

    J. Elevated temperature/fever

    K. Other findings indicative of the underlying cause

IV. **Diagnostic/laboratory findings**

    A. Although less commonly used today, 24-hr urine collection is used to evaluate the following:

        1. Polyuria (output greater than 300 ml/hr)

        2. Urine hypo-osmolality (dilute and odorless)

        3. Check glucose and creatinine as well

    B. Hypernatremia

    C. Decreased urinary specific gravity and urinary osmolarity

    D. Hypokalemia

    E. Hypercalcemia

    F. Increased serum osmolality

    G. Severe dehydration

    H. If central DI is suspected, a vasopressin (desmopressin) challenge test should be ordered.

        1. Desmopressin acetate (Stimate), 0.05–0.1 ml (5–10 µg) intranasally, or 1 µg SC or IV, is administered

        2. Urine volume is measured 12 hr before and after administration

        3. Sodium levels are checked for hyponatremia

        4. If the response is questionable or marginal, the dose is doubled

5. Patients with central DI have a positive test result (i.e., thirst markedly decreases, as well as polyuria; sodium usually remains normal).

6. The test result is negative in patients with nephrogenic DI (i.e., there is no improvement in the patient's clinical condition).

I. If the cause remains unclear, MRI may be used to check for a mass or lesion

V.   Management

A. Fluid replacement (oral or intravenous)
   1. Cornerstone of treatment
   2. Each 1-L water deficit is equal to a 3- to 5-mEq/L rise in serum sodium
   3. Calculate free water deficit = $0.6 \times$ weight in kilograms $\times$ (140/serum sodium mmol/L)
   4. Initiate intravenous fluid replacement with 0.9% normal saline until perfusion restored; then change to 0.45% normal saline, replacing ½ free water deficit in the first 12–24 hr
   5. Do not exceed 10–15 mEq/L/day serum sodium reduction; rapid correction can result in cerebral edema and death

B. Serum levels of glucose, blood/urea/nitrogen, potassium, sodium, calcium, plasma, and urine osmolarity should be monitored frequently.

C. For central DI, desmopressin (1-deamino-8-d-arginine vasopressin, exogenous ADH) should be used. This agent increases water reabsorption by the kidneys and has vasoconstrictive properties.
   1. Desmopressin, nasal solution 0.01% and nasal spray 0.01 mg/actuation (most commonly used as it is a metered dose), 10–40 mcg/day intranasally as a single daily dose or every 12 hr
   2. Desmopressin 1–4 mcg/day IV or SQ every 12–24 hr
   3. Desmopressin (0.1 or 0.2 mg tablets); initial dose is 0.05 mg (one-half of the 0.1 mg tablet) PO BID; maintenance dose is 0.1–0.8 mg/day in divided doses

D. Reduce aggravating factors such as corticosteroids. Increase water clearance to improve polyuria

E. Hydrochlorothiazide with a potassium supplement may be ordered for central and nephrogenic DI. Since hydrochlorothiazide is associated with various side effects such as weakness, low blood pressure, and nausea, the maximum dose should be limited to 50 mg/day.

F. Chlorpropamide (Diabinese) may be used to decrease thirst sensation in patients with continued hypernatremia, useful in partial central DI. Chlorpropamide may cause hypoglycemia and is generally less effective than desmopressin. The usual dose is 125–250 mg once or twice a day.

G. Nephrogenic DI may be managed with a combination of indomethacin-hydrochloride 25–50 mg daily, indomethacin-desmopressin, or indomethacin-amiloride; acutely, 50 mg of indomethacin every 8 hr is usually effective but is associated with more adverse effects than desmopressin.

H. Amiloride (Midamor) 5–20 mg daily may be divided in two doses; used to treat lithium-induced nephrogenic DI. This drug can cause hyperkalemia. Patients with kidney disease or diabetes, in particular, should closely monitor potassium levels when taking amiloride. In addition, regular measurements of lithium levels as well as a decrease in lithium dosage may be necessary due to the increased plasma levels of lithium.

BIBLIOGRAPHY

ACP PIER & AHFS DI® Essentials™. (2013). Philadelphia, PA: American College of Physicians.

Bagshaw, S. M., Townsend, D. R., & McDermid, R. C. (2009). Disorders of sodium and water balance in hospitalized patients. *Canadian Journal of Anesthesia, 56,* 151–167.

Elhassan, E. A., & Schrier, R. (2011). Hyponatremia: Diagnosis, complications, and management including V2 receptor antagonists. *Current Opinion in Nephrology and Hypertension, 20*(2), 161–168.

Fitzgerald P. A. (2013). Endocrine disorders. In M. A. Papadakis, S. J. McPhee, & M. W. Rabow (Eds.), *CURRENT medical diagnosis & treatment 2014* (53rd ed.). New York, NY: McGraw-Hill Education.

John, C. A., & Day, M. W. (2012). Central neurogenic diabetes insipidus, syndrome of inappropriate secretion of antidiuretic hormone, and cerebral salt-wasting syndrome in traumatic brain injury. *Critical Care Nurse, 32*(2), e1-e7; quiz e8. doi:10.4037/ccn2012904

Kelen, G. D., & Hsu, E. (2011). Fluids and electrolytes. In J. E. Tintinalli, J. S. Stapczynski, O. J. Ma, D. M. Cline, R. K. Cydulka, & G. D. Meckler (Eds.), *Tintinalli's emergency medicine: A comprehensive study guide* (7th ed.). New York, NY: McGraw-Hill Medical.

Melmed, S. (2013). Pituitary. In E. G. Nabel & D. D. Federman (Eds.), *ACP Medicine.* Philadelphia, PA: Decker Publishing Inc.

Pal, A., Karavitaki, N., & Wass, J. (2010). Disorders of the posterior pituitary gland. In D. A. Warrell, T. M. Cox, & J. D. Firth (Eds.), *Oxford textbook of medicine* (5th ed.). New York, NY: Oxford University Press.

Urden, L. D., Stacy, K. M., & Lourgh, M. E. (2014). *Thealan's critical nursing diagnosis* (7th ed.). St. Louis, MO: Elsevier.

Management of Musculoskeletal Disorders

CHAPTER 55

Arthritis

COLLEEN R. WALSH

OSTEOARTHRITIS

I. **Definition**
   A. Osteoarthritis (OA) is a progressive joint disorder that is characterized by slow destruction of the normal collagen architecture, which is followed by attempts of chondrocytes to produce replacement articular cartilage of joint surfaces
   B. OA is now classified as inflammatory because inflammatory changes occur as a result of synovial response to reactive new bone formation
   C. OA is classified as primary or secondary

II. **Etiology/incidence/predisposing factors**
   A. Thought to be "wear and tear" syndrome; 16 million affected in the U.S.
   B. Increased age: people older than age 60 have a 60% chance of developing OA
   C. Sex: both sexes are affected equally between the ages of 45 and 55
      1. After age 55, women are more likely to be affected
      2. Black women have twice the incidence of white women
      3. Men more often have OA in the hips; women have OA more often in the hands and fingers
   D. Genetics
      1. Evidence suggests that OA may be genetically inherited as an autosomal recessive trait
      2. Genetic/congenital conditions such as congenital hip dysplasia; increased incidence of Heberden's nodules in OA in distal interphalangeal (DIP) joint caused by a single gene that has not yet been identified
   E. Metabolic abnormalities such as Paget's disease

    F. Height and weight alterations such as abnormal height or increased weight-to-height ratio (i.e., obesity)

    G. Mechanical stressors such as repetitive microtrauma associated with sports injuries, ballet dancing, repetitive physical tasks

    H. Prior trauma, especially sprains, dislocations, and fractures that extend into the joint

    I. Chemicals, such as organic or heavy metals, that stimulate cartilage-injuring enzyme activity

    J. Neurologic disorders such as diabetic neuropathy, Charcot's, and neuropathic joints

    K. Hematologic/endocrine disorders such as hemochromatosis, hemophilia, and acromegaly

III. **Subjective findings**

    A. Pain in one or more joints, usually in weight-bearing joints, such as hips and knees, but also in central and peripheral joints such as fingers, hands, and wrists

    B. Stiffness of affected joints after prolonged sitting that dissipates upon arising

    C. "Grating" sensation during any range of motion (ROM); usually worsens as day progresses

    D. Feeling of instability, locking, or buckling of the knees, especially when climbing or descending stairs

    E. Fine motor skill deficits in the hands affect ability to perform routine ADLs

IV. **Physical findings**

    A. Bony induration or enlargement of affected joints; some effusions with warmth and redness

    B. Heberden's nodules—enlargements on DIP joints

    C. Bouchard's nodules—enlargements on proximal interphalangeal (PIP) joints

    D. Angular deformities of affected joints (valgus and varus), especially the knees

    E. Limited ROM with palpable/audible crepitus

    F. Pain on palpation of the joint line

V. **Laboratory/diagnostic findings**

    A. Plain x-rays show narrowing of joint space with cyst formations.

    B. Anteroposterior and lateral knee films should be taken bilaterally and standing to detect and measure degrees of varus and valgus deformity if present.

    C. Synovial fluid analysis reveals clear, yellow fluid with a normal WBC count (less than 1000/mm) and glucose levels that approximate patient's serum glucose

    D. No laboratory test is specific for OA; complete blood count and biochemical panel should be drawn to detect any hematologic or renal impairment when treatment with NSAIDs is considered.

E. Sedimentation rate may be elevated due to secondary inflammation from free floating intra-articular particles of cartilage

F. Bone scan, MRI, and CT should be considered if there is a question about infection, malignancy, or spur formations, or if compression or disruption of soft tissue structures is suspected.

VI. Management

A. Overall goals
  1. Relieve symptoms
  2. Maintain or improve function
  3. Limit disability as much as possible
  4. Avoid drug toxicity

B. Multidisciplinary team approach is best
  1. The American College of Rheumatology (ACR) Guidelines recommends the following therapy for the initial management of hand OA:
     a. Rest and joint protection: should obtain occupational therapy consultation for splinting and/or assistive devices to help with ADLs
     b. Heat and cold therapy; physical therapy evaluation
     c. Topical capsaicin
     d. Topical NSAIDs, including trolamine salicylate
     e. Oral NSAIDs, including COX-2 selective inhibitors
        i. Act by inhibiting the enzyme cyclooxygenase (COX), which is required for the synthesis of prostaglandins and thromboxanes
           (a) Two isoforms have been identified: COX-1 and COX-2
           (b) COX-1 is believed to be tissue-wide and is thought to protect the gastric mucosa
              1. COX-2 is induced mainly at the inflammation site
        ii. Older NSAIDs act by blocking both COX isoforms, leading to possible gastric ulceration. COX-2 drugs are selective, thus providing greater gastric protection.
           (a) Celecoxib (Celebrex), 100–200 mg PO daily
              1. Members of the FDA panel that have been reviewing COX-2 drugs unanimously agree that these drugs do cause heart problems in many patients.
              2. However, panel members also found that these drugs provide some benefit; therefore, they advised that there is no need to recall Celebrex at this time. The panel has recommended that Celebrex should carry the strictest form of warning, highlighted in a black box, on the label.

      f. Tramadol

      g. The ACR strongly recommends against the use of intra-articular therapies and opioids

      h. The ACR also recommends that persons older than 75 years should use topical rather than oral NSAIDs.

  2. The ACR Guidelines recommend the following therapy for the initial management of hip and knee OA:

      a. Weight reduction, if applicable

      b. Patients need to be enrolled in self-management programs

      c. Patients need to engage in cardiovascular aerobic exercises within their functional capabilities

      d. Alternative therapies such as tai chi and acupuncture

      e. TENS (transcutaneous external nerve stimulator)

      f. Referral to physical therapy for multimodal orthotics and assistive devices

      g. Acetaminophen

      h. Topical NSAIDs (for knee only)

      i. Tramadol

      j. NSAIDs

      k. Intraarticular corticosteroid injections

         i. Concurrent use of zafirlukast, fluconazole, and fluvastatin may increase serum concentration of celecoxib.

      l. The ACR recommends against the use of chondroitin sulfate and glucosamine as well as topical capsaicin.

      m. Surgical options: Refer to orthopedist for definitive surgical treatment

         i. Total joint replacement

         ii. Arthrotomy/arthroscopy for joint debridement

         iii. Osteotomy

         iv. Autogenous cartilage implantation and osteochondral grafting

RHEUMATOID ARTHRITIS

I.   **Definition**

    A. Rheumatoid arthritis (RA) is a chronic, systemic autoimmune disease of unknown origin that causes inflammation of connective tissue

    B. Synovium of joints is primarily affected first; then, the disorder spreads to articular cartilage, tendons, ligaments, and other soft tissues, including renal, cardiovascular, hematopoietic, and pulmonary structures. Systemic involvement occurs because of the disease process

II.   **Etiology/incidence/predisposing factors**

    A. Approximately 6 million people in the U.S. are affected; 75% are women, and the female-to-male ratio is 3:1. Two thirds of those affected have moderate to severe disease.

B. Cause is unknown; probably multifactorial, with genetic, environmental, hormonal, and reproductive components

C. Exposure to Epstein-Barr virus, bacteria, and mycoplasma

D. Autoimmune response in genetically predisposed individuals with defects in HLA-DR4, HLA-DQ, and HLA-DP areas of histocompatibility complex

E. Decreased reproductive hormones after birth exacerbate disease

F. The proinflammatory cytokine tumor necrosis factor-α (TNF-α) is thought to play a dominant role in the pathogenesis of RA.

G. The annual cost of treating patients with rheumatoid arthritis and other rheumatologic diseases is approximately $250 million.

III. **Subjective findings**

A. Symmetric joint and muscle pain that is usually worse in the morning and improves as the day progresses

B. Weakness, fatigue

C. Anorexia

D. Weight loss

E. Generalized malaise

IV. **Physical examination findings**

A. Articular

  1. Swelling of joints with a typical "boggy" feel on palpation; most frequently seen in metacarpophalangeal (MCP) joints, wrists, and PIP joints

  2. Warmth and redness of skin over affected joints

  3. Multiple, symmetric joint involvement

  4. Deformity of joints, especially PIP, DIP, and MCP of hands

  5. Multiple nodules on volar aspect of forearms

  6. Osteopenia of fingers occurs early in disease process

B. Extra-articular

  1. Pleural effusions

  2. Scleritis and episcleritis: inflammation of the sclerae and surrounding ophthalmologic structures

  3. Arteritis

  4. Pericarditis, conduction defects, myocarditis

  5. Splenomegaly (Felty's syndrome)

  6. Pulmonary nodules and fibrosis may be caused by disease or drugs used to treat disease

V. **Laboratory/diagnostic studies**

A. Granulocytopenia (Felty's syndrome): neutrophil count less than 500/μl

B. Anemia (hypochromic, microcytic)

  1. Low hemoglobin count (normal, 14–18 grams/dl in males and 12–16 grams/dl in females)

  2. Low serum ferritin and low or normal total iron-binding capacity

C. May have positive rheumatoid factor, although nonspecific

D. Antinuclear antibody may be elevated

E. Erythrocyte sedimentation rate is usually elevated

F. Radiographs reveal joint swelling, then progressive cortical thinning, osteopenia, and joint space narrowing.

G. Radiographs of cervical spine are needed to detect cervical spine instability due to atlantoaxial (C1-C2) subluxation

H. Synovial fluid: yellow, turbid fluid with friable mucin clot; elevated WBC up to 100,000/mm; normal glucose

I. RA is a clinical diagnosis, not a laboratory or radiologic diagnosis

J. See Table 55.1 for diagnostic studies commonly used in rheumatic diseases

VI. **Management**

A. Multidisciplinary team approach is best, with early aggressive treatment started as soon as diagnosis is made

B. "Traditional" stepwise pyramid for treatment of RA has now been rejected. Early diagnosis, referral, and treatment with disease-modifying antirheumatic drugs (DMARDs) have been advocated (Table 55.2)

C. Early referral to a rheumatologist is recommended

D. DMARDs used in treatment of RA

1. Methotrexate

2. Cyclosporine (unlabeled use therapy)

    a. Immunomodulatory agent that blocks the production and release of several cytokines, including interleukin-2

    b. Used for RA unresponsive to methotrexate and gold preparations

    c. Implications: may cause nephrotoxicity, which is dose dependent

3. Gold preparations

    a. Use determined by rheumatologist due to toxicity and/or lack of long-term benefit

    b. Auranofin, aurothioglucose, and aurothiomalate are parenteral preparations used for moderate to severe RA.

    c. Implications: can cause serious adverse effects, including thrombocytopenia, proteinuria, and hematuria

    d. Drugs should be ordered and monitored by a rheumatologist

4. Hydroxychloroquine

    a. Antimalarial drug whose mechanism of action is unknown

    b. Implications: low adverse effect profile, but a major possible adverse effect is retinal damage

    c. Drug should be ordered and monitored by a rheumatologist

5. Sulfasalazine

    a. Used for moderate RA, but mechanism of action is unknown

    b. Used in combination with methotrexate and cyclosporine

Table 55.1	Common diagnostic studies used in rheumatic diseases	
Test and Purpose	**Normal Value**	**Significance**
Antinuclear Antibody (ANA)		
• ANAs are gamma globulins that react to specific antigens • ANA titer indicates the presence of antibodies that are produced in response to the nuclear part of the white blood cell • If antibodies are present, further tests determine the type of ANA circulating in the blood	Titer 1:32 or less	• A small number of healthy adults have a positive ANA test • ANA levels may increase with age, even in those without immune disease • Positive titers (1:10–1:30) are associated with SLE, SS, dermatomyositis, and Sjogren's syndrome • The higher the titer, the greater the degree of inflammation • A negative test for ANA is strong evidence against the diagnosis of SLE
C4 Complement		
• Method to determine serum hemolytic complement activity • Complement is a protein that binds antigen-antibody complexes for purposes of lysis • Activation of the entire complement system leads to an inflammatory response that destroys/damages cells • When the number of antigen-antibody complexes increases markedly, complement is used for lysis, thus decreasing its availability	Men: 12–72 mg/dL Women: 13–75 mg/dL	• Increase in active inflammatory disease and in autoimmune disorders (rheumatoid spondylitis, JRA) • May be decreased in RA and SLE

Table 55.1	Common diagnostic studies used in rheumatic diseases	
Test and Purpose	**Normal Value**	**Significance**
Radioallergosorbent Test (RAST)		
Measures the quantity and increase of the antigen IgE present in the serum after exposure to a specific antigen	0.01–0.04 mg/dl	• Elevated with allergic reactions: asthma, hay fever, dermatitis • May be used to elevate suspected allergic responses in patients on gold therapy
HLA-B27 Antigen		

• Measures the presence of HLA-B27, which is used for tissue typing/tissue recognition
• Five series have been designated for HLA: A, B, C, D, DR, each with 10–20 distinct antigens
• Measure the values of immunoglobulins, serum antibodies produced by the plasma cells of the B lymphocytes
• Five classes:
  • IgA—protects mucous membranes from viruses and bacteria
  • IgM—first responder to appear after antigens enter body; produces antibody against rheumatoid factor
  • IgG—produces antibodies against bacteria, viruses, toxins
  • IgD—less active
  • IgE—less active
	• Titer greater than 1:32
	• IgA:
	  85–385 mg/dl
	• IgG:
	  565–1700 mg/dl
	• IgM:
	  55–370 mg/dl
	• IgD: trace
	• IgE: trace
		• Primary use is to predict the compatibility of donor/recipient tissues and platelets
		• HLA-B27 found in 80%–90% of those with AS and Reiter's syndrome. Also found in persons with the pauciarticular subgroup of JRA. Presence does not mean disease: HLA-B27 is also seen in 8% of the general population
		• Basic function of immunoglobulins is to neutralize toxic substances (antigens) to allow phagocytosis
		• Unique because of their genetic coding: each immunoglobulin interacts with other molecules
		• The recognition mechanism of the immunoglobulin forms the basis of the immune response
		• Increased levels are found in autoimmune diseases, specifically IgM (lupus, RA), IgG (RA)

Table 55.1	Common diagnostic studies used in rheumatic diseases	
Test and Purpose	**Normal Value**	**Significance**
Red Blood Cell Count		
Measures the number of circulating erythrocytes per cubic millimeter of blood	Men: 4.7–6.1 million (mn)/mm Women: 4.2–5.4 mn/mm	• Normal values vary according to age • When the value is greater than 10% below the normal value, the patient is considered anemic • Decrease in SLE, RA, chronic inflammation
Erythrocyte Sedimentation Rate (ESR)		
Measures the rate at which red blood cells settle out of unclotted blood in 1 hr	Wintrobe Men: 0–7 mm/hr Women: 0–25 mm/hr Westergren Men: 0–20 mm/hr Women: 0–30 mm/hr Higher elevations are seen in both men and women older than age 50	• Increased rate seen in inflammation and necrotic processes • Increase often seen in any inflammatory connective tissue disease • An increase often indicates increased inflammation, resulting in clustering of red blood cells, which makes them heavier than normal; the higher the sedimentation rate, the greater the inflammatory activity • Particularly useful as a guide to the management of the patient with RA • Decrease in salicylate toxicity • Falsely elevated with excessive exercise, anxiety, pain, or dehydration

Table 55.1	Common diagnostic studies used in rheumatic diseases		
Test and Purpose	**Normal Value**	**Significance**	
C-Reactive Protein (CRP)			
Indicates presence of abnormal plasma protein (glycoprotein) that appears as a nonspecific response to a variety of inflammatory stimuli	Trace to 6 mg/ml	• CRP is a nonspecific antigen- antibody reaction test to help determine the extent/severity of a disease process • Elevated measurements indicate active inflammation, both infectious and noninfectious • Elevated in RA, bacterial and viral infections, disseminated lupus erythematosus • In RA, the test becomes negative with successful therapy, indicating that the inflammatory reaction has disappeared, although the ESR may continue to be elevated	
LE Prep (LE Test)			
• Measures the number of LE cells, essentially a type of ANA • Should be repeated on 3 consecutive days to obtain the most accurate results	Negative	• Positive in 75%–80% of patients with SLE • Positive results may also be associated with RA and SS	
Rheumatoid Factor (RF)			
• Determines the measurement for RF, a macroglobulin (antibody) directed toward a gamma globulin (IgG) • Two tests are used: latex fixation and sheep red cell agglutination	1:160 or less considered significant in latex fixation 1:16 or less considered significant for agglutination titer	• Positive RF present in 70%–90% of persons with RA • Negative RF found in 10%–30% of patients with clinical diagnosis of RA • Positive RF may also suggest SLE or mixed connective tissue disease • The higher the titer (the number to the right of the colon), the greater the degree of inflammation • Titer is normally increased in older persons and in those who have multiple vaccinations or blood transfusions	

Table 55.2	Commonly Used Agents for the Treatment of Arthritis		
Drug	**Dosage**	**Adverse Effects**	**Comments**
Acetaminophen	1000 mg PO every 8 hr NOT to exceed 3000 mg/24 hr	pruritus, constipation, nausea, vomiting, headache, insomnia, agitation, atelectasis, exanthematous pustulosis, Stevens-Johnson Syndrome, toxic epidermal necrolysis, liver failure	• Analgesic and antipyretic properties • NO anti-inflammatory properties • Does not induce GI bleeding • Well tolerated and safe for all age groups • Available in many formulations (IV, PO, NG, PR) • Adjust dose in hepatic impairment, elderly • BBW: life-threatening cases of acute hepatic failure leading to liver transplant or death
Tramadol (Ultram)	50–100 mg PO every 6–8 hr Max: 400 mg/day	flushing, nausea, dizziness, somnolence, seizures, respiratory depression	• NOT chemically related to opiates • Reduce dose & frequency for renal or hepatic impairment • Avoid in patients with seizures • Withdrawal symptoms have been reported • As of August 2014, tramadol is a controlled substance (schedule IV)
Corticosteroids			
• Hydrocortisone (Cortef) • Prednisolone (Delta-Cortef) • Prednisone (Deltasone)	Highly individualized but the lowest dosage possible is 10 mg/day or less	nausea, hyperglycemia, psychosis, weight gain, osteoporosis, adrenal insufficiency, mask infections	• NOT used as chronic maintenance therapy • If required, use lowest effective dose • Work quickly to suppress acute flares • Taper dose after remission is achieved

Table 55.2 Commonly Used Agents for the Treatment of Arthritis

Drug	Dosage	Adverse Effects	Comments
Nonsteroidal Anti-Inflammatory Drugs (NSAIDs)			
aspirin*	325–650 mg PO 6 hr; Max: 3.9 grams/24 hr	**Central nervous system:** Headache, tinnitus, dizziness	Analgesic, antipyretic, and anti-inflammatory properties
diclofenac (Voltaren)	100–150 mg/day PO in 2–3 divided doses; Max: 200 mg/day	**Cardiovascular:** Fluid retention, hypertension, edema; Rare: myocardial infarction, heart failure	All agents are equally efficacious Do not use ASA in children = Reye's syndrome risk
diflunisal (Dolobid)	500–1000 mg PO BID; Max: 1500 mg/day	**Gastrointestinal:** Abdominal pain, dysplasia, nausea, vomiting Rare: ulcers or bleeding	Selection based on cost/availability/preference
etodolac (Lodine)	800–1200 mg/day PO in 2–4 divided doses; Max: 1200 mg/day	**Hematologic:** Rare: thrombocytopenia, neutropenia, aplastic anemia	ALL patients taking NSAID's should be evaluated for concurrent administration of proton pump inhibitor therapy to prevent GI complications
fenoprofen (Nalfon)	300–600 mg PO 3–4 times/day; Max: 3200 mg/day	**Hepatic:** Abnormal liver function tests; Rare: liver failure **Pulmonary:** Asthma **Skin:** Rash, pruritus	BBW: may cause an increased risk of serious cardiovascular thrombotic events
flurbiprofen (Ansaid)	200–300 mg/day PO in 2–4 divided doses; Max: 100 mg/dose; 300 mg/day	**Renal:** Renal insufficiency, renal failure, hyperkalemia, proteinuria	*available OTC
ibuprofen (Motrin, Advil)*	1200–3200 mg/day PO in 3–4 divided doses Max: 3200 mg/day		
indo-methacin (Indocin)	25 mg PO 2–3 times/day Max: 100 mg/dose; 200 mg/day		

Table 55.2	Commonly Used Agents for the Treatment of Arthritis		
Drug	**Dosage**	**Adverse Effects**	**Comments**
Nonsteroidal Anti-Inflammatory Drugs (NSAIDs)			
meclofenamate	200–400 mg/day PO in 3–4 divided doses; Max: 400 mg/day	**Central nervous system:** Headache, tinnitus, dizziness **Cardiovascular:** Fluid retention, hypertension, edema; Rare: myocardial infarction, heart failure **Gastrointestinal:** Abdominal pain, dysplasia, nausea, vomiting Rare: ulcers or bleeding **Hematologic:** Rare: thrombocytopenia, neutropenia, aplastic anemia **Hepatic:** Abnormal liver function tests; Rare: liver failure **Pulmonary:** Asthma **Skin:** Rash, pruritus **Renal:** Renal insufficiency, renal failure, hyperkalemia, proteinuria	Analgesic, antipyretic, and anti-inflammatory properties All agents are <u>equally efficacious</u> Do not use ASA in children = Reye's syndrome risk Selection based on cost/availability/preference ALL patients taking NSAID's should be evaluated for concurrent administration of proton pump inhibitor therapy to prevent GI complications BBW: may cause an increased risk of serious cardiovascular thrombotic events ***available OTC**
meloxicam (Mobic)	7.5 mg PO daily Max: 15 mg/day		
nabumetone (Relafen)	500–1000 mg/day PO 1–2 times/day Max: 2000 mg/day		
naproxen (Naprosyn, Aleve)*	250–500 mg PO BID Max: 1500 mg/day		
oxaprozin (Daypro)	600–1200 mg PO daily; Max: 1800 mg/day		
piroxicam (Feldene)	10–20 mg PO daily Max: 20 mg/day		
sulindac (Clinoril)	150 mg PO BID Max: 400 mg/day		
tolmetin (Tolectin)	200–600 mg PO TID Max: 1800 mg/day		
ketoprofen (Orudis)	150–300 mg/day PO in 3–4 divided doses Max: 300 mg/day		

Table 55.2	Commonly Used Agents for the Treatment of Arthritis		
Drug	**Dosage**	**Adverse Effects**	**Comments**
Nonsteroidal Anti-Inflammatory Drugs (NSAIDs)			
celecoxib (Celebrex)		back pain, peripheral edema, abdominal pain, dyspepsia, flatulence, dizziness, headache, insomnia, hypertension, MI	Analgesic, antipyretic and anti-inflammatory properties Efficacy equals that of the other NSAIDs Fewer endoscopic ulcers than most other NSAIDs (?) Renal toxicities similar to traditional NSAIDs Not recommended in renal or liver failure Screen for sulfa allergy BBW: may cause an increased risk of serious cardiovascular thrombotic events BBW: increased risk of serious GI adverse events, especially in the elderly
Topical Agents			
Disease-Modifying Antirheumatic Drugs (DMARD)			
methotrexate	7.5–15 mg PO or IM weekly	alopecia, photosensitivity, erythematous rashes, headache, drowsiness, aphasia, blurred vision, hemiparesis, paresis, seizures, fatigue, malaise, dizziness, elevated LFT's, abdominal pain, diarrhea, indigestion, nausea, stomatitis, vomiting, renal failure, agranulocytosis, thrombocytopenia	Monitor renal and hepatic function Give with folic acid 1 mg/day Risk of toxicity increased with use of alcohol, patient must refrain Follow CBC, UA, AST, BUN, and Cr every 6–8 wk during therapy

Table 55.2	Commonly Used Agents for the Treatment of Arthritis		
Drug	**Dosage**	**Adverse Effects**	**Comments**
Topical Agents			
Disease-Modifying Antirheumatic Drugs (DMARD)			
hydroxychloroquine (Plaquenil)	200–400 mg PO daily	Retinal or visual field changes CNS: vertigo, headaches, confusion; blood dyscrasias, skin rash, pruritus, skeletal muscle weakness, gastrointestinal distress	Gastrointestinal distress: Ophthalmic exam: baseline then every 6 months CBC: baseline and every 6–12 months Instruct patient to report any visual changes, unexplained bruising or bleeding, skin eruptions or weakness Inform patient that full efficacy may not be seen for 6 months
sulfasalazine (Azulfidine)	1 gram PO BID Max: 3 grams/day	Stomach pain, achiness, diarrhea, dizziness, headache, light sensitivity, itching, appetite loss, liver abnormalities, lowered blood count, nausea, vomiting, rash	Slow acting—take with food to decrease gastrointestinal upset; drink 8 glasses of water/day Monitor liver function, renal function, UA routinely
Topical Agents			
Disease-Modifying Antirheumatic Drugs (DMARD)†			
minocycline (Minocin)	100–200 mg PO daily	Tooth discoloration, dizziness, headache, fatigue, erythema multiforme, Stevens-Johnson Syndrome	Not FDA-labeled for this indication Limited to patients with low disease activity

Table 55.2	Commonly Used Agents for the Treatment of Arthritis		
Drug	**Dosage**	**Adverse Effects**	**Comments**
Disease-Modifying Antirheumatic Drugs (DMARD)			
leflunomide (Arava)	<u>Loading dose:</u> 100 mg PO daily for 3 days, followed by <u>Maintenance dose:</u> 10–20 mg PO daily	Diarrhea, elevated liver enzymes (ALT and AST), alopecia and rash	Monitor liver enzymes monthly initially Long half-life: greater than 2 weeks BBW: pregnancy must be excluded before the start of treatment, do not use in patients with acute or chronic liver disease Cholestyramine 8 grams PO TID for cases of toxicity
cyclosporine (Neoral, Sandimmune)	2.5 mg/kg/day PO 1–2 times/day	Bleeding, tender or enlarged gums, fluid retention hypertension, increase hair growth, loss of renal function, loss of appetite, trembling or shaking of hands, tremors	Can be used alone or in combination with methotrexate Monitor liver and renal function routinely Administer with food and encourage frequent mouth care may help alleviate tender and bleeding gums Monitor blood pressure and renal function Many drug-drug interactions

Table 55.2	Commonly Used Agents for the Treatment of Arthritis		
Drug	**Dosage**	**Adverse Effects**	**Comments**
Disease-Modifying Antirheumatic Drugs (DMARD)			
capsaicin cream (Capsin, Zostrix)	Apply to affected joint 3–4 times/day	erythema, application site pain, application site rash, pruritus, nausea, HTN	Advantages over systemic drugs: delivery at the site of insult, lower initial rates of systemic absorption, fewer systemic effects and patient preference Useful for osteoarthritis, neuropathic pain (capsaicin, lidocaine) Topical preparations safer than their oral agents (?)
diclofenac (Voltaren gel 1%)	Apply 4 grams to lower extremities 4 times daily; Apply 2 grams to upper extremities 4 times daily; Max: 8 grams/day to any single joint of upper extremity 16 grams/day to any single joint of lower extremity 32 grams/day total over all affected joints		
trolamine salicylate (Aspercreme 10%)	Apply to affected area 3–4 times/day	Erythema, skin irritation, tinnitus	
lidocaine 5% patch (Lidoderm)	Apply up to 3 patches to affected area/joint at one time, for up to 12 hr within a 24-hour period	hypotension, nausea, rash	

Table 55.2	Commonly Used Agents for the Treatment of Arthritis		
Drug	**Dosage**	**Adverse Effects**	**Comments**
Disease-Modifying Antirheumatic Drugs (DMARD)			
azathioprine (Imuran)	Initial: 1 mg/kg/day PO 1–2 times/day, may titrate by 0.5 mg/kg/day after 6–8 weeks and every 4 weeks if no response Max: 2.5 mg/kg/day Patients who do not respond in 12 weeks are probably refractory	Gastrointestinal: nausea, vomiting, hepatotoxicity Hematologic: leukopenia, thrombocytopenia, macrocytic anemia Serious infections: fungal, bacterial, protozoal infections secondary to immunosuppression, may be fatal Carcinogenesis: increase risk of neoplasia, especially in homograft patients, lymphoma	Take drug in divided doses with food Avoid infections; patient must notify doctor if pregnant or wishes to become pregnant Monitor blood counts every 4–6 weeks Therapeutic effects are not usually seen for 6–8 weeks

Table 55.2 Commonly Used Agents for the Treatment of Arthritis

Disease-Modifying Antirheumatic Drugs (DMARD): Biologic Agents

Anti-TNF Agents

Drug	Dosage	Adverse Effects	Comments
adalimumab (Humira)	40 mg SQ every other week	Injection site pain/reaction, rash, antibody development, antinuclear antibody positive, headache, sinusitis, erythema multiforme, Stevens-Johnson Syndrome, CHF, pancytopenia, thrombocytopenia, infection, liver failure	Evaluate patients for latent TB prior to initiating therapy BBW: increased risk for infections, some progressing to serious infections leading to hospitalization or death BBW: Lymphoma and other malignancies, some fatal, have been reported
infliximab (Remicade)	3 mg/kg IV over at least 2 hr given at weeks 0, 2 and 6, then every 8 weeks in combination with methotrexate Pre-medicate: antihistamine, acetaminophen, and/or corticosteroids	Injection site pain/reaction, rash, abdominal pain, nausea, headache, infection, fatigue, fever, drug-induced lupus erythematosus, pancytopenia, Thrombocytopenia	Evaluate for active TB and test for latent TB prior to initiating therapy Monitor liver/renal function and CBC every 6–8 weeks BBW: increased risk for infections, some progressing to serious infections leading to hospitalization or death BBW: Lymphoma and other malignancies, some fatal, have been reported

Table 55.2	Commonly Used Agents for the Treatment of Arthritis		
Drug	**Dosage**	**Adverse Effects**	**Comments**
Disease-Modifying Antirheumatic Drugs (DMARD): Biologic Agents			
Anti-TNF Agents			
Etanercept (Enbrel)	50 mg SQ weekly	Injection site reaction, infection, erythema multiforme, malignant melanoma, necrotizing fasciitis, primary cutaneous vasculitis, thrombocytopenia, seizure, optic neuritis	Evaluate for active TB and test for latent TB prior to initiating therapy BBW: increased risk for infections, some progressing to serious infections leading to hospitalization or death BBW: Lymphoma and other malignancies, some fatal, have been reported
Certolizumab Pegol (Cimzia)	Initial: 400 mg SQ (two SQ injections of 200 mg) once and then repeat at weeks 2 and 4 Maintenance: 200 mg SQ once every 2 weeks OR 400 mg SQ (two SQ injections of 200 mg) once every 4 weeks	Arthralgia, infection, cardiac dysrhythmia, congestive heart failure, hypertensive heart disease, myocardial infarction, pericardial effusion, pericarditis, erythema multiforme, erythema nodosum, Stevens-Johnson Syndrome, toxic epidermal necrolysis, urticaria, bowel obstruction, seizure, nephrotic syndrome, renal failure	Evaluate for active TB and test for latent TB and hepatitis B viral infection prior to initiating therapy Monitor liver/renal function and CBC every 6–8 weeks BBW: increased risk for infections, some progressing to serious infections leading to hospitalization or death BBW: Lymphoma and other malignancies, some fatal, have been reported

Table 55.2	Commonly Used Agents for the Treatment of Arthritis		
Drug	**Dosage**	**Adverse Effects**	**Comments**
Disease-Modifying Antirheumatic Drugs (DMARD): Biologic Agents Anti-TNF Agents			
golimumab (Simponi)	50 mg SQ once monthly in combination with methotrexate	Hypertension, injection site reaction, rash, elevated liver enzymes, dizziness, paresthesia, congestive heart failure, lupus erythematosus, erythema multiforme-like syndrome, optic neuritis, anaphylaxis, immune hypersensitivity reaction	Evaluate for active TB and test for latent TB and hepatitis B viral infection prior to initiating therapy Monitor liver/renal function and CBC every 6–8 weeks BBW: increased risk for infections, some progressing to serious infections leading to hospitalization or death BBW: Lymphoma and other malignancies, some fatal, have been reported
Disease-Modifying Antirheumatic Drugs (DMARD): Biologic Agents Non-TNF Agents			
abatacept (Orencia)	125 mg SQ weekly	Nausea, infection, hypersensitivity reactions, headache, exacerbation of chronic obstructive pulmonary disease, cellulitis, cancer	Evaluate for active TB and test for latent TB and hepatitis B viral infection prior to initiating therapy Concomitant use of biologic rheumatoid arthritis therapy (anakinra), tumor necrosis factor (TNF) antagonists, live vaccines or use of live vaccines within 3 months of discontinuation of abatacept is not recommended

Table 55.2	Commonly Used Agents for the Treatment of Arthritis		
Drug	**Dosage**	**Adverse Effects**	**Comments**
Disease-Modifying Antirheumatic Drugs (DMARD): Biologic Agents			
Non-TNF Agents			
rituximab (Rituxan)	1000 mg IV followed by a second 1000 mg IV dose 2 weeks later in combination with methotrexate every 24 weeks or based on clinical evaluation; no more often than every 16 weeks Pre-medicate: glucocorticoid (methylprednisolone 100 mg IV), antihistamine, and acetaminophen 30 minutes prior to each infusion	Hypotension, peripheral edema, night sweats, abdominal pain, diarrhea, nausea, vomiting, anemia, arthralgia, myalgia, asthenia, headache, dizziness, sensory neuropathy, infection, fever, pain, shivering, angioedema, tumor lysis syndrome, cardiac dysrhythmia, heart failure, Stevens-Johnson Syndrome, toxic epidermal necrolysis	Screen all patients for hepatitis B virus (HBV) prior to initiation of therapy *BBW:* fatal infusion reactions may occur within 24 hr of rituximab infusion; approximately 80% of fatal reactions occurred with first infusion

Table 55.2 Commonly Used Agents for the Treatment of Arthritis

Drug	Dosage	Adverse Effects	Comments
Disease-Modifying Antirheumatic Drugs (DMARD): Biologic Agents			
Non-TNF Agents			
tocilizumab (Actemra)	Weight less than 100 kg: 162 mg SQ every other week; increase to 162 mg SQ every week based on clinical response Weight 100 kg or greater: 162 mg SQ every week	Hypertension, Injection site reaction, rash, Diarrhea, abdominal pain, elevated liver enzymes, Dizziness, Headache, Gastrointestinal perforation, Neutropenia, thrombocytopenia, Anaphylaxis, Hypersensitivity reaction, cancer, infection	Evaluate for active TB and test for latent TB and hepatitis B viral infection prior to initiating therapy Baseline absolute neutrophil count (ANC) of 2000/mm(3) or greater and a platelet count of 100,000/mm(3) or greater are required before initiating tocilizumab Do not initiate in patients with baseline ALT or AST levels greater than 1.5 x upper limit of normal (ULN) BBW: increased risk for infections, some progressing to serious infections leading to hospitalization or death
anakinra (Kineret)	100 mg/day SQ; administer dose at approximately the same time every day	Injection site reaction, cardiorespiratory arrest, malignant melanoma, neutropenia, immune hypersensitivity reaction, infection, cancer	Concomitant use of tumor necrosis factor blocking agents is not recommended Live vaccines should not be administered concurrently Increases risk of new onset or reactivation of latent TB

       c. Implications: major toxicities include leukopenia, thrombocytopenia, hemolysis, agranulocytosis, aplastic anemia, and eosinophilic pneumonia

       d. Drug should be ordered and monitored by a rheumatologist

    6. Leflunomide

       a. Mechanism of action is to disrupt T-cell proliferation; indicated for moderate to severe RA

       b. Drug should be ordered and monitored by a rheumatologist

    7. Etanercept

       a. Acts by inhibiting the binding of TNF-α and TNF-β to the cell surface TNF receptor

       b. Can be used in conjunction with methotrexate and other DMARDs

       c. Orencia (abatacept)

    8. Monitor liver function studies at the onset of treatment with DMARDs and periodically thereafter because recent studies have revealed elevated LFTs in some patients

  E. Physical/occupational therapy for assistive devices and durable medical equipment

  F. New guidelines emphasize importance of screening for latent or overt tuberculosis prior to starting biological modifiers of disease (BMD)

    1. Tuberculin skin tests (TSTs)

    2. Interferon-release assays (IGRAs)

  G. Hepatitis and biological agents

    1. Not recommended in patients with untreated chronic hepatitis B and in treated patients with chronic hepatitis B and Child-Pugh classification B or higher (liver involvement)

  H. Surgery: refer to orthopedist

    1. Arthrotomy/arthroscopy for joint debridement

    2. Osteotomy

    3. Total joint replacement; hand joint replacement

GOUT

I.   **Definition**

  A. Inflammatory disorder that occurs in response to uric acid production that results in elevated levels of uric acid in the blood and other bodily fluids, including synovial fluid

  B. When uric acid concentrations rise to certain levels, crystallization occurs, and these insoluble precipitates cause inflammation, especially in the joints.

II.   **Etiology/incidence/predisposing factors**

  A. Defect in purine metabolism resulting in excessive formation of monosodium urate

  B. Impaired renal function due to excess uric acid or to crystallization of uric acid that results in decreased glomerular filtration rate

C. Although no data indicate specific incidence, evidence suggests that the number of persons affected worldwide is increasing as the Western diet is being introduced worldwide.

D. Foods that are high in purine, such as dairy foods, red meat, and certain shellfish, along with beer consumption, are thought to be factors in the development of gout

E. Activation of proinflammatory mediators adds to the inflammatory response

F. Within the joint, urate crystals react with neutrophils and monocytes, and these cause tissue damage that perpetuates the inflammatory process

G. G6PD inherited disorder with two main subtypes:
1. Type A
2. Mediterranean

III.   **Subjective findings**
A. Acute onset of painful joint, often the great toes
B. Patient reports pain at night
C. Flank pain due to renal calculi is described

IV.   **Physical examination findings**
A. Warm, swollen joint; often the first metatarsal
B. Fever
C. Leukocytosis
D. Elevated erythrocyte sedimentation rate
E. Tophi, usually on the helix of the ear
F. Limited joint motion in other joints due to impingement by urate crystals

V.   **Laboratory/diagnostic studies**
A. Elevated serum uric acid levels greater than 7 mg/dl
B. Joint aspiration reveals urate crystals seen under red lamp in the laboratory
C. Radiographs may reveal joint erosion; intravenous venous pyelogram or renal ultrasound may reveal renal stones

VI.   **Management**
A. The three NSAIDs that are FDA approved for the treatment of acute gout are naproxen, indomethacin, and Sulindac. For the acute stage, consider indomethacin, 50 mg PO every 8 hr for 1–2 weeks; then, gradually taper or naproxen, 500 mg BID for 5 days, or Sulindac, 200 mg PO every 12 hr for 7 days (refer to Pain chapter for more information on NSAIDs)

B. Colchicine may be given PO to those individuals who cannot tolerate NSAIDs; IV colchicine is no longer produced or approved in the United States. It is no longer considered a first-line treatment but is still used with dose modification. Give 1.6 mg PO at onset of flare, followed by 0.6 mg PO one hour later

1. Use with caution in patients with renal impairment; may be contraindicated if estimated GFR is less than 30 ml/min
2. Low-dose colchicine may be used for prophylaxis therapy
C. Corticosteroids may be given PO, IV, or SQ if the patient cannot tolerate either NSAIDs or colchicine
D. Any combination of drugs can be used if the patient cannot tolerate one therapeutic regimen or is unresponsive to monotherapy
E. Collect 24-hour urine for uric acid output
F. Start xanthine oxidase inhibitors after acute flare over
   1. Allopurinol, 100 mg PO daily until uric acid level is less than 6 mg/dl; depending on renal function, may give up to 800 mg PO daily
   2. Febuxostat, 40 mg PO daily, may be increased to 80 mg PO daily if serum uric acid levels less than 6 mg/dl are not achieved after 2 weeks
G. Initiate drugs that increase renal excretion of uric acid (uricosuric drugs) if xanthine oxidase inhibitors are contraindicated or if patient fails to achieve clinical relief.
   1. Probenecid, 250 mg PO twice a day for 7 days, then increase to 500 mg PO twice a day for 14 days. Continue to increase weekly by 500 mg per day increments until satisfactory control is achieved (Max dose: 2000 mg per day)
H. Biological modifiers of disease (BMD)
   1. Gout: Refractory to Conventional Therapy:
      a. Pegloticase (Krystexxa), 8 mg IV over no less than 2 hr every 2 weeks; premedicate with antihistamines and corticosteroids
   2. Not recommended for treatment of asymptomatic hyperuricemia
   3. Gout flare prophylaxis with an NSAID or colchicine one week before pegloticase initiation is recommended
   4. Monitor serum uric acid levels prior to infusions and consider discontinuing treatment if levels increase to above 6 mg/dl, particularly when 2 consecutive levels above 6 mg/dl are observed
   5. BBW: should be administered in healthcare settings and by healthcare providers prepared to manage anaphylaxis and infusion reactions
   6. Contraindicated in patients with G6PD deficiency

BIBLIOGRAPHY

Centers for Disease Control. *Osteoarthritis*. (2011). Retrieved from http://www.cdc.gov/arthritis/basics/osteoarthritis.htm

Dougados, M. & Hochberg, M. C. (2011). Management of osteoarthritis. In M. C. Hochberg, A. J. Silman, J. S. Smolen, M. E. Weinblatt, & M. H. Weisman (Eds.), *Rheumatology* (5th ed., pp. 1793–1799). Philadelphia, PA: Mosby/Elsevier.

Hochberg, M. C., Altman, R., April, K. T., Benkhalti, M., Guatt, G., McGowan, J., . . . Tugwell, P. (2012). American College of Rheumatology 2012 recommendations for the use of nonpharmacologic and pharmacologic therapies in osteoarthritis of the hand, hip, and knee. *Arthritis Care & Research, 64*(4), 465–474.

Khanna, D., Fitzgerald, J. D., Khanna, P. P., Bae, S., Singh, M. K., Neogi, T., . . . Terkeltaub, R. (2012). 2012 American College of Rheumatology guidelines for management of gout. Part 1: Systematic nonpharmacologic and pharmacologic therapeutic approaches to hyperuricemia. *Arthritis Care & Research, 64*(10), 1431–1446.

Khanna, D., Khanna, P. P., Fitzgerald, J. D., Singh, M. K., Sangmee, B., Neogi, T. (2012). 2012 American College of Rheumatology guidelines for management of gout. Part 2: Therapy and antiinflammatory prophylaxis of acute gouty arthritis. *Arthritis Care & Research, 64*(10), 1447–1461.

Lozada, C. J. (2013). *Osteoarthritis treatment and management.* Retrieved from http://emedicine.medscape.com/article/330487-treatment

Rothschild, B. M. (2013). *Gout and pseudogout treatment and management.* Retrieved from http://emedicine.medscape.com/article/329958-treatment

Singh, J. A, Furst, D. E., Bharat, A., Curtis, J. R., Kavanaugh, A. F, Kremer, J. M., . . . Saag, K. G. (2012). 2012 update of the 2008 American College of Rheumatology recommendations for the use of disease-modifying antirheumatic drugs and biologic agents in the treatment of rheumatoid arthritis. *Arthritis Care & Research, 4*(5), 625–639.

Stetka, B. S., & Kay, J. (2012). *New gout management guidelines: A quick and easy guide.* Retrieved from http://www.medscape.com/features/slideshow/gout

U. S. Food and Drug Administration. (2011). What is a serious adverse event? Retrieved from http://www.fda.gov/safety/medwatch/howtoreport/ucm053087. htm

CHAPTER 56

Subluxations and Dislocations

COLLEEN R. WALSH

SUBLUXATIONS

I. **Definition**
   A. Partial loss of articulation of bone ends within the joint capsule caused by partial displacement or separation of the bone end from its position in the joint
   B. Also defined as a partial dislocation, caused by disruption of the joint ligaments

II. **Etiology/incidence/predisposing factors**
   A. Trauma, usually blunt force
   B. Congenital
      1. Ehlers-Danlos syndrome
   C. Pathologic
   D. Neuromuscular diseases, such as muscular dystrophy, CVAs
   E. Inflammatory joint diseases, such as rheumatoid arthritis
   F. Ligamentous laxity: condition in which ligamentous structures are loose, stretched, or injured; can lead to injury or dislocation such as Ehlers-Danlos syndrome
   G. Often associated with fractures
   H. Common sites
      1. Acromioclavicular joint
      2. Shoulder
      3. Elbow
      4. Wrist
      5. Hip
      6. Knee
      7. Patella
      8. Ankle

9. Spine

III. **Subjective findings**
- **A.** Patient gives detailed description of mechanism of injury
- **B.** Pain over affected area
- **C.** Patient may give history of repeated subluxations with decreasing trauma associated with each subluxation

IV. **Physical examination findings**
- **A.** Swelling/ecchymosis around peripheral joints
- **B.** May have obvious joint deformity
- **C.** Loss of range of motion (ROM) at the affected joint
- **D.** Loss of movement or sensation distal to the affected joint

V. **Laboratory/diagnostic findings**
- **A.** Plain radiographs, CT, or MRI reveal area and extent of subluxation
- **B.** Complete blood count may show elevated WBC count (greater than 10,000 mm/L) as result of stress response to trauma

VI. **Management**
- **A.** Early reduction of subluxation; many reduce spontaneously
- **B.** Immobilization: cast, splint, sling, brace
- **C.** Physical therapy for muscle-strengthening exercises
- **D.** NSAIDs for pain and swelling
- **E.** Narcotics rarely needed, except in cases of multiple trauma

DISLOCATIONS

I. **Definition**
- **A.** Complete loss of articulation of bone ends within the joint capsule
- **B.** Caused by complete displacement or separation of the bone end from its position in the joint

II. **Etiology/incidence/predisposing factors**
- **A.** High-energy blunt force trauma
- **B.** Congenital
- **C.** Pathologic
- **D.** Neuromuscular diseases, such as muscular dystrophy
- **E.** Inflammatory joint diseases, such as rheumatoid arthritis
- **F.** Ligamentous laxity: condition in which ligamentous structures are loose, stretched, or injured; can lead to injury or dislocation
- **G.** Seen in all age groups but more frequent in those younger than age 35 due to sports and/or trauma
- **H.** Very commonly associated with fractures
- **I.** Common sites
    - **1.** Shoulder
        - **a.** Anterior: associated with humeral head fracture and labrum/rotator-cuff injury
        - **b.** Posterior: spontaneously due to ligament laxity
        - **c.** Superior: fall on outstretched arm (FOOSH)

      d. Inferior: neuromuscular disorder (e.g., CVA, brachial plexus injury)

  2. Elbow

      a. Radial-ulnar joint, "nursemaid's elbow" caused by pulling and distraction forces

      b. Radial-ulnar-humeral joint; FOOSH mechanism

      c. Radial head dislocation

  3. Wrist

      a. Dorsal dislocation: fall on pronated hand causing injury to the radial-ulnar joint and may have entrapped extensor tendons

      b. Volar dislocation: fall on supinated hand causing injury to the radial-ulnar joint

  4. Hip

      a. High energy impact often associated with acetabular fractures

      b. Anterior dislocation will have internal rotation of the hip

      c. Posterior dislocation will have external rotation of the hip

  5. Knee

      a. Anterior dislocation: loss of integrity of anterior cruciate ligament (ACL) usually caused by hyperextension

      b. Posterior dislocation: loss of integrity of posterior cruciate ligament (PCL) usually caused by "dash board" type impact

      c. Loss of integrity of both ACL and PCL medical emergency-unstable knee

  6. Ankle/foot

      a. Subtalar dislocation: medial dislocation is most commonly caused by inversion; foot and calcaneus are displaced medially

III. **Subjective findings**

  A. Pain over affected area, usually severe

  B. History of mechanism of injury

  C. Patient may complain of numbness and/or tingling distal to injury

IV. **Physical examination findings**

  A. Obvious joint deformity

  B. Shortening and abnormal posture of affected limb

  C. Swelling

  D. May see contusion or laceration over affected joint due to blunt force trauma

  E. Decreased or absent peripheral pulses distal to joint

  F. Decreased or absent ROM of joint or distal to joint

  G. Decreased or absent sensation distal to joint due to peripheral nerve damage/compression

  H. Paresthesia distal to the injury

V. **Laboratory/diagnostic findings**

  A. CBC

    1. WBC may be elevated because of stress response to trauma (greater than 10,000 mm/L)

2. Hgb/Hct may be low in response to hematoma formation or other bleeding

B. X-rays reveal dislocation
  1. Anteroposterior and lateral films should be ordered for all dislocations
  2. May consider oblique films for dislocations associated with fractures
  3. Inlet/outlet views for all pelvic trauma

C. CT scan is indicated for pelvic trauma to rule out hip or sacral fracture/dislocation

D. Always order ultrasound and/or arteriogram for posterior knee dislocation because of high incidence of popliteal artery injury

E. Consider compartment pressure measurements in knee dislocations with vascular compromise that are longer than 6 hr since injury

VI. **Management**

A. Early anatomic reduction is essential.
  1. Closed, manual reduction is primarily used in dislocations without fractures
  2. Surgical reduction may be necessary if fractures are associated with dislocation

B. Postreduction immobilization is essential
  1. Splints
  2. Casts
  3. Immobilizers
  4. External fixation devices for knee dislocations associated with vascular injury and repair
  5. Slings
  6. Elevation of extremity with application of cold compresses to reduce swelling

C. Surgical repair of ligamentous structures

D. Physical therapy for muscle-strengthening exercises

E. Occupational therapy for assistive devices if neurovascular injury occurs

F. NSAIDs: See Tables 54.1 and 54.2 for comprehensive list

G. May need skeletal muscle relaxant for severe muscle spasms
  1. Diazepam (Valium), 2–10 mg PO every 6–8 hr PRN
  2. Cyclobenzaprine (Flexeril), 10 mg PO three times a day PRN
  3. Metaxalone (Skelaxin), 800 mg PO three or four times a day PRN
  4. Methocarbamol (Robaxin), 500–750 mg PO every 6–8 hr, tizanidine (Zanaflex), 2 mg PO every 6 hr PRN
  5. Baclofen (Lioresal), 5 mg PO three times a day PRN
  6. Chlorzoxazone (Parafon Forte), 500 mg PO three times a day PRN
  7. Orphenadrine (Norflex), 100 mg PO twice a day PRN

H. Narcotics for short-term use; all narcotic agents have potential for dependency and can cause serious depression and/or sedation of the CNS except tramadol

1. Hydrocodone/acetaminophen combination (Norco), 5–325 mg tablets (1–2 tablets) PO every 4–6 hr PRN if severe pain or opioid tolerance

2. Oxycodone/acetaminophen combination (Percocet), 5–325 mg tablets (1–2 tablets) PO every 4–6 hr PRN if severe pain or opioid tolerance

3. Tramadol (Ultram), 100 mg PO every 6 hr PRN

4. Avoid carisoprodol (Soma) due to its addictive properties and central nervous system effects

I. Skeletal traction therapy in select cases

BIBLIOGRAPHY

Bollier, M., & Fulkerson, J. P. (2011). The role of trochlear dysplasia in patellofemoral instability. *Journal of the American Academy of Orthopaedic Surgery, 19*(1), 8–16.

Bussièrres, A. E., Peterson, C., & Taylor, J. A. (2011). Diagnostic imaging guideline for musculoskeletal complaints in adults—An evidence-based approach—Part 2: Upper extremity disorders. *Journal of Manipulative and Physiological Therapeutics, 31*(1), 2–32.

Crowther-Radulewicz, C. L., & McCance, K. L. (2010). Alterations of musculoskeletal function. In K. L. McCance, S. E. Heuther, V. L. Brasher, & N. S. Rote (Eds.), *Pathophysiology: The biological basis for disease in adults and children* (6th ed., pp. 1568–1643). Maryland Heights, MO: Mosby-Elsevier.

Diazepam. (2013).In Epocrates Essentials for Apple iOS (Version 4.4.1) [Mobile application software]. Retrieved August 19, 2014 from http://www.epocrates.com/products/

Kastell, B. (2013). The hip, femur, and pelvis. In L. Schoenly (Ed.), *Core curriculum for orthopaedic nursing* (7th ed., pp.549–570). Chicago, IL: National Association of Orthopaedic Nurses.

Levy, H. P. (2012). *Ehlers-Danlos Syndrome, hypermobility type.* Genetic Reviews Seattle (WA): University of Washington, Seattle; 1993–2013. Retrieved from http://www.ncbi.nlm.nih.gov/books/NBK1279/

McDevitt, K. A. (2013). Orthopaedic trauma. In L.Schoenly (Ed.), *Core curriculum for orthopaedic nursing* (7th ed., pp. 393–422). Chicago, IL: National Association of Orthopaedic Nurses.

Panni, A. S., Vasso, M., & Cerciello, S. (2013). Acute patellar dislocation. What to do? *Knee Surgery, Sports Traumatology, Arthroscopy: Official Journal of the ESSKA, 21*(2), 275–278.

Perez, R. A. (2013). The elbow. In L.Schoenly (Ed.), *Core curriculum for orthopaedic nursing* (7th ed., pp. 509–526). Chicago, IL: National Association of Orthopaedic Nurses.

Robaxin. (2013). In Epocrates Essentials for Apple iOS (Version 4.4.1) [Mobile application software]. Retrieved August 19, 2014 from http://www.epocrates.com/products/

Skelaxin. (2013). In Epocrates Essentials for Apple iOS (Version 4.4.1) [Mobile application software]. Retrieved August 19, 2014 from http://www.epocrates.com/products/Kahn-

Tschebulu, C., & Arya, R. (2014). Cervical spine injury. In F. J. Domino (Ed.), *The 5 minute clinical consult* (22nd ed., pp. 222–223). Philadelphia, PA: Lippincott Williams & Wilkins.

Walsh, C. R. (2009). Musculoskeletal injuries. In K. A. McQuillan, M. Flynn, M. B. Makic, & E. Whalen (Eds.), *Trauma nursing: From resuscitation through rehabilitation* (4th ed., pp. 735–777). Philadelphia, PA: Elsevier.

Walsh, C. R. (2009). Sign off on casting. *OR Nurse, 3*(5), 45–51.

Walsh, C. R. (2011). Musculoskeletal problems: Nursing management. In S. L. Lewis, M. M. Heitkemper, S. R. Dirksen, P. G. O'Brien, & L. Bucher (Eds.), *Medical-surgical nursing: Assessment and management of clinical problems* (8th ed., pp. 1620–1640). St. Louis, MO: Mosby.

Wheeless, C. R. (2013). *Wheeless Textbook of Orthopaedics*. Retrieved from http://www.wheelessonline.com

CHAPTER 57

Soft Tissue Injury

COLLEEN R. WALSH

I. Definition

A. Any injury that occurs in non-osseous structures of the musculoskeletal system

B. These soft tissues consist of:

1. Muscles
2. Ligaments
3. Tendons
4. Bursa
5. Cartilage
6. Skin, especially as it pertains to coverage over bones and joints

II. Classifications

A. Closed injuries

1. Contusions
2. Hematomas
3. Ecchymoses
4. Crush
5. Strains—muscles
6. Sprains—ligaments
   a. First degree—mild
   b. Second degree—moderate
   c. Third degree—severe, these often are complex, unstable injuries that must be referred to the physician for definitive care/surgery
7. Ruptures
   a. Both muscles and ligaments

   b. Need immediate referral to the physician for definitive care/surgery

   c. Characterized by:

    i. Instability

    ii. Inability to move injured extremity

    iii. Swelling

  8. Shearing injuries: Morel lesions are internal degloving injuries that most frequently occur in the subcutaneous tissues adjacent to the greater trochanter (Carroll)

B. Open

 1. Lacerations/tears

 2. Abrasions

 3. Avulsions

 4. Penetrating/puncture

 5. Amputations

III. **Etiology/incidence/predisposing factors**

A. Trauma

 1. Blunt

 2. Penetrating

 3. Rotational

 4. Shear forces

B. Exercise

C. Overuse syndromes

D. Sports

E. Autoimmune diseases such as systemic lupus erythematosus (SLE), scleroderma, and rheumatoid arthritis (RA)

F. Soft tissue injury commonly seen in all age groups; more frequent in those younger than age 35, commonly due to sports and/or trauma in this age group

G. Obesity

H. Age: elderly with increased risk for skin tears related to thinning of skin and co-morbid medical conditions/medications

IV. **Subjective findings**

A. Pain

B. Swelling

C. History of precipitating event

D. Feeling of instability of joint

V. **Physical examination findings**

A. Muscle tears/ruptures

 1. Decreased or absent range of motion (ROM) of joint/joints affected by the muscle

 2. Swelling with hematoma formation almost immediately after injury

 3. Ecchymosis of skin over muscle

    4. Palpable discontinuity of muscle belly with obvious defect on careful palpation

    5. Abnormal contour of muscle

    6. Complete instability of joint

    7. Inability to perform adequate examination because of pain and guarding by patient

    8. Neurovascular integrity should be monitored closely, owing to potential vascular disruption

B. Ligaments

    1. Sprains (stretching or tearing of ligaments)

       a. Pain on palpation and ROM

       b. Moderate swelling with decreased ROM

       c. Possible hematoma formation

       d. Lachman's test: possible knee laxity of the anterior/posterior cruciate ligaments during special maneuvers; sensation of the joint acting hypermobile during stressing maneuvers

         i. The examiner grasps the tibia with one hand while stabilizing the femur with the other hand

         ii. The patient relaxes the leg while the examiner holds the knee flexed at 30 degrees and pulls forward/pushes backward on the tibia

         iii. Excessive motion determines a positive sign

C. Strains (stretching or tearing of muscles or tendons)

    1. Swelling

    2. Possible hematoma formation

    3. Decreased or absent ROM of affected joint

    4. Limited examination due to pain and patient guarding

D. Cartilage

    1. Moderate swelling of joint, usually several hours after injury occurs

    2. Palpable and/or audible "click" during special maneuvers such as McMurray's test

       a. McMurray's test: indicates an injured/torn meniscus through production of a pronounced audible or palpable "click" during manipulation of the tibia with the knee flexed and then abruptly straightened

    3. Pain on palpation over joint lines

    4. Limited examination due to pain and patient guarding

E. Bursa

    1. Swelling of bursa with "boggy" feeling on palpation

    2. Erythema over bursa

    3. May see abrasion over bursa

    4. Possible decreased ROM caused by swelling

F. Skin

    1. Obvious laceration

    2. Puncture or penetrating object

    3. Avulsion of skin or body part

VI. **Laboratory/diagnostic findings**

  A. CBC

    1. Possible WBC elevation (greater than 10,000/mm), especially with bursitis

    2. Hgb and Hct may be decreased if large blood loss is associated with massive soft tissue injuries

  B. Joint aspiration of synovial fluid

    1. WBC—infection or inflammation

    2. RBC—bleeding into the joint

    3. Crystals—gout

  C. Plain x-rays may reveal soft tissue swelling

  D. Magnetic resonance imaging of joint, especially knee and shoulder, reveals location and degree of injury

VII. **Management**

  A. PRICE (protection, rest, ice, compression, elevation) of injured part

  B. Immobilization may be necessary, depending on location, severity, and type of injury

    1. Casts

    2. Splints

    3. Immobilizers

    4. Slings

    5. External fixation if fracture is associated with soft tissue loss for easier wound management

  C. Surgery may be necessary if:

    1. Rupture of tendons, muscles, or ligaments

    2. Grade III ligament sprains with joint instability

    3. Septic bursa: incision and drainage performed

    4. Wound closure with open, soft tissue injuries, depending on severity of tissue loss; goes upward in a ladder-like sequence:

      a. Primary closure

      b. Skin graft

      c. Local flap

      d. Regional flap

      e. Distant flap

      f. Free flap

  D. Physical therapy for muscle strengthening and ROM

  E. Pharmacologic interventions

    1. NSAIDs: See Arthritis chapter and Table 55.2

    2. May need skeletal muscle relaxant for severe muscle spasms

      a. Diazepam (Valium), 2–10 mg PO every 6–8 hr PRN

      b. Cyclobenzaprine (Flexeril), 10 mg PO 3 times a day PRN

      c. Metaxalone (Skelaxin), 800 mg PO 3 or 4 times a day PRN

      d. Methocarbamol (Robaxin), 500–750 mg PO every 6–8 hr

3. Opioids for short-term use
   a. Oxycodone/acetaminophen (Tylox, Percocet, Roxicet), 5–7.5 mg/325–500 mg (1–2 tablets) PO every 4–6 hr PRN
   b. Codeine/acetaminophen (Tylenol #3 or #4) 30–60 mg/300 mg (1–2 tablets) PO every 4–6 hr PRN
   c. Hydrocodone/acetaminophen (Lortab, Norco, Vicodin), 5–10 mg/300–500 mg (1–2 tablets) PO every 4–6 hr PRN
   d. Patient-controlled analgesia (PCA) pump for in-house patients, and consult Pain Management Services, if available
4. Broad-spectrum antibiotics for septic bursitis that will cover most common Gram-positive organisms
   a. Cephalexin (Keflex), 250–500 mg PO 4 times a day for 7–10 days
   b. Cefazolin (Ancef), 1 gram IV every 8 hr for 48–72 hr after incision and drainage; then continue with cephalexin (Keflex) for a total of 10 days of treatment
5. Aminoglycosides for suspected anaerobic, Gram-negative bacilli; immunocompromised patients and those with grossly contaminated wounds at greatest risk
   a. Gentamicin (Garamycin), 3–5 mg/kg/day IV
   b. Newest recommendations are that total dose should be given once a day to prevent renal impairment, although dosing every 8 hr is still common
   c. Duration of therapy is variable, depending on patient response
6. Antibiotic beads containing tobramycin, amikacin, or other antibiotics are placed into contaminated wounds to deliver antibiotics directly to infected tissue or bone
7. Hyperbaric oxygen therapy may be beneficial in wounds that require skin grafts or in wounds infected with anaerobic bacteria
8. Closed negative pressure wound dressings

BIBLIOGRAPHY

Carroll, J. F. (2010), *Morel-Lavallee Lesions*. MRI Web Clinic-June 2010. Retrieved from http://www.radsource.us/clinic/1006

Courtney, P., & Doherty, M. (2013). Joint aspiration and injection and synovial fluid analysis. Best practice and research. *Clinical Rheumatology, 27*(2), 137–169. doi:10.1016/j.berh.2013.02.005

Crowther-Radulewicz, C. L., & McCance, K. L. (2010). Alterations of musculoskeletal function. In K. L. McCance & S. E. Heuther (Eds.), *Pathophysiology: The biological basis for disease in adults and children*, (6th ed., pp. 1568–1643). Maryland Heights, MO: Mosby-Elsevier.

Davis, J., & Saulog-Wendel, P. (2013). The knee. In L.Schoenly (Ed.), *Core curriculum for orthopaedic nursing* (7th ed., pp. 571–586). Chicago, IL: National Association of Orthopaedic Nurses.

Dryden, M. S.(2010). Complicated soft tissue and skin infection. *Journal of Antimicrobial and Chemotherapy, 65*(suppl 3), iii35-iii44. doi:10.1093/jac/dkq302

Eagles, K., & Stevenson, H. J. (2014). Bursitis. In F. J. Domino (Ed.). *The 5 minute clinical consult* (22nd ed., pp. 190–191). Philadelphia, PA: Lippincott.

Williams Hill, K., & Ostrow, M. K. (2013). The foot and ankle. In L.Schoenly (Ed.), *Core curriculum for orthopaedic nursing* (7th ed., pp. 587–612). Chicago, IL: National.

Kunkler, C. E. (2013). Therapeutic modalities. In L.Schoenly (Ed.), *Core curriculum for orthopaedic nursing* (7th ed., pp. 233–262). Chicago, IL: National.

Lese, A. B. (2013). Soft tissue hand injury treatment and management. *Medscape Reference*. Retrieved from http://emedicine.medscape.com/article/826498-treatment.

Levy, D. B. (2013). Soft tissue knee injury. *Medscape Reference*. Retrieved from http://emedicine.medscape.com/article/826792-overview.

Matt, S. E., Johnson, L. S., Shupp, J. W., Kheirbek, T., & Sava, J. A. (2011). Management of fasciotomy wounds--does the dressing matter? *American Surgeon, 77*(12), 1656–1660.

McDevitt, K. A. (2013). Orthopaedic trauma. In L.Schoenly (Ed.), *Core curriculum for orthopaedic nursing* (7th ed., pp. 393–422). Chicago, IL: National Association of Orthopaedic Nurses.

Ogawa, T., Tanaka, T., Yanai, T., Kumagai, H., & Ochiai, N. (2013). Analysis of soft tissue injuries associated with distal radius fractures. *BMC Sports Science, Medicine and Rehabilitation, 5*(19). doi:10.1186/2052–1847–5-19. Retrieved from http://www.biomedcentral.com/2052–1847/5/19.

Parker, R. (2013). Orthopaedic complications. In L. Schoenly (Ed.), *Core curriculum for orthopaedic nursing* (7th ed., pp. 191–216). Chicago, IL: National Association of Orthopaedic Nurses.

Saziye, K., Mustafa, C., Ilker, U., & Afksendyios, K. (2011). Comparison of vacuum-assisted closure device and conservative treatment for fasciotomy wound healing in ischaemia-reperfusion syndrome: Preliminary results. *International Wound Journal, 8*(3), 229–236. doi:10.1111/j.1742–481X.2011.00773.x

Seah, R., & Mani-Babu, S (2010). Managing ankle sprains in primary care; What is best practice? A systematic review of the last 10 years of evidence. *British Medical Bulletin, 1*(97). doi:10.1093/bmb/ldq028

Soh, C. R., Pietrobon, R., Freiberger, J. J., Chew, S.T ., Rajgor, D., Gandhi, M.,
. . . Moon, R. E. (2012). Hyperbaric oxygen therapy in necrotising soft tissue
infections: A study of patients in the United States Nationwide Inpatient
Sample. *Intensive Care Medicine, 38*(7), 1143–1151. doi:10.1007/s00134–
012–2558–4

Walsh, C. R. (2009). Musculoskeletal injuries. In K. A. McQuillan, M. Flynn, M.
B. Makic, & E. Whalen (Eds.), *Trauma nursing: From resuscitation through
rehabilitation.* (4th ed., pp. 735–777). Philadelphia, PA: Elsevier.

Walsh, C. R. (2011). Musculoskeletal problems: Nursing management. In S. L.
Lewis, M. M. Heitkemper, S. R. Dirksen, P. G. O'Brien, & L. Bucher (Eds.).
Medical-surgical nursing: Assessment and management of clinical problems
(8th ed., pp. 1620–1640). St. Louis: Mosby.

CHAPTER 58

Fractures

I. **Definition:**
  A. Break or disruption in the continuity of a bone

II. **Classification-Gustillo**
  A. Closed: no break in skin over fracture
  B. Open: varying amounts of skin or soft tissue injury over fracture
    1. Type I: wound smaller than 1 cm, minimal contamination
    2. Type II: wound larger than 1 cm, moderate contamination; moderate, not extensive soft tissue damage with bony comminution
    3. Type III: high degree of contamination, severe fracture with instability, extensive soft tissue damage
      a. Type IIIA: soft tissue coverage is adequate; fracture is severely comminuted
      b. Type IIIB: extensive injury to or loss of soft tissue; moderate amount of periosteal stripping with exposed bone
      c. Type IIIC: any open fracture associated with arterial injury; not dependent on amount of skin or tissue loss
  C. Incomplete or complete
  D. Simple or comminuted
  E. Traumatic or pathologic
  F. Intra-articular or extra-articular
  G. Displaced or non-displaced
  H. Avulsion
  I. Buckle
  J. Stress
  K. Type of fracture line
    1. Transverse
    2. Spiral

3. Oblique
4. Comminuted
5. Longitudinal
6. Butterfly
7. Segmental
8. Impacted
9. Stellate
10. Salter Harris Classification- Growth plate-pediatric and adolescent fractures must be closely examined for evidence of growth plate fractures that, unless anatomically reduced, can result in abnormalities in longitudinal bone growth. Five major classifications:
    a. I - S: Straight across
    b. II - A: Above the physis (away from the joint)
    c. III - L: Lower (below) the physis
    d. IV - T: Through - fracture through metaphysis / physis / epiphysis
    e. V - R: Rammed (compression fracture)

III. **Etiology/incidence/predisposing factors**
   A. High-energy trauma, such as crush, blunt, or deceleration forces
   B. Rotational forces
   C. Osteoporosis/osteopenia
   D. Tumors of bone—either primary or metastatic
   E. Metabolic disorders, such as Paget's disease, rickets, and renal osteodystrophy
   F. Drugs, such as corticosteroids (prednisone) and phenytoin (Dilantin)
   G. Nutritional deficiencies, such as vitamin D, malabsorption syndromes, and inflammatory bowel diseases; alcoholism
   H. Infectious disorders, such as tuberculosis and osteomyelitis
   I. Congenital disorders
   J. Neuromuscular disorders, such as spinal cord injury and muscular dystrophy

IV. **Subjective findings**
   A. Pain is usually moderate to severe
   B. Patient gives history of traumatic event
   C. In patients with neuromuscular disorders in whom sensation is decreased or absent (especially spinal cord-injured patients with lesions above T7), may complain of headache. This could indicate autonomic dysreflexia in response to the noxious stimulus of pain.

V. **Physical examination findings may, but not always, include the following:**
   A. Pain on palpation over fracture site
   B. May have deformity of limb; not always immediately visible
   C. Palpable and audible crepitus
   D. May see diminished or absent distal pulses

E. Swelling

F. Ecchymosis or frank bleeding

G. Decreased or absent range of motion distal to fracture

H. Neurologic injury distal to fracture

I. Specific fracture findings: always determine the mechanism of injury
   1. Cervical spine: always treat as if fracture exists until proven otherwise
   2. Shoulder: inability to abduct or adduct arm
   3. Humerus (proximal): ecchymosis, deformity, inability to abduct arm
   4. Humerus (midshaft): neurovascular compromise, radial nerve palsy, abnormal positioning
   5. Humerus (distal): neurovascular compromise, inability to flex or extend the elbow
   6. Forearm (proximal): swelling, inability to flex or extend the elbow
   7. Forearm (midshaft): may have some swelling or tenderness on pronation/supination
   8. Forearm (distal): deformity around wrist, inability to flex or extend wrist
   9. Wrist: "dinner fork" deformity; inability to flex or extend wrist
   10. Hand/finger: pain; may have obvious deformity
   11. Hip, proximal femur: shortening with external rotation of leg
   12. Femur (midshaft, distal): possible shortening with internal or external rotation of leg
   13. Tibia (proximal): plateau fractures with swelling, or may be occult
   14. Tibia (midshaft): swelling; may see exposed bone or lacerations
   15. Tibia (distal): external/internal rotation of foot
   16. Ankle: malposition of foot, ecchymosis, swelling
   17. Foot/toe: ecchymosis, swelling
   18. Thoracic/lumbar spine: always treat as if a fracture exists until it is ruled out
   19. Pelvis: leg shortening, perineal ecchymosis, swelling or bleeding
       a. Maintain pelvic compression to decrease chance of fatal retroperitoneal bleeding

VI. **Laboratory/diagnostic findings**

A. Radiologic evidence of fracture
   1. Always order anteroposterior (AP) and lateral x-ray films
   2. Oblique films for complex fractures of humerus, femur, or ankle
   3. Mortise view of ankle fractures to check talus
   4. Three-dimensional and/or coronal and sagittal CT scan if pelvic or spinal fractures are found on plain films
   5. Inlet and outlet views of pelvis if fracture suspected
   6. MRI if spinal cord injury is suspected and the patient is clinically stable
   7. Swimmer's open mouth views of odontoid if CT scan not done

      8. May need dual-energy x-ray absorptiometry (DEXA) scan to determine amount of osteopenia/osteoporosis and to detect or treat impending fractures

  B. Leukocytosis without left shift-stress response to trauma

  C. Serial hemoglobin & hematocrits to monitor blood loss from fracture site(s)

  D. Urinalysis in crush injuries to check for myoglobinuria and blood in acute blunt or penetrating trauma

  E. Electrolytes (especially elevated K+ caused by necrosis of muscle tissue with rapid release of intracellular K+), lactate, and CPK

  F. Coagulation studies to evaluate blood clotting

  G. Type and screen or crossmatch for blood if long bone or pelvic fracture is present

  H. Continuous EKG monitoring required with crush injuries

  I. Arteriogram if diminished or absent distal pulses or evidence of active bleeding on CT

VII. **Management**

  A. Acute interventions

    1. Follow tenets of trauma care: ABC (airway, breathing, circulation) are first priority (current ATLS guidelines)

    2. Musculoskeletal examination is part of secondary survey

    3. Fluid resuscitation with normal saline or Ringer's lactate (no LR in crush injuries)

    4. Cover open wounds with saline dressings until the patient is taken to the operating room for debridement

    5. Early anatomic reduction of fracture is mandatory, with adequate immobilization of fracture after reduction

    6. Formal surgical irrigation and debridement of open fracture is mandatory for adequate healing and prevention of infection

    7. Pharmacologic therapy

      a. Any open fracture requires antibiotics

        i. Discontinue 24 hr after injury or surgery

      b. Cefazolin (Kefzol), 1 gram IV every 8 hr for Gram-positive coverage. If penicillin and cephalosporin allergies exist or there is concern/suspicion for MRSA, give vancomycin (Vancocin).

        i. Consult with pharmacy for dose/frequency to achieve vancomycin level of 10–15 mg/kg (or 15–20 mg/kg if there is concern for osteoporosis)

      c. Depending on the environment in which the injury occurred, may need to add gentamicin (Garamycin). Consult with pharmacist for appropriate pharmacokinetic dosing to achieve therapeutic levels and avoid toxicity

    d. Clindamycin (Cleocin), 600 mg IV every 8 hr if *Clostridium perfringens* and/or *C. tetani* is suspected or other anaerobic organism

    e. Opioids for pain:

        i. May use patient-controlled analgesia pump with morphine, hydromorphone (Dilaudid)

        ii. Oxycodone/acetaminophen (Tylox, Percocet, Roxicet), 5–7.5 mg/325–500 mg (1–2 tablets) PO every 4–6 hr PRN

        iii. Acetaminophen/codeine (Tylenol #¾) 30–60 mg/300 mg (1–2 tablets) PO every 4–6 hr PRN

        iv. Tramadol (Ultram), 100 mg PO every 6 hr PRN

        v. Hydrocodone/acetaminophen (Lortab, Norco, Vicodin), 5–10 mg/300–500 mg (1–2 tablets) PO every 4–6 hr PRN

    f. Tetanus toxoid if status unknown. Usually done in ER

    g. Patients with known osteoporosis and/or major risk factors may require appropriate therapy (i.e., alendronate, calcium) upon discharge, if not already taking prior to admission. Inquire as to history of gastroesophageal disease.

        i. Consult Fracture Liaison Service for medication recommendations as bisphosphonates, if available, can initially impair fracture healing by inferring with osteoclasts

  8. Percutaneous injection of bone morphogenic protein-2 into fracture site demonstrates accelerated fracture repair

  9. Percutaneous injection of bone cement in patients undergoing vertebroplasty

  10. May need renal hemodialysis, continuous renal replacement therapy (CRRT), or peritoneal dialysis in cases of severe crush syndrome for acute renal failure and nephrology should be consulted regarding these therapies

B. Reduction of fractures

  1. Referral to orthopedist for all fractures, except for minor, nondisplaced fractures

  2. Toe fractures can be "buddy-taped" to toes on either side of fracture to immobilize; this is primarily a comfort measure

  3. Radius/ulna fractures: can be placed in splint with Ace bandage wrap if simple hairline or greenstick fracture, but open reduction may be needed with internal fixation or external fixation

  4. Always order postreduction/splinting AP and lateral radiographs to check for displacement during splinting

  5. Always check neurovascular function and document before and after reduction of fractures

  6. Intramedullary rodding for closed femoral and tibial shaft fractures

  7. External fixation devices for open fractures requiring extensive soft tissue care

BIBLIOGRAPHY

Abel, L. E. (2013). Metabolic bone conditions. In L. Schoenly (Ed.), *Core curriculum for orthopaedic nursing* (7th ed., pp. 335–376). Chicago, IL: National Association of Orthopaedic Nurses.

Buckley, R. (2012). General principles of fracture care treatment and management. *Medscape Reference.* Retrieved from http://emedicine.medscape.com/article/1270717-treatment

Court-Brown, C. M., Aitken, S., Hamilton, T. W., Rennie, L., & Caesar, B. (2010). Nonoperative fracture treatment in the modern era. *Journal of Trauma, 69*(3), 699–707. doi:10.1097/TA.0b013e3181b57ace

Crowther-Radulewicz, C. L., & McCance, K. L. (2010). Alterations of musculoskeletal function. In K. L. McCance & S. E. Heuther (Eds.), *Pathophysiology: The biological basis for disease in adults and children*, (6th ed., pp. 1568–1643). Maryland Heights, MO: Mosby-Elsevier.

Devitt, J. & Khodaee, M. (2014). Stress fracture. In F. J. Domino (Ed.). *The 5 minute clinical consult* (22nd ed., pp. 1166–1167). Philadelphia, PA: Lippincott Williams.

Hoff, W. S., Bonadies, J. A., Cachecho, R., & Dorlac, W. C. (2011). EAST Practice Management Guidelines Work Group: Update to practice management guidelines for prophylactic antibiotic use in open fractures. *Journal of Trauma, 70*(3), 751–754.

Kahn-Kastell, B. (2013). The hip, femur, and pelvis. In L.Schoenly (Ed.), *Core curriculum for orthopaedic nursing* (7th ed., pp.549–570). Chicago, IL: National Association of Orthopaedic Nurses.

Kunkler, C. E. (2013). Therapeutic modalities. In L.Schoenly (Ed.), *Core curriculum for orthopaedic nursing* (7th ed., pp. 233–262). Chicago, IL: National Association of Orthopaedic Nurses.

Mauffrey, C., Bailey, J., Bowles, R., Price, C., Hasson, D., Hak, D., & Stahel, P. (2012). Acute management of open fractures: Proposal of a new multidisciplinary algorithm. *Orthopedics, 35,* 877–881. doi:10.3928/01477447–20120919–08

Musahl, V., Tarkin, I., Kobbe, P., Tzioupis, C., Siska, P. A., Pape, H. C., & Pauwels, W. (2009). New trends and techniques in open reduction and internal fixation of fractures of the tibial plateau. *The Bone & Joint Journal, 91*(4), 426–433.

McDevitt, K. A. (2013). Orthopaedic trauma. In L.Schoenly (Ed.), *Core curriculum for orthopaedic nursing* (7th ed., pp. 393–422). Chicago, IL: National Association of Orthopaedic Nurses.

Mehlman, C. T. (2012). Growth plate (physeal) fractures treatment and management. *Medscape Reference*. Retrieved from http://emedicine.medscape.com/article/1260663-treatment

Pearce, A. N. (2013). The spine. In L. Schoenly (Ed.), *Medscape Reference*. (7th ed., pp. 447–476). Chicago, IL: National Associatioin of Orthopaedic Nurses.

Shaller, T. M. (2012). Open fractures. *Medscape Reference*. Retrieved from http://emedicine.medscape.com/article/1269242-overview

Smalley, M. J. (2013). Pediatric and congenital disorders. In L. Schoenly (Ed.), *Core curriculum for orthopaedic nursing* (7th ed., pp. 263–320). Chicago, IL: National Association of Orthopaedic Nurses.

Walsh, C. R. (2009). Musculoskeletal injuries. In K. A. McQuillan, M. Flynn, M. B. Makic, & E. Whalen (Eds.), *Trauma nursing: From resuscitation through rehabilitation* (4th ed., pp. 735–777). Philadelphia, PA: Elsevier.

Walsh, C. R. (2011). Musculoskeletal problems: Nursing management. In S. L. Lewis, M. Heitkemper, S. R. Dirksen, P. G. O'Brien, & L. Bucher (Eds.), *Medical-surgical nursing: Assessment and management of clinical problems* (8th ed., pp.1620–1640). St. Louis, MO: Mosby.

Walsh, C. R. (2013). Musculoskeletal tumors. In L. Schoenly (Ed.), *Core curriculum for orthopaedic nursing* (7th ed., pp. 423–446). Chicago, IL: National Association of Orthopaedic Nurses.

Wheeless, C. R. (2013). External fixators for tibial fractures. *Wheeless Textbook of Orthopaedics*. Retrieved from http://www.wheelessonline.com/ortho/external_fixators_for_tibial_frx

Wheeless, C. R. (2013). Open fractures. *Wheeless Textbook of Orthopaedics*. Retrieved from http://www.wheelessonline.com/ortho/open_fractures

CHAPTER 59

Compartment Syndrome

COLLEEN R. WALSH

I. **Definition**
   A. Condition in which increased tissue pressure within a limited space compromises the circulation and function of the contents within that space
   B. A compartment consists of bone, blood vessels, nerves, muscles, and soft tissue lying within a fascial envelope. Fascia is a nonexpanding tissue that contributes to the syndrome.
   C. Of the body's 46 compartments, 38 are in the arms and legs
   D. Can also occur in the abdominal muscle compartments in trauma and/or surgical patients
II. **Etiology/incidence/predisposing factors**
   A. Incidence
      1. Compartment syndrome most common in men under the age of 35
      2. Fractures account for 75% of compartment syndromes with the tibia most often involved (compartment syndrome can occur in up to 10% of this type of fracture)
      3. Increased risk with comminuted fractures
   B. Space-limiting envelope
      1. Circumferential dressings
      2. Casts
      3. Splints
      4. Eschar and/or scars
   C. Increased intracompartmental contents owing to
      1. Bleeding/hemorrhage
      2. Coagulation disorders
      3. Iatrogenic

        a. Infiltrated intravenous sites

        b. Improper positioning

        c. Arterial blood gas punctures

    4. Venous pooling/obstruction

    5. Increased capillary filtration

        a. Trauma/surgery

        b. Crush syndrome

        c. Tissue ischemia/reperfusion injuries

        d. Thermal/electrical burns

        e. Snake/spider bites

        f. Intermittent swelling and fluid shifts in extremity compartments during exercise that return to baseline after cessation of the exercise event

        g. Supranormal trauma resuscitation

III.   **Subjective findings**

    A. Pain out of proportion to injury

    B. History of trauma event

    C. Complaints of paresthesias, decreased sensation in affected limb

    D. Feelings of "heaviness" in affected extremity

IV.   **Physical examination findings**

    A. The six Ps

        1. Pain on passive stretch of affected compartment

        2. Paresthesias along dermatomal patterns

        3. Paralysis of affected limb-late finding

        4. Pulses

            a. Early: bounding distal pulses as compensatory mechanism

            b. Late: pulselessness

            c. The traditional five (5) P's of acute ischemia in a limb are not clinically reliable; these may manifest only in late stages of compartment syndrome by which time extensive and irreversible soft tissue damage may have already taken place. Peripheral pulses and capillary refill may remain normal in upper extremity acute compartment syndrome.

        5. Pallor of affected limb late in course—rubor early in course of syndrome due to compensatory vasodilatation

        6. Polar/poikilothermia: limb becomes ice cold or the same temperature as the environment

            a. Swelling may not be evident by palpation or inspection, but affected limb or abdomen may feel tense to palpation

V.   **Laboratory/diagnostic findings**

    A. WBC count may be elevated (more than 14,000 cells/mcl)

    B. Electrolytes may demonstrate elevated K+ levels caused by tissue necrosis in which excess K+ is released

    C. ECG may reveal classic hyperkalemic changes with peaked T waves

    D. Urinalysis may show positive myoglobin

E. Creatine phosphokinase (CPK) and lactate dehydrogenase (LDH) levels elevated
   1. CPK levels: 1,000–5,000 units/ml
   2. LDH levels: greater than 330 units/L
   3. Myoglobinuria can also suggest compartment syndrome

F. Elevated levels of serum inflammatory mediators such as histamine and cytokines

G. Elevated compartment pressure readings (using the calculation of delta pressures)
   1. This is the diastolic blood pressure minus the compartment pressure.
      a. If the difference is less than 30, then acute compartment syndrome is present
      b. Normal compartment pressures 0–8 mmHg

H. Acute compartment syndrome is a clinical diagnosis that is based on a high index of suspicion, mechanism of injury, signs, and symptoms

I. Calculation formula to guide in treatment
   1. Tissue perfusion is proportional to the difference between the capillary perfusion pressure (CPP) and the interstitial fluid pressure, which is stated by the following formula:
   $LBF = (PA - PV)/R$. In the formula above, LBF is local blood flow, PA is local arterial pressure, PV is venous pressure, and R is local vascular resistance.

J. MRI useful in identifying the presence of increased intracompartment contents; may be used as an adjunct diagnostic tool

VI. Management

A. Nonsurgical
   1. There is no effective nonsurgical treatment
   2. Position limb at level of heart; do not elevate limb because blood flow is compromised as an effect of gravity
   3. Remove all bandages and casts (either bivalve, release one side of cast or complete removal of cast)
   4. May consider diuretics (i.e. furosemide), if necessary. Acetazolamide may be useful if urinary alkalinization is needed.
   5. Continuous neurovascular function checks
   6. Renal failure due to myoglobinuria not uncommon; hemodialysis or continuous renal replacement therapy (CRRT) used until acute renal failure resolves
   7. Continuous intracompartmental pressure monitoring has been shown to have a high sensitivity and specificity for acute compartment syndrome in tibial shaft fractures
   8. Administer anti-venom in cases of snake envenomation

    B. Surgical-emergent consultation as delay in fasciotomy increases morbidity
1. Fasciotomy of affected compartment
2. Delayed closure of fasciotomy wounds (5–7 days)
    a. Negative pressure wound vacuum dressings used along with oxygen therapy. Use of hyperbaric has been recently shown to be beneficial
3. Skin grafting procedures
4. Amputation may be necessary owing to sepsis from necrotic tissue
    C. Restorative
1. Functional splinting, especially ankle-foot orthosis (AFO) for lower extremity compartment syndrome to prevent heel cord shortening
2. Active/passive range of motion exercises
3. If amputation required, early prosthetic fitting and ambulation

BIBLIOGRAPHY

Crowther-Radulewicz, C. L., & McCance, K. L. (2010). Alterations of musculoskeletal function. In K. L. McCance & S. E. Heuther (Eds.), *Pathophysiology: The Biological Basis for Disease in Adults and Children* (6th ed., pp. 1568–1643). Maryland Heights, MO: Mosby-Elsevier.

King, T. W., Lerman, O. Z., Carter, J. J., & Warren, S. M. (2010). Exertional compartment syndrome of the thigh: A rare diagnosis and literature review. *Journal of Emergency Medicine, 39*(2), e93–e99.

Marshall, S. T., & Browner, B. D. (2012). Emergency care of musculoskeletal injuries. In: A. M. Townsend, R. D. Beauchamp, B. M. Evers, & K. L. Mattox (Eds.), *Sabiston Textbook of Surgery* (19th ed.). Philadelphia, PA: Saunders Elsevier.

Matt, S. E., Johnson, L. S., Shupp, J. W., Kheirbek, T., & Sava, J. A. (2011). Management of fasciotomy wounds--does the dressing matter? *American Surgeon, 77*(12), 1656–1660.

McDevitt, K. A. (2013). Orthopaedic trauma. In L. Schoenly (Ed.), *Core Curriculum for Orthopaedic Nursing* (7th ed., pp. 393–422). Chicago, IL: National Association of Orthopaedic Nurses.

McQueen, M. M., Duckworth, A. D., Aitken, S. A., & Court-Brown, C. M. (2013). The estimated sensitivity and specificity of compartment pressure monitoring for acute compartment syndrome. *Journal Bone and Joint Surgery American, 95*(8), 673–677.

Meehan, W. P. (2013). Chronic exertional compartment syndrome. In D. S. Basow (Ed.), *UpToDate*. Waltham, MA: UpToDate.

Rasul, A. T. (2013). Acute compartment syndrome. *Medscape Reference.* Retrieved from http://emedicine.medscape.com/article/307668-overview

Rasul, A. T. (2013). Fasciotomy for acute compartment syndrome. *Medscape Reference.* http://emedicine.medscape.com/article/2058838-overview

Stracciolini, A., & Hammerber, E. M. (2013) Acute compartment syndrome of the extremities. In D. S. Basow (Ed.), *UpToDate.* Waltham, MA: UpToDate.

Walsh, C. R. (2009). Musculoskeletal injuries. In K. A. McQuillan, M. Flynn, M. B. Makic, & E. Whalen (Eds.), *Trauma Nursing: From Resuscitation Through Rehabilitation.* (4th ed., pp. 735–777). Philadelphia, PA: Elsevier.

Wheeless, C. R. (2013). Compartment syndrome. *Wheeless Textbook of Orthopaedics.* Retrieved from http://www.wheelessonline.com/ortho/compartment_syndrome

CHAPTER 60

Back Pain Syndromes

COLLEEN R. WALSH

LOW BACK PAIN

I. **Definition**
   A. Low back pain (LBP) is any pain perceived by the patient as originating from the lumbosacral region of the spinal column
   B. Pain usually in the lower back that causes discomfort, limited range of motion, varying degrees of neurologic symptoms, and inability to participate in or perform activities of daily living
   C. May be localized or may radiate to lower extremities
   D. LBP is the leading cause of lost workdays in the United States and costs the U.S. economy $300 billion dollars a year. It is important to distinguish the causes of back pain because each back syndrome presents with varying symptoms, and treatment options differ for each of the four major syndromes
      1. Back strain
      2. Disk herniation—see next section, Herniated Disk
      3. Osteoarthritis/disk degeneration: osteophyte (bone spur) formation of vertebral bodies
      4. Spinal stenosis: narrowing of the spinal foramen leading to encroachment on spinal nerve roots

II. **Etiology/incidence/predisposing factors (see table 60.1)**
   A. Most Americans experience LBP at least once in their lives
   B. Common causes include the following:
      1. Mechanical strain
      2. Obesity
      3. Poor body mechanics
      4. Trauma
      5. Repetitive twisting, bending, or lifting

Table 60.1	Findings Suggesting Particular Disorder
Factor	**Possible disorder**
Age greater than 70	Degenerative disease or cancer
IV drug use	Epidural abscess, discitis, drug seeking
Immunosuppression	Abscess, discitis
Cancer history	Metastasis, primary
Progressive pain or weakness	CA, infection, degenerative, AVM
Worse at rest	CA, tumor, infection
Tearing or stabbing	Retroperitoneal disorder (renal, ureteral, pancreatic, aortic)
Fever	Infection
Weight loss	Infection, CA, PUD,
Night sweats	CA, TB, immunosuppression
Vascular symptoms	Vascular disorders (overlap with rheumatology)
Bowel or bladder dysfunction	CA (in males, usually prostate), AAA, mass
Saddle anesthesia	CA, mass
Medically inexplicable	Psychosomatic, malingering

Note: IV = intravenous; CA = cancer; AVM = arteriovenous malformations; PUD = peptic ulcer disease; TB = tuberculosis; AAA = abdominal aortic aneurysm.

6. Herniated lumbar disks
7. Spondylolysis: defect in neural arch of vertebral body
8. Spondylolisthesis: forward subluxation of vertebral body due to defect in the neural arch of the vertebral body
9. Spinal stenosis: narrowing of the spinal canal or the foramen in which spinal nerves exit the spinal cord
10. Degenerative disk disease
11. Osteoarthritis of the spine
12. Metastatic or primary tumors
13. Rheumatologic diseases such as ankylosing spondylitis

III. **Subjective findings**
    A. Pain in lower back region; may include radicular (radiating) component in affected nerve dermatome
    B. Numbness along specific dermatome
    C. Bowel, bladder, or sexual dysfunction
        1. If present, bowel/bladder dysfunction requires immediate referral for possible emergency surgical intervention.
    D. Cauda equina syndrome: gradual to sudden weakness and/or inability to lift or move legs; bowel and/or bladder incontinence or retention; and loss of or diminished sensation in legs
        1. May be first symptom of spinal cord compression from metastatic lesion to spine

2. Cauda equina syndrome is a surgical emergency and requires emergency referral.

IV. Physical examination findings

A. Back strain: paraspinal muscle spasms, listing to one side, decreased range of motion (ROM), positive bilateral straight leg raise test

1. Straight leg raise: with the patient in supine position, lift one leg at a time, forcefully dorsiflex the foot, and ask the patient if there is pain down the leg (radiculopathy)

2. Crossover straight leg raise: if the patient has a herniated disk, the crossover straight leg raise test will cause radicular pain down the affected leg, even if the other leg is raised

3. Simultaneous bilateral straight leg raise: this test reproduces the back pain but does not cause radicular pain

B. Herniated disk—see next section, Herniated Disk

C. Osteoarthritis: decreased ROM, muscle spasm, possible positive bilateral straight leg raise, but rarely with radicular component

D. Spinal stenosis: often called "neurogenic claudication"; caused by back, buttock, and leg pain during ambulation

1. Pain is relieved with rest and sitting: thought to be relieved by sitting when the spine is flexed and the spinal nerve roots have less compression and more room in which to traverse the spinal foramen

2. Positive straight leg raises with radicular component: often multilevel in lower lumbar spine

E. Weak rectal tone

V. Laboratory/diagnostic findings

A. Serum blood work usually within normal limits, except in cases where underlying rheumatologic diseases exist

B. Plain x-rays (anteroposterior [AP] and lateral) to rule out bony defects; scoliosis, bone spurs

C. MRI best for soft tissue structures; reveals disk bulge

D. CT scan for detailed bony imaging

E. Myelography of spine with or without CT scan to show filling defects along spinal nerve roots—currently not often used

VI. Management

A. Nonsurgical

1. Rest for 1–2 days only

2. Alternate ice/heat therapy

3. NSAIDs for mild to moderately severe injuries

a. Act by inhibiting the enzyme cyclooxygenase (COX), which is required for the synthesis of prostaglandins and thromboxanes

i. Two isoforms have been identified: COX-1 and COX-2

ii. COX-1 is found tissue-wide and is believed to protect gastric mucosa.

iii. COX-2 is induced primarily at the inflammation site.

      b. Older NSAIDs act by blocking both COX isoforms, leading to possible gastric ulceration. COX-2 drugs are selective, thus providing greater gastric protection.

      c. Acetaminophen (Tylenol) is not an NSAID, but exhibits similar analgesic properties

      d. See Chapter 55 (Table 55.2) for information on management with NSAIDs and acetaminophen

  4. May need antispasmodic for severe muscle spasms

      a. Diazepam (Valium), 2 mg every 6 hr PRN

      b. Cyclobenzaprine (Flexeril), 10 mg PO three times a day PRN

      c. Metaxalone (Skelaxin) 800 mg PO three times a day PRN

      d. Tizanidine (Zanaflex), 2 mg PO every 6 hr PRN

      e. Baclofen (Lioresal), 5 mg PO three times a day PRN

      f. Chlorzoxazone (Parafon Forte), 500 mg PO three times a day PRN

      g. Orphenadrine (Norflex), 100 mg PO twice a day PRN

      h. Methocarbamol (Robaxin), 500 mg PO every 6 hr PRN

  5. Opioids may be needed for short-term acute back strain to promote mobility

      a. Hydrocodone/acetaminophen 5 mg/325 mg (Norco), 1 tablet PO every 4 hr PRN for moderate pain, 2 tablets PO every 4 hr PRN for severe pain

      b. Oxycodone/acetaminophen 5 mg/325 mg (Percocet), 1 tablet PO every 4 hr PRN for moderate pain, 2 tablets PO every 4 hr PRN for severe pain

      c. Tramadol (Ultran) 50–100 mg, PO every 4–6 hr PRN

  6. Although not appropriate for acute pain relief, anticonvulsants (i.e., gabapentin, pregabalin) and antidepressants (i.e., duloxetine, venlafaxine) may be beneficial for pain that is neuropathic in origin

  7. Physical therapy for toning, strengthening muscles

  8. Weight loss program

  9. Epidural steroid injections: given with use of anesthesia directly into the affected nerved sheath; patient referred to pain management center for treatment

  10. Acupuncture shown to be effective in treating older adults who are not surgical candidates

  11. Self-management with health provider support effective for lower income individuals who do not have resources for formal physical therapy or back school programs

B. Surgical

  1. Foraminotomy and diskectomy for nerve root decompression in spinal stenosis

  2. Depending on number and level of disks, may require spinal fusion with bone grafts

  3. See next section, Herniated Disk

HERNIATED DISK

I.   Definition

   A. Bulging or protrusion of the nucleus pulposus through a defect in the annulus of cervical, thoracic, or lumbar intervertebral disks

   B. May encroach on peripheral nerves exiting the spinal cord

II.   Etiology/incidence/predisposing factors

   A. Degeneration of the nucleus pulposus, which is the portion of the disk that contains gelatinous material enclosed in a fibrous band

   B. Dehydration of the disk

   C. Trauma

   D. Forceful coughing or sneezing (e.g., Valsalva maneuver)

   E. Sedentary lifestyle

   F. Obesity

   G. Peak incidence at ages 35–45

   H. Ninety percent located at L4-L5 and L5-S1

III. Subjective findings

   A. Radicular pain along specific dermatomal pattern

   B. Numbness or sense of weakness along affected dermatome

   C. Bowel, bladder, or sexual dysfunction

      1. Requires immediate referral for possible surgical intervention

IV.   Physical examination findings

   A. All physical findings dependent on the spinal nerve root affected

   B. Decreased or absent reflexes innervated by specific nerve

   C. Atrophy of muscles innervated by affected nerve in chronic compression

   D. Antalgic gait; limp

   E. Proprioception (position sense) decreased

   F. Possible positive straight leg raise test: radicular or sciatic pain

   G. Limited ROM of spine

   H. Positive pelvic rock test: test for sacroiliac joint dysfunction

      1. Place one hand over each anterior-superior iliac spine, and attempt to "open and close" the pelvis

      2. Positive test if patient feels pain in either or both sacroiliac joints

V.   Laboratory/diagnostic findings

   A. Serum blood work is usually within normal limits

   B. Radiographic studies most commonly used

      1. AP and lateral plain x-rays of the spine

      2. CT scan with and without contrast dye; good for detecting bony defects in the spinal canal or foramen

      3. MRI scan with and without contrast dye; good for detecting soft tissue defects, such as herniated disks

      4. Myelogram: consists of injection of contrast dye into the spinal canal to detect filling defects in myelin sheaths

   C. Electromyelography (EMG): consists of stimulating various nerves with low-voltage electrical impulses to test for nerve innervation to muscles

Table 60.2	Neurologic Chart for Evaluation of Lower Extremity Pain			
Sign/Symptom	**L4**	**L5**	**S1**	**Cauda Equina**
Pain	Anterior thigh	Posterior leg	Posterior leg into ankle	Lower back, sciatic
Weakness	Knee extension Quadriceps	Ankle dorsiflexion Extensor hallucis longus and tibialis anterior	Ankle plantar flexion Gastro- cnemius	Lower extremities Multiple muscles ****Either incontinent or retaining stool/urine**
Numbness	Medial malleolus	Great toe interspace	Lateral foot	Saddle
Reflex absent/ motor	Knee	None	Achilles	Sphincter tone

Note. L4, L5 = Lumbar 4–5; S1 = Sacral vertebrae 1.

    D. Nerve conduction studies: also use electrical impulses to test amplitude and waveform of different spinal nerves

VI. **Specific lumbar nerve root findings—See Table 60.2**
    A. L4 root: indicative of pathology in the disk between L3 and L4
        1. Motor: quadriceps muscles weak and/or atrophic; difficulty extending the quadriceps of the knee
        2. Sensory: pain radiating into medial malleolus; numbness along the same path, especially the medial aspect of the knee
        3. Reflex: diminished or absent knee jerk
        4. Screening examination: have patient squat and rise
    B. L5 root: indicative of pathology in disk between L4 and L5
        1. Motor: weakness of the dorsiflexion mechanism of great toe and foot (extensor hallucis longus)
        2. Sensory: pain radiating into lateral calf; numbness of dorsum of foot and lateral calf and between first toe web space
        3. Reflex: none at this level
        4. Screening examination: have patient walk on heels of feet
    C. S1 root: indicative of pathology in disk between L5 and S1
        1. Motor: weakness of plantar flexion of great toe and foot
        2. Sensory: pain along buttocks, lateral leg, and lateral malleolus; numbness on lateral aspect of foot and in posterior calf (gastrocnemius muscles)
        3. Reflex: diminished or absent Achilles reflex
        4. Screening examination: have patient walk on toes

VII. Management
   A. Nonsurgical and Patient Education
      1. Functional bracing with an orthotic device
      2. Rest for 1–2 days only for mild disk bulges/herniations
      3. Physical therapy for muscle strengthening
      4. Alternate heat/ice therapy
      5. Weight loss program
      6. Education in proper body mechanics
      7. Transcutaneous electrical nerve stimulator
      8. NSAIDs for mild to moderately severe injuries
         a. Other classifications of drugs used include anticonvulsants and antidepressants
            i. See Chapter 55 (Table 55.2) for information on management with NSAIDs
         b. May need antispasmodic for severe muscle spasms
            i. Diazepam (Valium), 2 mg PO every 6 hr PRN
            ii. Cyclobenzaprine (Flexeril), 10 mg PO 3 times a day PRN
            iii. Metaxalone (Skelaxin), 800 mg PO 3 times a day PRN
            iv. Tizanidine (Zanaflex), 2 mg PO every 6 hr PRN
            v. Baclofen (Lioresal), 5 mg PO three times a day PRN
            vi. Chlorzoxazone (Parafon Forte), 500 mg PO three times a day PRN
            vii. Orphenadrine (Norflex), 100 mg PO twice a day PRN
            viii. Methocarbamol (Robaxin), 500 mg PO every 6 hr PRN
      9. Narcotics for short-term use
         a. Oxycodone/acetaminophen 5 mg/325 mg (Percocet), 1 tablet PO every 3 hr PRN
         b. Hydrocodone/acetaminophen 5 mg/325 mg (Norco), 1 tablet PO every 4 hr PRN
         c. Tramadol (Ultram), 100 mg PO every 6 hr PRN
         d. Many persons are afraid to take opioids for acute/chronic low back pain because of fear of "addiction"; they need support and reassurance that this is a very uncommon occurrence
      10. Epidural steroid injections: given with the use of anesthesia directly into the affected nerve sheath; patient referred to pain management center for treatment

   B. Surgical
     1. Laparoscopic diskectomy
     2. May require hemilaminectomy
     3. Depending on number and level of disks, spinal fusion with bone grafts may be required
     4. Investigational total disk replacement arthroplasty procedures are currently being carried out in select centers to prevent fusion and maintain normal biomechanical function of the lumbar spine
     5. Patients must be informed that neurologic function may not return for an unknown length of time post-surgery because of axonal changes due to prolonged nerve compression

BIBLIOGRAPHY

Choi, B. K., Verbeek, J. H., Tam, W. W., Jiang, J. Y. (2010). Exercises for prevention of recurrences of low-back pain. *Cochrane Database of Systematic Reviews 2010*: CD006555.

Chou, R., Loeser, J. D., Owens, D. K., Rosenquist, R. W., Atlas, S. J., Baisden, J., . . . Eric, M. (2009). Interventional therapies, surgery, and interdiscinaplinary rehabilitation for low back pain: An evidence-based clinical practice guideline from the American Pain Society. *Spine, 34*(10), 1066–1077.

Chou, R., & Huffman, L. H. (2009). Guideline for the evaluation and management of low back pain: Evidence review. *American Pain Society*. Glenview, IL: American Pain Society.

Crowther-Radulewicz, C. L., & McCance, K. L. (2010). Alterations of musculoskeletal function. In K. L. McCance & S. E. Heuther (Eds.), *Pathophysiology: The biological basis for disease in adults and children*, (6th ed., pp. 1568–1643). Maryland Heights, MO: Mosby-Elsevier.

Dahm, K. T., Brurberg, K. G., Jamtvedt, G., Hagen, K. B. (2010). Advice to rest in bed versus advice to stay active for acute low-back pain and sciatica. *Cochrane Database of Systematic Reviews 2010*: CD007612.

Kahn-Kastell, B. (2013). The hip, femur, and pelvis. In L.Schoenly (Ed.), *Core curriculum for orthopaedic nursing* (7th ed., pp.549–570). Chicago, IL: National Association of Orthopaedic Nurses.

Knight, C. L., Deyo, R. A., Staiger, T. O., & Wipf, J. E. (2013). Treatment of acute low back pain. *UpToDate*. Retrieved from http://www.uptodate.com/contents/treatment-of-acute-low-back-pain

Kunkler, C. E. (2013). Therapeutic modalities. In L.Schoenly (Ed.), *Core curriculum for orthopaedic nursing* (7th ed., pp. 233–262). Chicago, IL: National Association of Orthopaedic Nurses.

Pearce, A. N. (2013). The spine. In L. Schoenly (Ed.), *Core curriculum for orthopaedic nursing* (7ᵗʰ ed., pp. 447–476). Chicago, IL: National Associatioin of Orthopaedic Nurses.

Pinto, R. Z., Maher, C. G., Ferreira, M. L., Hancock, M., Oliveira, V. C., McLachlan, A. J., . . . Koes, B. (2012). Epidural corticosteroid injections in the management of sciatica: A systematic review and meta-analysis. *Annals of Internal Medicine, 157*(12), 865–877.

Wheeler, S. G., Wipf, J. E., Staiger, T. O., & Deyo, R. A. (2013). Approach to the diagnosis and evaluation of low back pain in adults. *UpToDate.* Retrieved from http://www.uptodate.com/contents/approach-to-the-diagnosis-and-evaluation-of-low-back-pain-in-adults

Management of Patients with Hematologic Disorders

CHAPTER 61

Anemias

LISA EVANS

INITIAL ANEMIA WORKUP

I. **Definition of anemia**

    A. Reduction in one or more of the major red blood cell (RBC) measurements:

        1. Hemoglobin (Hgb) concentration

        2. Hematocrit (Hct) percentage

        3. RBC count

    B. Anemia is gender specific

        1. Males Hgb less than 13.5 grams/dl or Hct less than 41%

        2. Females Hgb less than 12.0 grams/dl or Hct less than 36%

    C. Volume status affects Hgb, Hct, and RBC measurements; dependent on RBC mass and plasma volume

    D. Inability of the blood to supply adequate oxygen for proper functioning of the body

    E. Classified according to pathophysiologic basis, diminished production, accelerated loss of RBCs, or cell size

    F. Causes

        1. Decreased RBC production (lack of nutrients, bone marrow disorders, and hypothyroidism)

        2. Increased RBC destruction (inherited/acquired hemolytic anemias)

        3. Blood loss (obvious/occult/induced)

    G. Classification by RBC indices

        1. Morphology of RBCs (normal range)

            a. Mean corpuscular volume (MCV): 80–100 fl

            b. Mean corpuscular hemoglobin (MCH): 26–34 p/cell

            c. Mean corpuscular hemoglobin concentration: 32–36 grams/dl

II. **Incidence/predisposing factors**
  A. In a healthy person, approximately 1% of fully mature circulating RBCs are lost daily.
  B. Anemia is common among the elderly
    1. Occurs in more than 33% of outpatients
    2. Hgb and Hct decrease slightly with age but remain in the normal adult range
    3. Prevalence and incidence of mild anemia increases with age; affects 1/10 elderly individuals
  C. Anemia is a sign, not a diagnosis
    1. Search for treatable disorders
  D. Adults residing at higher altitudes have normal values that are higher than those of adults residing at lower altitudes
  E. Plasma volume expansion in fluid-retaining states can mimic the appearance of anemia; conversely, states of dehydration can mimic the appearance of a normal Hct when the patient may actually be anemic.
  F. Increased morbidity and mortality when associated with the following:
    1. Chronic kidney disease
    2. Malignancy
    3. Heart failure
    4. Rheumatoid arthritis
    5. HIV
    6. Inflammatory bowel disease
    7. Elderly individuals
    8. Hospitalized adults
      a. Occurs in 50% of hospitalized patients
      b. Occurs in 75% of elderly hospitalized patients
      c. Seen in 90% of patients in the intensive care unit by day 3

III. **Subjective/physical examination findings**
  A. Complaints are related to tissue hypoxia and may include the following:
    1. Dyspnea on exertion that previously had not caused problems
    2. Headaches
    3. Tinnitus
    4. Syncope
    5. Dizziness
    6. Fatigue, weakness
    7. Sleep disturbance
    8. Mood disturbance
    9. Impaired concentration
    10. Neurologic manifestations
    11. Increased frequency of angina pectoris
  B. Dementia or intermittent claudication may be exacerbated
  C. Anorexia and weight loss
  D. If anemia has developed very slowly, the patient may be asymptomatic

    E. Skin and mucous membrane pallor

    F. Tachycardia and increased pulse pressure (may be minimal if anemia is slow, progressive)

    G. Systolic ejection murmurs

    H. Venous hums

    I. Peripheral edema

    J. Retinal hemorrhages (flame like) in severe anemia associated with thrombocytopenia

    K. Jaundice

    L. Hepatosplenomegaly

    M. Arrhythmias

IV. **Laboratory/diagnostic findings**

    A. Initially, consider ordering the following:

        1. Complete blood count (CBC) with differential or Hct with MCV

        2. Reticulocyte count (absolute)

        3. Platelet count (or estimate of platelets on smear)

        4. Wright-stained blood smear

        5. Serum ferritin, serum iron, and total iron-binding capacity (TIBC)

V. **Evaluation/management**

    A. Diagnosis of the specific cause of anemia should be made before transfusion, if possible

    B. Evaluate Hgb and Hct against normal ranges of patient population

    C. Evaluate reticulocyte count

        1. Absolute reticulocyte count not elevated indicates anemia of marrow failure. This is the most common cause of anemia.

        2. Elevated absolute reticulocyte count indicates erythropoietic response to anemia and probable blood loss or hemolysis

    D. Evaluate peripheral blood smear for characteristics

    E. Classify RBC indices according to the size or MCV of erythrocytes

        1. Microcytosis is decreased MCV (less than 80 fl)

        2. Normocytosis is normal MCV (80–100 fl)

        3. Macrocytosis is increased MCV (greater than 100 fl)

    F. Classify RBCs by variation in size from normal red cell size using red cell indices in concert with red cell distribution width (RDW) rating

        1. Normal RDW is 11.5% to 14.5%

        2. Increased RDW may indicate anisocytosis resulting from a heterogeneous mix of cells or poikilocytosis from a variation in cell mix. The type of cell is then specified.

        3. RDW in conjunction with MCV can be helpful in identifying cause of anemia

    G. Consider bone marrow smear and biopsy. Interpretation requires a differential count of the following:

        1. Myeloid, lymphoid, erythroid series, and maturational characteristics

        2. Iron stain

H. Specific studies are indicated to rule out specific disease processes
1. Hgb electrophoresis (hemoglobinopathies, thalassemia syndromes)
2. Antiglobulin testing (hemolytic anemias)
3. Osmotic fragility test (hereditary spherocytosis)
4. Sucrose hemolysis test or acidified serum test (known as Ham test) (paroxysmal nocturnal hemoglobinuria)
5. Tests for RBC enzymes (hemolytic anemias, glucose-6-phosphate dehydrogenase deficiency, pyruvate kinase deficiency)
6. Serum iron and iron-binding capacity (iron deficiency anemia)
7. Folate and vitamin B12 measurements (megaloblastic anemias)

PERNICIOUS ANEMIA

I. **Definition**
   A. A megaloblastic anemia
   B. Caused by a lack of intrinsic factor (IF) produced by parietal cells of the gastric mucosa; this prevents vitamin B12 absorption, resulting in vitamin B12 deficiency
   C. Autoimmune in origin
II. **Incidence/predisposing factors**
   A. May be inherited as an autosomal recessive disorder
      1. More common in people of northern European ancestry
      2. Rare in African Americans and Asians
   B. May be caused by atrophic gastritis, antibodies to gastric parietal cells, or autoimmune histamine-fast achlorhydria
   C. Occurs in approximately 1% of people, usually adults older than 60 years
   D. Antibodies to IF are detected in approximately 50% of patients with the disease
   E. The patient may have or develop other associated autoimmune diseases including the following:
      1. Immunoglobulin (Ig)A deficiency
      2. Rheumatoid arthritis
      3. Graves' disease
      4. Myxedema
      5. Thyroiditis
      6. Idiopathic adrenocortical insufficiency
      7. Hypoparathyroidism
         a. Agammaglobulinemia
      8. Vitiligo
      9. Tropical sprue
      10. Celiac disease
      11. Crohn's disease
      12. Ileum and small intestine infiltrate disorders
   F. It takes approximately 3 years for liver stores of vitamin B12 to be depleted after absorption ceases.

G. Predisposition to gastric polyps and stomach cancer
H. Identification and early treatment is essential

III.   Subjective/physical examination findings

A. Patient is usually pale and may be mildly icteric
B. Abnormal reflexes
C. Babinski's sign is positive
D. Romberg's sign is positive
E. Vibratory sensation and proprioception are lost or decreased in lower extremities
F. Paresthesia and numbness of extremities
G. Ataxia
H. Sense of smell is lost or diminished
I. Patient may exhibit loss of glossal papillae with tenderness (smooth tongue)
J. Depression or dementia may be present
K. Splenomegaly
L. Tinnitus
M. Hepatomegaly
N. Tachycardia
O. Congestive heart failure
P. Weakness
Q. Asthenia
R. Bleeding gums
S. Nausea, appetite loss, and weight loss
T. Sore tongue in approximately 50% of patients
U. Paresthesias
V. Difficulty maintaining balance
W. Yellowish tinge to eyes and skin
X. Shortness of breath
Y. Decreased mental concentration
Z. Headache
AA. Depression
AB. Palpitations/chest pain

IV.   Laboratory/diagnostic findings

A. Vitamin B12 deficiency is a megaloblastic anemia
   1. Macrocyte with MCV is usually 110–140 fl but may be in normal range if concurrent with iron deficiency or thalassemia.
   2. RDW is increased
B. Hct may be 10–15 ml/dl or lower
C. Peripheral blood smears usually exhibit macro-ovalocytes, anisocytosis, and poikilocytosis with hypersegmented neutrophils present (more than four lobes, sometimes six lobes).
D. Reticulocyte count is usually reduced
E. In severe cases, pancytopenia is present with white blood cell and platelet count reduced

    F. Serum folate is usually increased in vitamin B12 deficiency

    G. Decreased serum vitamin B12 (Cbl) levels

        1. Greater than 300 pg/ml: normal, deficiency unlikely

        2. 200–300 pg/ml: borderline, deficiency possible

        3. Less than 200 pg/ml: low, deficiency likely

    H. Red cell folate is usually decreased in vitamin B12 deficiency

    I. Serum ferritin is increased

    J. Lactate dehydrogenase may be elevated. Often, it is mistakenly assumed that anemia is hemolytic.

    K. Consider ordering the following:

        1. Anti-IF and anti-parietal cell antibodies (presence affirms deficiency)

        2. Schilling test (used only when it is unclear why the patient is vitamin B12 deficient because of the expense of the testing due to radioactive agents)

        3. Gastric analysis for achlorhydria

        4. Serum concentration of homocysteine

        5. Methylmalonic acid levels

    L. Megaloblastosis of the bone marrow characteristically is present

V.   **Management**

    A. Parenteral vitamin B12, 1 mg SC daily for 7 days, 1 mg SC once a week for 1 month, then 1 mg SC monthly for the remainder of life

        1. Oral regimen of 2,000 µg load, then 1,000 µg daily may be equally effective

    B. Folic acid should not be given without vitamin B12 because of the potential for fulminant neurologic deficit

    C. Hypokalemia may coincide with the first week of vitamin B12 replacement

    D. Central nervous system signs and symptoms are reversible if of short duration (less than 6 months) and if replacement therapy is initiated aggressively and promptly

    E. Endoscopy every 5 years even if asymptomatic (opinion varies in the literature)

VITAMIN B12 DEFICIENCY

I.   **Definition**

    A. A megaloblastic anemia caused by deficiency of vitamin B12

    B. Usually results from a deficiency of hydrochloric acid or pancreatic enzymes that causes an inability to metabolize vitamin B12

II.   **Incidence/predisposing factors**

    A. Vegans and strict vegetarians are at risk

    B. Major cause is malabsorption that results from diseases of the ileum or enteritis

    C. Blind loop syndrome

    D. Drugs such as alcohol, anesthetics, metformin, nitrous oxide, and the antituberculosis drug para-aminosalicylic acid

    E. Hemodialysis

    F. Roux-en-Y gastric bypass

    G. Fish tapeworm (Diphyllobothrium latum)

    H. Because storage of vitamin B12 is normally high and body utilization is low, deficiency takes approximately 2–7 years to develop in the case of malabsorption.

    I. Nutritional vitamin B12 deficiency is rare in the United States

III. **Subjective/physical examination findings**

    A. Same as in pernicious anemia (see previous section)

IV. **Laboratory/diagnostic findings**

    A. Same as in pernicious anemia (see previous section), except as follows:

        1. Anti-IF and anti-parietal cell antibodies (specific for pernicious anemia)

        2. Schilling test (used only when it is unclear why the patient is vitamin B12 deficient, not to prove the existence of anemia, because of the expense of the test due to radioactive agents)

V. **Management**

    A. As in pernicious anemia (see previous section) if severe deficiency

    B. Treatment of underlying cause will normalize vitamin B12 levels

        1. In blind loop syndrome, adequate antimicrobial coverage achieved with 7- to 10-day course of the following:

            a. Rifaximin (1650 mg/day)

            b. Amoxicillin-clavulanate (30 mg/kg/day)

            c. Metronidazole (20 mg/kg/day)

            d. Norfloxacin (800 mg/day)

        2. For fish tapeworm (common in Scandinavian countries), give vitamin B12 alone or IF plus vitamin B12

    C. Oral supplementation in mega doses is reported with success in the literature

        1. 1000 mcg/day (see previous section about folate concerns)

        2. Inconsistencies in absorption reported in the literature (caution is recommended with "timed released" over-the-counter B12 therapy)

IRON DEFICIENCY

I. **Definition**

    A. State in which iron stores in the body are inadequate to preserve homeostasis (usually less than 12 mcg/L) and patient responds to iron therapy

    B. Microcytic anemia is characterized by small, pale RBCs and depleted iron stores

II. **Incidence/predisposing factors**

    A. Most common anemia worldwide

1. Accounts for 60% of anemias in patients older than 65 years
2. Usually mild but may become moderate or even severe
3. Present in 1%–2% of adults

B. Common causes:
   1. Blood loss
      a. Overt blood loss: hemorrhage, hemoptysis, and melena
      b. Occult blood loss: gastrointestinal and genitourinary tracts
   2. Decreased iron absorption
   3. Celiac disease
   4. Foods/medications
   5. Gastric or small bowel surgery without adequate iron supplements
   6. Blood donations
   7. Iron requirements increase during pregnancy, upsetting iron balance
   8. Long-term aspirin use may precipitate iron loss without documented lesion
   9. Menorrhagia or other uterine bleeding
   10. Chronic hemoglobinuria; traumatic hemolysis resulting from abnormally functioning cardiac valve
   11. Repeated pregnancies with breast feeding

III. **Physical examination/subjective findings**
   A. Pallor (skin and conjunctiva)
   B. Red and smooth tongue
   C. May have spoon-shaped, brittle nails (koilonychia)
   D. May have cheilosis (cracking corners of the mouth)
   E. Tachycardia
   F. Palpitations
   G. Peripheral paresthesias
   H. May have apical systolic "hemic" heart murmur
   I. Initially may be asymptomatic
   J. Fatigue
   K. Exertional dyspnea
   L. Dizziness
   M. Headache
   N. Exercise intolerance
   O. May develop pica (usually craving for substances such as ice, but may be for other items such as starch, paint, or clay)

IV. **Laboratory/diagnostic findings**
   A. Peripheral smear
   1. Staging of deficiency
      a. Stage 1: body stores depleted but laboratory test results may be normal
      b. Stage 2: hemoglobin possibly normal but iron stores depleted per laboratory test values
      c. Stage 3: iron depletion, slight anemia, and normal MCV

        d. Stage 4: severe iron deficiency, hypochromic RBCs, and low MCV with marked anemia

    2. Microcytosis, poikilocytosis, and hypochromia appear as deficiency worsens

B. Elevated RDW in the absence of any other RBC abnormalities is a major diagnostic indicator

C. Reticulocyte count is disproportionately decreased in relation to the degree of anemia

D. Ferritin level less than 10–12 mcg/dl; TIBC increased by more than 300 mcg/dl

E. Serum iron (usually low, less than 50 mg/dl) test ordered for transferrin saturation ratio (serum iron to TIBC); if ratio less than 15%, then iron deficiency is present

F. Platelet count may be elevated to as high as 1.5 million/mm

G. Bone marrow biopsy is indicated when the preceding are inconclusive

    1. Gold standard is bone marrow iron stain

    2. Decreased or absent marrow iron stores indicate deficiency

    3. Deficiency is reported as Prussian blue negative on bone marrow stain

H. Consider ordering the following:

    1. Stool

        a. For guaiac testing

        b. For ova and parasites

    2. Gastrointestinal endoscopy

    3. Clotting studies

V.   Management

A. Determine the cause and amount of blood loss, and treat the underlying disorder

B. Therapeutic trial of iron

    1. Oral ferrous sulfate, 300–325 mg 3 times a day 1 hr before meals for 6 months

    2. Enteric-coated or sustained-release iron preparations not well absorbed and should be avoided

C. For uncomplicated iron deficiency anemia, a polysaccharide iron complex (Hytinic, Niferex, Niferex-150, Nu-Iron, and Nu-Iron-150) may be considered

    1. These are associated with few adverse reactions.

    2. Dosage for adults: 50–100 mg of elemental iron 3 times a day

D. Follow-up in 3 weeks with CBC count

    1. Hgb should be normalized at 2 months

    2. Six months of treatment recommended to build iron stores

E. Transfusion of packed RBCs may be necessary if anemia is symptomatic (1 ml of transfused RBCs delivers 1 mg iron)

F. Sodium ferric gluconate complex (Ferrlecit) injection 62.5 mg/5 ml

1. Although anaphylaxis is not as frequent as with iron dextran, it may occur
   a. Rapid infusion may cause hypotension and flushing
   b. Epinephrine and resuscitation equipment should be readily available in the event of an anaphylactic reaction (lower incidence than with iron dextran)
2. 10 ml (125 mg elemental iron) is a common dosage that is repeated during eight sequential dialysis treatments for a total cumulative dose of 1 gram
3. Precise dosing may be determined (total of 1.5–2 grams) by calculating the decrease in volume of RBC mass and supplying 1 mg of iron for each milliliter volume below normal plus an additional 1 gram for iron storage
4. Test dose of dilute solution should be administered before full dosing and the patient observed for anaphylaxis

G. Parenteral iron intravenously or deep intramuscularly is reserved for intolerance of or noncompliance with oral supplements (gaining favor in the literature with newer and safer intravenous iron preparations).
   1. Anaphylaxis may occur
      a. A test dose of 0.5 ml should be given before therapy is initiated
      b. Diphenhydramine (Benadryl) and epinephrine should be readily available
   2. Painful injections should be given in large muscles of the buttocks
      a. Injections may stain the skin
      b. No more than 1 ml in each buttock per day should be given
   3. Intravenous administration may cause phlebitis
   4. Administration can be provided according to the following formula: milligrams of iron = {(normal Hgb - patient's Hgb) × weight (kg)} × 2.21 / 1,000
   5. Iron dextran (Imferon), 50 mg/ml, can be administered intramuscularly or intravenously; intravenous administration should not exceed 1 ml/min and 2 ml/day

H. Within 7–10 days, a reticulocyte response and increase in hematocrit should occur with either form of parenteral iron

I. Failure to respond to therapy within 5–8 weeks warrants evaluation for compliance, impaired absorption, gastric or bowel pathology, blood loss, or incorrect diagnosis

FOLIC ACID DEFICIENCY

I. **Definition**
  A. A megaloblastic anemia
  B. Decreased RBCs and hemoglobin content caused by impaired production related to decreased serum folate

II. **Incidence/predisposing factors**
  A. Usually a result of the following:
    1. Inadequate dietary intake
    2. Lack of absorption
    3. Inadequate conversion of folate to tetrahydrofolate
  B. Nutritional folate deficiency usually related to alcoholism, anorexia, older age with inadequate dietary intake, or special diet
  C. Malabsorption of folic acid found with celiac disease, tropical sprue, and gluten-sensitive enteropathy
  D. Increased utilization of folic acid during pregnancy, malignancy, or hemolysis
  E. May be drug-induced by the following agents:
    1. Methotrexate
    2. Pyrimethamine
    3. Phenytoin
    4. Alcohol
    5. Isoniazid
    6. Oral contraceptives
  F. Normal body store of folate is 5,000–20,000 µg
  G. Clinical signs of folate deficiency may be noted in approximately 4 months

III. **Subjective/physical examination findings**
  A. Fatigue
  B. Pallor
  C. Mouth/tongue pain
  D. Symptoms may not be present until anemia is severe
  E. Patient may show signs of malnutrition
  F. Patient may or may not show the following:
    1. Glossitis
    2. Stomatitis
    3. Gastrointestinal symptoms
    4. Hyperpigmentation
    5. Infertility
    6. Orthostatic hypotension
    7. Weight loss
  G. Neurologic symptoms are less common but do occur

IV. **Laboratory/diagnostic findings**
  A. Serum folate concentration
    1. Greater than 4 ng/ml: can rule out folate deficiency

2. Less than 2 ng/ml: diagnostic of folate deficiency (in absence of fasting/anorexia)

B. RBC folate is a better indicator of tissue levels; less than 150 ng/ml is diagnostic for folate deficiency

C. MCV is usually greater than 115 fl or may gradually increase over several months to years and remain in the normal range

D. Serum concentration of homocysteine will be elevated

V. Management

A. Care should be taken to ensure a correct diagnosis

B. Administration of folate can exacerbate the neurologic symptoms of untreated vitamin B12 deficiency

C. Oral folate, 1–5 mg/day for 3–4 months

D. Folate should be given along with vitamin B12 when both are deficient

E. After initiation of folate

1. Peak of reticulocytosis occurs in 6–8 days, followed by a slow increase in Hgb
2. Total correction should be seen within 2 months

ANEMIA OF CHRONIC DISEASE (ACD)

I. Definition

A. An anemia that

1. Is gradual in onset
2. Is usually normochromic and normocytic, can occasionally be hypochromic and microcytic
3. Accompanies
   a. Chronic infection or chronic inflammation
   b. Acute or chronic immune activation (rheumatoid arthritis)
   c. Chronic kidney disease and/or end stage renal disease
   d. Underlying malignancies
   e. May also be seen with severe trauma, diabetes mellitus, and advanced age
4. Resolves when the underlying disorder clears

B. Reduction in RBC production by bone marrow due to:

1. Abnormal iron metabolism and reduced absorption from gastrointestinal tract
2. Inability to increase erythropoiesis in response to anemia
3. Decrease in production of erythropoiesis
4. Shortening of red cell life-span

II. Incidence/predisposing factors

A. Second most common anemia after iron deficiency

1. Accompanies any chronic infection
2. Seen with inflammation, particularly connective tissue (immune) disorders
3. Common in
   a. Acute inflammatory disorders

          b. Protein-energy malnutrition

          c. Burns

          d. Myocardial infarction

    B. Seen with

      1. Chronic renal disease

      2. Liver disease with or without alcoholism

      3. Endocrine disorders

          a. Hypothyroidism

          b. Hypopituitarism

          c. Hypogonadism

          d. Hyperparathyroidism

    C. Anemia develops within 1–2 months of onset of illness

    D. Degree of anemia usually coincides with severity of the underlying disease

    E. Usually manifests in individuals in whom primary disease is obvious

    F. Any infection due to a bacterium or a fungus that lasts longer than 2 weeks can cause anemia

    G. Commonly confused with iron deficiency anemia

III. **Subjective findings**

    A. Frequently occurs without symptoms

    B. If anemia is severe, the patient may report the following:

      1. Fatigue

      2. Shortness of breath

      3. Weight loss

      4. Light-headedness

      5. Loss of appetite

    C. The patient may report only symptoms related to the underlying chronic disease.

IV. **Physical examination findings are primarily those of the underlying disease**

V. **Laboratory/diagnostic findings**

    A. Mild to moderate anemia with Hgb concentration less than 10 grams/dl is extremely unusual

    B. RBCs are usually normocytic and normochromic but occasionally are hypochromic and microcytic

    C. Reticulocyte count is less than 1% or a low absolute number

    D. Normal or increased iron stores differentiate ACD from iron deficiency anemia

      1. Serum ferritin is usually high in ACD (greater than 100 ng/ml)

      2. TIBC is usually depressed in ACD (less than 250 µg/ml)

    E. RBC morphology varies very little from normal: RDW is usually normal in ACD

    F. Sideroblasts are absent in bone marrow, but iron stores are normal or increased

G. Leukocytosis and thrombocytosis are often seen in the peripheral smear if infection or malignancy is present.

H. Consider ordering erythrocyte sedimentation rate to assess the severity of inflammation associated with the underlying chronic illness

VI. **Management**

A. First-line therapy directed at the identification and treatment of underlying disease. If the disorder is reversible, anemia should resolve.

B. In premenopausal women, a therapeutic trial of oral iron may be given with reevaluation of CBC in 2–3 weeks to rule out iron deficiency anemia.

1. A 1.5 gram/dl or greater rise in Hgb concentration should have occurred

2. Failure warrants further investigation

3. Not appropriate for postmenopausal women or men of any age

C. No specific therapy exists. Oral iron alone is of no benefit in this anemia.

D. Recombinant human erythropoietin (e.g., Epogen, EPO, and Procrit) is used for individuals with chronic diseases such as renal disease/failure and rheumatoid arthritis to promote hematopoiesis

1. Dosage for adults is individualized: starting dose is 50–100 units/kg SC 3 times per week

a. Can also dose to equivalent of 30,000–40,000 units SC 1 time per week

2. Nondialysis or continuous peritoneal dialysis patients may receive doses subcutaneously or intravenously

3. Dose is adjusted in 2–8 weeks in accordance with response to therapy

4. Target Hct range, 30–33 ml/dl (maximum, 36 ml/dl)

5. Hct should not increase by more than 4 points during any 2-week period to reduce risk of hypertension or seizures

6. Concurrent administration of supplemental iron is recommended to ensure adequate iron stores to achieve/maintain hemoglobin levels, to target the following:

a. Transferrin saturation greater than 20%

b. Serum ferritin greater than 100 ng/ml

THALASSEMIA

I. **Definition**

A. A group of inherited disorders that are the result of defective production of the globin portion of hemoglobin; characterized by hypochromic and microcytic anemia

B. Cooley's anemia is the name commonly used for severe thalassemia (thalassemia major)

II. **Incidence/predisposing factors**

A. The word thalassemia is derived from the Greek word for "sea"

1. The disorder was first recognized in Mediterranean coastal regions among individuals of Italian or Greek ancestry.
2. Worldwide distribution of thalassemia is associated with that of malignant malaria.
3. Thalassemia affords a protective effect against *Plasmodium falciparum* malaria in indigenous areas.

B. Many genetic mutations make up the β-thalassemia syndromes. General classifications include the following:
1. Thalassemia minor
2. Thalassemia intermedia
3. Thalassemia major (Cooley's anemia), or homozygous β-thalassemia

C. α-thalassemia is classified into four types:
1. Silent carrier state: α-thalassemia-2 trait (asymptomatic)
2. Mild, microcytic, and hypochromic anemia: α-thalassemia-1 trait
3. Moderately severe hemolytic anemia usually not requiring chronic transfusions; three genes affected
4. Nonfunctional: all four genes affected; results in hydrops fetalis and Bart's hemoglobin

D. The most common form is thalassemia trait
1. Represented in the heterozygous form of α- or β-thalassemia
2. In areas where the thalassemia trait is common, the homozygous form is more prevalent.

E. In the United States, β-thalassemia is most prevalent among ethnic groups originating from the Mediterranean area and parts of Africa and Asia.

F. In the United States, α-thalassemia is the most prevalent among patients of Asian ancestry.

G. Gallstones occur in 15% of patients older than 15 years

III. Physical examination/subjective findings

A. Hepatosplenomegaly

B. Cardiac failure/dilatation

C. Jaundice

D. Cooley's anemia facies (marked osteoporosis and cortical thinning)
1. Erythroid overgrowth of the marrow may distort the bones of the head, face, rib cage, and pelvis
2. Predisposed to pathologic fractures of long bones and vertebrae

E. Growth retardation with delayed or absent adolescent growth spurt and delayed menarche, oligomenorrhea, or amenorrhea
1. Delayed secondary sexual characteristics
2. Hypogonadism

F. Heterozygous β-thalassemia silent carriers

G. Pallor

H. Fatigue

I. Dark urine

J. Poor growth

IV. **Laboratory/diagnostic findings**

A. Hallmark is microcytic and hypochromic anemias

B. Usually manifests as a decrease in Hgb, Hct, MCV, and MCH in conjunction with normal to increased RBC, normal to mildly decreased mean corpuscular hemoglobin concentration, and normal RDW

C. Wright stain

   1. Homozygous β-thalassemia and double heterozygous non-α-thalassemia exhibit extreme anisocytosis and poikilocytosis with bizarre shapes, target cells, and ovalocytes and large numbers of nucleated RBCs.

   2. Heterozygous β-thalassemia

      a. Exhibits hypochromic and microcytic cells with mild to moderate anisocytosis and poikilocytosis

      b. Target cells are frequent, with basophilic stippling

D. Indirect bilirubin level

   1. Increased in thalassemia major and thalassemia intermedia

   2. Ranges from 1–6 mg/dl

   3. Indirect bilirubin levels in thalassemia intermedia exceed those in thalassemia major.

E. Osmotic fragility of red cells—may be used as inexpensive screening for thalassemia carrier state

F. Hgb electrophoresis is used to confirm the diagnosis—cellulose acetate electrophoresis is preferred to starch gel electrophoresis or citrate agar gel electrophoresis

   1. HbA2: if elevated, consistent with heterozygous β-thalassemia

   2. HbF: if HbF and HbA2 levels are normal, microcytosis with minimal or no anemia suggests α-thalassemia

G. Genetic testing: restriction endonuclease mapping of α-globin genes is the only definitive test for α gene deletion

   1. Expensive and time consuming

   2. Usually reserved for special circumstances involving prenatal diagnosis

H. Consider ordering the following:

   1. Evaluation of iron status to rule out iron deficiency anemia and assess for iron load

      a. Serum iron level

      b. TIBC

      c. Serum ferritin level

   2. Free erythrocyte protoporphyrin if lead poisoning suspected

I. Skull x-ray may show "hair on end" appearance in a patient with homozygous β-thalassemia

V. **Management**

A. Severe β-thalassemia

   1. Blood transfusion support

      a. Each unit of packed RBCs contains approximately 200 mg iron

      b. Multiple transfusions predispose a patient to manifestations of hemochromatosis at an early age

      c. Patients with thalassemia intermedia, who may not receive transfusions, are also at risk, but at a later age

  2. Iron chelation therapy with severe β-thalassemia

      a. Deferoxamine (Desferal), 2–6 grams given parenterally 5–6 nights a week, with 30–40 mg excretion of iron daily in older patients

        i. Usually given IM

        ii. Abdominal subcutaneous pump infusion slowly more than 8–12 hr nightly is most effective.

      b. Chelation therapy via a Hickman catheter at 3–4 grams/day more than 18–20 hr may be self-administered by well-motivated patients

  3. Goal for Hgb levels: 9–10 grams/dl with chelation therapy

  4. Concurrent administration of vitamin C (150–250 mg/day) orally may enhance iron excretion

      a. Use cautiously with older patients

      b. May enhance iron toxicity

B. Observation for leukopenia and thrombocytopenia as indicators for splenic enlargement and potential need for splenectomy

C. Allogeneic bone marrow transplantation

GERONTOLOGY CONSIDERATIONS

I.   **Considerations for the elderly**

  A. Anemia is common in older adults

  B. Prevalence of 8%–25% in elderly population in the United States

  C. Nursing home residents at increased risk

  D. Hospitalized older adults with highest prevalence rates

  E. Tends to be milder form of anemia with Hgb greater than 10 grams/dl

  F. Increased morbidity and mortality associated with lower extremes of Hgb less than 12 grams/dl

  G. Impaired function

    1. Physical

    2. Mental

      a. Impaired cognitive function, depression, and decreased quality of life

  H. Causes of anemia-multifactorial

    1. May be associated with underlying renal insufficiency, myelodysplasia, and nutritional deficiency, among others

  I. Should undergo standard evaluation for anemia and identification of underlying cause

BIBLIOGRAPHY

Alleyne, M., Horne, M. K., & Miller, J. L. (2008). Individualized treatment of iron deficiency anemia. *American Journal of Medicine, 121*(11), 943–948. doi:http://dx.doi.org/10.1016/j.amjmed.2008.07.012

Annibale, B., Lahner, E., & Delle Fare, G. (2011). Diagnosis and management of pernicious anemia. *Current Gastroenterology Reports, 13*(6), 518–524. doi:10.1007/s11894–011–0225–5

Cullis, J. O. (2011). Diagnosis and management of anemia of chronic disease: Current status. *British Journal of Hematology, 154*(3), 289–300. doi:10.1111/j.1365–2141.2011.08741.x

Goddard, A. F. (2011). *Guidelines for the management of iron deficiency anaemia.* Great Britain: British Society of Gastroenterology.

Haines, D., Martin, M., Carson, S., Oliveros, O., Green, S., Coates, T., . . . Vichinsky, E. (2013). Pain in thalassaemia: The effects of age on pain frequency and severity. *British Journal of Hematology, 160*(5), 680–687.

John, S., & Hoegerl, C. (2009). Nutritional deficiencies after gastric bypass surgery. *Journal of the American Osteopathic Association, 109*(11), 601–604.

McEvoy, M. T., & Shander, A. (2013). Anemia, bleeding, and blood transfusions in the ICU: Causes, risks, costs, and new strategies. *American Journal of Critical Care, 22*(6). doi:http://dx.doi.org/10.4037/ajcc2013729

Oberley, M. J., & Yang, D. T. (2013). Laboratory teting for cobalamin deficiency in megaloblastic anemia. *American Journal of Hematology, 88*(6), 522–526. doi:10.1002/ajh.23421

Price, E. A., Mehra, R., Holmes, T. H., & Schrier, S. L. (2011). Anemia in older persons: Etiology and evaluation. *Blood Cells, Molecules and Diseases, 46*(2), 159–165. doi:10.1016/j.bcmd.2010.11.004

Quigly, E. M., & Abu-Shanab, A. (2010). Small intestinal bacterial overgrowth. *Infectious Disease Clinics of North America, 24*(4), 943–959.

Raman, G. (2012). *Quality of reporting in systematic reviews of implantable medical devices.* Rockville, MD: Agency for Healthcare Research and Quality.

Richards, J. B., & Stapleton, R. D. (2014). *Non-pulmonary complications of critical care: A clinical guide.* New York, NY: Springer.

Stabler, S. P. (2013). Vitamin B12 deficiency. *New England Journal of Medicine, 368,* 149–160. doi:10.1056/NEJMcp1113996

Tettamanti, M., Lucca, U., Gandini, F., Recchia, A., Mosconi, P., Apolone, G., . . . Riva, E. (2010). Prevalence, incidence and types of mild anemia in the elderly: The "Health and Anemia" population-based study. *Haematologica, 95*(11), 1849–1856. doi:10.3324/haematol.2010.023101

Theurl, I., Aigner, E., Theurl, M., Nairz, M., Seifer, M., Schroll, A., . . . Weiss G. (2009). Regulation of iron hemostasis in anemia of chronic disease and iron deficiency anemia: Diagnostic and therapeutic implications. *Blood, 113*(21), 5277–5286. doi:10.1182/blood-2008–12–195651

Yuan, J. X. (2011). *Textbook of pulmonary vascular disease.* New York, NY: Springer.

CHAPTER 62

Sickle Cell Disease/Crisis

LISA EVANS

I.   Definition

  A. Inherited autosomal recessive disorder

    1. Defect in hemoglobin molecule; specifically, a variant in β globin polypeptide

      a. HbF (fetal hemoglobin) replaced by HbA (adult hemoglobin) during postnatal period

      b. HbS (sickle) is inherited variant of HbA

    2. Hemoglobin S

      a. Variants of β globin gene (HbS)

      b. Disease expression occurs with inheritance of 2 copies of HbS or HbS and another copy of β globin variant

        i. Sickle cell trait (HbS)

          (a) HbS and HbA

          (b) Usually no expression of disease

          (c) Can have milder expression of disease under extreme circumstances (high altitude/increased temperature/decreased oxygen supply)

    3. Sickle cell disease (SS)

      a. HbS and HbS

      b. Moderate to severe hemolytic anemia in first months of life

    4. Hemoglobin sickle C disease (SC)

      a. HbS and HbC

      b. Moderate to severe hemolytic anemia

      c. Increased risk for splenomegaly, retinal disease, and aseptic necrosis

    5. Sickle/β thalassemia (SA)

      a. HbS and β thalassemia

      b. Manifestations vary, depending on degree of thalassemia

B. Abnormal properties conveyed to sickle cell erythrocytes by mutant sickle cell hemoglobin

   1. Hemoglobin polymerization leading to erythrocyte rigidity, distortion to sickle shape, and vaso-occlusion

   2. Hallmark of disease is vaso-occlusive phenomena and hemolytic anemia

   a. Sickle cell anemia (SS) is uncompensated hemolytic anemia with shortened red blood cell (RBC) survival (16 days versus 120 days normally); increased RBC production (erythropoiesis) is insufficient to balance the increased rate of destruction.

   b. Characterized by hemolytic anemia, dactylitis, and acute episodic "crisis"

   i. Episodic crisis

   (a) Vaso-occlusive (most common) leading to tissue ischemia and acute pain

   (b) Acute chest syndrome

   (c) Sequestration crisis

   (d) Aplastic crisis

   (e) Increased risk for stroke, organ damage, bacterial infections, and complications from blood transfusions

II. **Incidence/predisposing factors**

A. In the United States, African Americans are primarily affected. Persons of Mediterranean, Asian, Caribbean, South and Central American, and East Indian origin may also be affected.

   1. Worldwide, sickle cell disease is most common in areas where malaria is endemic.

   2. Sickle cell trait confers a protective effect against *Plasmodium falciparum* malaria

   a. HbS affects 2.5 million people in the United States and 300 million worldwide

   b. One in 12 African Americans affected

   3. Sickle cell disease

   a. 90,000–100,000 individuals within the United States, millions worldwide

   b. Sickle cell disease (SS):1 in 375 individuals

   c. Sickle C disease (SC): 1 in 835 individuals

   d. Sickle B/β thalassemia (SA): 1 in 1,667 individuals

   4. Higher survival rates among children leading into adulthood

   5. Early identification is critical; universal screening of all newborns within United States

B. Hospitalizations

   1. Associated with acute crisis and pain issues

   2. One third of patients with SS rarely have pain

   3. One third are hospitalized for pain 2–6 times a year

   4. One third have six or more pain-related hospitalizations per year

   C. Common neurologic complications occur in 25% of SS patients.
      1. Transient ischemic attacks, stroke (intracranial hemorrhage), unexplained coma, and epilepsy
      2. Twenty-four percent of individuals will have overt stroke by age 25 years
      3. Higher incidence of neurocognitive decline
   D. Infection is leading cause of morbidity and mortality for SS patients
      1. Due to splenic dysfunction
      2. Bacterial infections: *Streptococcus pneumoniae* and *Haemophilus influenzae*
      3. Viral infections: H1N1; parvovirus
   E. Pain is most common phenomena for individuals
      1. Chronic pain
      2. Acute pain episodes—typically managed at home, presentation to emergency department (ED) when pain no longer manageable

III. Subjective/physical examination findings
   A. Symptoms usually relate to increased cell viscosity and subsequent vaso-occlusion that result in the following:
      1. Generalized pain in long bones and joints
      2. Fever, fatigue, and malaise
      3. Abdominal pain, nausea, vomiting, and decreased appetite
      4. Swelling in hands, feet, and joints
      5. Priapism
   B. Depression (particularly in adolescents—due to low self-esteem, delays in maturation, and chronic pain crises)
   C. Chronic hemolytic anemia
   D. Tachycardia
   E. Fever
   F. Tachypnea
   G. Splenomegaly
      1. Frequently seen with (SC)
      2. Usually nonpalpable with (SS)
   H. Hepatomegaly
   I. Jaundice
   J. Cardiomegaly
   K. Retinopathy
   L. Adolescents may exhibit physical immaturity
      1. Delay in secondary sexual characteristics with delayed menarche
      2. Delayed adolescent growth in both height and weight
      3. Decreased physical endurance compared with peers
   M. Leg ulcers near the medial or lateral malleolus may occur spontaneously or as the result of trauma

IV. Laboratory/diagnostic findings
   A. Hemoglobin electrophoresis will confirm the following:
      1. Hemoglobin genotype (cellulose acetate and citrate agar gel) for sickle cell disease
      2. Hemoglobin F (fetal) and A2 for presence of thalassemia

B. SS patients are anemic; hematocrit is usually 20–30 ml/dl

C. Reticulocyte count is markedly elevated (10%–25%); if not, then anemia source other than sickle cell disease should be sought

D. White blood cell count is usually elevated (12,000–15,000 µg/L)

E. Sickle cells (5%–50%) are found on the peripheral blood smear

F. Diagnosis is confirmed by hemoglobin electrophoresis
1. Hemoglobin S usually constitutes approximately 85% to 95% of Hgb
2. Hemoglobin A will not be present in homozygous S disease
3. Hemoglobin F levels are variably increased (high Hgb F is associated with more benign disease)

G. Elevated levels of
1. Serum unconjugated (indirect) bilirubin
2. Serum transaminase
3. Alkaline phosphatase

H. Serum creatinine level is lower than normal (unless in renal failure) because of the increased glomerular filtration rate of the kidneys, which cannot concentrate urine

I. Urine may contain protein

J. Decreased levels of
1. Plasma protein C
2. Plasma protein S

K. Elevated levels of
1. Factor VIII activity
2. von Willebrand factor antigen
3. Thrombin

L. Thrombocytosis

M. Howell-Jolly bodies and target cells may be present with hyposplenism

N. Transcranial Doppler ultrasonography is recommended for children and adolescents to identify those at high risk for stroke

O. Consider the following:
1. Ordering x-ray studies of painful bones
2. To rule out aseptic necrosis, the following may need to be obtained:
   a. CT scan
   b. MRI
3. Fever
   a. Blood cultures
   b. Complete blood count with differential

V. **Management**

A. Acute pain episodes
1. Prompt treatment within 30 min of arrival to ED
   a. Morphine, 0.1–0.15 mg/kg
   b. Hydromorphone, 0.02–0.05 mg/kg
   c. Continual reassessment

       d. Hospitalization warranted if pain does not improve

       e. If hospitalization is warranted,

          i. Parenteral analgesics with Dilaudid/Morphine/Fentanyl

          ii. Patient-controlled analgesia

          iii. Oral opioids for breakthrough pain

  2. Ensure adequate fluid volume status

       a. Normal saline (NS) boluses to maintain hemodynamic stability and reduce viscosity

          i. Avoid fluid overload

       b. If signs and symptoms of dehydration and no hypovolemic shock,

          i. 0.5–1 L of NS

       c. Maintenance fluids

          i. ¼ or ½ NS infusion

          ii. Encourage oral intake

B. Administer oxygen to hypoxic patients with partial pressure of oxygen in arterial blood (PaO_2) less than 60–70 mmHg. Use humidified O_2, 40%

C. Give nonopioid analgesics such as nonsteroidal anti-inflammatory drugs or acetaminophen

  1. May be given for mild to moderate pain

  2. Evaluate renal function, adjust accordingly

D. Continuous release analgesics appropriate

E. Alternative drugs, usually used in combination with analgesics, include:

  1. Antihistamines

  2. Tricyclic antidepressants

F. Use phenothiazines for nausea and vomiting

G. Acute vaso-occlusive crises are managed with exchange transfusions

H. Consider blood transfusions for the following:

  1. Symptomatic anemia

  2. Acute events

  3. Preoperatively for major surgeries

  4. Acute sepsis/meningitis

  5. Prevention of recurrent stroke

  6. Chronic hypoxia

  7. Recurrent and chronic symptomatic anemia

I. Hospitalization is indicated for

  1. Persistent pain unrelieved by analgesics for longer than 8 hr

  2. Sepsis and persistent fever

  3. Central nervous system disorders

       a. Increased lethargy

       b. Headaches

    4. Acute chest syndrome
      a. EKG
      b. Complete blood count
      c. Chest x-ray/chest CT scan
      d. Blood and sputum cultures
    5. Oxygen supplementation
    6. Surgical emergency
    7. Pregnancy-related complications
    8. Priapism (may require exchange transfusion or surgical shunting by urologist)

J. Preventive measures and chronic disease management for the adult should include the following:
    1. Folic acid, 1 mg PO, daily
    2. If elevated velocities are observed with transcranial Doppler ultrasonography in high-risk patients, consider long-term transfusion to prevent stroke.
    3. Pneumococcal, hepatitis, and influenza vaccines
    4. Foot care and protective shoes may prevent chronic leg ulcers
    5. Annual and repeated health care visits PRN, with two to three visits a year for patients older than age 30 years (as dictated by patient status)
    6. Annual retinal evaluation is begun at school age; if no sickle cell-related findings, repeat visits as adult every 2–3 years
    7. History of priapism should be sought at each visit, with early treatment provided
    8. Ongoing chelation therapy for patients with iron overload
      a. Deferoxamine mesylate (Desferal) for intramuscular, intravenous, and subcutaneous administration
      b. Deferasirox (Exjade) for oral administration
    9. Routine exchange transfusion to increase oxygen-carrying capacity while decreasing viscosity and complications related to hemolysis

K. Genetic counseling should be offered
    1. Birth control options should be presented to adolescents with sickle cell disease
    2. Oral contraceptives are not contraindicated

L. Patients should avoid temperature extremes and physical overexertion that leads to dehydration

M. In (SS), aliphatic butyrate salts and hydroxyurea increase the level of fetal hemoglobin
    1. Hydroxyurea, 500–750 mg/day, is used to reduce the occurrence of painful crises; long-term safety is unclear
    2. Erythropoietin is mentioned in the literature on sickle cell disease, but effective dosage schedules are unclear

N. Successful cure of (SS) has been accomplished with hematopoietic cell transplantation—mostly true in children, higher mortality rates in adults

BIBLIOGRAPHY

Booth, C., Inusa, B., Obaro, S. K. (2009). Infection in sickle cell disease: A review. *International Journal of Infectious Diseases, 14*(1), e2-e12.

Chapman, S., & Robinson, G. (2009). *Oxford handbook of respiratory medicine* (2nd ed.). Oxford: OUP Oxford.

Darbari, D. S., Neely, M., van den Anker, J., & Rana, S. (2011). Increased clearance of morphine in sickle cell disease: Implications for pain management. *Journal of Pain, 12*(5), 531–538. doi:10.1016/j.jpain.2010.10.012

Hoffman, R., & Benz, E. J. (2013*). Hematology* (6th ed.). London: Elsevier Health Sciences.

Hsieh, M. M., Fitzhugh, C. D., & Tisdale, J. F. (2011). Allogeneic hematopoeitic stem cell transplant for sickle cell disease: The time is now. *Blood, 118*(5).

Kato, J. G, Hebbel, R. P, Steinberg, M. H., & Gladwin, M. T. (2009). Vasculopathy in sickle cell disease: Biology, pathophysiology, genetics, translational medicine, and new research directions. *American Journal of Hematology, 84*(9), 618–625. doi:10.1002/ajh.21475

Knight, J. A. (2010). Sickle cell disease. In J. Knight (Ed.), *Salem health genetics & inherited conditions* (pp. 1121–1125). Pasadena, CA: Salem Press.

Knight-Madden, J. M., Barton-Gooen, A., Weaver, S. R., Reid, M., & Greenough, A. (2013). Mortality, asthma, smoking, and acute chest syndrome in young adults with sickle cell disease. *Lung, 191*(1), 95–100. doi:10.1007/s00408–012–9435–3

Lanzkrou, S., Carroll, C. P., & Haywood, C. (2013). Mortality rates and age at death from sickle cell disease: U.S., 1979–2005. *Public Health Reports, 128*(2), 110–116.

McGann, P. T., Nero, A. C., & Ware, R. E. (2013). Current management of sickle cell anemia. *Cold Spring Harbor Perspectives in Medicine, 3*(8). doi:10.1101/cshperspect.a011817

Meremikwu, M. M., & Okomo, U. (2011). Sickle cell disease. *Clinical Evidence, 2011*(2402). Retrieved from http://www.ncbi.nlm.nih.gov/pmc/articles/PMC3217656/

Rees, D. C., Williams, T. N., & Gladwin M. T. (2010). Sickle-cell disease. *Lancet, 376*(9757), 2018–2031. doi:10.1016/S0140–6736(10)61029-X

Yusuf, H. R, Lloyd-Puryear, M. A., Grant, A. M., Parker, C. S., Creary, M. S., & Atrash, H. K. (2011). Sickle cell disease [Supplement 4]. *American Journal of Preventative Medicine, 41*(6), S376-S383.

CHAPTER 63

Coagulopathies

LISA EVANS

IDIOPATHIC THROMBOCYTOPENIC PURPURA (ITP)

I. **Definition**
   A. Autoimmune disorder
      1. B cells produce IgG autoantibodies
      2. Directed against platelet membrane
      3. Increase platelet destruction
      4. Inhibit platelet production
   B. Isolated thrombocytopenia
   C. No apparent associated conditions present (i.e., systemic lupus erythematosus and chronic lymphocytic leukemia)
   D. Classifications
      1. Primary: no identifiable underlying cause
      2. Secondary: immune mediated and associated with underlying disorder
      3. Chronic: lasting greater than 12 months
      4. Refractory: failure to respond, relapse occurs after splenectomy

II. **Incidence/predisposing factors**
   A. In children
      1. Usually precipitated by a viral illness
      2. Self-limiting
      3. Results in bruising and mucosal bleeding
   B. In adults
      1. Usually chronic
      2. Requires periodic treatment
   C. Disease of young persons: women ages 20–40 years outnumber men 2:1
   D. Spontaneous recovery occurs in only 5% of adult cases

E. Thrombocytopenia may be induced by the following:
  1. Heparin (most common cause in hospitalized patients)
  2. Sulfonamides
  3. Thiazides
  4. Quinine
  5. Cimetidine
  6. Gold
F. Thrombocytopenic purpura is a common secondary manifestation of
  1. Systemic lupus erythematosus in 14% to 26% of patients
  2. Chronic lymphocytic leukemia
G. Approximately two thirds of patients require no further treatment after splenectomy; response is achieved within 10 days
H. Thirteen thousand new cases of adult ITP are believed to occur each year in the United States.

III. **Subjective/physical examination findings**
A. Presenting complaint is usually mucosal or epidermal bleeding
  1. Epistaxis
  2. Oral bleeding
  3. Menorrhagia
  4. Purpura
  5. Petechiae
  6. Menorrhagia
B. Patient is usually systemically well
C. Patient is afebrile and usually appears well, with no abnormal findings on examination except those related to bleeding
D. Spleen is nonpalpable

IV. **Laboratory/diagnostic findings**
A. Thrombocytopenia is the hallmark of the disease; may be fewer than 20,000 platelets per microliter
B. No definitive test for ITP exists; diagnosis occurs by exclusion
C. Other hematopoietic cell lines are normal, although platelets are enlarged (megathrombocytes)
D. Ten percent of patients have coexistent autoimmune hemolytic anemia (Evans syndrome)
  1. Anemia, reticulocytosis, and spherocytes are seen on peripheral smear
  2. No fragmented cells (schistocytes) should be seen
E. Antinuclear antibody testing may point to an autoimmune process
F. Consider ordering the following:
  1. Monoclonal antibody immobilization of platelet antigens
    a. Considered the most sensitive and specific antibody test
    b. IgG platelet antibodies are present in 90% of patients
  2. Bone marrow biopsy (normal or increased megakaryocytes) to exclude myelodysplasia

3. Peripheral blood smear to confirm the automated count and to rule out ethylenediaminetetraacetic acid artifact from the test
   a. Platelet clumping may be seen in a purple-top tube with ethylenediaminetetraacetic acid
   b. Platelet count should be repeated with a blue-top tube with sodium citrate or a green-top tube with heparin
4. WinRho, also called anti-D antibody therapy, consists of concentrated antibodies that bind to the Rh antigen on red blood cells. It works only in Rh-positive individuals born to Rh-negative mothers. It helps increase platelet count but may cause anemia. Determine blood type, specifically Rh status, if WinRho treatment (described subsequently) is considered as a treatment option.

V. **Management**

A. Treatment may not be needed until the platelet count is less than 20,000/μl, unless the patient is symptomatic
   1. Initial treatment consists of prednisone, 1–2 mg/kg/day
   2. Bleeding often diminishes within 1 day of treatment initiation
   3. Elevation of platelets is usually seen within a week
B. High-dose intravenous gamma globulin (1 gram/kg for 1 or 2 days) is highly effective
   1. Very expensive treatment (approximately $5,000)
   2. Usually produces response in 1–5 days (90%) that only lasts 1–2 weeks
   3. Usually reserved for emergency situations
   4. In HIV-related ITP, gamma globulin (2 mg/kg/day in divided doses) is preferred to steroids
C. Splenectomy is highly effective
   1. Indicated when prednisone therapy fails
   2. Pneumococcal vaccine should be considered several weeks before splenectomy to minimize complications from sepsis
D. Chemotherapy is used for those who fail to respond to splenectomy and prednisone therapy
   1. Danazol, 600 mg/day in 2–4 divided doses, for 2 months, or
   2. Immunosuppressive agents
      a. Vincristine, 1–2 mg for adults for 5–7 days, 3 courses
      b. Vinblastine, 0.1 mg/kg, maximum dose 10 mg, for 5–7 days, 3 courses
      c. Azathioprine, 50–250 mg (average, 150 mg) for 3–26 months (average, 10 months)
      d. Cyclophosphamide, 50–200 mg/day for 1–9 months; used in refractory cases
E. Thrombopoiesis stimulating agents
F. Platelet transfusion is used only in cases of life-threatening bleeding
G. WinRho for Rh-positive individuals with ITP born to Rh-negative mothers

1. 10 mg/kg of body weight followed by daily doses of 20 mg/kg until either their platelet count increases to a minimum of 20,000–30,000/mm² or hemoglobin levels decrease greater than 2 grams/dl, which indicates anemia.

H. Most serious complication of ITP: spontaneous intracranial hemorrhage
   1. Less than 1% of patients are afflicted with this disorder
   2. Patients are at risk when platelet count is lower than 5000/µl

HEPARIN-INDUCED THROMBOCYTOPENIA (HIT)

I.   **Definition**
   A. Thrombocytopenia induced by heparin
   B. Produces arterial and venous thrombosis
   C. Categories:
      1. Functional: fall in platelet count within 1–4 days after heparin initiation, returns to normal with discontinuation of heparin (most common)
      2. Immunologic fall in platelet count within 5–10 days after heparin initiation; immune-mediated disorder, this type has a higher incidence of thromboembolic events.
      3. IgG autoantibody formation against heparin-platelet factor 4 complex

II. **Incidence/predisposing factors**
   A. Most common type of drug-induced thrombocytopenia
   B. Most common cause of thrombocytopenia in hospitalized patients
   C. Occurs with low molecular weight heparin and with unfractionated heparin, but occurs more often with unfractionated heparin
   D. Occurs more frequently in surgical patients
      1. Surgical performance measure include DVT/VTE prophylaxis
      2. Patients who undergo cardiopulmonary bypass receive a large heparin load

III. **Subjective/physical examination findings**
   A. Often initially asymptomatic
   B. May develop symptoms related to arterial or venous thromboses
   C. Related to location of venous or arterial thromboses
   D. Skin necrosis at injection site
   E. Anaphylactic reaction after intravenous or subcutaneous heparin injection

IV. **Laboratory/diagnostic findings**
   A. Suspect HIT if platelets have fallen greater than 50% from previous value, even if absolute thrombocytopenia does not exist
   B. Tests used to detect HIT include the following:
      1. Heparin-induced platelet aggregation assay: with 90% sensitivity and 100% specificity, measures platelet aggregation optically

2. Serotonin release assay along with heparin-induced platelet aggregation assay is considered HIT testing reference standard
3. Platelet C serotonin release assay: test is difficult, time consuming, and requires radioactive isotopes; 94% sensitive and 100% specific
4. Heparin PF4 enzyme-linked immunosorbent assay: immunologic test, depends on direct detection of heparin-induced antibodies

C. Additional considerations
   1. Utilize the American Society of Hematology's 2009 Clinical Practice Guidelines on the Evaluation and Management of HIT. "The 4 T's" provides a clinical probability scoring model based on the following:
      a. The extent of thrombocytopenia
      b. Timing of thrombocytopenia
      c. Presence of thrombosis
      d. Thrombocytopenia, other causes
      e. A score of 4 or higher indicates an intermediate to high risk of HIT

V.   Management

A. Hematology referral for suspected cases
B. The key lies in recognition of the syndrome and discontinuation of heparin because of the high risk of associated thrombosis
C. Direct thrombin inhibitors should be substituted as alternative forms of anticoagulation, when indicated, as follows:
   1. Danaparoid: adjust dose based on weight and renal function
      a. Initial bolus dosing or accelerated initial infusion
      b. Followed by maintenance infusion
   2. Argatroban: initiate infusion of 2 µg/kg/min
      a. Hepatic impairment: initiate dose at 0.5 µg/kg/min
      b. Does not require renal adjustment
      c. Adjust Partial Thromboplastin Time to steady-state of 1.5–3 times baseline (not to exceed 100 seconds)
      d. Therapeutic aPTT levels often achieved within 1–3 hr
      e. Check aPTT 2 hr after initiation of therapy
   3. Bivalirudin (Angiomax): initiate infusion of 0.15 µg/kg/hr
      a. Adjust to steady-state aPTT of 1.5–2.5 times baseline
      b. Can be adjusted for renal/hepatic impairment
   4. Fondaparinux: weight based
      a. Use with caution in renal impairment (creatinine clearance, 30–50 ml/min)
      b. Contraindicated with creatinine clearance less than 30 ml/min
   5. Transition to warfarin when the following conditions are met:
      a. Properly anticoagulated with thrombin specific inhibitor, overlap with warfarin until international normalized ratio (INR) is at goal
      b. Platelet count has increased to over 150,000

    c. Start with less than 5 mg/day: dosing for target goal INR of 2.0–3.0

    d. Minimum of 5 days overlapping therapy with thrombin inhibitor and warfarin before discontinuing thrombin inhibitor

DISSEMINATED INTRAVASCULAR COAGULATION (DIC)

I.   **Definition**

    A. Acquired coagulation disorder (with hemorrhage and thrombosis) that occurs as a secondary process concomitant with a pathophysiologic disease or a clinical state

    B. Hemorrhagic syndrome

       1. Caused by consumption of many coagulation factors and platelets

       2. An abnormal stimulus results in the formation of excess thrombin, which, in turn, causes the following:

          a. Fibrinogen consumption

          b. Irreversible platelet aggregation

          c. Activation of the fibrinolytic system

    C. Other names

       1. Consumptive coagulopathy

       2. Diffuse intravascular coagulation

II.   **Incidence/predisposing factors**

    A. Infection is the most common cause; 10% to 20% of cases are caused by gram-negative sepsis

    B. Often associated with

       1. Obstetric complications

       2. Malignant neoplasms

       3. Liver disease

       4. Trauma

       5. Burns

    C. Transfusion of ABO-incompatible red blood cells

III. **Subjective/physical examination findings**

    A. Bleeding complications are most common

       1. The patient may exhibit mild symptoms, such as oozing from venipuncture sites or wounds

       2. Typically, bleeding occur from multiple sites

    B. The patient may complain of bleeding that is

       1. Oral

       2. Gingival

       3. Gastrointestinal

       4. Genitourinary

    C. Acute DIC

       1. Tachycardia

       2. Hypotension

       3. Edema

    D. Other possible findings

1. Spontaneous bruising
2. Gastrointestinal bleeding
3. Respiratory tract bleeding
4. Hematuria
5. Persistent bleeding at venipuncture sites or wounds
6. Skin necrosis
7. Venous thromboembolism

E. Thrombosis
   1. May be superficial or deep venous (Trousseau syndrome)
   2. Digital ischemia and gangrene may be the most common forms
   3. Thrombosis is most common in patients with cancer

IV. **Laboratory/diagnostic findings**

A. No single laboratory test is diagnostic; clinical states are not static

B. International Society of Thrombosis and Hematology (ISTH) "Diagnostic scoring system for overt DIC" 2009 may be used to aid in diagnosis. It is a five-step algorithm to calculate DIC score. It has a 91% sensitivity and 97% specificity.

C. Of the fibrin degradation products, the D-dimer is the most sensitive.

D. Hypofibrinogenemia is also a very important finding (limited disorders cause this finding)

E. Acute uncompensated DIC (active hemorrhage evident)
   1. Thrombocytopenia—platelet count less than 150,000/µl universal finding
   2. Prothrombin time (PT) and aPTT are prolonged by 70% and 50%, respectively
   3. Fibrinogen, factor V, and factor VII levels are low
   4. Fragmented red blood cells (schistocytes) are found on peripheral blood smear

F. Subacute DIC
   1. PT and aPTT are usually normal
   2. Fibrinogen levels are usually normal
   3. Thrombocytopenia and an elevated D-dimer may be the only abnormal laboratory values

G. Chronic or compensated DIC
   1. Elevated fibrin degradation product levels (FDPs greater than 45 µg/ml, or present in greater than 1:100 dilution)
   2. D-Dimer is most sensitive (positive at greater than 1:8 dilution) for differentiating DIC from primary fibrinolysis

H. Consider ordering the following:
   1. Blood cultures to rule out sepsis
   2. Repeat fibrinogen levels and partial thromboplastin time (PTT)
      a. Initially, fibrinogen levels may be normal in DIC because fibrinogen half-life is approximately 4 days.
      b. Diagnosis is confirmed by rapidly falling fibrinogen levels

> **3.** Factor VIII (usually in the normal range in coagulopathy associated with liver disease alone)

V. Management

A. Hematology referral for suspected cases

B. Diagnose and correct the underlying cause

  1. Correct hypotension

  2. Control sepsis

  3. Deliver placenta or dead fetus

C. When risks of hemorrhagic complications are significant, maintenance of blood volume and hemostatic function is indicated.

  1. Packed red blood cells

  2. Replacement therapy by platelet transfusion (goal: platelet count of 30,000–50,000/μl)

  3. Cryoprecipitate

   a. Goal: plasma fibrinogen level of 150 mg/dl

   b. One unit cryoprecipitate increases fibrinogen level by approximately 6–8 mg/dl

   c. Administration of 15 units raises the level from 50–150 mg/dl

  4. Fresh frozen plasma every 30 min in severe DIC

D. Supportive treatment includes prevention of hypoxemia and hemodynamic compromise

E. Heparin therapy is controversial but is considered appropriate, with thrombosis or fibrin deposition producing acral cyanosis. A dose of 500–750 units per hour is usually sufficient, but this cannot be effective if antithrombin III levels are depleted.

  1. Antithrombin III levels should be measured

  2. Fresh frozen plasma or concentrates of antithrombin III should be used to raise levels more than 50%.

  3. When heparin is used, it is not necessary to prolong the PTT

  4. Success is measured by increasing fibrinogen levels and declining fibrin degradation products

F. Temperature also has an effect on coagulation factor enzymes. The literature suggests that each decrease of 1 degree Celsius reduces activities by approximately 10% (particularly the interaction of von Willebrand factor with platelet glycoprotein Ib/Ix).

G. Five new approaches are available for measuring coagulation:

  1. Platelet function analyzer (PFA-100)

   a. Substitute for bleeding time

   b. Used for diagnosing different types of von Willebrand disease

   c. Distinguishing von Willebrand disease from platelet function

  2. Waveform analysis (in bleeding disorders and hemophilia)

  3. Thrombin generation test (used to monitor treatment in hemophilia)

  4. Overall hemostasis potential

  5. Thrombelastography

BIBLIOGRAPHY

American Society of Hematology. (2011). *Evidenced-based practice guidelines for immune thrombocytopenia*. Retrieved from http://www.hematology.org/Practice/Guidelines/2934.aspx

Cuker, A., & Crowther, M. A. (2013). Clinical practice guideline on the evaluation and management of adults with suspected HIT. *American Society of Hematology*. Retrieved from http://www.hematology.org/Practice/Guidelines/2934.aspx

Favaloro, E. J. (2010). Laboratory testing in disseminated intravascular coagulation. *Seminars in Thrombosis and Hemostasis, 36*(4), 458–467. doi:10.1055/s-0030–1254055

Levi, M., Toh, C. H., Thachel, J., & Watson, H. G. (2009). Guidelines for the diagnosis and management of disseminated intravascular coagulation. *British Journal of Haematology, 145*(1), 24–33.doi:10.1111/j.1365–2141.2009.07600.x

Levi, M., & van der Poll, T. (2013). Disseminated intravascular coagulation: A review for the internist. *Internal and Emergency Medicine, 8*(1), 23–32. doi:10.1007/s11739–012–0859–9

Linkins, L., Dans, A. L., Moores, L. K., Bona, R., Davidson, B. L., Schulman, S., & Crowther, M. (2012). Treatment and prevention of heparin-induced thrombocytopenia: Antithrombotic therapy and prevention of thrombosis (9th ed.): American College of Chest Physicians Evidence-Based Clinical Practice Guidelines [Supplement]. *Chest, 14*(2), e495s-e550s. doi:10.1378/chest.11–2303

Provan, D., Stasi, R., Newland, A. C., Blanchette, V. S., Bolton-Maggs, P., Bussel, J. B., . . . Kuter, D. J. (2010). International consensus report on the investigation and management of primary immune thrombocytopenia. *Blood, 115*(2), 168–186. doi:10.1182/blood-2009–06–225565

Management of Patients with Oncologic Disorders

CHAPTER 64

Leukemias

JACQUELINE RHOADS

ACUTE LYMPHOCYTIC LEUKEMIA

I.   Definition
   A. Malignancy that causes hematopoietic progenitor cells to lose their ability to mature normally and differentiate
   B. Cells proliferate in uncontrolled fashion and ultimately replace normal bone marrow, leading to decreased production of normal red blood cells (RBC), white blood cells (WBC), and platelets

II. Incidence/predisposing factors
   A. No clear cause; suggested greater incidence in benzene and petroleum product exposure
   B. Slightly higher incidence in populations of European descent
   C. Constitutes 80% of all childhood leukemias, with peak onset at ages 3–7 years, and 20% of adult leukemias; incidence of second peak at age 60 years
   D. Acute lymphocytic leukemia (ALL) is the most common cancer and the leading cause of death in children younger than 15 years.
   E. Survivors of ALL are at risk for late sequelae of secondary brain tumors
   F. Childhood ALL survivors are at greater risk for reduced growth (secondary to cranial irradiation and resultant decreased bone mass), learning disabilities, and osteoporotic fractures in later life.

III. Subjective/physical examination findings
   A. Usually sudden onset of acute illness for days or weeks
   B. Fever
   C. Anorexia
   D. Fatigue
   E. Bone and joint pain

    F. Dyspnea

    G. Gum hypertrophy and gingival bleeding

    H. Epistaxis

    I. Angina

    J. Pale, with purpura and petechiae

    K. Generalized lymphadenopathy

    L. Gingival hypertrophy

    M. Stomatitis

    N. Hepatosplenomegaly

    O. Bone tenderness, particularly in the sternum and tibia

IV. **Laboratory/diagnostic findings**

    A. Pancytopenia with circulating blasts is the hallmark of the disease

    B. Blasts present in the peripheral smear in 90% of cases

    C. Bone marrow is usually hypercellular; diagnosis requires that more than 30% of cells are blasts. (The World Health Organization has proposed changing the threshold between myelodysplastic syndrome and acute myelogenous leukemia [AML] to 20% marrow blasts and deleting the category of refractory anemia with excess blasts in transformation.)

    D. Anemia occurs in most patients; decreases in RBCs and in hemoglobin (Hgb), and hematocrit (Hct) levels range from mild to severe

    E. Platelets are usually decreased but may be in the normal range

    F. Bone marrow biopsy is often essential for establishing the diagnosis owing to the variability of preceding factors

    G. Hyperuricemia and azotemia are present

    H. Terminal deoxynucleotidyl transferase is present in 95% of cases

    I. Consider ordering the following:

        1. Immunophenotyping by fluorescent-activated cell sorter (FACS) with monoclonal antibodies directed at leukemia-specific antigens at the time of diagnosis. Monoclonal antibodies may be used to define other phenotypes of ALL.

            a. Primitive B-lymphocyte antigens include CD19 and sometimes CD10

            b. T-cell ALL is diagnosed by the finding of CD2, CD5, and CD7

        2. Cytogenetic studies (prognostic value)

            a. Hyperdiploid states: more favorable prognosis

            b. Unfavorable prognosis found with Philadelphia chromosomes t(9;22) and t(4;11).

        3. Bone marrow stains

            a. Periodic acid-Schiff—positive

            b. Sudan black—negative

            c. Myeloperoxidase—negative

            d. Terminal deoxynucleotidyl transferase—positive

        4. Chromosome analysis

5. Multiparametric flow cytometry (confirms light microscopy diagnosis; may be useful for relapse prediction)
6. Electron microscopy (rarely used except in poorly differentiated leukemia)
7. Molecular genetic studies
8. Screening lumbar puncture (if central nervous system [CNS] involvement)

V. **Management**

A. Hematology/oncology referral for suspected cases
B. Treatment is usually supportive or is designed to eradicate leukemic cell mass. Stem cell transplant is the goal whenever possible.
   1. Cures are infrequent except in children
   2. In adults, expect at least a 25% disease-free 5-year survival, and with aggressive regimens, a 35% to 40% 5-year survival
C. Supportive care may include the following, when indicated. For Ph-positive patients, tyrosine kinase inhibitors (TKIs) will be part of the induction therapy.
   1. Transfusion of RBCs or platelets
   2. Hydration
   3. Aggressive antibiotic therapy for infection
   4. Allopurinol, 100–200 mg PO 3 times a day, to prevent hyperuricemia and renal damage; should be initiated before marrow-ablative chemotherapy is initiated
   5. Acetazolamide, 500 mg/day, to promote alkalinization of urine
D. If patient remains uremic, consider dialysis before initiation of chemotherapy
E. Chemotherapy
   1. Given according to protocols
   2. Divided into three phases:
      a. Remission induction
      b. Postremission therapy consolidation
      c. CNS prophylaxis
   3. Remission induction therapy
      a. Initial treatment is combination chemotherapy plus TKI if Ph-positive or a clinical trial
      b. A number of combinations are used
         i. Usual drugs include vincristine, prednisone, cyclophosphamide, vincristine, doxorubicin, dexamethasone, cytarabine, methotrexate, vincristine, imatinib, or dasatinib as the TKIs.
         ii. Intrathecal methotrexate with l-asparaginase is another standard combination; intrathecal methotrexate ± cytarabine ± corticosteroids is standard
      c. Maintenance therapy usually includes 6-mercaptopurine and methotrexate

4. Postremission therapy consolidation
   a. Short courses of further chemotherapy are given
   b. Usually, chemotherapy agents not used to initiate therapy, such as the following:
      i. High-dose methotrexate
      ii. Cyclophosphamide
      iii. Cytarabine
      iv. TKIs in Ph-positive patients
   c. Common maintenance therapies
      i. Daily low dose of 6-mercaptopurine, or
      ii. Weekly or biweekly doses of methotrexate
      iii. TKIs in Ph-positive patients with nelarabine preferred in refractory T-cell ALL
5. CNS prophylaxis: intrathecal methotrexate alone or in combination with radiation therapy
   a. CNS relapse is much higher in ALL than in AML
F. Bone marrow transplantation should be considered at the time of first relapse or second remission
G. M.D. Anderson Cancer Center has reported a regimen for relapsed ALL that alternates four cycles of fractionated high-dose cyclophosphamide, vincristine, doxorubicin, and dexamethasone with four cycles of high-dose cytosine-arabinoside/daunorubicin (HDAC) and high-dose methotrexate.

VI. Definition

A. Malignancy of hematopoietic progenitor cell
B. An acute leukemia very similar to ALL, distinguished by morphologic examination and cytochemistry that differentiates myeloblasts from lymphoblasts
C. The classification of AML encompasses four major categories:
   1. AML with recurrent genetic abnormalities
   2. AML with multilineage dysplasia
   3. Therapy-related AML
   4. AML not otherwise categorized
D. The required bone marrow or peripheral blood blast percentage for the diagnosis of AML has been recently reduced from 30% (French-American-British classification) to 20% (World Health Organization classification, 2001).

VII. Incidence/predisposing factors

A. No clear cause
B. Chromosomal abnormalities are found in most patients with acute leukemias
C. Increased incidence in patients with Down syndrome
D. Predominant type of acute leukemia in adults: 80% of acute leukemias in individuals older than 20 years
E. Incidence increases with age: median age is 67 years

F. Increased incidence of associated disseminated intravascular coagulation (DIC), especially with acute promyelocytic leukemia (M3 variant)

VIII.   **Subjective/physical examination findings**
- A. Bleeding
- B. Shortness of breath
- C. Easy bruising
- D. Fever
- E. Anorexia/weight loss
- F. Fatigue
- G. Headache
- H. Bone and joint pain
- I. Bone tenderness—particularly in the sternum and tibia
- J. Therapy related (secondary AML) is a consequence of prior cancer treated with cytotoxic agents for solid tumor or hematologic cancers and is rising as survivorship from cancers has risen
- K. Environmental exposure to petrochemicals and or ionizing radiation
- L. Increased incidence of DIC especially with acute promyelocytic leukemia (M3 variant)
- M. Occasional lymphadenopathy
- N. Hepatosplenomegaly
- O. Stomatitis and gingival hypertrophy
- P. Purpura, petechiae, and overt bleeding
- Q. Signs of infection

IX.   **Laboratory/diagnostic findings**
- A. Pancytopenia with circulating blasts
- B. Anemia in most patients; RBCs, Hgb and Hct levels, and platelets, usually decreased
- C. Most patients have at least mild thrombocytopenia; approximately 25% have severe thrombocytopenia (fewer than 20,000 platelets per microliter).
- D. Granules visible in blast cells
- E. Presence of Auer rods
- F. Many myeloblasts
- G. Monocytic lineage can be established by the finding of butyrate esterase
- H. DIC: Presents as an elevation in PT, PTT, fibrin degradation products, and D-dimer. The fibrinogen level is decreased
- I. Consider ordering the following:
    1. Human leukocyte antigen (HLA) typing at time of diagnosis in preparation for possible bone marrow transplantation
    2. Immunophenotyping by FACS with monoclonal antibodies directed at leukemia-specific antigens at time of diagnosis
        a. Favorable prognostics found with t(8;21), t(15;17), and inv(16)(p13;q22)

        b. Unfavorable prognostics found with monosomy 5 and 7 and complex abnormalities

   3. Bone marrow stain: result in AML is Sudan black positive and myeloperoxidase positive

   4. Uric acid

   5. Metabolic profile

   6. PT, PTT, fibrinogen, fibrin split products, and fibrin D-dimers

X. **Management**

  A. Treatments include chemotherapy, other drugs, radiation therapy, stem cell transplants, and targeted immune therapy. Once the leukemia is in remission, you need additional treatment to make sure that it does not come back (National Cancer Institute, National Institutes of Health).

  B. Hematology/oncology referral for suspected cases

  C. Supportive care includes

   1. Transfusion of RBCs or platelets

   2. Hydration

   3. Aggressive antibiotic therapy for infection

   4. Acetazolamide, 500 mg/day, to produce alkalinization of urine

   5. Allopurinol, 100–200 mg PO 3 times a day, to prevent hyperuricemia and renal damage

  D. If patient remains uremic, consider dialysis before initiating chemotherapy

  E. Chemotherapy is divided into remission induction therapy and consolidative and maintenance therapy. Chemotherapy is given according to protocols.

   1. Remission induction therapy options include one of the following equivalent combination chemotherapy regimens:

      a. Dose-intensive cytarabine-based induction therapy

      b. Cytarabine + daunorubicin

      c. Cytarabine + idarubicin

      d. Cytarabine + daunorubicin + thioguanine; cytarabine + daunorubicin + cladribine

      e. Mitoxantrone + etoposide; cytarabine + 5-azacytidine + decitabine

      f. Treatment of CNS leukemia, if present: intrathecal cytarabine or methotrexate

   2. Consolidative and maintenance therapy

      a. Cytarabine-based combination if tolerated

      b. Mitoxantrone + daunorubicin

      c. Mitoxantrone + idarubicin

      d. High-dose Ara-C, 1–3 grams/m^2 of body surface area, BID preferred

      e. Therapy for M3 subtype is initiated with retinoic acid, then is followed by consolidative and maintenance therapy with traditional agents (making the M3 diagnosis is crucial)

F. Bone marrow transplantation should be considered at the time of first relapse or second remission (reserved for "salvage" therapy). Bone marrow transplantation should be considered after induction therapy and each surveillance visit or change of treatment visit.

CHRONIC LYMPHOCYTIC LEUKEMIA

I.   Definition

  A. A chronic leukemia characterized by abnormal B lymphocytes and often generalized lymphadenopathy. In patients presenting predominately with blood and bone marrow involvement, it is called chronic lymphocytic leukemia (CLL); in those predominately with enlarged lymph nodes, it is called small lymphocytic lymphoma.

II.   Incidence/predisposing factors

  A. Most common type of leukemia in older adults

  B. Primarily a disease of the elderly

     1. Ninety percent of patients are older than 50 years

     2. Median age is 65 years

     3. Poorer prognosis with increased age

  C. Usually slow progression of disease, occasionally progressive

  D. Origin is unknown; first-degree relatives of patients with CLL have 3 times the normal risk of developing the disease and who have relatives of Russian or Eastern European Jewish decent

  E. Farmers have an increased incidence of CLL

  F. Men are more often affected than women (2:1)

  G. Associated with warm antibody autoimmune hemolytic anemia

  H. Median survival is approximately six years

  I. Clinical stage is strongest predictor of survival

III. Subjective/physical examination findings

  A. Frequently asymptomatic

  B. As disease progresses, patient may have

     1. Fatigue, malaise, and lethargy

     2. Anorexia/weight loss

     3. Early satiety

     4. Weight loss

     5. Occasionally, patients who exhibit infection have notable lymph node enlargement.

     6. Painless swelling of the lymph nodes in the neck, underarm, stomach, or groin

     7. Pain or a feeling of fullness below the ribs

  C. Fever is rare

  D. Patients with CLL have a strong reaction to insect bites, but this phenomenon has not been explained.

  E. Lymphadenopathy is present in 80% of patients

     1. Cervical, supraclavicular, and axillary nodes are most often involved

    2. Nodes are usually mobile and nontender and have a rubbery feel

  F. Hepatosplenomegaly is present in 50% of patients

  G. Progressive weight loss

  H. Patients may exhibit nodular or diffuse skin infiltrations

IV. **Laboratory/diagnostic findings**

  A. Lymphocytosis is a hallmark of the disease

    1. Minimum level is greater than 5,000/μl

    2. Usual range is 40,000–150,000/μl

  B. Lymphocytes constitute 75% to 98% of circulating cells

  C. Smudge cells are usually seen on peripheral smear

  D. Hypogammaglobulinemia is present in 50% of cases, more commonly in advanced disease.

  E. Immunoglobulin (Ig)G, IgA, or IgM levels are low in 25% of patients at diagnosis; with disease progression, levels are low in 50% to 70% of patients

  F. Consider ordering the following when diagnosis is uncertain:

    1. Immunophenotyping by FACS with monoclonal antibodies directed at leukemia-specific antigens at time of diagnosis

      a. B-lymphocyte lineage marker CD19 with T-lymphocyte marker CD5 observed only in CLL and mantle cell lymphoma

      b. Mutated forms of the immunoglobulin gene seen in indolent forms of CLL (low levels of surface antigen CD38); do not express the zeta-associated protein (ZAP-70)

      c. Poorer prognosis found in unmutated IgV genes and with high levels of ZAP-70

    2. Bone marrow biopsy

      a. More than 30% lymphocytes seen in disease

      b. Focal or diffuse infiltration can be seen on core biopsies

      c. Extent of marrow infiltration correlates directly with prognosis

  G. Rai system (prognostic staging)

    1. Stage 0, lymphocytosis only

    2. Stage I, lymphocytosis plus lymphadenopathy

    3. Stage II, organomegaly

    4. Stage III, anemia

    5. Stage IV, thrombocytopenia

V. **Management**

  A. Hematology/oncology referral for suspected cases

  B. History, physical examination, peripheral blood counts, and lymphocyte morphology are usually all that are required to diagnose CLL in the clinical setting.

  C. No specific therapy for patients in early disease, but patients are monitored carefully—"watchful waiting"

    1. Treatment is usually not initiated until symptoms occur

    2. Fatigue and malaise occasionally necessitate treatment

D. Monitor for lymphadenopathy, anemia, and thrombocytopenia; these require therapy, whether or not symptoms occur

E. Chemotherapy is given according to guidelines and are based on Rai stage, age (younger or older than 70 years), and present or absence of deletions at 11q and 17p. Chemotherapy is often combined with a targeted therapy drug (usually a monoclonal antibody) and/or an immunotherapy drug.

 1. If younger than 70 years

  a. FCR—fludarabine, cyclophosphamide, rituximab

  b. FR—fludarabine and rituximab

  c. PCR—pentostatin, cyclophosphamide, rituximab

  d. Bendamustine ± rituximab

  e. Consider stem cell transplant after induction for those younger than 65 years

 2. If 70 years and older

  a. Chlorambucil ± rituximab

  b. Bendamustine ± rituximab

  c. Alemtuzumab

  d. Lenalidomide

 3. If frontline treatment is not successful or relapse occurs, then the combination of drugs is changed or patient may be switched to one of the more aggressive lymphoma chemotherapy treatments per guidelines.

 4. Clinical guidelines indicate that fludarabine is now preferred by many as initial therapy, as opposed to its prior place as second-line therapy.

  a. Although studies have not shown significant differences in overall survival rates, a higher response rate that is more complete and lasting has been achieved with fludarabine.

  b. Fludarabine (Fludara), 25–30 mg/m^2/day for 5 days, every 4 weeks for 4–6 months

 5. Fludarabine in combination with rituximab, a chimeric monoclonal anti-CD20 antibody, has been shown to improve survival in CLL.

 6. Standard therapy has been chlorambucil (Leukeran), 0.6–1 mg PO every 3–6 weeks.

  a. Dosage is adjusted on the basis of development of thrombocytopenia or neutropenia, with maintenance continued for 6–12 months

  b. May be given on a pulsed schedule (0.5–2 mg/kg) over 1–4 days every 4 weeks, or every 2 weeks at half the dosage

  c. This treatment has been well tolerated, effective, and convenient and is often the first choice for elderly patients.

F. Cytoxan, Oncovin, and prednisone regimen (used less often)

 1. Cyclophosphamide (Cytoxan), 100–300 mg/m^2 PO on days 1 through 5

    2. Vincristine (Oncovin), 2 mg IV on day 1

    3. Prednisone, 100 mg PO on days 1 through 5

G. Other commonly used agents include:

    1. Cladribine ([2-chloro-2'-deoxyadenosine] Leustatin)

    2. Pentostatin ([2'-deoxycoformycin] Nipent)

H. Stage 0 or I disease median survival has increased to 10–15 years

I. Stage III or IV disease median survival is 2 years

J. Splenectomy in very select cases

K. Radiation is usually limited to localized nodal masses that are refractory to chemotherapy

L. Supportive care

    1. Annual influenza vaccine

    2. Pneumococcal vaccine every 5 years—Prevnar preferred

    3. Avoid all live vaccines including Zoster

CHRONIC MYELOGENOUS LEUKEMIA

I.   **Definition**

    A. Disorder characterized by myeloid cell overproduction; abnormal cells overcome and replace normal hematopoiesis

    B. Distinguished by the presence of Philadelphia chromosome in the leukemic cells (reciprocal translocation between the long arms of chromosomes 9 and 22); the translocated pieces form a fusion gene BCR/ABL protein that leads to leukemia

    C. Clonal stem cell disorder

    D. Also known as chronic granulocytic leukemia or chronic myeloid leukemia

II.   **Incidence/predisposing factors**

    A. Accounts for 7% to 15% of adult leukemias

    B. Primarily a disorder of middle age

        1. Median age is 67 years

        2. May occur in patients as young as 10 years or as old as 80 years

    C. Ionizing radiation exposure increases risk of chronic myelogenous leukemia (CML). Atomic bomb survivors have a dose-related increased incidence of CML that peaks 5–12 years after exposure.

    D. Etiology is unknown. Chromosomal abnormality is invariably associated with disease

    E. Children of parents with CML have no greater incidence than is found in the general population.

    F. Median survival has been 3–4 years, but with the addition of targeted agents, more than 80% are in remission at 4 years. Since targeted agents, patients may expect to have a "normal" life span if the respond to the TKIs.

III.   **Subjective/physical examination findings**

    A. Insidious onset

    B. Fatigue

    C. Early satiety

    D. Weight loss

    E. Diminished exercise tolerance

    F. Common after disease progression

        1. Low-grade fever

        2. Dizziness

        3. Irritability

        4. Increased sweating/night sweats

        5. Abdominal fullness (left upper quadrant)

        6. Bone pain

        7. Blurred vision

        8. Respiratory distress

        9. Splenomegaly in 60% of cases

        10. Bone pain/sternal tenderness

        11. Hepatomegaly (less common)

        12. Bleeding and infection may be present in blast crisis

IV.   **Laboratory/diagnostic findings**

    A. Hallmark of CML is WBC elevation (15,000–500,000/µl; frequently 150,000/µl at initial diagnosis). Blasts are usually less than 5%

    B. Diagnosis established with the presence of BCR/ABL gene detected in the peripheral blood with the use of polymerase chain reaction; polymerase chain reaction also provides predictive power of disease progression

    C. Hgb and Hct levels initially are normal; they may decrease with disease progression

    D. Platelets may be increased initially; they will decrease with disease progression

    E. Vitamin B12 serum levels are usually elevated (sometimes to more than 10 times normal levels)

    F. Lactate dehydrogenase (LDH) and uric acid levels may be elevated

    G. Philadelphia chromosome is present in peripheral blood or bone marrow (bone marrow examination is not necessary for diagnosis).

    H. Characteristic finding is low to absent leukocyte alkaline phosphatase (LAP), also called neutrophilic alkaline phosphatase (NAP) (normal: males, 22–124 units/L; females, 33–149 units/L)

V.   **Management**

    A. Hematology/oncology referral for suspected cases

    B. Immediate therapy is not indicated unless

        1. WBC count is lower than 200,000/µl, or

        2. Evidence indicates

            a. Priapism

            b. Confusion

            c. Venous thrombosis

            d. Visual blurring

            e. Dyspnea

    C. Therapy is started immediately with the tyrosine kinase inhibitor of imatinib, which is a selective inhibitor of BCR-ABL

D. However, other therapy may be used based on BCR-ABL KD mutation status after imatinib failure or intolerance.
   1. The first would be to change to a different tyrosine kinase inhibitor such as nilotinib or bosutinib
   2. Omacetaxine can be considered after the resistance or intolerance to two TKIs has occurred
   3. Hematopoietic stem cell transplant is considered based on TKI response and patient's clinical condition
E. Supportive therapy includes:
   1. Hydration
   2. Allopurinol, 100 mg 3 times a day, for hyperuricemia
   3. For symptomatic leukocytosis, hydroxyurea or apheresis can be used in addition to the TKI.
   4. For symptomatic thrombocytosis, hydroxyurea, antiaggregants, anagrelide, or apheresis can be used.
F. Treatment with a TKI continuous with evaluation at month 3 and 6 then every 6 months
   1. Evaluate toxicities and patient compliance at each evaluation in addition to response by bone marrow evaluation
   2. Drugs that induce or inhibit the CYP3A4 or CYP3A5 enzymes may alter therapeutic effects of all the TKIs. Proton pump inhibitors may alter plasma levels of bosutinib.
   3. TKI has many toxicities beside the usual hematological seen with chemotherapy and include increase liver function test, fluid retention, muscle cramping, skin rash, prolong QT intervals, pulmonary hypertension, or diarrhea.
      a. For toxicities: stop the TKI
      b. Correct the toxicity
      c. Notify the oncologist who will determine when or if the TKI should be resumed
G. Imatinib mesylate (Gleevec), a BCR-ABL tyrosine kinase inhibitor, is the drug of choice in the management of patient with CML in other countries and is yielding promising results in current studies in the U.S.
H. Allogeneic bone marrow transplantation (usually sibling matched) is the only curative therapy. Treatment is as follows:
   1. More effective in younger patients
      a. In the early chronic phase
      b. With matching, related donor
   2. Usually available for those younger than age 60 years with a matching sibling donor
I. Median survival without bone marrow transplantation is 3–4 years
J. Long-term survival rate for adults with transplantation is 60%, but 1-year mortality rate is increased owing to transplantation adverse effects

BIBLIOGRAPHY

Malek, S. (2013). *Advances in Chronic Lymphocytic Leukemia*. Boston, MA: Springer US.

Diehl, V. (2014). *Hodgkin's lymphoma, an issue of hematology/oncology clinics*. Amsterdam: Elsevier.

Harmening, D. (2009). *Clinical hematology and fundamentals of hemostasis* (5th ed.). Philadelphia, PA: F. A. Davis Co.

Hashad, D. (2012). *Cancer management*. Rijeka: InTech.

Leung, L. L. K. (2013). Disseminated intravascular coagulation. In E. G. Nabel (Ed.), *ACP medicine*. Philadelphia, PA: Decker Publishing.

Levi, M., & Seligsohn, U. (2010). Disseminated intravascular coagulation. In E. Beutler, T. Kipps, K. Kaushanksy, M. Lichtman, J. Prchal, & U. Seligsohn (Eds.), *Williams hematology* (8th ed., pp. 2101–2120). New York, NY: McGraw-Hill.

McPhee, S. J., & Papadakis, M. A. (2011). *Current medical diagnosis & treatment 2011* (50th ed.). New York, NY: McGraw-Hill Medical.

National Cancer Institute, National Institutes of Health. (2013). *Adult acute lymphoblastic leukemia treatment*. Retrieved from http://www.cancer.gov/cancertopics/pdq/treatment/adultALL/healthprofessional

National Cancer Institute, National Institutes of Health. (2013). *Adult acute myeloid leukemia treatment*. Retrieved from http://www.cancer.gov/cancertopics/pdq/treatment/adultAML/healthprofessional

National Cancer Institute, National Institutes of Health. (2013). *Childhood acute myeloid leukemia/other myeloid malignancies treatment*. Retrieved from http://www.cancer.gov/cancertopics/pdq/treatment/childAML/healthprofessional

National Cancer Institute, National Institutes of Health. (2013). *Childhood acute lymphoblastic leukemia treatment*. Retrieved from http://www.cancer.gov/cancertopics/pdq/treatment/childALL/healthprofessional

National Cancer Institute, National Institutes of Health. (2013). *Chronic lymphocytic leukemia treatment*. Retrieved from http://www.cancer.gov/cancertopics/pdq/treatment/CLL/healthprofessional

National Cancer Institute, National Institutes of Health. (2013). *Chronic myelogenous leukemia treatment*. Retrieved from http://www.cancer.gov/cancertopics/pdq/treatment/CML/healthprofessional

National Cancer Institute, National Institutes of Health. (2013). *Hairy cell leukemia treatment*. Retrieved from http://www.cancer.gov/cancertopics/pdq/treatment/hairy-cell-leukemia/healthprofessional

National Comprehensive Cancer Network. (2013). *Acute lymphoblastic leukemia*. Retrieved from http://www.nccn.org/professionals/physician_gls/PDF/aml.pdf

National Comprehensive Cancer Network. (2013). *Acute myeloid leukemia*. Retrieved from http://www.nccn.org/professionals/physician_gls/PDF/aml.pdf

National Comprehensive Cancer Network. (2013). *Chronic myelogenous leukemia*. Retrieved from http://www.nccn.org/professionals/physician_gls/PDF/cml.pdf

National Comprehensive Cancer Network. (2013). *Non-Hodgkin's lymphomas*. Retrieved from http://www.nccn.org/professionals/physician_gls/PDF/nhl.pdf

Perry, M. C. (2012). *Perry's the chemotherapy source book* (5th ed.). Philadelphia, PA: Wolters Kluwer Health/Lippincott Williams & Wilkins.

Popat, U. R., & Abraham, J. (2011). *Leukemia*. New York, NY: DemosMedical.

Rodgers, G. M. (2009). Acquired coagulation disorders. In D. A. Arber, J. Foerster, B. Glader, J. P. Greer, R. T. Means, Jr., F. Praskevas, & G. M. Rodgers (Eds.), *Wintrobe's clinical hematology* (12th ed., pp. 1425–1464). Philadelphia, PA: Lippincott, Williams and Wilkins.

Washburn, L. (2011). CME Chronic lymphocytic leukemia: The most common leukemia in adults. *Journal of the American Academy of Physician Assistants, 24*(5), 54–58.

CHAPTER 65

Lymphoma

JENNA RUSH

STAGING

I. **Ann Arbor Staging Classification is the anatomic staging system that parallels non-Hodgkin lymphoma (NHL) and Hodgkin disease.**

    A. Stage I: single lymph node or single extralymphatic origin

    B. Stage II: two or more lymph node regions or extralymphatic sites on the same side of the diaphragm

    C. Stage III: involvement of lymph node regions or extralymphatic sites on both sides of the diaphragm

    D. Stage IV: diffuse or disseminated involvement of more than one extralymphatic organ with or without associated lymph node involvement. Bone marrow involvement confers Stage IV designation.

II. **Cotswold modifications of the Ann Arbor Classification system**

    A. Bulky disease (X) (thoracic ratio of maximum transverse mass diameter) 33% or more of the internal transverse thoracic diameter (e.g., Stage IX)

    B. Number of anatomic regions involved should be indicated by a subscript (e.g., II_3).

    C. Stage III may be subdivided into the following:

        1. III_1, with or without splenic, hilar, celiac, or portal nodes

        2. III_2, with para-aortic, iliac, or mesenteric nodes

    D. Staging should be identified as clinical stage or pathological stage

    E. New category of response to therapy, unconfirmed/uncertain complete remission, can be designated following persistent radiologic abnormalities of uncertain significance.

III. **Revised European American Lymphoma Classification (REAL)**

    A. B-cell neoplasms

1. Precursor B-cell neoplasms; precursor B-lymphoblastic leukemia/lymphoma
2. Peripheral B-cell neoplasms
   a. B-cell chronic lymphocytic leukemia/prolymphocytic leukemia/small lymphocytic lymphoma
   b. Lymphoplasmacytoid lymphoma/immunocytoma
   c. Mantle cell lymphoma
   d. Follicle center lymphoma, follicular lymphoma
   e. Provisional cytologic grades
      i. Grade I: small cell
      ii. Grade II: mixed small and large cell
      iii. Grade III: large cell
      iv. Provisional subtype: diffuse, predominantly small cell type
   f. Marginal zone B-cell lymphoma
      i. Extranodal (mucosa-associated lymphoid tissue type with B cells that are usually IGM and Bcl-2 positive but not always)
      ii. Provisional subtype: nodal and sometimes called monocytoid B-cell lymphoma secondary to the presence of that type of B-cells
   g. Provisional entity: splenic marginal zone lymphoma characterized by the presence of circulating villous lymphocytes
   h. Hairy cell leukemia
   i. Plasmacytoma/plasma cell myeloma
   j. Diffuse large B-cell lymphoma; subtype: primary mediastinal (thymic) B-cell lymphoma
   k. Burkitt lymphoma
   l. Provisional entity: high-grade B-cell lymphoma, Burkitt-like
B. T-cell and putative natural killer (NK) cell neoplasms
   1. Precursor T-cell neoplasms; precursor T-lymphoblastic lymphoma/leukemia
   2. Peripheral T-cell and NK cell neoplasms
      a. T-cell chronic lymphocytic leukemia/prolymphocytic leukemia
      b. Large granular lymphocytic leukemia
         i. T-cell type
         ii. NK cell type
      c. Mycosis fungoides/Sézary syndrome
      d. Peripheral T-cell lymphomas, unspecified
         i. Provisional cytologic categories
            (a) Medium-sized cell
            (b) Mixed medium-sized and large cells
            (c) Large cell

　　　(d) Lymphoepithelioid cell
　ii. Provisional subtype: hepatosplenic gamma delta T-cell lymphoma
e. Angioimmunoblastic T-cell lymphoma, formerly known as angioimmunoblastic T-cell lymphoma with dysproteinemia
f. Angiocentric lymphoma
g. Intestinal T-cell lymphoma, which involves the small bowel (enteropathy-associated location) and also presents with celiac disease
h. Adult T-cell lymphoma/leukemia
i. Anaplastic large cell lymphoma (ALCL)
　i. CD30+ type
　ii. T-cell type
　iii. Null cell type
j. Provisional entity: ALCL, Hodgkin-like

C. Hodgkin disease
1. Lymphocyte predominance
2. Nodular sclerosis (NS)
3. Mixed cellularity (MC)
4. Lymphocyte depletion (LD)
5. Provisional entity: lymphocyte-rich classic Hodgkin disease

IV. **World Health Organization (WHO) Classification of Lymphoid Neoplasm (modified from REAL: Gold Standard)**

A. B-cell neoplasm
1. Precursor B-cell neoplasm
a. Precursor B-lymphoblastic leukemia/lymphoma (precursor B-cell acute lymphoblastic leukemia)
2. Mature (peripheral) B-cell neoplasm
a. B-cell chronic lymphocytic leukemia/small lymphocytic lymphoma
b. B-cell prolymphocytic leukemia
c. Lymphoplasmacytic lymphoma
d. Splenic marginal zone B-cell lymphoma (with or without villous lymphocytes)
e. Hairy cell leukemia
f. Plasma cell myeloma/plasmacytoma
g. Extranodal marginal zone B-cell lymphoma (with or without monocytoid lymphocytes)
h. Nodal marginal zone B-cell lymphoma (with or without monocytoid lymphocytes)
i. Follicular lymphoma
j. Mantle cell lymphoma
k. Diffuse large B-cell lymphoma
l. Burkitt lymphoma/Burkitt cell leukemia

B. T-cell and NK cell neoplasms

1. Precursor T-cell neoplasm
   a. Precursor T-lymphoblastic lymphoma/leukemia (precursor T-cell acute lymphoblastic leukemia)
2. Mature (peripheral) T/NK cell neoplasm
   a. T-cell prolymphocytic leukemia
   b. T-cell granular lymphocytic leukemia
   c. Aggressive NK cell leukemia
   d. Adult T-cell lymphoma/leukemia (human T-lymphotropic virus [HTLV-1])
   e. Extranodal NK/T-cell lymphoma, nasal type
   f. Enteropathy-type T-cell lymphoma
   g. Hepatosplenic gamma delta T-cell lymphoma
   h. Subcutaneous panniculitis-like T-cell lymphoma
   i. Mycosis fungoides/Sézary syndrome
   j. ALCL, T/null cell, primary cutaneous type
   k. Peripheral T-cell lymphoma, not otherwise characterized
   l. Angioimmunoblastic T-cell lymphoma
   m. ALCL, T/null, primary systemic type

V. **International Prognostic Index**
   A. Prognostic factors (one point for each)
      1. Older than 60 years
      2. Performance status greater than 2
      3. Elevated lactate dehydrogenase (LDH)
      4. Extranodal sites greater than 2
      5. Stage II or IV
   B. Total points predict risk category (e.g., category predicts poor long-term survival)
      1. Low (0 or 1)
      2. Low-intermediate (2)
      3. High-intermediate (3)
      4. High (4 or 5)

VI. **Eastern Cooperative Oncology Group performance status**
   A. Grade 0: fully active predisease performance
   B. Grade 1: restricted in physical strenuous activity, able to perform light or sedentary activities
   C. Grade 2: ambulatory, capable of self-care but unable to carry on work activities; up and about 50% of waking hours
   D. Grade 3: capable of only limited self-care; confined to care more than 50% of waking hours
   E. Grade 4: completely disabled; unable to perform activities of daily living; confined to bed or chair
   F. Grade 5: dead

NON-HODGKIN LYMPHOMA

I. **Definition**
   A. Heterogeneous group of lymphocytic cancers predominantly of B-cell origin (85%–90%) and lacking the Reed-Sternberg cells that produce a diverse group of malignancies

II. **Incidence/predisposing factors**
   A. NHL results from the transformation of B and T natural killer cells (NK). Also, aberrant rearrangements of IG and TCR genes are present. Chromosomal and gene changes play an important part in prognosis and treatment.
   B. Median age for all types is 66 years
   C. Forty-five percent higher in males than females
   D. The United States has the highest rate in the world—69,740 new cases last year and 19,020 deaths
   E. Incidence in HIV infection has fallen with the development of highly active antiretroviral therapy
   F. Incidence is increased with viruses and bacteria
      1. Epstein-Barr virus
      2. HTLV-1
      3. Hepatitis C
      4. *Helicobacter pylori* in the stomach associated with mucosa-associated lymphatic tissue
   G. Associated with warm-antibody autoimmune hemolytic anemias (AIHAs)
   H. Because lymphomas are extensive at diagnosis, associated oncological emergencies such as superior vena cava syndrome and cardiac tamponade should be anticipated, diagnosed, and treated

III. **Subjective/physical examination findings**
   A. Lymphadenopathy—painless, widespread, or isolated
   B. Most patients are asymptomatic
   C. Fever
   D. Night sweats
   E. Weight loss
   F. Abdominal fullness (mass or bowel obstruction common seen in Burkitt lymphoma)
   G. Skin ulcers
   H. Lymphadenopathy, isolated or widespread, painless
   I. Extranodal sites of disease (skin ulcers). Eighty percent of indolent lymphomas manifest as Stage IV disease (usually with bone marrow involvement)
   J. Splenomegaly
   K. Hepatomegaly

IV. **Laboratory/diagnostic findings**
   A. Tissue biopsy of the largest node or involved organ that is accessible is required, but not definitive in diagnosis

1. Biopsy should be reviewed by a pathologist experienced in the diagnosis of hematologic malignancy
2. Excisional biopsy is preferred for initial diagnosis. Aspirates do not allow examination of nodal architecture which is critical to diagnosis.

B. Peripheral blood is usually normal on light microscopy

C. Molecular profiling is required for determination of gene expression

D. High-grade lymphomas may consist of malignant cells in spinal fluid

E. Classification into three categories:
   1. Indolent lymphomas: small, well-differentiated cells
   2. Aggressive lymphomas: larger, more immature cells
   3. Highly aggressive lymphomas: larger, immature cells with diffuse pattern of growth

F. The recent REAL classification and WHO system lend themselves to immunophenotypic studies and cytogenetic/molecular genetic studies. Recent guidelines report that adequate immunophenotyping is needed to establish diagnosis and appropriate treatment

G. Consider ordering the following:
   1. Labs: complete blood count with differential and erythrocyte sedimentation rate (may help to follow clinical course), Hepatitis panel, HIV, and flow cytometry
   2. LDH determination; useful marker for tumor bulk
   3. CT scan of chest and abdomen to aid in staging, or positron emission tomography scans
   4. Bone marrow biopsy (site specific and whether bilateral is under debate)
   5. Lumbar puncture and cerebral spinal fluid cytology (if central nervous system involvement suspected)

V.   Management

A. Hematology/oncology referral for suspected cases

B. Treatment is determined by histologic type of the lymphoma and the age and underlying condition of the patient

C. Timing of treatment, drugs to be used, and therapeutic goals vary among individual patients

D. Treatment may be deferred until the patient is symptomatic in low-grade but not in high-grade lymphoma

E. Chemotherapy—historically most important modality, frequently combined with immunotherapy
   1. Leads to remission but not cure in low-grade lymphoma
   2. Accompanied by palliative therapy
   3. Bendamustine + Rituximab (NCCN Guidelines Non-Hodgkin's Lymphoma, p. 37 of 452)
   4. CHOP: cyclophosphamide, hydroxydaunomycin/doxorubicin (Adriamycin), vincristine (Oncovin), and prednisone given every 14 or 21 days until remission or not tolerated. Dosage is based on patient condition and body mass index. Often in conjunction with rituximab (RCHOP)

5. CVP: cyclophosphamide, vincristine, and prednisone given every 14 or 21 days until remission or not tolerated. Often in conjunction with rituximab (RCVP)

F. Radiotherapy or surgical resections may be key in certain cases

G. Biological and targeted treatments—monoclonal antibodies and recombinant agents also used

1. Rituximab, an unconjugated monoclonal antibody, was found to produce greater responses and longer remissions. However, patients build up a tolerance to the antibody and become resistant.

2. Other monoclonal antibodies are as follows:

   a. Approved by the Food and Drug Administration
      i. CD20 ibritumomab, tositumomab, and ofatumumab
      ii. CD52 alemtuzumab

   b. Undergoing investigational trials:
      i. CD20 afutuzumab—approved for chronic lymphocytic leukemia but not lymphoma
      ii. CD23 lumiliximab

   c. Immunotherapy with lenalidomide usually given with rituximab

   d. Stem cell transplants, traditionally may be used in recurrent or refractory disease and in high-risk diagnosis

   e. Radioimmunotherapy is used by tagging the monoclonal antibody to a radioisotope

3. Immunomodulatory agents and small molecular inhibitors: approved by the Food and Drug Administration for a subtype of NHL (mantle cell lymphoma), and ibrutinib and lenalidomide are under investigation

VI. Prognosis

A. Prognosis is poorer if the patient is unable to receive full treatment doses because of age or underlying conditions. Five-year survival rate is 60%. Long-term quality of life can be affected by late treatment-related adverse effects such as cardiomyopathy and neuropathy.

B. Observe patients undergoing treatments for sepsis

1. Usually caused by Gram-negative bacteria, such as *Escherichia coli, Klebsiella spp.*, and *Pseudomonas spp.*

2. Endogenous flora usually causes infection in these patients, particularly if they are asplenic

HODGKIN LYMPHOMA

I. Definition

A. A group of cancers characterized by the presence of Reed-Sternberg giant cells in a background of benign inflammatory cells or fibrosis

II. **Incidence/predisposing factors**
  A. The cause is unclear; infection, genomic alterations, deregulation of growth factor gene, and immune defects are postulated
  B. Median age is 68 years. Cases are rare before 30 years of age
  C. More than 75% of all newly diagnosed patients can be cured with combination chemotherapy and/or radiation therapy (RT)
  D. History of infectious mononucleosis increases the likelihood that Hodgkin lymphoma (HL) will occur (Epstein-Barr)
  E. In the United States, Caucasians account for 90% of cases
  F. Primary Hodgkin disease is the most common cause of mortality in the first 15 years, and secondary malignant neoplasms are the cause of death after 15 years.
  G. Associated with warm antibody AIHAs
  H. Because lymphomas are often diffuse at diagnosis, superior vena cava syndrome and cardiac tamponade should be anticipated, diagnosed, and treated

III. **WHO classification**
  A. Classical HL
    1. NS HL (3%–8% of cases)
      a. Nodular growth pattern
      b. With or without diffuse areas
      c. Rare Reed-Sternberg cells
    2. Lymphocyte-rich classical HL
    3. MC HL
    4. LD HL
  B. Nodular lymphocyte-predominant HL

IV. **Subjective/physical examination findings**
  A. Manifests as a painless mass, usually in the neck
  B. Patients may exhibit no symptoms (Group A)
  C. Group B symptoms include the following:
    1. Unexplained fever of 101°F or 38.3°C
    2. Drenching night sweats
    3. Weight loss of 10% or more in the previous 6 months
  D. Milder versions of the preceding symptoms may be seen
  E. Generalized pruritus, weakness, and malaise (unusual)
  F. Approximately 90% of cases manifest as painless, nontender cervical lymphadenopathy
  G. Can manifest in the adolescent or young adult as a large mediastinal mass on chest x-ray (fewer than 20% of cases)
  H. The patient may have generalized pruritus

V. **Laboratory/diagnostic findings**
  A. The hallmark is the presence of Reed-Sternberg cells on lymph node biopsy. Needle aspiration or needle biopsies are not adequate for diagnosis.
  B. Molecular profiling needed for examination of gene expression

C. Anatomic staging is based on regions involved and the presence or absence of symptoms.
   1. Stage I: one lymph node involved
   2. Stage II: two lymph nodes involved on one side of diaphragm
   3. Stage III: lymph nodes involved on both sides of diaphragm
   4. Stage IV: disseminated disease with bone marrow or liver involvement
   5. Stage A: no constitutional symptoms
   6. Stage B: constitutional symptoms (see Subjective/Physical Examination Findings section)
D. Histopathologic (Rye) classification of Hodgkin disease
   1. Lymphocyte predominance
   2. NS
   3. MC
   4. LD
E. Anergic to typical skin antigen tests such as those of mumps and *Candida*. If the patient previously had a positive response to a tuberculin test, the response is now negative.
F. To facilitate staging, consider ordering the following:
   1. Chest x-ray
      a. About half of patients exhibit mediastinal adenopathy, often detected on routine chest x-ray
      b. Observe for pleural effusions
   2. CT of thorax, abdomen, and pelvis
   3. Complete blood count, erythrocyte sedimentation rate, Coombs' test, liver function tests, and albumin, LDH, calcium, and uric acid levels
   4. Lymphangiography and gallium scan
   5. Bilateral bone marrow biopsy (for patients with inadequate or equivocal lymphangiogram)
   6. Bone scan
   7. Consider the need for staging laparotomy if therapy will be changed by documentation of subdiaphragmatic disease

VI. Management
A. Hematology/oncology referral for suspected cases. Delays in receiving appropriate therapy are associated with high medicolegal liability.
B. RT is the treatment of choice for nonbulky Stage IA/IIA disease
   1. Ninety-five percent complete remission with limited disease
   2. Associated with unwanted effects, such as secondary malignancies
   3. Goal is lowest effective dose of RT
C. Consider ovarian transposition by laparoscopy to prevent iatrogenic ovarian failure and increase the possibility of pregnancy in the future
D. Patients with advanced Hodgkin disease (late Stage II, Stage III, or Stage IV) should receive the following:

1. CHOP—cyclophosphamide, doxorubicin, vincristine, and prednisone ± rituximab (RCHOP)
2. CVP—cyclophosphamide, vincristine, and prednisone ± rituximab (RCVP)
3. EPOCH—cyclophosphamide, doxorubicin, etoposide, vincristine, and prednisone ± rituximab
4. ABVD—Adriamycin (doxorubicin), bleomycin, vinblastine, and dacarbazine (ABVD) +/- radiation therapy
5. BEACOPP—bleomycin, etoposide, doxorubicin (Adriamycin), cyclophosphamide, vincristine (Oncovin), procarbazine, and prednisone; will require GCSF granulocyte colony stimulating factor to prevent leukopenia
   a. Usual regimen includes four cycles of escalated BEACOPP followed by four cycles of standard BEACOPP
6. Dosing is based on body mass index and condition of the patient
7. Gemcitabine—pulmonary toxicity can be severe when used with ABVD or BEACOPP; thus, baseline LFTs are essential
   a. High response rate

E. Anti-CD30 monoclonal antibodies (brentuximab vedotin)
   1. Excellent response rate when CD30 antigen expressed on both Reed-Sternberg cells in HL and malignant cells of anaplastic large cell NHL

F. Increased risk of pulmonary fibrosis with ABVD

G. Concurrent radiation/chemotherapy may be avoided out of concern for increases in late secondary leukemias or solid malignancies, except in cases with massive mediastinal involvement. Such treatments also have a higher risk of cardiomyopathies.

H. Tumor bulk and stage appear to be the most important prognostic factors
   1. The presence of Group B symptoms is a poor prognostic factor
   2. Low hematocrit (Hct) and high LDH levels are associated with higher rates of relapse

I. Positron emission tomography scans may distinguish between residual tumor and fibrosis post treatment

J. Preoperative pneumococcal vaccine for splenectomy patients with daily prophylactic oral antibiotics and patient education regarding precautions for febrile illnesses

K. Relapsed patients who have received allogenic (usually sibling match) bone marrow transplants have shown a lower relapse rate compared with autologous (previously harvested from patient) stem cell recipients

L. Observe for sepsis
   1. Usually caused by Gram-negative bacteria, such as *E. coli*, *Klebsiella spp.*, and *Pseudomonas spp.*
   2. Endogenous flora usually causes infection in these patients, particularly if they are asplenic

BIBLIOGRAPHY

Abramson, R. H., Advani, C. B., Andreadis C. B., Bartlett N., Bellam N., Byrd J. C., . . . Zafar, N. (2011). Non-Hodgkin's lymphomas. *Journal of the National Comprehensive Cancer Network, 9*(5), 484–560.

Borchmann, P., Engert, A., Monsef, I., Rancea, M., Skoetz, N., & Will, A. (2013). Fifteenth biannual report of the cochrane haematological malignancies group—Focus on non-Hodgkin's lymphoma. *Journal of the National Cancer Institute, 105*(15), 1159–1170. doi:10.1093/jnci/djt165

Chiu, B. C., Evens, A. M., Gordon, L. I., Rosen, S. T., Tsang, R., & Winter, J. N. (2009). Non-Hodgkin lymphoma. In K. A. Camphausen, W. J. Hoskins, R. Pazdur, & L. D. Wagman (Eds.), *Cancer management: A multidisciplinary approach: Medical, surgical and radiation oncology* (12th ed.). New York, NY: C.M.P. Healthcare Media.

Coiffier, B., & Younes, A. (2013). *Lymphoma: Diagnosis and treatment (current clinical oncology).* New York, NY: Springer.

Ershler, W. B., & Longo, D. L. (2009). Non-Hodgkin's and Hodgkin's lymphomas and myeloma. In J. B. Halter, J. G. Ouslander, M. E. Tinetti, S. Studenski, K. P. High, & S. Asthana (Eds.), *Hazzard's geriatric medicine and gerontology* (6th ed.). New York, NY: McGraw-Hill.

Foon, K. A., & Lichtman, M. A. (2010). General considerations of lymphoma: Epidemiology, etiology, heterogeneity, and primary extranodal disease. In J. T. Prchal, K. Kaushansky, T. J. Kipps, M. A. Lichtman, J. T. Prchal, & U. Seligsohn (Eds.), *Williams hematology* (8th ed.). New York, NY: McGraw-Hill.

National Cancer Institutes, National Institute of Health. (2013). *Hodgkins lymphoma.* Retrieved from http://www.cancer.gov/cancertopics/types/Hodgkin

National Cancer Institutes, National Institute of Health. (2013). *Non-Hodgkins lymphoma.* Retrieved from http://www.cancer.gov/cancertopics/pdq/treatment/adult-non-hodgkins/HealthProfessional/page3

National Comprehensive Cancer Network. (2013). *Hodgins lymphoma.* Retrieved from http://www.nccn.org/professionals/physician_gls/PDF/aml.pdf

National Comprehensive Cancer Network. (2013). *Non-Hodgins lymphoma.* Retrieved from http://www.nccn.org/professionals/physician_gls/PDF/aml.pdf

Westin, J., Hagemeister, F. B., Reed, V. K., & Fanale, M. (2011). Hodgkin lymphoma. In H. M. Kantarjian, R. A. Wolff, & C. A. Koller (Eds.), *The MD Anderson manual of medical oncology* (2nd ed). Retrieved November 29, 2013, from http://www.accessmedicine.com/content.aspx?aID=8302526

CHAPTER 66

Other Common Cancers

COLLEEN R. WALSH

LUNG CANCER

I. **General comments/incidence/predisposing factors**

    A. Leading cause of cancer deaths among men and women in the United States

    B. Accounts for 13.4% of all new cancers

    C. More people die from lung cancer than from colon cancer, breast cancer, and prostate cancer combined.

    D. In 2010, 201,144 people were diagnosed with lung cancer, and 158,248 people died from it.

    E. Increased incidence with the following:

        1. Tobacco smoking

            a. Women who smoke have a greater risk of developing small cell rather than squamous cell lung cancer.

            b. Men who smoke have a similar risk for small and non-small cell types.

        2. Secondhand smoke

        3. Ionizing radiation

        4. Occupational exposure (may be additive or synergistic to tobacco)

            a. Asbestos

            b. Chromium

            c. Nickel

            d. Hydrocarbons

            e. Chloromethyl ether

    F. Less well-established risks include the following:

        1. Air pollution

        2. Vitamins A and E deficiencies

        3. Cigar and pipe use

G. Average age of people found to have lung cancer is 60 years—unusual in those younger than 40 years

H. If found and treated early, before lymph node or other organ involvement, the 5-year survival rate is 42%

II. **Subjective findings**

A. In all, 10% to 25% of patients are asymptomatic at the time of diagnosis

B. Symptomatic lung cancer is generally advanced disease

C. May have nonspecific complaints such as:
1. Weight loss
2. Chest pain
3. Dyspnea
4. Loss of appetite

D. Symptoms confined to the lungs
1. Cough
2. Hemoptysis
3. Hoarseness
4. Wheezing
5. Dyspnea
6. Sputum production with or without fever
7. Chest pain
8. Recurring infections such as bronchitis and pneumonia

III. **Physical examination findings**

A. Central tumors may obstruct the following areas of the lungs:
1. Segmental (left has eight segments, right has ten segments)
2. Lobar (left has two lobes, right has three lobes)
3. Mainstem bronchi (also cause atelectasis and postobstructive pneumonitis)

B. Peripheral tumors may cause no abnormalities on physical examination

C. Tumor invasion of pleural surface may cause pleural effusion

D. Disease confined to the chest may include the following physical findings:
1. Stridor, hoarseness
2. Changes on physical examination related to atelectasis
3. Consolidation
4. Diaphragm paralysis or effusion
5. Superior vena caval obstruction
   a. Cyanosis
   b. Engorgement of neck veins
   c. Lack of pulsations
   d. Enlarged neck circumference
   e. Pericardial disease
   f. Tamponade

E. Lymphadenopathy, hepatomegaly, and clubbing are present in approximately 20% of patients.

F. Horner syndrome may be present
   1. Horner syndrome is the result of neurologic damage to cervical nerve
   2. It presents as unilateral miotic pupil, ptosis, and facial anhidrosis (inadequate perspiration).
G. Pancoast syndrome may be present
   1. Associated with tumor in apex of the lung
   2. Symptoms include neuropathic pain in the arm and atrophy of the muscles of the arm and hand caused by brachial plexus and sympathetic ganglia tumor
H. Malignant pleural effusions associated with bronchogenic carcinoma

IV. **Laboratory/diagnostic findings**
A. The only definitive test is biopsy
B. Chest x-ray presentation varies with cell type
C. Comparison with old films is extremely valuable
   1. Central lesions tend to be
      a. Squamous cell carcinoma
      b. Small cell carcinoma (SCC)
   2. Peripheral lesions tend to be
      a. Adenocarcinoma
      b. Large cell carcinoma
      c. Bronchoalveolar cell carcinoma
   3. Cavitation tends to be
      a. Squamous cell carcinoma
      b. Large cell carcinoma
   4. Early mediastinal-hilar involvement is usually indicative of small cell carcinoma
D. Sputum cytology 80% in centrally located lesions, less than 20% in peripheral nodules
E. Bronchoscopy may be used to obtain tissue for histologic confirmation
F. Percutaneous needle aspiration
G. Pleural fluid, approximately 40% to 50% in malignant pleural effusion
H. Mediastinal exploration (rare)
I. Open biopsy is used only occasionally to confirm diagnosis when less invasive diagnostics are negative, or the lesion is inaccessible for other diagnostic modalities

V. **Major treatments**
A. Refer to oncology specialist
B. Therapy dependent on
   1. Cell type
   2. Premorbid condition
   3. Underlying lung function
C. SCC
   1. Almost always treated with chemotherapy
   2. Accounts for approximately 20% of all lung cancers

3. Other names for small cell lung cancer are oat cell cancer and small cell undifferentiated

D. SCC staged most often as
1. Limited stage—one lung and in lymph nodes on the same side of the chest
   a. Surgery first option
   b. Chemotherapy second option with a cisplatin or carboplatin-based regimen with etoposide or irinotecan as the second drug
   c. SCC commonly spreads to the brain
   d. Patients treated with chemotherapy with or without radiation usually experience remission, although only temporarily
   e. Survival rates for limited-stage SCC treated with chemotherapy and radiation are 60% at 1 year, 30% at 2 years, and 10% to 15% by 5 years.
2. Extensive stage—both lungs, with spread to lymph nodes on the other side or to distant organs
   a. Very poor prognosis when left untreated
   b. Carboplatin or cisplatin and etoposide are the chemotherapy drugs usually used
   c. Radiation therapy is sometimes used
   d. Survival is 20% to 30% at 1 year, 5% by two years, and 1%–2% by 5 years

E. Non-small cell carcinoma (NSCC) is the most common type of lung cancer; it occurs in about 80% of lung cancers and includes:
1. Squamous cell adenocarcinoma
2. Bronchoalveolar cell
3. Large cell
4. Adenosquamous cell

F. NSCC staged with TNM system
1. TNM: tumor, nodes, metastases
2. Described in roman numerals 0 through IV (0 through 4); the lower the number, the less the cancer has spread
3. Stage 0—limited to lining of air passages
   a. Usually treated surgically with segmentectomy or wedge resection
   b. Usually does not require chemotherapy
   c. Usually does not require radiation
4. Stage I—invaded lung tissue
   a. Usually involves lobectomy
   b. Patient may receive radiation therapy although tumors not particularly sensitive
   c. Five-year survival with surgery approximately 60%
5. Stage II—invasion of lung tissue expanded
   a. Treatment usually the same as in Stage I

       b. Five-year survival rates approximately 35% for patients with surgery

  6. Stage IIIA—treatment depends on location of cancer in the lung and whether it has spread to lymph nodes

       a. Surgery may be used alone

       b. Chemotherapy or radiation therapy may be provided although tumors not particularly sensitive

       c. Brachytherapy (selective placement of radioactive source in contact with or implanted into tumor tissues) may be recommended

       d. Five-year survival range is 10% to 20%, or better if without lymph node metastases

  7. Stage IIIB—cancer has spread too widely to be completely removed surgically

       a. May require chemotherapy or radiation although tumor not particularly sensitive

       b. Five-year survival rate is 10% to 20%

  8. Stage IV—cancer has spread to distant organs

       a. Cure is not possible

       b. Therapy is palliative

       c. Chemotherapy may prolong life

       d. One-year survival is approximately 20% to 25%

G. Localized disease commonly treated based on mutational analysis of the tumor when known and the three main mutations preformed are EGFR, KRAS, and ALK

  1. KRAS mutation has shown to cause primary resistance to tyrosine kinase inhibitor therapy.

  2. EGFR and ALK most commonly are mutually exclusive

  3. EGFR positive disease is treated with erlotinib or afatinib as frontline therapy and both are tyrosine kinase inhibitors.

  4. If mutational analysis not known, then chemotherapy is given with a platinum-based combination of either cisplatin or carboplatin with another drug such as etoposide, docetaxel, gemcitabine, vinorelbine, or paclitaxel.

H. Advanced disease commonly treated with:

  1. Cisplatin if not already given

  2. Pemetrexed

  3. Any drugs used in frontline therapy that the patient has not previously been given

  4. Bevacizumab may be also be added to the chemotherapy

I. Surgical resection may involve solitary nodule in localized disease Stages I to IIIA.

J. Radiation therapy considered for nonsurgical candidates

K. Stage IIIB or IV usually receives

  1. Palliative radiation

    2. Experimental chemotherapy clinical trials protocols

L. Therapeutic thoracentesis (if symptomatic) used with malignant pleural effusions

M. Decision algorithms for lung cancer detection and treatment were published in 2012

    1. Stereotactic body irradiation treatment can be used for curative purposes

    2. Low-dose helical computerized tomography is now recommended as a screening tool in persons with several risk factors including long-term smokers

    3. Many insurance companies will still not approve

COLORECTAL CANCER

I.   **General comments/predisposing factors**

A. Second most common cause of cancer (excluding skin cancer) in males and females in the United States

    1. In the United States in 2010, 131,607 people were diagnosed with colorectal cancer, and 52,045 people died from it.

B. Ninety-five percent of colorectal cancers are adenocarcinomas

C. Increased incidence in the following:

    1. Those who are older than 50 years

    2. Those with a personal history of

        a. Colorectal cancer

        b. Colorectal adenomas

        c. Inflammatory bowel disease

        d. Peutz-Jeghers syndrome

        e. Breast cancer

        f. Ovarian cancer

        g. Endometrial cancer

        h. Prostate cancer

        i. Hereditary nonpolyposis colon cancer

        j. High-fat or low-fiber diet

    3. Those with a family history of

        a. Colorectal cancer

        b. Cancer family syndrome

        c. Gardner syndrome

II.   **Subjective findings**

A. Often asymptomatic until disease is advanced

B. Bowel-specific symptoms include

    1. Change in bowel habits

    2. Bloody rectal discharge

    3. Abdominal discomfort

    4. Straining during a bowel movement

C. Systemic symptoms are frequently insidious and may include

    1. Fatigue

2. Weight loss
3. Anemia
4. Nausea
5. Loss of appetite
6. Jaundice if extensive liver involvement

III.   Physical examination findings
   A. Often, external examination of the abdomen is unrevealing
   B. Abdominal examination may reveal
      1. Abdominal tenderness
      2. Discrete mass may be palpated, dependent on tumor location and size
   C. Digital rectal examination, combined with stool guaiac testing, is the most important part of the physical examination

IV.   Laboratory/diagnostic findings
   A. Screening tests, recommended to begin at age 50 years by both the American Cancer Society and the National Comprehensive Cancer Network, include the following:
      1. Fecal occult blood testing (FOBT)
      2. Digital rectal examination (DRE)
      3. Flexible sigmoidoscopy
      4. Colonoscopy
      5. Double-contrast barium enema
   B. If there is reason to suspect colon or rectal cancer on history and physical examination regardless of age, the following should be considered:
      1. DRE
      2. FOBT
      3. Colonoscopy
      4. Biopsy
      5. CBC
   C. Clinician may consider serum carcinoembryonic antigen (CEA)
      1. Not recommended for screening
      2. Useful in monitoring effectiveness of therapy after surgery
      3. Elevation suggests recurrence
   D. CT may be ordered
   E. Chest x-ray also may be ordered

V.   Evaluation for metastasis may include
   A. CT-guided needle biopsy
   B. MRI
   C. Positron emission tomography
   D. Angiography
   E. Consultation with an enterostomal therapist
   F. Bone scan

VI.   Major treatments in general include
   A. Surgery (treatment of choice)

1. Prior to surgery, treatments include the following:
   a. Liver function tests
   b. CEA level
   c. Colonoscopy
   d. Chest film
2. Liver resection along with targeted chemotherapy shown to increase life span after diagnosis

B. Chemotherapy, which in part will be influenced by mutations or lack of mutations in KRAS, EGFR, and BRAF V600E. The lack of mutation is called wild type. Also, KRAS and BRAF with mutations have a less favorable prognosis.
   1. First-line will have a 5-FU based with oxaliplatin, leucovorin, and irinotecan
   2. Bevacizumab can be added based on patient's risk profile
   3. 5-FU is usually only used as a single agent when given intra-arterially to hepatic metastases
   4. Cetuximab or panitumumab can be used only with KRAS wild type
   5. Regorafenib, a VEGFR inhibitor, can be used if EGFR positive
   6. Frequently, leucovorin and oxaliplatin are used with 5-FU to enhance its effectiveness.
   7. Levamisole HCl (Ergamisol) is used to reduce the rate of tumor recurrence

C. Radiation therapy
   1. Not primary treatment
   2. May be used in conjunction with surgical excision of Stage B2 and Stage C rectal tumors
   3. Owing to extensive lymphatic drainage in the rectum, rectal tumors tend to metastasize to regional lymph nodes early
   4. Radiation therapy inhibits metastasis

D. See algorithms for therapy for different stages of colorectal cancer on the American Cancer Society website at www.cancer.org, or on the National Comprehensive Cancer Network website at www.ncc.org.

BREAST CANCER

I. **General comments/predisposing factors**
   A. Most common nonskin malignancy in females in the United States
   B. Second only to lung cancer as cause of death in women
      1. In the United States in 2010, 206,966 women were diagnosed with breast cancer, and 40,996 women died from the disease.
   C. Increased incidence in the following:
      1. Age older than 50 years, with mean and median ages of 60 and 61 years
      2. Personal history of the following:
         a. Breast cancer

> > **b.** Colon cancer
> > **c.** Endometrial cancer
> > **d.** Ovarian cancer
> > **e.** Nulliparity, low parity, or late first pregnancy
> > **f.** Older than 30 years at first live birth
> > **g.** Early menarche, younger than 12 years
> > **h.** Menopause after age of 50 years
> > **i.** Cellular atypia or lobular carcinoma in situ on breast biopsy
> > **j.** Dense breast tissue
> > **k.** Radiation to breast or chest at moderate or high doses
> > **3.** Family history of
> > > **a.** Breast cancer
> > > **b.** Cancer family syndrome
> **D.** Genetic mutations associated with breast cancer include:
> > **1.** BRCA1
> > **2.** BRCA2

II. Subjective findings
> **A.** Palpable, usually painless, breast lump is detected by the patient in most palpable breast cancers
> **B.** Nipple discharge (particularly if bloody and unilateral)
> **C.** Focal breast pain with inflammation of the skin over the breast area may be associated with cancer but may also be associated with other benign breast conditions.
> **D.** Less frequent symptoms include the following:
> > **1.** Breast pain
> > **2.** Nipple discharge
> > **3.** Erosion
> > **4.** Retraction
> > **5.** Enlargement
> > **6.** Itching of the nipple
> > **7.** Redness
> > **8.** Generalized hardness
> > **9.** Enlargement of the breast
> > **10.** Shrinking of the breast

III. Physical examination findings
> **A.** Early findings
> > **1.** Single mass
> > **2.** Nontender
> > **3.** Firm to hard mass with ill-defined margins
> > **4.** Mammographic abnormalities
> > **5.** No palpable mass
> **B.** Dominant breast masses should be considered highly suspicious for breast cancer
> **C.** Increased suspicion because of the following conditions:
> > **1.** Mass is hard or fixed to the overlying skin

    2. Overlying skin is dimpled or retracted

    3. Unilateral bloody nipple discharge from the breast with the mass

    4. New onset of inverted nipple with or without evidence of mass

    5. Axillary adenopathy present (inconclusive finding)

    6. Breast enlargement, redness, edema, and pain

    7. Laboratory/diagnostic findings

D. Confirmation of breast cancer requires cytologic or histologic finding

    1. Fine needle aspiration (a negative finding is not conclusive to rule out cancer)

    2. Core needle biopsy

    3. Open excisional biopsy is used in conjunction with planned surgical intervention

    4. Stereotactically guided core needle biopsy may also be used with occult nonpalpable breast lesions detected by mammography

E. A consistently elevated erythrocyte sedimentation rate may be the result of disseminated cancer

F. Liver and bone metastases may be associated with serum alkaline phosphatase elevation

G. Hypercalcemia may be present in advanced disease; it provides an indication for bone scan

H. Tumor markers used to follow the disease process include the following:

    1. Serum CEA

    2. Serum CA 27 29

I. Breast ultrasonography is used to distinguish fluid-filled cysts from solid tumor

J. Breast tissue biopsy may be evaluated with the following:

    1. Tumor hormone receptor (estrogen receptor [ER]/progesterone receptor [PR]) testing

        a. ERs

        b. PRs

        c. Primary tumors that are receptor positive have a more favorable response to therapy.

    2. Human epidermal growth factor receptor (HER)-2/neu testing

    3. Cancer cell division

        a. S-phase fraction (SPF)

        b. Ki-67

K. Types of breast cancer include the following:

    1. Carcinoma in situ (confined to ducts or lobules without invasion of surrounding tissues or organs)

        a. Lobular carcinoma in situ usually does not become an invasive cancer

        b. Ductal carcinoma in situ is the most common type of noninvasive breast cancer

2. Infiltrative (or invasive) ductal carcinoma is the most common of all breast cancers
3. Infiltrative (or invasive) lobular carcinoma
4. Medullary carcinoma
5. Colloid carcinoma
6. Tubular carcinoma
7. Inflammatory breast carcinoma
8. Adenoid cystic carcinoma

IV. **Major treatment**
   A. Immediate referral of suspected cases for biopsy
   B. Treatment can be curative or palliative
   C. Management of breast cancer is multifaceted and is based on patient preference, medical expertise, and characteristics of the breast cancer
   D. Lumpectomy
      1. Breast-conserving surgery
      2. Used in select women to remove the mass and limited surrounding tissue
   E. Modified radical mastectomy/partial radical mastectomy
      1. Removal of the breast
      2. Axillary dissection
      3. Preservation of the pectoral muscles except in total radical mastectomy
   F. Adjuvant therapy initially affects quality of life but is considered transient and minor overall
      1. Indicated for positive axillary nodes such as the following:
         a. Combination chemotherapy for women younger than 50 years. If older, the risk versus the benefit will be considered.
         b. Tamoxifen or some type or aromatase inhibitor for women older than 50 years
   G. Melphalan and fluorouracil can be used.
      1. Postmenopausal women with estrogen receptor-positive tumors
      2. Adjuvant therapy indicated for negative axillary nodes
      3. May not require adjuvant therapy if tumor is smaller than 1 cm
   H. Preferred chemotherapy regimens are as follows:
      1. Doxorubicin/cyclophosphamide followed by paclitaxel
      2. Docetaxel and cyclophosphamide for those patients who cannot tolerate doxorubicin
   I. Trastuzumab or pertuzumab will be added to regimens for HER-2-positive tumors
   J. Radiation therapy is another available option, should staging require more intensive treatment; it is often used with stem cell transplantations

K. Decision algorithms for the different stages of breast cancer are available on the American Cancer Society website at www.cancer.org, and on the National Comprehensive Cancer Network website at www.nccn.org.

CERVICAL CANCER

I. **General comments/predisposing factors**

A. Cervical cancer was once one of the most common causes of cancer death for American women, but it is much less common today. Approximately 12,000 women per year are diagnosed in the United States with squamous cell comprising 80%–90% of cervical cancers.

B. When combined with cancers of the corpus uteri, cervical cancer is the fourth most common nonskin malignancy among females in the United States.

C. Infection with human papillomavirus (HPV) types 16, 18, 31, 33, 35, 45, 51, 52, and 56 has been strongly linked with cervical cancer. HPV 16 is the most carcinogenic accounting for approximately 55%–60% of cervical cancers.

D. Increased incidence with the following:
  1. Early age at first intercourse
  2. Multiple sexual partners
  3. A promiscuous male partner
  4. History of genital warts
  5. Folate deficiency
  6. Immunosuppression
  7. Low socioeconomic status
  8. Lapse of more than 5 years since last Pap smear
  9. Smoking

II. **Subjective findings**

A. Usually asymptomatic

B. Postcoital spotting

C. Abnormal uterine bleeding and vaginal discharge

D. Bloody or purulent, odorous, nonpruritic discharge may appear after invasion

E. Late symptoms include
  1. Bladder dysfunction
  2. Rectal dysfunction
  3. Fistulas and pain

III. **Physical examination findings**

A. Direct visualization of the cervix
  1. Should begin when woman first engages in sexual intercourse
  2. Should be performed every 1–3 years on the basis of risk factors

B. Cervical lesions may be visible on inspection as tumors or ulcerations

IV. **Laboratory/diagnostic findings**

  A. The Papanicolaou (Pap) smear interpretation most often used is the Bethesda Classification System. The Pap smear report is divided into three sections:

  1. The first section of the report is a statement of sample adequacy reported as follows:

    a. Satisfactory for evaluation

    b. Satisfactory for evaluation, but limited by (a reason is supplied in the report)

    c. Unsatisfactory for evaluation

  2. The second section of the Bethesda system report contains one of the following:

    a. Within normal limits

    b. Benign cellular changes

    c. Epithelial cell abnormalities

  3. The third section is the description of diagnoses that further explains benign cellular changes or epithelial cell abnormalities

    a. Benign cellular changes are further explained as reactive changes related to inflammation or infection

    b. Epithelial changes are further divided

      i. Squamous cell abnormalities

        (a) Atypical squamous cells of undetermined significance

        (b) Low-grade squamous intraepithelial lesions

        (c) High-grade squamous intraepithelial lesions (this also includes squamous carcinoma in situ)

        (d) Squamous cell carcinoma

      ii. Glandular cell abnormalities

        (a) Benign endometrial cells

        (b) Atypical glandular cells of undetermined significance

        (c) Adenocarcinoma in situ and adenocarcinoma

  4. With vaginal smears only—a fourth section on the Pap smear includes an evaluation of hormonal patterns related to patient age and history

  B. An abnormal Pap smear requires consultation with a physician to determine the best procedure for follow-up.

  C. Repeated Pap smear and colposcopy are common methods of follow-up

  D. Follow-up is variable depending on findings on the cytopathology report

  E. Acetic acid wash of the cervix is used as an adjunct to the Pap smear, with whitened areas recommended to undergo colposcopy

  F. Colposcopy is used

  1. To identify abnormal areas and extent of lesions

2. To obtain biopsy specimen

V. **Major treatments**

A. Dysplasia on Pap smear warrants colposcopic examination of the cervix

B. Management is dependent on specific findings of the following:
   1. Lesion grade
   2. Size and involvement of the endocervical canal

C. The following therapies may be provided:
   1. Cryotherapy—freeze/burn of abnormal cells
   2. Laser ablation—laser is used to burn abnormal cells or to remove a small piece of tissue for study
   3. Low-voltage loop electroexcision (loop electrosurgical excision procedure/loop excision of the transformation zone)—thin, electrically heated wire is used as a "knife" to remove tissue
   4. Cone biopsy—a cone-shaped piece of tissue is removed from the cervix by surgery or laser knife
   5. Simple hysterectomy—surgical removal of the uterus, with tissue near the uterus such as parametria and uterosacral ligaments left in place. The vagina and pelvic lymph nodes also are not removed.
   6. Radical hysterectomy—removal of uterus, parametria, and uterosacral ligaments
   7. Pelvic exenteration—removal of all of the organs and tissues removed in radical hysterectomy, along with bladder, vagina, rectum, or part of the colon
   8. Radiation therapy
      a. External beam radiation—radiation from outside the body
      b. Brachytherapy—radioactive source placed in contact with surface of tumor or inserted into tumor
   9. Chemotherapy
      a. Cisplatin-based chemotherapy is recommended alone or in combination
      b. Other chemotherapy drugs include paclitaxel, topotecan, and gemcitabine as primary treatment

D. Follow-up
   1. Every 4–6 months for 1–2 years
   2. Repeat colposcopy is done for recurrent abnormalities

E. Atypia on the Pap smear may warrant colposcopy
   1. Patient may be treated for an infection
   2. Reexamined with Pap smear in 3–4 months
   3. Persistent atypia warrants colposcopy

F. Common therapies include the following:
   1. Carcinoma in situ (Stage 0)—in women who have completed their childbearing, total hysterectomy is the treatment of choice
   2. Invasive carcinoma
      a. Stage IA

> **i.** Simple extrafascial hysterectomy
>
> **b.** Stage IB and Stage IIA
> > **i.** Radical hysterectomy
> > **ii.** Radiation therapy
>
> **c.** Stage IIB, Stage III, and Stage IV cancers are treated with radiation therapy
>
> **d.** Radical surgery without radiation is the preferred mode of therapy in younger women

G. Decision algorithms for cervical cancer are available on the American Cancer Society website at www.cancer.org and at the National Comprehensive Cancer Network website at www.nccn.org.

H. Gardasil, the HPV vaccine approved by the Food and Drug Administration for use in young women and teenage girls, is now available for those who have not been exposed to the HPV virus. This vaccine is given in a series of three injections, similar to the hepatitis B vaccine.

OVARIAN CANCER

I. **General comments/incidence/predisposing factors**

A. Leading cause of death from gynecologic cancer and the fifth most common cause of cancer deaths among women; 20,000 women in the United States each year are diagnosed with ovarian cancer

B. Sixth most common nonskin malignancy in females in the United States

C. Half of all ovarian cancers are found in women older than 65 years

D. Increased incidence of ovarian cancer in those with the following:

> **1.** Personal history of
> > **a.** Breast cancer
> > **b.** Endometrial cancer
> > **c.** Colon cancer
> > **d.** Infertility or use of fertility drugs
> > **e.** Nulliparity
> > **f.** Perineal talc exposure
> > **g.** BRAC1 and BRAC2 genetic markers
> > **h.** KRAS oncogene
>
> **2.** Family history of
> > **a.** Ovarian cancer
> > **b.** Breast cancer
> > **c.** Endometrial cancer
> > **d.** Colon cancer

E. Oral contraceptive use, a single full-term pregnancy, tubal ligation, hysterectomy, and breast feeding may reduce risk in women, including those with a family history of ovarian cancer.

F. Epithelial ovarian carcinomas account for approximately 85% to 90% of ovarian cancers. Carcinomas are divided into the following types:

1. Serous
2. Mucinous
3. Endometrioid
4. Clear cell

G. Germ cell tumors can be cancerous, although most are noncancerous. The most common germ cell tumors are as follows:
   1. Teratoma—can be subdivided into the following:
      a. Mature teratoma, which is also referred to as dermoid cyst (which may contain a variety of benign tissues such as bone and teeth) and usually occurs during the teens to the 40s
      b. Immature teratoma—cancerous form that occurs in girls and young women, usually younger than 18 years
   2. Dysgerminoma—most common ovarian cancer germ cell; represents only approximately 2% of all ovarian cancers
   3. Endodermal sinus tumor (yolk sac tumor) and choriocarcinoma—very rare tumors that usually grow and spread rapidly but respond to chemotherapy. They usually occur in girls and young women.
   4. Stromal tumors—account for approximately 5% of ovarian cancers. They can occur in young women, but about half occur in women older than 50 years.

II. **Subjective findings**
   A. Frequently asymptomatic
   B. When symptoms appear, they usually indicate more advanced disease and may include the following:
      1. Abdominal bloating
      2. Early satiety or anorexia
      3. Dyspepsia
      4. Pelvic pressure or pain
      5. Frequent urination
      6. Constipation
      7. Leg pain
      8. Unusual vaginal bleeding is a rare sign

III. **Physical examination findings**
   A. Pelvic mass
   B. Abdominal distention
   C. Pleural effusion
   D. Ascites
   E. Adenopathy
   F. Cachexia

IV. **Laboratory/diagnostic findings**
   A. Pelvic examination
   B. Pelvic transvaginal ultrasonography
   C. Color flow Doppler of ovarian vessels
   D. Serum tumor markers for epithelial tumors

        1. CA125 (also known as OC-125)

        2. CA72

        3. CA15–3

        4. α-l-fucosidase levels

        5. Serum inhibin levels (elevated with mucinous-type tumors)

        6. Serum He4

   E. Germ cell tumors

        1. Serum beta-human chorionic gonadotropin (hCG), or

        2. Elevated alpha-fetoprotein levels with various germ cell tumors

   F. Preoperative staging tests may include the following:

        1. Chest x-ray

        2. CBC and serum chemistries

        3. Intravenous pyelogram

        4. Cystoscopy

        5. Proctoscopy

        6. MRI

        7. CT

        8. Barium enema

   G. Surgery: definitive diagnosis is made by histology on a surgical specimen

V.   **Major treatments**

   A. Surgery (laparotomy) may be used to

        1. Stage the lesion

        2. Debulk the tumor

        3. Relieve bowel obstruction

   B. Early-stage disease

        1. Includes Stage I (well differentiated)

        2. Includes Stage II (moderately differentiated)

        3. Usually involves no further treatment

   C. Stage I, Grade III; Stage II; and Stage IIIA are often managed with the following:

        1. Systemic chemotherapy (melphalan [Alkeran])

        2. Intraperitoneal chromic phosphate (32P)

        3. Whole abdomen radiation therapy

   D. Advanced disease may be managed with the following:

        1. Systemic chemotherapy

            a. Cisplatin or carboplatin

            b. Other drugs in combination with a platinum drug or alone are paclitaxel, docetaxel, gemcitabine, and doxorubicin

            c. Bevacizumab may be added to the chemotherapy

        2. Intraperitoneal chemotherapy

        3. Biologic response modifiers

        4. Autologous bone marrow transplantation

        5. Hormonal therapy

   E. Palliative therapies include the following:

    1. Surgery to debulk the tumor
    2. Radiation
    3. Drainage of ascites or pleural effusion
  F. Follow-up usually involves the following:
    1. Serial CA125 levels to assess disease process
    2. Possible follow-up laparotomy to assess for residual disease

PROSTATE CANCER

I. General comments/predisposing factors
  A. Most common nonskin malignancy
  B. The second leading cause of cancer mortality among men in the United States
    1. Approximately 238,590 new cases of prostate cancer will be diagnosed, and approximately 29,720 men will die of prostate cancer
  C. Increased incidence in the following:
    1. Men older than 50 years
    2. Those of African American descent
    3. Those with a family history of
      a. Prostate cancer
      b. Breast cancer
      c. Endometrial cancer
      d. Colon cancer
    4. Men with a personal history of
      a. Colon cancer
      b. High-fat diet
      c. Occupational exposure to cadmium or rubber
      d. Green tea, selenium, and vitamins A, B6, C, and E may reduce prostate cancer risk
  D. Prostate-specific antigen (PSA) screening should be offered annually to men 50 years or older.
  E. Awareness of the patient's consumption of the following medications/herbs is important because these can lower PSA levels and produce a normal PSA level in some cases of early prostate cancer. These medications include the following:
    1. Finasteride (Proscar or Propecia)
    2. Androgen-receptor blockers
    3. Saw palmetto
    4. PC-SPES (Latin "spes," hope; PC = prostate cancer)

II. Subjective findings
  A. Initially, usually asymptomatic
  B. Local symptoms: rapid onset usually due to urinary tract obstruction; symptoms include:
    1. Nocturia
    2. Urgency

3. Frequency
4. Hesitancy

C. Regional symptoms
1. Lower extremity edema
2. Hematuria

D. Systemic symptoms
1. Low back pain due to lumbar sacral spinal metastasis
2. Weakness
3. Weight loss

III. **Physical examination findings**
A. DRE findings
1. Prostatic nodule
2. Induration
3. Enlargement
4. Asymmetry

B. DRE can be normal

C. The patient may present with the following:
1. Hydronephrosis
2. Adenopathy
3. Back pain due to metastasis
4. Biopsy revealing "adenocarcinoma of unknown primary"

IV. **Laboratory/diagnostic findings**
A. PSA greater than 4 ng/ml is abnormal; the use of age-specific reference ranges is somewhat controversial, but these are still used clinically

B. The age-specific normal reference ranges for PSA for men, based on a previous PSA of less than 4 ng/ml, are as follows:
1. Ages 40–49 years, level lower than 2.5 ng/ml
2. Ages 50–59 years, level lower than 3.5 ng/ml
3. Ages 60–69 years, level lower than 4.5 ng/ml
4. Ages 70–79 years, level lower than 6.5 ng/ml

C. Normal PSAs are present in approximately 40% of cases of prostate cancer

D. Prostatic acid phosphatase may be used to evaluate for nonlocalized disease

E. Bone scans generally are not indicated with PSA less than 10 ng/ml and no bone pain

F. Transrectal ultrasonography is used to evaluate the prostate for biopsy

G. Transrectal biopsy or aspiration with biopsy is required for diagnosis

H. Lymph node biopsy may be obtained through
1. Incisional biopsy or
2. Fine needle aspiration

I. A percent-free PSA may be ordered for borderline range PSA values. A low percent-free PSA suggests the presence of cancer and the need for biopsy.

J. The following may be ordered for cancer staging:

1. CT
2. MRI
3. Radionuclide bone scan
K. The most common prostate cancer grading system is the Gleason system, which ranges from 1–5.
    1. Primary and secondary grades are summed to yield 2–10
    2. The higher the score, the poorer the prognosis
V. **Major treatments**
    A. Localized prostate cancer
        1. "Watchful waiting"
            a. Palliative therapy for symptomatic/metastatic progression
        2. Radical prostatectomy is reserved for patients with greater than 10-year life expectancy
            a. Radical retropubic approach
            b. Perineal approach
        3. Radiation therapy is reserved for poor surgical candidates
            a. External beam radiation for localized cancer only
            b. Brachytherapy (internal radiation)—is less effective than external beam but has less toxic side effects to bladder and rectum
        4. Cryotherapy (new therapy)
    B. Regional or metastatic prostate cancer
        1. Chemotherapy
            a. First line will be docetaxel
            b. Abiraterone acetate with prednisone or enzalutamide or cabazitaxel after docetaxel
            c. Other drugs with limited responses include paclitaxel, carboplatin, vinorelbine, etoposide, doxorubicin, estramustine, and mitoxantrone.
            d. If patient has bone metastases, denosumab or zoledronic acid are added to therapy
        2. Palliative therapy includes the following:
            a. Transurethral resection/incision of the prostate (TURP/TUIP)
            b. Stents
            c. Hormonal therapy
            d. Bilateral orchiectomy
            e. Medical orchiectomy
            f. Radiation therapy
            g. Chemotherapy
    C. Follow-up: 3- to 6-month intervals with DRE and PSA
    D. For clinical guidelines for specific therapies related to stages of prostate cancer, see the American Cancer Society website at www.cancer.org, or the National Comprehensive Cancer Network website at www.nccn.org.

BLADDER CANCER

I. **General comments/incidence/predisposing factors**
  A. Fourth most common cancer in males in the United States and tenth among women
  B. Mean age at diagnosis is 65 years
  C. Reduced levels of serum carotene and serum retinol are seen in patients with bladder cancer
  D. Increased incidence associated with the following:
    1. Cigarette smoking
    2. Exposure to industrial dyes or solvents
    3. High dietary fat
    4. Race and gender—more common in Caucasians and men
    5. Chronic bladder irritation and infection
    6. Positive history of bladder cancer or other urothelial carcinomas
    7. Bladder birth defects
    8. Genetics and family history
    9. Chemotherapy and radiation therapy
    10. Arsenic—repeated exposure
    11. Low fluid consumption
  E. Reduced incidence associated with the following:
    1. Soy protein and garlic
    2. Administration of vitamins A, B6, C, E, and selenium
    3. Nonsteroidal anti-inflammatory drugs may inhibit the development of bladder cancer
II. **Subjective findings**
  A. May be asymptomatic in early disease
  B. Hematuria
    1. Gross or microscopic
    2. Chronic
    3. Intermittent
  C. Irritative voiding symptoms such as urinary frequency and urgency
III. **Physical examination findings**
  A. Masses detected on bimanual examination
  B. Hepatomegaly or supraclavicular lymphadenopathy may be present in metastatic disease
  C. Lymphedema of lower extremities may be present owing to metastases to pelvic lymph nodes
  D. Pyuria, occasionally
IV. **Laboratory/diagnostic findings**
  A. Urinalysis may show hematuria in most cases
  B. Azotemia associated with ureteral obstruction
  C. Anemia may be present owing to blood loss
  D. Urine tests to detect recurrent bladder cancer after treatment

1. Urine cytology—very effective in detecting high-grade bladder cancers but will miss many papillary urothelial neoplasms of low malignancy
2. BTA (tumor marker)—looks for specific proteins in the urine indicative of recurrent bladder cancer cells
3. NMP22 (tumor marker)—also looks for protein specific to recurrent bladder cancer cells
4. BTA and NMP22 are more sensitive than urine cytology in detecting low-grade cancers such as papillary urothelial neoplasms
5. Other markers currently being tested include HA-HAase, CYFRA21–1, and an antibody to whole cells called immunocyte

E. Exfoliated cells from normal and abnormal urothelium are seen in voided urine specimens
1. Cytology is sensitive to detection of exfoliated cells but may be enhanced by flow cytometry

F. Filling defects may be detected by the following:
1. Intravenous urography
2. Ultrasonography
3. CT
4. MRI

G. Diagnosis and staging of cancer confirmed by the following:
1. Cystoscopy
2. Biopsy
3. Transurethral resection

H. Grading based on the following:
1. Size
2. Pleomorphism
3. Mitotic rate
4. Hyperchromatism
5. World Health Organization classifications include low grade (Grades I and II) and high grade (Grade III).

I. Staging based on the following:
1. Extent of regional metastases
2. Distant metastases

V. **Major treatments**
A. Treatment
1. Transurethral resection
   a. Initial form of treatment
   b. Muscle-infiltrating cancers require more aggressive therapy
2. Partial cystectomy
   a. Solitary lesions
   b. Bladder diverticulum
3. Radical cystectomy removes the following:
   a. In men
      i. Bladder

    ii. Prostate
    iii. Seminal vesicles
    iv. Surrounding fat
    v. Peritoneal attachments
   b. In women
    i. Uterus
    ii. Cervix
    iii. Urethra
    iv. Anterior vaginal vault
    v. Ovaries
    vi. Bladder
   c. Bilateral pelvic lymph node dissection may be accomplished at the same time in both men and women
   d. Urinary diversion may also be performed
 B. Intravesical immunotherapy—agents delivered directly into the bladder by a urethral catheter usually BCG or interferon
 C. Intravesical chemotherapy
   a. Mitomycin
   b. Thiotepa
   c. Doxorubicin
 D. Chemotherapy
   1. Cisplatin-based combination chemotherapy is commonly used
   2. Chemotherapy may be used before surgery or postoperatively in an attempt to preserve the bladder
 E. Radiotherapy
   1. External beam radiotherapy is generally well tolerated
   2. Ten to fifteen percent of patients develop bladder, bowel, or rectal complications
 F. Decision algorithms for bladder cancer are available on the American Cancer Society website at www.cancer.org, and on the National Comprehensive Cancer Network website at www.nccn.org.

ENDOMETRIAL CANCER

I. **General comments/predisposing factors**
 A. Cancer of the endometrium is the most common cancer of the female reproductive organs
 B. Increased incidence with the following:
   1. Women 50–70 years old
   2. Menopause (75%)
   3. Obesity, especially upper body fat
   4. Unopposed exogenous estrogen
   5. History of infertility or nulliparity
   6. Diabetes
   7. Polycystic ovaries with prolonged anovulation
   8. Extended use of tamoxifen for the treatment of breast cancer

9. Personal or family history of ovarian or breast cancer
10. Higher socioeconomic status
11. Prior pelvic radiation therapy

C. Whites are 70% more likely to develop endometrial cancer than are African Americans.

D. The 5-year survival rate is 84% for all types of endometrial cancer, collectively.

II. **Subjective findings**

A. Postmenopausal bleeding should be treated as endometrial cancer until proven otherwise.

B. Abnormal bleeding is the presenting sign in 80% of cases

C. Lower abdominal pain or pressure

D. Back pain (rare)

E. Lower extremity edema may manifest as the result of metastasis

F. Weight loss

III. **Physical examination findings**

A. Usually, findings are normal on examination of the following:
1. Vagina
2. Uterus
3. Cervix

B. Enlarged uterus or pelvic mass may be present with advanced disease

C. Cervical stenosis

D. Pyometra

E. Mucosanguineous vaginal discharge may be present in cervical and vaginal metastases

F. Bladder or rectal mass may be a presentation of regional metastasis

IV. **Laboratory/diagnostic findings**

A. Endometrial biopsy (EMB), a first-line procedure in the office, may consist of
1. Endocervical sampling
2. Endometrial sampling

B. EMB provides an adequate sample in 90% to 95% of cases.

C. Dilatation and curettage has a higher sensitivity, especially when combined with EMB; the detection rate approaches 100%

D. Transvaginal uterine ultrasonography determines the thickness of the endometrium.

E. Hysteroscopy with directed biopsy may be required for staging of occult cancer.

F. Routine Pap smear
1. May detect cancer as "endometrial cells"
2. Insensitive diagnostic tool

G. Serial serum CA125 may be used to determine cancer recurrence.

V. **Major treatments**
  A. Extrafascial total abdominal hysterectomy with wide vaginal cuff
    1. Salpingo-oophorectomy
    2. Retroperitoneal lymph node sampling
  B. Radical hysterectomy
    1. Salpingo-oophorectomy
    2. Retroperitoneal lymph node dissection with cervical involvement
  C. Radiation may be used in the uterine cavity or externally before surgery in Grade II or Grade IIIA and may be concurrent with chemotherapy in Stage III.
  D. Radiation also is used for recurrences
  E. Vaginal brachytherapy for high-risk Stage IA or Stage IB
  F. In advanced or recurrent disease,
    1. Continuous nonestrogenic progesterone derivatives are used and evaluated every 3 months
    2. Combination chemotherapy is recommended with two of the following cisplatin, paclitaxel or doxorubicin. Carboplatin can be used in patients who cannot tolerate cisplatin.
  G. Common follow-up schedules include the following:
    1. Every 2 months for the first year
    2. Every 3 months for the second year
    3. Every 4 months for the third year
    4. Every 4 months for the fourth year
    5. Every 6 months for the fifth year
    6. Then, annually
    7. Breast examination every 6 months
    8. Mammogram annually
    9. Cytologic smears from the vaginal apex
      a. Every 6 months for 5 years
      b. Then annually
      c. May require vaginal lubrication and plastic vaginal dilator, particularly if radiation has been used
  H. Specific additional recommendations may be found on various websites, including the American Cancer Society website at www.cancer.org, and the National Comprehensive Cancer Network website at www.nccn.org.

BIBLIOGRAPHY

Alberg, A. J., Brock, M. J., Ford, J. G., Samet, J. M., & Spivack, S. D. (2013). Epidemiology of lung cancer: Diagnosis and management of lung cancer, 3rd ed: American College of Chest Physicians Evidence-Based Clinical Practice Guidelines. *Chest, 143*(Suppl. 5), e1S-e29S. doi:10.1378/chest.12–2345

American Cancer Society. (2013). *Bladder cancer*. Retrieved from http://www.cancer.org/cancer/bladdercancer/detailedguide/bladder-cancer-treating-general-info

American Cancer Society. (2013). *Endometrial cancer.* Retrieved from http://www.cancer.org/cancer/endometrialcancer/

American Cancer Society. (2013). *Prostate cancer.* Retrieved from http://www.cancer.org/cancer/prostatecancer/detailedguide/prostate-cancer-key-statistics

Centers for Disease Control. (2013). *Breast cancer.* Retrieved from http://www.cdc.gov/cancer/breast/

Centers for Disease Control. (2013). *Breast cancer treatment.* Retrieved from http://www.cdc.gov/cancer/breast/basic_info/treatment.htm

Centers for Disease Control. (2013). *Cervical cancer.* Retrieved from http://www.cdc.gov/cancer/cervical/

Centers for Disease Control. (2013). *Colorectal cancer.* Retrieved from http://www.cdc.gov/cancer/colorectal/

Centers for Disease Control. (2013). *Lung cancer.* Retrieved from http://www.cdc.gov/cancer/lung/

Centers for Disease Control. (2013). *Ovarian cancer.* Retrieved from http://www.cdc.gov/cancer/ovarian/

Jacobson, F. L., Austin, J. H., Field, J. K., Jett, J. R., Keshavjee, S., MacMahon, H., . . . Jaklitsch, M. T. (2012). Development of the American Association for Thoracic Surgery guidelines for low-dose computed tomography scans to screen for lung cancer in North America: Recommendations of the American Association for Thoracic Surgery Task Force for Lung Cancer Screening and Surveillance. *Thoracic and Cardiovascular Surgery, 144*(1), 25–32. doi: 10.1016/j.jtcvs.2012.05.059

Kemeny, N. E. (2013). Treatment of metastatic colon cancer: "The times they are a-changing." *Journal of Clinical Oncology, 31*(16), 1913–1916. doi:10.1200/JCO.2013.49.4500

National Cancer Institute. (2013). *General information about non-small cell lung cancer (NSCLC).* Retrieved from http://www.cancer.gov/cancertopics/pdq/treatment/non-small-cell-lung/healthprofessional/page1

National Collaborating Centre for Cancer. (2011). *Lung cancer. The diagnosis and treatment of lung cancer (Clinical guideline no. 121).* London, UK: National Institute for Health and Clinical Excellence (NICE).

Moorman, P. G. (2012). Genetic markers for ovarian cancer risk. Are we closer to seeing a clinical impact. *Personalized Medicine, 9*(6), 565–567.

National comprehensive Cancer Network. (2013). Non-small cell lung cancer. *Clinical Practice Guidelines in Oncology* (Version 2.2014). Retrieved from http//www.nccn.org/profressionals/physician_gls/PDF/nhl/pdf.

National comprehensive Cancer Network. (2013). Small cell lung cancer. *Clinical Practice Guidelines in Oncology* (Version 2.2014). Retrieved from http//www.nccn.org/profressionals/physician_gls/PDF/nhl/pdf

National comprehensive Cancer Network. (2013). Bladder cancer. *Clinical Practice Guidelines in Oncology* (Version 2.2014). Retrieved from http//www.nccn.org/profressionals/physician_gls/PDF/nhl/pdf

National comprehensive Cancer Network. (2013). Breast cancer. *Clinical Practice Guidelines in Oncology* (Version 2.2014). Retrieved from http//www.nccn.org/profressionals/physician_gls/PDF/nhl/pdf

National comprehensive Cancer Network. (2013). Endometrial cancer. *Clinical Practice Guidelines in Oncology* (Version 2.2014). Retrieved from http//www.nccn.org/profressionals/physician_gls/PDF/nhl/pdf

National comprehensive Cancer Network. (2013). Colon cancer. *Clinical Practice Guidelines in Oncology* (Version 2.2014). Retrieved from http//www.nccn.org/profressionals/physician_gls/PDF/nhl/pdf

National comprehensive Cancer Network. (2013). Cervical cancer. *Clinical Practice Guidelines in Oncology* (Version 2.2014). Retrieved from http//www.nccn.org/profressionals/physician_gls/PDF/nhl/pdf

National comprehensive Cancer Network. (2013). Ovarian cancer. *Clinical Practice Guidelines in Oncology* (Version 2.2014). Retrieved from http//www.nccn.org/profressionals/physician_gls/PDF/nhl/pdf

National comprehensive Cancer Network. (2013). Prostate cancer. *Clinical Practice Guidelines in Oncology* (Version 2.2014). Retrieved from http//www.nccn.org/profressionals/physician_gls/PDF/nhl/pdf

Saslow, D. (2012). *American Cancer Society, American Society for Colposcopy and Cervical Pathology and American Society for Clinical Pathology Screening Guidelines for the prevention and early detection of cervical cancer.* Retrieved from www.ncbi.nlm.nih.gov/pubmed/22431528

Schmidlin, E. J., Sundaram, B., & Kazerooni, E.A. (2012). Computed tomography screening for lung cancer. *Radiology Clinics of North America, 50*(5), 877–894. doi:10.1016/j.rcl.2012.06.008

Stephenson, A. J. (2013). Bladder cancer treatment: Invasive bladder. *UpToDate. Beyond the basics.* Retrieved from http://www.uptodate.com/contents/bladder-cancer-treatment-invasive-cancer-beyond-the-basics

U.S. Cancer Statistics Working Group. (2013). *United States Cancer Statistics: 1999–2010 incidence and mortality web-based report. Atlanta, GA: Department of Health and Human Services, Centers for Disease Control and Prevention, and National Cancer Institute.* Retrieved from http://www.cdc.gov/uscs

Management of Patients With Immunologic Disorders

CHAPTER 67

HIV/AIDS and Opportunistic Infections Among Older Adults

DAVID A. MILLER • THOMAS W. BARKLEY, JR.

HIV BACKGROUND INFORMATION

I. **HIV infection is not a barrier to living beyond the age of 50.**
    A. Between 2008 and 2011, incidence rates of HIV infection for those 50–54 remained stable, while incidence rates for those 55–64 years decreased.
    B. The greatest rise in incidence of HIV infection between the years 2008–2010 was among those 65 years and over.
    C. The prevalence of AIDS during 2008–2010 increased for those 65 years and older, decreased for those 60–64 years of age, and remained stable for those 50–59 years of age.
    D. Overall survival decreases if HIV is diagnosed after the age of 45 years of age, unless the patient has been previously, routinely tested.
    E. Approximately 11% of new HIV infections occur in patients aged 50 years or older, and is the fastest growing population HIV infected group in the United States

II. **Older individuals with HIV infection, with or without a stage 3 diagnosis of AIDS, often have co-morbidities that require treatment.**

III. **Virtually all of the current antiretroviral medications have been approved by the FDA based upon studies in individuals younger than 50 years old.**
    A. Older HIV-infected individuals require special monitoring to prevent significant drug-drug interactions, including with over-the-counter medications, herbals, and dietary supplements.

IV. **Current therapy for HIV infection, and its major complicating secondary illnesses (opportunistic diseases)—as well as for prevention of these secondary illnesses—undergoes frequent changes in current standards of care.**

   A. The provider of care to these patients is cautioned to check the most current standards. The Centers for Disease Control and Prevention issues regular updates to guidelines for care; these are available in printed media and on the Internet (see the references at the end of this chapter).

HIV INFECTION

I. **Etiology/incidence**

   A. HIV infection and AIDS are common; approximately 35 million persons infected worldwide

   B. The incidence of HIV infection varies among groups

   1. Heterosexually acquired HIV infection is frequent in Africa and Asia, and the incidence of heterosexually acquired HIV infection is rising in Western societies as well.

   2. In Western nations, men who have sex with men, illicit use of injected drugs, and congenital spread have been responsible for most HIV infections to date. Data among the elderly population is similar.

II. **Course of infection and important pathophysiologic markers**

   A. Retroviral infection by one of the strains of the human immunodeficiency virus

   B. HIV infects cells that express the CD4 receptor, including:

   1. Macrophages

   2. CD4+ T lymphocytes

   3. Langerhans' cells of the skin

   4. Macrophages in the CNS

   5. Other protected reservoirs, including the intestinal wall

   C. HIV infection is chronic and progressive

   1. Initially, a rapid increase occurs in the number of viral particles in the blood.

   2. During a period of clinical latency, which can be prolonged, the number of viral particles in each milliliter of blood (known as the viral load) is relatively low but detectable.

   3. During the development of symptomatic HIV disease and AIDS, the viral load increases and the number of CD4 lymphocytes measurable in the blood decreases.

   D. Therapy against HIV infection may alter the rate of progression to advanced immunodeficiency.

1. Recent data show that persons with HIV disease and AIDS live longer than in the past, and that combinations of antiretroviral medications (known collectively as antiretroviral therapy [ART] and in the past as highly active antiretroviral therapy, or HAART), along with appropriate management have clearly reduced mortality from HIV disease and opportunistic diseases that characterize AIDS.

DOCUMENTING HIV DISEASE

I. **Medical history: It is important to discuss these issues with all elderly patients, rather than to assume that they are not at risk.**
   A. Review of significant risk factors
      1. Documented risk factors for viral transmission
         a. Men who have sex with men
         b. Men and women who have unprotected sex with multiple partners
         c. Men and women who exchange sex for money or drugs, or who have sex partners who do
         d. Sexual partners of HIV-infected individuals; note that sexual transmission through rectal, vaginal, and oral sex has been documented
         e. Persons who are being treated for sexually transmitted infections (STIs)
         f. Persons who share equipment used to inject drugs
         g. Receipt of a blood transfusion in the early or mid-1980s, prior to screening of the blood supply (unlikely among persons over the age of 50)
         h. Transmission via blood in health care settings, including
            i. Accidental needlestick
            ii. Splashing of blood onto wounds
            iii. During dental procedures
      2. No other evidence of transmission has occurred during the pandemic.
   B. Current symptoms
      1. Acute retroviral syndrome
         a. Flulike illness
            i. Fever
            ii. Chills
            iii. Fatigue
            iv. Diffuse erythematous rash
         b. Serologic tests for HIV may be indeterminate, negative, or positive, depending on the length of time that has passed since the initial infection.
         c. HIV viral load measures are clearly elevated, and the CD4+ T-lymphocyte count is within normal range or reduced

       d. Often missed clinically because of rapid resolution without the need for acute medical care

       e. When documented, clearly dates the onset of infection

2. Latent HIV infection—the "asymptomatic phase"

       a. Few or no signs or symptoms of HIV-related illness; patient may have persistent generalized lymphadenopathy

       b. Positive enzyme-linked immunosorbent assay (ELISA) and Western blot for HIV infection

       c. Variable HIV viral load and CD4+ T-lymphocyte count over time

3. Symptomatic HIV disease (formerly AIDS-related complex)

       a. Fever, chills, diarrhea, unintended weight loss

       b. Appearance of non-AIDS-defining infections that are normally kept quiescent by an intact immune system, including

             i. Shingles (herpes zoster)

             ii. Thrush (candidiasis)

                  (a) Oral

                  (b) Mucocutaneous

                  (c) Vaginal

            iii. Frequent bacterial infections

       c. Laboratory evidence of declining CD4+ T-lymphocyte count or increasing HIV viral load

4. AIDS

       a. Measurable immunodeficiency, with the appearance of one of many AIDS indicator illnesses or opportunistic infections (see later section, Prophylaxis Against Opportunistic Infections); common opportunistic organisms include, among others (others listed later in this chapter):

             i. *Pneumocystis jiroveci* (formerly *P. carinii*)

             ii. *Cryptosporidium parvum*

            iii. *Candida albicans*

       b. The CD4+ T-lymphocyte count is typically below 500/mcl

       c. AIDS is diagnosed in the absence of opportunistic disease if the CD4+ T-lymphocyte count is below 200/mcl

5. Advanced HIV infection

       a. Category of HIV disease in which the CD4+ T-lymphocyte count is below 50/mcl

       b. Symptoms include:

              i. Wasting

             ii. Periodic fevers

            iii. Fatigue

       c. Single or multiple opportunistic infections may occur

       d. If this phase is documented during therapy for HIV infection, the prognosis is generally poor.

CLINICAL EVALUATION OF THE PATIENT AT RISK FOR HIV INFECTION

I. **Serologic testing**
   A. Screening tests
      1. ELISA for HIV (oral and/or blood sample)
         a. Initial test to screen for antibodies to HIV
         b. Requires seroconversion (process in which patient's HIV status changes from HIV negative to HIV positive), which occurs approximately 3 weeks to 6 months after exposure to the virus. Thus, enough time must have elapsed since exposure for antibodies to be detected on the ELISA so an accurate result can be obtained.
      2. Rapid screening tests are also available that determine results in less than 30 minutes.
         a. In general, these tests are not as reliable as ELISA because of higher rates of false-positive results.
         b. However, these are most useful in urgent care situations
            i. Hospital emergency rooms
            ii. After HIV exposure in health care settings
            iii. When the patient is not likely to return for screening results
            iv. Other settings such as clinics, small blood banks, etc.
         c. These tests include
            i. Saliva test (OraQuick—also available as a serum/blood test)
            ii. Urine test (Calypte HIV Urine Enzyme Immunoassay [EIA])
            iii. Blood tests
               (a) OraQuick Advance Rapid HIV 1 and 2 Antibody Test
               (b) Reveal Rapid HIV-1 Antibody Test
               (c) Uni-Gold Recombigen HIV Test
               (d) Multispot HIV-1/HIV-2 Rapid Test
               (e) Alere Determine HIV-½ Ag/Ab Combo test (can determine antibody presence and the presence of the HIV-1 p24 antigen)
         d. These tests have not replaced the ELISA in screening for HIV infection, although all are reasonably sensitive and specific.
      3. One kit is currently FDA approved and is available for patients to use at home.
         a. Home Access Express Test
         b. Counseling is given by telephone to those with positive results.
   B. Confirmatory tests for HIV infection

1. Western blot test
   a. Screens for the presence of antibodies against HIV
   b. Used after a positive result is determined by ELISA
   c. Relies on the detection of several different antibodies, including antibodies against envelope proteins of the HIV; to be considered indicative (positive) for HIV infection, at least two of the following should be present:
      i. gp160/120
      ii. gp41
      iii. p24
   d. Indeterminate tests, in which only one antibody is measurable, should be reevaluated in 4–6 weeks.
2. HIV DNA may be checked by polymerase chain reaction (PCR), or HIV RNA may be checked by PCR (quantitative) if the Western blot test yields indeterminate results; however, these tests require more time (days) and are more costly.

II. **Current and past health, social, sexual, and family histories, along with**
   A. Complete physical examination
      1. Specifically, height and weight (for BMI); fundoscopic; oral, skin, abdomen (liver, spleen), genitalia, and neurological
      2. Central obesity and frailty are being recognized more commonly among elderly patients with HIV infection.
      3. Racial disparities are more common among patients over the age of 50 than in the younger population of HIV infected individuals, especially among Blacks and Hispanic women.
   B. Full medication reconciliation (including herbals, vitamins, over-the-counter medications, and dietary supplements)
   C. Prior medication intolerance and allergies
      1. Sulfa allergies, particularly, since sulfa drugs may be used for prophylaxis against opportunistic disease, and because individuals treated with darunavir may exhibit cross-sensitivity to sulfa drugs
   D. Assessment of comorbidities, including hyperlipidemia, diabetes mellitus, coronary artery disease, and others related to tobacco use
   E. Discussions with the patient and family regarding health-care planning, end-of-life care, determination of the patient's mental capacity, palliative care, and advanced directives/durable power of attorney should be held during the course of management of the patient.

III. **HIV Prevention**
   A. Traditional
      1. Condoms
         a. Male: current evidence suggests that risk of seroconversion is lowered by consistent use
         b. Female: effective against many STDs, but unknown effectiveness with heterosexual spread of HIV

2. Male circumcision
   a. Heterosexual transmission in circumcised males was reduced by over 50% in several trials within Africa; because of the cell composition and fragility, foreskin is especially prone to HIV infection

B. Pre-Exposure prophylaxis (PrEP)
   1. Groups for who PrEP should be considered:
      a. PrEP is recommended as a preventative option for sexually-active adult men who have sex with men (MSM) at substantial risk of HIV infection.
      b. PrEP is recommended as one prevention option for adult injection drug users (IDU) at substantial risk of HIV infection.
      c. PrEP should be discussed with heterosexually-active women and men whose partners are known to have HIV infection (HIV discordant couples) as one of several options to protect the uninfected partner during conception and pregnancy so that an informed decision can be made in awareness of what is known and unknown about the benefits and risks of PrEP for mother and fetus.
   2. Combination regimen for PrEP
      a. Tenofovir, 300 mg daily, and
      b. Emtricitabine, 200 mg daily

C. Post-Exposure prophylaxis (PEP)
   1. Consists of a 28 day course of a 3 drug regimen
   2. Preferred regimen is emtricitabine/tenofovir (Truvada) and raltegravir

IV. **Initial laboratory evaluation of the HIV-infected patient**
A. CBC count
B. CD4+ cell count (CD4+ T lymphocyte, or "helper" lymphocyte, is a target cell for HIV infection), measured in cells per microliter (cells/mcl)
C. HIV RNA level, quantitative (viral load)
   1. Inflammatory processes, including other infections, may increase the viral load, and interpretation should always consider this fact, even when repeated viral load testing is conducted after therapy has begun.
   2. Drug resistance to one, or more than one, of the antiretroviral medications used as ART, and non-adherence to ART, should also be considered if the viral load remains elevated or rises after therapy has begun.
D. HIV resistance testing
   1. Drug resistance testing is recommended at entry into HIV care, regardless of whether therapy is initiated immediately or deferred.
   2. Genotypic testing is recommended as the preferred resistance testing to guide therapy in antiretroviral-naïve patients.

3. The action of phenotypic to genotypic testing is generally preferred for persons with known or suspected complex drug-resistance mutation patterns, particularly to protease inhibitors.

E. Syphilis testing (Venereal Disease Research Laboratory [VDRL] or rapid plasma reagin [RPR])

F. Hepatitis screening (A, B, and C)

G. Serum chemistry evaluation, including lipid profile and liver profile

H. Vitamin D level
   1. Severe vitamin D deficiency has been documented, related to the intensity and levels of inflammation, important among elderly patients at risk for osteoporosis.

I. Tuberculosis skin test (results are positive with induration of 5 mm or greater)

J. Pap smear/gynecologic evaluation

K. Chest x-ray

L. Other testing
   1. Toxoplasmosis serology (to assist in the differential diagnosis of CNS lesions)
   2. Cytomegalovirus (CMV) serology, especially for those at apparent low risk for CMV infection (CMV is a blood-borne pathogen)
   3. Glucose-6-phosphate dehydrogenase (G6PD) levels (especially in men of Mediterranean background and possibly in men of African heritage as well) prior to dapsone, primaquine, and sulfonamide therapy, which is associated with severe hemolysis in G6PD-deficient individuals
   4. Varicella antibody testing to determine prior infection (in patients unable to recall prior disease) with chicken pox or shingles in the event that a significant exposure occurs in the future
   5. If use of abacavir (Ziagen) is considered, testing for the HLA-B*5701 is recommended to reduce the risk of development of delayed hypersensitivity to abacavir and signs and symptoms of fever, rash (including toxic epidermal necrolysis), gastrointestinal symptoms, and respiratory complaints.

INITIATION OF ANTIRETROVIRAL THERAPY (ART)

I. **Referral to infectious disease specialist**
   A. Primary care providers without HIV experience should identify experts in their regions, preferably an infectious disease specialist, who will be available for consultation when needed.

II. **Asymptomatic patients**
   A. Debate continues in clinical practice as to when it is best to start ART
   1. Current trends favor starting antiretroviral therapy once a patient becomes aware of HIV-positive status, thereby reducing viral load.

2. However, decisions regarding when to start therapy should be considered within the context of each patient/clinical presentation, including potential issues of accessibility to care (e.g., homeless, adherence, etc.)
3. Antiretroviral therapy (ART) is recommended for all HIV-infected individuals to reduce the risk of disease progression (Rating of Recommendations: A = Strong; B = Moderate; C = Optional; Rating of Evidence: I = Data from randomized controlled trials; II = Data from well-designed nonrandomized trials or observational cohort studies with long-term clinical outcomes; III = Expert opinion).
   a. The strength of and evidence for this recommendation vary by pretreatment CD4 T lymphocyte (CD4) cell count: CD4 count less than 350 cells/mm (AI); CD4 count 350–500 cells/mm (AII); CD4 count greater than 500 cells/mm (BIII).
4. ART also is recommended for HIV-infected individuals for the prevention of transmission of HIV.
   a. The strength of and evidence for this recommendation vary by transmission risks: perinatal transmission (AI); heterosexual transmission (AI); other transmission risk groups (AIII).
5. Patients starting ART should be willing and able to commit to treatment and understand the benefits and risks of therapy and the importance of adherence (AIII). Patients may choose to postpone therapy, and providers, on a case-by-case basis, may elect to defer therapy on the basis of clinical and/or psychosocial factors.

III. **Symptomatic patient (with or without AIDS-defining illness; acute retroviral syndrome)**
   A. Treat, regardless of CD4+ cell count or viral load measurement
   B. Follow 2014 Treatment Guidelines

ANTIRETROVIRAL THERAPY (ART)

I. **Regimen considerations**
   A. Table 67.1 depicts current FDA-approved medications for HIV/AIDS.
   B. ART involves combination therapy, that is, the use of three or more antiretroviral agents from different drug classes.
   C. It is strongly believed that although management of HIV/AIDS is within the scope of practice of the acute care nurse practitioner (ACNP), patients should be closely monitored and followed by an experienced expert HIV/AIDS specialist health care provider. That is, extreme caution should be taken when one is considering adjusting or changing HIV/AIDS medication regimens in clinical practice unless the nurse practitioner is an experienced HIV/AIDS specialist. This will be particularly true for elderly patients who are on multiple medications for comorbid conditions, in whom drug-drug interactions with ART medications, especially protease inhibitors are included (e.g., simvastatin).

Table 67.1	Currently Marketed Antiretroviral Medications	
Generic Name	**Trade Name**	**Abbreviation**
Nucleoside and Nucleotide Reverse Transcriptase Inhibitors (NRTI)		
Abacavir	Ziagen	ABC
Didanosine	Videx	ddI
Emtricitabine	Emtriva	FTC
Lamivudine	Epivir	3TC
Stavudine	Zerit	d4T
Tenofovir	Viread	TDF
Zidovudine	Retrovir, AZT	ZDV
Non-Nucleoside Reverse Transcriptase Inhibitors (NNRTI)		
Delavirdine	Rescriptor	DLV
Efavirenz	Sustiva	EFV
Etravirine	Intelence	ETR
Nevirapine	Viramune	NVP
Rilpivirine	Edurant	RPV
Protease Inhibitors (PI)		
Atazanavir	Reyataz	ATV
Darunavir	Prezista	DRV
Fosamprenavir	Lexiva	FPV
Indinavir	Crixivan	IDV
Lopinavir	Kaletra (RTV/LPV)[a]	LPV
Nelfinavir	Viracept	NFV
Ritonavir	Norvir	RTV
Saquinavir	Invirase	SQV
Tipranavir	Aptivus	TPV
Integrase Inhibitors (INSTI)		
Dolutegravir	Tivicay	DTG
Raltegravir	Isentress	RAL
Elvitegravir[b]	Stribild	EVG
Fusion Inhibitor		
Enfuvirtide	Fuzeon	ENF
CCR5 Antagonist		
Maraviroc	Selzentry	MVC

[a]Lopinavir currently available only in co-formulation with ritonavir

[b]EVG currently available only in co-formulation with cobicistat (COBI)/TDF/FTC

D. Practitioners are encouraged to assess each patient's reconciled medication list with any new medications prescribed as ART or as prophylaxis against opportunistic diseases.

Table 67.2	Currently recommended regimens to be used as first-line medications for ART
Regimen	**Included drugs**
Optimal approaches:	Three medications, often two NRTIs ("backbone" of therapy), along with either a "boosted" protease inhibitor (PI + ritonavir), or a NNRTI, or an integrase inhibitor.
Recommended combination therapy irrespective of baseline viral load or CD4+ lymphocyte count	NNRTI-based regimen: EFV/TDF/FTC PI-based regiments: ATV/r plus TDF/FTC DRV/r plus TDF/FTC Integrase Inhibitor-based regimens: DTG plus ABC (for patients who are HLA-B*5701 negative)/3TC DTG plus TDF/FTC EVG/cobi/TDF/FTC (if CrCl is greater than 70 ml/min) RAL plus TDF/FTC

Note. 3TC = lamivudine; ABC = abacavir; ART = antiretroviral therapy; ARV = antiretroviral; ATV/r = atazanavir/ritonavir; cobi = cobicistat; CrCl = creatinine clearance; DRV/r = darunavir/ritonavir; DTG = dolutegravir; EFV = efavirenz; EVG = elvitegravir; FTC = emtricitabine; INSTI = integrase strand transfer inhibitor; LPV/r = lopinavir/ritonavir; NNRTI = non-nucleoside reverse transcriptase inhibitor; NRTI = nucleoside reverse transcriptase inhibitor; PI = protease inhibitor; RAL = raltegravir; RPV = rilpivirine; RTV = ritonavir; TDF = tenofovir disoproxil fumarate.

II.   Follow-up of Initial ART

A. CD4+ cell count and HIV viral load determination 4–6 weeks after initiation and every 3–6 months thereafter until the viral load is fully suppressed or is undetectable. A rise in CD4+ lymphocyte count and reduction in HIV viral load is anticipated. Elderly patients may improve their CD4+ lymphocyte counts and viral load levels more slowly than younger patients. Once the viral load is suppressed, the CD4+ lymphocyte count need only be checked if the viral load becomes elevated again (Panel, 2014).

B. Patient counseling about the need to faithfully adhere to the prescribed medication regimen and to attend scheduled follow-up visits is mandatory.

   1. The need for adherence and follow-up visits should be reiterated at each visit. Repeat medication reconciliation is suggested at each follow-up visit.

   2. A half log rise in the viral load or a significant drop in the CD4+ cell count warrants consideration for revision of ART.

   3. Depending on the opportunistic infection, prophylaxis against opportunistic infections should be continued once started, or when the CD4+ lymphocyte count exceeds a level recommended by current evidence.

4. Current recommendations may alter prophylaxis therapy if patients has significant immunologic stability or improvement in immunodeficiency (see Prophylaxis Against Opportunistic Infections section)

5. Elderly patients initiated on tenofovir (Ziagen) should have regular (monthly) tests of glomerular filtration (eGFR; creatinine; BUN) to assure altered renal function (i.e., creatinine clearance less than 50 cc/hr) is not occurring due to the drug.

III. Treatment for patients who are deteriorating during ART therapy deterioration is measured by deteriorating CD4+ cell count, a verified half log rise in the viral load, or the appearance of an opportunistic infection during ART therapy.

A. Refer to an HIV/AIDS or infectious disease specialist for consideration of revision of ART

B. Drug resistance testing may be used to determine whether a patient's dominant HIV strain is still sensitive to current ART.

1. Genotypic testing looks for known patterns of mutations in the reverse transcriptase or viral protease genes.

2. This testing may therefore guide changes in ART if needed

3. Routine genotypic or phenotypic testing provides information relevant for selecting appropriate alternative regimens. There currently is no evidence that elderly patients with HIV differ from younger patients in this regard. Genotypic or phenotypic testing may provide relevant information in selecting appropriate alternative regimens.

PROPHYLAXIS AGAINST SELECT OPPORTUNISTIC INFECTIONS (2013 Guidelines)

I. Recommendations for Select Opportunistic Infections

A. Tuberculosis, based on a positive screening test for latent tuberculosis infection (LTBI) (which may include tuberculin skin test [TST] or interferon-gamma release assays [IGRA]), on recent exposure to a person infected with active TB, or on previously inadequately treated TB: Isoniazid, 300 mg PO with pyridoxine, 50 mg PO daily for 9 months

B. *Pneumocystis jiroveci* (formerly *P. carinii*), based on a rapidly declining CD4+ cell count or an absolute CD4+ cell count of less than 200 cells/mcl:

1. Trimethoprim-sulfamethoxazole (TMP/SMX) DS, 1 tablet PO daily, or aerosolized pentamidine, 300 mg, via nebulizer monthly, or atovaquone, 1500 mg PO daily

2. Patients whose CD4+ T-lymphocyte counts rise above 300 cells/mcl for over 3 months while on ART may stop primary prophylaxis (i.e., no prior *P. jiroveci* [*carinii*] pneumonia [PCP])

3. Secondary prophylaxis (i.e., patients with history of PCP) should continue prophylaxis
   a. TMP-SMX DS 1 tablet PO daily or
   b. Aerosolized pentamidine 300 mg via nebulizer every month or
   c. Atovaquone 1500 mg PO daily

C. Toxoplasmosis, based on CD4+ count less than 100 cells/mcl and positive immunoglobulin G (Ig) serology
   1. TMP/SMX as above for PCP or dapsone, 50 mg daily plus pyrimethamine, 50 mg weekly; leucovorin, 25 mg weekly or atovaquone 1500 mg PO (with or without pyrimethamine 25 mg plus leucovorin 10 mg) daily
   2. Patients whose CD4+ T-lymphocyte counts rise above 200 cells/mcl for 3 months in response to ART may stop primary prophylaxis against toxoplasmosis.
   3. Secondary prophylaxis may be considered to be discontinued if patient successfully completes initial therapy, remains free of signs/symptoms of TE, and has a CD4+ count above 200 cells/mcl for more than 6 months in response to ART therapy.

D. Mycobacterium avium, based on CD4+ cell count below 50 cells/mcl
   1. Azithromycin (Zithromax), 1200 mg once weekly, or clarithromycin (Biaxin), 500 mg BID
   2. In patients whose CD4+ T-lymphocyte count is higher than 100 cells/mcl for 3 months may stop primary prophylaxis against *M. avium*
   3. Patients who have had active *M. avium* infection, especially bacteremia, should complete therapy for their primary infection and then receive secondary prophylaxis, as listed above. Although some clinicians would stop this secondary prophylaxis, others would treat indefinitely. May be considered to be discontinued if patient has completed more than 12 months of therapy, shows no signs/symptoms of MAC disease, and has a CD4+ count greater than 100 cells/mcl for more than 6 months in response to ART therapy.

E. There are other opportunistic infections that may require prophylaxis (i.e. *Histoplasma*, Coccidioidomycosis, Penicilliosis)

II. **Vaccinations recommended**

A. Hepatitis B, based on finding anti-hepatitis B core antigen negative
   1. Recombivax HB, 10 mcg IM, or Engerix-B, 20 mcg IM, on three separate occasions, at 3, 6, and 12 months
   2. Assess antibody response, especially if CD4+ counts rise above 200 cells/mcl

B. Inactivated influenza vaccine (all patients): 0.5 ml IM annually in October or November
   1. May cause the viral load to increase temporarily and is contraindicated in HIV-infected patients

2. Viral load determinations should be done prior to administration of the vaccine or upon waiting several weeks after the vaccine.
3. Live-attenuated influenza vaccine is contraindicated in HIV-infected patients

C. Hepatitis A vaccination for HAV-susceptible patients with chronic liver disease, are injection drug users, or men who have sex with men (MSM), especially those with chronic hepatitis C infection
1. Havrix, 0.5 ml IM on two occasions 6 months apart
2. The CDC has recommended Havrix for all men who have sex with men who are seronegative for hepatitis A.

D. Pneumococcal vaccine (for all patients), 0.5 mL IM once
1. Revaccination can be recommended for patients whose initial CD4+ T-lymphocyte count was less than 200 cells/mcl and rises to above that level. Revaccination should also be considered (after 5 years) for patients who have other comorbid conditions, including chronic heart, lung, and kidney disorders, and diabetes, according to current Advisory Committee on Immunization Practices/Centers for Communicable Diseases annual recommendations.

E. Tdap vaccine: one time administration as an adult instead of Td
F. Varicella zoster virus vaccination should be considered for all elderly patients whose CD4+ T lymphocyte counts are over 200 cells/mcl

AIDS DEFINING CONDITIONS

I. An HIV serology screening should be done in all patients who present with the conditions listed in this section (signs/symptoms/treatment included for most common opportunistic infections)

A. Candidiasis of the esophagus, trachea, bronchi, or lungs
1. Symptoms are referable to the region of the body affected
2. Severe disease may require IV therapy: amphotericin B, 0.5–1 mg/kg/day; fluconazole (Diflucan), 200–400 mg/day
3. Milder disease may respond to fluconazole, 200 mg/day PO

B. Cervical cancer, invasive
C. Coccidioidomycosis, extrapulmonary
D. Cryptococcosis, extrapulmonary
1. Meningitis
   a. Manifestations may include fever, headache, and altered level of consciousness
   b. Treatment: Liposomal amphotericin B 3–4 mg/kg IV daily + flucytosine 25 mg/kg PO GID for at least 2 weeks, followed by fluconazole, 400 mg/day PO for at least 8 weeks; followed by secondary prophylaxis at 200–400 mg/day
2. Pulmonary/disseminated disease; depends on the severity of the disease, severe manifestation is treated the same as for meningitis

      a. Fluconazole, 200–400 mg/day, followed by secondary prophylaxis at 200 mg/day

E. Cryptosporidiosis with diarrhea for over 1 month

F. Cytomegalovirus of any organ, excluding liver, spleen, and lymph nodes

G. Herpes simplex mucocutaneous outbreak lasting longer than 1 month, or of the bronchi, lungs, or esophagus

    1. Treatment of severe disease: acyclovir (Zovirax), 400 mg PO 5 times a day for 7 days

    2. Secondary prophylaxis should be offered to patients with recurrences of herpes outbreak: acyclovir, 400 mg BID

H. Histoplasmosis, extrapulmonary

I. HIV-Associated dementia

J. HIV-Associated wasting

K. Isosporiasis, with diarrhea for longer than 1 month

L. Kaposi's sarcoma in a patient younger than age 60

M. Lymphoma, brain, in a patient younger than age 60

N. Lymphoma, non-Hodgkin's, of B-cell origin, or immunoblastic lymphoma

O. *Mycobacterium avium* or *Mycobacterium kansasii* infection with dissemination

P. *Mycobacterium tuberculosis* infection, disseminated

Q. *Mycobacterium tuberculosis* infection, pulmonary

    1. For symptoms, findings, diagnosis, and treatment, see Restrictive (Inflammatory) Lung Diseases and Heart Failure chapter

R. Nocardiosis

S. *Pneumocystis jiroveci (carinii)* pneumonia

    1. Moderately high fever (e.g., 103°F), nonproductive cough, and dyspnea, often out of proportion to radiographic findings; may progress to respiratory failure with acute respiratory distress syndrome

    2. Diagnosis, definitive: silver stains of bronchial washings or biopsies. Some clinicians elect to treat empirically.

    3. Treatment

        a. Trimethoprim, 15–20 mg/kg/day with sulfamethoxazole, 75–100 mg/kg/day IV every 6–8 hr, changing to oral TMP/SMX (2 double-strength tablets three times a day) for a total of 21 days of therapy

        b. Corticosteroids (prednisone, 40 mg BID or Solu-Medrol, 40 mg IV every 12 hr) are indicated for moderately severe or severe disease (PaO_2 [partial pressure of oxygen in arterial blood] less than 70 on room air), with the dose tapered as the disease responds to antimicrobial therapy.

    T. Pneumonia, recurrent bacterial
        1. For symptoms, findings, diagnosis, and treatment, see Lower
           Respiratory Tract Pathogens chapter
    U. Progressive multifocal leukoencephalopathy
    V. Salmonella septicemia, recurrent (non-typhoid)
    W. Strongyloidosis, outside the gut
    X. Toxoplasmosis, internal organ
    Y. CD4+ cell count less than 200 cells/mcl

BIBLIOGRAPHY

Aberg, J. A., Gallant, J. E., Ghanem, K. G., Emmanuel, P., Zingman, B. S., & Horberg, M. A. (2014). Primary care guidelines for the management of persons infected with HIV: 2013 update by the HIV Medicine Association of the Infectious Diseases Society of America. *Clinical Infectious Disease, 58*(1), 1–10. doi:10.1093/cid/cit757

Ansemant, T., Mahy, S., Piroth, C., Ornetti, P., Ewing, S., Guilland, J-C., . . . Piroth, L. (2013). Severe hypovitaminosis D correlates with increased inflammatory markers in HIV infected patients. *BioMed Central Infectious Diseases, 13*(7). doi:10.1186/1471–2334–13–7

Arcangelo, V. P., & Peterson, A. M. (Eds.). (2013). *Pharmacotherapeutics for advanced practice: A practical approach* (3rd ed.). Philadelphia, PA: Lippincott Williams & Wilkins.

Bartlett, J. G. (2013). Considerations prior to initiating antiretroviral therapy. In D. S. Basow (Ed.), *UpToDate*. Waltham, MA: UpToDate.

Bartlett, J. G. (2013). Selecting antiretroviral regimens for the treatment naïve HIV-infected patient. In D. S. Basow (Ed.), *UpToDate*. Waltham, MA: UpToDate.

Brooks, J. T., Buchacz, K., Gebo, K. A., & Mermin, J. (2012). HIV infection and older Americans: The public health perspective. *American Journal of Public Health, 102*(8), 1516–1526. doi:10.2105/AJPH.2012.300844

Cahill, S., & Valadéz, R. (2013). Growing older with HIV/AIDS: New public health challenges. *American Journal of Public Health, 103*(3), e7-e15. doi:10.2105/AJPH.2012.301161

Campanelli, C. M. (2012). American Geriatrics Society updated Beers criteria for potentially inappropriate medication use in older adults. *Journal of the American Geriatrics Society, 60*(4), 616–631. doi:10.1111/j.1532–5415.2012.03923.x

Campo, J. W., Jamjian, C., & Boulston, C. (2012). HIV antiretroviral drug resistance. *Journal of AIDS & Clinical Research, S5*. doi:10.4172/2155–6113. S5–002

Centers for Disease Control and Prevention. (2013). *HIV surveillance report, 23*. Retrieved November 15, 2013, from http://www.cdc.gov/hiv/pdf/ statistics_2011_HIV_Surveillance_Report_vol_23.pdf

Centers for Disease Control and Prevention. (2013). *Pre-exposure prophylaxis*. Retrieved March 26, 2014, from http://www.cdc.gov/hiv/prevention/research/ prep/

Centers for Disease Control and Prevention. (2014). *Male circumcision*. Retrieved March 26, 2014, from http://www.cdc.gov/hiv/prevention/research/ malecircumcision/

Cianelli, R. [Editorial]. (2010). HIV: A health-related disparity among older Hispanic women. *Hispanic Health Care International, 8*(2). doi:10.1891/1540–4153.8.2.58

Darque, A., Enel, P., Ravaux, I., Petit, N., & Retornaz, F. (2012). Drug interactions in elderly individuals with the human immunodeficiency virus. *Journal of the American Geriatric Society, 60*(2), 382–384.

Food and Drug Administration (FDA). (2013). *DetermineTM HIV-½ Ag/ Ab combo*. Retrieved November 29, 2013, from http://www.fda.gov/ downloads/BiologicsBloodVaccines/BloodBloodProducts/ApprovedProducts/ PremarketApprovalsPMAs/UCM364698.pdf

Food and Drug Administration. (2013). *Antiretroviral drugs used in the treatment of HIV infection*. Retrieved Nov. 21, 2013, from http://www.fda. gov/forconsumers/byaudience/forpatientadvocates/hivandaidsactivities/ ucm118915.htm

Hansten, P. D., & Horn, J. R. (2013). *The top 100 drug interactions: A guide to patient management* (2013 edition). Freeland, WA: H&H Publications.

Henry J. Kaiser Family Foundation. (2013). *The global HIV/AIDS epidemic*. Retrieved November 20, 2013, from www.kff.org/global-health-policy/fact- sheet/the-global-hivaids-epidemic/

Katzung, B. G., Masters, S. B., & Trevor, A. J. (Eds.). (2012). *Basic & clinical pharmacology* (12th ed.). New York, NY: McGraw-Hill.

Landovitz, R. J., & Currier, J. S. (2009). Postexposure prophylaxis for HIV infection. *New England Journal of Medicine, 361*, 1768–1775.

Linley, L., Prejean, J., An, Q., Chen, M., & Hall, H. I. (2012). Racial/ethnic disparities in HIV diagnoses among persons aged 50 years and older in 37 US states, 2005–2008. *American Journal of Public Health, 102*(8), 1521–1534.

Liu, A., Cohen, S., Follansbee, S., Cohen, D., Weber, S., Sachdev, D., & Buchbinder, S. (2014). Early experiences implementing pre-exposure prophylaxis (PrEP) for HIV prevention in San Francisco. *Public Library of Science Medicine, 11*(3). doi:10.1371/journal.pmed.1001613

Panel on Antiretroviral Guidelines for Adults and Adolescents. (2014). *Guidelines for the use of antiretroviral agents in HIV-1-infected adults and adolescents.* Retrieved June 23, 2014, from http://aidsinfo.nih.gov/ContentFiles/ AdultandAdolescentGL.pdf

Sabharwal, C. J., & Casau-Schulhof, N. (2013). In D. S. Basow (Ed.), *UpToDate.* Waltham, MA: UpToDate.

Sankar, A., Nevedal, A., Neufeld, S., Berry, R., & Luborsky, M. (2011). What do we know about older adults and HIV? A review of social and behavioral literature. *AIDS Care, 23*(10), 1187–1207.

Shar, K., Hilton, T. N., Myers, L., Pinto, J. F., Luque, A. E., & Hall, W. J., (2012). A new frailty syndrome: Central obesity and frailty in older adults with the human immunodeficiency virus. *Journal of the American Geriatrics Society, 60*(3), 545–549. doi:10.1111./j.1532–5415.2011.03819.x

Smith, D. K., Martin, M., Lansky, A., Mermin, J., & Choopanya, K. (2013). Update to interim guidance for preexposure prophylaxis (PrEP) for the prevention of HIV infection: PrEP for injecting drug users. *Morbidity and Mortality Weekly Report, 62*(23), 463–465.

Test Texas HIV Coalition. (2013). *ICD Coding for HIV/AIDS.* Retrieved November 16, 2013, from http://testtexashiv.org/documents/ICD_Coding_for_ HIV_AIDS_2.pdf

University of Miami Ethics Programs. (2013). *Geriatrics: Decision-making, autonomy, valid consent and guardianship.* Retrieved November 27, 2013, from http://www.miami.edu/index.php/ethics/projects/geriatrics_and_ethics/ decision-making_autonomy_valid_consent_and_guardianship/

University of Miami Ethics Programs. (2013). *Geriatrics: End-of-life issues.* Retrieved November 27, 2013, from http://www.miami.edu/index.php/ ethics/ projects/geriatrics_and_ethics/end-of-life_issues/

U.S. Department of Health and Human Services. (2014). *Panel on opportunistic infections in HIV-infected adults and adolescents.* Guidelines for the prevention and treatment of opportunistic infections in HIV-infected adults and adolescents: Recommendations from the Centers for Disease Control and Prevention, the National Institutes of Health, and the HIV Medicine Association of the Infectious Diseases Society of America. Retrieved from http://aidsinfo.nih.gov/contentfiles/ lvguidelines/adult_oi.pdfNote.

Wamai, R. G., Morris, B. J., Bailis, S. A., Sokal, D., Klausner, J. D., Appleton, R., . . . Banerjee, J. (2011). Male circumcision for HIV prevention: Current evidence and implementation in sub-Saharan Africa. Journal of International AIDS Society, 14(49). doi:10.1186/1758-2652-14-49

CHAPTER 68

Autoimmune Diseases

LISA A. JOHNSON • THOMAS W. BARKLEY, JR.

GIANT CELL ARTERITIS

I. **Definition**
   A. Systemic panarteritis of the medium-sized and large arteries, usually the temporal artery or the aorta
   B. Believed to represent the extreme spectrum of polymyalgia rheumatica
      1. Polymyalgia rheumatica is a clinical diagnosis based on pain and stiffness in the shoulder and pelvic girdle region. Often associated with malaise, weight loss, and fever
      2. Headache, jaw claudication, scalp tenderness, and throat pain are classic symptoms
      3. Considered a medical emergency
      4. Untreated temporal arteritis may result in irreversible blindness.
      5. Untreated aortic arteritis may result in the serious or life-threatening sequela of aortic occlusion.

II. **Etiology/incidence/predisposing factors**
   A. Vascular endothelial cells become "activated" and
      1. Act as antigen-presenting cells and sources of cytokine production
      2. Interact with immune-competent cells, and
      3. Express adhesion molecules, promoting leukocyte binding and aggregation.
   B. Occurs most commonly in adults older than 50 years
   C. Slightly more common in women than in men
   D. Approximately 50% of patients with giant cell arteritis also have polymyalgia rheumatica.
   E. Patients are 17 times more likely to develop thoracic aortic aneurysms (typically occurs 7 years after diagnosis)

III.   Subjective findings
   A. Persistent headache
   B. Localized scalp tenderness on palpation
   C. Jaw claudication
   D. Visual impairment (particularly diplopia or amaurosis fugax)
   E. Throat pain
   F. Arm claudication

IV.   Physical examination findings
   A. Difficulty talking
   B. Fever (giant cell arteritis accounts for 15% of all cases of fever of unknown origin in patients older than 65 years)
   C. Temporal artery may be large, nodular, tender, pulseless, or normal
   D. Blindness (from anterior ischemic optic neuropathy)
   E. Asymmetry of pulses in arm, aortic regurgitation, bruits nears the clavicle, or unequal upper extremity blood pressures suggest the involvement of the aorta or major branches.

V.   Laboratory/diagnostic findings
   A. Computed tomography angiography can confirm the diagnosis by demonstrating arterial narrowing
   B. Normal white blood cell count between 6,000 and 10,000/ml (before prednisone is initiated)
   C. Elevated erythrocyte sedimentation rate (ESR); typically above 50 mm/hr
   D. C-reactive protein elevation (not always present)
   E. Interleukin 6 is the most sensitive but not widely used
   F. Biopsy of the affected artery is the gold standard
      1. Positive biopsy result confirms the diagnosis
      2. False-negative biopsy result can occur. If clinical suspicion is strong, the patient should be treated, regardless of the negative result.
   G. Aortogram as indicated by the clinical presentation of aortic aneurysm or occlusion
   H. Reactive thrombocytosis with mild normochromic and normocytic anemia

VI.   Management
   A. Should begin prednisone immediately upon clinical diagnosis
      1. Do not wait for biopsy
      2. Biopsies obtained 1–2 weeks after initiation of prednisone are reliable
   B. Intravenous methylprednisolone, 1 gram daily for 3 days in patients with visual loss
   C. Prednisone, 40–60 mg/day for 6 weeks to 2 months
   D. Prednisone may be tapered after 6 weeks to 2 months if symptoms have subsided

E. Falling ESR may be used as a guide for beginning tapering, but tapering should not start sooner than 6 weeks after initiation of therapy, regardless of ESR

F. Educate patient regarding signs and symptoms of recurrence; patients are at greater risk for recurrence

SYSTEMIC LUPUS ERYTHEMATOSUS (SLE)

I. **Definition**
   A. A chronic, inflammatory, autoimmune disorder that may affect multiple body systems
   B. Clinical signs and symptoms are caused by trapping of antigen/antibody complexes in capillaries or visceral structures, or by autoantibody-mediated destruction of host cells
   C. Clinical course is characterized by exacerbations and remissions. The disease may be mild or rapidly fatal.

II. **Etiology/incidence/predisposing factors**
   A. Must rule out drug-induced lupus; hydralazine, methyldopa, quinidine, chlorpromazine, and isoniazid are among many of the potential drugs that cause drug-induced lupus, which resolves when offending drug is stopped.
   B. A variety of stimuli are thought to trigger aberrant function of T and B cells in a genetically predisposed host.
      1. Sex hormones
      2. Ultraviolet radiation
      3. Infection
      4. Stress
   C. Autoantibody and immunoglobulin production is increased
   D. Eighty-five percent of patients with SLE are women
   E. SLE occurs most often in African-American women
   F. An increased familial risk has been noted

III. **Clinical findings**
   A. Joint symptoms with or without synovitis often the earliest symptom (nonerosive arthritis)
   B. Systemic features: fever, malaise, weight loss, and anorexia
   C. Skin lesions (malar or discoid rash present in less than 50% of patients)
   D. Oral and nasopharyngeal ulcers
   E. Ocular changes (photophobia, conjunctivitis, blurring, and blindness)
   F. Heart failure from myocarditis and hypertension, cardiac arrhythmias, and mesenteric vasculitis
   G. Pericarditis, pleural effusions, pleurisy, pneumonia, and restrictive lung disease
   H. Glomerulonephritis and chronic kidney disease
   I. Abdominal pain (postprandial), ileus, and peritonitis

J. Cognitive impairment, psychosis, depression, neuropathies, strokes, and seizures

IV. Laboratory/diagnostic findings

    A. Serum antinuclear antibody is present in virtually all patients and is sensitive, but not specific; titers less than 1:160 are usually false-positives.

    B. A variety of other laboratory tests may show abnormalities, but not with 100% frequency.

        1. Anemia (hemoglobin less than 12 grams/dl)

        2. Leukopenia (white blood cell count less than 4,000/mm)

        3. Positive anticardiolipin antibody test

        4. Positive direct Coombs test

        5. Proteinuria

        6. Hematuria

        7. Antibody to native DNA

        8. Antibody to Sm

        9. False-positive serology for syphilis

        10. Thrombocytopenia less than 100,000

        11. Antiphospholipid antibodies

        12. Hypocomplementemia

    C. No specific test is diagnostic; a collection of clinical findings and laboratory tests are the basis of diagnosis

V. Management

    A. Treatment is supportive; no curative management strategies are currently available

    B. Sunscreen for photosensitivity

    C. Topical corticosteroid creams or lotions for rashes are used primarily for discoid lupus, not systemic disease control.

    D. Nonsteroidal anti-inflammatory drugs for minor joint symptoms (see Table 55.2 for NSAID agents/dosing)

    E. Hydroxychloroquine, 200–400 mg PO daily, to help prevent flares

        1. Maximal effects may not be seen for 6 months

    F. Prednisone, 1–2 mg/kg/day for serious manifestations and during flares. Taper to low doses during disease inactivity.

    G. Pulsed steroid therapy for life-threatening exacerbations

        1. Methylprednisolone 500–1,000 mg IV daily for 3–6 days, followed by 60 mg oral prednisone daily

        2. Requires consultation with a rheumatologist

    H. Patients need hospitalization if worsening glomerulonephritis, myelitis, pulmonary hemorrhage, or severe infections, especially if the patient is on immunosuppressant therapy

    I. Calcium supplementation 1,200 mg/day, along with multivitamin containing vitamin D, 800–1,000 IU/day, for patients on long-term systemic corticosteroid therapy

J. Warfarin (Coumadin) to achieve an international normalized ratio of 2–3 for patients with anticardiolipin antibodies

K. Cytotoxic drugs for serious/life-threatening manifestations (i.e., lupus nephritis); requires rheumatologist consultation

L. Patient education

    1. Rest/activity balance

    2. Sun avoidance or appropriate protection

    3. Smoking cessation

BIBLIOGRAPHY

Hellman, D. B., & Imboden, J. B. (2013). Rheumatologic and immunologic disorders. In S. J. McPhee, M. A. Papadakis, & L. M. Tierney (Eds.), *Current medical diagnosis and treatment* (53rd ed.). New York, NY: McGraw Hill/ Appleton & Lange.

Hahn, B. H. (2012). Systemic lupus erythematosus. In A. Fauci, E. Braunwald, D. L. Kaspar, S. L. Hauser, D. L. Longo, J. L. Jameson, J. Loscalzo (Eds.), *Harrison's principles of internal medicine* (18th ed.). New York, NY: McGraw-Hill.

Johns Hopkins antibiotic guide. Retrieved from http://www.hopkinsguides.com/ hopkins/ub

Washington University School of Medicine Department of Medicine. (2010). In C. Foster, N. Mistry, S. Sharma, & P. Peddi (Eds.), *Washington manual of medical therapeutics* (33rd ed.). Philadelphia, PA: Lippincott, Williams, & Wilkins.

Management of Patients with Miscellaneous Health Problems

CHAPTER 69

Integumentary Disorders

DONNA GULLETTE · THOMAS W. BARKLEY, JR.

GENERAL

I. **History**
  A. Presenting complaint
    1. Presenting lesion
    2. Onset and progression
  B. Past and present systemic disorders
  C. Family history
    1. Blood relatives (genetic or infectious diseases)
    2. Are household contacts affected similarly?
      a. Include information regarding pets in the home environment
  D. Drug history (Table 69.1)
    1. Question carefully about medications that have been taken within the past month, as well as commonplace routine medications taken on a regular basis that otherwise may be forgotten
    2. Question about which treatments have already been tried, including over-the-counter remedies, and how successful they were
  E. Occupation and leisure activities, in particular, any activities that have been adopted recently or near the time of onset of symptoms
  F. Travel—within or outside of the country
II. **Morphology**
  A. Skin lesions are categorized according to the configuration of the lesions or identifying characteristics (Figure 69.1)
  B. Various terms are applied to skin changes (Table 69.2)
  C. Skin eruptions or exanthems are divided into three groups:
    1. Macular and maculopapular lesions
    2. Vesicular or bullous lesions
    3. Pustular, petechial, or purpuric lesions
    4. Figure 69.2 describes various types and shapes of skin lesions

Table 69.1	Drug-Related Skin Disorders
Disorder	**Drugs**
Acne	Corticosteroids, isoniazid
Bullous lesions	Barbiturate overdose, penicillamine, sulfonamides
Eczematous dermatitis	Antibiotics, methyldopa, phenylbutazone, sulfonamides
Erythema multiforme	Barbiturates, hydantoins, penicillin, salicylates, sulfonamides, sulfonylureas
Erythema nodosum	Contraceptives, sulfonamides
Exfoliative dermatitis	Allopurinol, gold, indomethacin, phenylbutazone
Lichenoid eruption	Chloroquine, chlorpropamide, mepacrine, quinidine, quinine, thiazides
Photosensitivity	Amiodarone, nalidixic acid, sulfonamides, tetracycline
Pigmentation	Chloroquine, heavy metals, mepacrine
Psoriasiform rash	Gold, methyldopa
Purpura	Cytotoxic drugs, meprobamate, quinidine, quinine
Systemic lupus erythematosus	Hydralazine, isoniazid, penicillamine, procainamide
Urticaria	Aspirin, imipramine, penicillin, serum, toxoid, vaccines

Table 69.2	Glossary of Skin Changes
Bulla	Large vesicle, more than 0.5 cm in diameter
Comedone	Plug of keratin and sebum wedged in a dilated pilosebaceous orifice
Crust	Accumulated dried exudate
Excoriation	Superficial (epidermal) abrasion caused by scratching
Lichenification	Area of increased epidermal thickening with exaggerated skin markings, caused by constant rubbing (e.g., atopic eczema)
Macule	Flat, circumscribed area of skin discoloration
Nodule	Circumscribed, palpable area of the skin that is more than 0.5 cm in diameter and appears in part or wholly within the dermis
Papule	Circumscribed, palpable elevation of the skin, less than 1 cm in diameter
Patch	Large macule, more than 2 cm in diameter
Plaque	Circumscribed, disk-shaped elevated area of the skin, more than 1 cm in diameter
Purpura	Extravasation of blood in the skin that causes macules and papules (approximately 2 mm in diameter); larger spots are called ecchymoses

Table 69.2	Glossary of Skin Changes
Pustule	Visible collection of pus
Scales	Visible and often palpable, whitish flakes due to aggregation of dried/diseased shed epidermal cells
Scar	Area of fibrous tissue that replaces the lost epidermis
Stria	Streak-like, linear, atrophic, pink, purple, or white lesion caused by stretching of the skin
Telangiectasia	Visible dilatation of a small cutaneous blood vessel
Ulcer	Loss of epidermis and part or whole of the dermis
Vesicle	Visible accumulation of fluid beneath the epidermis (less than 0.5 cm in diameter)
Wheal	Circumscribed, elevated area of cutaneous edema

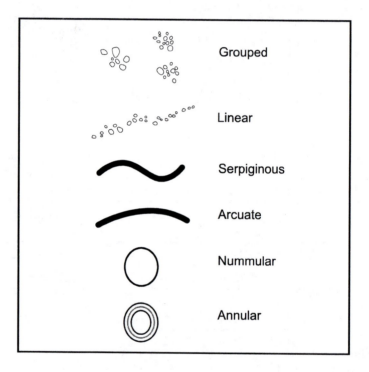

Figure 69.1. Various configurations of skin lesions. From *Fitzpatrick's Color Atlas and Synopsis of Clinical Dermatology* (7th ed.), by K. Wolff, R. A. Johnson, and A. Saavedra, 2013, New York: McGraw-Hill.

III. Physical examination

A. It is necessary to examine the entire skin, including nails, scalp, palms, soles, and mucous membranes. The patient is examined undressed in an area with good lighting.

1. Most important part of the assessment in relation to skin cancer or moles

B. Identify morphology, configuration, and distribution of any lesions

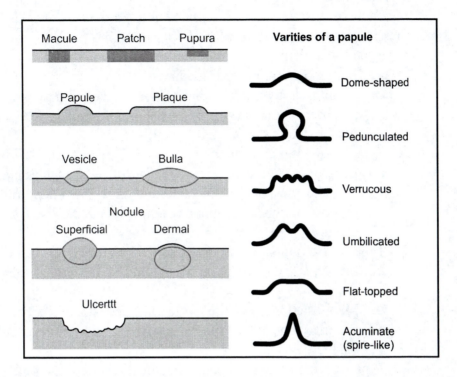

Figure 69.2. Various types and shapes of skin lesions. From *Fitzpatrick's Color Atlas and Synopsis of Clinical Dermatology* (7th ed.), by K. Wolff, R. A. Johnson, and A. Saavedra, 2013, New York: McGraw-Hill.

    C. Use a magnifying glass to view the surfaces of lesions
    D. Examine for secondary changes of skin lesions
        1. Comedones
        2. Crusting
        3. Excoriation
        4. Lichenification
        5. Scales
        6. Scarring
        7. Telangiectasis

DERMATITIS MEDICAMENTOSA (DRUG ERUPTION)

I.   **Definition**
    A. Onset is an abrupt, widespread, and symmetric erythematous eruption
        1. Drug eruptions are caused by immunologic or nonimmunologic mechanisms.
        2. Eruptions are provoked by systemic or topical administration of a drug.
        3. May resemble inflammatory skin condition
    B. True allergic drug reactions involve prior exposure to the offending drug and require minimal doses to elicit a reaction.
    C. Most allergic reactions have skin manifestations

II. **Incidence/predisposing factors**

A. See Table 69.1 for reactions associated with particular drug classes

B. Classification of adverse cutaneous drug reactions

1. Type I—immediate-type immunologic reaction
    a. Immunoglobulin (Ig) E mediated
    b. Manifested by urticaria and angioedema of skin or mucosa, edema of other organs, and fall in blood pressure (anaphylactic shock)

2. Type II—cytotoxic reaction
    a. Drug or causative agent causes lysis of cells, such as platelets or leukocytes, or may, by combination with another drug, produce antibodies (immune complexes) that cause lysis or phagocytosis

3. Type III—serum sickness, drug-induced vasculitis
    a. IgG or, less commonly, IgM, antibodies are formed against a drug
    b. Manifested by vasculitis, urticaria-like lesion, arthritis, nephritis, alveolitis, hemolytic anemia, thrombocytopenia, and agranulocytosis

4. Type IV—morbilliform (exanthematous) reaction
    a. Cell-mediated immune reaction
    b. Sensitized lymphocytes react with the drug, releasing cytokines that bring on a cutaneous inflammatory response
    c. Drug eruption with eosinophilia and systemic syndromes (DRESS)
        i. A serious allergic drug reaction producing systemic involvement that can present as hepatitis, eosinophilia, pneumonia, lymphadenopathy, and nephritis
        ii. Symptoms may last 2–6 weeks after beginning the medication; most commonly associated with antiepileptics, β-blockers, and allopurinol medications (Godara, Hirbe, Nassif, Otepka, & Rosenstock, 2013).

C. Amoxicillin, TMP-SMZ, and either ampicillin or penicillin medications are the most common causes of urticaria and maculopapular allergic skin reactions

D. Cephalosporins are associated with reactions in 5%–15% of penicillin-sensitive patients. Carbapenems have a reported 15%–30% cross-reactivity with PCN-allergic patients.

1. Third-generation cephalosporins may be less likely to react than first-generation cephalosporins.

E. "Red man" syndrome associated with vancomycin often responds to slowing of infusion rate

F. ACE inhibitors are associated with chronic cough and angioedema

G. β-blockers can precipitate asthma and should not be given to patients at risk for anaphylaxis because β-blockers may block the action of epinephrine.

H. Anticonvulsants and sulfonamides are the most common causes of toxic epidermal necrolysis and Stevens-Johnson syndrome.

I. Radiocontrast media and opioids may simulate mast cell histamine release through a non-IgE-mediated mechanism.

    1. Only 20%–30% have repeat reactions

III. Subjective findings

    A. Abrupt onset

    B. Usually with bright confluent erythema

    C. May have facial edema or central facial involvement

    D. May have swelling of the tongue

    E. Often with itching

    F. May have fever and/or chills

    G. Skin reaction usually symmetric in distribution

    H. May have arthralgias or symptoms of arthritis

    I. May have accompanying shortness of breath, wheezing, and hypotension

    J. False history of drug reaction may be due to patient misunderstanding, such as the following:

        1. Specific drug reactions are not inherited

        2. Undetermined reactions of childhood may not be reproducible in adult life

        3. Common adverse effects, such as nausea, vomiting, or weight gain, may be mistaken for allergy

        4. When a true allergic reaction has not actually occurred, the patient's records should be corrected.

    K. A detailed, accurate account of a drug reaction should be documented

IV. Physical findings

    A. Bright confluent erythema is the common presentation

    B. Urticaria and angioedema imply mast cell degranulation. If an IgE-mediated mechanism was the cause, a repeat reaction is likely.

    C. May have morbilliform and maculopapular (exanthematous) eruptions

        1. The most common type of cutaneous drug reaction and most often on trunk than extremities

        2. May develop exfoliative dermatitis, especially if drug is not discontinued

    D. May have eczematoid rash

    E. May have photodermatitis

    F. Reactions involving other systems may include the following:

        1. Hemolytic anemia

        2. Liver or kidney dysfunction

        3. Serum sickness (rash, fever, and malaise)

V.   Laboratory/diagnostic findings
  A. Diagnosis is usually made on the basis of clinical findings alone
  B. Routinely ordered blood work is usually of no value in diagnosis
  C. Eosinophil count greater than 1,000/µl: lymphocytosis with atypical lymphocytes
  D. Consider ordering the following:
    1. Liver function tests (not usually done)
    2. Skin biopsies (may be of value in confirming diagnosis)
    3. Allergy skin testing (should not be done while skin is flared—may yield false-positive results)
    4. Patch and photo testing (may reveal contact or photodermatitis —not commonly done)
    5. Challenge dosing, preferably orally, if an anaphylactic reaction seems unlikely
    6. Serum level and hepatic/renal monitoring when indicated
VI.   Management
  A. Withdrawal of the drug may be the only treatment necessary
  B. Treatment is aimed at symptoms
  C. Epinephrine 1:1,000, 0.5–1 ml IV or SQ may provide rapid temporary relief from urticaria and angioedema. Dosage may be repeated after 20 min and PRN up to three doses
    1. In life-threatening situations, use 0.5–1 mg of a 1:10,000 solution of epinephrine IV or ET or IO
  D. Give oral or IV antihistamine
    1. Diphenhydramine (Benadryl), 25–50 mg IV every 6 hr for 3–5 days, may follow epinephrine
    2. Ranitidine, H2 blocker, 50 mg IV once, followed by 150 mg PO twice a day for 3 days if necessary
  E. Corticosteroids are generally not indicated if the offending agent is discontinued. In severe cases, use systemic corticosteroids and taper very slowly
    1. Prednisone (or equivalent), 1 mg/kg (or 40–60 mg) PO daily for up to 7 days
  F. Wheezing may be treated with the use of inhaled bronchodilators or inhaled β-2 agonists
  G. Treatment of dermatitis varies according to the stage of presentation, ranging from topical application comfort measures to hospitalization for extensive blistering eruptions, such as toxic epidermal necrolysis, which may result in erosions and superficial ulcerations that require hospitalization as for burns.
  H. For more serious anaphylactoid reactions, see Management of the Patient in Shock
  I. Morbilliform rashes and serum sickness may require 1–2 weeks of treatment with antihistamines or systemic corticosteroids.
  J. Corticosteroid use in Stevens-Johnson syndrome is controversial

1. Extensive blistering resulting in erosions or ulcerations requires hospital admission and care similar to that provided for burn patients.

K. Prevention of drug reactions
1. Use alternative drug in a different class
2. Premedication does not prevent true IgE-mediated reactions but may be successful for non-IgE-mediated reactions, for example:
   a. Prednisone, 50 mg at 13 hr, 7 hr, and 1 hr or hydrocortisone, 200 mg IV at 13 hr, 7 hr, and 1 hr before radiocontrast media
   b. Diphenhydramine, 50 mg IV/PO 1 hr before drug
   c. Some sources indicate ranitidine, 50 mg
3. Desensitization may be successful but may be temporary

L. Follow-up
1. Patient education: a written list of drugs most likely to cause problems should be given to the patient
2. Avoid unnecessary medications
3. Medical warning bracelet should be worn by the patient who has a history of life-threatening reactions, and he or she should have an epinephrine injection kit

CELLULITIS

I. **Definition**
A. Diffuse spreading infection of the dermis and subcutaneous tissues
B. Caused by Gram-positive cocci (group A β-hemolytic streptococci and *Staphylococcus aureus*)

II. **General comments/incidence/predisposing factors**
A. A break in the integrity of the skin/dermis almost always precedes this infection
B. Cellulitis may be noted in proximal tissue adjacent to a necrotic area such as an abscess
C. The following predispose a patient to cellulitis:
1. Prior trauma
2. Underlying skin lesion
3. Diabetes
4. Pedal edema
5. Venous and lymphatic compromise
6. Injection drug use
D. Cellulitis most commonly involves the lower extremities
E. Cellulitis predisposes a patient to recurrent infection
F. Cellulitis of the lower extremities of the elderly is often complicated by deep vein thrombosis
G. Gram-negative rods, such as *Escherichia coli*, may also be causative
H. Gram-negative bacilli, such as *Serratia, Proteus, Enterobacter,* and fungi (*Cryptococcus neoformans*), often cause cellulitis in neutropenic and immunosuppressed patients.

I. *Haemophilus influenzae* is usually responsible for facial or upper extremity cellulitis, especially in children

J. Streptococci and staphylococci are predominant agents in patients with diabetes mellitus, but if the condition is associated with infected ulceration of the skin, anaerobic bacteria and Gram-negative rods are probably also present.

K. Occupational exposure to cellulitis of the hands occurs in fish and meat handlers
   1. *Erysipelothrix rhusiopathiae* for fish, meat, or poultry handlers
   2. *Aeromonas*—Gram-negative bacillus; freshwater exposure
   3. *Vibrio*—saltwater exposure

III. **Subjective findings**

A. The trauma site within several days of occurrence often exhibits the following:
   1. Tenderness
   2. Pain
   3. Swelling
   4. Erythema
   5. Warmth

B. Symptoms intensify rapidly and spread

C. Fever, chills, and malaise may be present

D. Should septicemia develop, may develop hypotension followed by shock

IV. **Physical findings**

A. Erythema with indistinct margins; warmth and tenderness of the skin

B. Enlargement and tenderness of regional lymph nodes are common

C. Linear streaks of erythema and tenderness indicate lymphatic spread (lymphangitis)

D. Patches of erythema and tenderness may occur a few centimeters proximal to the edge of the infection.

E. Lymph node enlargement and lymphatic streaking (lymphangitis) confirm the diagnosis of cellulitis.

V. **Laboratory/diagnostic findings**

A. The infecting organism is usually not identified, and identification may not be necessary

B. Blood and lysis cultures of the leading edge of infection rarely yield the pathogen

C. Blood cultures and skin site cultures may be taken when patients have:
   1. Failed response to standard therapy
   2. Other serious medical problems
   3. Ulcers or abscesses
   4. Lymphedema
   5. Buccal or periorbital cellulitis
   6. Infection associated with salt or freshwater
   7. High fever and chills

      8. Immunodeficiency

VI.   **Differential diagnosis**

    A. Two potentially life-threatening diagnoses should be ruled out because they can appear similarly to cellulitis in their presentation:

      1. Deep venous thrombosis and

      2. Necrotizing fasciitis: suspect in patients with a very toxic appearance, such as the following:

        a. Bullae

        b. Crepitus

        c. Anesthesia of the involved skin

        d. Overlying skin necrosis

        e. Evidence of rhabdomyolysis (elevated creatine phosphokinase)

        f. Disseminated intravascular coagulation

VII.   **Management**

    A. Antibiotic coverage for both streptococci and staphylococci are generally appropriate choices. For the outpatient without concomitant serious illness or comorbid conditions, the following may be given:

      1. Penicillin V-K, 500 mg PO four times a day for 5 days

      2. Cephalexin, 500 mg PO every 6 hr for 5 days

      3. Dicloxacillin, 250 or 500 mg PO four times a day for 5 days

      4. If allergic to penicillin:

        a. Erythromycin, 250 mg PO four times a day

        b. Erythromycin ethylsuccinate, 400 mg PO four times a day

        c. Clindamycin, 300 mg PO four times a day (expensive) for 5 days

      5. CA-MRSA

        a. Doxycycline, 100 mg PO twice a day

        b. TMP-SMX, double strength 1 tablet PO twice a day

        c. Clindamycin, 300 mg PO four times a day for 5 days

        d. Linezolid, 600 mg PO twice a day

      6. MSSA

        a. Penicillin V-K, 500 mg PO four times a day for 5 days

        b. Cephalexin, 500 mg PO every 6 hr for 5 days

        c. Dicloxacillin, 250 or 500 mg PO four times a day for 5 days

        d. Therapy should be given for 5 days or if afebrile 3–5 days.

    B. Patients who appear toxic or who have underlying disease that causes impaired immune response should be hospitalized. IV antibiotics administered in inpatient therapy may include:

      1. Nafcillin or oxacillin, (Nafcil, Unipen), 1–2 grams IV every 4 hr

      2. Cefazolin (Ancef), 1 gram IV every 8 hr

      3. MRSA (inpatient) Vancomycin, consult with pharmacy for dose/frequency to achieve vancomycin level of 10–15 µg/ml

        a. Treat until afebrile, then outpatient treatment with:

          i. Linezolid, 600 mg PO twice a day

        ii. Doxycycline, 100 mg PO twice a day

        iii. Clindamycin, 300 mg or 450 mg PO four times a day

        iv. Trimethoprim/sulfamethoxazole, 1 or 2 DS tablets PO twice a day

    4. For immunocompromised patients

        a. Hospitalization and empiric antibacterial therapy with vancomycin (consult with pharmacy for dose/frequency to achieve vancomycin level of 10–15 μg/ml) plus:

            i. An antipseudomonal antibiotic: cefepime, 1 gram IV every 12 hr

            ii. A carbapenem: imipenem-cilastatin, 500 mg IV every 6 hr or meropenem, 1 gram IV every 8 hr

            iii. Piperacillin-tazobactam, 3.375 grams IV every 6 hr

C. When specific causative agents are suspected, therapy may include the following:

    1. *Erysipelothrix*: penicillin

    2. *Vibrio* species: doxycycline plus ceftriaxone or cefotaxime

    3. *Aeromonas hydrophila*: doxycycline plus ceftriaxone or cefotaxime

D. Immobilization and elevation of the affected limb may be initially helpful

E. Moist heat may help to localize the infection

F. Follow-up is necessary to ensure eradication of infection

G. When an accompanying tinea skin infection is present, topical antifungal creams, such as terbinafine hydrochloride 1% and butenafine 1%, should be used.

H. Long-term, low-dose antibiotic therapy (e.g., penicillin G, 250–500 mg orally BID) may be indicated in select patients who have recurrence of cellulitis.

HERPES ZOSTER (SHINGLES)

I. **Definitions**

A. Reactivation of latent varicella-zoster virus (human herpesvirus type 3, VZV), usually of the sensory neurons

B. Characterized by unilateral pain and is present 48 hr before rash

C. A vesicular or bullous eruption limited to a single dermatome, or may involve two or three dermatomes

II. **Incidence/predisposing factors**

A. Patient is usually older than 50 years

B. Impaired immune system, Hodgkin disease, HIV infection, therapeutic radiation, local trauma, surgery stress, spinal cord tumors, lymphoma, fatigue, and age are predisposing factors

C. Postherpetic neuralgia is pain persisting for more than 1 month post-rash; increases with aging

III. **Subjective findings**
   A. Prodromal symptoms of pain (stabbing, pricking, sharp, boring, penetrating, lancinating, and shooting), burning, itching, or a dull ache in the affected dermatome precedes eruptions by 3–5 days (range, 1–14 days).
   B. Malaise, fever, and headache are noted in approximately 5% of patients
   C. The patient may experience allodynia, a heightened sensitivity to mild stimuli
   D. The patient may be afebrile or may have low-grade fever

IV. **Physical examination findings**
   A. Lymphadenopathy may occur 1–2 days before development of vesicles
   B. Grouped vesicles appear on an erythematous, tender base, usually unilaterally along a sensory nerve group. Two or more contiguous dermatomes may be involved. Noncontiguous dermatomal zoster is rare.
   C. Occasionally, one to three vesicles may cross the midline or appear in other areas
   D. Papules appear within 24 hr and progress to vesicles and bullae within 48 hr, then to pustules with cloudy fluid within 96 hr. Crusts form in 7–10 days and fall off after 2–3 weeks. New lesions continue to appear for up to 1 week.
   E. Ophthalmologic referral immediately if first branch of the trigeminal nerve (tip of nose) is involved even if the patient has no ophthalmologic symptoms

V. **Laboratory/diagnostic findings**
   A. Rarely needed because clinical presentation is enough
   B. Electrocardiogram is ordered during prodromal phase to rule out ischemic heart disease
   C. In addition, imaging studies are ordered in the prodromal phase to rule out organic, pleural, pulmonary, or abdominal disease.
   D. VZV antigen detection: clinical findings are confirmed by direct fluorescent antibody obtained from the vesicle base or fluid (77%–82% sensitivity)
   E. Tzanck test is positive in 75% of cases (least sensitive test, does not distinguish between herpes simplex and herpes zoster)
   F. Viral culture may require up to 2 weeks and is positive in 44% of cases (20% sensitivity, 100% specificity)
   G. Polymerase chain reaction technique, when clinically available, can confirm within 24 hr; collected on unstained slide made for Tzanck smear (94%–95% sensitivity, 100% specificity)

VI. **Management**
   A. Ophthalmic zoster is heralded by vesicles on the side and tip of the nose. When ophthalmic zoster is encountered, refer to an ophthalmologist because of potential complications.

B. High-risk groups with the need for physician referral include patients with Hodgkin's disease or AIDS
   1. "50–50–50" rule can be applied as a guide for antiviral therapy:
      a. 50 hr or less since onset of lesions
      b. 50 years or older
      c. More than 50 lesions
C. Acyclovir (Zovirax), 800 mg PO five times a day, can accelerate healing of skin lesions and decrease the duration of acute pain, particularly if given within 48 hr of onset of the rash. Dosing should be adjusted for those with kidney impairment.
D. Severely immunocompromised patients should receive acyclovir, 10 mg/kg IV every 8 hr for 7–10 days, ideally started within 48 hr of onset. Oral therapy may be substituted after 3 days if good responsiveness to IV therapy is noted. Adjust dose for patients with renal impairment.
E. Alternative drugs include the following:
   1. Famciclovir (Famvir), 500 mg PO three times a day. Adjust dose for patients with renal impairment
   2. Valacyclovir (Valtrex), 1,000 mg TID. The duration of treatment is 7–10 days, depending on the severity of the outbreak. Adjust dose for patients with renal impairment.
   3. Foscarnet (Foscavir), 90 mg/kg IV every 12 hr for immunocompromised patients who do not respond to acyclovir
   4. Only acyclovir is available for intravenous administration
   5. Varicella vaccine recommended to be given in two doses to adults without prior evidence of immunity, except for pregnant or immunocompromised patients.
F. Minimizing pain with opioid analgesics is indicated
   1. Intractable pain may warrant suicidal precautions
   2. Nonopioid analgesics, such as acetaminophen, may reduce the pain of zoster.
G. Application of moist dressing (water, saline, and Burow's solution) for 15 min four times a day or soothing baths with baking soda added to the water aid in alleviating pain
H. Oral corticosteroids, such as prednisone, have not been proven to prevent postherpetic neuralgia.
I. Hydroxyzine (Atarax), 25–50 mg PO three times a day, may be used for relief of pruritus
J. Many agents have been used to treat postherpetic neuralgia pain. According to the literature, many of these preparations are inappropriate and provide only minor relief, if any. Medications specifically effective for the treatment of neuropathic pain should be employed.

1. Lidocaine topical patch 5% (Lidoderm), apply up to 3 patches at one time for up to 12 hr within a 24 hr period (12 hr on, 12 hr off). Adjust dose for those with renal impairment

2. Pregabalin (Lyrica), 50 mg three times a day (150 mg/day); may be increased to 300 mg/day within 1 week; maximum dose is 100 mg three times a day (300 mg/day). Caution: adjust dose in patients with decreased renal function

3. Other agents that may be useful include the following:
   a. Topical anesthetics such as 5% Lidoderm topical patches
   b. Capsaicin cream, 0.075% 3–4 times daily (use only with unopened lesions)
      i. Advise patient to avoid touching mucous membranes, eyes, or contact lenses after use
      ii. Instruct patient to wash hands with soap and water immediately after applying the topical cream, unless hand area is being treated
   c. Capsaicin patch 8% (Qutenza)-consult package insert for special instructions on application, a single 30 min application of up to 4 patches every 3 months PRN; do not apply more frequently than every 3 months
   d. Analgesics/opioids
      i. Oxycodone (immediate release) 5 mg PO three times a day, titrate dose to pain relief. Once pain relief is attained, may convert to a sustained-release preparation.
      ii. Tramadol (Ultram), 50 mg PO three times a day, may titrate up to 100 mg four times a day; adjust dose for liver or renal impairment
   e. Tricyclic antidepressants
      i. Desipramine or nortriptyline, 25 mg PO at bedtime, may titrate up to 150 mg/day

K. Intrathecal methylprednisolone, reserved for those unresponsive to other therapies and should consult with pain management specialist. Healthcare workers with no immunity (those who have not had varicella or who have not received the varicella vaccine) and pregnant women should avoid exposure to active cases. Contagion rate is low, but chicken pox can be elicited in contacts who have never been exposed.

L. The most common complication of herpes zoster is postherpetic neuralgia (longer than 30 days after lesions have healed). Follow patients until pain is resolved—usually within 1 year

SKIN CANCER

I. **Definition**

    A. Basal cell carcinoma (BCC) is the most common type and occurs more often in fair-skinned individuals in sun-exposed areas. General presentation is a papule or nodule with a central scab or eroded area. The nodule has a waxy, "pearly" appearance.

        1. Locally invasive

        2. Slowly evolving growing to 1–2 cm in diameter over the years

        3. Destructive

        4. Limited capacity to metastasize

    B. Squamous cell carcinoma (SCC)

        1. Non-healing ulcer or wart-like nodule

        2. May develop from actinic keratosis

        3. Malignant tumor of epithelial keratinocytes (skin and mucous membrane)

        4. Capacity to metastasize

        5. Usually the result of exogenous carcinogens

II. **Etiology/incidence/predisposing factors**

    A. BCC is the most common form of cancer

        1. Sun exposure before age 14 years predisposes to development of BCC

        2. Arsenic exposure increases risk for superficial multi-centric BCC 30–40 years later

        3. BCC is rare in brown- and black-skinned persons

        4. Usually develops in sun-exposed areas, especially face and neck

    B. SCC is the second most common skin cancer in Caucasians and the most common skin cancer in African Americans.

        1. Male-to-female ratio, 2:1

        2. Smokers have an increased risk for lip involvement

        3. Occurs more frequently on the legs of females

        4. Slowly evolving cancer

        5. Penile SCC is more common (20%) in developing countries, with only 1% reported in the United States.

        6. Human papillomavirus is associated with increased incidence of SCC

    C. Commonalities of BCC and SCC include the following:

        1. Occur most frequently on skin with the highest degree of sun exposure

        2. White-skinned persons with poor tanning capacity are at highest risk, but BCC and SCC can occur with other skin types.

III. **Subjective findings**

    A. BCC may manifest as waxy, pearly nodules with telangiectatic vessels; papules; non-healing ulcers; scabbed lesions; or visual or scaly plaques

    B. SCC should be suspected in any lesion that is scaly, red, hard, nodular, crusty, or does not heal; usually asymptomatic

IV. **Physical examination findings**
  A. BCC can present in several forms
    1. Nodule or papule ulcerative tumor
        a. Small, pearly, or translucent, waxy papule that enlarges peripherally and develops a central depression that may be ulcerated or scaly
        b. Borders are translucent, elevated, and shiny with fine telangiectasias
    2. Superficial BCC: erythematous scaly macule or patch with an elevated threadlike border
  B. SCC tumors
    1. Appear as firm, skin-colored to reddish-brown nodules on damaged skin
    2. May arise out of actinic keratoses
    3. Central ulceration may be present
    4. Scaling and crusting may be present
    5. Heaped-up edges of lesions appear fleshy rather than clear
    6. Seventy percent occur on the head and neck
    7. Lesions on the lower lip appear as firm, whitish macules (leukoplakia) with possible central ulceration
    8. Lip, oral cavity, tongue, and genital SCCs have greater rates of metastasis and require special management
V. **Laboratory/diagnostic findings**
  A. Suspected BCC or SCC lesions should be biopsied, shaved, or punch biopsied
  B. Raised lesions can be examined through simple superficial shave biopsy
  C. Small lesions with distinct borders (2–10 mm) can be excised by punch biopsy in cases where tissue loss is acceptable
  D. Large lesions require incisional biopsies, a small punch (2–3 mm), or a shave biopsy. Punch biopsies are not appropriate because electrodesiccation and curettage is the ultimate treatment.
  E. Confirmation of the diagnosis is made histologically
VI. **Management**
  A. Referral/consultation to a dermatologist
  B. Lesion should be shaved, biopsied, or punch biopsied. Curettage and electrodesiccation for BCC lesions smaller than 1 cm in diameter and in non-facial area
    1. The technique of three cycles of curettage and electrodesiccation is the gold standard; it consists of three scraping and burning cycles performed in a single sitting (becomes a more difficult procedure if punch biopsy has previously been performed).
    2. This is not indicated for head and neck lesions
    3. Appropriateness for use with SCC varies in the literature

C. Cryosurgery: for superficial BCC lesions, except around nose, ears, eyelids, forehead, and temples. Not appropriate for SCC. Less control of tissue destruction

D. Tissue must be microscopically evaluated to ensure clear borders; technique is appropriate for BCCs and SCCs when removed by excision.

E. Radiotherapy is infrequently used in BCC. It is usually reserved for very large lesions. Recurrent lesions after radiation are generally more aggressive and difficult to treat.

F. Referral for fresh tissue microscopically controlled excision (Mohs) surgery is indicated for head/neck or cosmetically prominent location, or for areas difficult to treat, such as eyelids, inner canthus, nose, ears, lips, genitalia, or fingers. It is indicated for both SCC and BCC.

G. Systemic agents are not indicated for treatment of uncomplicated BCC or SCC.

H. Prophylaxis therapy for BCC includes:
   1. 5-Fluorouracil, cover lesions with 5% cream or solution BID for 3–6 weeks up to 10–12 weeks for superficial BCC when surgical methods are less appropriate; avoid sun exposure
   2. Imiquimod (Aldara), apply once daily 5 times per week for 6 weeks; apply at bedtime and leave on skin for 8 hr: For superficial BCC on trunk, neck, or extremities when surgical methods are less appropriate and follow-up is assured

I. Follow-up for 5 years required for patients with BCC to detect new or recurrent lesions

J. Topical application of sunscreen is recommended for prevention

MELANOMA

I. **Definition**
   A. Tumor characterized by dark pigmentation; may be flat or raised; irregular borders; may be red, black, or bluish in color; size greater than 6 mm
   B. Malignant melanomas develop from benign melanocytic cells

II. **Etiology/incidence/predisposing factors**
   A. Malignant melanoma is the leading cause of death from skin disease
   B. Prevention—avoidance of blistering solar radiation and the use of sunscreen, especially during adolescent years—is the key to cure
   C. The worldwide incidence of melanoma increases with proximity to the equator.
   D. Highest incidence is between ages 30 and 50 years. Median age at diagnosis is 45 years.
   E. Family history of melanoma in parents, children, or siblings increases risk
   F. Increased risk if a person has fair skin, freckling, blue eyes, and blond hair

G. Twice the risk if sunburned at a young age

H. Those with increased number of nevi are at greatest risk

I. The most common sites in males are head, neck, and trunk; lower extremities represent the most common site in females

III. Subjective findings

A. May manifest with any change in pigmented lesion, including the following:

    1. Bleeding and ulceration are ominous signs

    2. Scaling

    3. Texture change and irregular boarder

    4. Size change greater than 6 mm

    5. Development of inflammation

    6. Color change

    7. Itching

IV. Physical examination findings

A. Six signs of malignant melanoma (ABCDEE changes):

    1. Asymmetric shape

    2. Border irregularity

    3. Color variegation

    4. Diameter is usually large (greater than 6 mm)

    5. Elevation is almost always present.

    6. Enlargement or increase in the size of the lesion is probably the most important sign

B. Primary malignant melanomas may be classified into the following types:

    1. Superficial spreading malignant melanoma

        a. The most common type

        b. Primarily a disease of Caucasians

    2. Lentigo maligna melanoma (on sun-exposed skin, older individuals)

    3. Nodular malignant melanoma

    4. Acral lentiginous melanoma

        a. On the palms, soles, and nail beds

        b. More common among darkly pigmented people

    5. Malignant melanoma on mucous membranes

    6. Miscellaneous forms

        a. Amelanotic (non-pigmented) melanoma

        b. Melanomas arising from blue nevi (rare)

        c. Congenital and giant nevocytic nevi

V. Laboratory/diagnostic findings

A. Surgical biopsy is the only form of appropriate diagnostic procedure.

    1. A full-thickness total excisional biopsy specimen with 1- to 2-mm borders is preferred and must be sent for pathologic specimen.

    2. Melanoma should never be curetted, electrodesiccated, or shaved

B. Lesions are staged by the pathologist (Clark staging):

1. Level 1—confined to epidermis (in situ) (recommended margin, 0.5 cm)
2. Level 2—invasion of papillary dermis
3. Level 3—invasion of interface of papillary and reticular dermis
4. Level 4—invasion of reticular dermis
5. Level 5—invasion of subcutaneous fat

C. Lesion may also be staged by the pathologist with the use of Breslow staging:
1. Thin: less than 0.75 mm depth of invasion (recommended margin, 1 cm)
2. Intermediate: 0.76–3.99 mm depth of invasion (recommended margin, 2 cm)
3. Thick: greater than 4 mm depth of invasion

VI. Management

A. Suspicion of malignant melanoma should always be referred to a dermatologist owing to the potential for metastasis and death
B. Follow up every 3–6 months with skin examinations
C. Patient should be instructed to self-examine skin weekly
D. Treatment of melanoma is based on stage
1. Melanoma less than 1 mm thick: wide excision with a 1-cm margin. Routine elective lymph node dissection is not usually recommended for this group.
2. Melanoma measuring 1–4 mm in thickness or Clark level IV thickness of lesions: wide excision with 2-cm margins recommended. Sentinel nodal biopsy is usually recommended. Preoperative lymphatic mapping is used to identify draining patterns.
3. Melanoma measuring more than 4 mm in thickness: at least 2 cm recommended for margins
E. Adjuvant therapy: consult hematology/oncology specialist
1. α-interferon, as determined by dermatology/oncology specialist as part of chemotherapy, may be indicated for high-risk melanomas
F. Strong recommendation for referral of intermediate-risk and high-risk patients to centers with expertise

BIBLIOGRAPHY

Berger, T. G. (2013). Dermatologic disorders. In M. A. Papadakis, S. J. McPhee, & M. W. Rabow (Eds), *Current medical diagnosis and treatment* (52nd ed., pp. 94–158). New York, NY: McGraw Hill/Appleton & Lange.

Cassidy, S. B., & Allanson, J. E. (2010). *Management of genetic syndromes* (3rd ed.). Hoboken, NJ.: Wiley-Blackwell.

Centers for Disease Control. (2014). *Recommended adult immunization schedule: United States 2014*. Retrieved from http://www.cdc.gov/vaccines/schedules/downloads/adult/adult-combined-schedule.pdf.

Gilbert, D. N., Moellering, R. C., Eliopoulos, G. M., Chambers, H. F., & Saag, M. S. (2013). *The Sanford guide to antimicrobial therapy 2013* (43rd ed.). Sperryville, VA: Antimicrobial Therapy, Inc.

Godara, H., Hirbe, A., Nassif, M., Otepka, H., & Rosenstock, A. (2013). *The Washington manual of medical therapeutics* (34th ed). Philadelphia, PA: Wolters Kluwer, Lippincott Williams & Wilkins.

Herpes zoster vaccine options for consideration. (2013). Toronto, Ont.: Public Health Ontario.

Kundu, R. V., & Patterson, S. (2013). Dermatologic conditions in skin of color: Part 1. Special considerations for common skin disorders. *American Family Physician, 87*(12), 850–856.

Kundu, R. V., & Patterson, S. (2013). Dermatologic conditions in skin of color: Part II. Disorders occuring predominantly in skin of color. *American Family Physician, 87*(12), 859–865.

National Cancer Instititue. (2013). *Basal cell carcinoma of the skin treatment*. Retrieved from http://www.cancer.gov/cancertopics/pdq/treatment/skin/HealthProfessional/page4.

Sharfman, W. H. (2012). *Melanoma*. New York, NY: Demos Medical Pub.

Stevens, D. L., Bisno, A. L., Chambers, H. F., Dellinger, E. P., Goldstein, E. J., Gorbach, S. L., . . . Wade, J. C. (2014). Practice guidelines for the diagnosis and management of skin and soft tissue infections: 2014 update by the Infectious Diseases Society of America. *Clinical Infectious Diseases, 59*(2), e10-e52.

Sym, D., Jabonillo, R., & Lim, J. (2013) Postherpetic neuralgia: Treatment and prevention strategies. *US Pharmacist*. Retrieved from http://www.uspharmacist.com/continuing_education/ceviewtest/lessonid/108941

Wolff, K., Johnson, R. A, & Saavedra, A. (2013). *Fitzpatrick's color atlas and synopsis of clinical dermatology* (7th ed.). New York, NY: McGraw-Hill.

CHAPTER 70

Ectopic Pregnancy and Sexually Transmitted Infections

ANGELA STARKWEATHER • THOMAS W. BARKLEY, JR.

ECTOPIC PREGNANCY

I. **Definition**
   A. Implantation of the fertilized ovum in tissue other than the endometrium
   B. The most common implantation site is the fallopian tube

II. **Etiology/incidence/predisposing factors**
   A. Any condition that prevents or retards passage of the fertilized ovum into the uterus, such as the following:
      1. Pelvic inflammatory disease (PID), sexually transmitted infections (STIs), especially *Neisseria gonorrhoeae* and *Chlamydia trachomatis* salpingitis
      2. History of endometriosis
      3. Prior tubal or uterine surgery related to adhesions
      4. Use of a contraceptive intrauterine device (IUD)
      5. Congenital anomalies associated with diethylstilbestrol
      6. Tubal tumors
      7. Infertile women treated with ovulation-inducing drugs, such as clomiphene citrate (Clomid)
      8. Postabortal and puerperal infections
      9. Prior tubal pregnancy
      10. Previous tubal sterilization
      11. Cigarette smoking
   B. Most common cause of maternal mortality in the first trimester
   C. Leading cause of maternal mortality in the United States; of every 100 women who were known to conceive, 2 had an ectopic pregnancy

III. **Subjective findings**
   A. Early
      1. Missed or delayed menses, followed by continuous intermittent vaginal bleeding typically dark in color
      2. The nature, duration, and intensity of pain vary considerably
      3. Sudden, sharp, and stabbing abdominal pain, diffuse pelvic pain, referred neck or shoulder pain
   B. Late
      1. Fainting, vertigo, dizziness
      2. Nausea, vomiting, diarrhea
      3. Right or left pelvic pain
IV. **Physical examination findings with rupture and intra-abdominal hemorrhage**
   A. Signs of hypovolemic shock—hypotension, skin pallor, and tachycardia
   B. Temperature may or may not be changed.
   C. Ecchymotic blueness around umbilicus (Cullen sign)
   D. Uterine size is generally normal; uterus is sometimes displaced to the side
   E. Palpation of adnexal mass
   F. Bimanual examination is very painful with cervical motion tenderness
   G. Unilateral abdominal tenderness with rebound
V. **Laboratory findings/diagnostic findings**
   A. Decreased hemoglobin and hematocrit with mild leukocytosis
   B. Absence of an intrauterine gestational sac with human chorionic gonadotropin (β-hCG) concentration of 1500 mIU/ml or greater is suggestive of ectopic pregnancy
   C. Culdocentesis (aspiration of the cul-de-sac) when ultrasonography is not available; aspiration of nonclotting blood is considered positive
   D. Pregnancy test: β-hCG radioimmunoassay is usually below normal for estimated gestational age in ectopic pregnancies.
VI. **Management**
   A. Ectopic pregnancy should always be a priority as a differential diagnosis in any woman of childbearing age with an acute abdomen
   B. Salpingectomy: per outpatient laparoscopy
   C. Linear salpingostomy: unruptured tube greater than 2 cm
   D. Outpatient nonsurgical treatment with methotrexate (amethopterin) therapy
   E. Methotrexate is a folic acid antagonist
      1. Criteria:
         a. Less than 6 weeks pregnant
         b. Unruptured tubal mass smaller than 3.5 cm
         c. No embryonic cardiac motion
         d. No active renal or hepatic disease
         e. No evidence of thrombocytopenia or leukopenia

    f. Hemodynamic stability

2. Pretreatment medical workup should consist of baseline laboratory values and diagnostic tests
   a. Transvaginal ultrasound to determine the presence or absence of extrauterine gestational sac
   b. Quantitative: β-hCG level
   c. Liver function (serum glutamic-oxaloacetic transaminase)
   d. Renal function: BUN and creatinine
   e. Blood type, Rh factor, and presence of antibodies
   f. CBC
   g. Bone marrow function tests

3. Absolute contraindications to methotrexate:
   a. Existence of an intrauterine pregnancy
   b. Immunodeficiency
   c. Sensitivity to methotrexate
   d. Moderate to severe anemia, leukopenia, or thrombocytopenia
   e. Hemodynamically unstable
   f. Active pulmonary or peptic ulcer disease
   g. Clinically important hepatic or renal dysfunction
   h. Breastfeeding
   i. Evidence of tubal rupture

4. Single dose regimen:
   a. Methotrexate 50 mg/m^2 IM single dose; consider repeat dose (50 mg/m^2) every 7 days based on hCG levels
   b. Leucovorin rescue is not required with the single dose protocol, even if multiple doses are given

5. Multiple dose regimen:
   a. Methotrexate, 1 mg/kg IM every other day for 7 days; if hCG has dropped more than 15% from last dose, stop therapy and start surveillance
   b. Leucovorin, 0.1 mg/kg PO every other day for 8 days; start use the day after initial methotrexate dose; stop therapy when methotrexate is discontinued

6. Additional management
   a. Central venous line if hemodynamically unstable, use Ringer lactate or normal saline; run at rate appropriate for patient's hemodynamic condition
   b. Blood transfusions, packed red blood cells as indicated for low hemoglobin/hematocrit
   c. Maintain urinary output of 30 ml/hr
   d. Cefoxitin (Mefoxin), 2 grams IV single dose for empiric Gram-negative and positive coverage
   e. Oxycodone/acetaminophen (Percocet) every 4 hr PRN for pain. Give morphine sulfate, 2.5–10 mg IV every 2–6 hr PRN, to a hospitalized patient.

   f.   Do not administer PO treatment
   g.   Rho(D)-negative unsensitized patient to receive intramuscular injection of Rho(D) immune globulin (RhIG)
      i.   50 mcg for patients 12 weeks gestation or less
      ii.   300 mcg for patients 13 weeks gestation or more
   h.   Biweekly hCG is required (with a drop in hCG after 7 days); 1500 mIU/ml β-hCG is considered normal. Monitor until β-hCG levels become undetectable
   i.   Advise patients not to take vitamins with folic acid until complete resolution of the ectopic pregnancy/while on methotrexate
   j.   Avoid sun exposure

PID SALPINGITIS

I.   **Definition**
   A.   Acute or chronic inflammation of the upper female genital tract caused by bacterial infection
II.   **Etiology/incidence/predisposing factors/morbidity**
   A.   One million cases of PID reported annually in the United States
   B.   Polymicrobial causation
   C.   Most common causative organisms are *N. gonorrhoeae* and *C. trachomatis* (exogenous)
   D.   Other etiologic agents
      1.   Normal vaginal flora (anaerobes)
         a.   Such as *Haemophilus influenzae* and *Gardnerella*
         b.   Streptococci
         c.   Enteric Gram-negative rods
         d.   *Mycoplasma hominis*
      2.   Trauma
      3.   Surgery
   E.   Predisposing risk factors
      1.   Sexually active women with multiple partners
      2.   Younger than 25 years
      3.   Reduced socioeconomic status
      4.   Sexual exposure to a partner with urethritis
      5.   Low educational attainment
      6.   First 3 weeks after placement of an IUD
      7.   Douching
      8.   Menses: incidence increases with onset or cessation of menses
      9.   Smoking: alters the protective nature of cervical mucus
      10.   Substance abuse
      11.   Pelvic surgery
      12.   Prior history of PID or cervicitis
   F.   Complications
      1.   Infertility

2. Tubal pregnancy
3. Chronic pelvic pain due to adhesions
4. Recurrent PID
5. Tubo-ovarian abscess
6. Pelvic abscess and rupture
7. Infectious perihepatitis (Fitz-Hugh and Curtis syndrome)

G. Morbidity
   1. Infertility
   2. Chronic pelvic pain
   3. Ectopic pregnancy

III. **Subjective findings**

A. Early (up to 1 week)
   1. Clinical presentation varies widely; many women have atypical or no symptoms
   2. Lower abdominal pain
   3. Menstrual cramping
   4. Low-grade fever
   5. Malaise

B. Late symptoms
   1. Severe lower abdominal pain
   2. Temperature greater than 101.4°F (38.6°C)
   3. Increased foul, purulent vaginal discharge
   4. Dyspareunia and painful defecation

IV. **Physical examination findings**

A. Mucopurulent cervical or vaginal discharge
B. Friable cervix (bleeding)
C. Uterine and cervical motion tenderness (Chandelier sign: marked tenderness of the cervix, uterus, and adnexa)
D. Abdominal rebound tenderness or guarding
E. Infectious perihepatitis, Fitz-Hugh and Curtis syndrome (i.e., right upper quadrant abdominal pain)

V. **Laboratory findings/diagnostic findings**

A. Assess the following:
   1. Last normal menstrual period
   2. STI history
   3. Contraceptive use
   4. Sexual history
   5. Pregnancy test
   6. Drug allergy

B. Centers for Disease Control and Prevention (CDC) Diagnostic Criteria for PID
   1. Minimum criteria for diagnosing PID in any sexually active female with one of the following:
      a. Uterine/adnexal tenderness
      b. Cervical motion tenderness

2. Additional criteria
   a. Oral temperature higher than 101°F (38.3°C)
   b. Abnormal cervical/vaginal mucopurulent discharge; white blood cells (WBCs) noted on vaginal microscopy
   c. Elevated erythrocyte sedimentation rate
   d. Elevated C-reactive protein
   e. Laboratory evidence of gonococcal or chlamydial infection
   f. Leukocytosis (WBC count greater than 10,000/mm)
3. Definitive criteria for diagnosing PID
   a. Histopathologic evidence on endometrial biopsy
   b. Tubo-ovarian abscess on transvaginal sonography
   c. Laparoscopic abnormalities consistent with PID (diagnosis confirmed in 60% of cases)

VI. Management

A. Early detection and aggressive treatment of STIs and lower genital tract infections essential in prevention of PID
B. CDC guidelines for treatment of acute PID
   1. Parenteral inpatient treatment
      a. Regimen A
         i. Cefotetan, 2 grams IV every 12 hr, or cefoxitin sodium (Mefoxin), 2 grams IV every 6 hr plus
         ii. Doxycycline (tetracycline), 100 mg IV or PO every 12 hr for 10–14 days
         iii. When tubo-ovarian abscess is present, clindamycin or metronidazole with doxycycline can be used for continued therapy rather than doxycycline alone because this regimen provides more effective anaerobic coverage.
      b. Regimen B
         i. Clindamycin hydrochloride (Cleocin), 900 mg IV every 8 hr plus
         ii. Gentamicin sulfate (Garamycin) loading dose intravenous or intramuscular (2 mg/kg body weight) followed by a maintenance dose (1.5 mg/kg every 8 hr until discharge)
            (a) Patients with renal impairment should consult with a pharmacist for appropriate pharmacokinetic dosing to achieve therapeutic levels and avoid toxicity.
         iii. Regimens are continued until at least 24–48 hr after significant clinical improvement. Then follow-up with doxycycline, 100 mg PO every 12 hr for 14 days, or clindamycin, 450 mg PO four times a day for 10–14 days.
   2. CDC-recommended regimens for outpatient treatment of PID
      a. Regimen A
         i. Ceftriaxone, 250 mg IM in a single dose plus

      ii. Doxycycline, 100 mg PO two times a day for 14 days, with or without,

      iii. Metronidazole, 500 mg PO two times a day for 14 days

    b. Regimen B

      i. Cefoxitin sodium (Mefoxin), 2 grams IM plus probenecid (Benemid), 1 gram PO in a single dose concurrently plus

      ii. Doxycycline (tetracycline), 100 mg PO BID for 14 days with or without metronidazole, 500 mg PO two times a day for 14 days

    c. Regimen C

      i. Other parenteral third-generation cephalosporin (e.g., ceftizoxime and cefotaxime) plus doxycycline, 100 mg PO two times a day for 14 days with or without metronidazole, 500 mg PO two times a day for 14 days

C. CDC recommendations for hospitalization

  1. Surgical emergencies: rule out ectopic pregnancy or appendicitis

  2. Coexisting pregnancy

    a. HIV infected with low CD4 counts

    b. Adolescent

    c. Immunosuppressed

    d. Nausea, vomiting, and fever

    e. Dehydration

    f. Pelvic and tubo-ovarian abscess suspected

  3. Unable to tolerate or follow an outpatient regimen

  4. Failed to respond clinically to oral antimicrobial therapy within 72 hr

D. Additional considerations

  1. Notification and prompt treatment of sexual partners

  2. Counseling on safer sex practices and high-risk behaviors

  3. Screening for other STIs

  4. Testing for cure within 7 days of completion of therapy

  5. Rescreening in 4–6 weeks for *C. trachomatis* and *N. gonorrhoeae*

  6. Removal of IUD

  7. Testing for HIV

  8. In-hospital treatment only with parenteral antibiotics for pregnant women

E. Other treatments

  1. Warm sitz baths for 10–15 minutes PRN for pain

  2. No douching

  3. Use of sanitary napkins

  4. Avoidance of sexual intercourse for 7 days

  5. Bed rest in a semi-Fowler position

  6. Over-the-counter pain medications, such as acetaminophen (Tylenol)

  7. Adequate hydration (6–8 glasses of water daily)

  8. Condoms

VAGINITIS

I. **Definition**
   A. Vaginitis is characterized by a vaginal discharge, vulvar itching, and irritation and a vaginal odor
II. **Etiology/incidence/complications**
   A. Etiology
      1. The three most common diseases diagnosed among women with these symptoms include:
         a. Bacterial vaginosis
         b. Vulvovaginal candidiasis
         c. Trichomoniasis
      2. Other causes of vaginal discharge or irritation include:
         a. Normal physiologic variation
         b. Allergic reactions
         c. Herpes simplex virus
         d. Mucopurulent cervicitis
         e. Atrophic vaginitis
         f. Vulvar vestibulitis
         g. Foreign bodies
         h. Desquamative inflammatory vaginitis
   B. Over 1.1 million people diagnosed with trichomoniasis in the United States each year
   C. Complications
      1. Cervicitis
III. **Subjective findings**
   A. Vaginal discharge
   B. Vulvar itching and irritation
   C. Vaginal odor
   D. May be asymptomatic
IV. **Physical examination findings**
   A. Visual inspection of the vaginal discharge
      1. Color
      2. Viscosity
      3. Adherence to vaginal walls, and
      4. Presence of an odor
   B. Speculum examination
         a. Bacterial vaginosis
            i. Discharge is homogenous, adherent, thin, milky white, malodorous, and foul fishy
         b. Candidiasis
            i. Discharge is thick, clumpy, white like cottage cheese
            ii. Clinical findings may include inflammation and erythema

        c. Trichomoniasis
- i. Discharge is frothy, gray or yellow/green, and malodorous
- ii. Cervical petechiae may be present and is known as "strawberry cervix"

C. Laboratory/diagnostic findings
1. Bacterial vaginosis
   a. Amsel criteria
      - i. Vaginal pH greater than 4.5; most sensitive but least specific
      - ii. Presence of clue cells on wet mount
      - iii. Positive amine, "whiff" or "fishy odor" test
      - iv. Homogenous, nonviscous, milky-white discharge adherent to the vaginal walls
2. Candidiasis
   a. 10% KOH Wet Prep, saline wet mount, or Gram stain —visualization of pseudohypha and/or budding yeast
3. Trichomoniasis
   a. Wet mount—motile trichomonads seen
   b. Vaginal pH greater than 4.5
   c. Culture
   d. Nucleic acid amplification test; considerably more sensitive than culture

V. **Management**

A. CDC recommended regimens for adolescents and adults
1. Bacterial vaginosis
   a. Metronidazole, 500 mg PO twice a day for 7 days or metronidazole gel 0.75% one full applicator (5 grams) intravaginally, once a day for 5 days or clindamycin cream 2%, one full applicator (5 grams) intravaginally at bedtime for 7 days
   b. Alternative regimen: tinidazole, 2 grams PO once daily for 2 days or tinidazole, 1 gram PO once daily for 5 days; clindamycin, 300 mg PO BID for 7 days; or clindamycin ovules, 100 mg intravaginally once at bedtime for 3 days
2. Candidiasis
   a. Oral agent: fluconazole, 150 mg oral tablet in a single dose
   b. Intravaginal agents: butoconazole 2% cream, 5 grams intravaginally for 1–3 days depending on the product selected (OTC vs Rx); nystatin 100,000-units vaginal tablet, 1 tablet for 14 days; terconazole 0.4% cream, 5 grams intravaginally for 7 days; terconazole 0.8% cream, 5 grams intravaginally for 3 days; or terconazole, 80 mg vaginal suppository, 1 suppository for 3 days

3. Trichomoniasis
   a. Metronidazole, 2 grams PO in a single dose or tinidazole, 2 grams PO in a single dose
   b. Alternative regimen: metronidazole, 500 mg PO twice a day for 7 days
B. CDC recommended regimens for pregnancy
   1. Metronidazole, 500 mg PO twice a day for 7 days
   2. Metronidazole, 250 mg PO three times a day for 7 days
   3. Clindamycin, 300 mg PO twice a day for 7 days
C. CDC follow-up guidelines
   1. Encourage disclosure of diagnosis to sexual partner and referral for treatment
   2. Test of cure is not recommended by CDC
   3. Tell patient to avoid sexual activity until therapy has been completed and patient and partner are both asymptomatic (approximately 7 days)
   4. Patient counseling and education should cover the nature of the disease, transmission issues, and risk reduction

CHLAMYDIA TRACHOMATIS INFECTION

I. **Definition**
   A. Chlamydia is a parasitic STI that produces serious reproductive tract complications in persons of either sex.
II. **Etiology/incidence/complications**
   A. Etiology
      1. Causative organism, *C. trachomatis*
         a. An obligate, intracellular parasite
         b. This organism can live only inside of cells; therefore, transfer of body fluids is necessary for transmission.
      2. Incubation period thought to be 10–30 days
   B. Incidence
      1. More than 3 million new cases annually
      2. Age
         a. Commonly seen in either sex in those younger than 25 years
         b. Most common in women ages 15–19 years
      3. Annual screening recommended for the following populations:
         a. Sexually active adolescents
         b. Nonusers of contraceptive devices
         c. Those who have had one or more sexual partners within the previous 3 months
         d. Those who are pregnant
         e. Those undergoing an abortion
   C. Complications
      1. Women
         a. PID

      i. Pelvic abscess (ovarian)

      ii. Involuntary infertility

      iii. Ectopic pregnancy

    b. Abnormal Pap smear with mucopurulent cervicitis

    c. Late-onset postpartum endometritis

  2. Men

    a. Epididymitis

    b. Reiter syndrome (primarily young men)

      i. Urethritis

      ii. Conjunctivitis

      iii. Arthritis

      iv. Skin lesions

  3. Newborn

    a. Conjunctivitis

    b. Pneumonia

III. **Subjective findings**

  A. Female

    1. Often asymptomatic (70%–80%)

    2. Intramenstrual spotting

    3. Postcoital bleeding

    4. Lower abdominal pain

    5. Painful urination (dysuria)

    6. Painful intercourse (dyspareunia)

    7. Mucopurulent endocervical discharge

  B. Male

    1. Often asymptomatic (25%–50%)

    2. Painful urination (dysuria)

    3. Thick, cloudy penile discharge

    4. Unilateral testicular pain and swelling

IV. **Physical examination findings**

  A. Vital signs: temperature higher than 100°F (37.7°C) when infection has progressed to PID

    1. Abdominal assessment

      a. Guarded referred pain

      b. Rebound tenderness

    2. External genitalia inspection

      a. Edema

      b. Ulcerations

      c. Lesions

      d. Excoriations

      e. Erythema

    3. Speculum examination

      a. Vaginal walls reddened

      b. Cervical erythema and friability

      c. Mucopurulent cervical discharge may or may not be present

      d. Cervical erosion (cervical lips inflamed and eroded)

  4. Bimanual examination

      a. Cervical motion tenderness (i.e., Chandelier sign)

      b. Adnexal tenderness and fullness

      c. Uterine tenderness

  5. Male inspection

      a. Scanty mucoid discharge

      b. The meatus edge is red, everted, and edematous.

      c. Unilateral testicular pain

V.   **Laboratory/diagnostic findings**

  A. McCoy cell culture is the gold standard for diagnosis.

    1. Advantages

      a. Most specific (100%) with acceptable sensitivity (70%–80%)

      b. Detects infection with small numbers of organisms present

      c. Findings are positive if mature inclusion bodies are found in cells on microscopic examination.

    2. Disadvantages

      a. Method technically difficult

      b. Specific transport and storage requirements for test

      c. Takes 2–6 days to obtain results

  B. Non-culture tests

    1. Advantages

      a. Sensitivity of test is 70%–90%

      b. Results available sooner than culture test

      c. Less influenced by storage and transport

    2. Disadvantages

      a. Most are less than 99% specific.

      b. False-positives in low-risk populations

    3. Types available

      a. Direct immunofluorescent monoclonal antibody stain

      b. Enzyme-linked immunosorbent assay

      c. Nucleic acid hybridization test (DNA probe); sensitivities and specificities vary

      d. Rapid enzyme immunoassay (i.e., chlamydiazyme)

    4. Other relevant laboratory tests

      a. Wet mount: polymorphonuclear cells present

      b. If history indicates, testing for syphilis and gonorrhea (coinfection high)

      c. HIV testing

      d. Hepatitis B testing

VI.   **Management**

  A. CDC recommended regimens for adolescents and adults

    1. Azithromycin (Zithromax), 1 gram single dose PO (safety for persons younger than age 15 and in pregnancy not established) or doxycycline, 100 mg PO BID for 7 days

    B. Alternative regimens
       1. Erythromycin base (E-Mycin), 500 mg PO four times a day for 7 days or
       2. Erythromycin ethylsuccinate (EES), 800 mg PO four times a day for 7 days or
       3. Ofloxacin (Floxin), 300 mg PO BID for 7 days (not active against Treponema as patient will be at increased risk for syphilis) or
       4. Levofloxacin, 500 mg PO for 7 days
    C. CDC recommended regimens for pregnancy
       1. Azithromycin (Zithromax), 1 gram PO in a single dose or
       2. Amoxicillin (Amoxil), 500 mg PO three times a day for 7 days
    D. Alternative regimens for pregnancy
       1. Erythromycin base (E-Mycin), 250 mg PO four times a day for 14 days or
       2. EES, 400 mg PO four times a day for 14 days or
       3. EES, 800 mg PO four times a day for 7 days or
       4. Erythromycin base, 500 mg PO four times a day for 7 days
    E. CDC follow-up guidelines
       1. If symptoms persist or reinfection is suspected, timely treatment of sexual partner is essential
       2. All sex partners of patients whose last sexual contact with the patient was within 60 days before onset of symptoms or diagnosis of infection should be evaluated and treated for *N. gonorrhoeae* and *C. trachomatis* infections.
       3. Test of cure not routinely required by CDC guidelines but, if done, should occur 3 weeks after treatment
       4. Tell patient to avoid sexual activity until cured
       5. Tell patient to use condoms
       6. Report to health department

GONORRHEA

I.   **Definition**
    A. Classic bacterial STI that prefers columnar and pseudostratified epithelium and can be symptomatic or asymptomatic in men and women

II. **Etiology/incidence/predisposing factors**
    A. Causative organism is *N. gonorrhoeae*
       1. Gram-negative, intracellular, nonmotile, diplococcal bacterium
       2. Cultured from the genitourinary tract, oropharynx, or anorectum of men and women
    B. The CDC reports that in the United States, an estimated 700,000 new infections with *N. gonorrhoeae* occur each year
    C. Incidence in the population is approximately 1%–13.3%
    D. Incubation period averages 3–7 days (range, 1–14 days)

    E. Male-to-female transmission is 80%–90% after exposure; female-to-male transmission is as low as 20% after exposure

    F. Possible serious complications

       1. PID

       2. Ectopic pregnancy

       3. Infertility

       4. Perihepatitis (Fitz-Hugh and Curtis syndrome)

       5. Disseminated gonococcal infection

       6. Epididymitis

III. **Subjective findings**

    A. Females: 80% asymptomatic

       1. Early symptoms

          a. Dysuria and frequency

          b. Malodorous and mucopurulent vaginal or urethral discharge

          c. Labial pain and swelling

          d. Lower abdominal discomfort

          e. Pharyngitis

       2. Later symptoms

          a. Fever

          b. Abnormal menstrual periods

          c. Increased dysmenorrhea

          d. Nausea and vomiting

          e. Joint pain and swelling

    B. Males: usually symptomatic

       1. Early symptoms

          a. Dysuria with frequency

          b. Whitish urethral discharge

          c. Pharyngitis

       2. Later symptoms

          a. Yellow-greenish, profuse, purulent urethral discharge with meatal edema and erythema

         b. Epididymitis

         c. Lower abdominal pain (proctitis)

IV. **Physical examination findings**

    A. Fever often present

    B. Abdominal examination

       1. Guarding

       2. Referred pain

       3. Rebound pain

       4. Hyperperistalsis

    C. Pelvic examination

       1. Inspect Bartholin and Skene glands for tenderness, enlargement, or discharge

       2. Urethral discharge

       3. Vaginal wall discharge or redness

   4. Cervix
      a. Mucopurulent discharge and friability
      b. Most common site of infection in women
   5. Adnexal tenderness and masses, uterine tenderness, and cervical motion and tenderness per bimanual examination
D. Throat and endocervical culture, if oral and vaginal sex practiced
E. Men
   1. Inspect for erythema and edema in the penile shaft
   2. Purulent urethral discharge
   3. If anal sex is practiced, perform rectal examination for tenderness and discharge

V. Laboratory/diagnostic findings

A. Endocervical and throat culture for *N. gonorrhoeae* with the use of modified Thayer-Martin medium is the cornerstone of diagnosis.
B. Non-simplified DNA probe test (in remote areas)
C. Cervical culture or antigen detection of *C. trachomatis*
D. Lipase chain reaction of cervical specimen
E. Test all patients for syphilis
F. Offer HIV testing.
G. Differential diagnoses
   1. Chlamydia
   2. Appendicitis
   3. Ectopic pregnancy
   4. PID
H. Elevated WBC count
I. Elevated erythrocyte sedimentation rate
J. Examine male patient at least 1 hr after voiding

VI. Management

A. CDC recommendation for treatment of adults with uncomplicated gonococcal infections of cervix, urethra, throat, and rectum
   1. Ceftriaxone (Rocephin), 250 mg single dose IM and either azithromycin 1 gram PO as a single dose or doxycycline, 100 mg PO BID for 7 days
B. CDC recommended regimens for pregnancy
   1. Azithromycin (Zithromax), 2 gram PO if cephalosporin cannot be tolerated
C. Patients should be instructed to refer sex partners for evaluation and treatment
D. All sex partners of patients whose last sexual contact with the patient was within 60 days before onset of symptoms or diagnosis of infection should be evaluated and treated for *N. gonorrhoeae* and *C. trachomatis* infections.
E. If the patient's last sexual intercourse was greater than 60 days before the onset of symptoms or diagnosis, the patient's most recent sex partner should be treated.

F. Patients should be instructed to avoid sexual intercourse until cure is established

G. Follow-up

    1. Test for cure is not recommended by CDC unless symptoms recur, exacerbate, or do not resolve. Reevaluation 3 months after treatment is recommended by the CDC.

    2. Any gonococci isolated should be tested for antimicrobial susceptibility.

H. Persons with disseminated gonococcal infection should be hospitalized for initial therapy

I. Report to health department

HERPES SIMPLEX VIRUS

I.   **Definition**

    A. Recurrent, incurable viral infection of the genital or orofacial skin or epithelia characterized by transient, fluid-containing eruptions on a slightly raised erythematous base

    B. There are two strains of the herpes simplex virus (HSV): HSV-1 and HSV-2. These strains are quite different (50% difference in genome). Differences include the following:

      1. Sensitivity to viral drugs

      2. Ability to cause specific disease in other organs

II.   **Etiology/incidence/predisposing factors**

    A. Etiology

      1. Organism is a double-stranded DNA virus

      2. Both HSV-1 and HSV-2 may be excreted by asymptomatic persons

      3. Can cause oral or genital lesions

      4. Approximately 50 million persons in the United States have genital HSV infection

        a. HSV type 1

          i. Commonly causes herpes labialis (cold sores) and herpes keratitis

          ii. Acute gingivostomatitis: occurs in both children and adults

          iii. Causes 25% of primary genital infections (oral sex, kissing)

          iv. Incubation period ranges from 2–7 days

          v. Lesions heal within 3 weeks

          vi. Milder recurrences that diminish in frequency

          vii. HSV-1 is more common; tends to occur earlier in life

        b. HSV type 2

          i. Causes 90% of genital herpes infections

          ii. Tends to cause more severe and recurrent episodes and occurs later in life

   iii. Incubation period is from 2–7 days; lesions heal in 2–3 weeks

   iv. Recurrent episodes vary greatly from person to person

   v. Symptoms vary from person to person

   vi. Most recurrent infections are milder, and lesions heal faster

 B. Incidence

  1. Use of HSV-2-specific antibody test shows that one third of sexually active adults have serologic evidence of HSV-2

  2. Less than 5% have a history of HSV

  3. Up to 1 million new HSV-2 infections may be transmitted each year in the United States

  4. Approximately 45 million individuals are infected with HSV-2

 C. Predisposing factors/causes

  1. Caused by close physical contact, usually sexual (vaginal, anal, or oral) with infected person who is shedding virus

  2. Multiple sexual partners

  3. Use of alcohol or drugs before and during sexual activity

  4. Improper use of condoms

III. **Subjective findings: genital herpes (primary infection)**

 A. Flulike symptoms

  1. Fever

  2. Fatigue

  3. Headache

  4. Pharyngitis

  5. Myalgia

  6. Backache

 B. Itching, pain, urine retention, constipation, and lower extremity weakness

 C. Dysuria

 D. Hyperesthesia (unusual sensitivity to sensory stimuli)

IV. **Physical examination findings**

 A. Genital herpes (primary infection)

  1. Small, multiple painful vesicles or pustules distributed over external genitalia

  2. More common in genital area

  3. Painful ulcerating papules (all lesions are contagious)

  4. White-gray area of necrosis on cervix

  5. Inguinal lymphadenopathy

  6. Vaginal discharge

  7. Extragenital cutaneous lesions on hips and buttocks

 B. Recurrent genital herpes

  1. Precipitated by trauma, menses, stress, illness, fever, and overexposure to the sun

  2. Prodrome of local burning, itching, or tingling

3. Recurrent disease symptoms generally milder
4. Eruption of lesions over course of 3 days that resolve in 7–10 days
5. Viral shedding occurs around days 4–7
6. Recurrences are due to reactivation of virus already present in the nerve endings.

V. Laboratory/diagnostic findings

A. Tzanck smear
   1. Immediate diagnosis: 85%–95% sensitivity and 95% specificity
   2. Collecting specimen:
      a. Unroof vesicular lesion and scrape the base; it is not the fluid that you are testing
      b. Transfer specimen to glass slide; fix immediately
      c. Positive smear shows giant cells with eosinophilic inclusion bodies
B. HSV culture (confirmatory test of choice)
   1. Results available in 3–7 days
   2. Expensive and time consuming
C. POCkit HSV-2 (rapid test): serum test
D. Enzyme-linked immunosorbent assay and Western blot are highly accurate

VI. Management: CDC recommendations for palliative management options

A. No cure for disease; duration of symptoms and infectivity is reduced by drug therapy
B. First primary episode
   1. Acyclovir (Zovirax), 400 mg PO three times a day for 7–10 days, or until healing is complete (contraindicated in patients with acute or chronic renal involvement) or
   2. Acyclovir, 200 mg PO five times a day for 7–10 days or
   3. Famciclovir, 250 mg PO three times a day for 7–10 days or
   4. Valacyclovir, 1 gram PO BID for 7–10 days
   5. Extensive counseling regarding the following:
      a. Natural history of genital herpes and sexual transmission
      b. Methods to reduce sexual transmission
         i. Use of condoms to prevent viral transmission even without lesions because of viral shedding
      c. Potential recurrent episodes
   6. CDC recommended regimens for pregnancy
      a. Doxycycline, 100 mg PO twice a day for at least 3 weeks until all lesions have completely healed
C. Recurrent infections
   1. Acyclovir is not routinely indicated in immunocompromised patients.
   2. If used, institute acyclovir during prodrome or within 2 days of onset of lesions

3. Recommended regimens for episodic recurrent infection:
    a. Acyclovir (Zovirax), 400 mg PO three times a day for 5 days or
    b. Acyclovir (Zovirax), 800 mg PO three times a day for 2 days or
    c. Acyclovir (Zovirax), 800 mg PO BID for 5 days or
    d. Valacyclovir (Valtrex), 500 mg PO BID for 3 days or
    e. Valacyclovir (Valtrex), 1 gram PO once a day for 5 days or
    f. Famciclovir (Famvir), 125 mg PO BID for 5 days
    g. Famciclovir (Famvir), 1000 mg PO BID for 1 day
    h. Famciclovir (Famvir), 500 mg once, followed by 250 mg BID for 2 days
4. Suppressive treatment is often offered to clients with evidence of more than six episodes of herpes infection per year
    a. Asymptomatic viral shedding: ~10% of patients with genital herpes experience asymptomatic viral shedding
        i. Valacyclovir, 1 gram PO every day is recommended for suppressive therapy; if fewer than 9 recurrences per year, 500 mg PO every day may be administered
        ii. Acyclovir, 400 mg PO twice a day
        iii. Famciclovir, 250 mg PO twice a day
    b. Provisions for effective contraception should be made
D. Complications
    1. Secondary infections
    2. Keratitis (keep fingers away from eyes)
    3. Meningitis
    4. Encephalitis
    5. Pneumonitis
    6. Hepatitis
E. Follow-up: PRN
F. Education: always use acyclovir (Zovirax) in full doses to avoid resistance

HUMAN PAPILLOMAVIRUS (HPV)

I. **Definition**
A. HPV infection occurs at the basal cell layer of stratified squamous epithelial cells and can cause genital warts, cervical cellular abnormalities, and cancer.
B. Low-risk types (nononcogenic types)
    1. Associated with genital warts and benign/low grade cervical cellular changes
    2. Most genital warts caused by HPV types 6 and 11
    3. Recurrent respiratory papillomatosis (rare) is associated with HPV types 6 and 11
C. High-risk types (oncogenic types)

1. Associated with low- and high-grade cervical cellular changes and dysplasia as well as anogenital (rare) cancers
2. HPV types 16 and 18 account for 70% of cervical cancers

II. **Etiology/incidence/predisposing factors**
   A. A double-stranded DNA virus that belongs to the *Papillomaviridae* family
   B. Incubation period varies.
      1. Weeks to months for genital warts
      2. Months to years for cervical cellular abnormalities
   C. Each year, 14.1 million new cases of sexually transmitted HPV occur in the United States.
   D. Most common STD; estimated that every sexually active man and woman will acquire genital HPV at some point in their life

III. **Subjective findings**
   A. Usually transient without clinical manifestations or sequelae
   B. Genital warts visualized without magnification
      1. Condylomata acuminata—cauliflower like
      2. Smooth papules
      3. Flat papules
      4. Keratotic warts
         a. Warts commonly occur in areas of coital friction
         b. When warts occur on the cervix and rectum, they should be treated by an expert

IV. **Laboratory/diagnostic findings**
   A. Diagnosis of genital warts is usually made by visual inspection.
   B. Biopsy may be needed because of the following:
      1. Diagnosis is uncertain
      2. Patient is immunocompromised
      3. Warts are pigmented, indurated, or fixed
      4. Lesions do not respond or worsen with standard treatment
      5. There is persistent ulceration or bleeding
   C. Cervical Pap test is recommended for all sexually active women

V. **Management**
   A. Left untreated, visible genital warts regress spontaneously or persist with or without proliferation
   B. Current therapies may reduce infectivity but do not eradicate; treatment ameliorates symptoms and cosmetic concerns
   C. No evidence that genital warts are associated with development of cervical cancer
      1. Infection with several HPV types (particularly HPV-16 and HPV-18) is considered the major risk factor for development of cervical neoplasia; HPV-6 and HPV-11 are most commonly associated with development of low-grade dysplasia manifested as genital warts

   2. Women who have received the HPV vaccine should continue routine cervical cancer screening.
D. Patient applied:
   1. Sinecatechins ointment 15%; apply a 0.5 cm strand of ointment topically 3 times daily to each external genital and perianal warts; continue treatment until complete clearance of warts, but no longer than 16 weeks
   2. Imiquimod 5% cream; apply topically to affected area three times per week until total clearance or up to a MAX duration of 16 weeks; apply at bedtime and leave on skin for 6–10 hr
   3. Podofilox 0.5% solution or gel; apply solution to gel topically every 12 hr in the morning and evening for 3 days, then withhold for 4 days; repeat cycle up to four times
E. Provider applied: cryotherapy with liquid nitrogen or cryoprobe, podophyllin resin 10%–25% in a compound tincture of benzoin, trichloroacetic acid or bichloroacetic acid 80%–90%, or surgical removal
F. Follow-up
   1. Partner exam not necessary; no data to indicate that reinfection plays a role in recurrences
   2. Genital warts are especially infectious; beneficial to use approaches to reduce risk of transmission
   3. HPV vaccine can protect against HPV infection types not already acquired; all women aged 9–26 years are recommended to receive HPV vaccination regardless of prior history of HPV infection.
      a. Cervarix (bivalent vaccine) or Gardasil (quadrivalent vaccine), 0.5 mL IM for three doses at 0, 1–2, and 6 months; both vaccines are indicated for preventing cervical pre-cancers and cervical cancer in females 9–26 years of age; in addition, Gardasil is indicated for the prevention of genital warts caused by HPV-16 and -18 in males between the ages of 9 and 25 years.

SYPHILIS

I.   **Definition**
   A. Systemic STI that progresses through distinct stages
      1. Primary
      2. Secondary
      3. Latent
      4. Tertiary
II. **Etiology/incidence/predisposing factors**
   A. Causative organism is the bacterium *Treponema pallidum*, a strict anaerobic spirochete
   B. Incubation period varies
      1. Typically, 10–90 days

    2. Average, 21 days

C. Case rate of 3/100,000 people in the United States

D. Incidence: 200,000 new cases reported annually; rates have increased

E. This type of bacterium is capable of infecting any organ or tissue in the unborn and is transported to various sites via the bloodstream.

F. Infection occurs at the site of inoculation: A small abrasion or sore results

III. **Subjective/physical examination findings**

  A. Primary syphilis

    1. Chancre

      a. Classic finding is a painless and indurated ulcer, "sore," or lesion

      b. Usually appears approximately 3–4 weeks after exposure

      c. Heals spontaneously in 1–5 weeks

    2. Regional lymphadenopathy

  B. Secondary syphilis (stage of dissemination)

    1. Flulike symptoms

      a. Low-grade fever

      b. Headache

      c. Sore throat

      d. Malaise

      e. Generalized arthralgia

      f. Systemic disease

    2. Maculopapular rash on palms and soles of feet 2–6 weeks after infection; this heals spontaneously in 4–10 weeks

    3. Patchy alopecia

    4. Condyloma lata (wartlike lesions) in mouth, throat, and cervix

    5. Genital lesions are highly infectious and are transmitted by direct contact.

    6. Untreated lesions resolve in 3–12 weeks

  C. Latent syphilis: often asymptomatic and lasts 2–20 years

    1. Early latency: Infection lasting less than 1 year may be infectious.

    2. Late latency: Infection lasting longer than 1 year is noninfectious.

    3. Blood test remains positive for antibodies to *T. pallidum*

  D. Tertiary (late) syphilis may take one of several forms

    1. Gummatous syphilis (soft granulomatous tumor of the tissues)

    2. Cardiovascular syphilis (rare)

    3. Neurosyphilis

IV. **Laboratory/diagnostic findings**

  A. Positive dark-field microscopic examination and direct fluorescent antibody test of lesion exudate are definitive tests for diagnosing early syphilis.

  B. Nontreponemal serologic test

  C. Venereal Disease Research Laboratory (VDRL) and rapid plasma reagin (RPR) tests become positive 1–2 weeks after chancre formation.

   1. VDRL and RPR tests can be negative in up to 30% of patients at an initial visit for primary syphilis.
D. Treponemal specific tests
   1. Treponemal antibody absorption test (fluorescent treponemal antibody absorbed) or microhemagglutination assay for antibodies to *T. pallidum* is positive
   2. False-positive test occurs with many other diseases
   3. Most commonly used test
   4. Treponemal tests remain positive for life after treatment.
   5. All reactive serologic tests require confirmation with a treponemal test
E. Both nontreponemal and treponemal tests become reactive within 3 weeks after chancre has occurred
F. Secondary: all serologic tests are positive
G. Latent: serologic tests are positive

V. **Management: Treatment is stage specific**
A. Early primary, secondary, and early latent: benzathine penicillin G (Bicillin L-A), 2.4 million units IM, single dose
B. Late latent syphilis or syphilis of unknown duration: benzathine penicillin G (Bicillin L-A), 7.2 million units IM given as 2.4 million units per week for 3 weeks
C. Tertiary disease, excluding neurosyphilis: benzathine penicillin G, 7.2 million units IM given as 2.4 million units IM weekly for 3 weeks
D. Neurosyphilis: aqueous crystalline penicillin G, 18–24 million units/day IV (3–4 million units IV every 4 hr or continuous infusion for 10–14 days); if compliance with therapy can be ensured, the following alternative regimen may also be considered:
   1. Procaine penicillin G (Wycillin), 2.4 million units per day IM, plus probenecid, 500 mg PO four times a day for 10–14 days
E. Exposure (sexual contact with persons with infectious syphilis): as for early disease
F. If penicillin allergy exists, desensitize and then treat with penicillin (see CDC guidelines)
G. CDC recommended regimens for pregnancy: treat with penicillin regimen appropriate for their stage of infection
H. Follow-up
   1. Clinical and serologic follow-up at 3 and 6 months after treatment
   2. If symptoms persist or recur with a sustained fourfold increase in the nontreponemal test titer compared with baseline or previous titer, suspect failed treatment or reinfection: retreat after HIV testing
   3. Some experts recommend CSF examination
   4. Recommended retreatment regimen: Wycillin, 2.4 million units IM given 1 week apart for 3 consecutive weeks, unless CSF examination indicates that neurosyphilis is present
I. Management of sex partners: treat presumptively
J. Report to health department

BIBLIOGRAPHY

Del Rio, C., Hall, G., Homes, K., Soge, O., Hook, E. W., Kirkcaldy, R. D., . . . Bolan, G. (2012). Update to CDC's sexually transmitted diseases treatment guidelines, 2010: Oral cephalosporins no longer a recommended treatment for gonococcal infections. *Morbidity and Mortality Weekly Report, 61*(31), 590–594.

Centers for Disease Control and Prevention. (2010). *Sexually transmitted diseases treatment guidelines*. Retrieved from http://www.cdc.gov/std/treatment/2010/toc.htm

Centers for Disease Control and Prevention. (2011). *Diseases characterized by genital, anal, or perianal ulcers*. Retrieved from http://www.cdc.gov/std/treatment/2010/genital-ulcers.htm#syphpreg

Centers for Disease Control and Prevention. (2011). *Diseases characterized by vaginal discharge*. Retrieved from http://www.cdc.gov/std/treatment/2010/vaginal-discharge.htm

Centers for Disease Control and Prevention. (2011). *Gonococcal infections*. Retrieved from http://www.cdc.gov/std/treatment/2010/gonococcal-infections.htm.

Centers for Disease Control and Prevention. (2011). *Sexually transmitted disease surveillance*. Retrieved from http://www.cdc.gov/std/stats11/toc.htm

Goodwin, T. M. (2010). *Management of common problems in obstetrics and gynecology* (5th ed.). Chichester, West Sussex: Wiley-Blackwell.

Kirkcaldy, R. D., Bolan, G. A., & Wasserheit, J. N. (2013). Cephalosporin-resistant gonorrhea in North America. *Journal of the American Medical Association, 309*(2), 185–187.

CHAPTER 71

Eye, Ear, Nose, and Throat Disorders

DAVID A. MILLER • THOMAS W. BARKLEY, JR. • CHARLENE M. MYERS

SIGNS AND SYMPTOMS THAT SUGGEST PROBLEMS OF THE EYES, EARS, NOSE, AND THROAT

I.   **Eyes**
  A. Halos around lights in surrounding darkness: cataracts and glaucoma
  B. Loss of central vision: macular degeneration
  C. Loss of peripheral vision: glaucoma and retinal detachment
  D. Pain: glaucoma, foreign body, and corneal abrasion
  E. Sudden change in vision: retinal detachment, foreign body, corneal abrasion, optic neuritis, temporal arteritis, migraine headaches, TIA or stroke, tumor, etc.

II. **Ears**
  A. Loss of hearing: presbycusis, drug toxicity (aminoglycosides, aspirin, and furosemide), Ménière's disease, acoustic neuroma, stroke, polyarteritis nodosa, autoimmune disorders (lupus), viral infection (herpes simplex virus, adenovirus, mononucleosis, diabetes, meningitis, multiple sclerosis, etc.).

III. **Nose**
  A. Posterior epistaxis

IV. **Mouth**
  A. Burning in mouth, oral cavity: vitamin B12 deficiency; stomatitis; ill-fitting dentures and bridges
  B. Xerostomia: dehydration; drugs with anticholinergic activity (antidepressants, diuretics, and antipsychotics); salivary gland dysfunction following radiation therapy
  C. Loss of taste: drugs (antihistamines; antidepressants); oral infection (candidiasis)

V. Throat

    A. Swallowing disorders: esophageal stricture, malignancy, foreign body, stroke

CONJUNCTIVITIS

I. Definition

    A. Common, generally acute, painful inflammation with or without infection of the conjunctiva (palpebral or bulbar), but not involving the cornea or deeper structures of the eye (aka "pinkeye")

    B. Can be chronic, but most cases are acute, and many are infectious, can be bilateral or unilateral

II. Etiology/predisposing factors

    A. Spread by direct inoculation via fingers or droplets

    B. Bacterial

        1. *Staphylococcus aureus*

        2. *Pseudomonas*

        3. *Haemophilus influenzae*

        4. *Streptococcus pneumoniae*

        5. *Moraxella*

        6. Gonorrhea and chlamydia

    C. Viral

        1. Commonly adenovirus

        2. Herpes virus (may be vision threatening)

    D. Allergens/hypersensitivity to the following:

        1. Pollen

        2. Dust

        3. Contact lenses

        4. Dyes

        5. Ophthalmic drops

        6. Make up

    E. Trauma (chemical and ultraviolet flash burns)

    F. Keratoconjunctivitis sicca (dry eye)

    G. Parasitic infestation (pediculosis pubis)

    H. Systemic disease

        1. Reiter syndrome

        2. Behçet's syndrome

        3. Temporal arteritis

        4. Thyroid exophthalmos

        5. Sjogren syndrome

    I. May accompany other eye disorders

        1. Keratitis

        2. Uveitis

        3. Acute angle-closure glaucoma

    J. Medication adverse effects (e.g., antihistamines and anticholinergics)

    K. Environmental insults (wind, heat, sun, and smoke)

III. Subjective/physical examination findings
   A. Redness or excessive tearing (sense of a foreign body in the eye)
   B. Swelling or itching
   C. History of allergenic/infectious/traumatic exposure
   D. Discharge
   E. Visual acuity (see Laboratory/Diagnostic Findings section)
   F. Edema of external eye or lid
   G. Extraocular movement, visual fields, pupillary response, cornea, and anterior chamber are usually normal. The presence of photophobia rules out conjunctivitis.
   H. Conjunctival injection/swelling (chemosis)/foreign body
      1. While wearing gloves, evert the upper lid by rolling it externally along the cotton end of a swab and inspect for foreign bodies or papillary changes.
         a. Normal internal lid is pink and smooth.
         b. With injection, "bumpy" flesh or cobblestone appearance (i.e., giant papillary conjunctivae) indicates tissue changes induced by chronic irritation, as from the following:
            i. Poor hygiene
            ii. Improper use of extended wear contacts
            iii. Allergic response to ophthalmic solutions
      2. Examine for obvious foreign body
   I. Drainage may be purulent or serous. If intent is to culture, a specimen should be taken before drops or irrigation is instilled.
IV. Laboratory/diagnostic findings
   A. Decreased visual acuity may indicate a more serious condition
   B. Consider culture of secretions: Giemsa stain for possible infection with chlamydia or gonorrhea
V. Management
   A. Nonpharmacological
      1. Eye compresses—cool for itching/irritation; warm for crusting
      2. Discontinue wearing contact lens and eye makeup until resolved.
   B. Rule out corneal abrasion or foreign body
      1. Instill topical anesthetic (2 drops tetracaine [Pontocaine], 0.5%, or proparacaine, 0.5%)
      2. Stain the eye with fluorescein with the use of drops or paper
      3. Examine under ultraviolet light or slit lamp
   C. Bacteria
      1. Topical antibiotic ophthalmic solutions or ointments
         a. Gentamicin (Garamycin), 3 mg/ml solution, 1–2 drops every 4 hr while awake for 5 days; if severe, may be increased to 2 drops every 1–2 hr; 0.3% solution, apply ½ inch ribbon 2–3 times a day
         b. Neomycin (Neosporin), 1–2 drops solution every 1–6 hr; or ointment ½ inch ribbon every 3–4 hr; for 7–10 days

       c. Polymyxin, apply ointment every 3–4 hr for 7–10 days

       d. Sulfacetamide sodium (Sodium Sulamyd), 10% solution, 1–2 drops into affected eye every 2–6 hr while awake; or ointment ½ inch ribbon every 3–8 hr; for 7–10 days

       e. Ofloxacin (Ocuflox), 0.3% solution, 1–2 drops into affected eye every 1–6 hr depending on severity

  2. Note: a 15% potential for an adverse reaction to neomycin-containing products (Neosporin) has been reported

D. In the presence of other systemic disease, treat the underlying condition accordingly (e.g., otitis media: typically treated with synthetic penicillin with or without clavulanate or a macrolide regimen)

E. Chlamydia

  1. Oral tetracycline or erythromycin, 250 mg 4 times a day, or doxycycline, 100 mg BID, for 3–4 weeks or

  2. Single dose of azithromycin, 1 gram PO

  3. Local antibiotics generally are not indicated

F. Gonorrhea

  1. Single dose of ceftriaxone, 1 gram IM

  2. Note: gonococcal conjunctivitis should be confirmed by Gram stain and culture

  3. Patients suspected of ophthalmic infection should be immediately referred to an ophthalmologist because of the risk of corneal perforation

G. Allergy

  1. Vernal type occurs seasonally (typically in the spring) and affects adolescents and young adults predominantly. Atopic keratoconjunctivitis affects older adults more commonly and may manifest with lid structural changes and blepharitis (with or without bacterial infection).

  2. Over-the-counter: naphazoline, instill 1–2 drops of 0.012% or 0.1% ophthalmic solution into each eye every 3–4 hr or 4 times daily, PRN

  3. H1-receptor antagonists:

       a. Ketotifen, 0.025%, 2 drops 2–4 times a day

       b. Loratadine, 10 mg PO, once daily

       c. Fexofenadine, 180 mg PO, once daily

       d. Cetirizine, 5–10 mg PO, once daily

  4. NSAIDs:

       a. Ketorolac tromethamine, 2 drops every 6 hr

  5. Topical mast cell stabilizers, cromolyn, vasoconstrictors, and antihistamines should be considered for vernal type

  6. Ophthalmic corticosteroids should be considered for acute exacerbations. Note: Cataracts, glaucoma, and worsening of infections, such as herpes, may occur with use of steroids.

7. If pertinent, and allergy to contacts or contact solution is suspected, discontinue agent and refer to ophthalmologist. Change in contact type or cleaning solution (e.g., hydrogen peroxide based), discontinuance of one or both, or simply a more judicious cleaning protocol may be indicated.

H. Herpes simplex virus—refer to ophthalmologist

CORNEAL ABRASION

I. **Definition:**
   A. Disruption of the epithelium of the cornea (the clear, anterior covering of the eye)

II. **Etiology/incidence/predisposing factors**
   A. Usually associated with chemical, burn, or mechanical trauma (including foreign body)
   B. Very common
   C. Result of outdoor activity, occupational hazards and lack of using proper eye protection (e.g., welding, painting, and construction)

III. **Subjective/physical examination findings**
   A. Intense pain associated with the vast sensory nerve supply of the eye
   B. A sense of foreign body in the eye
   C. Report of redness or discharge of the conjunctiva
   D. History of decreased visual acuity or vision may be unchanged
   E. Complaint of tearing
   F. Photophobia
   G. Decrease in visual acuity
      1. Except in trauma involving emergency need for irrigation of the eye, visual acuity should be the initial measure of vision.
      2. When a Snellen chart is unavailable, gross evaluation, such as a finger count, can be used
      3. Instill a topical anesthetic such as tetracaine (Pontocaine) ophthalmic drops (1–2 drops)
      4. Avoid repeated use of eye anesthetics, which may result in further injury and delayed healing
   H. Inspect for other signs of trauma (foreign body) by everting the lid
      1. Note positive findings with location
      2. See Conjunctivitis section for lid eversion procedure
   I. Fluorescein staining of the cornea
      1. May reveal disruptions in the corneal epithelium
      2. Appears as increased uptake (pooling) of dye when the area is illuminated by a Wood lamp or ultraviolet (blue) light

IV. **Management**
   A. Refer to an ophthalmologist
   B. Apply antibiotic ointment (preferred by many clinicians and patients) or solution, such as the following:

1. Gentamicin ophthalmic ointment 0.3%, apply a ½ inch ribbon to the affected eye(s) 2–3 times a day, or solution 3 mg/ml, 1–2 drops into affected eye every 2–3 hr while awake or

2. Sulfacetamide sodium, 10% ointment, apply a ½ inch ribbon to the affected eye(s) every 3–8 hr for 7–10 days, or solution, apply 1–2 drops every 2–6 hr

3. Cycloplegic or mydriatic drops (e.g., isopto atropine [Atropisol], isopto, and tropicamide [Mydriacyl]) may be prescribed for 24 hr (until recheck by clinician) to promote analgesia and healing. Caution regarding glaucoma: Adverse effect of ciliary and papillary dilatation is increased ocular pressure. Do not use in patient with angle-closure conditions.

C. Apply a soft eye patch (or soft contact lens bandage); dressing should be removed within 24 hr by clinician

D. Update tetanus immunization if indicated

E. Reevaluate in 24 hr, at which time healing should be complete

F. Refer to ophthalmologist for removal of foreign bodies or for failed initial management

DIABETIC RETINOPATHY

I. **Definition**
A. Ocular disease of the retina resulting from systemic diabetes

II. **Etiology/incidence/predisposing factors**
A. Most common cause of blindness in the United States
B. Inhibition of aldose reductase pathways results in increased blood flow and pressure, thereby diminishing the integrity of the blood-retina barrier
   1. Entry of large cells into the extracellular space of the retina causes macular edema
   2. Microaneurysms, intraretinal microvascular leaking, and hemorrhage may result, leading to scarring and proliferation of new capillary vessels and ischemia of existing retinal vasculature
   3. Smoking, uncontrolled hyperglycemia, and hypertension are associated with greater risk

III. **Subjective/physical examination findings**
A. Symptoms that may be present are as follows:
   1. Flashing lights in peripheral visual fields
   2. Blurred vision
   3. "Cobwebs"
   4. Black spots
   5. Loss of central vision
   6. Difficulty with color perception
B. Sudden loss of vision, funduscopic examination may reveal exudates (hard or soft) and microaneurysms seen as dot and flame hemorrhagic markings

C. Hard, bright-yellow markings may be noted arising from lipid transudation via leaky capillaries

D. Soft exudates produced by infarcted nerve tissue appearing as pale, yellow, irregular; cotton wool spots may be present

IV. **Laboratory/diagnostic findings**

A. Retinopathy is associated with poor glycemic control

B. Sustained glucose levels greater than 130 mg/dl have been associated with an increase in microvascular complications

C. Hypertension increases risk

V. **Management**

A. Refer to an ophthalmologist

   1. Macular edema can be ascertained only via stereoscopic examination or by fluorescein angiography

   2. Visual acuity is not a sufficient indicator of retinopathy

B. Laser photocoagulation for focal macular edema

C. Vitrectomy and laser therapy, as indicated

D. Tight glycemic control is paramount

E. Management of blood pressure

F. Smoking cessation

RETINAL DETACHMENT

I. **Definition**

A. Separation of the neural retina from the choroid after trauma, hemorrhage, increased intraocular pressure, or transudation of fluid leaving the retina without oxygen and nourishment

II. **Etiology/incidence/predisposing factors**

A. Trauma

B. Intraocular/intracerebral mass

C. Uveitis (inflammation of the iris)

D. Annually, 10 out of every 100,000 persons suffer a retinal detachment without rhegmatogenous tear (tear with fluid between retinal layers).

E. In all, 1%–3% of patients undergoing cataract surgery suffer a retinal detachment

F. The following are associated with chronic retinal detachment:

   1. Diabetes mellitus

   2. Sickle cell anemia

   3. Myopia and cataract extraction

III. **Subjective/physical examination findings**

A. Sudden onset of painless visual changes, floaters, blurred vision, light flashes

B. As detachment becomes pervasive, a "curtain" may obscure part or all of the field of vision.

C. Large detachments may produce a Marcus Gunn pupil (afferent pupil that reacts more consensually than directly)

D. Elevations of the retina related to tears

E. Exudative, bullous elevation without tears

IV. Management

   A. Immediate referral to an ophthalmologist for evaluation and treatment, such as the following:

   1. Diathermy—application of alternating electrical current that creates heat and coagulates the tissue, causing scleral shrinkage with subsequent necrosis

   2. Cryotherapy/cryopexy—freezing the area around the hole to help reattach the retina

   3. Scleral buckling—sewing a silicone rubber or sponge to the sclera over the affected area that indents the wall of the eye and relieves some of the force caused by the vitreous tugging on the retina

   4. Photocoagulation—using a laser to burn around the tear, creating scarring that welds the retina to the underlying tissue

   5. Pneumatic retinopexy—injection of a bubble of air or gas into the vitreous that floats against the retinal tear and seals it

   6. Vitrectomy—removal of vitreous along with any tissue that is tugging on the retina; air, gas, or liquid is then injected into the vitreous space to reattach the retina

   B. If the detachment is a result of traumatic insult, patch the eye with a metal shield (i.e., Fox eye shield).

CENTRAL AND BRANCH RETINAL ARTERY OBSTRUCTION

I. Definition

   A. Abrupt blockage of the central retinal artery or its branches, causing sudden visual loss or loss of visual fields

   B. Permanent partial or complete visual loss may ensue without immediate intervention

II. Etiology/predisposing factors

   A. Causes

   1. Thrombosis

   2. Embolism

   3. Arteritis of the central retinal artery

   B. Associated with the following:

   1. Migraine

   2. Advancing age

   3. History of vasculitis

   4. Atrial fibrillation

   5. Diabetes

   6. Hypertension

   7. Inflammatory conditions (temporal arteritis, syphilis, Lyme disease, etc.)

   8. Coagulopathies (sickle cell disease, Hodgkin's disease, anemia, platelet or clotting factor abnormalities, oral contraceptives, etc.)

III. **Subjective/physical examination findings**
   A. Sudden, painless, gross visual loss (monocular), or visual field loss
   B. Amaurosis fugax (ipsilateral, intermittent monocular blindness) is associated with ipsilateral carotid disorder and is a harbinger of impending stroke.
   C. Intraocular hemorrhage can occur in patients on antiplatelet and anticoagulant therapy. Patients should be asked if they have ever experienced this in the past, since this may not directly be an ophthalmological disorder.
   D. Visual loss may be central (if fovea is affected) or peripheral
   E. Partial dilatation of the pupil, which is sluggishly reactive to direct light but may have a normal consensual response
   F. Funduscopic examination
      1. May reveal a pale, opaque fundus and a characteristic "cherry-red spot" at the fovea (bifurcation of the arteries where emboli is most likely to become lodged)
      2. Retina may be edematous
      3. Arterial vessels may appear pale and bloodless

IV. **Laboratory/diagnostic findings**
   A. Elevated erythrocyte sedimentation rate associated with giant cell arteritis
   B. Consider testing to evaluate for coagulopathies in appropriate patients (antitreponemal antibody, antiphospholipid antibody, ANA, RF, serum protein electrophoresis, hemoglobin electrophoresis, PT, PTT, fibrinogen, protein C and S, antithrombin III, and factor V Leiden)
   C. CBC for anemia, polycythemia, and platelet disorders
   D. Fasting blood sugar, HgbA1c, cholesterol, triglycerides, and lipid panel for atherosclerotic disease
   E. Blood cultures for bacterial endocarditis and septic emboli
   F. Fluorescein angiography
   G. Visual acuity, visual field examination

V. **Management**
   A. Immediate consultation with an ophthalmologist
   B. Intermittent digital massage of the anterior chamber by gentle pressure over the eyelid may be sight saving. If an embolus can be dislodged, retinal ischemia can be relieved.
   C. Consider rebreathing CO_2 per air-tight mask or bag to decrease alkalosis
   D. Consider intravenous anticoagulant (e.g., heparin, 10,000 units)
   E. Treatment of underlying comorbidities such as carotid and cardiac disease causing emboli, hypertension, migraine, oral contraceptive use, thrombophilia, and so forth

GLAUCOMA

I.   Definition

  A. Disorder of progressive visual loss. Typically, peripheral vision decreases first, then central vision; can result in blindness.

  B. Optic neuropathy usually associated with elevated intraocular pressure (open-angle glaucoma) causing vascular resistance, causing decreased vascular perfusion of the optic nerve leading to ischemia that can lead to partial or complete blindness

II.   Etiology/incidence/predisposing factors

  A. Primarily of two types:

  1. Chronic open angle (wide) (most common) or

  2. Acute or chronic closed angle (narrow)

  B. Primary open-angle glaucoma accounts for nearly two thirds of all cases and results from increased intraocular fluid production with decreased removal.

  C. Secondary or induced glaucoma, resulting from the following:

  1. Prolonged steroid use

  2. Uveitis

  3. Cataracts

  4. Tumor

  5. Trauma

  D. Obstruction of the outflow of aqueous humor from the ciliary body through the trabecula and the canal of Schlemm produces increased intraocular pressure, which leads to atrophy of the optic nerve head.

  E. Risk factors

  1. Advancing age

  2. Heredity (Asians are more likely to have normal intraocular pressure in open-angle glaucoma)

  3. Myopia

  4. African-American ethnicity (open-angle glaucoma more common in Blacks than Whites)

  5. Corticosteroid therapy

  6. Trauma

  7. Family history

III.   Subjective/physical examination findings

  A. In open-angle glaucoma, visual changes occur slowly, with decreasing peripheral vision noted over time.

  1. Photophobia and visual blurring may occur

  2. Headache and halos around lights are atypical, although a unilateral headache, in conjunction with visual changes on the same side as the headache, may occur

  B. In secondary glaucoma, such as from ophthalmic corticosteroid use, elevated intraocular pressure may be produced in just 2 weeks.

  C. In acute closed-angle glaucoma, symptoms develop rapidly.

1. The patient complains of intense eye pain and visual disturbances (halos around lights), with nausea and vomiting
2. Note: although pain is common with closed-angle glaucoma, painless variants may be distinguished only by a fixed pupil

D. Inspect for external signs such as redness, tearing, lid deformities, foreign body, proptosis, or ptosis, and for corneal clouding

E. A "hard eye" may be palpated in acute glaucoma

F. Observe changes in pupillary response, reactivity, symmetry, and accommodation

G. Visual acuity may remain normal

H. Examine for increased intraocular pressure (IOP) by measuring IOP with Schiøtz tonometer or Goldmann applanation tonometer
   1. Never apply the tonometer to an infected or possibly infected eye
   2. Increased IOP is defined as pressure greater than 23 mmHg
   3. In acute angle-closure glaucoma, IOP may be 40–80 mmHg
   4. With specialized equipment, corneal thickness, retinal photography, and automatic visual fields testing

I. Observe for decreased peripheral vision with confrontation test

J. Funduscopy
   1. Optic disc may appear irregular with notching of the physiologic cup or "cupping"
   2. Observe for increased cup-to-disc ratio

IV. Management

A. Acute open-angle glaucoma requires immediate initiation of medication and referral to an ophthalmologist for surgical treatment.

B. Chronic glaucoma requires consult/referral to an ophthalmologist for examination and monitoring of the condition
   1. Prostaglandin analogs (first-line therapy)
      a. Bimatoprost (Lumigan), latanoprost (Xalatan), tafluprost (Zioptan), travoprost (Travatan), unoprostone (Rescula)
   2. β-blocking agents (first-line therapy)
      a. Betaxolol (Betoptic), levobunolol (Betagan), carteolol (Ocupress), metipranolol (OptiPranolol), timolol (Betimol, Timoptic)
      b. Use with caution in pulmonary disease, bradycardia, heart failure, and heart block
   3. α-2 adrenergic agonists (second-line therapy, adjunct therapy)
      a. Apraclonidine (Lopidine), brimonidine (Alphagan)
   4. Carbonic anhydrase inhibitor (second-line therapy, adjunct therapy)
      a. Brinzolamide (Azopt), dorzolamide (Trusopt), acetazolamide (Diamox), methazolamide (Neptazane)
      b. Oral agents: indicated only when failing to respond to or tolerate maximum topical therapy due to adverse effect profile
   5. Parasympathomimetic agents (limited role in therapy)

       a. Carbachol (Miostat), echothiophate iodide (Phospholine Iodide), pilocarpine (Isopto Carpine)

       b. Use decreased significantly because of local ocular adverse effects and/or frequency of dosing

       c. Reserved primarily for patients who are either not responding to or are intolerant of other therapy due to serious ocular and systemic toxic effects

    6. Sympathomimetic agents (limited role in therapy)

       a. Dipivefrin HCl (Propine)

       b. Clinical use has decreased dramatically since the advent of better tolerated and more efficacious agents

C. Non-pharmacological treatment options include laser surgery or trabeculectomy.

D. Follow up 3–4 weeks after beginning medication

E. Closed-angle glaucoma is an ophthalmologic emergency

    1. Consult an ophthalmologist as soon as the diagnosis is suspected

    2. Followed every 3 months by ophthalmologist

BELL'S PALSY

I.   **Definition**

    A. Sudden onset of unilateral facial paralysis or weakness

    B. Generally self-limiting, with restoration of health in a matter of weeks

II.   **Etiology/incidence/predisposing factors**

    A. Idiopathic

    B. Probably involves inflammation of cranial nerve VII near the stylomastoid foramen

    C. Affects individuals across the life span without gender preference

    D. Affects 25 in 100,000 persons in the United States annually

    E. Clinical appearance often correlates with periods of stress, viral infection, or fatigue

    F. Familial tendency

    G. Increased incidence in the following:

       1. Hypertension

       2. Diabetes

       3. Viral infection: herpes simplex, herpes zoster, Epstein-Barr virus, cytomegalovirus, coxsackievirus, adenovirus, and influenza B

       4. Ramsay Hunt syndrome (herpes zoster oticus occurs when shingles infection affects the facial nerve near one ear, which can cause permanent facial paralysis and hearing loss in the affected ear)

       5. Demyelinating disease

       6. Sarcoidosis

       7. Lyme disease

          a. Increased incidence of recurrence

    H. May be related to cold exposure

III. Subjective/physical examination findings

    A. Unilateral paralysis of the face

        1. Affects the eyebrow, eyelid, and/or mouth

        2. Although paralysis may mimic symptoms of cerebrovascular accident, only facial muscle involvement is noted

    B. Taste impairment

    C. Ipsilateral pain in ear, cheek, and face

    D. Weakness of upper and lower face

    E. Inability to close the eyelids

    F. May be drooling as the result of mouth paralysis

    G. Abnormal corneal reflex on the affected side

    H. Hyperacusis (increased hearing sensitivity)

    I. Normal facial sensation or may have pain in or behind the ear

    J. Taste disturbance

    K. Herpetic lesions around ear/face

    L. The corneal reflex (blink test) is abnormal in 100% of cases

    M. Excessive tearing or dry eye

IV. Laboratory/diagnostic findings

    A. Diagnostic testing is nonspecific; diagnosis is one of exclusion

    B. A lumbar puncture is not typically needed but may reveal elevated levels of CSF protein and cells.

    C. Consider tests to confirm other diagnoses such as:

        1. CT, MRI (rule out tumor)

        2. Lyme titer (if history of tick exposure)

        3. Audiogram to rule out cranial nerve VIII involvement (not associated with Bell's palsy)

V. Management

    A. Eye care, including moisturizers such as Artificial Tears or Tears Naturale, PRN

    B. Eyelids may have to be taped closed to prevent external trauma.

    C. Consider referral to a physical therapist for evaluation, exercise, and stimulation to reduce the risk of contractures of the paralyzed muscles

    D. The use of steroids is indicated to decrease inflammation around cranial nerve VII.

        1. In the early stages of illness (before day 10 of onset)

        2. Tapered regimen of methylprednisolone (Medrol Dosepak):

            a. Day 1: 8 mg PO before breakfast; 4 mg after lunch and after dinner; 8 mg at bedtime

            b. Day 2: 4 mg PO before breakfast, after lunch, and after dinner; and 8 mg at bedtime

            c. Day 3: 4 mg PO before breakfast, after lunch, after dinner, and at bedtime

            d. Day 4: 4 mg PO before breakfast, after lunch, and at dinner

            e. Day 5: 4 mg PO before breakfast and at bedtime

            f. Day 6: 4 mg PO before breakfast

3. Antiviral drugs, such as acyclovir or valacyclovir, may stop the progression of the infection if a virus is the cause.
E. Explain to the patient that the disorder is usually self-limiting and that most cases begin to resolve in 4–6 weeks with complete resolution in 6 months

OTITIS EXTERNA

I. **Definition**
   A. Painful inflammation of the external auditory canal and auricle
   B. Commonly known as "swimmer's ear"
   C. Does occur in the elderly, but more common in younger persons

II. **Etiology/incidence/predisposing factors**
   A. Five times more common among swimmers
   B. More common in humid, warm environments
   C. Bacteria
      1. *Pseudomonas aeruginosa* (the most common pathogenic organism)
      2. *Staphylococcus aureus* (the most common organism in the outer ear)
      3. *Proteus vulgaris*
      4. *Streptococcus*
   D. Fungi (especially *Candida*) secondary to prolonged otic antibiotic use
   E. Trauma: scratching of the external canal with bobby pins, ear plugs, or other foreign objects
   F. Allergic reaction to drugs, including topical neomycin, topical benzocaine, and topical propylene glycol
   G. Viral

III. **Subjective/physical examination findings**
   A. Pain: severity increases with manipulation of the tragus or the pinna
   B. Decreased hearing or sense of fullness in the ear
   C. Fever
   D. Lymphadenitis (generally preauricular/postauricular and anterior cervical triangle)
   E. Itching
   F. Canal and outer ear edema
   G. Otorrhea, which may be as follows:
      1. Purulent
      2. Bloody
      3. Serous
      4. Yellow/orange cerumen mixture
      5. Tympanic membrane is normal or may be erythematous or dull
   H. Tenderness on palpation of the auricle, pinna with movement

IV. **Management**
   A. Gentle suction and removal of debris from the external canal
   B. Once the ear canal is free of debris, administer appropriate drops

1. Combined antibiotic and steroid solution such as Cortisporin Otic, 4 drops in affected ear 3–4 times a day, or Cipro HC otic, 3 drops BID for 7 days
2. Antimicrobial solution, such as TobraDex, 2 drops BID for 7 days
3. Zoto-HC drops, 3 drops BID for 7 days

C. A cotton gauze wick may be inserted into the canal if severe edema is present (remove within 2–3 days of insertion).
D. Oral antibiotic if based upon cultures taken
   1. Ciprofloxacin, 750 mg twice a day, may be required if infection extends outside the ear canal or if treating malignant otitis externa
E. Warm compresses to outer ear
F. Consider corticosteroids (Medrol Dosepak), 5-day tapering dose, to reduce edema and pain
G. Oral analgesics, such as acetaminophen, nonsteroidal anti-inflammatory drugs (NSAIDs), may need opioids (such as hydrocodone/acetaminophen).
H. A 50/50 combination of rubbing alcohol and white vinegar may be applied to the affected ear after swimming or bathing as a preventive measure.
I. Follow-up in 1 week

OTITIS MEDIA

I. **Definition**
   A. Infectious or inflammatory process within the middle ear
   B. May be acute or chronic, suppurative, or serous in nature

II. **Etiology/incidence/predisposing factors**
   A. Eustachian tube dysfunction or congestion that prevents effective drainage of the middle ear
   B. Infectious causative agents typically are respiratory bacteria:
      1. *Streptococcus pneumoniae*
      2. *Haemophilus influenzae*
      3. *Moraxella catarrhalis*
      4. *Staphylococcus aureus*
   C. A neoplasm may occlude the eustachian tube, causing a buildup of serous fluid.

III. **Subjective/physical examination findings**
   A. Throbbing pain
   B. Hearing loss (conductive)
   C. Vertigo and nausea
   D. Severe ear pain with sudden relief usually indicates tympanic membrane rupture with immediate release of fluid into the middle ear cavity
   E. Otorrhea may be pulsatile
   F. Red, dull, and bulging tympanic membrane (serous fluid may be amber in color)

G. A fine, black line (fluid meniscus) indicates a partially-filled cavity

H. Air bubbles may be visible beyond the tympanic membrane

I. Bony landmarks are obscured

J. Hole in tympanic membrane in severe cases if rupture occurs

K. Tympanic membrane retracted, opaque, and dull with decreased movement (in otitis media with effusion)

IV. Management

    A. Antibiotics (oral course for 10 days)

        1. Amoxicillin (Amoxil), 500 mg PO every 12 hr or 250 mg every 8 hr (for mild to moderate AOM); 875 mg PO every 12 hr or 500 mg every 8 hr (for severe AOM); duration of 7 days

            a. If allergic to penicillin, trimethoprim-sulfamethoxazole (Bactrim), 80/400 mg 2 tablets PO BID for 10 days, or azithromycin (Zithromax), 500 mg PO on first day followed by 250 mg PO on days 2–5

        2. Cefdinir (Omnicef), 600 mg daily for 5 days

        3. Cefuroxime, 500 mg PO twice a day

        4. Cefpodoxime, 100–200 mg PO twice a day

    B. If perforation occurs, Cortisporin Otic, 4 drops topically 3 times a day for 7 days

    C. Analgesics PRN for pain—OTC acetaminophen or NSAIDs, opioids only if needed. Topical analgesic, Auralgan, is effective to relieve pain for a non-perforated, non-draining otitis media.

    D. Refer to ENT for recurrent acute otitis media (3–4 times in 6 months) or chronic otitis media (3 months or more bilaterally; or 6 months or more unilaterally); if perforation of tympanic membrane, hearing loss of 20 dB or more following treatment.

VERTIGO

I. Definition

    A. False sensation of movement (either you or your surroundings), usually associated with disequilibrium

    B. Disequilibrium is a sense of light-headedness or of being off-balance without movement

    C. Severe vertigo is also associated with nausea and vomiting, in addition to trouble standing or walking

II. Etiology/incidence/predisposing factors

    A. Viral syndromes (e.g., vestibular neuronitis)

    B. Labyrinthitis

    C. Labyrinthine hydrops (Ménière disease)

    D. Vascular disease/spasm—may occur from thrombosis or disruption in an artery or vein

    E. Damage to cranial nerve VIII

        1. Meningitis

        2. Trauma

          3. Tumors
- F. Damage to brain stem nuclei
    1. Encephalitis
    2. Brain abscess
    3. Hemorrhage
    4. Multiple sclerosis
- G. Other conditions
    1. Tertiary syphilis
    2. Alcohol intoxication
    3. Drugs (e.g., antihypertensives, sedatives, hypnotics, and narcotics)
    4. Cardiac arrhythmia
    5. Hypoglycemia
    6. Thyroid disorders
    7. Anemia
    8. Diabetes mellitus
    9. Dehydration
- H. Cerebellar (vertebrobasilar)
    1. Transient ischemic attack
    2. Cerebrovascular accident

III. **Subjective/physical examination findings**
- A. Sensation of movement/rotation
- B. Light-headedness/"faint feeling"
- C. Sense of floating, swimming
- D. Tinnitus
- E. Hearing impairment
- F. Nausea, vomiting
- G. "Full" sensation in ear
- H. Nystagmus
- I. Carotid bruits
- J. Positional hypotension
- K. Conductive hearing loss
- L. Positive Romberg sign
- M. Note: no objective findings may be reported

IV. **Laboratory/diagnostic findings**
- A. Thyroid-stimulating hormone to rule out hypothyroidism
- B. Hematocrit to rule out anemia
- C. Fasting blood glucose level
- D. Electrolytes and therapeutic drug levels
- E. Consider alcohol level, drug screen
- F. Venereal Disease Research Laboratory or rapid plasma reagin
- G. Audiogram/tympanogram evaluation
- H. Refer to specialist for possible inner ear testing
- I. Consider CT or MRI of the brain, carotid Doppler studies, Holter monitor

V.   Management
    A. Treat symptomatically
    B. Medication reconciliation and stopping unnecessary medications
    C. Bed rest during acute attacks
    D. Vestibular exercises to facilitate CNS compensation
    E. Vestibular suppressants
        1. Meclizine (Antivert), 25–100 mg PO divided every 6 hr
        2. Diazepam (Valium), 2.5–5 mg PO at bedtime (low dose for shortest duration only if absolutely needed)
        3. Scopolamine (Transderm Scope patch), apply 1 patch every 3 days
    F. Low-salt diet in combination with diuretics if Ménière disease is suspected
    G. Antiemetics
        1. Ondansetron (Zofran), 4–8 mg PO every 12 hr;
        2. Metoclopramide (Reglan), 10 mg every 6 hr; or
        3. Promethazine (Phenergan), 12.5–25 mg PO (tablet) or per rectum (suppository) every 4 hr PRN for nausea and vomiting (caution regarding side effects and risk of falls in the elderly)

ALLERGIC RHINITIS

I.   Definition
    A. An immunoglobulin (Ig) E-mediated reaction to an antigen (allergen) that occurs after previous exposure to the same substance
    B. May be seasonal or perennial

II.   Etiology/incidence/predisposing factors
    A. Seasonal
        1. Occurs at the same time every year
        2. Varying pollens, depending on geographic region
        3. Common offenders:
            a. Trees
            b. Grasses
            c. Ragweed
    B. Perennial
        1. Occurs year round
        2. Associated with indoor inhalants
        3. Common offenders
            a. Dust mites
            b. Mold spores
            c. Animal dander
    C. Other aggravating factors:
        1. Cigarette smoke
        2. Temperature changes
        3. Chemical irritants
            a. Perfume
            b. Candles

    c. Industrial chemicals
   4. Air pollutants
   5. Foods

III. **Subjective/physical examination findings**
  A. Clear nasal drainage
  B. Nasal congestion/pressure
  C. Sneezing
  D. Excessive postnasal drainage causing sore throat and cough
  E. Facial swelling/puffiness under the eyes
  F. Itching of nose and eyes
  G. Headache
  H. Decreased smell and taste
  I. Clear rhinorrhea
  J. Pale, edematous mucous membranes
  K. Enlarged, blue-boggy turbinates
  L. Mouth breathing
  M. "Allergic shiners"—dark circles under the eyes
  N. "Allergic salute"—rubbing of the nose upward, causing a horizontal crease
  O. Allergic conjunctivitis

IV. **Laboratory/diagnostic findings**
  A. Consider referring to an allergist for antigen testing

V. **Management**
  A. Avoidance of allergens
  B. 1st generation antihistamines
   1. Diphenhydramine (Benadryl), 25–50 mg PO every 4–6 hr; maximum 300 mg/day
   2. Brompheniramine (Dimetapp), 4 mg PO every 4–6 hr
   3. Chlorpheniramine (Chlor-Trimeton), 4 mg PO every 4–6 hr; maximum 24 mg/day
   4. All equally effective
   5. Limited ability to reverse acute allergic symptoms
   6. Caution with alcohol and other CNS depressants; some patients experience paradoxical excitation
  C. Non-sedating antihistamines, or 2nd/3rd generation antihistamines (all PRN or for exacerbations)
   1. Azelastine (Astelin) nasal spray, 1–2 sprays per nostril BID
   2. Cetirizine (Zyrtec), 10 mg PO daily
   3. Desloratadine (Clarinex), 5 mg PO daily
   4. Fexofenadine (Allegra), 60 mg PO BID, or 180 mg PO daily
   5. Levocetirizine (Xyzal), 2.5–5 mg PO daily
   6. Loratadine (Claritin) 10 mg PO daily
   7. Olopatadine (Patanase), 2 sprays per nostril BID
   8. Most effective when taken prophylactically to prevent allergic symptoms

      9. Limited ability to reverse acute allergic symptoms

      10. Considered less effective than 1st generation agents

  D. Topical corticosteroid nasal sprays

      1. Fluticasone (Flonase), 2 sprays daily for exacerbations

      2. Budesonide (Nasacort, Rhinocort), 1 spray per nostril once daily; maximum 4 sprays per nostril once a day

      3. Beclomethasone (Beconase AQ), 1−2 sprays in each nostril, 2 times daily

      4. Drugs of choice for allergic rhinitis, minimal adverse effects

      5. All equally effective

      6. May take 3−4 weeks to achieve peak response

      7. Most effective when taken in advance of expected allergen exposure

  E. Miscellaneous agents

      1. Cromolyn (NasalCrom nasal spray), 1 spray per nostril 3−6 times a day

      2. Ipratropium (Atrovent nasal spray), 2 sprays per nostril (42 mcg) 2−3 times a day

      3. Montelukast (Singulair), 10 mg PO daily

      4. Limited effectiveness and less efficacy than other agents

      5. May take 4 weeks to achieve peak response

  F. May use a corticosteroid (dexamethasone long-acting [Decadron-LA]) 8 mg IM, or Medrol Dosepak, for acute episodes

  G. Oral decongestants may be used in conjunction with antihistamines

  H. Provide environmental counseling

EPISTAXIS

I. **Definition**

  A. Spontaneous bleeding from the nose

  B. May be minor or may indicate a serious disease process

  C. Commonly seen from Kiesselbach's plexus in the anteroinferior septum

II. **Etiology/incidence/predisposing factors**

  A. In all, 90% of cases occur at Kiesselbach's plexus

  B. More common in winter months

  C. Forceful expiration

      1. Sneezing

      2. Coughing

  D. Trauma

      1. Blow to the nose

      2. Fracture

      3. Picking the nose

      4. Foreign bodies

  E. Drying or thinning as the result of oxygen use and nasal sprays

  F. Infectious/allergic sinusitis, rhinitis, and systemic infection

G. Nasopharyngeal fibroma, angioma, and malignant tumors

H. Hypertension

I. Coagulopathies (including iatrogenic)

J. Change in atmospheric pressure

III. Subjective/physical examination findings

A. History of bleeding from the nose

B. May be none

C. Acute bleeding from nasal fossa or posterior nasopharynx

D. Site of bleeding

1. Anterior bleed—Kiesselbach's plexus

2. Posterior bleed—inspect for active bleeding from the posterior oropharynx

3. Multiple oozing points may be evident

E. Ulcerations or erosions of tissue/septal wall

F. Blood pressure may be normal or elevated

IV. Laboratory/diagnostic findings

A. Sinus series to rule out sinusitis, tumor, and angiofibroma

B. May consider CBC, prothrombin time/partial thromboplastin time, or bleeding time studies to rule out coagulopathy

C. Other laboratory studies as indicated for suspected underlying diseases (e.g., allergy testing)

V. Management

A. Position the patient with head erect and elevated

B. Provide reassurance

C. Clear blood from nostrils

1. Remove clots with gentle suctioning, and visualize point of bleed

2. Observe closely for foreign object

D. Saturate a cotton ball with oxymetazoline (Afrin), and gently insert it into the site of bleeding

E. Apply gentle pressure by compressing the nasal alae together just below the bridge for 10–15 min

F. Examine nostril for bleeding site

G. Apply topical lidocaine anesthetic (4% solution, 1–5 mg; maximum 4.5 mg/kg); then touch the site with a silver nitrate stick until the vessel ends are completely cauterized (painful!)

H. If unable to cauterize, insert nasal packing

I. If the bleeding is uncontrollable or occurs from a posterior site, immediate referral to an ear, nose, and throat specialist is indicated. Posterior bleeding can be difficult to control and may require cauterization with silver nitrate stick, electrocautery or balloon inflation compression.

SINUSITIS

I. Definition

A. Infection/inflammation of the paranasal sinus mucous membrane

B. May be acute (lasting less than 4 weeks) or chronic (occurring 3 or more times a year)

II. Etiology/incidence/predisposing factors

A. Viruses cause one fifth of cases

B. In all, 1%–3% of upper respiratory infections involve sinusitis

C. Common organisms:

  1. *Haemophilus influenzae*

  2. *Streptococcus pneumoniae*

  3. *Moraxella catarrhalis*

  4. Various anaerobes

D. Recurrent disease may be due to irritants, allergens, bacteria, or fungi

E. Anatomic blockage of sinus openings

F. Nasal polyps, masses, or neoplasms

G. Prolonged nasal intubation or prolonged use of nasogastric tubes

III. Subjective/physical examination findings

A. Recent upper respiratory infection

B. Pain/pressure over face, nose, cheeks, and teeth

C. Often confused with toothache

D. Purulent/blood-tinged nasal drainage

E. Headache, increased pain in supine or bending position, and sense of fullness in the head

F. Nasal congestion

G. Generalized malaise

H. Orbital pain or visual disturbances indicate a more serious problem. Immediately refer to ENT for swelling of forehead or orbital areas, severe pain, or visual disturbance.

I. Fever may not be present in the elderly patient

J. Localized tenderness over the sinuses

K. Facial edema

L. Swollen, reddened turbinates

M. May have nasal septal deviation

N. Foul smelling nasal or postnasal drainage

IV. Laboratory/diagnostic findings

A. Sinus series reveals clouding or thickening of sinus cavity; air-fluid levels may be seen.

B. For chronic sinusitis or for hospitalized patients, CT of the sinuses is indicated.

C. In chronic manifestation, culture the drainage to determine the causative organism.

V. Management

A. Antibiotics (guide by cultures especially for chronic sinusitis)

  1. Amoxicillin/clavulanate (Augmentin), 500 mg PO 3 times a day or 875 mg PO twice a day for 7–10 days

    a. Improved quality of life was the only positive outcome in a recent study

        b. Augmentin may be superior for those greater than 65 years when used in doses of 2 grams BID for *S. pneumoniae* causing the sinusitis

   2. Macrolides are no longer recommended due to the high rate of resistance of *S. pneumoniae* to these agents.

   3. Doxycycline, 100 mg PO twice a day, and a respiratory fluoroquinolone (levofloxacin or moxifloxacin) are reasonable alternatives for patients allergic to penicillin

        a. Levofloxacin, 500–750 mg PO daily, or

        b. Moxifloxacin, 400 mg PO daily

   4. The addition of corticosteroids to the antibiotics has not been convincingly shown to improve therapeutic outcomes

B. Analgesics (judicious use of NSAIDs and narcotics among the elderly)

   1. Acetaminophen (Tylenol), 650 mg PO every 4 hr 3–4 times daily (maximum 4 grams daily) with caution given to not use any other acetaminophen-containing products

PHARYNGITIS

I.   **Definition**

   A. Inflammation of the pharynx

   B. Usually associated with tonsillitis

   C. Can be acute or chronic

II.   **Etiology/incidence/predisposing factors**

   A. Viral (the most common cause in all adults)

      1. Influenza A and influenza B

      2. Adenovirus

      3. Enterovirus

   B. Bacterial (less common in adults)

      1. Group A β-hemolytic streptococcus (GABHS)

      2. *Haemophilus influenzae*

      3. *Neisseria gonorrhoeae*

      4. *Mycoplasma*

   C. Fungal: *Candida albicans* is commonly seen in immunosuppressed patients

   D. Pharyngitis may be associated with the following:

      1. Esophageal reflux

      2. Allergic rhinitis

      3. Sinusitis

      4. Carcinoma

III.   **Subjective/physical examination findings**

   A. Sore or painful throat

   B. Dysphagia

   C. Fever/chills

   D. Malaise/myalgia

   E. Viral

1. Edema of lymphoid tissue in the posterior oropharyngeal wall—elevated oval islands
2. Pale, boggy mucosae of the posterior pharynx, palatial petechiae
3. Painful ulcers/blistering in oral cavity/pharynx
4. Posterior cervical lymphadenopathy

F. Streptococcal (GABHS)
   1. Bright red, edematous pharyngeal mucosa
   2. White or yellow exudate
   3. Fever greater than 101°F
   4. Anterior cervical lymphadenopathy

G. Candidal
   1. Shiny, white, and raised patches located on the following:
      a. Posterior pharynx
      b. Tongue
      c. Buccal mucosa
   2. Patches may have erythematous rims (red base).

IV. **Laboratory/diagnostic findings**
   A. Rapid strep antigen screen
   B. Throat culture to identify the offending pathogen, if rapid strep is negative WBC and cell differential counts
   C. Mono spot for suspicion of mononucleosis
   D. If indicated, culture for chlamydia infection and/or gonorrhea

V. **Symptomatic therapy is important, even if the patient expects an antibiotic.**
   A. Pain relief
      1. Lozenges, for soothing relief; available over-the-counter. Use PRN
      2. Throat sprays, for soothing relief; available over-the-counter
      3. Warm salt water gargle
      4. Systemic analgesics: acetaminophen and NSAIDs (brief use only)
      5. Glucocorticoids are not recommended

VI. **Treatment: antimicrobial therapy based on the finding of GABHS only**
   A. Benzathine penicillin (Bicillin L-A), 1.2 million units IM single dose, or penicillin V (Pen-Vee K), 500 mg PO 2 times a day for 10 days
   B. Cephalexin, 500 mg PO BID for 10 days
   C. Cefadroxil, 1000 mg PO daily, for 10 days
   D. Clindamycin, 300 mg PO three times a day for 10 days
   E. Azithromycin, 500 mg PO daily for 5 days
   F. Clarithromycin, 250 mg PO BID for 10 days
   G. Consider antiulcer agents for gastric reflux
      1. Omeprazole (Prilosec), 20 mg PO daily
      2. Lansoprazole (Prevacid), 15–30 mg PO daily
      3. Rabeprazole (Aciphex), 20 mg PO daily
      4. Pantoprazole (Protonix), 40 mg PO daily
      5. Esomeprazole (Nexium), 20 mg PO daily

6. Dexlansoprazole (Dexilant), 30 mg PO daily

H. Analgesics, such as acetaminophen (Tylenol), 650 mg PO every 4 hr, PRN, with caution given to not use any other acetaminophen-containing products

I. For Candida

   1. Nystatin (Mycostatin), 100,000 U/ml, take 4–6 ml swish and swallow 4 times a day (only for mild oropharyngeal disease, as esophageal involvement requires systemic treatment) or

   2. Fluconazole (Diflucan), 200 mg PO initially, and then 100 mg daily for at least 2 weeks

EPIGLOTTITIS/SUPRAGLOTTITIS

I. **Definition**

   A. Inflammation of the mucous membrane of the epiglottis that results in acute airway obstruction

   B. Potentially life-threatening condition

   C. Swelling of the laryngeal entrance obstructs air flow to and from the lungs

II. **Etiology/incidence/predisposing factors**

   A. Commonly caused by *H. influenzae* infection, but other organisms are possible, including penicillin-resistant *S. pneumoniae*, β-hemolytic streptococci, and *S. aureus*, facts that govern empiric antibiotic therapy

   B. Seen more often in males

   C. Recent upper airway infection

III. **Subjective/physical examination findings**

   A. Change in voice

   B. Dysphagia

   C. Dyspnea

   D. Anxious—the patient may appear exhausted or lethargic

   E. Fever

   F. Sore throat

   G. Muffled or hoarse voice; if severe, stridor

   H. Drooling

   I. Do not examine the pharynx until:

      1. Lateral soft tissue x-rays have been obtained and

      2. Emergency airway equipment is available (to prevent or treat laryngospasm)

IV. **Laboratory/diagnostic findings**

   A. Lateral soft tissue neck x-ray (taken with caution) reveals a swollen epiglottis that is posteriorly displaced

   B. CT scan of the neck may be needed

   C. Arterial blood gas analysis

   D. Chest x-ray

   E. CBC, blood cultures

   F. Direct laryngoscopy by a specialist

V. Treatment

A. Management is guided by the apparent severity of respiratory distress. Consult an otolaryngologist and an anesthesiologist early

B. Immediately prepare for monitoring, IV infusion, transport to ER

C. Monitor vital signs, oxygen saturation

D. Protect the airway. Airway access may be best obtained in the operating room with administration of anesthesia.

E. Prepare for possible surgical opening of the airway

F. Initial empiric therapy after cultures and smears have been submitted.

   1. Third-generation cephalosporin (ceftriaxone or cefotaxime) and an anti-staphylococcal, anti-MRSA agent (clindamycin or vancomycin)

      a. Vancomycin dose is adjusted to achieve vancomycin level of 10–15 mg/L

      b. Clindamycin, 600 mg IV every 8 hr

      c. Ceftriaxone (Rocephin), 1–2 grams intravenously every 24 hr, OR

      d. Cefotaxime (Claforan), 1–2 grams IV every 8 hr, AND

      e. Piperacillin/tazobactam 3.375 grams IV every 6 hr; or cefotaxime/ceftriaxone plus clindamycin or vancomycin

   2. Clinical improvement usually occurs within 48–72 hr of the institution of antibiotic therapy

TEMPOROMANDIBULAR JOINT DISORDER

I. Definition

A. Group of symptoms involving pain in the temporomandibular joint (TMJ), decreased range of motion, and jaw clicking, especially with chewing

II. Etiology/incidence/predisposing factors

A. Rheumatoid arthritis

B. TMJ synovitis

C. Trauma

D. Ill-fitting dentures

E. Intra-articular disk disease

F. Approximately half of the population is affected, although most are untreated

G. Oromandibular dysfunction

H. Recent dental work

III. Subjective/physical examination findings

A. TMJ pain

B. TMJ clicking or popping with movement

C. Headache

D. Jaw locking/spasm of masseter muscles

E. Earache

F. TMJ tenderness

G. TMJ click with range of motion

H. Cervical or cranial tenderness

I. Dental malocclusion

J. Dental erosion from bruxism (teeth grinding)

IV.   Laboratory/diagnostic findings

A. In advanced cases, consider x-rays of the TMJ, which may reveal bone abnormalities.

B. CT, MRI, and arthrography all may show soft tissue and bony changes at an earlier stage than x-rays

C. A positive test for rheumatoid arthritis factor (RF) may rule out a diagnosis of TMJ disorder.

V.   Management

A. NSAIDs (caution regarding chronic use due to potential for reduced renal function; take with meals)

1. Ibuprofen, 200–600 mg 4 times a day for 5 days

2. Naproxen, 500 mg PO initially, followed by 250 mg PO 3–4 times a day

B. Local heat PRN

C. Soft diet

D. Consider referral for surgery in severe conditions

E. Consider referral for trigger point injections or arthroscopy

TRIGEMINAL NEURALGIA (TIC DOULOUREUX)

I.   Definition

A. Neuralgia (pain and pressure) along the fifth cranial nerve

B. The trigeminal nerve, which arises from the pons, is a mixed nerve with many branches

C. Symptoms depend on the branch affected

II.   Etiology/incidence/predisposing factors

A. Idiopathic

B. Surgery and autopsy suggest a compressive origin

C. Affects 16 out of 100,000 persons annually

D. Both genders are affected, but most sources note a female preference

E. Increased incidence after age 50 years

F. Pain occurs in paroxysms and may last for hours

G. The right side is most often affected

H. May be triggered by ordinary events such as brushing the teeth, chewing, and exposure to wind or cold

I. Can occur in multiple sclerosis

III.   Subjective/physical examination findings

A. Intense bouts of pain along the affected tract

B. Symptoms tend to be unilateral

C. Intractable lip, cheek, gum, or facial pain

D. Pain described as "lightning flashes"

E. Facial flushing

F. Salivation

G. Headache

H. The neurologic examination is normal, except a sensory defect may be found with cranial nerve V on the affected side.

IV. **Laboratory/diagnostic findings**

A. CT to rule out neoplasm

B. MRI for cranial nerve V abnormalities

C. ESR to rule out temporal arteritis

V. **Management**

A. Carbamazepine (Tegretol), 100–1200 mg/day (monitor liver enzymes and serum drug levels; caution for potential drug-drug interactions in the elderly), use lowest effective dose

B. If the patient is unable to tolerate carbamazepine, then phenytoin, 300–600 mg/day,

   1. Monitor drug levels; many drug-drug interactions

C. Lamotrigine (Lamictal), 100–400 mg per day

D. Adjunctive therapy with baclofen, 5–20 mg 3–4 times a day (maximum, 80 mg daily)

E. Consider neurosurgical consultation for possible exploration for patients who fail to respond to pharmacological management.

   1. Recently, posterior fossa exploration has revealed anomalous vascular structures, resulting in nerve compression. Relief of symptoms has occurred with decompression and release. However, surgery is not appropriate in multiple sclerosis.

BIBLIOGRAPHY

American Geriatrics Society 2012 Beers Criteria Update Expert Panel. (2012). American Geriatrics Society updated criteria for potentially inappropriate medication use in older adults. *Journal of the American Geriatrics Society*. doi:10.1111/j.1532–5415.2012.03923.x

Arcangelo, V. P., & Peterson, A. M. (Eds.). (2013). *Pharmacotherapeutics for advanced practice: A practical approach* (3rd ed.). Philadelphia, PA: Lippincott Williams & Wilkins.

Carter, J. E. (2013). Anticoagulant, antiplatelet, and fibrinolytic (thrombolytic) therapy in patients at high risk for ocular hemorrhage. In D. S. Basow (Ed.), *UpToDate*. Waltham, MA: UpToDate.

Cash, J. C., & Glass, C. A. (Eds.). (2011). *Family practice guidelines* (2nd ed.). New York, NY: Springer Publishing Company.

Centers for Medicare and Medicaid Services. (2013). *2014 ICD-10 PCS and GEMs*. Retrieved November 25, 2013, from http:///www.cms.gov/Medicare/Coding/ICD10/2014-ICD-10-PCS.html

Chow, A. W., & Doron, S. (2013). Evaluation of acute pharyngitis in adults. In D. S. Basow (Ed.), *UpToDate*. Waltham, MA: UpToDate.

Domino, F., Raldor, R. A., Grimes, J. A., & Golding, J. (2013). *The 5-minute clinical consult 2014*. Philadelphia, PA: Lippincott Williams and Wilkins.

Epocrates Online. (2014). Retrieved January 31, 2014, from https://online.epocrates.com

Food and Drug Administration. (2013, March 12). *FDA drug safety communication: Azithromycin (Zithromax or Zmax) and the risk of potentially fatal heart rhythms*. Retrieved November 25, 2013, from http://www.fda.gov/downloads/Drugs/DrugSafety/UCM343347.pdf

Garlington, W., & High, K. (2013). Evaluation of infectioun in the older adult. In D. S. Basow (Ed.), *UpToDate*. Waltham, MA: UpToDate.

Gilbert, D. N., Moellering, R. C., & Eliopoulos, G. M. (Eds.). (2013). *The Sanford guide to antimicrobial therapy 2013*. Sperryville, VA: Antimicrobial Therapy.

Givre, S., & Van Stavern, G. P. (2013). Amaurosis fugax (transient monocular or binocular visual loss). In D. S. Basow (Ed.), *UpToDate*. Waltham, MA: UpToDate.

Goguen, L. A. (2013). External otitis: Pathogenesis, clinical features, and diagnosis. In D. S. Basow (Ed.), *UpToDate*. Waltham, MA: UpToDate.

Goldman, L, & Shafer, A. I. (Eds.) (2012). *Goldman's Cecil medicine* (24th ed.). Philadelphia, PA: Saunders.

Hansten, P. D., & Horn, J. R. (2013). *The top 100 drug interactions: A guide to patient management (2013 edition)*. Freeland, WA: H&H Publications.

Hwang, P. H., & Getz, A. (2013). Acute sinusitis and rhinosinusitis in adults: Treatment. In D. S. Basow (Ed.), *UpToDate*. Waltham, MA: UpToDate.

Jacobs, D. S. (2013). Open-angle glaucoma: Epidemiology, clinical presentation, and diagnosis. In D. S. Basow (Ed.), *UpToDate*. Waltham, MA: UpToDate.

Katzung, B. G., Masters, S. B., & Trevor, A. J. (Eds.). (2012). *Basic & clinical pharmacology* (12th ed.). New York, NY: McGraw-Hill.

Limb, C. J., Lustig, L. R., & Klein, J. O. (2013). Acute otitis media in adults (suppurative and serous). In D. S. Basow (Ed.), *UpToDate*. Waltham, MA: UpToDate.

Longo, D. L., Kasper, D. L., Jameson, J. L., Fauci, A. S., Hauser, S. L., & Loscalzo, J. (Eds.) (2011). *Harrison's principles of internal medicine* (18th ed.). New York, NY: McGraw Hill.

Mandell, G. L., Bennett, J. E., & Dolin, R. (2010). *Principles and practice of infectious diseases* (7th ed.). Philadelphia, PA: Churchill Livingston.

Stead, W. (2013). Symptomatic treatment of acute pharyngitis in adults. In D. S. Basow (Ed.), *UpToDate*. Waltham, MA: UpToDate.

Woods, C. R. (2013). Epiglottitis (supraglottitis): Clinical features and diagnosis. In D. S. Basow (Ed.), *UpToDate*. Waltham, MA: UpToDate.

Woods, C. R. (2013). Epiglottitis (supraglottitis): Treatment and prevention. In D. S. Basow (Ed.), *UpToDate*. Waltham, MA: UpToDate.

CHAPTER 72

Headache

DONNA L. GULLETTE • THOMAS W. BARKLEY, JR. • CHARLENE M. MYERS

I. **Definition**

   A. Subjective sensation of pain involving any part of the head, including the scalp, face (including the orbitotemporal area), sinuses or teeth, and cranium or cerebrum; with or without associated symptoms (aura)

   B. Headache pain is one of the most common reasons patients seek medical intervention.

   C. Headaches are either a primary or secondary disorder.

II. **Etiology/predisposing factors**

   A. Most common headaches are benign

      1. Overall, 90% are primary and may be attributed to either tension type, cluster, or migraine headache; primary headaches are reoccurring.

      2. Approximately 10% are related to organic disorders

   B. Headache is caused by vasodilation/constriction of blood vessels being a secondary effect of "cortical depression and neuropeptide release." Neuronal depolarization → neuropeptides release → nerve ganglion → neurogenic inflammation → vasodilation → pain/headache

   C. About one third of patients with brain tumors present with a chief complaint of headache

   D. Headache occurs at any age but primarily during the peak productive years of 25–55 years of age for both men and women

   E. Migraine headaches have a 3:1 female-to-male ratio

   F. Cluster headaches occur predominantly in middle-aged men.

   G. Three categories of primary headaches include: cluster, migraine, and tension type.

H. Secondary headaches include the following:
  1. Acute new-onset headaches or uniquely severe headaches may be caused by:
    a. Acute angle-closure glaucoma
    b. Encephalitis
    c. Giant cell arteritis
    d. Idiopathic intracranial hypertension
    e. Intracerebral hemorrhage
    f. Meningitis
    g. Sinusitis
    h. CNS mass lesion
      i. Hemorrhage
      ii. Hematoma
      iii. Tumor
    i. Metabolic causes
    j. Benign causes, such as:
      i. Hangover
      ii. Caffeine withdrawal
      iii. Eyestrain
      iv. Analgesic overuse
      v. Hormones (e.g., estrogen)
      vi. Nitrates
      vii. Proton pump inhibitors
    k. Subarachnoid hemorrhage
  2. Intermittent discrete headaches may be caused by
    a. Cervical spondylosis
    b. Pseudotumor cerebri
    c. Tic douloureux
    d. CNS mass lesions (as in the preceding section)
  3. Chronic persistent headaches may result from the same causes as intermittent discrete headaches.
I. Red flags in headache (Table 72.1)
J. Overview of subarachnoid hemorrhage (Table 72.2)

III. **Subjective/physical examination findings**
A. Obtain the individual's headache attack profile.
  1. Prodromal symptoms (preceding the headache)
  2. Time of peak and severity of symptoms
  3. Duration of symptoms
  4. Precipitating factors
  5. Associated symptoms
  6. Alleviating symptoms
  7. Review of history that predisposes to QT interval prolongation:
    a. History of unexplained syncopal episodes
    b. Structural heart disease on a variety of cardioactive medications

Table 72.1	Red Flag Findings with Cause for Headache
Red Flags	**Possible cause**
Neurologic signs or symptoms Changes in mental status Weakness, diplopia, papilledema, focal neurologic deficits	Encephalitis, subdural hematoma, subarachnoid hemorrhage, intracerebral hemorrhage, tumor, mass, increased intracranial pressure
Thunderclap headache (peaks within seconds)	Subarachnoid hemorrhage
Progressively worsening headache	Secondary headache
Cancer or immunosuppression	Brain infection, metastases, HIV infection, AIDS
Meningismus	Meningitis, subarachnoid hemorrhage, subdural empyema
Red eye and halos around lights	Acute angle-closure glaucoma
Systemic symptoms (e.g., fever, weight loss)	Sepsis, thyrotoxicosis, cancer
Onset of headache after age 50	Increased risk of serious cause (e.g., tumor, giant cell arteritis)
Combination of fever, weight loss, visual changes, jaw claudication, temporal artery tenderness, and proximal myalgias	Giant cell arteritis
Pulsatile tinnitus	Idiopathic intracranial hypertension

Table 72.2	Overview of subarachnoid hemorrhage	
Etiology	Cerebral aneurysm rupture	
	Cerebral arteriovenous malformation	
Signs and symptoms	"Worst headache of my life" with sudden onset, no precipitating factors, no relief with OTC analgesia	
	Altered consciousness	
	Mental status changes, confusion, and irritability	
	Nuchal rigidity, low back pain	
	Nausea and vomiting	
	Photophobia	
	Seizures	
	Cranial nerve abnormalities	
	Motor or sensory deficits	

Table 72.2	Overview of subarachnoid hemorrhage
Diagnosis	Obtain a noncontrast head CT scan with or without a lumbar puncture. Negative CT and lumbar puncture rules out subarachnoid hemorrhage (SAH). Cerebral angiography should be considered if findings are in doubt. Lumbar puncture is mandatory if there is evidence of SAH despite a normal head CT.
	Routine serum blood work includes CBC, BUN, creatinine, glucose, electrolytes, prothrombin time, international normalized ratio, activated partial thromboplastin time, basic metabolic panel, hemoglobin A1C
Treatment	To prevent further hemorrhage and secondary complications such as acute hydrocephalus, cerebral vasospasm, delayed cerebral ischemia, increased intracranial pressure, seizures, and cardiac dysrhythmias.
	Prevention of vasospasm: Intravascular volume expansion with crystalloid or colloid solution Induced hypertension with norepinephrine, dopamine, or phenylephrine Balloon angioplasty Administer via IV if possible; if unsuccessful, intra-arterial administration of vasodilators such as nicardipine, milrinone, nimodipine, verapamil, and nitroprusside
	Pharmacological Management: Stool softeners—avoid Valsalva maneuver Morphine sulfate to reduce fluctuations and prevent rebleeding PUD prophylaxis Nimodipine (Nimotop), 60 mg PO every 4 hr for 21 days Phenobarbital, 30–60 mg PO or SQ every 6 hr PRN for sedation Heparin, 5000 units SQ every 8–12 hr Phenytoin (Dilantin), 100 mg PO TID

      c. Renal or liver disease-related altered drug clearance

B. Obtain the history of prior headaches
    1. Variables (as in the headache attack profile)
    2. Family history of headaches or sudden death in family members
    3. Correlation or relationship of headaches to particular events/activities

C. See Table 72.4 for comparison of types of headache characteristics

D. No gold standard exists for diagnosis of the more common headache categories; diagnosis is based on clinical assessment.

E. Criteria for diagnosis of common migraine without aura represents 80% of attacks
    1. Duration of 4–72 hr
    2. Must have at least two of the following:
       a. Unilateral location—can be generalized or lateralized
       b. Pulsating or throbbing quality
       c. Moderate to severe intensity
       d. Aggravated by routine physical activity

    e. Interferes with activities of daily living
3. At least one of the following:
    a. Nausea or vomiting
    b. Photophobia, osmophobia, and/or phonophobia
4. At least five attacks that fulfill the preceding criteria listed in 1, 2, and 3
5. No evidence of organic disease

F. Criteria for diagnosis of classic migraine with aura
1. Pain is preceded by at least one of the following neurologic symptoms, which gradually develops over 5–60 min:
    a. Visual: combination of field defects and luminous visual hallucinations
        i. Scintillating scotoma
        ii. Fortification spectra
        iii. Unformed light flashes—photopsia
        iv. Hemianopsia
        v. Geometric visual patterns
        vi. Occasional hallucinations
    b. Somatosensory disturbance of face or arms
        i. Paresthesia
        ii. Numbness
        iii. Clumsiness
        iv. Weakness in a circumscribed area
        v. Speech disturbance
2. No evidence of organic disease

G. Criteria for diagnosis of tension-type headache
1. At least two of the following:
    a. Viselike or tightening and pressure (non-pulsating) quality
    b. Bilateral mild to moderate pain that is generalized
    c. Pericranial tenderness at back of head or neck
    d. Not aggravated by routine physical activity
    e. Not associated with focal neurologic symptoms
2. Both of the following:
    a. No nausea or vomiting
    b. Photophobia and phonophobia absent or only one present
3. No evidence of organic disease

H. Criteria for diagnosis of cluster headache:
1. Severe unilateral, periorbital, supraorbital, or temporal pain lasting 15–180 min
2. At least one of the following on the headache side:
    a. Reddened conjunctiva
    b. Facial sweating
    c. Lacrimation
    d. Miosis
    e. Ipsilateral nasal congestion

    f. Rhinorrhea

    g. Horner syndrome (ptosis of eyelid, miosis or constriction of pupil, and anhidrosis or reduced sweat secretion)

   3. Bouts last 4–8 weeks and may occur several times during the year

IV.   Management of primary headaches (Table 72.3)

Table 72.3 Characteristics of Primary Headaches		
	Migraine	**Cluster headache**	**Tension headache**
Pain location	Unilateral (60%)	Unilateral	Bilateral
	Bilateral (40%)	Behind the right or left eye	"Headband" configuration
Pain quality	Throbbing	Throbbing Sometimes piercing	Non-throbbing
Pain severity	Moderate to severe	Severe	Mild to moderate
Duration	4 hr to 3 days	15 min to 2 hr[a]	30 min to 7 days[b]
Impact of activity	Worsens pain	None	None
Associated symptoms	Nausea, vomiting, photophobia, phonophobia	Conjunctival redness, lacrimation, nasal congestion, rhinorrhea, ptosis, miosis—all on the same side as the headache	Uncommon
Usual time of onset	Early morning	Nighttime	Daytime
Preceded by aura	Yes, in 30%	No	No
Triggers	Many; see Table 72.8	Usually unidentified	Tension, anxiety
Gender prevalence	More common in females (3:1)	More common in males (5:1)	Slightly (10%) more common in females
Family history	Likely	Unlikely	Unlikely
Impact on daily life	Often substantial	Usually substantial	Minimal

Note. [a]Headaches occur in clusters that typically consist of one or more headaches, lasting 15 minutes to 2 hr each day for 2–3 months, with a headache-free interval between each cluster. [b]Chronic tension headaches occur at least 15 days out of the month for 6 months or longer

V. **Evidence-based guidelines for prevention of migraine (Table 72.4)**

VI. **Evidence-based guidelines for pharmacologic management of migraines (Table 72.5)**

VII. **Additional agents**

  A. Triptans should be used only in patients who are not at risk for coronary disease; for information on clinical pharmacology of the triptans, see Table 72.6

   1. Eletriptan (Relpax) for acute migraines

   2. The various triptans are similarly effective; if one does not work, another may

  B. A stratified approach to pharmacologic management is recommended

   1. Start low and build up slowly with a course or a full trial that lasts 1–2 months

   2. Such an approach allows the patient to choose among several treatment options, depending on the severity of the attack

  C. Consider the following:

   1. Administer tricyclic antidepressants if depression is associated with headache

    a. The patient may see improvement without evidence of depression

    b. Use standard dosing

   2. Avoid calcium channel blockers in patients of childbearing age (these drugs may induce infertility)

   3. Baseline ECG if antiemetics such as prochlorperazine, 5 mg; promethazine, 25 mg; or droperidol, 0.625 mg every 4 hr or 1.25 mg, are used because of the potential for prolongation of the QT interval

VIII. **Factors that can precipitate migraine headache (Table 72.7)**

IX. **Triggers of migraine headachaches (Table 72.8)**

Table 72.4	Management of primary headache	
Primary Headache	**Pharmacologic management**	**Nonpharmacologic management**
Tension type	Acetaminophen Aspirin Nonsteroidal anti-inflammatory drugs (ibuprofen, ketoprofen, and naproxen); NSAIDs are more effective than acetaminophen for tension type headaches; Ketorolac IM is effective for in-office or inpatient	Heat, ice, massage of neck and temples, rest and relaxation techniques, exercise, and regular sleep Follow-up in 2 weeks to monitor progress Consultation with a physician if conservative treatment fails or clinical depression is suspected
Migraine	*Acute attack*-a simple analgesic, such as aspirin, acetaminophen, ibuprofen, or naproxen, taken immediately, may abort the headache Butorphanol tartrate nasal spray (Stadol NS), 1 mg (1 spray) in one nostril, repeat 2nd dose in 60 min Cafergot combination (ergotamine maleate 1 mg + caffeine 100 mg), 1–2 tablets at onset, may repeat 1 tablet every 30 min up to 6 tablets (if attack includes nausea/vomiting, Cafergot suppositories [one half to one containing 2 mg of ergotamine tartrate], inhalers [0.36 mg per puff], and ergotamine SL [2 mg tablets are available with a maximum of 6 mg/24 hr and 10 mg/week]) Dihydroergotamine mesylate (DHE 45), 0.5–1 mg IV, or 1–2 mg SC/IM; repeat every hour PRN to maximum of 3 mg. Maximum of 3 mg/24 hr and 6 mg/week. Nasal spray, 0.5 mg (one spray) in each nostril, repeat after 15 min. (4 sprays, 2 mg total). Serious/life-threatening peripheral ischemia on black box warning.	• Diet counseling (see Table 72.8) • Lifestyle modification (weight loss, smoking cessation, and nutritional diet) has been shown to decrease episodes in frequent migraine sufferers. • During attacks, patient should stay in a dark, quiet environment and rest. • Warm baths may help patient to relax. • Follow-up at regular intervals to assess effectiveness of treatment (initially, every 2 weeks for 2 months; then, every month for 6 months and PRN if treatment successful) • Consultation with physician if patient does not respond to traditional management, or if condition worsens

Table 72.4 Management of primary headache

Primary Headache	Pharmacologic management	Nonpharmacologic management
Migraine	Triptans include: sumatriptan, zolmitriptan, naratriptan, rizatriptan, almotriptan, eletriptan, and frovatriptan. Eletriptan, naratriptan, and rizatriptan are oral preparations. • All are effective for treatment of acute migraines. • Sumatriptan (Imitrex), 6 mg • SQ to rapidly abort the headache; may repeat once in 2 hr; maximum 12 mg/24 hr. 25–100 mg PO; may repeat once in 2 hr; maximum 200 mg/24 hr. 5–20 mg IN; may repeat once in 2 hr; maximum 40 mg/24 hr. 6.5 mg (1 patch) TD over 4 hr to upper arm/thigh; may apply 2nd patch 2 hr after activation of 1st; maximum 13 mg (2 patches)/24 hr • Zolmitriptan (Zomig), 1.25–5 mg PO; may repeat after 2 hr, maximum 10 mg/24 hr. 2.5–5 mg IN, may repeat dose in 2 hr; maximum 10 mg/24 hr. • Naratriptan (Amerge), 1 or 2.5 mg PO, may repeat once after 2 hr; maximum 5 mg/24 hr • Rizatriptan (Maxalt), 5 or 10 mg PO, may repeat once after 2 hr; maximum 30 mg/24 hr • Almotriptan (Axert), 6.25–12.5 mg PO, may repeat once after 2 hr; maximum 25 mg/24 hr • Eletriptan (Relpax), 20 or 40 mg PO, may repeat once after 2 hr; maximum 80 mg/24 hr • Frovatriptan (Frova), 2.5 mg PO, may repeat once after 2 hr; maximum 7.5 mg/24 hr	

Table 72.4	Management of primary headache	
Primary Headache	**Pharmacologic management**	**Nonpharmacologic management**
Migraine	**Prophylaxis** (should be considered if patient has attacks more often than 2 or 3 times per month, treatments may not be FDA labeled for migraine prophylaxis)-indicated if headaches are frequent, long-lasting, or account for significant degree of disability **β-blockers:** Propranolol (Inderal), 20 mg TID (max 320 mg/24 hr) Metoprolol (Lopressor), 50 mg daily (max 200 mg/24 hr) **Antiepileptics:** Valproic acid (Depacon), 250 mg BID (max 2000 mg/24 hr) Topiramate (Topamax), 25 mg daily (max 100 mg/24 hr) **Antidepressants:** Amitriptyline (Elavil), 10–150 mg/24 hr Venlafaxine (Effexor), 75 mg/24 hr (max 150 mg/24 hr) Onabotulinumtoxin A (Botox), 155 units as 5 units (0.1ml) IM into each of 31 sites divided across 7 head/neck muscle areas. 20 units in 4 frontalis muscle sites, 10 units in 2 corrugator muscle sites, 5 units in 1 procerus muscle site, 30 units in 6 occipitalis muscle sites, 40 units in 8 temporalis muscle sites, 30 units in 6 trapezius muscle sites, and 20 units in 4 cervical paraspinal muscle sites. Retreatment every 12 weeks.	

Table 72.4	Management of primary headache	
Primary Headache	**Pharmacologic management**	**Nonpharmacologic management**
Cluster	*Acute attack:* Sumatriptan (Imitrex), 6 mg SQ to rapidly abort the headache; may repeat once in 2 hr; maximum 12 mg/24 hr. 25–100 mg PO; may repeat once in 2 hr. 5–20 mg IN; may repeat once in 2 hr; maximum 200 mg/24 hr. 6.5 mg (1 patch) TD over 4 hr to upper arm/thigh; may apply 2nd patch 2 hr after activation of 1st; maximum 13 mg (2 patches)/24 hr (see above) Zolmitriptan, 2.5–5 mg IN, may repeat dose Dihydroergotamine mesylate (DHE 45), 1 mg IV/IM/SQ/IN, repeat in 1 hr intervals until 3 mg (2 mg IV)/24 hr. Max 6 mg/week. Not routine regimen, evidence is limited. Ergotamine tartrate aerosol (0.36 mg/puff)—up to 6 puffs/attack. 100% oxygen inhalation (7 L/min for 15 min)	Lifestyle modification and supportive care are of limited benefit for these patients, because there are few known precipitating factors for a bout of attacks. During a bout, some patients report that alcohol, stress, glare, or ingestion of certain foods will precipitate an attack, but this is highly individual. Patients are certainly advised to avoid anything that they feel worsens their condition. Follow-up should be provided at regular intervals during treatment: pacing of visits will vary depending on the patient's pattern of remissions and bouts.

Table 72.4 Management of primary headache

Primary Headache	Pharmacologic management	Nonpharmacologic management
Cluster	Prophylaxis: Verapamil, 240–480 mg/day Lithium carbonate, 150–600 mg/day Topiramate, 50–200 mg/day Valproic acid, 500–2000 mg/day Avoidance of medication overuse: Medication overuse headache (MOH) = analgesic rebound headache All acute symptomatic medications used to treat headaches have the potential for causing MOH. Degree of risk differs depending upon the specific class of medication-high-risk medications include opioids, butalbital-containing analgesics, triptans and low-risk includes NSAIDs.	

Table 72.5 Classification of migraine preventive therapies (available in the United States)

Level A: Medications with established efficacy (greater than 2 Class I studies)	Level B: Medications are probably effective (1 Class I or 2 Class II studies)	Level C: Medications are possibly effective (1 Class II study)	Level U: Inadequate or conflicting data to support or refute medication use	Other: Medications that are established as possibly or probably ineffective
				Established as not effective
Antiepileptic drugs (AEDs)	Antidepressants/SSRI/SSNRI/TCA	ACE inhibitors	Carbonic anhydrase inhibitor	AEDs
Divalproex sodium	Amitriptyline	Lisinopril	Acetazolamide	Lamotrigine
Sodium valproate	Venlafaxine	Angiotensin receptor blockers	Antithrombotics	
				Probably not effective
Topiramate	β-blockers	Candesartan	Acenocoumarol	
β blockers	Atenolol	α-agonists	Coumadin	Clomipramine[a]
Metoprolol	Nadolol	Guanfacine	Picotamide	Clonidine
Propranolol	Triptans (MRM[b])	AEDs	Antidepressants/SSRI/SSNRI	Acebutolol[a]
Timolol[a]	Naratriptan[b] Zolmitriptan[b]	Carbamazepine	Fluvoxamine[a]	Clonazepam[a]
Triptans (MRM[b])		β Blockers	Fluoxetine	Nabumetone[a]
Frovatriptan[b]		Nebivolol	AEDs	Oxcarbazepine
		Pindolol[a]	Gabapentin	Telmisartan
		Antihistamines	TCAs	
		Cyproheptadine	Protriptyline[a]	
		Nicardipine	β-blockers	

Table 72.5	Classification of migraine preventive therapies (available in the United States)			
Level A: Medications with established efficacy (greater than 2 Class I studies)	Level B: Medications are probably effective (1 Class I or 2 Class II studies)	Level C: Medications are possibly effective (1 Class II study)	Level U: Inadequate or conflicting data to support or refute medication use	Other: Medications that are established as possibly or probably ineffective
Antiepileptic drugs (AEDs)	Antidepressants/SSRI/SSNR/TCA	ACE inhibitors	Carbonic anhydrase inhibitor	Established as not effective
			Bisoprolol[a]	
			Ca++ blocker	
			Nifedipine[a]	
			Nimodipine	
			Verapamil	
			Direct vascular smooth muscle relaxants	
			Cyclandelate	

Note: ACE = angiotensin-converting enzyme; MRM = menstrually related migraine; SSNR = selective serotonin-norepinephrine reuptake inhibitor; SSRI = selective serotonin reuptake inhibitor; TCA = tricyclic antidepressant; Ca ++ blocker = calcium channel blocker. Adapted with permission from "Evidence-based guideline update: Pharmacologic treatment for episodic migraine prevention in adults; Report of the Quality Standards Subcommittee of the American Academy of Neurology and the American Headache Society," by S.D. Silberstein, S. Holland, and F. Freitag, 2012, Neurology, 78, pp. 1337–1345.[c]

[a] Classification based on original guideline and new evidence not found for this report. [b] Short-term prophylaxis of MRM. [c] Information listed in this table provides guidelines from 2000.

Table 72.6	Evidence-based guidelines for episodic migraine therapies			
Group 1: Proven pronounced statistical and clinical benefit	Group 2: Moderate statistical and clinical benefit	Group 3: Statistically but not proven clinically *or* clinically but not proven statistically effective	Group 4: Proven to be statistically or clinically ineffective	Group 5: Clinical and statistical benefits unknown
Acetaminophen plus aspirin plus caffeine PO	Acetaminophen plus codeine PO	Butalbital, aspirin, caffeine PO	Acetaminophen PO	Dexamethasone IV
Aspirin PO	Butalbital plus aspirin, caffeine, codeine PO	Ergotamine PO	Chlorpromazine IM	Hydrocortisone IV
Butorphanol IN	Butorphanol IM	Ergotamine plus caffeine PO	Granisetron IV	
Dihydroergotamine (DHE) SC, IM, IV	Chlorpromazine IM, IV	Metoclopramide IM, PO	Lidocaine IV	
DHE IV plus antiemetic	Diclofenac K, PO			
DHE IN	Ergotamine plus caffeine, pentobarbital			
Ibuprofen PO	Belafolline PO			
Naproxen sodium PO	Flurbiprofen PO			
Naratriptan PO	Isometheptene compound PO			
Prochlorperazine IV	Ketorolac IM			

Table 72.6	Evidence-based guidelines for episodic migraine therapies			
Group 1: Proven pronounced statistical and clinical benefit	**Group 2: Moderate statistical and clinical benefit**	**Group 3: Statistically but not proven clinically *or* clinically but not proven statistically effective**	**Group 4: Proven to be statistically or clinically ineffective**	**Group 5: Clinical and statistical benefits unknown**
Rizatriptan PO	Lidocaine IN			
Sumatriptan SC, IN, PO	Meperidine IM, IV			
Zolmitriptan PO	Methadone IM			
	Metoclopramide IV			
	Naproxen PO			
	Prochlorperazine IM, PR			

Note: Adapted with permission from "Practice parameter: Evidence-based guidelines for migraine headache (an evidence-based review)" by S.D. Silberstein, 2000, *Neurology, 55,* pp. 754–762.

Table 72.7	Clinical pharmacology of the triptans					
Drug	Route	Onset, min	Duration	Half-life, hr	Dosage	Comments
Sumatriptan	Oral	30–60	Short	2.5	25, 50, or 100 mg May repeat in 2 hr Maximum 200 mg/24 hr	First triptan (Imitrex) available; most widely used and best understood
	Nasal	15–20			5 or 20 mg May repeat in 2 hr Maximum 40 mg/24 hr	Only triptan available in IN and SC formulations, which act faster than oral triptans
	SC	10–15			6 mg May repeat in 1 hr Maximum 12 mg/24 hr	
Almotriptan (Axert)	Oral	30–120	Short	3.1	6.25 or 12.5 mg May repeat in 2 hr Maximum 25 mg/24 hr	Incidence of chest discomfort (pain, tightness, pressure) is lower than with other triptans Safe for use with MAO inhibitors
Frovatriptan (Frova)	Oral	120–180	Long	26	2.5 mg May repeat in 2 hr	Longest half-life and slowest onset, but also lowest rate of headache recurrence Decrease dose if combined with propranolol Safe for use with MAO inhibitors

Table 72.7	Clinical pharmacology of the triptans					
Drug	**Route**	**Onset, min**	**Duration**	**Half-life, hr**	**Dosage**	**Comments**
Naratriptan (Amerge)	Oral	60–180	Long	6	1 or 2.5 mg May repeat in 4 hr Maximum 5 mg/24 hr	Available in melt-in-the-mouth tablets that can be taken without water Safe for use with MAO inhibitors
Rizatriptan (Maxalt)	Oral	30–120	Short	2–3	5 or 10 mg May repeat in 2 hr Maximum 30 mg/24 hr	May be the most consistently effective triptan Decrease dose if combined with propranolol.
Zolmitriptan (Zomig)	Oral	45	Short	3	2.5 or 5 mg May repeat in 2 hr Maximum 10 mg/24 hr	Available in melt-in-the-mouth tablets that can be taken without water.

Note. MAO = monoamine oxidase. Adapted with permission from Pharmacology for Nursing Care (5th ed.) by R.A. Lehne, 2004, St. Louis: Elsevier Saunders.

Table 72.8	Triggers for Migraine Headaches
Emotions	Anticipation
	Anxiety
	Depression
	Excitement
	Frustration
	Stress
Food Ingredients	Aspartame (e.g., diet sodas and artificial sweeteners)
	Monosodium glutamate (e.g., Chinese food and canned soups)
	Nitrates (e.g., cured meats)
	Phenylethylamine (e.g., chocolate)
	Tyramine (e.g., aged cheeses and Chianti wine)
	Yellow food coloring
Drugs	Alcohol
	Analgesics (excessive use or withdrawal)
	Caffeine (excessive use or withdrawal)
	Cimetidine
	Cocaine
	Estrogen (e.g., oral contraceptives)
	Nitroglycerin
Other Factors	Carbon monoxide
	Hormonal changes in women
	Flickering lights, glare
	Loud noises
	Hypoglycemia
	Change in altitude or barometric pressure
	Altered sleep pattern (excessive sleep or sleep deprivation)

Note. Adapted with permission from Pharmacology for Nursing Care, (5th ed.), by R.A. Lehne, 2004, St. Louis: Elsevier Saunders.

BIBLIOGRAPHY

Aminoff, M. J., & Kerchner, G. A. (2013). Nervous system disorders. In M. A. Papadakis, S. J. McPhee, & M. W. Rabow (Eds.), *Current medical diagnosis and treatment* (52nd ed., pp. 962–1036). New York, NY: McGraw Hill.

Ashkenazi, A., & Schwedt, T. (2011). Cluster headache—acute and prophylactic therapy. *Headache, 51*(2), 272–286.

Bajwa, Z., & Sabahat, A. (2013). Acute treatment of migraine in adults. In *UpToDate*. Retrieved from http://www.uptodate.com/contents/acute-treatment-of-migraine-in-adults?source=search_lt&search=Acute+treatment+of+migraine+in+adults&selectedTitle=1%7E150

Bucelli, R. C., & Ances, B. (2014). Neurologic disorders. In H. Godara, A. Hirbe, M. Nassif, H. Otepka, & A. Rosenstock (Eds.), *The Washington manual of medical therapeutics* (34th ed., pp. 946–986). Philadelphia, PA: Wolters Kluwer, Lippincott, Williams, & Wilkins.

Cutrer, M. (2013). Evaluation of the adult with headache in the emergency department. In *UpToDate*. Retrieved from http://www.uptodate.com/contents/evaluation-of-the-adult-with-headache-in-the-emergency-department?source=search_t&search=Evaluation+of+the+adult+with+headache+in+the+emergency+department&selectedTitle=1%7E150

Hainer, B. L., & Matheson, E. M. (2013, May 15). Approach to acute headaches in adults. *American Family Physician, 87*(10), 665–738.

Lehne, R. A. (2010). *Study guide, pharmacology for nursing care* (7th ed.). St. Louis, MO: Saunders/Elsevier.

May, A. (2013). Cluster headache: Treatment and prognosis. In *UpToDate*. Retrieved from http://www.uptodate.com/contents/cluster-headache-treatment-and-prognosis?source=search_t&search=cluster+headache%3A+treatment+and+prognosis&selectedTitle=1%7E54

Olesen, J., & Ramadan, N. (2010). *Headache care, research, and education worldwide*. Oxford, UK: Oxford University Press.

Schwedt, T., & Dodick, D. (2012). Thunderclap headache. In *UpToDate*. Retrieved from http://www.uptodate.com/contents/thunderclap-headache?source=search_result&search=Thundercap+headache&selectedTitle=1%7E150

Silberstein, S. D., Holland, S., & Freitag, F. (2012). Evidence-based guideline update: Pharmacologic treatment for episodic migraine prevention in adults: Report of the Quality Standards Subcommittee of the American Academy of Neurology and the American Headache Society. *Neurology, 78*, 1337–1345. doi:10.1212/WNL.0b013e3182535d20

Silberstein, S. D., Holland, S., & Freitag, F. (2012). Evidence-based guideline update: NSAIDs and other complementary treatments for episodic migraine prevention in adults: Report of the Quality Standards Subcommittee of the American Academy of Neurology and the American Headache Society. *Neurology, 78*, 1346–1353. doi:10.1212/WNL.0b013e3182535d0c

Singer, R., Ogilvy, C., & Rordorf, G. (2013). Treatment of aneurysmal subarachnoid hemorrhage. In *UpToDate*. Retrieved from http://www.uptodate.com/contents/treatment-of-aneurysmal-subarachnoid-hemorrhage?source=search_t&search=treatment+of+aneurysmal+subarachnoid+hemmorrhage&selectedTitle=1%7E150

Singer, R., Ogilvy, C., & Rordorf, G. (2013). Clinical manifestations and diagnosis of aneurysmal subarachnoid hemorrhage. In *UpToDate*. Retrieved from http://www.uptodate.com/contents/clinical-manifestations-and-diagnosis-of-aneurysmal-subarachnoid-hemorrhage?source=search_t&search=clinical+manifestations+and+diagnosis+of+aneur-ysmal+subarachnoid+hemmorrhage&selectedTitle=1%7E150

Singh, A., & Soares, W. E. III. (2012). Management stragtegies for acute headache in the emergency department. *Emergency Medicine Practice, 14*(6), 1–24. Retrieved from https://www.ebmedicine.net/topics.php?paction=showTopic&topic_id=315

Taylor, F. (2013). Tension-type headache in adults: Acute treatment. In *UpToDate*. Retrieved from http://www.uptodate.com/contents/tension-type-headache-in-adults-acute-treatment?source=search_t&search=Tension+type+headache+in+adutls%3A+acute+treatment&selectedTitle=1%7E150

SECTION TWELVE

Common Problems
in Acute Care

CHAPTER 73

Fever

LORRIS J. BOUZIGARD • THOMAS W. BARKLEY, JR. • CHARLENE M. MYERS

I.   **Definition**
   A. Elevation of body temperature above the normal daily physiologic variation
   B. Body temperature higher than 100°F (37.8°C) orally or greater than 100.8°F (38.2°C) rectally
   C. Cardinal manifestation of infectious and noninfectious disease origins

II. **Fever of undetermined/unknown origin (FUO)**
   A. Body temperature 101°F (38.3°C) or above rectally for 3 weeks or longer without an apparent cause, despite extensive investigation for at least 1 week in patients without neutropenia or immunosuppression

III. **Pathophysiology**
   A. Fever begins with the production of one or more of a group of cytokines from monocyte-macrophages in response to exogenous pyrogenic substances.
   B. Immunologic mediators also play a role in the pathophysiology of fever
      1. Interleukin 1 (primary)
      2. Tumor necrosis factor
      3. Interleukin 6
      4. Interferon gamma
   C. Cytokines interact with receptors in the hypothalamus, causing the production and release of prostaglandins (mainly prostaglandin 2); this raises body temperature by initiating the production of cyclic adenosine monophosphate; this production of cyclic adenosine monophosphate resets the thermoregulatory set point of the hypothalamus.

IV. **Causes**
  A. Infection
  1. Bacterial
      a. Bacteremia, sepsis
      b. Pneumonia (community-acquired pneumonia, hospital-acquired pneumonia, healthcare-associated pneumonia, and aspiration), bronchitis, sinusitis, empyema, and tuberculosis
      c. Urinary tract infections (rarely cause FUO), prostatitis, and pyelonephritis
      d. Cellulitis, phlebitis, and decubitus ulcers
      e. Colitis, cholecystitis, cholangitis, diverticulitis, and bacterial hepatitis
      f. Abscesses (various locations, most often located intra-abdominally); considered as a cause of FUO
      g. Endocarditis (rarely causes FUO)
      h. Osteomyelitis
      i. Bacterial infections of prosthetic devices
          i. Heart valve
          ii. Pacemaker
          iii. Joint replacement
          iv. Venous access catheter
      j. Meningitis, encephalitis
      k. Other bacterial infections
  2. Viral
      a. Viral hepatitis
      b. HIV from opportunistic infections, associated malignancies, or HIV itself
      c. Epstein-Barr virus (can cause prolonged febrile illness)
      d. Herpes/varicella virus (simplex, zoster)
      e. Cytomegalovirus (can cause prolonged febrile illness)
      f. Common cold, influenza, parainfluenza, adenovirus, and Rous sarcoma virus
  3. Rickettsia
      a. Rocky Mountain spotted fever
      b. Q fever
  4. Fungal (antibiotics, immunosuppression, and intravascular devices expose patients to opportunistic fungi)
      a. Candidiasis
      b. Histoplasmosis
      c. Cryptococcosis
      d. Aspergillosis
  5. Parasitic
      a. Malaria
      b. Toxoplasmosis

      6. Chlamydia

B. Autoimmune/collagen vascular disease/vasculitis

      1. Temporal and giant cell arteritis

      2. Rheumatoid arthritis

      3. Systemic lupus erythematosus

      4. Polyarteritis nodosa

      5. Wegener granulomatosis

      6. Sarcoidosis

C. Central nervous system (CNS) disease

      1. Head trauma

      2. Mass (space-occupying lesion)

      3. Subarachnoid hemorrhage

      4. Seizures

D. Malignancy

      1. Lymphoma/leukemia

      2. Renal cell carcinoma

      3. Hepatocellular carcinoma

      4. Colon carcinoma

      5. Metastatic malignancies, especially to bone or liver

E. Cardiovascular disease

      1. Myocardial infarction and pulmonary embolism

      2. Thrombophlebitis, deep vein thrombosis, acute vasculitis

      3. Dissection of aortic aneurysm

      4. Mesenteric ischemia

      5. Myxoma

F. GI disease

      1. Inflammatory bowel disease

          a. Ulcerative colitis

          b. Crohn's disease (most common GI cause of FUO)

      2. Alcoholic and granulomatous hepatitis

      3. Pancreatitis

      4. Hepatic cirrhosis with active hepatocellular necrosis

      5. Whipple disease

G. Drug/medication induced

      1. Amphetamines, cocaine, lysergic acid diethylamide

      2. Monoamine oxidase inhibitors and tricyclic antidepressants

      3. Quinidine and procainamide (Pronestyl)

      4. Methyldopa (Aldomet)

      5. Isoniazid

      6. Antimicrobials

H. Familial Mediterranean fever

I. Tissue injury

J. Hematoma

K. Factitious fever

1. Occurs in patients about to undergo extensive or invasive procedures
2. Most common among young people in health professions
3. Consider the presence of psychiatric problems

L. Heatstroke

M. Malignant hyperthermia from inhalation anesthetics and succinylcholine (Anectine)

N. Malignant neuroleptic syndrome
   1. Phenothiazines
   2. Haloperidol (Haldol)
   3. Fluoxetine (Prozac)
   4. Clozapine (Clozaril) and olanzapine (Zyprexa)
   5. Metoclopramide (Reglan)

O. Exercise

P. Microcrystalline arthritis
   1. Gout
   2. Pseudogout

Q. Surgery

R. Blood products (reaction)

S. Endocrinopathies
   1. Thyrotoxicosis/hyperthyroidism
   2. Pheochromocytoma
   3. Adrenal insufficiency

T. Reaction to IM injection

U. Hemorrhage into the following:
   1. CNS
   2. Retroperitoneum
   3. Joint
   4. Lung
   5. Adrenals

V. Hypertriglyceridemia

V. **Diagnostic approach to adults with fever**

A. History
   1. Collect information on general/nonspecific complaints such as the following:
      a. Localizing symptoms
      b. Fever and chills
      c. Sweats/night sweats
      d. Weight loss
      e. Arthralgias and myalgias
   2. Chronology of symptoms in relation to the use of medications (prescription, over-the-counter, and herbal) and surgical/dental procedures
   3. Comorbidities
      a. Diabetes

        b. HIV

        c. Immunosuppression

        d. Neutropenia

        e. Malignancy

        f. Renal failure

        g. Sickle cell anemia

4. Travel history and geographic areas in which the patient has lived

5. Household pets

6. Hobbies

7. Use of tobacco, marijuana, intravenous drugs, alcohol, or other illicit drugs

8. Trauma, animal bites, and insect bites (especially tick)

9. Previous blood transfusion

10. Immunizations

11. Drug allergies or hypersensitivities

12. Ethnic origin

13. History of psychiatric disorders

14. Exact nature of any prosthetic materials or implanted devices

15. Careful occupational history with special attention to exposures to the following:

        a. Animals

        b. Toxic fumes

        c. Potential infectious agents

        d. Possible antigens

16. Other febrile or infected individuals in the home, workplace, or school

17. Sexual orientation and practices to include use or lack of precautions

18. Dietary practices

19. Any recent dental care and last dental visit

20. Family history, especially of the following:

        a. Tuberculosis

        b. Infectious disease

        c. Arthritis

        d. Collagen vascular disease

B. Physical examination

  1. Vital signs

  2. Perform frequent physical examinations to identify any new findings that may direct diagnostic workup

  3. Special attention paid to the following:

        a. Skin and mucous membranes

        b. Lymph nodes

        c. Head, ears, eyes, nose, and throat

        d. Nail beds

        e. Cardiovascular system

      f. Chest

      g. Abdomen

      h. Nervous system

      i. Prostate, penis, and scrotum in male

      j. Pelvic examination in female

   4. Invasive line insertion sites

   5. Be aware of any changes from a previous examination

   6. Clinical manifestations of fever:

      a. May be asymptomatic

      b. Sensation of warmth or flushing

      c. Malaise and fatigue

      d. Hypothalamic activity, through somatic efferent nerves, causes increased muscle tone that generates heat and raises body temperature even further.

      e. Shaking chills or rigors

      f. Mild inability to concentrate; confusion, delirium, or even stupor (especially in the elderly or debilitated)

      g. Increased cardiac output

      h. Tachycardia

      i. Angina or heart failure in patients with underlying heart disease due to high-output stress

C. Basic laboratory studies and diagnostic procedures

   1. Complete blood count may show the following:

      a. Anemia

      b. Leukocytosis with a shift to the left (bacterial)

      c. Leukopenia (viral)

      d. Bandemia

   2. Urinalysis to rule out urinary tract infection and tumors of the urinary tract

   3. Blood chemistries

      a. Serum glucose helpful with unsuspected or undiagnosed diabetes mellitus

      b. Liver function tests help to determine obscure sources of fever

   4. Erythrocyte sedimentation rate (lacks sensitivity and specificity, but elevation warrants additional testing)

   5. Cultures and analysis

      a. Blood: two sets (aerobic and anaerobic). Consider peripheral draws as well as from central lines or arterial lines looking for line contamination

      b. Urine

      c. Sputum

      d. Stool: especially looking for *Clostridium difficile*

      e. Invasive line catheter tips

      f. Cerebrospinal fluid

      g. Peritoneal fluid

h. Liver biopsy

i. Bone marrow aspiration

j. Lymph node biopsy

6. Immunologic serologies

   a. HIV

   b. Anti-DNAase B titers (rheumatic fever and other streptococcal infections)

   c. Heterophile test to rule out infectious mononucleosis

   d. Widal titers to rule out salmonella

   e. Antinuclear antibody and rheumatoid factors

   f. Other immunologic studies as indicated by other causes of fever

7. Imaging

   a. Chest radiography or abdominal ultrasonography

   b. CT scans

      i. Used if ultrasonography reveals nothing in a patient with signs and symptoms suggestive of an intra-abdominal process

      ii. Intravenous pyelogram may be more sensitive in some instances

      iii. Because there is no reason to perform both MRI and CT on these patients, an MRI is not recommended.

   c. Endoscopy (upper and lower)

      i. To assess for the following:

         (a) Crohn's disease

         (b) Biliary tract disease

         (c) GI tumor

      ii. Barium enema or upper GI series also may be needed

   d. Radionuclide studies

      i. Ventilation-perfusion scans or thin-sliced spiral CT is needed to diagnose a pulmonary embolus

      ii. Some cases may require pulmonary angiography

   e. Echocardiography helps in the diagnosis of cardiac tumor or endocarditis

   f. Invasive procedures and biopsy are the final methods of diagnosing an FUO

      i. Biopsy specimens may be taken from enlarged, accessible lymph nodes or from the bone marrow

      ii. An exploratory laparotomy may be indicated when noninvasive testing suggests an intra-abdominal process

   g. PDG-PET/CT: sometimes can be used for the workup on FUO; however, it serves limited usefulness in the acute care setting for most patients

VI. Treatment

A. Initial approach to treatment of fever in an acute care setting should include a thorough evaluation to establish the cause of fever

    1. Fever in the ICU/CCU, acute care, long-term care patient can be due to infection from a variety of sources, including the following:

        a. Intravenous sites

        b. Nasogastric tubes

        c. Urinary catheters

        d. Surgical incisions

        e. Endotracheal tubes (pulmonary)

        f. Deep vein thrombosis/pulmonary embolism

    2. A thorough evaluation of the possible underlying causes of fever is paramount in making accurate treatment decisions

B. Pharmacological therapy

    1. Antibiotics (see Table 73.1)

        a. If practitioner initiates antibiotic coverage before establishing an infectious cause, it is necessary to begin with empiric broad-spectrum antibiotic therapy, taking into consideration local antibiotic resistance patterns (see Infections chapter).

        b. Once the source of fever/infection is identified via diagnostic tests/laboratory assessments, initial antibiotic therapy should be adjusted according to the clinical situation for more definitive therapy.

    2. Antifungals—empiric (see Infections chapter)

        a. Febrile neutropenia: caspofungin, 70 mg IV on day 1, then 50 mg IV daily, micafungin, 100 mg IV every 24 hr, or voriconazole, 6 mg/kg IV every 12 hr for one day, followed by 3 mg/kg IV every 12 hr

        b. Febrile non-neutropenic critical care patients

            i. Fluconazole, 800 mg IV for one dose, then 400 mg IV every 24 hr (preferred first-line agent unless azole resistance is suspected)

            ii. Echinocandin (micafungin 100 mg every 24 hr), (preferred agent if suspect azole-resistant strains)

            iii. Amphotericin B, 0.5–1 mg/kg IV every 24 hr or amphotericin B Lipid Complex 3–5 mg/kg IV every 24 hr (amphotericin is the agent of choice for *Cryptococcosis*)

            iv. Itraconazole, 200 mg PO/NG daily BID

Table 73.1	Empiric Treatment Recommendations for Common Adult Infections		
Infection Site	**Suspected Pathogen**	**Initial Empiric Therapy**	**Comments**
CNS			
Community Acquired	*S. pneumoniae* *N. meningitidis* *H. influenzae*	Cefotaxime + vancomycin	Suspect Listeria: add ampicillin Maintain vancomycin trough level at 15–20 mg/L Consult with a pharmacist for appropriate pharmacokinetic dosing to achieve therapeutic levels and avoid toxicity
Neurosurgery or Head Trauma	*S. aureus* Enterobacteriaceae Resistant GNB *S. pneumoniae*	Cefepime + vancomycin	Maintain vancomycin trough level at 15–20 mg/L Consult with a pharmacist for appropriate pharmacokinetic dosing to achieve therapeutic levels and avoid toxicity
LUNG			
Community Acquired	*S. pneumoniae* *H. influenzae* *M. catarrhalis* Atypical	Cefotaxime + macrolide or doxycycline	Suspect aspiration: add metronidazole
Hospital Acquired	Enterobacteriaceae Resistant GNB *S. aureus* / MRSA Anaerobes	Cefepime OR piperacillin/ tazobactam + tobramycin + vancomycin	Maintain vancomycin trough level at 15–20 mg/L Consult with a pharmacist for appropriate pharmacokinetic dosing to achieve therapeutic levels and avoid toxicity
GU			
Community Acquired	Enterobacteriaceae Enterococci	Cefotaxime +/- ampicillin	

Table 73.1	Empiric Treatment Recommendations for Common Adult Infections		
Infection Site	**Suspected Pathogen**	**Initial Empiric Therapy**	**Comments**
ABDOMEN			
Community Acquired	Enterobacteriaceae *B. fragilis* Enterococci *Streptococcus* spp.	Cefotaxime + metronidazole	
Hospital Acquired or Post-operative intra-abdominal or pelvic surgery	Enterobacteriaceae Resistant GNB Enterococci *B. fragilis*	Piperacillin/tazobactam + tobramycin	Suspect *C. diff*: add oral metronidazole Consult with a pharmacist for appropriate pharmacokinetic dosing to achieve therapeutic levels and avoid toxicity
Hospital Acquired	Resistant GNB Enterococci	Cefepime OR piperacillin/ tazobactam + tobramycin	Consult with a pharmacist for appropriate pharmacokinetic dosing to achieve therapeutic levels and avoid toxicity
FEVER WITH NEUTROPENIA			
	Enterobacteriaceae Resistant GNB Staphylococci Enterococci	Cefepime OR Piperacillin/tazobactam + tobramycin	Suspect gram positive source: add vancomycin Consult with a pharmacist for appropriate pharmacokinetic dosing to achieve therapeutic levels and avoid toxicity

Table 73.1 Empiric Treatment Recommendations for Common Adult Infections

Infection Site	Suspected Pathogen	Initial Empiric Therapy	Comments
SKIN			
Community Acquired	Streptococci (Group A) S. aureus (consider community onset MRSA)	Cellulitis: cefazolin or oxacillin Furunculosis or abscess, suspect community onset MRSA: vancomycin + incision and drainage when possible Necrotizing fasciitis: Penicillin G + clindamycin Suspected mixed infection: cefotaxime + clindamycin	Consult with a pharmacist for appropriate pharmacokinetic dosing to achieve therapeutic levels and avoid toxicity
Hospital Acquired or Diabetic	Streptococci Staphylococci Enterobacteriaceae Resistant GNB B. fragilis	Superficial or no ulcer: see skin above Uncomplicated diabetic foot: Cefotetan + vancomycin Health-care associated or limb-threatening: Piperacillin/tazobactam ± tobramycin + vancomycin	Consult with a pharmacist for appropriate pharmacokinetic dosing to achieve therapeutic levels and avoid toxicity

Note. GNB = Gram-negative bacteria; MRSA = methycillin-resistant *Staphylococcus aureus.*

3. Antipyretic therapy
   a. Pharmacological
      i. Acetaminophen, 650 mg PO/NG/PR every 4 hr PRN for fever, not to exceed 3000 mg/24 hr
         (a) Note that critically ill patients have decreased GI function that may affect acetaminophen metabolism
         (b) Fever also hinders GI function
         (c) Peak concentration is attained faster and overall plasma concentration is higher when acetaminophen is administered via nasogastric tube as compared with rectal administration
         (d) Note that maximum change in temperature occurs earlier with acetaminophen than with ibuprofen
   C. Nonpharmacological
      1. Cooling blankets are often used to treat the critically ill with fever
         a. Limited research supports this practice
         b. Cooler temperatures may not be most effective for promoting heat loss because they decrease blood flow to the skin
         c. Patients are more comfortable when blankets are set at a higher temperature, which decreases the effectiveness of the cooling blanket
      2. For extreme cases of hyperthermia, patients may be immersed in an ice water bath until body temperature decreases to the normal range

VII. **Geriatric considerations**
   A. The elderly have increased susceptibility to infections as well as an increased risk of mortality and morbidity due to the presence of comorbid health conditions and low physiologic reserves associated with the natural biologic changes of the aging process (limited hypothalamic ability to permit endogenous pyrogens to exert its effect on the CNS).
   B. The elderly often have a blunted or absent fever response necessitating prevention, prompt recognition, and timely administration of empirical antimicrobials paramount.
   C. Signs and symptoms in the geriatric populations are more nonspecific and subtle
   D. A robust fever to infection usually points to a serious bacterial or viral infection
   E. The most common causes of fever in the geriatric population include the following:
      1. Connective-tissue diseases such as rheumatoid arthritis, polymyalgia rheumatica, temporal arteritis, Wegener granulomatosis, polyarteritis nodosa, and sarcoidosis
      2. Malignancies such as colon cancer, lymphoma, and leukemia

3. Infections such as intra-abdominal infections and tuberculosis (see Infections chapter)
4. Medication effect

F. Blood cultures tend to have lower diagnostic yield

BIBLIOGRAPHY

Beers, M. H., Porter, R. S., Jones, T. V., & Kaplan, J. L. (2011). *The Merck manual of diagnosis and therapy* (19th ed.). Whitehouse Station, NJ: Merck.

Cornely, O. A., Bassetti, M., Calandra, T., Garbino, J., Kullberg, B. J., Lortholary, O., . . . Ullmann, A. J. (2012). ESCMID guideline for the diagnosis and management of Candida diseases 2012: Non-neutropenic adult patients. *Clinical Microbiology and Infection, 18*(Suppl. 7), 19–37.

Davaro, R. E., & Glew, R. H. (2011). Approach to fever in the intensive care patient. In R. S. Irwin and J. M. Rippe (Eds.), *Irwin and Rippe's intensive care medicine* (7th ed). Philadelphia, PA: Lippincott Williams & Wilkins.

Dinarello, C. A., & Porat, R. (2011). Fever and hyperthermia. In D. L. Longo, D. L. Kasper, J. L. Jameson, A. S. Fauci, S. L. Hauser, and J. L. Loscalzo (Eds.), *Harrison's principles of internal medicine* (18th ed.). New York, NY: McGraw-Hill.

Heppner, H. J. (2013). Infections in the elderly. *Critical Care Clinics, 29*(3), 757–774.

High, K. P., Bradley, S. F., Gravenstein, S., Mehr, D. R., Quagriarello, V. J., Richards, C., and Yoshikawa, T. T. (2009). Clinical practice guideline for the evaluation of fever and infection in older adult residents of long-term care facilities: 2008 update by the Infectious Disease Society of America. *Journal of the American Geriatrics Society, 57*, 375–394.

Kaya, A., Ergul, N., Kaya, S. Y., Kilic, F., Yilmaz, M. H., Besirli, K., and Osaras, R. (2013). The management and diagnosis of fever of unknown origin. *Expert Review of Anti-infective Therapy, 11*(8), 805–815.

Kouijer, I. J., Bleeker-Rovres, C. P., & Oyen, W. J. G. (2013). FDG-PET in fever of unknown origin. *Seminars in Nuclear Medicine, 43*, 333–339.

McPhee, S. J., Papadakis, M. A., & Rabow, M. W. (Eds.). (2013). *Current medical diagnosis and treatment* (52nd ed.). New York, NY: McGraw Hill/Appleton & Lange.

CHAPTER 74

Pain

MARCIE NOMURA • THOMAS W. BARKLEY, JR. • CHARLENE M. MYERS

I. Definition

  A. Pain is defined as "an unpleasant sensory and emotional experience associated with actual or potential tissue damage, or described in terms of such damage. While it is unquestionably a sensation in part or parts of the body, it is always unpleasant and therefore, an emotional experience" (International Association for the Study of Pain [IASP], 1986)

  1. Pain is always subjective

II. Classification—there are many ways to classify pain, most often simply grouped into three types:

  A. Acute pain

  1. Caused by injury to the body (i.e., surgical pain or trauma)

  2. Treatment is definitive due to clear source of injury

  3. Duration usually short (less than 6 months)

  4. Generally resolves on its own as healing occurs

  B. Noncancer or persistent (chronic) pain

  1. Persistent or intermittent pain that is generally prolonged (6 months or longer)

  2. Rarely resolves on its own

  3. Examples include arthritis pain, postherpetic neuralgia, diabetic neuropathy, or back pain

  C. Cancer pain

  1. Can be acute or chronic pain (longer than 3 months duration)

  2. Because it is related to the cancer itself or the cancer treatment, it usually has a definable etiology

  3. Pain can also be grouped by its likely pathology

D. Nociceptive pain results from the normal physiologic functions that lead to the perception of noxious stimuli through transduction, transmission, perception, and modulation

1. Transduction is when noxious stimuli activate the release of intracellular "excitatory" substances that activate nociceptors.
   a. Examples of these substances include serotonin, substance P, histamine, prostaglandin, and bradykinin
2. Transmission involves moving the pain message from the peripheral nerve endings through the dorsal root ganglia to the spinal cord and into the ascending tract to the brain.
   a. Many opioid receptors (e.g., μ and κ) are located on the substantia gelatinosa in the dorsal horn of the spinal cord.
   b. Many complex neurophysiologic and neurochemical mechanisms occur within the dorsal horn, releasing a variety of transmitters such as glutamate, neurokinins, and substance P.
   c. Glutamate binds to the N-methyl d-aspartate (NMDA) receptor, which promotes the transmission of pain.
3. Perception is the conscious awareness of pain. The thalamus allows the body to perceive pain.
4. Modulation is the inhibition of pain impulses and involves the release of endogenous opioids serotonin and norepinephrine.

E. There are two types of nociceptive pain:

1. Somatic pain that arises from the bone, muscle, joint, skin, and connective tissue usually aching or throbbing in quality and is well localized
2. Visceral pain begins from the visceral organs, such as the gastrointestinal tract, pancreas, and liver.
   a. Tumor involvement in an organ capsule usually causes aching and fairly well-localized pain.
   b. Pain in a hollow organ cannot be localized and causes intermittent cramping pain.

F. Neuropathic pain results from abnormal processing by the peripheral and central nervous systems. A new definition states, "neuropathic pain is pain arising as a direct consequence of a lesion or disease affecting the somatosensory system."

1. Centrally generated pain involves the dysregulation or injury of the peripheral, central, or autonomic nervous system (e.g., phantom limb pain, burning pain below a spinal cord lesion, or pain associated with complex regional pain syndrome).
2. Peripherally generated pain is associated along the distribution of nerves or an injury to the peripheral nerves (e.g., diabetic neuropathy, postherpetic neuralgia, trigeminal neuralgia, or nerve entrapment).

III. Assessment
  A. Thorough pain assessment requires a comprehensive evaluation of the following:
    1. Description of pain explains the quality and can help the clinician diagnose the underlying mechanism of pain
      a. Somatic pain: patients may describe their pain as "sore," "sharp," or "stabbing"
      b. Neuropathic pain: "burning," "electric shock," or "pins and needles" is characteristic of neuropathic pain
        i. Ask "What does the pain feel like?" and "What words describe the pain?"
        ii. The treatment options for somatic pain and neuropathic pain are very different; therefore, it is important to assess a patient's description of pain accurately.
    2. Duration and onset of pain. Ask your patient whether the pain is continuous, intermittent, breakthrough, or end of dose. This can assist in the decision making regarding the frequency of dosing analgesics.
      a. Pain is considered continuous if it is present for half a day or more
      b. Ask "When did the pain start?" "How long does the pain last?" and "How often does the pain occur?"
    3. Location: have the patient point to the area(s) of discomfort
      a. Ask "Where is the pain?" and "Does it radiate to other parts of your body?"
    4. Alleviating/aggravating factors: determine whether there are specific activities, emotions, or other conditions that may aggravate the pain
      a. Ask "What makes the pain worse?" and "What makes the pain better?"
      b. Patients may know which treatments are most beneficial for them from past experience, whether it be pharmacological and/or nonpharmacological options
    5. Intensity: patient's self-report of pain is the gold standard for assessment; a pain scale is often used for grading intensity of pain. There are many pain measurement scales that are available; the clinician must choose the appropriate tool for the patient based on cognitive function, culture, language, and developmental age.
      a. The most commonly used self-report pain scale is the numerical rating scale (NRS), which rates pain from 0 (no pain) to 10 (worse possible pain).
      b. For children, the most common self-report pain scale is the Wong-Baker FACES scale. Studies have also shown the FACES tool is also effective for use with the cognitively impaired older adult patient population.

    c. The most recommended self-report scale for use in clinical practice with cognitively intact adolescents, adults, and older adults includes a combined NRS and FACES scale (Figure 74.1)

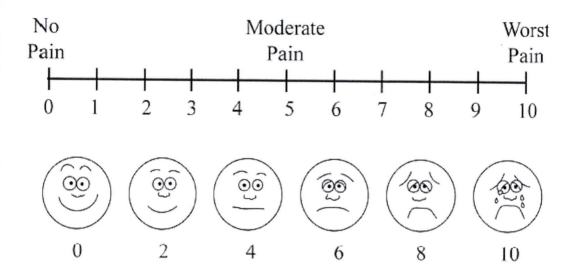

Figure 74.1. Combined numerical rating scale and FACES scale. Adapted from Hockenberry-Eaton, M. J., Wilson, D., & Winkelstein, M. L. (2005). *Wong's essentials of pediatric nursing*, (7th ed., p. 1259). St. Louis, MO: Mosby. Used with permission.

    d. For critically ill patients incapable of self-reporting pain, a recent study found a pain observational tool that includes four areas: facial expression, movement, muscle tension, and ventilator compliance were found to have the highest reliability and validity when used with nonverbal critically ill adults.

6. Associated signs and symptoms: unrelieved pain can lead to numerous negative physiological and psychological consequences due to the sympathetic nervous system activation, which may include the following:

    a. Glucose intolerance, insulin resistance, and hyperglycemia

    b. Tachycardia, hypertension, myocardial oxygen consumption, and hypercoagulability

    c. Decreased tidal volumes and alveolar ventilation leading to atelectasis and pneumonia

    d. Delayed gastric emptying and decreased intestinal activity

    e. Immobility, sleep disturbances, anxiety, anorexia, fatigue, and depression

        i. Patients with chronic pain may not exhibit these physical or clinical signs of pain

IV. **Management**

  A. Pharmacological therapy is the mainstay of treatment for acute pain and cancer pain in all age-groups. The World Health Organization proposed a stepwise ladder approach for the management of cancer pain in the 1980s, endorsed by the American Pain Society in 1992 and the Agency for Health Care Policy and Research in 1994.

  1. Patients do not necessarily progress through each level of pain intensity; a postoperative patient may begin with severe pain and beginning with Step 3 treatments is appropriate.

  B. Nonopioid analgesics (Step 1 for mild pain): useful in the management of acute and chronic pain due to surgery, trauma, arthritis, and cancer

  1. Acetaminophen: has analgesic properties and does not damage GI mucosa; watch for hepatotoxicity (maximum of 3000 mg/24 hr, depending on institution)

  2. Aspirin (acetylsalicylic acid): invented in 1897; it is one of the oldest nonopioid analgesics, risk for serious gastrointestinal effects, has been largely replaced by newer nonsteroidal anti-inflammatory drugs (NSAIDs)

  3. NSAIDs: useful for pain that involves inflammation since acetaminophen and opioids do not possess anti-inflammatory properties. All NSAIDs can produce adverse GI effects, can be minimized by taking with food. Also available in parenteral form ketorolac (Toradol) and topical form such as diclofenac (Voltaren, Flector, and Pennsaid)

  C. Opioid analgesics (Step 2 for mild to moderate pain and Step 3 for severe pain): should be added to nonopioids to manage acute pain and cancer-related pain that does not respond to nonopioids alone; carefully monitor nonopioid maximum dosage if combination opioids are used

  1. Mu agonist opioids

  a. Morphine: the standard of comparison for opioid analgesics, multiple routes of administration, start with lower doses in older adults; use with caution in patients with renal failure; M3G is primary metabolite of morphine and is renally excreted. Extended release form is also available (MS Contin, Kadian, Avinza)

  b. Hydromorphone (Dilaudid): alternative to morphine but slightly shorter duration, also multiple routes of administration, mostly used for moderate to severe pain

  c. Fentanyl: fast-acting opioid with a short half-life primarily used for severe acute pain, but can be prolonged when administered at a steady state parenterally. The use of fentanyl (Duragesic) transdermal patch is not recommended for acute pain. Preferred for managing breakthrough pain (BTP) for cancer-related pain, available in transmucosal lozenges (Actiq), buccal tablet/soluble film (Fentora, Onsolis), sublingual tablet/spray (Abstral, Subsys), and nasal spray (Lazanda)

  d. Hydrocodone: available in combination with acetaminophen or ibuprofen; use for mild to moderate pain (e.g., Norco, Vicodin, and Vicoprofen)

  e. Oxycodone: available both as a single entity (e.g., Oxycodone IR, Roxicodone) to treat severe pain and in combination with acetaminophen (e.g., Percocet, Percodan) to treat mild to moderate pain. Also available in extended release (OxyContin)

  f. Codeine: limited usefulness, usually available in combination with acetaminophen (e.g., Tylenol #3), but analgesia is shown to be inferior to NSAIDs

  g. Meperidine (Demerol): no longer recommended for use in pain management due to accumulation of its metabolite, normeperidine, a CNS excitotoxin than can produce tremors, myoclonus, and generalized seizures. Also not recommended in the treatment of sickle cell disease because of renal impairment; normeperidine is renally excreted

  h. Methadone (Dolophine): a unique opioid because it has both mu agonist and NMDA receptor antagonist properties. NMDA receptor antagonism has been shown to produce additional analgesia independent of opioids and can also provide relief of neuropathic pain. Very long half-life (15–60 hr), often used to treat severe pain in patients who are opioid tolerant. Black box warning: QT interval prolongation

  i. Oxymorphone: available in both short- and long-acting forms (e.g., Opana, Opana ER) and I (Numorphan) Naloxone (Narcan) is a mu opioid antagonist and is used to reverse/treat opioid overdose. It has a rapid onset of action (2 min) and is given intravenously. Mix 0.4 mg (1 ampule) with 10 ml normal saline, never give naloxone undiluted or too rapidly as this may cause a dangerous increase in sympathetic activity and rebound severe pain

 2. Dual mechanism analgesics

    a. Tramadol (Ultram): synthetic opioid analgesic used for moderate to moderately-severe pain by weakly binding to the mu opioid receptor and inhibiting serotonin and norepinephrine reuptake. Also available in combination with acetaminophen (Ultracet)

    b. Tapentadol (Nucynta): newer drug, also with dual mechanism of action as tramadol, and can be used for moderate to severe acute pain. Comparison studies have shown tapentadol to be as effective as oxycodone

  3. Agonist-antagonist opioids

    a. Buprenorphine: the only partial mu agonist with a high affinity for the mu opioid receptor; it powerfully binds to the mu receptor but does not produce the same effects as a full mu agonist such as morphine. It is therefore not used for severe escalating pain but is approved to treat opioid addiction. Available as a sublingual (Subutex and Suboxone), intravenous (Buprenex), and transdermal patch (Butrans)

    b. Other medications include butorphanol (Stadol), dezocine (Dalgan), and nalbuphine (Nubain) are less utilized

D. Adjuvant analgesics

  1. Multimodal therapy was first proposed in the 1990s, which uses several classes of analgesics to treat the different pain mechanisms. This may allow lower doses of each medication for the desired effect, thus decreasing the risk of side effects, especially those caused by mu agonist opioids

  2. Anticonvulsants

    a. Gabapentin (Neurontin): classified as an anticonvulsant, along with pregabalin (Lyrica), is a first line treatment for neuropathic pain and is increasingly added as a regimen for postoperative pain. Mechanism of action is heightening the calcium channel current and increasing synthesis of the neurotransmitter γ-aminobutyric acid. Side effects include sedation, ataxia, and fatigue

    b. Pregabalin (Lyrica): faster onset than gabapentin although studies show patients with more adverse effects (e.g., sedation, dizziness, and vomiting); as a result, gabapentin is recommended as a first-line agent for neuropathic pain

    c. Other examples include carbamazepine (Tegretol), topiramate (Topamax), valproic acid (Depakote), and oxcarbazepine (Trileptal)

  3. NMDA receptor antagonists

    a. Ketamine: a dissociative anesthetic with analgesic, sedative, and amnesic properties. It is given at low doses to treat refractory neuropathic and postoperative pain; when used in conjunction with other analgesics, ketamine can have a significant opioid dose-sparing effect. Usually limited for use by anesthesia and pain management teams

    b. Other examples are memantine (Namenda), amantadine (Symmetrel), and dextromethorphan (antitussive)

4. Topical anesthetics: in addition to topical NSAIDs, there are several types of topical anesthetics that can penetrate the skin and produce effective analgesia

    a. Topical lidocaine 5% patch (Lidoderm), lidocaine gel, lidocaine/prilocaine (EMLA) cream, and plain lidocaine cream (LMX-4)

    b. Capsaicin is a molecule found in all hot peppers and when applied topically desensitizes nociceptive nerve endings in the skin, available in low and high concentrations (e.g., capsaicin patch Qutenza)

    c. Other topical creams containing soothing materials such as menthol, camphor, or homeopathic ingredients (e.g., Zepol, Flexall, Traumeel)

5. Skeletal muscle relaxants

    a. Used to treat musculoskeletal pain although may have excessive sedative effects when given in conjunction with mu agonist opioids

    b. Carisoprodol (Soma), cyclobenzaprine (Flexeril), metaxalone (Skelaxin), and methocarbamol (Robaxin) are centrally acting muscle relaxants

    c. Baclofen (Lioresal) activates γ-aminobutyric acid receptors in order to decrease the release of neurotransmitters and amino acids. Abruptly stopping baclofen may lead to seizure activity

    d. Tizanidine (Zanaflex) is approved in the United States for treatment of spasticity related to multiple sclerosis, spinal cord injury, and neuropathic pain

        i. Benzodiazepines, such as clonazepam (Klonopin) and diazepam (Valium), are also used for centrally mediated muscle relaxation, but be very cautious when used along with mu agonist opioids as this may lead to excessive sedation. Not recommended for use in older patients.

6. α-2 adrenergic agonists

    a. Labeled as nonspecific, multipurpose analgesics for acute and persistent pain

    b. Clonidine (Catapres) is administered as a tablet or transdermal patch, used to treat continued sympathetic pain symptomatology and neuropathic pain

    c. Dexmedetomidine (Precedex) is used primarily in the critical care setting for sedation and not for analgesic purposes

    d. Tizanidine (Zanaflex) is also a centrally acting muscle relaxant also with α-2 receptor agonist properties

  7. Antidepressants

    a. Used as an adjuvant analgesic in patients with persistent neuropathic pain including diabetic neuropathy, postherpetic neuralgia, fibromyalgia, persistent headaches, and some chronic back pain. Recommended in the early treatment of fibromyalgia, studies show significant improvement in pain, fatigue, depression, and sleep disturbances. Not typically used in the treatment of acute pain. Divided into two major groups:

    b. Tricyclic antidepressants include tertiary amines such as amitriptyline (Elavil) and imipramine (Tofranil), secondary amines that include desipramine (Norpramin) and nortriptyline (Aventyl and Pamelor), and triazolopyridine (Trazodone).

    c. Second-generation antidepressants are subdivided into serotonin norepinephrine reuptake inhibitors, tetracyclic compounds, and selective serotonin reuptake inhibitors.

      i. Serotonin norepinephrine reuptake inhibitors: bupropion (Wellbutrin), duloxetine (Cymbalta), venlafaxine (Effexor), and milnacipran (Savella)

      ii. Tetracyclic compound: mirtazapine (Remeron)

      iii. Selective serotonin reuptake inhibitors: fluoxetine (Prozac), paroxetine (Paxil), and sertraline (Zoloft)

  8. Corticosteroids

    a. Primarily utilized in the cancer population, in addition to its anti-inflammatory effect, corticosteroids are also beneficial in the treatment of nausea, malaise, anorexia, and overall quality of life. Seldom used in the treatment of severe pain in the acute care setting.

V. **Analgesic delivery devices**

  A. Patient-controlled analgesia (PCA): one of the most common and patient-preferred methods of delivering intravenous opioids, it allows for patients to treat their pain by self-administering doses of analgesics through a programmable infusion pump. PCA pumps are mostly used to treat acute pain. Some facilities may require an anesthesia or pain management consult to order a PCA.

    1. Three most common medications used in a PCA are morphine, hydromorphone, and fentanyl

    2. The Institute for Patient Safety and the Joint Commission has identified specific patient groups who are at increased risk for PCA and warrant additional monitoring if PCA is used:

      a. Infants and small children

      b. Older patients who are confused

    c. Patients who have asthma

    d. Obese patients

    e. Patient who have sleep apnea

    f. Patients taking other medications with sedating effects, such as skeletal muscle relaxants, antiemetics, and benzodiazepines

B. Epidural analgesia: recommended for patients who undergo significant surgeries, such as a thoracotomy, large abdominal surgeries, joint replacement surgery, and multiple rib fractures as a result of trauma. A catheter is placed into the epidural space at the level of the surgery or injury, and then analgesia is delivered through the catheter with an infusion pump. Epidural catheters are typically placed and managed by anesthesia and/or pain management service.

    1. Three most common medications used in an epidural are morphine (Duramorph), hydromorphone, and fentanyl at significantly lower doses than if given parenterally

    2. Local anesthetics (e.g., bupivacaine and ropivacaine) are often added into the epidural solution to allow a reduced dose of opioids and decrease the likelihood of opioid adverse effects such as respiratory depression, nausea, sedation, and pruritis

    3. Epidural analgesia can be administered by clinician bolus injection, continuous infusion, and as patient-controlled epidural analgesia (PCEA), often in combination

        a. With epidural analgesia, the opioid diffuses through the dura mater where it makes contact with mu and kappa opioid receptors on the substantia gelatinosa in the dorsal horn.

C. Peripheral local anesthetic catheters: one of the newer techniques for acute pain management, a catheter is threaded through a needle inserted into the targeted nerve site by an anesthesiologist

    1. The catheter is connected to an infusion device filled with a local anesthetic, usually bupivacaine and ropivacaine. Local anesthetics can also be administered as multiple single bolus injections during the postoperative period.

    2. Studies have found a high rate of patient satisfaction with this method, and patients use less opioids, have less pain, and have a decreased hospital length of stay.

D. Nerve blocks

    1. Steroids with or without local anesthetic can be injected into the targeted nerve site (e.g., intercostal, epidural, facet, and sympathetic) at the bedside and under fluoroscopy

    2. Local anesthetic (e.g., bupivacaine and ropivacaine) can be injected into the surgical or procedural area and block the involved nerves. The disadvantages of this technique are most blocks last 6–8 hr and patients will experience increased pain when the block wears off.

E. Intrathecal pump

1. Used for long-term persistent cancer and noncancer pain, a catheter attached to a programmable pump is inserted by a surgeon or an anesthesiologist specialized in pain management into the intrathecal space. Not used for acute pain.
2. Various analgesics are used in combination to reach the desired analgesic effect, including morphine, hydromorphone, fentanyl, bupivacaine, clonidine, ziconotide (Prialt), and baclofen (Lioresal)

VI. **Considerations**

A. Nonpharmacological therapy: pain guidelines from multiple professional organizations recommend combining nonpharmacological methods along with medication management
   1. Physical therapy: focuses on physical aspects of pain
      a. Transcutaneous/percutaneous electrical nerve stimulation: electrical stimulation causes the release of endogenous opioids such as endorphins
      b. Superficial heat or cold treatment
   2. Cognitive behavioral therapy: can be used to promote rest and relaxation, decrease anxiety, and strengthen coping skills
   3. Complementary/alternative medicine
      a. Acupuncture: a 2012 study showed equivalent postoperative surgical pain relief, as with the use of a PENS unit, both decreased pain levels and reduced need for opiates
      b. Herbal medication
      c. Aromatherapy, massage
      d. Healing touch or therapeutic touch (endorsed by the American Holistic Nursing Association)

B. Older patients: reduce starting doses of opioids by 25%–50% and frequently monitor for adverse effects

C. Patients with chronic pain or opioid tolerance
   1. Should be taking their usual home doses of opioids for chronic pain in addition to medications to treat acute pain
   2. Doses of opioids may need to be increased by 25%–50% to treat acute pain

D. Opioid-induced hyperalgesia: created when increasing doses of opioid results in increasing sensitivity to pain to a normally unpleasant stimulus
   1. Allodynia: when pain is produced by a non-noxious stimulus (e.g., light touch and gentle massage), common in neuropathic pain
   2. Suspect opioid-induced hyperalgesia when rapidly increasing (usually high) doses of opioids fail to relieve pain and patients even report worsening pain at the original or at other sites
   3. Recommended treatment includes opioid dose reduction, opioid rotation, use of an NMDA receptor antagonist, and use of a COX-2 selective NSAID (Celebrex)

        a. Opioid rotation: the process of switching an opioid-tolerant patient to an alternative opioid; it is recommended to reduce the starting dose of the new opioid equianalgesic dose by 25%–50% to prevent overdosing

E. Protective analgesia: an aggressive, continuous approach where multimodal treatments are initiated in the preoperative (known as preemptive analgesia), intraoperative, and postoperative periods; directed at the prevention of persistent neuropathic postsurgical pain syndromes

F. Opioid dosing

   1. Consider around-the-clock (ATC) dosing, continuous infusion, or use of an extended release opioid if pain is continuous (12 hr or longer) to achieve a steady state opioid plasma level

        a. The use of ATC dosing should always be accompanied by a short-acting opioid for breakthrough pain

   2. Intermittent and breakthrough pain is treated with an as-needed (prn) approach

VII. **Useful approximate equianalgesic opioid dosing equivalent conversions (Table 74.1)**

   A. Equianalgesic doses contained in this chart are approximate and should be used only as a guideline. Dosing must be titrated to individual response.

Table 74.1	Approximate Equianalgesic Opioid Dosing Equivalents					
Medication	**Onset (min)**	**Half-life (hr)**	**Duration (hr)**	**Parenteral Dose**	**Oral dose**	**Oral-to-parenteral ratio**
Codeine	10–30 (IM) 30–60 (PO)	3–4	4–6		200 mg	
Fentanyl	Immediate (IV) 12–24 (trans patch)	1–6	1–2 72 (trans patch)	100 µg		
Hydrocodone	10–20 (PO)	3–4	4–6		30 mg	
Hydromorphone	less than 5 (IV) 15–30 (PO)	2–4	4–6	1.5 mg	7.5 mg	5:1
Meperidine	less than 5 (IV) 10–15 (IM/SQ/PO)	3–4	2–4	75 mg	300 mg	4:1
Methadone	10–20 (IV) 30–60 (PO)	15–60	4–6 (acute) greater than 8 (chronic)	10 mg	20 mg	2:1 (chronic) 1:1 (acute)
Morphine	less than 5 (IV) 15–60 (PO)	2–4	3–6 Long acting: 12	10 mg	20–30 mg (ATC dosing) 60 mg (single dose)	3:1 (chronic) 6:1 (acute)
Oxycodone	10–15 (PO)	3–4	4–6 Long acting: 12		20–30 mg	

Note. Equianalgesic doses contained in this chart are approximate and should be used only as a guideline. Dosing must be titrated to individual response. There is often incomplete cross-tolerance among these drugs. It is, therefore, recommended to begin with a 50% lower dose than the equianalgesic dose when changing drugs and then titrate to a safe/effective response. Dosing adjustments for renal or hepatic insufficiency, cytochrome P450 drug interactions, genetics, and other conditions or medications that affect drug metabolism, kinetics or response may also be necessary. Also consider pain control at time of switch. In general, use cautious dosing for elderly or debilitated patients and patients with renal or hepatic impairment. Some products have specific dosing recommendations for these populations.

Table 74.2	Pharmacological Agents for Pain		
Drug	**Dosage**	**Adverse Effects**	**Comments**
acetaminophen	PO/NG/PR/IV 325–650 q 4 hr or 1000 mg q 8 hr NOT to exceed 3000 mg/24 hr	pruritus, constipation, nausea, vomiting, headache, insomnia, agitation, atelectasis, exanthematous pustulosis, Stevens-Johnson Syndrome, toxic epidermal necrolysis, liver failure	Indication: mild to moderate pain Analgesic and antipyretic properties NO anti-inflammatory properties Does not induce GI bleeding Well tolerated and safe for all age groups Available in many formulations (IV, PO, NG, PR) Adjust dose in hepatic impairment, elderly BBW: Life-threatening cases of acute hepatic failure leading to liver transplant or death
tramadol (Ultram)	50–100 mg PO q 6–8 hr Max: 400 mg/day	flushing, nausea, dizziness, somnolence, seizures, respiratory depression	Indication: moderate to moderately severe pain NOT chemically related to opiates Reduce dose & frequency for renal or hepatic impairment Avoid in patients with seizures Withdrawal symptoms have been reported As of August 2014, tramadol is a controlled substance (schedule IV)
Nonsteroidal Anti-Inflammatory Drugs (NSAIDs)			
aspirin*	325–650 mg PO q 6 hr; Max: 3.9 grams/24 hr	headache, tinnitus, dizziness fluid retention,	Indication: Mild to moderate pain
diclofenac (Voltaren)	100–150 mg/day PO in 2–3 divided doses; Max: 200 mg/day	hypertension, edema, myocardial infarction, heart failure, abdominal	Analgesic, antipyretic and anti-inflammatory properties All agents are equally efficacious

Table 74.2	Pharmacological Agents for Pain		
Drug	**Dosage**	**Adverse Effects**	**Comments**
diflunisal (Dolobid)	500–1000 mg PO BID; Max: 1500 mg/day	pain, dysplasia, nausea, vomiting, ulcers or bleeding, thrombocytopenia, neutropenia, aplastic anemia, abnormal liver function tests, asthma, rash, pruritus, renal insufficiency, renal failure, hyperkalemia, proteinuria	Do not use ASA in children = Reye's syndrome risk
etodolac (Lodine)	800–1200 mg/day PO in 2–4 divided doses; Max: 1200 mg/day		Selection based on cost/availability/preference
fenoprofen (Nalfon)	300–600 mg PO 3–4 times/day; Max: 3200 mg/day		ALL patients taking NSAID's should be evaluated for concurrent administration of proton pump inhibitor therapy to prevent GI complications
flurbiprofen (Ansaid)	200–300 mg/day PO in 2–4 divided doses; Max: 100 mg/dose; 300 mg/day		BBW: May cause an increased risk of serious cardiovascular thrombotic events *available OTC
ibuprofen (Motrin, Advil)*	1200–3200 mg/day PO in 3–4 divided doses Max: 3200 mg/day		
indomethacin (Indocin)	25 mg PO 2–3 times/day Max: 100 mg/dose; 200 mg/day		[a]Ketorolac: total duration of use of PO/IV/IM dosing is not to exceed 5 days
ketoprofen (Orudis)	150–300 mg/day PO in 3–4 divided doses Max: 300 mg/day		Max dose age over 65 is 60 mg/day (IV/IM)
ketorolac (Toradol)[a]	15–30 mg IV/IM q 6 hr Max: 120 mg/day 10 mg PO q 6 hr Max: 40 mg/day		

Table 74.2	Pharmacological Agents for Pain		
Drug	**Dosage**	**Adverse Effects**	**Comments**
meclofenamate	200–400 mg/day PO in 3 to 4 divided doses; Max: 400 mg/day		
meloxicam (Mobic)	7.5 mg PO daily Max: 15 mg/day		
nabumetone (Relafen)	500–1000 mg/day PO 1–2 times/day Max: 2000 mg/day		
naproxen (Naprosyn, Aleve)*	250–500 mg PO BID Max: 1500 mg/day		
oxaprozin (Daypro)	600–1200 mg PO daily; Max: 1800 mg/day		
piroxicam (Feldene)	10–20 mg PO daily Max: 20 mg/day		
sulindac (Clinoril)	150 mg PO BID Max: 400 mg/day		
tolmetin (Tolectin)	200–600 mg PO TID Max: 1800 mg/day		

Table 74.2	Pharmacological Agents for Pain		
Drug	**Dosage**	**Adverse Effects**	**Comments**
celecoxib (Celebrex)	100–200 mg PO BID or 200–400 mg PO daily Max: 400 mg/day	back pain, peripheral edema, abdominal pain, dyspepsia, flatulence, dizziness, headache, insomnia, hypertension, MI	Analgesic, antipyretic and anti-inflammatory properties Efficacy equals that of the other NSAIDs Fewer endoscopic ulcers than most other NSAIDs (?) Renal toxicities similar to traditional NSAIDs Not recommended in renal or liver failure Screen for sulfa allergy BBW: May cause an increased risk of serious cardiovascular thrombotic events BBW: increased risk of serious GI adverse events, especially in the elderly
Topical Agents			
capsaicin cream (Capsin, Zostrix)	Apply to affected joint 3–4 times/day	erythema, application site pain, application site rash, pruritus, nausea, HTN	Indication: Monotherapy for select patients, Adjunct to systemic medication Localized neuropathic and musculoskeletal pain
capsaicin 8% patch (Qutenza)	Apply for 60 minutes and repeat every 3 months or as warranted by the return of pain (not more frequently than every three months)		Advantages over systemic drugs: delivery at the site of insult, lower initial rates of systemic absorption, fewer systemic effects and patient preference

Table 74.2	Pharmacological Agents for Pain		
Drug	**Dosage**	**Adverse Effects**	**Comments**
diclofenac (Voltaren gel 1%)	Apply 4 grams to lower extremities 4 times daily; apply 2 grams to upper extremities 4 times daily; Max: 8 grams/day to any single joint of upper extremity 16 grams/day to any single joint of lower extremity 32 grams/day total over all affected joints		Useful for osteoarthritis, neuropathic pain (capsaicin, lidocaine) Topical preparations safer than their oral agents (?)
trolamine salicylate (Aspercreme 10%)	Apply to affected area 3 to 4 times/day	erythema, skin irritation, tinnitus	
lidocaine 5% patch (Lidoderm)	Apply up to 3 patches to affected area/joint at one time, for up to 12 hr within a 24-hour period	hypotension, nausea, rash	
Opioids			
morphine (morphine IR, MS Contin SR, Avinza ER, Kadian ER)	Oral IR: 15–30 mg q 4 hr prn pain SR: 15–30 mg q 8–12 hr ER: 30 mg daily IV/SQ 2–10 mg IV q 4 hr prn pain	behavioral restlessness, tremulousness, hyperactivity, respiratory depression, nausea, vomiting, increased ICP, postural hypotension,	Indication: Moderate to severe pain DOC for severe pain, chronic pain (cancer) Selection of agent and dose should be individualized by patient; initial dose selection must take into account patient's prior analgesic treatment experience and risk factors for addiction, abuse and misuse

Table 74.2	Pharmacological Agents for Pain		
Drug	**Dosage**	**Adverse Effects**	**Comments**
hydromorphone (Dilaudid)	PO: 2–4 mg q 4 hr prn pain IV/SQ: 0.5–1 mg q 4 hr prn pain	constipation, urinary retention, sedation, pruritus, urticaria	Due to substantial inter-patient variability in relative potency of different opioid products, including differences in extended-release morphine products, when converting it is recommended to underestimate a patient's 24-hour oral morphine requirements and provide rescue mediation as needed
fentanyl (Duragesic, Actiq**)	IV/SQ: 25–50 mcg q 2 hr prn pain Transdermal: 25 mcg q 72 hr Lozenge: 200 mcg q 4 hr prn pain		All opioids are not created equal All have potential to cause tolerance, dependence, addiction and/or withdrawal
hydrocodone (Norco)	5 mg (1 tablet) PO q 4 hr prn pain		
oxycodone (Percocet, OxyContin)	IR: 5 mg (1 tablet) PO q 4 hr prn pain SR: 10 mg PO q 12 hr		Long acting formulations NOT appropriate for acute pain Fentanyl patch and lozenge: for use in opioid-tolerant patients only
levorphanol (Levo-Dromoran)	PO: 2 mg q 6 hr prn pain IV: 1 mg q 4 hr prn pain		**Actiq may be dispensed only to patients enrolled in the TIRF REMS Access program
methadone (Dolophine)	PO: 2.5–5 mg q 8 hr IVPB: 2.5–5 mg q 8 hr		Methadone: due to its highly variable and prolonged half-life, methadone has the highest risk among opioids of overdose and accumulation during initial titration to effect (as steady state levels are approached) and during dose adjustment in chronic use
oxymorphone (Opana, Opana ER)	PO IR: 5–10 mg q 4 hr prn pain ER: 5 mg q 12 hr IV: 0.5 mg q 4 hr prn pain		
tapentadol (Nucynta, Nucynta ER)	IR: 50–100 mg PO q 4 hr prn pain ER: 50 mg PO q 12 hr		Methadone is associated with the risk of QT interval prolongation and Torsade de pointes

Table 74.2	Pharmacological Agents for Pain		
Drug	**Dosage**	**Adverse Effects**	**Comments**
Mixed Opioid Agonist-Antagonists			
buprenorphine/naloxone (Suboxone)	16 mg/4 mg PO daily	drowsiness, dizziness, light-headedness, euphoria, nausea, clammy skin, sweating, insomnia, abdominal pain, constipation, respiratory depression, shock	Indication: Moderate to severe pain Chronic pain Do not administer any partial agonist/drug with mixed opioid receptor actions to patients receiving pure agonist drugs: reduction of analgesia or precipitation of explosive abstinence syndrome Butorphanol/pentazocine: labor pain, migraine Buprenorphine: management of opioid dependence
butorphanol (Stadol)	1–2 mg IV/IM q 4 hr prn pain		
nalbuphine (Nubain	10 mg IV/SQ q 4 hr prn pain Max: 160 mg/day		
pentazocine (Talwin)	30 mg IV/SQ q 4 hr prn pain Max 360 mg/day		
Opioids Antagonist			
naloxone (Narcan)	0.4–2 mg IV, repeat every 2–3 minutes as needed	muscle/joint pain, sleep anxiety, headache, nervousness, withdrawal symptoms, vomiting	Indication: Reversal of opioid; acute opioid overdose Naloxone: DOC for acute opioid overdose Naloxone: short duration of action requires repeated dosing or continuous infusion Naltrexone: long duration of action; primarily used as a maintenance drug for addicts in treatment programs: alcohol dependence/opioid dependence
naltrexone (Vivitrol)	380 mg IM gluteal injection every 4 weeks		

Table 74.2	Pharmacological Agents for Pain		
Drug	**Dosage**	**Adverse Effects**	**Comments**
Antidepressants			
duloxetine (Cymbalta)	30–60 mg PO daily Max: 60 mg/day	diaphoresis, constipation, decrease in appetite, diarrhea, nausea, xerostomia, dizziness, headache, insomnia, somnolence, fatigue, HTN	Indication: Neuropathic pain (first line); fibromyalgia; chronic low back pain
venlafaxine (Effexor)	75–225 mg PO daily		
amitriptyline (Elavil)	25 mg PO qhs Max: 200 mg/day		Duloxetine/venlafaxine preferred over SSRI Adjust dose in hepatic and renal impairment
desipramine (Norpramin)	25 mg PO qhs Max: 150 mg/day		No TCAD FDA labeled for pain Not for acute pain
fluoxetine (Prozac)	20–60 mg PO daily Max: 60 mg/day		Numerous drug-drug interactions
Anticonvulsants			
gabapentin (Neurontin)	100–300 mg PO daily titrate up to TID dosing to max of 3600 mg/day	peripheral edema, increased appetite, weight gain, constipation, xerostomia, asthenia, ataxia, dizziness, headache, incoordination, blurred vision, diplopia, disturbance in thinking, euphoria	Indication: Neuropathic pain; fibromyalgia; chronic low back pain; trigeminal neuralgia
pregabalin (Lyrica)	50 mg PO TID Max: 300 mg/day		Gabapentin/pregabalin: DOC for neuropathic pain Evidence of efficacy not as robust for other agents
carbamazepine (Tegretol)	100 mg PO BID Max: 1200 mg/day		Lamotrigine (acute/chronic pain): A systematic review of lamotrigine for acute and chronic pain concluded that it does not have a place in the treatment of pain, given other more effective therapies Carbamazepine/oxcarbazepine: first-line for trigeminal neuralgia Many drug-drug interactions

Table 74.2	Pharmacological Agents for Pain		
Drug	**Dosage**	**Adverse Effects**	**Comments**
Skeletal Muscle Relaxants			
baclofen (Lioresal)	5 mg PO TID prn muscle spasm	drowsiness, dizziness, dry mouth, sedation, ataxia, light-headedness, somnolence, urinary retention, hypotension, bradycardia	Indication: adjunct therapy only
carisoprodol (Soma)	250 mg PO TID prn muscle spasm		Use lower initial dose in geriatrics
chlorzoxazone (Parafon Forte)	500 mg PO TID prn muscle spasm		Reduce dose for liver or renal impairment
cyclobenzaprine (Flexeril),	10 mg PO TID prn muscle spasm		Avoid carisoprodol (Soma) due to its addictive properties and increased potential for central nervous system effects
metaxalone (Skelaxin),	800 mg PO TID prn muscle spasms		Carisoprodol is a controlled substance (schedule IV)
methocarbamol (Robaxin),	500 mg PO q 6 hr prn muscle spasms		
orphenadrine (Norflex)	100 mg PO BID prn muscle spasm		
tizanidine (Zanaflex)	2 mg PO q 6 hr prn muscle spasm		

Table 74.2	Pharmacological Agents for Pain		
Drug	**Dosage**	**Adverse Effects**	**Comments**
Miscellaneous			
ziconotide (Prialt)	Intrathecal: Initial: no more than 2.4 mcg/day titrate by up to 2.4 mcg/day at intervals of no more than 2–3 times per week Max: 19.2 mg/day	peripheral edema, constipation, diarrhea, loss of appetite, nausea, taste sense altered, vomiting, spasms, abnormal gait, amnesia, articulatory dyspraxia, asthenia, ataxia, confusion, dizziness, dysarthria, headache, memory impairment, somnolence, tremor, vertigo, anxiety, hallucinations	Indication: Severe chronic pain; intrathecal analgesia in patients with refractory chronic pain Reserved for patients with no other reasonable options for pain control Contraindicated in patients with a preexisting history of psychosis Monitor all patients frequently for evidence of cognitive impairment, hallucinations or changes in mood or consciousness; discontinue therapy in the event of serious neurological or psychiatric signs or symptoms BBW: neurologic impairment and psychiatric symptoms

BIBLIOGRAPHY

American Society of Anesthesiologists (ASA) Committee on Standards and Practice Parameters. (2012). Practice guidelines for acute pain management in the perioperative setting: An updated report by the American Society of Anesthesiologists Task Force on Acute Pain Management. *Anesthesiology, 116*(2), 248–273.

American Society of Anesthesiologists Task Force on Chronic Pain Management. (2010). Practice guidelines for chronic pain management: An updated report by the American Society of Anesthesiologists Task Force on Chronic Pain Management and the American Society of Regional Anesthesia and Pain Medicine. *Anesthesiology, 112*(4), 810–833.

Benzon, H. T. (2014). *Practical management of pain* (5th ed.). Philadelphia, PA: Mosby.

Caraceni, A., Hanks, G., Kaasa, S., Bennett, M. I., Brunelli, C., Cherny, . . . Zeppetella, G. (2012). Use of opioid analgesics in the treatment of cancer pain: Evidence-based recommendations from the EAPC. *The Lancet Oncology, 13*(2), e58–e68.

Cedars-Sinai Medical Center. (2013). *Pain management reference card* (6th ed.). Los Angeles, CA: Department of Pharmacy Services.

D'Arcy, Y. (2010). An update on new pain medications. *Nursing, 40*(11), 63–64.

D'Arcy, Y. (2011). New criteria for assessing and treating neuropathic pain. *Nursing, 41*(12), 61–62.

D'Arcy, Y. (2011). New thinking about postoperative pain management. *ORNurse, 5*(6), 29–36.

D'Arcy, Y. (2012). Treating acute pain in the hospitalized patient. *Nurse Practitioner, 37*(8), 23–30.

Gavronsky, S., Koeniger-Donohue, R., Steller, J., & Hawkins, J. W. (2012). Postoperative pain: Acupuncture versus percutaneous electrical stimulation. *Pain Management Nursing, 13*(3), 150–156.

Pasero, C., & McCaffery, M. (2011). *Pain assessment and pharmacologic management*. St. Louis, MO: Mosby Elsevier.

Stites, M. (2013). Observation pain scales in critically ill adults. *Critical Care Nurse, 33*(3), 68–78.

Therapeutic Research Center. (2012, August). PL detail-document: Equianalgesic dosing of opioids for pain management. *Pharmacist's Letter/Prescriber's Letter.* Retrieved from http://www.nhms.org/sites/default/files/Pdfs/Opioid-Comparison-Chart-Prescriber-Letter-2012.pdf

ADDITIONAL RESOURCES

American Society of Anesthesiologists (ASA) Committee on Standards and Practice Parameters. (2012). Practice guidelines for acute pain management in the perioperative setting: An updated report by the American Society of Anesthesiologists Task Force on Acute Pain Management. *Anesthesiology, 116*(2). 248–273.

American Society of Anesthesiologists Task Force on Chronic Pain Management. (2010). Practice guidelines for chronic pain management: An updated report by the American Society of Anesthesiologists Task Force on Chronic Pain Management and the American Society of Regional Anesthesia and Pain Medicine. *Anesthesiology, 112*(4). 810–833.

CHAPTER 75

Psychosocial Problems in Acute Care

PAULA K. VUCKOVICH

VIOLENCE

I. Definitions
- **A.** Violence: direct verbal or physical attack on another person
- **B.** Assault: threat to do another person physical harm
- **C.** Abuse: a pattern of improper or violent treatment
    1. Physical
    2. Emotional
    3. Sexual
    4. Psychological
    5. Financial

II. Etiology/predisposing factors
- **A.** History of aggressive or violent behavior (single best predictor)
- **B.** Anger/frustration/hostility at healthcare providers/system
- **C.** Psychosis, mood disorders, and anxiety/panic
- **D.** Substance abuse
- **E.** Poor impulse control
- **F.** Domestic and personal problems
- **G.** Acute or chronic brain disorders, such as
    1. Seizures
    2. Subdural hematoma
    3. Dementia
    4. Stroke
- **H.** Undiagnosed or inadequately managed medical problem, such as
    1. Diabetes
    2. Renal failure
    3. Pain

III.   Subjective findings

   A. Acutely violent person

      1. Agitation

      2. Frustration/anger/rage

      3. Anxiety/fear

      4. May experience intolerable sense of needs being unmet/despair/suicidal thoughts

   B. Abuser

      1. Increased anxiety, confusion, depression, agitation, and verbal threats

      2. Guilty feelings and remorse after a violent episode

      3. Controlling behavior toward the abused

   C. Abused person

      1. Evasion of questions about injuries

      2. Depression, anxiety, refusal to talk about problems, and fear

      3. Shame, low self-esteem, self-blame, and guilt

IV.   Physical examination findings

   A. Acutely assaultive person often, but not always, displays:

      1. Hyperactivity

         a. Restlessness

         b. Pacing, if ambulatory

      2. Increasing physical tension

         a. Clenched jaw and fist

         b. Rigid posture

         c. Increased pulse/blood pressure

      3. Verbal cues

         a. Verbal abuse, profanity, and argumentativeness

         b. Loud voice

         c. Altered pitch

         d. Very soft voice, forcing others to strain to listen

         e. Stone silence

      4. Alcohol on the breath

   B. Abused person may have the following:

      1. Scars (including burn or bite marks), lacerations, and poorly healed old fractures

      2. Bruises (particularly on the inner aspects of the arms and legs, fingerprint or odd shapes)

      3. Vaginal or anal lacerations, bruises and sores, peritoneal pain, and signs of a sexually transmitted infection (STI)

      4. Hypertension, hyperventilation, tachycardia, and other physical signs of acute or chronic anxiety

V.   Laboratory/diagnostic assessment

   A. Assaultive person

      1. Blood/urine drug screen and blood alcohol level (to rule out substance abuse)

2. Electrolytes (to rule out fluid and electrolyte imbalance)
3. Metabolic panel (to rule out metabolic/hormonal problems)
4. CT scan of the head (to rule out subdural hematoma, or to investigate brain tumor in sudden, unprovoked violent episode)
5. Electroencephalography (to rule out seizures in sudden, unprovoked violence)

B. Abused person
1. Assess for life-threatening injury
2. X-ray injured areas to detect fractures versus old or healing fractures
3. Venereal disease research laboratory and other tests as indicated for STIs

VI. Management

A. Assaultive person
1. Summon police if armed with weapons; alert other staff before trying to talk down if no weapons
2. Address with respect, offering food, beverage, and assistance in resolving problems nonviolently
3. Maintain adequate distance and relaxed but ready body posture; induce to sit with you, if possible
4. Speak in quiet, calm voice, listening more than talking; allow but do not force eye contact
5. Medication (given immediately if acutely agitated); avoid intramuscular medication if patient is willing to accept oral medication (see Tables 75.3 and 75.4)
   a. Lorazepam (Ativan), 2 mg (1 mg if frail or older than 65) PO, IM, or IV
   b. Olanzapine ODT (Zydis), 5 mg PO once, or risperidone (Risperdal M-tab), 2 mg oral, rapid dissolving formulation (1 mg if frail or older than 65), or Olanzapine (Zyprexa), 10 mg (5 mg if frail or older than age 65) PO
   c. Haloperidol (Haldol), 5 mg (2 mg if frail or older than 65) PO
   d. Haloperidol (Haldol), 5 mg IM (2.5 mg if frail or older than 65) or IV STAT if IV only feasible method of administration
      i. Although injectable haloperidol is approved by the FDA only for intramuscular injection, there is considerable evidence from the medical literature that intravenous administration of haloperidol is a relatively common "off-label" clinical practice, primarily for treatment of severe agitation. Higher doses and intravenous administration of haloperidol appear to be associated with a higher risk of QT prolongation and Torsades de pointes (TdP). Because of this risk of TdP and QT prolongation, ECG monitoring is recommended if haloperidol is given intravenously.

Table 75.3	Pharmacologic Agents for Anxiety		
Agent	**Initial Dosage**	**Adverse Effects**	**Comments**
Benzodiazepines			
alprazolam (Xanax)	0.25 mg PO TID Max: 4mg/day	drowsiness, sedation, lethargy, ataxia, confusion	Alprazolam, Lorazepam, diazepam effective for situational anxiety Preferred agent for insomnia caused by anxiety Many other applications: seizures, EtOH withdrawal, adjunct to anesthesia, nausea Adjust dose for liver/renal dysfunction Some agents have active metabolites Antidote: flumazenil (Romazicon)
clonazepam (Klonopin)	1 mg PO daily Max: 4 mg/day		
lorazepam (Ativan)	0.5 mg PO BID Max: 10 mg/day		
diazepam (Valium)	2 mg PO QID Max: 40 mg/day		
oxazepam (Serax)	10 mg PO TID Max: 120 mg/day		
Serotonin Receptor Agonist			
buspirone (Buspar)	7.5 mg PO BID Max: 60 mg/day	nausea, dizziness, nervousness, headache, somnolence, tachycardia, heart failure, MI, CVA	Many drug-drug interactions Slow onset of action (14 days) Adjust dose for liver or renal impairment Not a controlled substance
Antidepressant agents			
duloxetine (Cymbalta)	30 mg PO daily Max: 120 mg/day	nausea, dry mouth, insomnia, somnolence, headache, anxiety, GI disturbances, dizziness, anorexia, fatigue, sexual dysfunction, suicidal ideation, serotonin syndrome, SJS	Effective for: General anxiety disorder Panic disorder Social Anxiety disorder Post Traumatic Stress Disorder Obsessive-compulsive disorder
escitalopram (Lexapro)	10 mg PO daily Max: 20 mg/day		
paroxetine (Paxil)	20 mg PO daily Max: 50 mg/day		
sertraline (Zoloft)	50 mg PO daily Max: 200 mg/day		

Table 75.3	Pharmacologic Agents for Anxiety		
Agent	**Initial Dosage**	**Adverse Effects**	**Comments**
Antidepressant agents continued			
venlafaxine (Effexor, Effexor XR)	37.5 mg PO BID 37.5 mg PO daily Max: 225 mg/day	insomnia, nausea, dry mouth, constipation, hypertension, dizziness, somnolence, sweating, agitation, blurred vision, headache, tremor, vomiting, drowsiness, increased appetite, sexual dysfunction, suicidal ideation, serotonin syndrome	

  e. Ziprasidone (Geodon), 20 mg IM (10 mg if frail or older than 65)

 6. Physical restraints (when no other way to prevent physical harm)

  a. Should be used (if on protocol) only as a last resort and by trained personnel

  b. Multiple, less restrictive interventions to control behavior must be tried (and later documented) before restraints are applied

 7. Hospitalize the individual psychiatrically if a danger to self or others

 8. Correct underlying medical problems, or seek consultation with a psychiatrist

 9. Legal duty requires that threatened individuals should be warned if a person voices harmful intent against another individual's life and that authorities should be notified if a child, a dependent adult, or an elderly person is abused (in some states, one has a duty to report any domestic violence if the victim comes to your attention with acute injury).

B. Abused person

 1. Screen all clients for the possibility of domestic violence: ask whether they have ever been emotionally or physically hurt in an intimate relationship; also ask if they are afraid of anyone close to them. If the answer is "yes" to either question, ask for specifics and ask about current situation. If current abuse exists, do the following:

  a. Problem-solve to encourage the person to avoid being harmed

  b. Discuss all options, including staying with the abuser, because some individuals will not leave the abuser initially

      c. Assist to identify resources such as friends, family members, and others who may give aid and shelter

      d. Refer to social services or to a battered person's program

DEPRESSION

I. **Definition**

    A. Depressed mood, diminished interest in normal activity, fatigue, feelings of worthlessness, and impaired concentration nearly every day

    B. The depressed person may or may not be suicidal or homicidal

II. **Etiology/predisposing factors/risk factors**

    A. Depression, the most common psychiatric diagnosis, is frequently undertreated

    B. May be caused by the following:

      1. Imbalance in levels of neurotransmitters or hormones

      2. Negative perception of life events (chronic stress, multiple losses, or significant trauma)

      3. General medical disorders/medication adverse effects

    C. Significant precursors of depression

      1. Family or personal history of depression/suicide attempts

      2. Recent bad news or perceived failure

      3. Chronic conditions or medical conditions with poor prognosis

      4. Loss of significant others

      5. Lack of a support system

    D. Suicidal risk must be assessed

      1. Elderly white males with medical problems who lack social supports are at greatest risk

      2. Hopelessness, suicidal thoughts with a plan, history of prior attempts or suicide of someone close, and lack of internal and external resources are the most significant predictors of risk

      3. Good and Nelson developed a useful way to remember assessment of suicide risk with the following mnemonic: SUICIDAL

        a. S: sex (males are more successful at suicide; females make a greater number of attempts)

        b. U: unsuccessful attempts (past attempt history, reasons for attempts)

        c. I: identified family members or friends with a history of successful suicide

        d. CI: chronic illness history

        e. D: depression, drug abuse, and drinking

        f. A: age of the patient (the elderly are more often successful; teenagers make a greater number of attempts)

        g. L: lethal method available (guns are most lethal, followed by hanging and intentional drug overdose)

      4. If you identify any of these signs, you must ask using a nonjudgmental matter-of-fact approach:

    a. Have you ever thought about death or dying?
    b. Have you ever thought that life was not worth living?
    c. Have you ever thought about ending your life?
    d. Have you ever attempted suicide?
    e. Are you currently thinking about ending your life?
    f. What are your reasons for wanting to die and your reasons for wanting to live?

III. **Subjective findings**
    A. Feelings of:
        1. Hopelessness (most predictive of suicide risk)
        2. Increased/decreased appetite

Table 75.1	Pharmacologic Agents for Depression		
Agent	**Initial Dosage**	**Adverse Effects**	**Comments**
Selective Serotonin Reuptake Inhibitors (SSRIs)			
citalopram (Celexa)	20 mg PO daily Max: 40 mg/day	nausea, dry mouth, insomnia, somnolence, headache, anxiety, GI disturbances, dizziness, anorexia, fatigue, sexual dysfunction, suicidal ideation, serotonin syndrome, SJS	Generally considered as first line therapy Many applications: OCD, anxiety, PTSD, others Well tolerated, but many drug-drug interactions **Black Box Warning:** increased risk of suicidal thinking/behavior[a] Onset of effect: 4–6 weeks
escitalopram (Lexapro)	10 mg PO daily Max: 20 mg/day		
fluoxetine (Prozac)	20 mg PO daily Max: 80 mg/day		
fluvoxamine (Luvox)	50 mg PO daily Max: 300 mg/day		
paroxetine (Paxil)	20 mg PO daily Max: 50 mg/day		
sertraline (Zoloft)	50 mg PO daily Max: 200 mg/day		
vilazodone (Viibryd)	10 mg PO daily Max: 40 mg/day		
Serotonin-norepinephrine Reuptake Inhibitors (SNRIs)			
duloxetine (Cymbalta)	20 mg PO BID Max: 120 mg/day	insomnia, nausea, dry mouth, constipation, hypertension, dizziness, somnolence, sweating, agitation, blurred vision, headache, tremor, vomiting, drowsiness, increased appetite, orthostatic hypotension, sexual dysfunction, suicidal ideation, serotonin syndrome	Other applications: pain disorders, fibromyalgia Several drug-drug interactions **Black Box Warning:** suicidal thinking/behavior[a] Withdrawal syndrome if stopped abruptly Onset of effect: 4–6 weeks
desvenlafaxine (Pristiq)	50 mg PO daily Max: 50 mg/day		
venlafaxine (Effexor, Effexor XR)	37.5 mg PO BID 37.5 mg PO daily Max: 225 mg/day		

Table 75.1	Pharmacologic Agents for Depression		
Agent	**Initial Dosage**	**Adverse Effects**	**Comments**
Serotonin Antagonists			
nefazodone (Serzone)	100 mg PO BID Max: 600 mg/day	insomnia, nausea, dry mouth, constipation, dizziness, somnolence, sweating, agitation, blurred vision, headache, tremor, vomiting, drowsiness, increased appetite, orthostatic hypotension, sexual dysfunction, suicidal ideation, serotonin syndrome, QTc prolongation	Several drug-drug interactions **Black Box Warning**: suicidal thinking/behavior[a] Withdrawal syndrome if stopped abruptly Other applications: insomnia (trazodone) Onset of effect: 4–6 weeks
trazodone (Desyrel)	50 mg PO TID Max: 400 mg/day		
Atypical Antidepressants			
bupropion (Wellbutrin, Wellbutrin SR, Wellbutrin XL)	100 mg PO TID 150 mg PO BID 150 mg PO daily Max: 450 mg/day	insomnia, nausea, dry mouth, dizziness, somnolence, sweating, agitation, blurred vision, headache, tremor, vomiting, drowsiness, weight gain, orthostatic hypotension, sexual dysfunction, suicidal ideation, serotonin syndrome, seizures	Several drug-drug interactions **Black Box Warning**: suicidal thinking/behavior[a] Withdrawal syndrome if stopped abruptly Bupropion lowers the seizure threshold Onset of effect: 4–6 weeks
mirtazapine (Remeron)	15 mg PO daily Max: 45 mg/day		
Monoamine Oxidase Inhibitors (MAOIs)			
isocarboxazid (Marplan)	10 mg PO BID Max: 40 mg/day	dry mouth, constipation, urinary retention, blurred vision, sedation, confusion, arrhythmias, insomnia, nausea, anorexia, drowsiness, orthostatic hypotension, sexual dysfunction, serotonin syndrome, suicidal ideation	Reserved for depression unresponsive to other agents Many drug-drug and drug-food (tyramine: HTN crisis) interactions **Black Box Warning**: suicidal thinking/behavior[a] Onset of effect: 4–6 weeks
phenelzine (Nardil)	15 mg PO TID Max: 90 mg/day		
tranylcypro -mine (Parnate)	10 mg PO TID Max: 60 mg/day		

Table 75.1	Pharmacologic Agents for Depression		
Agent	**Initial Dosage**	**Adverse Effects**	**Comments**
Tricyclic Antidepressants (TCAs)			
amitriptyline (Elavil)	25 mg PO TID Max: 300 mg/day	dry mouth, constipation, urinary retention, blurred vision, sedation, confusion, arrhythmias, insomnia, nausea, dizziness, somnolence, sweating, agitation, headache, tremor, vomiting, drowsiness, weight gain, orthostatic hypotension, sexual dysfunction, suicidal ideation	Several drug-drug interactions Other applications: pain disorders, fibromyalgia **Black Box Warning**: suicidal thinking/behavior[a] Onset of effect: 4–6 weeks
amoxapine (Asendin)	50 mg PO BID Max: 300 mg/day		
desipramine (Norpramin)	50 mg PO BID Max: 300 mg/day		
doxepin (Sinequan)	25 mg PO daily Max: 300 mg/day		
imipramine (Tofranil)	25 mg PO TID Max: 300 mg/day		
nortriptyline (Aventyl, Pamelor)	25 mg PO TID Max: 150 mg/day		

3. Decreased libido
4. Helplessness
5. Worthlessness
6. Guilt

B. Lack of energy

C. Sleep disturbances, particularly early morning awakening or oversleeping

D. Psychomotor agitation/retardation

E. Thoughts of death or suicide

F. The patient may have auditory hallucinations saying, "You deserve to die," or telling client to kill self

IV. **Physical findings**

A. Poor physical hygiene, unkempt appearance, poor posture, and overweight/underweight

B. Diarrhea or impaction

C. Only complaints may involve abdominal or chest pain without a physical cause

D. Physical symptoms may be overreported or underreported

V. **Laboratory/diagnostic assessment (rule out underlying medical problems)**

A. Thyroid function studies to rule out hypothyroidism

B. Vitamin B12 and folate levels

C. Blood glucose level to rule out diabetes

D. Complete blood count (CBC) to detect anemia, infection, or other problems

    E. The patient must undergo an electrocardiogram (ECG) before starting tricyclic antidepressants (tricyclics may exacerbate existing conduction problems).

    F. A thorough evaluation of renal function should be done before initiating lithium (lithium is excreted through the kidneys and may reach toxic blood levels if renal function is poor).

    G. Drug screen or blood alcohol level, as appropriate (drug effects may mimic depressive symptoms)

VI.   **Management**

    A. Prior to initiation of management, diagnosis of depression must be confirmed. Patients with underlying bipolar disorder that are prescribed antidepressants may experience a manic episode.

    B. If the patient is a danger to self or others, hospitalize and refer to a psychiatrist

    C. Treat any underlying medical problems

Table 75.2	Pharmacologic Agents for Bipolar Disorder		
Agent	**Initial Dosage**	**Adverse Effects**	**Comments**
lithium (Eskalith, Lithobid)	300 mg PO BID	headache, lethargy, fatigue, recent memory loss, nausea, vomiting, anorexia, abdominal pain, diarrhea, dry mouth, muscle weakness, hand tremors, leukocytosis, nephrogenic diabetes insipidus	Many drug-drug interactions Monitor drug levels Target range: 0.6–1.4 mEq/L Reduce dose in renal impairment Salt (Na) affects lithium reabsorption in the kidney
Anti-convulsant Agents			
carbamazepine (Tegretol)	200 mg PO BID Max: 1600 mg/day	dizziness, ataxia, somnolence, headache, nausea, diplopia, blurred vision, sedation, drowsiness, nausea, vomiting, prolonged bleeding time, SJS, Toxic epidermal necrolysis, bone marrow suppression	Listed agents are FDA labeled for bipolar Other anti-seizure agents?? Many drug-drug interactions Monitor drug levels: Carbamazepine target level: 4–12 mcg/ml Valproic acid target level: 50–125 mcg/mL
lamotrigine (Lamictal)	25 mg PO daily x 2 weeks, then 50 mg PO daily x 2 weeks then 100 mg PO daily x 1 week then 200 mg PO daily Max: 400 mg/day		
valproic acid (Depakote)	250 mg PO TID Max: 60 mg/kg/day		

Table 75.2	Pharmacologic Agents for Bipolar Disorder		
Agent	**Initial Dosage**	**Adverse Effects**	**Comments**
Antipsychotic Agents			
aripiprazole (Abilify)	15 mg PO daily Max: 30 mg/day	tachycardia, sedation, dizziness, headache, light-headedness, somnolence, anxiety, hostility, insomnia, nausea, dry mouth, constipation, akathisia, extrapyramidal symptoms, neuroleptic malignant syndrome, QTc prolongation, weight gain, diabetes	Effective as monotherapy or adjunct therapy
olanzapine (Zyprexa)	10 mg PO daily Max: 20 mg/day		
quetiapine (Seroquel)	50 mg PO daily Max: 800 mg/day		
risperidone (Risperdal)	2 mg PO daily Max: 6 mg/day		
ziprasidone (Geodon)	40 mg PO BID Max: 160 mg/day		

Table 75.4	Pharmacologic Agents for Acute Psychosis/Delirium		
Agent	**Dosage**	**Adverse Effects**	**Comments**
olanzapine (Zyprexa)	5 mg PO ONCE or 10 mg IM ONCE then 5 mg PO daily (or PRN) Max: 40 mg/day	Monitor for electrocardiographic changes QT interval prolongation and arrhythmias Extrapyramidal side effects Lowers seizure threshold Hyperglycemia Peripheral edema Causes sedation	Discontinue in patients with QTc higher than 500 msec
quetiapine (Seroquel)	50 mg PO ONCE then 50 mg PO BID (or PRN) Max: 800 mg/day		
risperidone (Risperdal)	2 mg PO ONCE then 2 mg PO daily (or PRN) Max: 6 mg/day		

Table 75.4	Pharmacologic Agents for Acute Psychosis/Delirium		
Agent	**Dosage**	**Adverse Effects**	**Comments**
haloperidol (Haldol)	2.5–5 mg PO ONCE or 5 mg IV* ONCE then 2.5–5 mg IV/ PO q 6 hr prn agitation	Monitor for electrocardiographic changes QT interval prolongation and arrhythmias Extrapyramidal side effects Neuroleptic malignant syndrome (rare) Lowers seizure threshold **Black box warning:** increased mortality in elderly with dementia-related psychosis Causes sedation	Avoid/discontinue in patients with QTc higher than 500 msec See warning on intravenous administration below[a]

Note. [a]Although injectable haloperidol is approved by the FDA only for intramuscular injection, there is considerable evidence from the medical literature that intravenous administration of haloperidol is a relatively common "off-label" clinical practice, primarily for treatment of severe agitation. Higher doses and intravenous administration of haloperidol appear to be associated with a higher risk of QT prolongation and Torsades de pointes (TdP). Because of this risk of TdP and QT prolongation, ECG monitoring is recommended if haloperidol is given intravenously.

D. If not suicidal/homicidal/hallucinating, the patient may be referred for outpatient psychotherapy to be provided by a mental health professional.

E. Counsel the patient that depression is a very treatable condition with the use of medication and psychotherapy

F. Useful mnemonic for counseling mildly depressed patients or other patients with self-limiting emotional conditions: BATHE

　1. B: background (allow the patient time to tell about the problem, with healing expression of feelings)

　2. A: affect (elicit affect/feelings, e.g., "How do you feel about that?")

　3. T: trouble (find out the most disturbing thing about the problem by asking, "What was most troubling about the situation?")

　4. H: handling (assess coping: "How have you been handling the situation?")

　5. E: empathy (acknowledge the difficulty of the situation, and commend the patient for his strength in handling the problem)

G. Pharmacological treatment (all antidepressants are equally effective; approximately 67% of people respond, 6–8 weeks is required for full effect) (see Table 75.1)

　1. Selective serotonin reuptake inhibitors (SSRIs)

    a. Citalopram (Celexa) or escitalopram (Lexapro), isomer of citalopram. Use cautiously in the elderly and in those with history of hepatic disease; may cause QT prolongation: get baseline ECG and liver functions at initiation of therapy

    b. Sertraline (Zoloft), preferred for elderly because of shorter half-life

    c. Fluoxetine (Prozac), 48 hr half-life

    d. Most commonly prescribed treatment owing to the following:

        i. Low danger of overdose

        ii. More favorable adverse effect profiles (e.g., low cardiac conduction problems)

2. Selective norepinephrine and serotonin reuptake inhibitors, mirtazapine, or bupropion may be used for those who have not had adequate improvement with SSRIs.

    a. Venlafaxine (Effexor, Effexor XR), divided or evening dosing may be preferred because of sedation

    b. Duloxetine (Cymbalta)

        i. Use cautiously in elderly patients, history of glaucoma, hepatic impairment, or alcohol abuse

3. Tricyclic antidepressants and monoamine oxidase inhibitors are not used as often as in the past owing to worsened adverse effect profiles and high overdose potential.

4. Bipolar disorder

    a. Three major types:

        i. Bipolar I disorder: manic or mixed episode that may be accompanied by depression

        ii. Bipolar II disorder: depression episode shifting with hypomanic episode

        iii. Cyclothymic disorder: fluctuations between hypomania and mild depression

    b. Treatment options:

        i. Treated with lithium carbonate, divalproex sodium (Depakote), or lamotrigine (Lamictal) (antidepressants are not recommended as first-line treatment if patient is known to have bipolar disorder) (see Table 75.2)

        ii. Treatment with these drugs should be implemented by a psychiatrist or a psychiatric nurse practitioner

5. Supplement with anxiolytic or low-dose antipsychotic if agitated because all these medications take many days to have a noticeable effect on depression.

SUBSTANCE USE DISORDER

I. **Definition**

    A. Prolonged use of alcohol or another mood-altering substance resulting in emotional or physical reliance on the substance to deal with normal life stress

B. Substance abuse may result in physical and emotional dependence on the drug

II. **Etiology/predisposing factors/risk factors**

    A. Substance abuse may be caused by specific alterations in opiate receptors and neurotransmitters, learned coping mechanisms, or genetic predisposition.

    B. Alcohol is the most frequently encountered drug of abuse owing to its low cost and high level of availability.

    C. Frequently substance abusers mix alcohol with other drugs; this can make withdrawal difficult

    D. Withdrawal from central nervous system (CNS) depressants and from alcohol has the potential for a fatal outcome. Alcohol withdrawal may progress into potentially fatal delirium tremens (DTs) if treatment for withdrawal is not initiated (a 5%–10% mortality rate is associated with DTs, even if treated)

    E. Cannabis, CNS stimulants, opiates, hallucinogens, and inhalants/solvents

        1. Commonly abused drugs that can be stopped abruptly without life-threatening results

        2. Although opiate withdrawal is uncomfortable physically, it is not fatal

III. **Subjective findings**

    A. Symptoms vary according to the substance abused

    B. Most persons who abuse drugs look for the mood-altering features of the substance or the recreational/euphoric/hallucinogenic effects

IV. **Physical examination findings**

    A. Physical findings vary according to the substance ingested (withdrawal from CNS depressants can be delayed because of residual in body fat, with symptoms appearing 5–8 days after the last dose)

    B. Withdrawal syndrome from alcohol is common and is a serious medical concern

        1. Early symptoms of alcohol withdrawal include the following:

            a. Elevated temperature, blood pressure, and pulse

            b. Anxiety

            c. Diaphoresis

        2. If untreated, the patient may progress to delirium tremens, with the following symptoms:

            a. Auditory/visual hallucinations

            b. Seizures

            c. Death

    C. Currently, which patient will go into DTs can be predicted only by monitoring of vital signs

V. **Laboratory/diagnostic assessment**

    A. Blood/urine drug screen to determine the substance(s) abused; this information will govern medical management

B. Blood alcohol level to determine approximate blood alcohol content. Individuals who have abused alcohol over many years may have high blood alcohol levels yet still go into withdrawal if they experience a sudden drop in their usual alcohol intake/blood alcohol level.

C. Liver function studies (to detect elevated liver enzymes, which indicate liver damage) including ammonia level (to determine risk for alcohol-induced hepatic encephalopathy)

D. General chemistry for electrolytes to monitor decreased levels of potassium, sodium, and magnesium

E. Serum amylase levels (to detect pancreatitis)

F. Complete blood count (to reveal infectious processes, gastrointestinal bleeding, and anemia)

G. Carbohydrate-deficient transferrin to detect prolonged ingestion of high amounts of alcohol

H. CAGE screening test for alcohol dependence:
  1. C: Have you ever felt the need to cut down on your drinking?
  2. A: Have people annoyed you by criticizing your drinking?
  3. G: Have you ever felt guilty about your drinking?
  4. E: Have you ever had a drink first thing in the morning to steady your nerves or get rid of a hangover (eye-opener)?

I. Addiction Research Foundation Clinical Institute Withdrawal Assessment (CIWA-Ar) (Table 75.5)
  1. The CIWA-Ar is an assessment tool that has been developed to measure potential for withdrawal.
  2. A score of less than 10 is considered to indicate a mild withdrawal that does not require medication
  3. A score greater than 10 with or without a history of withdrawal indicates that medication is needed

VI. **Management**

A. Possible pharmacological therapy for alcohol withdrawal
  1. More than 125 regimens for the treatment of alcohol withdrawal have been published. Practitioners should use the regimen approved by their institution. Regimens may include:
     a. Symptom-triggered (if staff is trained to assess with Clinical Institute Withdrawal Assessment for Alcohol [CIWA])
     b. Fixed schedule therapy (for settings where staff is not fully trained to assess CIWA)
  2. Individual medical status of all patients must be considered and their vital signs monitored before and during withdrawal

B. Intravenous medication used for DTs (see Table 75.3)
  1. Rehydration up to several liters of saline per day as indicated
  2. Treat hypertension and tachycardia, monitor on telemetry or cardiac monitoring
  3. Correction of electrolyte imbalance if needed
  4. Hypoglycemia prevention

Table 75.5 Clinical institute withdrawal assessment for alcohol

Withdrawal effects from least to most serious								
Nausea/ vomiting	No N/V	Mild nausea, no vomiting			Intermittent nausea with dry heaves			Constant nausea, frequent dry heaves and vomiting
Tactile disturbance	None	Very mild itching, pins and needles, burning or numbness	Mild itching, pins and needles, burning or numbness	Moderate itching, pins and needles, burning or numbness	Moderate severe hallucinations	Severe hallucinations	Extremely severe hallucinations	Continuous hallucinations
Tremor	No tremor	Not visible but can be felt fingertip to fingertip			Moderate, with patient's arm extended			Severe, even with arms not extended
Auditory disturbance	Not present	Very mild harshness or ability to frighten	Mild harshness or ability to frighten	Moderate harshness or ability to frighten	Moderately severe hallucinations	Severe hallucinations	Extremely severe hallucinations	Continuous hallucinations
Paroxysmal sweats	No sweat visible			Beads of sweat obvious on forehead				Drenching sweats
Visual disturbance	Not present	Very mild sensitivity	Mild sensitivity	Moderate sensitivity	Moderately severe hallucinations	Severe hallucinations	Extremely severe hallucinations	Continuous hallucinations

Table 75.6 Clinical institute withdrawal assessment for alcohol

Withdrawal effects from least to most serious

Anxiety	No anxiety, at ease	Mildly anxious			Moderately anxious, or guarded, so anxiety is inferred			Equivalent to acute panic states, as seen in severe delirium or acute schizophrenic reactions
Headache	Not present	Very mild	Mild	Moderate	Moderately severe	Severe	Very severe	Extremely severe
Agitation	Normal activity	Somewhat more than normal activity			Moderately fidgety and restless			Paces back and forth during most of the interview, or constantly thrashes about
Orientation/ clouding of sensorium	Oriented, can do serial addition	Cannot do serial additions or is uncertain about date	Disoriented for date by no more than two calendar days	Disoriented by date for more than two calendar days	Disoriented for place and/or person			

5. Thiamine, 100 mg IV, PO, or IM daily for at least 3 days, multivitamin 1 tablet PO daily

6. Diazepam (Valium) or lorazepam (Ativan) can be used as a slow intravenous push to sedate and to prevent withdrawal seizures. The following regimen of intravenous medication is given until the patient is calm:

    a. Lorazepam, 0.1 mg/kg at 2.0 mg/min

    b. Diazepam, 0.15 mg/kg at 2.5 mg/min

7. After the patient is calm, doses are individualized according to the patient's needs and tolerance to the effects of the medication, with care taken to not depress respirations.

C. Oral medication used for mild to moderate withdrawal symptoms (see Table 75.3)

    1. Alcohol withdrawal

        a. Lorazepam (Ativan), 2 mg PO every 2 hr as needed for withdrawal symptoms (individualize dose). Use CIWA-Ar every 1–2 hr to determine need (see Table 75.6)

        b. Second 48 hr: reduce dose and decrease frequency; after 96 hr, discontinue

        c. In patients with liver impairment

            i. Lorazepam (Ativan), 2 mg PO every 2 hr PRN for withdrawal symptoms

            ii. However, the dose must be slowly tapered over several days, owing to rapid excretion

    2. Sedative/hypnotic withdrawal

        a. Benzodiazepines

            i. Although a Cochrane review of the evidence-based management of benzodiazepine withdrawal recommends the use of phenobarbital because of its high overdose potential, it is reserved for hospitalized patients only. Current literature suggests the following for treatment of benzodiazepine withdrawal:

                (a) Treatment of withdrawal/detoxification in patients physically dependent on benzodiazepines is similar to treatment of alcohol withdrawal; chlordiazepoxide (Librium), 50 mg PO 3 times a day, or lorazepam (Ativan), 2 mg PO 3 times a day. Maintain initial dosage for 5 days, gradually taper over an additional 5 days. Longer durations may be required/necessary depending on severity of withdrawal symptoms

        b. Barbiturates

        i. Abuse problems with barbiturates are similar to benzodiazepines. Withdrawal from barbiturates should be handled similarly to interventions for the abuse of alcohol and benzodiazepines

  3. Opiate withdrawal

    a. Well managed with clonidine (Catapres), 0.1 mg PO four times a day (can titrate if needed to maximum of 1 mg/day for 2–4 days after cessation of opioids, then taper and discontinue by 7–10 days), or through patch and symptom management of gastrointestinal pain, insomnia, and anxiety with appropriate medications.

      i. Clonidine patches:

        (a) 50 kg: two clonidine TTS-1 (0.1 mg/24 hr) patches

        (b) 50–91 kg: two TTS-2 (0.2 mg/24 hr) patches

        (c) Greater than 91 kg: two or three TTS-2 (0.2 mg/24 hr) patches

D. Referral to mental health and 12-step recovery groups (e.g., Alcoholics Anonymous and Narcotics Anonymous) is very important. For sedative/hypnotic/opiate withdrawal, refer to substance abuse specialist

ANXIETY

I. **Definition**

  A. Subjective acute or chronic state of emotional discomfort and apprehension that mobilizes physiologic general adaptation to stress

II. **Etiology/incidence/predisposing factors**

  A. Anxiety is an emotional and physiologic response to stress

  B. Anxiety is a common response to medical problems and surgery

III. **Subjective findings**

  A. Commonly reported symptoms

    1. Restlessness/muscle tension

    2. Problems falling asleep

    3. Apprehension/worry/fear

    4. Depression

    5. Agitation/irritability

    6. Feeling threatened

    7. Overwhelmed/out of control

    8. Panic

  B. Physical complaints

    1. Diarrhea

    2. Urinary frequency/urgency

    3. Indigestion/vomiting

    4. Dry mouth

    5. Muscle stiffness

    6. Headache

       7. Racing heart/palpitations

IV.   **Physical examination findings**

    A. Acute manifestations

      1. Trembling

      2. Diaphoresis

      3. Vital signs elevated

      4. Pupils dilated

    B. Chronic problems

      1. Hypertension

      2. Muscular tension

V.   **Management**

    A. First rule out physical causes of anxiety or restlessness such as:

      1. Decreased oxygen saturation

      2. Pain that is insufficiently controlled

    B. Listening to a patient's concerns can relieve mild anxiety

    C. Benzodiazepines, such as lorazepam, can be used to relieve anxiety on a short-term basis (intravenous administration requires hospital protocol and constant monitoring) (see Table 75.3)

      1. Benzodiazepines should be used with caution in the elderly because they may cause confusion and agitation

    D. Buspirone (BuSpar) or a selective serotonin reuptake inhibitor are preferred over benzodiazepines when the patient has an established diagnosis of an anxiety disorder or major depressive disorder; does not provide immediate relief (see Table 75.3)

    E. Refer the patient to a mental health specialist for chronic anxiety, which can be treated by cognitive therapy or biofeedback

CRISIS INTERVENTION

I.   **Definition**

    A. Method of brief counseling to help individuals, families, or groups to cope with stressors

    B. Crisis can occur when individuals encounter medical problems or life-threatening situations

    C. Patients, family members, and hospital staff can develop an emotional crisis as a result of being faced with overwhelming issues.

    D. Individuals in crisis may or may not have preexisting mental health problems

II.   **Etiology/predisposing factors/risk factors**

    A. Common causes of crisis

      1. Sudden illness

      2. Loss of body parts

      3. Loss of ability to carry out normal life roles

      4. Threat of death

      5. Accidents

      6. Financial or relationship problems

    B. Individuals with a history of poor coping skills or emotional rigidity are particularly vulnerable

III. **Subjective findings**

    A. Anger (often with medical personnel)

    B. Denial of problem

    C. Depression

    D. Increased anxiety

    E. Slowed thought processes

    F. Difficulty with problem-solving

IV. **Management**

    A. Listen to the patient's concerns; the goal is to encourage use of coping skills that have been successful in the past

    B. Ask about thoughts and feelings; determine the patient's perceptions. Assist to develop realistic perceptions (use cognitive restructuring to reduce "catastrophizing")

    C. Focus on the present, and elicit available social supports

    D. Have the patient further clarify and focus on solving the current problem

    E. Discuss who or what agency may assist in meeting the patient's needs; clarify with the patient what must be done to resolve the problem

    F. Help the patient to make a realistic plan for problem resolution as well as contingency plans

    G. Refer to social services or other agencies as appropriate to the situation

    H. Medication is not used with individuals who do not have emotional problems owing to its hindering effect on problem-solving abilities

GRIEF

I. **Definition**

    A. Emotional state that occurs in response to the actual or perceived loss of a significant person, animal, or object in a person's life

    B. Acute grief lasts up to several weeks; however, the grieving process can take years to resolve

    C. Dysfunctional grief occurs when the grieving person cannot carry out normal activities of daily living (ADLs) after 3 months

II. **Etiology/incidence/predisposing factors**

    A. Most people have experienced grief over a loss

    B. Predisposing factors include the following:

        1. Emotional closeness

        2. Positive quality of a relationship

        3. Prior experiences with loss

    C. Support of significant others may ameliorate; lack of support may result in dysfunctional grieving

    D. Chronic stress-related medical problems may worsen

III. **Subjective findings**

    A. Extreme emotional pain/depression (common)

B. Physical pain and exhaustion/sleeping problems
C. Relief over the end of suffering
D. Remorse/guilt
E. Emptiness
F. Sense of loss of control or loss of direction and purpose
G. Anger
H. Feeling abandoned (common)/loss of part of identity
   1. Anxiety (common)
I. Dreaming about, and preoccupation with, the image of the lost (common)
J. Suicidal and homicidal thoughts and psychosis (not as common, but suicide risk should be assessed)

IV. **Physical examination findings**
A. Disheveled appearance
B. Poor eye contact
C. Depressed affect

V. **Management**
A. Listening to the grieving person is the best method of providing early therapy
B. Referral to local grief support groups can aid recovery
C. Medication is not recommended in early grief
D. Dysfunctional grief sometimes results in depression; the patient may need a psychiatric referral for antidepressant medication or psychotherapy if grief is prolonged or disabling, or causes suicidality

SEXUALITY

I. **Definition**
A. Expression of a person's identification and feelings about intimacy, sexual attraction, and identity as a human being

II. **Principles**
A. Humans have inherent needs for love and closeness
B. Both heterosexual and homosexual displays of affection can cause negative reactions depending on the situation and persons involved
C. Homosexual orientation is viewed as an alternative way of being, possibly genetically based, rather than as an illness or disorder.
D. Patients may express sexual feelings toward health care providers
E. Patients may have complex relationships with significant others (e.g., adulterous lovers and homosexual affairs) that may cause guilt, embarrassment, depression, or other feelings.
F. It is important for the health care provider to be nonjudgmental about the patient's relationships or focus of affection.

III. **Subjective findings/physical examination findings**
A. Sexual assessment
   1. Discuss whether the patient has any concerns about sexual function

2. Inquire about significant others who may be involved with the patient

3. Explore whether the person is involved with multiple sexual partners, which may predispose to sexually transmitted infections (STIs)

4. Discuss safer sex or contraceptive practices and history of STIs

5. Assess whether the patient is comfortable with his or her sexual orientation

B. Symptoms of STIs: observe for discharges, lesions, or other indications

IV. **Laboratory/diagnostic assessment**

A. HIV and other STI testing may require patient consent; provide counseling if test results are positive

V. **Management**

A. Empathy, support, and listening to patients facilitate expression of sexual concerns, problems with sexual performance, and other sexuality issues

B. Referral to an HIV support group and counseling improves survival rates

C. Refer to an internist, urologist, obstetrician-gynecologist, or psychiatrist PRN for workup of sexual dysfunction

DELIRIUM IN THE ACUTE CARE SETTING

I. **Definition**

A. The acute onset of confusion, excitement, incoherent speech, and agitation

B. Delirium is sometimes confused with psychosis, mood disorder, and dementia (see Table 75.6)

II. **Etiology/incidence/predisposing factors/risk factors**

A. Causes of delirium

1. Central nervous system disease

2. Systemic disease

3. Interaction effects of withdrawal or intoxication from drugs or toxic agents (such as mercury or other heavy metals)

B. Approximately 30% of intensive care patients develop delirium

C. Risk factors for development of delirium include the following:

1. Age: young children and those older than 60 years

2. Preexisting brain damage or dementia

3. History of alcoholism

4. Diabetes

5. Malnutrition

6. Cancer

D. Estimated mortality rate in 3 months is 23% to 33%

III. **Subjective findings**

A. Onset is acute, and symptoms worsen at night (see Table 75.5, Essential Features).

Table 75.6	Comparison of delirium with dementia	
	Delirium	**Dementia**
Onset	Sudden; days or weeks. Associated with a physical stressor	Gradual; months or years
Essential Features	Clouded sensorium, irritability and anxiety, misperception of sensory stimuli, possible hallucinations, lucid periods, alternating with confusion, suspiciousness, agitation	Memory loss, decreased intellectual functioning (confabulation and circumstantiality), loss of executive function
Causes	Toxins, alcohol/drug abuse, CNS or cardiac infarction, hypoxia, head trauma, adverse effects of medications, infections, electrolyte imbalance, poor nutrition, anesthesia, tumors, endocrine problems, impactions in the elderly	Neurotransmitter deficit, cortical atrophy, ventricular dilatation, cerebrovascular accident (multi-infarct dementia), Lewy bodies, Alzheimer's disease, Parkinson's disease, Huntington's chorea
Age	Any age	Usually older than 60 years

Note: CNS = central nervous system.

    B. Impaired memory, thinking, and judgment
    C. Clouding of consciousness, inattention, and disorientation
    D. Also usually present are the following:
        1. Perception disturbances
        2. Incoherent speech
        3. Disrupted sleep
        4. Poor insight
        5. Fear or acute anxiety
IV.   **Physical examination findings**
    A. Assessment may reveal the underlying medical cause
    B. Findings often reflect underlying medical conditions and may include some of the following:
        1. Arrhythmia, bradycardia, or tachycardia
        2. Cardiomegaly
        3. Papilledema
        4. Fever
        5. Hypotension or hypertension
        6. Carotid bruits
        7. Enlarged thyroid
        8. Liver enlargement
        9. Positive Babinski sign
      10. Pupil dilation

C. In delirium, cognitive decline is rapid, as opposed to dementia, in which onset of symptoms is often long and gradual, and the history of mental deterioration is progressive.

V. Laboratory/diagnostic assessment

A. Complete blood count with differential, thyroid function studies, sexually transmitted infection tests, electrolyte and serum amylase levels, and hepatic profile

B. Urinalysis

C. Blood and urine drug screens

D. Electrocardiography

E. Chest x-ray

F. Electroencephalography (slowed or focal activity usually indicates delirium)

G. Lumbar puncture for analysis of cerebral spinal fluid to rule out tertiary syphilis

   1. CT scan of the brain to rule out subdural hematoma or infarcts

H. Mini-mental state examination (verbal and written screening test of memory, ability to think abstractly, and motor and cognitive functions)

VI. Management

A. Treating the underlying medical condition is vital to resolving delirium

B. Failure in resolving delirium may rapidly lead to long-term cognitive impairment; just treating the agitation and psychosis is insufficient.

C. Efforts to reduce anxiety and agitation, including the maintenance of patient comfort, the attention to clinical needs, the provision of adequate analgesia, the frequent reorientation, and the optimization of the environment to maintain normal sleep patterns, should be attempted before administering sedatives or antipsychotics.

D. Acute psychotic agitation (see Tables 75.3 & 75.4)

   1. Lorazepam (Ativan); olanzapine (Zyprexa), 2.5 mg for patient with dementia, PO (use rapid dissolving) or IM; haloperidol (Haldol)*

   2. Subsequent doses should be given every 1–2 hr until the patient is calm: resume if agitation recurs. (Note: This is for rapid tranquilization only and has no benefit in rapidly reducing psychosis.)

   3. Benzodiazepines may worsen delirium, especially in the elderly, although lorazepam, 2 mg (1 mg if frail, small stature, or older than 65) IV bolus, is sometimes used for treatment of delirium

   4. If the patient is lucid, oral quetiapine (Seroquel), olanzapine (Zyprexa), risperidone (Risperdal), or haloperidol (Haldol), may be given; management with the lowest effective dose is preferred if the client is elderly and/or dementia has been diagnosed.

E. Patient should be constantly supervised until agitation clears and should be monitored closely until stable

F. Medical, neurologic, and psychiatric consultations

1. Although injectable haloperidol is approved by the FDA only for intramuscular injection, there is considerable evidence from the medical literature that intravenous administration of haloperidol is a relatively common "off-label" clinical practice, primarily for treatment of severe agitation. Higher doses and intravenous administration of haloperidol appear to be associated with a higher risk of QT prolongation and Torsades de pointes (TdP). Because of this risk of TdP and QT prolongation, ECG monitoring is recommended if haloperidol is given intravenously.

ACUTE AGITATION (PSYCHOSIS RELATED TO MENTAL ILLNESS)

I. **Definition**
   A. Symptoms of fear, irrational responses, and hyperactivity related to schizophrenia or bipolar disorder
   B. Patients with established psychiatric diagnoses present to acute care settings with the same illnesses as are seen in the general population
   C. Assess first for physical reasons for symptoms
   D. Persons with preexisting mental illness are vulnerable to delirium

II. **Etiology/incidence/predisposing factors**
   A. Schizophrenia occurs in approximately 1% of the population, as does bipolar disorder
   B. Persons with well-managed psychiatric illness may experience an exacerbation when under extreme stress (such as a serious illness)
   C. Stress can precipitate a first episode of schizophrenia or mania
   D. Persons who have difficulty with reality testing may have trouble understanding the acute care situation and may respond with confusion, fear, or anger
   E. Persons who are taking certain psychiatric medications (olanzapine particularly) may be admitted with new-onset diabetes

III. **Subjective findings**
   A. Schizophrenia
      1. Verbal responses when no one is present (auditory hallucinations of voices)
      2. Fear with no apparent precipitant
      3. Physical restlessness
      4. Incoherent responses to questions
      5. Disorientation to person or place
   B. Mania
      1. Rapid, pressured speech, and racing thoughts
      2. Physical hyperactivity
      3. History of not sleeping
      4. Extreme impatience
      5. Insistence on directing treatment
      6. Anger and aggression when thwarted

IV. **Management**

A. After ruling out physical causes, inquire about psychiatric history and medications. (Resume patient's prior-to-admission medication regimen/chronic medication as soon as clinically appropriate)

B. Use simple language to provide one statement, question, or direction at a time

C. Explain everything you do

D. Respond to irrational behavior with calm, firm direction

E. Refer for psychiatric evaluation

F. Olanzapine (Zydis), 5 mg PO once or quetiapine (Seroquel) 50 mg PO once, may be useful for acute agitation

BIBLIOGRAPHY

American Foundation for Suicide Prevention. (2013). *Risk factors and warning signs*. Retrieved from http://www.afsp.org/preventing-suicide/risk-factors-and-warning-signs

American Geriatrics Society. (2012). American Geriatrics Society updated beers criteria for potentially inappropriate medication use in older adults. *Journal of the American Geriatrics Society, 60*(4), 616–631. doi:10.1111/j.1532–5415.2012.03923.x

American Psychiatric Association. (2013). *Diagnostic and statistical manual of mental disorders* (5th ed.). Washington, DC: American Psychiatric Publishing.

American Psychiatric Association. (2010). *Practice guideline for the treatment of patients with major depression* (3rd ed.). Retrieved from http://psychiatryonline.org/content.aspx?bookid=28&sectionid=1667485

Barr, J., Fraser, G. L., Puntillo, K., Ely, E. W., Gélinas, C., Dasta, J. F., . . . American College of Critical Care Medicine. (2013). Clinical practice guidelines for the management of pain, agitation, and delirium in adult patients in the intensive care unit. *Critical Care Medicine,41*(1), 278–280. doi:10.1097/CCM.0b013e3182783b72

Boyd, M. A. (2013). *Psychiatric nursing: Contemporary practice* (5th ed.). Philadelphia, PA: Lippincott Williams & Wilkins.

Center for Substance Abuse Treatment (2009). *Detoxification and substance abuse training manual*. Rockville, MD: Substance Abuse and Mental Health Services Administration.

DiPiro, J., Talbert, R. L., Yee, G., Matzke, G., Wells, B., & Posey, L. M. (2011). *Pharmacotherapy: A pathophysiologic approach* (8th ed.). New York, NY: McGraw-Hill.

Halter, M. J. (2014). *Varcarolis' foundations of psychiatric mental health nursing practice*. St Louis, MO: Elsevier.

Juve-Udina, M.-E., Perez, E. Z., Padres, N. F., Samartino, M. G., Garcia, M. R., Creus, M. C., . . . Calvo, C. M. (2013). Basic nursing care: Retrospective evaluation of communication and psychosocial interventions documented by nurses in the acute care setting. *Journal of Nursing Scholarship, 46*(1), 65–72.

Kneisl, C. R., & Trigoboff, E. (2013). *Contemporary psychiatric-mental health nursing* (3rd ed.). Upper Saddle River, NJ: Pearson.

Pandharipande, P. P., Girard, T. D., Jackson, J. C., Morandi, A., Thompson, J. L., Pun, B. T., . . . BRAIN-ICU Study Investigators. (2013). Long-term cognitive impairment after critical illness. *New England Journal of Medicine, 369*, 1306–1316.

Patel, S. C., & Jakopac, K. A. (2012). *Manual of psychiatric nursing skills*. Sudbury, MA: Jones & Bartlett.

Rees, J. P. (2009). *Substance withdrawal syndrome*. New York, NY: Nova Biomedical Books.

Rhoads, J., & Murphy, P. M. (2013). *Nurses'clinical consult to psychopharmacology*. New York, NY: Springer.

Suicide Prevention Resource Center. (2011). *Is your patient suicidal? Emergency department poster kit*. Retrieved from http://www.sprc.org/for-providers/emergency-departments

Townsend, M. C. (2014). *Essentials of psychiatric mental health nursing* (6th ed.). Philadelphia, PA: FA Davis.

Tintinalli, J. E., Stapczynski, J., Ma, O. J., Cline, D. M., Cydulka, R. K., & Meckler, G. D. (2011). *Tintinalli's emergency medicine: A comprehensive study guide* (7th ed.). New York, NY: McGraw-Hill.

Tusaie, K. R., & Fitzpatrick, J. J. (Eds.) (2012). *Advanced practice psychiatric nursing*. New York, NY: Springer.

U.S. Preventive Services Task Force. (2013). *Screening and behavioral counseling interventions in primary care to reduce alcohol misuse*. Retrieved from http://www.uspreventiveservicestaskforce.org/uspstf/uspsdrin.htm

Videbeck, S. (2013). *Psychiatric-mental health nursing* (6th ed.). Philadelphia, PA: Lippincott Williams & Wilkins.

CHAPTER 76

Management of the Patient in Shock

VALERIE K. SABOL • ROBERT BLESSING •
THOMAS W. BARKLEY, JR. • CHARLENE M. MYERS

SHOCK

I. **Definition**
   A. Acute syndrome of organ and system dysfunction precipitated by failure of the circulation to meet metabolic needs
   B. Inadequate or inappropriately distributed tissue perfusion results in generalized cellular hypoxia and is often referred to as shock states
   C. Shock can develop within minutes or hours of an initial insult and, if not promptly reversed, can rapidly progress to death

II. **Pathophysiology**
   A. The primary physiologic disturbance is impaired cellular function due to decreased blood flow and an inability to meet metabolic demands.
   B. In shock states, oxygen consumption is greater than oxygen delivery, resulting in cellular hypoxia and dysfunction.
   C. Reduced oxygen and nutrient supply → anaerobic metabolism → production of acid (lactic and pyruvic) → decreased adenosine triphosphate (ATP) and reduced energy
      1. Acid further depresses cellular function
      2. As pH decreases, powerful enzymes (proteolytic) released from the cell destroy the cell membrane and digest the cellular contents. Once integrity of the cell membrane is lost, cellular changes are irreversible.
   D. Activation of the inflammatory response → release of proinflammatory cytokines (e.g., tumor necrosis factor - α, interleukin-1) and endothelial vasodilating oxygen free radicals, protease, nitric oxide, and other inflammatory mediators

Table 76.1	Hemodynamic alterations in shock states				Distributive
Parameter/ normal range	**Hypovolemic**	**Cardiogenic**	**Obstructive**	**Sepsis**	**Anaphylactic and Neurogenic**
Cardiac output, 4–8 L/minute	Low	Low	Low	High, then low	Low
Cardiac index, 2.5–4.5 L/minute/m²	Low	Low	Low	High, then low	Low
Right atrial pressure, 0–8 mmHg	Low	High	High	Low, then high	Low
Pulmonary artery diastolic pressure, 6–12 mmHg	Low	High	High	Low, then high	Low
Pulmonary capillary wedge pressure, 6–12 mmHg	Low	High	High	Low, then high	Low
Systemic vascular resistance, 800–1200 dynes/sec/cm⁻⁵	High	High	SVR low PVR high	Low	Low
Mixed venous oxygen saturation, 60%–80%	Low	Low	High	High, then low	Low

Note. L/minute/m² = liter per minute per square meter; mmHg = millimeter of mercury; PVR = pulmonary vascular resistance; SVR = systemic vascular resistance. From "Introduction to Critical Care Nursing" by M. L. Sole, D. Klein, and M. Moseley, 2012, *Hemodynamic alterations in shock states*, p. 6e. Copyright 2012 by Saunders. Adapted with permission.

III. Classification of Shock
 A. Hypovolemic
 B. Cardiogenic
 C. Obstructive (extracardiac)
 D. Distributive
  1. Sepsis
  2. Anaphylaxis
  3. Neurogenic

IV. Etiology
 A. Cardiac output falls dependent on cause (see Table 76.1)
  1. Decreased cardiac contractility, as from
   a. Acute myocardial infarction
   b. Cardiomyopathy
   c. Congestive heart failure
   d. Valvular failure (e.g., stenosis, regurgitation)
  2. Decreased circulating volume, as from
   a. Hypovolemia
   b. Hemorrhage
  3. Obstruction of central blood flow due to compression of the heart or great vessels
  4. Altered vascular resistance, such as vasodilatation and decreased peripheral vascular resistance, resulting in venous pooling and inadequate venous return, which leads to relative hypovolemia, as from
   a. Anaphylaxis
   b. Sepsis
   c. Neurologic disorders
 B. Compensatory mechanisms are activated.
  1. Nervous system compensation: Decreased cardiac output (CO) and blood pressure (BP) stimulate pressoreceptors (baroreceptors) to send impulses to the vasomotor center of the medulla. Here, the sympathetic nervous system (SNS) is stimulated, and norepinephrine is discharged:
   a. Increased activity of sweat glands
   b. Increased respiratory rate (RR) and depth
   c. Heart:
    i. Increased heart rate (HR) and increased force of contraction, which in turn, increase cardiac output (CO) and blood pressure (BP)
    ii. Vasodilatation of coronary arteries helps increase oxygenation to the heart muscle.
    iii. Vasodilatation of skeletal muscle vasculature
    iv. Dilatation of pupils

      v. Vasoconstriction of vasculature in skin, GI tract, and kidneys; this increases BP and enhances venous return, thus increasing CO and BP; vasoconstriction shunts blood to priority organs (e.g., brain, heart)

  2. Hormonal compensation

    a. SNS stimulation activates the anterior pituitary to release adrenocorticotropic hormone (ACTH)

    b. The adrenal cortex is activated to increase glucocorticoids in the liver; this enhances glycogenolysis and, in turn, serum glucose.

    c. The adrenal cortex also promotes the release of aldosterone, which increases Na reabsorption and, in turn, H_2O reabsorption.

    d. This results in increased fluid volume, enhances CO, and decreased urine output.

  3. Chemical compensation

    a. Pulmonary blood flow is reduced because of decreased CO, resulting in ventilation/perfusion abnormalities; some alveoli contain O_2 (adequate ventilation) but do not have adequate blood flow through the capillary bed (poor perfusion).

    b. Low oxygen tension stimulates chemoreceptors in the aorta and the carotid arteries, leading to increased rate and depth of respirations → hyperventilation → CO_2 blown off → respiratory alkalosis → vasoconstriction of cerebral vessels along with decreased O_2 tension → cerebral hypoxia and ischemia

V. Stages of Shock

A. Nonprogressive Stage—Stage I

  1. Early changes occur at cellular level

  2. No real obvious signs or symptoms (i.e., relatively normal vital signs and tissue perfusion)

B. Progressive Stage—Stage II

  1. Compensatory mechanisms that maintain normal perfusion begin to fail and circulatory and metabolic derangements become more pronounced

  2. Cellular function

    a. Arteriolar vasoconstriction → decreased capillary blood flow → decreased O_2 to cells → decreased ATP → increased anaerobic metabolism → local metabolic acidosis

  3. Capillary dynamics

    a. Capillary hydrostatic pressure increases: precapillary sphincters dilate in response to acidosis; this allows blood to flow freely into the capillary bed, while the postcapillary sphincter remains constricted, which causes accumulation of blood in the capillaries and pushes fluid into the tissues

    b. Protein leaks out, leading to decreased colloid osmotic pressure

    c. The result is decreased intravascular volume → interstitial edema → increased viscosity of blood → increased resistance to flow → capillary sludging → further impairment of flow

    d. Decreased volume and impaired flow → decreased venous return and decreased CO → decreased BP → decreased coronary artery perfusion → ischemia → arrhythmia or infarction

    e. Decreased CO perpetuates SNS response

4. Systemic circulation

    a. Blood is shunted to priority organs (i.e., brain, heart)

    b. Weak or absent pulses and cold extremities reflect severe vasoconstriction

    c. Decreased peripheral circulation may lead to ischemia of distal extremities, which provides new ports of entry for microbes

    d. A serum lactate level that remains elevated after initial resuscitation is a poor prognostic indicator

5. Specific organ systems

    a. Brain

        i. Decreased cerebral blood flow leads to decreased level of consciousness (LOC)

    b. Kidneys

        i. Urine output of less than 0.5 ml/kg/hr is considered a sign of shock; urine output decreases as the result of reduced renal perfusion → ischemia → acute tubular necrosis → acute renal failure

    c. GI system

        i. Prolonged decreased perfusion may lead to a paralytic ileus or ulceration with an increased incidence of hemorrhage and a decreased line of defense → translocation of bacteria into the bloodstream

        ii. Decreased perfusion to the GI musculature → slowing of intestinal activity → decreased bowel sounds, distention, nausea, constipation, and high residuals of enteral feedings

    d. Liver

        i. Kupffer cells cannot perform phagocytosis → decreased line of defense

        ii. Impaired metabolic activities (such as gluconeogenesis, glucolysis, and fat metabolism)

        iii. Buildup of waste products (ammonia, lactic acid)

        iv. Liver cells eventually become ischemic and die, resulting in an initial increase aspartate aminotransferase (AST), alanine aminotransferase (ALT), and lactate, dehydrogenase (LDH). Elevated bilirubin and jaundice may persist while other liver enzyme levels may begin to decline.

    e. Pancreas

        i. Cells become ischemic and release myocardial depressant factor (MDF), which directly depresses myocardial contractility

        ii. Increases in amylase and lipase are caused by pancreatic ischemia

    f. Lungs

        i. The most significant respiratory complication is acute respiratory distress syndrome (ARDS).

            (a) Reduced pulmonary blood flow and increased pulmonary

            (b) Vascular resistance → increased pulmonary capillary permeability → increased interstitial edema → atelectasis and alveolar edema (noncardiogenic pulmonary edema)

            (c) Decreased surfactant → atelectasis

            (d) Decreased compliance → hypoventilation and hypoxemia that is refractory to oxygen therapy

6. Clinical signs and symptoms of Stage II

    a. Decreased LOC

    b. Decreased pulse pressure

        i. Systolic blood pressure decreases in relation to decreased stroke volume (SV)

        ii. Diastolic blood pressure increases in relation to increased vasoconstriction (narrowed pulse pressure)

    c. Tachycardia (may exceed 150 beats/min)

    d. Weak and thready pulse

    e. Decreased filling time and decreased coronary artery perfusion may lead to myocardial ischemia and arrhythmia

    f. Decreased cellular metabolism leads to reduced temperature and heat production

    g. Skin pale or cyanotic, cold and clammy

        i. Capillary filling time (CFT) exceeds 3 seconds

    h. Possible jaundice

    i. Decreased urine output

    j. Increased RR, hypoventilation, rales/rhonchi, resonance leading to dullness

    k. Bowel sounds decreased or absent; possible paralytic ileus; bowel sounds may increase if bleeding occurs

C. Irreversible Stage—Stage III

1. The final, irreversible stage of shock, resulting in several vicious cycles

2. Cardiac failure
   a. Coronary perfusion decreases because of increased HR, decreased SV, decreased BP, and lack of perfusion pressure
   b. Contractility is impaired in relation to decreased O_2 delivery, MDF, and acidotic state
   c. CO falls further, resulting in decreased coronary perfusion

3. Acidosis is present in relation to
   a. Poor tissue perfusion, which results in impaired cellular function
   b. Poor renal perfusion, resulting in retention of waste products
   c. Respiratory failure

4. Acidosis results in
   a. Decreased contractility and in turn decreased CO
   b. Loss of vasomotor tone → fluid shift → relative hypovolemia
   c. Leads to additional impairments in tissue perfusion, renal function, and respiratory function

5. Aberrations in blood clotting
   a. Acidosis, decreased intravascular volume, and sluggish capillary flow → further impairment of flow → increased risk for clot formation
   b. May lead to disseminated intravascular coagulation (DIC)

6. Inadequate cerebral blood flow
   a. If cerebral perfusion pressure (CPP) falls, severe ischemia occurs → sympathetic discharge → increased deleterious effects; the patient progresses from being drowsy, confused, and lethargic to a state of unresponsiveness
   b. If ischemia continues, function of vital centers of the brain is depressed
   c. Vasomotor center fails: loss of sympathetic tone → severe decrease in BP → decreased HR, lethal decrease in tissue perfusion → decreased cerebral flow → increased cerebral ischemia → death

VI.   Laboratory Findings in Shock

A. Hyperglycemia

1. Early: increased early in shock as the result of sympathetic stimulation

2. Late: decreased late in shock because of depletion of body glycogen stores and decreased liver function

B. Arterial blood gases

1. Hypoxemia

2. Metabolic acidosis, often with respiratory alkalosis

3. Base deficit elevated, indicating inadequate tissue perfusion

C. Lactate level elevated, indicating inadequate tissue perfusion

D. Total protein and albumin: decreased as the result of leakage from capillaries and decreased synthesis in liver cells

E. BUN and Creatinine
   1. Increased as the result of renal ischemia and the development of acute tubular necrosis (ATN)

F. Sodium
   1. Early: increased early as the result of increased aldosterone that causes renal retention of sodium
   2. Late: increased or decreased late because of ATN

G. Potassium
   1. Early: decreased as the result of increased aldosterone, which causes renal excretion of potassium
   2. Late: increased because of acidosis, cell necrosis, and decreased renal function

H. Chloride
   1. Early: decreased as the result of an alkalotic state and HCO_3 excess
   2. Late: increased because of acidotic state and HCO_3 deficiency

I. Liver enzymes and bilirubin: initially increased because of cell necrosis, may decline with cell death (bilirubin may remain elevated)

J. Creatine phosphokinase (CPK): increased as the result of necrosis of muscle or heart cells

K. Amylase/lipase: increased as the result of necrosis of pancreatic cells

L. Blood cultures: may be positive

M. Hemoglobin/hematocrit
   1. Early in shock: may be increased as the result of fluid leakage from capillaries (hemoconcentration) without adequate fluid resuscitation. Otherwise, decreases when blood loss occurs

N. WBC count: increased because of the body's response to inflammation

O. Platelet count: decreased as the result of platelet aggregation and microemboli

P. Prothrombin time (PT)/partial thromboplastin time (PTT): may be abnormal in cases of liver injury/dysfunction or endovascular injury (e.g., DIC)

Q. Urine measurements
   1. Creatinine clearance: decreased because of impaired renal excretion caused by ATN
   2. Osmolality/specific gravity: may be decreased because of inability of the kidney to concentrate urine

VII. **Universal Management of Shock**
   A. Maintain airway and ventilation.
      1. Continuous O_2 saturation (via pulse oximetry) and frequent ABGs
      2. Administer supplemental O_2 for treatment or prevention of hypoxemia

3. Mechanical ventilation may be necessary to facilitate gas exchange

B. Hemodynamic monitoring (e.g., arterial line, pulmonary artery catheter, echocardiogram and continuous real-time non-invasive hemodynamic monitoring) is a critical tool for assessment of various types of shock; information can be obtained regarding fluid status, contractility of the heart, and effectiveness of vasoactive agents (see Table 76.2)

C. Circulation goals
   1. Maintain hemodynamic support for adequate tissue perfusion and adequate cellular metabolism (e.g., maintain MAP greater than 65 mmHg in sepsis)
   2. Mixed venous oxygen saturation (SvO_2) greater than 65%
   3. Euvolemia (e.g., monitor jugular venous pressure [JVP], central venous pressure [CVP], Stroke/Volume Variation [SVV] and Intake/Output)

D. Fluid therapy
   1. Fluid replacement for cellular nutrition and restoration of tissue perfusion
   2. IV fluids help to restore intravascular volume, maintain oxygen-carrying capacity, and establish hemodynamic stability, which is required for optimal tissue perfusion
   3. Type and amount depend on type of shock, the patient's medical problems, and availability of fluid
   4. Access (e.g., large bore peripheral IVs, intraosseous [IO], central venous catheters [CVC])
   5. Fluid challenges are often given to determine the patient's response
   6. Typically, fluid boluses may be required for initial resuscitation
   7. Monitor urine output: goal greater than 0.5 ml/kg/hr
   8. Judicious use of IV fluids with patients in cardiogenic shock

E. Correct acid-base imbalance
   1. Metabolic acidosis
      a. In severe cases (pH less than 7.10), $NaHCO_3$ may be administered to increase pH to between 7.20 and 7.25, although this treatment remains controversial
      b. Overcorrection of acidosis may precipitate alkalosis
   2. Respiratory acidosis
      a. Mechanical ventilation can be used to assist in "blowing off" excessive CO_2
      b. Mild permissive hypercapnia may be indicated as a lung protective strategy (e.g., keep plateau pressure less than 30 cm H_2O)
   3. Respiratory alkalosis
      a. Maintain ventilator setting to obtain pH goals

F. Pharmacologic treatment: depends on type of shock; different drugs are addressed under each type of shock (see Tables 76.2, 76.3, 76.4, and 76.5)

Table 76.2	Clinical Use of Vasoactive Agents

Selecting a Vasopressor:
No large randomized, well controlled trials to guide the pharmacologic management of hypotension.
Use of vasopressors and positive inotropes is generally based on data from small, often poorly controlled clinical studies.
Selection of the appropriate vasoactive agent should be made on a case by case basis with attention to the known or suspected underlying cause of hypotension.

Hypotension of Unknown Etiology:
For severe hypotension (SBP less than 70), a more potent adrenergic agent such as norepinephrine should be considered.
Dopamine in moderate to high doses may be a reasonable first choice given its combined positive inotropic and vasopressor effects.

Reduced Systemic Vascular Resistance:
The most common clinical situation encountered in the ICU setting: hypotensive patient with peripheral vasodilation and low SVR due to sepsis.
Given the superior potency of norepinephrine and data demonstrating worsening splanchnic perfusion with high dose dopamine, norepinephrine is emerging as the agent of choice for vasodilatory shock in sepsis.
Dopamine may be used as an alternate agent or in cases in which positive inotropic effects are desirable.
Difficult to assess the efficacy of phenylephrine relative to older agents, although its peripheral selectivity and lack of chronotropic effects make it a useful agent in cases of tachycardia or tachyarrhythmias.
Epinephrine is the least selective of the catecholamines and may be added for refractory shock.
Vasopressin is emerging as an alternative to adrenergic agents or in combination.
The ideal vasopressor remains controversial.

Hypotensive Patient With Significant Cardiac Pump Dysfunction:
Dobutamine is the inotropic agent of choice.
With cardiogenic shock and concomitant vasodilation, however, a drug with pressor action is usually needed (dopamine alone or in combination with dobutamine).
For patients with septic shock and myocardial dysfunction, dobutamine can be added to norepinephrine or dopamine for added inotropic support.
For acutely decompensated heart failure, concomitant vasopressor therapy may also be necessary.
Although no single agent is universally superior, dobutamine's ease of use and better side-effect profile, along with milrinone's pharmacokinetic considerations, render milrinone as a secondary agent.
In select situations, milrinone and dobutamine may be used in combination when an adequate cardiac index cannot be obtained with either agent alone.
An important consideration for use of milrinone over dobutamine in ADHF, however, is for patients admitted on β-blocker therapy where there effects of milrinone are not antagonized.

Table 76.3	Inotropic Agents						
Drug	**Dose**	**HR**	**MAP**	**PCWP**	**CO**	**SVR**	**Adverse Effects/Comments**
Dobutamine	2.5–20 mcg/kg/min Increase/decrease by 1 mcg/kg/min at intervals no longer than every 30 minutes Titration parameter: CO; CI	0/+	0	-	+	-	Arrhythmogenic, may potentiate hypokalemia, myocardial ischemia, hypotension/vasodilation Preferred vasoactive agent to treat cardiogenic shock with low output and increased afterload Septic shock with myocardial dysfunction may require norepinephrine plus dobutamine Higher doses may be required for patients previously on β-blockers
Milrinone	Loading dose: 50 mcg/kg over 10 minutes followed by Continuous infusion: 0.125–0.75 mcg/kg/min Increase/decrease by minimum of 0.125 mcg/kg/min at intervals no longer than Q 6 hr Titration parameter: CO; CI	0/+	0/-	-	+	-	Arrhythmogenic, thrombocytopenia, myocardial ischemia, hypotension/vasodilative Loading dose is frequently omitted Reduce dose for renal impairment Requires slower titration compared with dobutamine

Note. + = increase; - = decrease; 0 = no change; HR = heart rate; MAP = mean arterial pressure; PCWP = pulmonary capillary wedge pressure; CO = cardiac output; SVR = systemic vascular resistance.

Table 76.4	Vasodilating Agents			
Drug	**Indication**	**Onset of Action**	**Dosing**	**Comments**
Nitroglycerin	Antianginal for ischemic pain AMI / CHF Hypertensive urgency with ACS	2–5 min	*IV Bolus:* 12.5–25 mcg if no SL or spray given *Continuous Infusion:* 5–300 mcg/min Titrate by 5–10 mcg/min every 5 min to max of 300 mcg/min Titration parameter: SBP, angina	Preferred agent for pre-load reduction Little or no effect on after-load (SVR) Agent of choice for heart failure patients with ischemic component Tolerance may occur within 24–48 hr No phosphodiesterase inhibitors within 24 hr or tadalafil within 48 hr May increase ICP, use with caution in hypertensive encephalopathy Hypotension, flushing, headache, dizziness
Nitroprusside	Hypertensive urgency/emergency CHF (↓ afterload)	Immediate	*Continuous Infusion:* 0.1–5 mcg/kg/min (max: 10 mcg/kg/min) Increase/decrease rate by minimum of 0.5 mcg/kg/min at intervals no longer than Q 15 minutes Titration parameter: SBP, MAP	Primarily utilized in patients with significantly elevated SVR When treatment is prolonged (greater than 24–48 hr) or when renal insufficiency is present, risk of cyanide and thiocyanate toxicity is increased May cause hypotension, CO_2 retention Bradyarrhythmia, hypotension, palpitations, tachyarrhythmia

Table 76.5 Vasopressor Agents*

Drug	Dose	HR	MAP	PCWP	CO	SVR	Adverse Effects/Comments
Norepinephrine	2–40 mcg/min (0.01–0.5 mcg/kg/min) Increase/decrease rate by minimum of 1 mcg/min at intervals no longer than every 30 minutes Titration parameter: MAP; SBP Usual target: MAP greater than 65 OR SBP: 80–100	+	+	+	+	++	Arrhythmias, tissue/myocardial ischemia Most potent vasoconstrictor Drug of first choice for most types of shock
Epinephrine	1–10 mcg/min (0.01–0.2 mcg/kg/min) Increase/decrease rate by minimum of 1 mcg/min at intervals no longer than every 5 minutes Titration parameter: MAP; SBP Usual target: MAP greater than 65 OR SBP: 80–100	+	+	+	++	+	Tachyarrhythmias, tissue ischemia, myocardial ischemia, hyperglycemia Second line or adjunct agent for refractory hypotension First-line for cardiopulmonary resuscitation and anaphylactic shock

Table 76.5	Vasopressor Agents*						
Drug	**Dose**	**HR**	**MAP**	**PCWP**	**CO**	**SVR**	**Adverse Effects/Comments**
Dopamine	0.5–5 mcg/kg/min	0	0	0	0/+	-	Tachycardia, arrhythmias, myocardial ischemia
	5–10 mcg/kg/min	+	+	0	+	0	
	Greater than 10–20 mcg/kg/min	+	+	+	+	++	Dosage-dependent effects vary by individual and have not been reproduced in critically ill patients
	Increase/decrease rate by minimum of 1 mcg/kg/min at intervals no longer than every 30 minutes						May be considered first line agent for select patients (i.e., depressed LV function, bradycardia)
	Titration parameter: MAP; SBP						
	Usual target: MAP greater than 65 OR SBP: 80–100						

Table 76.5	Vasopressor Agents*						
Drug	**Dose**	**HR**	**MAP**	**PCWP**	**CO**	**SVR**	**Adverse Effects/ Comments**
Phenylephrine	50–400 mcg/min (0.5–5 mcg/kg/min) Increase/decrease rate by minimum of 10 mcg/min at intervals no longer than every 15 minutes Titration parameter: MAP; SBP Usual target: MAP greater than 65 OR SBP: 80–100	0	+	0/+	0	++	Reflex bradycardia, decreased renal perfusion Second-line agent Uses: non-cardiogenic hypotension Vasoconstrictor effect similar to norepinephrine Caution use in renal impairment
Vasopressin	0.04 units/min	0	+	0	0	+	Myocardial ischemia, tissue necrosis, and end organ ischemia (doses greater than 0.04 units/minute) Primary use is adjunct therapy Doses greater than 0.04 units/min may lead to cardiac arrest

Note. + = increase; - = decrease; 0 = no change; HR = heart rate; MAP = mean arterial pressure; PCWP = pulmonary capillary wedge pressure; CO = cardiac output; SVR = systemic vascular resistance. *Administration through a central line is preferred for all vasopressor agents

G. Surgical treatment may be necessary to correct underlying etiology (e.g., hemorrhage, valvular disease, resection of obstructive tumor)

H. Nutritional support

1. Patients in shock require increased caloric intake because of their stress state, in which nutritional stores are depleted, resulting in protein catabolism

2. Early nutritional support has been found to preserve the normal immune and defense functions of the GI tract, thereby preventing movement of bacteria and endotoxin across the mucosal barrier and into the systemic circulation

TYPES OF SHOCK

I. **Hypovolemic**

A. Blood volume is inadequate to maintain adequate circulation

B. Caused by exogenous or endogenous loss of circulating volume

C. Associated with a blood volume deficit of at least 15%–25%

D. Etiology

1. Hemorrhagic

   a. Traumatic

      i. Long-bone fractures, which can result in a large amount of blood loss

      ii. Ruptured liver/spleen

      iii. Lacerations of great vessels

   b. Non-traumatic

      i. GI Bleed

      ii. Hemorrhagic pancreatitis

2. Non-hemorrhagic

   a. Impaired venous return caused by obstruction of vena cava

   b. GI losses, as from

      i. Vomiting

      ii. Diarrhea

      iii. Poor oral intake

      iv. Large nasogastric tube aspirate

      v. Fistulas

   c. Renal losses: excessive diuresis may occur in certain conditions (e.g., diabetes insipidus, syndrome of inappropriate ADH [SIADH], Addison's disease) or related to diuretic therapy

   d. Exudative lesions or burns

   e. Excessive diaphoresis

E. Clinical manifestations specific to hypovolemic shock

1. Increased HR, decreased BP

2. Decreased CVP, CO, CI, pulmonary artery pressure (PAP), pulmonary artery occlusion pressure (PAOP)

3. Postural hypotension (Systolic Blood Pressure [SBP] decrease of 20 mmHg or more or heart rate increase of 20 beats/min or more)
4. Flat neck veins

F. Up to 10% of blood volume lost: may produce no symptoms because of compensatory mechanisms or slight tachycardia

G. Less than 15% blood volume lost, patient may exhibit the following:
1. Slight hypotension
2. HR normal or less than 100 beats/min
3. Capillary filling time less than 3 seconds
4. Anxiety or changes in sensorium
5. Orthostasis
6. Urine output adequate (greater than 0.5 ml/kg/hr)

H. 15%–30% blood volume lost; patient may exhibit:
1. MAP greater than 65 mmHg
2. Decreased pulse pressure
3. Tachycardia
4. Cool skin with pallor
5. Poor capillary filling time (greater than 3 seconds)
6. Lethargic, weak
7. Decreased urine output (less than 0.5 ml/kg/hr)
8. RR

I. More than 40% blood volume lost; patient may exhibit the following:
1. Moderate to severe hypotension (MAP less than 65 mmHg)
2. Tachycardia
3. Cold, cyanotic skin
4. LOC severely compromised
5. Oliguria

J. Management specific to hypovolemic shock (see Universal Management of Shock section)
1. Vasopressors are contraindicated until circulating volume has been restored
2. Fluid challenges: 250–500 ml (or greater) bolus of Ringer's lactate or normal saline; repeat boluses if BP or CVP remains low
3. Fluid replacement
   a. Blood/blood products
      i. Transfuse PRN depending on severity of shock
      ii. One unit of packed red blood cells (PRBCs) should increase hematocrit by approximately 3 ml/dl and hemoglobin by 1 gram/dl
      iii. When transfusing blood products, one must consider coagulation factors when not using whole blood (e.g., fresh frozen plasma [FFP] and cryoprecipitate)

        (a) FFP may be indicated to replace clotting factors with the exception of platelets. FFP should be ordered to restore coagulation factors when massive transfusions are required

        (b) Platelets may also be needed to control bleeding that is the result of a low platelet count or platelet dysfunction

  b. Crystalloids

    i. Initial fluid of choice in resuscitation of severe sepsis and septic shock

      (a) Crystalloids are inexpensive, convenient to use, and relatively free of adverse effects, but they are rapidly distributed across intravascular and interstitial cell spaces.

      (b) The two most common crystalloid solutions are Ringer's lactate and normal saline.

      (c) Ringer's lactate contains physiologic concentrations of sodium, chloride, calcium, potassium, and lactate in water and is effective as a volume expander and buffer in the presence of acidosis.

      (d) Normal saline (0.9% sodium chloride in water) increases plasma volume and is used most frequently when no loss of blood has occurred

          1. Usually requires volumes 2–4 times that of colloid to achieve an equivalent hemodynamic response

          2. Be aware that volume expansion is transient and that fluid will accumulate in the interstitial spaces, which may result in pulmonary edema

  c. Colloids (albumin)

    i. Recommended with severe sepsis and septic shock when patients require substantial amounts of crystalloids

    ii. Colloids produce a greater and more sustained increase in plasma volume with associated improvements in cardiovascular function and O_2 transport.

    iii. Plasma protein fractions, such as albumin and Plasmanate, are given when volume loss is caused by plasma rather than blood, such as in burns, third spacing, peritonitis, and bowel obstruction.

    iv. Synthetic plasma expanders are also effective in increasing plasma volume

    v. Monitor patient for adverse effects such as pulmonary edema, coagulopathies, and anaphylactic reactions

4. Military antishock trousers (MAST)

      a. MAST is an external counterpressure device that may be applied to assist with major organ perfusion, although its use is controversial

      b. MAST is useful in trauma patients to help splint fractures of the pelvis and long bones and to tamponade a bleed; compression redistributes blood flow from the peripheral circulation, which increases venous return and results in vital organ perfusion

II. Cardiogenic shock

A. Impaired ability of the heart to pump effectively, resulting in decreased SV and CO and inadequate tissue perfusion; cardiogenic shock consists of decreased cardiac output and evidence of tissue hypoxia in the presence of adequate intravascular volume

B. Results from ineffective contractility caused by the following:

    1. Acute myocardial infarction (AMI)

    2. Arrhythmias

    3. Congestive heart failure (CHF)

    4. Myocardial contusion

    5. Dissecting aortic aneurysm

    6. Surgical or spontaneous damage to valves or valvular heart disease such as:

      a. Acute mitral regurgitation

      b. Rupture of the interventricular septum

      c. Rupture of the free wall

      d. Large right ventricular infarction

    7. Myocarditis

    8. End-stage cardiomyopathy

    9. Septic shock with severe myocardial depression

    10. Any form of severe myocardial damage

C. Clinical findings specific to cardiogenic shock

    1. Increased PAP, PAOP, and SVR; CVP may or may not be elevated, depending on whether the right ventricle is involved, or whether volume from the left side of the heart has backed up into the right side

    2. Decreased SV, CO, and CI; a CI of less than 1.8 L/min/m^2 suggests cardiogenic shock

    3. Left ventricular ejection fraction (EF) significantly reduced on echocardiogram less than 30% if shock due to left ventricular failure; right ventricular failure can be seen on echocardiogram as well

    4. Pulmonary congestion: rales/rhonchi, decreased PaO_2 (partial pressure of oxygen in arterial blood), decreased $PaCO_2$ (partial pressure of carbon dioxide in arterial blood; early), increased $PaCO_2$ (late), and decreased mixed venous O_2 (MVO_2)

5. S3/S4 heart sounds, possibly palpable precordial thrill, rapid/faint pulse, possibly a systolic murmur of mitral regurgitation or ventricular septal defect
6. Peripheral edema
7. Distended neck veins
8. Signs of decreased tissue perfusion
   a. Oliguria
   b. Clouded sensorium
   c. Cool/mottled skin
9. Cardiogenic shock is diagnosed after documentation of myocardial dysfunction and exclusion/correction of such factors as hypovolemia, hypoxia, and acidosis

D. Diagnostic tests
   1. ECG to evaluate for ischemia or arrhythmia; echocardiogram should be performed immediately; the latter test provides information on overall and regional systolic and diastole function and can lead to rapid diagnosis of mechanical causes of shock such as ischemia, hypovolemia, obstruction due to valvular stenosis or tumor
   2. Other diagnostic tests usually include chest x-ray (cardiomyopathy, aortic abnormalities, ABGs, electrolytes (abnormalities may cause arrhythmia), CBC (anemia may cause ischemia), cardiac enzymes, and brain natriuretic peptide (BNP) (elevated in acute heart failure), left and right heart catheterization (to assess coronary arteries, degree of valvular disease and hemodynamics)
   3. Hemodynamic monitoring may be useful for excluding volume depletion, right ventricular infarction, and mechanical complications. Closely monitor CVP, PAOP, CO/CI, SVR, and SVV

E. Management of cardiogenic shock (See Universal Management of Shock section)
   1. Goal is improvement of contractility and CO
   2. Initial approach should include fluid resuscitation unless pulmonary edema is present
   3. Electrolyte abnormalities should be corrected; hypokalemia and hypomagnesemia are predisposing factors to ventricular arrhythmia, and acidosis can decrease contractile function.
   4. Pharmacologic treatment (see Tables 76.2 to 76.5)
      a. Inotropic agents
         i. Dopamine
         ii. Dobutamine
         iii. Milrinone
         iv. Vasodilating agents
      b. Agents to Reduce Afterload

        i. Nitroprusside

        ii. Vasopressor agents

    c. Agents to reduce preload; may be necessary for BP support in patients with cardiogenic shock

        i. Vasopressin: may be considered first in this patient population because it does not induce arrhythmias and is not a catecholamine

        ii. Norepinephrine: slow titration is necessary to avoid overly aggressive vasoconstriction (increases SVR causing a decrease in CO/CI) in the setting of left ventricular depression

        iii. Dopamine: may be used first-line owing to its positive inotropic action

        iv. Epinephrine: used primarily as adjunct/second-line therapy

        v. Phenylephrine: considered third-line because of vasoconstriction; may reduce/increase oxygen demand and compromise renal perfusion in this patient population

        vi. Nitroglycerin

        vii. Diuretics (see chapter on Heart Failure)

5. Counter-pulsation (intra-aortic balloon pump)

    a. Increases pump efficiency

    b. Augments diastolic pressure

    c. Increases coronary end-organ perfusion

    d. Reduces afterload

    e. Reduces myocardial oxygen demand

    f. Impella device

    g. Mechanical circulatory support (left ventricular assistive devices)

6. Revascularization—pathophysiologic considerations and clinical trials favor aggressive mechanical revascularization for patients with cardiogenic shock caused by an AMI acute myocardial infarction

III. Obstructive (Extracardiac) Shock

  A. Due to obstructive of flow in the cardiovascular circuit and characterized by either impairment of diastolic filling or excessive afterload

  B. Results from obstruction of central blood flow due to compression of the heart or great vessels, as from:

    1. Direct venous obstruction

      a. Intrathoracic obstructive tumors

    2. Increased intrathoracic pressure

      a. Tension pneumothorax

      b. High ventilator pressure (e.g., PEEP)

    3. Decreased cardiac compliance

        a. Constrictive pericarditis
        b. Cardiac tamponade
    4. Increased ventricle afterload
        a. Aortic dissection
        b. Pulmonary embolus
        c. Abdominal distention
        d. Constrictive pericarditis
        e. Acute pulmonary hypertension
C. Clinical findings, diagnostic tests, and management as per underlying etiology

IV. Distributive shock

A. Includes septic, neurogenic, and anaphylactic shock; all of these types of shock involve vasodilatation and loss of vasomotor tone resulting in venous 'pooling' of blood, and decreased venous return, leading to decreased cardiac output and inadequate tissue perfusion

B. Septic shock
    1. Sepsis is defined as a systemic inflammatory response syndrome (SIRS) plus infection.
        a. Activation of complement, clotting, and kinin systems occurs, as does release of vasoactive mediators from damaged tissues
        b. The initial manifestation of infection is an overwhelming inflammatory response
        c. A systemic cascade is activated by local release of bacteria, toxins, or other inflammatory mediators.
    2. Sepsis is a common cause of death in the ICU
    3. Systemic inflammatory response to the introduction of infective organisms into the bloodstream that alter vascular tone, resulting in relative hypovolemia
    4. Infection begins the vicious cycle of coagulation and inflammation
    5. Causative organisms include:
        a. Bacterial—Gram-negative bacilli
            i. *Escherichia coli*
            ii. *Klebsiella pneumoniae*
            iii. *Enterobacter*
            iv. *Proteus*
            v. *Pseudomonas*
            vi. *Serratia*
            vii. Meningococci
        b. Bacteria—Gram-positive organisms
            i. Staphylococci (*Staphylococcus aureus, S. epidermidis, S. saprophyticus*)
            ii. Streptococci (*Streptococcus pyogenes, S. agalactiae, S. anginosus, S. faecalis, S. bovis, S. viridans, S. pneumoniae*)

         iii. Clostridia (*Clostridium perfringens, C. tetani, C. difficile, C. botulinum*)

         iv. Bacteroides

    c. Viral

    d. Fungal

6. Nosocomial infections in the critically ill are a major cause of sepsis

    a. Predisposing factors include:

         i. Malnutrition

         ii. Instrumentation with catheters/invasive procedures

         iii. Trauma

         iv. Surgical wounds

         v. Advanced age

         vi. Immunosuppressive therapy (e.g., cytotoxics, corticosteroids)

         vii. Neoplastic diseases

         viii. Chronic diseases (e.g., diabetes mellitus, renal failure)

         ix. Extended hospital stays

    b. Sites of infection

         i. Genitourinary (GU) tract (most common cause of sepsis in the elderly)

         ii. Respiratory tract

         iii. Wounds

         iv. Invasive devices such as peripheral or central intravenous catheters or urinary catheters

         v. Meninges

         vi. GI tract

             (a) Overuse of broad-spectrum antibiotics has led to resistant strains of bacteria and increased incidence of infection and sepsis

7. Diagnostic testing specific to septic shock

    a. Leukocytosis (with a shift to the left) or leukopenia

    b. Thrombocytopenia +/- DIC

    c. Other inflammatory markers

         i. Procalcitonin more than two standard deviations above normal value

         ii. C-reactive protein (CRP) more than two standard deviations above normal value

    d. May have evidence organisms in blood cultures

    e. Chest x-ray to rule out pneumonia

    f. Urine culture and sensitivity

    g. Culture and sensitivity of wounds or invasive catheters

8. Management of septic shock (See Universal Management of Shock section)

    a. Initial Resuscitation (goals during first 6 hr of resuscitation)

     i. CVP = 8–12 mmHg

     ii. MAP greater than 65 mmHg

     iii. Urine output greater than 0.5 ml/kg/hr

     iv. SvO_2 greater than 65% or $ScvO_2$ greater than 70%

  b. Diagnosis

     i. Cultures as clinically appropriate before antimicrobial therapy if no significant delay (greater than 45 min) in the start of antibiotics

9. Pharmacologic treatment (see Table 76.5)

     (a) Fluid/Volume resuscitation

     (b) Normal saline or Ringer's lactate is essential prior to vasopressor use

  a. Antimicrobial therapy should be given within the hour in hypotensive patient

     i. Administration of effective IV antimicrobials within first hr of recognition of shock. Regimen should be reassessed daily for potential de-escalation

     ii. When choosing empirical therapy, clinicians should be cognizant of virulence and growing prevalence of MRSA and resistance to broad-spectrum β-lactams and carbapenems among Gram-negative bacilli in some communities/healthcare settings. Within regions of highly prevalent drug-resistant organisms, empiric therapy that is adequate to cover these pathogens is warranted.

     iii. One of the following:

       (a) Cefepime, 2 grams IV every 8 hr plus metronidazole, 500 mg IV every 8 hr; piperacillin/tazobactam, 4.5 grams IV every 6 hr; or Imipenem, 500 mg IV every 6 hr or meropenem, 1 gram IV every 8 hr, PLUS

       (b) Gentamicin/tobramycin/amikacin: consult with pharmacist for appropriate pharmacokinetic dosing to achieve therapeutic levels and avoid toxicity PLUS

       (c) Vancomycin: consult with pharmacist for dose/frequency to achieve vancomycin level of 15–20 mcg/ml or linezolid, 600 mg IV every 12 hr

     iv. Immunosuppressed patients: antibiotic coverage for atypical pathogens is recommended

  b. Hemodynamic support

  c. Vasopressor agents (see Tables 76.2 and 76.5)

     i. May be indicated when volume resuscitation has failed to correct hypotension and CVP goal has been met

     ii. Titrate agents to keep MAP to at least 65 mmHg

        (a) Norepinephrine: recommended as the first-choice vasopressor

        (b) Vasopressin: adjunct agent

        (c) Epinephrine: adjunct agent; first-line for ACLS

        (d) Dopamine: alternative pressor agent in select patients (e.g., depressed LV function, bradycardia)

        (e) Phenylephrine: not recommended except in patients with serious dysrhythmias, high cardiac output states, or salvage therapy (see Table 76.5)

        (f) Antipyretics/cooling blanket will help to reduce body temperature and metabolic demands

        (g) Inotropic agents (see Table 76.3)

        (h) Dobutamine

    d. Closed space infections (e.g., abscess, infected bowel, infected uterus, inflamed gallbladder) require surgical drainage

    e. Corticosteroids

        i. IV hydrocortisone is not recommended as a treatment of adult septic shock if adequate fluid resuscitation and vasopressor therapy are able to restore hemodynamic stability. If this is not achievable, hydrocortisone, 200 mg/day, may be initiated and tapered off when vasopressors are no longer required (per the 2012 Surviving Sepsis Guidelines).

C. Neurogenic shock

    1. Produced by a disturbance in the nervous system that causes massive vasodilatation due to interruption in or loss of sympathetic innervation

    2. Spinal shock is a sudden neurophysiologic phenomenon that results from damage (structural or biochemical) to the spinal cord tissue that causes temporary or permanent, complete or near-complete segmental interruption of neurotransmission (loss of control or reflex activity below the level of the lesion); duration of spinal shock usually ranges from 24 hr to 12 weeks

D. Pathophysiology

    1. Loss of sympathetic vasoconstrictor tone

    2. Blood volume is normal

    3. Cardiac function is normal (unless underlying cardiac disease)

E. Causes

    1. Injury or disease of the spinal cord or brain stem

    2. High levels of spinal anesthesia

    3. Vasomotor center depression

    4. Drugs that block sympathetic activity

F. Clinical manifestations specific to neurogenic shock

    1. Hypotension: due to significant vasodilatation

    2. Bradycardia: caused by loss of sympathetic tone in the heart

3. Hypothermia
4. Warm, dry skin due to venodilatation and resulting in venous pooling and loss of sweat response below the level of the lesion
5. Decreased SVR, stroke volume, and venous return (decreased CVP) caused by loss of sympathetic vasoconstrictor tone below the level of the lesion in arterioles, precapillaries, and venules
6. Hyporeflexic/areflexic

G. Management of neurogenic shock (See Universal Management of Shock section)
   1. Refer to Neurologic Trauma chapter for detailed management of spinal cord injuries
   2. Treat or remove cause if possible
   3. Careful fluid administration ensures adequate tissue perfusion (systolic blood pressure less than 90 mmHg, urine output less than 0.5 ml/kg/hr, and decreased LOC are indicators of poor perfusion)
   4. It is essential to differentiate neurogenic shock from hypovolemic shock. Both conditions result in hypotension, but patients who are in neurogenic shock manifest warm, dry skin and bradycardia, whereas those in hypovolemic shock have cool, moist skin and tachycardia due to compensatory mechanisms.
   5. Vasopressor agents (see Tables 76.2 and 76.5)
      a. Norepinephrine: recommended as the first-choice vasopressor
      b. Vasopressin: adjunct agent
      c. Epinephrine: adjunct agent; first-line for ACLS
      d. Dopamine: alternative pressor agent in select patients (e.g., depressed LV function, bradycardia)
      e. Phenylephrine: not recommended except in patients with serious dysrhythmias, high cardiac output states, or salvage therapy (see Table 76.5)
   6. For symptomatic bradycardia in which LOC, urine output, and BP are decreased, atropine 0.5–1 mg IV push and/or external pacing may be indicated
   7. As with all shock states, prognosis is dependent on underlying process

H. Anaphylactic shock
   1. The result of an immediate hypersensitivity reaction severe antibody/antigen response leads to decreased tissue perfusion and initiation of general shock response; anaphylaxis involves one or both of two features: respiratory difficulty and hypotension, which can manifest as fainting, collapse, or unconsciousness
   2. Causes
      a. Foods such as nuts, fish, shellfish, dairy products, legumes, eggs, fruits, and berries
      b. Food additives such as dyes and monosodium glutamate

        c. Diagnostic agents such as allergen extracts, vaccines, and radiocontrast media

        d. Blood products

        e. Environmental agents such as latex, pollen, mold spores, animal products, and dust

        f. Drugs, common culprits: antibiotics, acetylsalicylic acid, narcotics, dextran, anesthetic agents, muscle relaxants, and barbiturates

        g. Venom

I. Clinical manifestations

        a. Cardiovascular: hypotension, tachycardia, arrhythmias

        b. Respiratory: bronchospasm, laryngeal edema, patient describes "lump in throat", dysphasia, hoarseness, dyspnea, stridor, wheezing, rales/rhonchi, hypoxia

        c. Cutaneous: pruritus, erythema, urticaria, angioedema (swelling)

        d. CNS: restlessness, uneasiness, apprehension, feeling of impending doom, anxiety, decreased LOC

        e. GI: nausea and vomiting, diarrhea, abdominal cramps, metallic taste

        f. Hemodynamics: decreased CO, CI, CVP, PAOP, and SVR

J. Management of anaphylactic shock (See Universal Management of Shock section)

    1. Speed of treatment is essential

    2. Immediate administration of epinephrine (adrenaline) IM or subcutaneously, 0.5–1 mg (0.5–1 ml); additional doses may be required if improvement is not evident; epinephrine should be given to all patients with respiratory difficulty or hypotension

        a. Inhaled epinephrine is effective for mild to moderate laryngeal edema but would not be given if IM/SQ epinephrine has already been given as first-line treatment; it is not a substitute for IM/SQ epinephrine.

        b. Give IV epinephrine if circulation is already compromised in 1 mg (1:10,000 = 10 ml) slow IV push

        c. Do not wait to establish IV line; may give via endotracheal tube: 2–2.5 times (2–2.5 mg) the usual dose of 1 mg/10 ml epinephrine solution; use oxygen-valve reservoir bag, or "manually bag" patient several sufflations after administration

        d. Give 0.1–0.5 mg of 1 mg/10 ml epinephrine; repeat in 10-min intervals until the desired effect is achieved, or until adverse effects occur

    3. Maintain airway: intubate if necessary and administer supplemental O_2; tracheostomy may be necessary in those with severe obstruction that makes intubation not possible

4. Deliver antihistamine (diphenhydramine, 50 mg IV [or PO] single dose; may need up to 100 mg, not to exceed 400 mg/day) to block histamine effects
5. In anaphylaxis, H1 antihistamines may relieve itching, flushing, urticaria, angioedema, and nasal and eye symptoms.
6. H2 Blockers: i.e., ranitidine 50 mg IV
7. An H2 blocker, administered concurrently with an H1 blocker (antihistamine), potentially contributes to decrease in flushing, headache, and other symptoms.
8. May use albuterol for bronchospasm
9. Although helpful for lower respiratory tract symptoms/asthmatic patients, β-2 agonists should not be substituted for epinephrine because they have minimal α-1 adrenergic agonist vasoconstrictor effects and do not prevent/relieve laryngeal edema and upper airway obstruction, hypotension, or shock.
10. Expand vascular volume with Ringer's lactate infusion
11. Corticosteroids: methylprednisolone (Solu-Medrol) 125–250 mg/IV or hydrocortisone [Hydrocortone], 200 mg slow IV to decrease inflammation
12. Outside of an asthma or "inflammatory" clinical setting, a Cochrane systematic review failed to identify any evidence from randomized, controlled trials to confirm effectiveness of glucocorticoids in anaphylaxis treatment; raised concerns that they are often inappropriately used as first-line medications in place of epinephrine
13. Inotropic agents (see Tables 76.2 and 76.3)
14. Dobutamine
15. Vasoconstrictor agents (see Tables 76.2 and 76.5)
    a. Norepinephrine: recommended as the first-choice vasopressor
    b. Vasopressin: adjunct agent
    c. Epinephrine: adjunct agent; first-line for ACLS
    d. Dopamine: alternative pressor agent in select patients (e.g., depressed LV function, bradycardia)
16. Phenylephrine: not recommended except in patients with serious dysrhythmias, high cardiac output states, or salvage therapy
17. The keys to management are awareness, early recognition (consider in differential diagnosis), and quick treatment; anaphylaxis is easily treatable, and patients can make a complete recovery

V. **Evaluation**
A. Prompt assessment and diagnosis is important in the management of patients with shock
B. Ongoing evaluation of interventions is critical for positive patient outcomes; an interdisciplinary team-approach is key to providing optimal care to patients and their families

BIBLIOGRAPHY

Anwaruddin, S., Martin, J. M., Stephens, J. C., & Askari, A. T. (2012). *Cardiovascular Hemodynamics*. New York, NY: Humana Press.

Arnold, J. J., & Williams, P. M. (2011). Anaphylaxis: Recognition and management. *American Family Physician, 84*(10), 1111–1118.

Backer, D. D., Aldecoa, C., Nijmi, H., & Vincent, J. L. (2012). Dopamine versus norepinephrine in the treatment of septic shock: A meta-analysis. *Critical Care Medicine, 40*(3), 725–730.

Beloncle, F., Meziani, F., Lerolle, N., Radermacher, P., & Asfar, P. (2013). Does vasopressor therapy have an indication in hemorrhagic shock. *Annals of Intensive Care, 3*(13).

Cannesson, M., & Pearse, R. (2014). *Perioperative hemodynamic monitoring and goal directed therapy: From theory to practice*. New York, NY: Cambridge University Press.

Casserly, B., Read, R., & Levy, M. M. (2011). Hemodynamic monitoring in sepsis. *Critical Care Nursing Clinics of North America, 23*(1), 149–169. doi:10.1016/j.ccell.2010.12.009

Dabbagh, A., Esmailian, F., & Aranki, S. F. (Eds.). (2014). *Postoperative critical care for cardiac surgical patients* (pp. 41–72). New York, NY: Springer-Verlag Berlin Heidelberg.

Dellinger, R. P., Levy, M. M., Rhodes, A., Annane, D., Gerlach, H., Opal, S. M., . . . Moreno, R. (2012). Surviving Sepsis Campaign: International guidelines for management of severe sepsis and septic shock. *Intensive Care Medicine, 39*(2), 165–228. doi:10.1007/ s00134–012–2769–8

Faix, J. D. (2013). Biomarkers of sepsis. *Critical Reviews of Clinical Laboratory Science, 50*(1), 23–36. doi:10.3109/10408363.2013.764490

Feng, H. (2011). *Clinical management*. New York, NY: Springer

Gardenhire, D. S. (2011). *Rau's respiratory care pharmacology* (8th ed.). Maryland Heights, MO: Mosby.

Garg, S., Singhal, S., Sharma, P., & Jha, A. A. (2012). Inotropes and vasopressors: Review of physiology and clinical use. *Pulmonary and Respiratory Medicine, 2*(5).

Gauer, R. (2013). Early recognition and management of sepsis in adults: The first six hours. *American Family Physician, 88*(1), 44–53.

Guerin, C., Reignier, J., Richard, J. C., Beuret, P., Gacouin, A., Boulain, T., . . . Ayzac, L. (2013). Prone positioning in severe acute respiratory distress syndrome. *New England Journal of Medicine, 368*(23), 2159–2168. doi:10.1056/NEJMoa1214103

Gibson, J., & Nordby, D. B. (2014). Managing hemodynamics. *Nursing Critical Care, 9*(4), 12–16.

Havel, C., Arrich, J., Losert, H., Gamper, G., Mullner, M., & Herkner, H. (2011). Vasopressors for hypotensive shock. *The Cochrane Library, 5*(CD003709). doi:10.1002/14651858

Johnston, M. C., & Knight, J.E. (2012) *Septic shock: Symptoms, management and risk factors (Emergency and intensive care medicine).* Hauppage, NY: Nova Science Pub Inc.

Levy, M. M., Dellinger, R. P., Townsend, S. R, Linde-Zwirble, W. T., Marshall, J. C., Bion, J., . . . Surviving Sepsis Campaign. (2010). The Surviving Sepsis Campaign: Results of an international guideline-based performance improvement program targeting severe sepsis. *Critical Care Medicine, 38*(2), 367–374.

Levy, M., & van der Poll, T. (2010). Inflammation and coagulation. *Critical Care Medicine, 38,* 526–534.

Martin-Loeches, I., de Haro, C., Dellinger, R. P., Ferrer, R., Phillips, G. S., Levy, M. M., & Artigas, A. (2013). Effectiveness of an inspiratory pressure-limited approach to mechanical ventilation in septic patients. *European Respiratory Journal, 41*(1), 157–164. doi:10.1183/09031936.00221611

Martindale, R. G., McClave, S. A., Vanek, V. W., McCarthy, M., Roberts, P., Taylor, B., . . . Society of Critical Care Medicine (2009). Guidelines for the provision and assessment of nutrition support therapy in the adult critically ill patient: Society of Critical Care Medicine and American Society for Parenteral and Enteral Nutrition: Executive summary. *Critical Care Medicine, 37,* 1757–1761.

Nattachai, A., & Boyd, J. H., (2014). Serious adverse events associated with vasopressin and norepinephrine infusion in septic shock. *Critical Care Medicine, 42*(8), 1812–1820.

Nduka, O., & Parrillo, J. E. (2011). The pathophysiology of septic shock. *Critical Care Nursing Clinics of North America, 23*(1), 41–66. doi:10.1016/j.ccell.2010.12.003

O'Donnell, M., & Nacul, F. (2012). *Surgical intensive care medicine.* New York, NY: Springer.

Patel, G. P., & Balk, R. A. (2012). Systemic steroids in severe sepsis and septic shock. *American Journal of Respiratory and Critical Care Medicine, 185*(2), 133–139. doi:10.1164/rccm.201011–1897CI

Rech, M. A., Prasse, M., & Patel, G. (2011). Use of vasopressors in septic shock. *Journal of Clinical Outcomes Management Abstract, 18,* 273–277.

Reinhart, K., & Bloos, F. (2011). Pathophysiology of sepsis and multiple organ dysfunction. In J. Vincent, E. Abraham, F. Moore, P. Kochanek, & M. Fink (Eds.), *Textbook of Critical Care* (pp. 983–991). Philadelphia, PA: Saunders.

Senzaki, H. (2012). *Hemodynamics: Monitoring, theory and applications (Cardiology research and developments)*. Hauppage, NY: Nova Science Pub Inc.

Simons, F. E. R., Ardusso, L. R. F., Bilo, M. B., El-Gamal, Y. M., Ledford, D. K., Ring, J., . . . World Allergy Organization. (2011). World Allergy Organization guidelines for the assessment and management of anaphylaxis. *World Allergy Organization Journal, 4,* 13–37.

Terry, C. L., & Weaver, A. L. (2011). *Critical care nursing demystified*. New York, NY: McGraw Hill Publishing.

U. S. Food and Drug Admininstration (FDA) (2011, Oct. 15). *FDA Drug Safety Communication: Voluntary market withdrawal of Xigris (drotrecogin alfa [activated]) due to failiure to show a survival benefit*. Retrieved from http://www.fda.gov/Drugs/DrugSaftey/ucm277114.htm

Vasu, T. S., Cavallazzi, R., Hirani, A., Kaplan, G., Leiby, B., & Marik, P. E. (2012). Norepinephrine or dopamine for septic shock: Systematic review of randomized clinical trials. *Journal of Intensive Care Medicine, 27*(3), 172–178. doi:10.1177/0885066610396312

Wacker, C., Prkno, A., Brunkhorst, F. M., & Schlattmann, P. (2013). Procalcitonin as a diagnostic marker for sepsis: A systematic review and meta-analysis. *Lancet Infectious Disease, 13*(5), 426–435. doi:10.1016/s1473–3099(12)70323–7

CHAPTER 77

Nutritional Considerations

PAULA MCCAULEY • THOMAS W. BARKLEY, JR. • CHARLENE M. MYERS

I. Nutritional assessment
  A. Basic laboratory measurements
  1. Serum albumin
     a. Less than 3.5 grams/dl indicates protein malnutrition
     b. Half-life is 20 days; synthesis requires adequate amino acids and hepatic function
     c. Expect edema if less than 2.7 grams/dl
     d. Values skewed if liver or renal disease, heart failure, or inflammation
     e. Albumin is a principal drug carrier; dosage may need adjustment
  2. Pre albumin
     a. Normal concentration 20–50 mg/dl
        i. 10–15 grams/dl moderate depletion
        ii. Less than 10 grams/dl severe depletion
     b. Half-life of 2 days; reflect changes in nutritional status more quickly than albumin; trends are important
     c. Affected by renal, hepatic dysfunction, hydration status, and inflammation
  3. Transferrin or total iron binding capacity (TIBC)
     a. Normal concentration, 170–250 mg/dl
        i. 151–200 mg/dl mild depletion
        ii. 100–150 mg/dl moderate depletion
        iii. Less than 100 mg/dl severe depletion
     b. Half-life of 8–10 days; reflect changes more quickly than albumin; trends are important

        c. Synthesized in the liver

        d. Values can be skewed in liver disease, renal disease, congestive heart failure, or inflammation

        e. Concentration is influenced by iron status

        f. Can be calculated using TIBC as follows:

            i. $(TIBC \times 0.76) + 18$

    4. Hemoglobin

        a. Low levels (less than 12 grams/dl for women and 13.5 grams/dl for men) can indicate lack of iron or protein

        b. Inadequate oxygen perfusion to cells results in decreased energy production and affects many tissue functions, including healing and growth

    5. Hematocrit: a volume measurement that verifies hemoglobin level

    6. Lymphocyte

        a. Depressed level indicates lack of immune function/increased susceptibility to infection

        b. Steroid use can decrease count

B. Clinical observations (used to support laboratory data; not diagnostic)

    1. Skin free of color irregularities, smooth

    2. Mucous membranes smooth, pink, and moist

    3. Hair shiny, not easily plucked

    4. Musculature toned, some fat present

    5. Skeleton: erect posture

    6. Nails regularly shaped, free of ridges; rapid cellular turnover is noted in the above areas; nutritional deficiencies become obvious earlier

C. Dietary evaluation (used to evaluate food intake; supportive of other data)

    1. Twenty-four-hour recall (all foods and beverages consumed within the previous 24 hr)

    2. Three- and five-day food diaries

        a. List of all foods and beverages consumed within a specified time period

        b. Encourage patient to eat as he/she has eaten previously

        c. Can also include occurrence of symptoms

    3. Food frequency records: how often one eats a particular food or group of foods

    4. Patient interviews for diet history

        a. Likes and dislikes

        b. Intolerance

        c. Allergies

        d. Eating patterns

II.   **Ideal body weight (IDBW) calculations**

  A. Men

    1. One hundred six pounds allowed for first 5 ft of height

    2. Six pounds added for each inch over 5 ft

    3. Adjust 10% of total for frame (skeleton) size

        a. Add 10% for large frame

        b. Subtract 10% for small frame

        c. No adjustment for medium or average frame

B. Women

    1. One hundred pounds allowed for first 5 ft of height

    2. Five pounds added for each inch over 5 ft

    3. Adjust for frame size by 10% as for men

C. Individuals less than 5 feet in height

    1. Consult published tables for appropriate weight for height

III. **Determining nutritional needs**

A. Stressed patients first receive nutritional support in the flow or second stage of the stress response; correct fluid and electrolyte imbalances only in the first or ebb phase

B. Kilocalories per kilogram of body weight; use actual or desired weight depending on goal of therapy; consult dietitian for additional information

    1. Average adult requirement is 30 kcal/kg or 13 kcal/lb of body weight/24 hr

        a. Usually, stressed individuals require 25–30 kcal/kg

        b. For weight gain, 35 or more kcal/kg is appropriate

    2. For weight loss, 25 kcal/kg; 1 lb of body weight is equivalent to 3500 kcal; one kilogram is equivalent to 7700 kcal

    3. Elevated body temperature

        a. Seven percent increase in kilocalories/24 hr required for each degree above 98.6°F

        b. Thirteen percent increase in kilocalories for each degree higher than 98.6°F (37°C)

C. Fluid requirements

    1. One milliliter of fluid/kcal/24 hr (30–35 ml/kg of body weight) is usual; water, decaffeinated beverages, popsicles, flavored gelatin, and so forth are good sources; milk is 50% water

    2. Needs increase with elevation in vital signs, use of drains, nausea/vomiting, diarrhea, and so forth; increase by 150 ml/24 hr for each degree rise in body temperature above normal

D. Protein requirements

    1. Protein required per day ranges from 0.8–2 grams/kg of body weight

    2. Most stressed patients require 1.5 grams or more per kilogram of body weight

    3. Renal and hepatic diseases usually necessitate lower levels of protein because of the inability of the body to convert ammonia to urea in the liver or to excrete urea via the kidneys; protein is the primary source of all nitrogenous waste products

      4. Protein is needed for tissue growth and maintenance; should account for approximately 20% of daily kilocalories

      5. Protein is worth 4 kcal/gram; excessive protein intake increases the amount of nitrogenous waste—urea—that must be excreted through the urine

  E. Carbohydrate needs

      1. Account for largest proportion of kilocalories in most diets: approximately 50% of daily need

      2. More oxygen (and release of more carbon dioxide) is required than for protein or fat; patients with compromised respiratory function would benefit from less than average carbohydrate content.

      3. Carbohydrate consists of 4 kcal/gram

  F. Fat or lipid needs

      1. Fat has the lowest respiratory quotient or uses the least amount of oxygen and produces the least amount of carbon dioxide.

      2. Substituting fat for carbohydrates can reduce stress on the respiratory system, particularly if the patient has minimal lung capacity.

      3. Fats consist of 9 kcal/gram

  G. Vitamin and mineral requirements

      1. Use the recommended dietary allowance (RDA) as a guide; consult a dietitian for individual needs

      2. Beware of over-supplementation; the liver and kidneys must process and excrete excessive vitamins; 10 times the RDA is a megadose, and this amount should be regarded as a medication rather than a supplement

  H. Electrolyte needs

      1. Replace deficits

      2. Beware of excessive amounts (exceeding the RDA), especially in renal disease, or during the first or ebb stage of the stress response when acute renal failure may be present

IV. Food guide

  A. Choose the My Plate (myplate.com) pattern of adhering to dietary guidelines for Americans. My Plate illustrates the five food groups using a familiar mealtime visual, a place setting: fruits, vegetable, grains, protein foods, and dairy.

      1. The amount of food from all groups depends on age, sex, and level of physical activity.

      2. Half of the plate should be fruits and vegetables

      3. Grains: ½ of grains should be whole grains

      4. Dairy: milk, yogurt, and cheese

      5. Protein foods: lean proteins, meat, poultry, fish, dry beans, eggs, and nuts

      6. Oils

      7. Balance calories with physical activity to manage weight

8. Enjoy your food, but eat less
9. Avoid oversized portions
10. Consume fewer foods with sodium (salt), saturated fats, trans fats, cholesterol, added sugars, and refined grains
11. Compare sodium in foods like soup, bread, and frozen meals—and choose foods with lower numbers
12. Drink water instead of sugary drinks

V. Nutritional support

A. Initiation of feeding for the acutely ill patient; before initiation of feedings, assessment should include evaluation of weight loss and previous nutrient intake before admission, level of disease severity, comorbid conditions, and function of the gastrointestinal (GI) tract

1. Decisions regarding types of nutritional support rely on the following guidelines:
   a. The GI tract is nonfunctional; parenteral (vascular) feeding is appropriate
   b. The GI tract is functional
   c. Enteral nutrition (EN) (any feeding that uses the GI tract) is the preferred form of feeding. If the gut works, use it! Prevention of transmigration of GI bacteria through the intestinal wall to the bloodstream and resulting sepsis is dependent on the presence of food in the GI tract; consult a dietitian.

2. Oral support: feeding administered through the mouth. Often referred to as progressive diets or a progressive regimen; when a patient can tolerate clear liquids, he is then advanced to full liquids and, with GI toleration, to more complex foods.

3. Clear liquids
   a. Liquids or foods that become liquid in the mouth and, when held to the light, are clear, or one can see through them
   b. Includes flavored gelatin, ice, popsicles, carbonated beverages, meat broths, sherbet, sorbets, and tea
   c. Neither caffeinated nor decaffeinated coffee is included because coffee increases gastric acid production
   d. Indications for use include postsurgery, nausea and vomiting, and minimal GI residue, as seen before GI surgery
   e. Incomplete nutritionally, so should be used for a minimal time if only means of nutritional support

4. Full liquids
   a. All foods on a clear liquid diet plus milk and dairy products
   b. Fluid milk, plain yogurt, ice cream, cream soups, and hot cereals such as cream of wheat
   c. Indications for use include anorexia, previous clear liquid diet, and so forth
   d. Can be nutritionally complete

5. Soft
   a. Foods that are soft in texture and easy to digest
   b. Lean, tender meat; potatoes, rice; cooked vegetables and fruits
   c. Mechanical soft usually refers to a pureed or blended diet for those who have difficulty chewing.
   d. Indications for use include situations in which energy conservation is important, as well as previous GI upsets, including nausea, vomiting, flatus, and cramping
   e. Nutritionally complete
6. Regular
   a. Follows USDA guidelines for My Plate
7. Supplemental formula feedings
   a. Commercially prepared formulas are offered between meals or as a meal substitute to provide additional kilocalories or additional amounts of a nutrient such as protein.
   b. Usually better accepted if served cold and with a drinking straw
   c. Should be sipped for at least 20 min to avoid GI discomfort
   d. Examples of commonly used formulas include Ensure by Ross Products and Isocal by Mead Johnson

B. EN should be initiated in the acutely ill patient who is unable to maintain volitional intake
   1. Consult/referral to dietitian, nutrition support team, and/or metabolic support team
   2. EN is the preferred route of feeding
   3. Enteral feeding should be started early within the first 24–48 hr following admission and should be advanced toward goal over the next 48–72 hr
   4. In the setting of hemodynamic compromise, EN should be withheld until the patient is fully resuscitated and/or stable.
   5. Neither the presence nor the absence of bowel sounds or the presence of flatus or stool is required for the initiation of enteral feeding
   6. Gastric or small bowel feeding is acceptable. Acutely ill patients should be fed via an enteral access tube placed in the small bowel if high risk for aspiration or showing intolerance to gastric feeding.
   7. Withholding enteral feeding for repeated high gastric residual volumes alone may be a sufficient reason to switch to small bowel feeding
   8. If the patient is expected to need support for longer than 6 weeks, use an enterostomal tube
   9. If the patient is expected to need support for less than 6 weeks, use a transnasal tube
   10. If the patient is at risk for aspiration, use duodenal placement for the tube

11. The same products used for supplemental feedings are usually appropriate for EN. These products either have intact nutrients or are not predigested; they require a fully functional GI tract.
12. Enteral routes
    a. Nasogastric tubes
        i. End of tube located in the stomach
        ii. Most similar to route of normal digestion
        iii. Acid reflux common
        iv. Lack of integrity of gastric mucosa contraindicates use
    b. Nasoduodenal tubes
        i. End of tube is located in the duodenum
        ii. Acid reflux or aspiration is less common than with gastric tubes
        iii. May require a hydrolyzed or elemental formula, one that is at least partially predigested. Examples include Vivonex Plus by Sandoz Nutrition and Peptamen by Clintec.
    c. Nasojejunal tubes
        i. Tube placement in the jejunum
        ii. Formula type depends on the area of the jejunum that is to be used: intact for the upper portion and hydrolyzed for the mid to lower portion
    d. Enterostomies: surgically created openings from the exterior to the GI tract for long-term use (more than 6 weeks), or when transnasal tube is inappropriate
        i. Esophagostomy
        ii. Ostomy in esophagus with tube end located in stomach
        iii. Intact or blenderized formulas appropriate
    e. Gastrostomy
        i. Opening into the stomach
    f. Percutaneous endoscopic gastrostomy
        i. Created with use of an endoscope; often, procedure occurs at the bedside with local anesthesia
        ii. Can be used for feeding within 24 hr
        iii. Intact formula appropriate
    g. Jejunostomy
        i. Percutaneous endoscopic jejunostomy is an extension of percutaneous endoscopic gastrostomy
        ii. See nasojejunal tube information above for formula choice
13. Rate of feeding:
    a. Bolus
        i. Usually administered with a large syringe
        ii. Volume of 250–500 ml given over 10–20 min every 4–6 hr

          iii. Least likely to be well tolerated

    b. Intermittent

          i. Volume of 100–400 ml allowed to flow by gravity for 20–40 min every 2–4 hr

    c. Continuous

          i. Requires the use of an infusion pump

          ii. Administered over 18–24 hr; best tolerated

          iii. Elevate the head of the patient's bed when administering feedings and for 30–40 min after the feeding

          iv. Do not administer iron preparations or insulin through a nasointestinal tube; consult the pharmacist regarding other medications that can be used to avoid drug-nutrient interactions; flush the tubing before and after giving medications

          v. Most commercial tube feeding formulas contain 80% water by volume; 1 ml of water for every kilocalorie, a 2,000 ml/24 hr volume would contain 1,600 ml of water; the remaining 400 ml must be given additionally; water used to flush the tubing before and after feeding contributes to the day's allowance.

  14. Complications of enteral support

    a. GI complications such as diarrhea, constipation, cramping, and gastric retention are fairly common. Manipulate the fiber content of the formula for stool consistency. If there is evidence of diarrhea, soluble fiber-containing or small peptide formulations may be utilized.

    b. Osmolarity of the formula can also be a factor

    c. Formula is best tolerated at room temperature

    d. Ensure that hydration is adequate

    e. Monitor regularly for metabolic complications such as hyperglycemia and electrolyte imbalances

    f. Be aware of drugs, their adverse effects, and potential interactions with nutrients

    g. Consult a dietitian and a pharmacist for additional information on problem solving

C. Parenteral nutrition support (use of the vascular system to deliver nutrients); may be used with enteral feedings or as sole nutritional support; consult pharmacist for content of the solutions

  1. Consult/referral to dietitian, nutritional support team, or metabolic support team

  2. In the patient who was previously healthy before acute illness with no evidence of protein calorie malnutrition, use of PN should be reserved and initiated only after the first 7 days of hospitalization (when EN is not available).

3. If there is evidence of protein-calorie malnutrition on admission and EN is not feasible, it is appropriate to initiate PN as soon as possible following admission and adequate resuscitation.

4. If a patient is expected to undergo major upper GI surgery and EN is not feasible, PN should be provided under very specific conditions: If the patient is malnourished, PN should be initiated 5–7 days preoperatively and continued into the postoperative period.

5. PN should not be initiated in the immediate postoperative period but should be delayed for 5–7 days (should EN continue not to be feasible)

6. PN therapy provided for a duration of less than 5–7 days would be expected to have no outcome effect and may result in increased risk to the patient.

7. If unable to meet energy requirements (100% of target goal calories) after 7–10 days by the enteral route alone, consider supplemental PN

8. Concentrations of dextrose greater than 10% require a central line

9. Peripheral parenteral nutrition (PPN)
   a. Limited to 10–14 days because of vein infiltration

10. Central parenteral nutrition or total parenteral nutrition
    a. Usually administered by using the jugular or subclavian vein to access the superior vena cava
    b. For anticipated support longer than 10–14 days

11. Considerations when administering parenteral support:
    a. Monitor blood glucose every 6 hr
    b. Monitor electrolytes, CBC, Ca, Phos, Mg, LFTs, as well as triglyceride levels
    c. Infuse fat emulsions slowly
    d. Involve pharmacist, dietitian, and physician in planning parenteral support
    e. Trend nutritional laboratory results a minimum of weekly

12. Complications of parenteral nutritional support are many and varied
    a. Metabolic complications, such as hyperglycemia and hypercapnia, may result, along with those involving the GI tract and the liver.
    b. High risk for infection due to high glycemic content
    c. Risk of pancreatitis with lipid infusion

BIBLIOGRAPHY

Baron, R. B. (2013). Nutritional disorders. In M. A. Papadakis, S. J. McPhee, M. W. Rabow, & T. G. Berger (Eds.), *CURRENT medical diagnosis & treatment 2014*. New York, NY: Lange Medical Books.

Bedi, N. M., & Robinson, M. K. (2012). Nutrition and metabolic support. In J. Matloff, D. D. Dressler, D. J. Brotman, & J. S. Ginsberg (Eds.), *Principles and practice of hospital medicine*. New York, NY: McGraw Hill.

Druyan, M. E., Compher, C., Boullata, J. I., Braunschweig, C. L., George, D. E., Simpser, E., . . . American Society for Parenteral and Enteral Nutrition Board of Directors. (2012). Clinical guidelines for the use of parenteral and enteral nutrition in adult and pediatric patients: Applying the GRADE system to development of A.S.P.E.N. Clinical Guidelines. *Journal of Parenteral and Enteral Nutrition, 36*(1), 77–80.

Heimburger, D. C. (2012). Malnutrition and nutritional assessment. In D. L. Longo, A. S. Fauci, D. L. Kasper, S. L. Hauser, J. L. Jameson, & J. Loscalzo (Eds.), *Harrison's principles of Internal Medicine* (18th ed.). New York, NY: McGraw Hill.

U.S. Department of Agriculture, Center for Nutrition Policy and Promotion. (2011). *Dietary Guidelines for Americans, 2010* (7th ed.). Retrieved from http://www.nutrition.gov/smart-nutrition-101/dietary-guidelines-americans

U.S. Department of Agriculture. (2014). *MyPlate and food pyramid resources*. Retrieved from http://www.nutrition.gov/smart-nutrition-101/myplate-food-pyramid-resources

CHAPTER 78

Fluid, Electrolyte, and Acid–Base Imbalances

R. MICHAEL CULPEPPER • THOMAS W. BARKLEY, JR. • CHARLENE M. MYERS

HYPONATREMIA

I.   **Definition**
  A. Decreased serum sodium (Na) of less than 135 mEq/L; normal range is 135–145 mEq/L
  B. Hypotonic hyponatremia (low serum osmolality [SOsm])
     1. State of body water excess; both intra- and extracellular fluid (ECF) dilution
     2. Clinical signs arise from cellular water excess, causing cell swelling
  C. Isotonic hyponatremia (normal SOsm)
     1. Laboratory artifact; extreme hyperlipidemia or hyperproteinemia displaces water in lab sample
     2. Body water is normal and patients are asymptomatic
  D. Hypertonic hyponatremia (high SOsm)
     1. Dilution of extracellular fluid sodium by water movement from cells into high concentrations of nonsodium solute (e.g., glucose, mannitol)
     2. Clinical signs are those of primary disorder, not redistribution of body water

II. **Etiology/incidence/predisposing factors**
  A. 1%–4% prevalence in hospitalized patients
  B. Renal water excretion is less than water intake
     1. Decreased glomerular filtration forming less urine overall
     2. Impaired formation of dilute urine (e.g., diuretic effect) or disease
     3. Non-osmotic antidiuretic hormone (ADH) release concentrating urine

C. Hypervolemic hyponatremia: edematous state of excess total body sodium content, with or without hemodynamic deficiency, that stimulates ADH secretion

    1. Congestive heart failure, hepatic cirrhosis, or nephrotic syndrome

D. Hypovolemic hyponatremia: state of deficient total body sodium content, with or without hemodynamic insufficiency, that stimulates ADH secretion

    1. Blood loss

    2. Gastrointestinal (GI) fluid loss: nasogastric suction, emesis, or diarrhea

    3. Renal fluid loss: excess diuresis or aldosterone deficiency

    4. Skin fluid loss: excess sweating or burns

E. Euvolemic hyponatremia

    1. State of normal body sodium content

    2. Edema-free and normal hemodynamic state with autonomous ADH secretion or reduced renal water formation

        a. Syndrome of inappropriate ADH (SIADH)

        b. Diuretics, especially thiazides in elderly females

        c. Renal failure, acute or chronic

        d. Cortisol deficiency

        e. Hypothyroidism

        f. Water ingestion exceeding capacity for renal water excretion per unit time; primary polydipsia (psychogenic) and forced water intake (marathoners)

        g. Beer potomania: inadequate solute (salt) intake; kidney cannot make the quantity of dilute urine needed to excrete a large fluid (beer) intake

III. Subjective findings

A. Neurologic symptoms related to brain swelling from water excess; severity roughly parallels fall in serum sodium ; more pronounced with acute (hours to 1–2 days) versus chronic (more than 2 days to weeks) development of hyponatremia

B. Correlation with serum sodium

    1. Serum Na = 120–125 mEq/L

        a. Acute: nausea, malaise, gait instability

        b. Chronic: none to gait instability (fall risk in elderly)

    2. Serum Na = 110–120 mEq/L

        a. Acute: headache, confusion, lethargy, nausea

        b. Chronic: occasionally none to mild confusion or lethargy

    3. Serum Na less than 110 mEq/L

        a. Acute: nausea, seizures, coma

        b. Chronic: rarely none, greater confusion or lethargy

IV. Physical examination findings

A. General neurologic depression, rarely focal neurologic findings

B. Major findings may reflect the disorder that caused hyponatremia

   C. Cardiovascular focus: hyper- or hypovolemia may stimulate ADH
      release
      1. Hypervolemia: edema, ascites, pulmonary crackles, cardiac gallop,
         jugular venous distension
      2. Hypovolemia: postural fall in blood pressure and rise in pulse;
         jugular venous collapse
      3. Euvolemia: normal hemodynamic exam

V.   **Laboratory/diagnostic findings**
   A. Hypotonic hyponatremia
      1. Serum Na less than 135 mEq/L and SOsm less than 270 mOsm/kg
         (normal, 280–295 mOsm/kg; SOsm ≈ 2 × Serum Na)
      2. Urine osmolality (UOsm): pathological if less than serum
         osmolality in hyponatremic state
         a. UOsm less than 100 mOsm/L: water intake at rate or volume
            that exceeds normal renal water excretion
         b. UOsm greater than 100 mOsm/L: ADH effect or decrease in
            renal ability to form water free of solutes
      3. Urine sodium (UNa)
         a. UNa less than 20 mEq/L
            i. Decreased renal blood flow
            ii. Seen in hypervolemic or hypovolemic states
         b. UNa greater than 40 mEq/L
            i. SIADH
            ii. Diuretics
            iii. Renal failure
            iv. Hypothyroidism
            v. Adrenal insufficiency
   B. Isotonic hyponatremia
      1. Serum Na less than 135 mEq/L, SOsm 280–290 mOsm/kg
      2. Extreme hyperlipidemia (triglycerides greater than
         1000–1500 mg/dl) or hyperproteinemia (protein greater than
         12–15 grams/dl), as in multiple myeloma
      3. Plasma water sodium is normal (obtained after separation of
         non-soluble lipid or protein from serum)
   C. Hypertonic hyponatremia
      1. Serum Na less than 135 mEq/L, SOsm greater than 290 mOsm/kg
      2. Hyperglycemia: each 100 mg/dl increment in serum glucose above
         100 mg/dl decreases serum Na by approximately 1.6 mEq/L
         (e.g., for serum glucose, 900 mg/dl), serum Na falls by
         8 × 1.6 mEq/L, or by 13 mEq/L
      3. Infusion of mannitol or glycerol causes the same phenomenon

VI.   **Management**
   A. Only hypotonic hyponatremia requires treatment directed at serum
      sodium itself

1. Therapy is guided by symptoms, level of serum sodium, and rapidity of development
2. Rate of correction of serum sodium is critical; overcorrection or very rapid rise in serum sodium may inflict further CNS injury, as seen in the syndrome of pontine myelinolysis

B. Seizures or coma with serum Na less than 120 mEq/L, acute or chronic
   1. Infuse 3% hypertonic saline at a rate to increase serum Na by 1–2 mEq/L/hr until Na rises by 12–15 mEq/L, or to a level of 120 mEq/L
   2. Maximum correction rate is 8–12 mEq/L/24 hr, or 25 mEq/L/48 hr
   3. Example: Na^+ mEq required = $0.5 \times$ body weight (kg) $\times$ (120 − serum Na)
      a. 80-kg patient with serum Na 107 mEq/L: Na required = $(0.5 \times 80) \times (120 - 107) = 520$ mEq
      b. Infuse 1 L 3% saline (Na = 513 mEq/L) over 6–12 hr; would acutely correct hyponatremia to $\approx$ 120 mEq/L in this patient

C. Moderate symptoms or serum Na less than 115 mEq/L, especially acute onset: infuse 3% saline as above, or treat on the basis of volume status (below)

D. Mild or no symptoms
   1. Hypovolemic state: infuse 0.9% normal saline (NS) at a rate to correct volume deficiency; ADH secretion stops, and kidneys excrete excess water
   2. Hypervolemic state: administer loop diuretic furosemide (Lasix), 40–80 mg IV or PO
   3. ADH secretion stops, and kidneys excrete excess water

E. All cases: restrict water or total fluid intake to 1000 ml/24 hr or less

F. Discontinue drugs that enhance sodium excretion

G. Associated hypokalemia: supplement potassium PO or intravenous PRN

H. Underlying condition
   1. Hypothyroidism: thyroid replacement
   2. Adrenal insufficiency: cortisol therapy
   3. SIADH: treatment directed at blocking ADH effect in kidney
      a. Conivaptan—use in hospitalized patients diagnosed with hypervolemic or euvolemic hyponatremia only; 20-mg IV loading dose and continuous IV infusion 20–40 mg over 24 hr for maximum of four days; discontinuation of hypertonic saline and fluid restriction may cause hypotension and/or hypokalemia; no adjustment required in geriatric patients

        b. Tolvaptan—use in hypervolemic or euvolemic hyponatremia patients only; initiate in hospital, titrate as outpatient; oral administration 15-mg starting dose titrated to maximum of 60 mg/day; maximum use of 30 days; discontinuation of hypertonic saline and fluid restriction may cause hepatic injury; monitor transaminase (ALT, AST) levels

        c. Demeclocycline—150–300 mg PO Q 6 hr for longterm therapy; photosensitizing drug; limit sun exposure with use

  I. Monitor serum Na every 2–4 hr in all symptomatic patients

HYPERNATREMIA

  I. **Definition**

    A. Increased serum Na greater than 146 mEq/L

    B. Hypernatremia always indicates hyperosmolality, a deficit of total body water

  II. **Etiology/incidence/predisposing factor**

    A. Occurs in 0.3%–1% of hospitalized patients

    B. Combination of excess water loss and inability to acquire water; more common in debilitated elderly, those with debility following CVA, and infants

    C. Primary water loss

      1. Central (pituitary) diabetes insipidus; lack of ADH secretion

      2. Nephrogenic (renal) diabetes insipidus; failed response to ADH

    D. Water loss in excess of sodium loss

      1. Renal osmotic diuresis

        a. Glucosuria of diabetes mellitus

        b. Mannitol or glycerol infusion

        c. High urea excretion in catabolic states (e.g., burn)

      2. GI fluid loss

        a. Persistent diarrhea or emesis

        b. Postsurgical drainage

      3. Cutaneous fluid loss

        a. Burns

        b. Profuse sweating

    E. Excess hypertonic saline solutions

      1. Hypertonic sodium bicarbonate ($NaHCO_3$) infusion for cardiopulmonary resuscitation (CPR) or lactic acidosis

      2. Hypertonic sodium chloride (NaCl) (3% saline) infusion

  III. **Subjective findings**

    A. Mostly neurologic

      1. Related to brain cell shrinkage from water loss

      2. Severity is relative to degree and rapidity of development of hypernatremia

    B. Correlation with serum sodium

      1. Serum Na 146–150 mEq/L; often asymptomatic

2. Serum Na 151–160 mEq/L
   a. Acute: nausea, weakness, lethargy, confusion, or irritability
   b. Chronic: none to mild CNS symptoms
3. Serum Na greater than 160 mEq/L
   a. Acute: stupor, coma
   b. Chronic: moderate to more severe CNS symptoms

C. Thirst/polydipsia: appropriate response in alert patients
D. Polyuria/nocturia
   1. Indicative of renal basis
   2. Occurs with diabetes insipidus or osmotic diuresis (glucosuria in hyperglycemia)

IV. **Physical examination findings**
A. CNS depression, rare focal neurologic findings
B. Hypotension, tachycardia, or oliguria in volume-depleted states
C. Major findings may reflect primary disorder that causes hypernatremia

V. **Laboratory/diagnostic findings**
A. Serum Na greater than 146 mEq/L: SOsm greater than 300 mOsm/L
B. Urine osmolality (UOsm)
   1. UOsm less than 300 mOsm/L: central or nephrogenic diabetes insipidus
   2. UOsm = 300–400 mOsm/L: suggests osmotic diuresis
   3. UOsm greater than 400 mOsm/L: gastrointestinal, cutaneous, or insensible fluid (water) loss
C. Serum ADH levels during hypernatremia occasionally useful
D. Water deprivation test; requires constant patient monitoring
   1. Withhold all fluid intake
   2. Monitor blood pressure (BP), serum sodium, and urine osmolality
   3. When urine osmolality is nearly constant (less than 30 mOsm/L change for 2–3 hr),
      a. Inject aqueous vasopressin (AVP) 5 units subcutaneously or
      b. Inject desmopressin (DDAVP) 4 mcg subcutaneously
      c. Measure urine volume and urine osmolality after 1 hr
   4. Central diabetes insipidus: increase in urine osmolality to 600–700 mOsm/L
   5. Nephrogenic diabetes insipidus: little or no increase in urine osmolality

VI. **Management**
A. Rapid lowering of serum sodium indicated for acute, symptomatic hypernatremia; chronic hypernatremia must be treated more slowly
   1. For acute hypernatremia: serum sodium concentration should be corrected no faster than 1–2 mEq/L/hr to avoid cerebral edema
   2. For chronic hypernatremia: serum sodium concentration should be corrected at a maximum rate of 0.5 mEq/L/hr
B. Estimate water deficit at approximately $0.4 \times$ Body wt (kg) $\times$ [(serum Na/140) − 1]

C. Discontinue or reduce any excess saline solution administration
D. Replace water at rate calculated to reduce serum sodium by approximately 1 mEq/L/hr in acute hypernatremia; in chronic hypernatremia, to reduce serum sodium by approximately one half of excess above 140 mEq/L over 24 hr
E. Enteral therapy: oral water preferable replacement in conscious patients
F. Intravenous therapy
1. Mild volume depletion
   a. Intravenous 5% dextrose in water (D5W)
   b. Avoid hyperglycemia/glucosuria to prevent further renal water loss
2. Moderate volume depletion
   a. Intravenous one-half normal saline (0.45% NS)
   b. Saline component restores ECF volume
   c. Free water component repletes body water
3. Severe volume depletion
   a. Intravenous 0.9% NS
   b. Follow with ½ NS (0.45% NS) or D5W when cardiovascular state has been stabilized
G. Monitor serum sodium every 2–4 hr in acute hypernatremia, every 4–6 hr in chronic hypernatremia
H. Treat diabetes insipidus, if present (see Diabetes Insipidus chapter)

HYPOKALEMIA

I. **Definition**
   A. Decreased serum potassium (K) concentration: K less than 3.5 mEq/L; normal is 3.5–5.5 mEq/L
   B. Serum levels may fall as the result of body loss or due to cellular uptake of potassium from extracellular fluids

II. **Etiology/incidence/predisposing factors**
   A. Renal potassium loss
   1. Diuretics
      a. Pharmacological: acetazolamide, loop diuretics (furosemide), thiazides
      b. Osmotic: mannitol, glycerol, glucose in diabetics
   2. Mineralocorticoid excess
      a. Primary hyperaldosteronism of adrenal disease
      b. Secondary aldosterone excess in hypovolemic states
      c. Secondary aldosterone excess in renovascular hypertension
   3. Renin-secreting tumor
   4. Cushing's syndrome or adrenal hyperplasia
   5. Exogenous mineralocorticoid effect: high-dose prednisone therapy, fludrocortisone, authentic licorice ingestion
   6. Renal tubular disorders

        a. Renal tubular acidosis (RTA), types I and II

        b. Bartter's, Gitelman's, or Liddle's syndrome

    7. Hypomagnesemia

  B. Nonrenal potassium loss

    1. Emesis and nasogastric suction; both GI and renal losses may occur

    2. Diarrhea, especially laxative abuse, and secretory diarrheas

  C. Potassium uptake into cells

    1. Insulin therapy: common in the treatment of diabetic ketoacidosis

    2. Catecholamine excess: epinephrine or β-adrenergic therapy (albuterol)

    3. Metabolic diseases

        a. Familial periodic paralysis

        b. Thyrotoxic paralysis

  D. Inadequate dietary potassium intake: rare as sole cause

  E. Occurs in up to 20% of hospitalized patients and in 10%–40% of outpatients who are taking diuretics (incidence correlates with diuretic dose)

III.   **Subjective findings**

  A. Skeletal muscle cramps, tenderness, and weakness; leg weakness may ascend with eventual diaphragmatic paralysis in extreme hypokalemia

  B. Paralytic ileus; abdominal distension, nausea, emesis

  C. Cardiac palpitations; varied cardiac arrhythmias; high risk with digoxin treatment

  D. Polyuria and polydipsia; inability to concentrate urine in chronic hypokalemia

IV.   **Physical examination findings**

  A. Muscle tenderness or weakness

  B. Cardiac rhythm changes including premature atrial or ventricular beats

V.   **Laboratory/diagnostic findings**

  A. Serum potassium less than 3.5 mEq/L

  B. Electrocardiogram: T wave flattening, appearance of U wave

  C. Urinary K excretion

    1. Greater than 25 mEq/L/24 hr: renal potassium wasting

    2. Less than 25 mEq/L/24 hr: nonrenal potassium losses

  D. Increased serum bicarbonate (HCO_3): suggests mineralocorticoid excess

  E. Serum magnesium (Mg)

    1. Normal is 1.5–2.5 mg/dl

    2. Decreased in up to 40% of hypokalemic patients

VI.   **Management**

  A. Discontinue drugs that enhance potassium excretion

  B. Body deficits are poorly correlated with serum K; estimate 100 mEq K loss for each 0.3mEq/L decrease in serum K less than 4.0 mEq/L

C. Intravenous potassium chloride (KCl), potassium phosphate (KPO_4), and potassium acetate: patients with cardiac arrhythmias (especially on digitalis therapy) or hepatic encephalopathy, or those unable to take oral potassium
   1. Maximum solution concentration based on vein irritation
      a. Peripheral vein infusion: 40 mEq/L solution
      b. Central vein infusion: 60 mEq/L solution
         i. Rate of infusion: maximum 10–20 mEq/hr; continuously monitor ECG
D. Oral potassium; chloride salt most effective, especially in metabolic alkalosis
   1. KCl (K–Lor and others):
      a. Acute—maximum single oral dose of 40–60 mEq with repeat measurement of serum K in 4 hr, then repeat PRN
      b. Chronic—10–40 mEq/day in 1–2 doses
   2. KCl extended-release (K-Dur, Micro-K Extencaps), dose as above
E. Potassium-sparing diuretics: usually given in combination with other diuretics
   1. Spironolactone (Aldactone), 25–100 mg PO daily
   2. Amiloride (Midamor), 5 mg PO daily
   3. Eplerenone (Inspra), 25–50 mg PO daily
F. High-potassium diet: nuts, dried fruits, tomatoes, potatoes, oranges

HYPERKALEMIA

I. **Definition**
   A. Increased serum potassium concentration
      1. Serum potassium greater than 5.5 mEq/L
      2. Normal is 3.5–5.5 mEq/L
   B. Serum levels may rise from decreased renal excretion, decreased cellular uptake, or increased cellular release of potassium
II. **Etiology/incidence/predisposing factors**
   A. Decreased renal excretion
      1. Renal failure, acute or chronic
      2. Decreased aldosterone synthesis
         a. Adrenal insufficiency
         b. Heparin therapy
      3. Decreased renal aldosterone effect
         a. Potassium-sparing diuretics
         b. Certain renal diseases (e.g., diabetic, obstructive, or sickle cell nephropathies)
   B. Renin-angiotensin system disruption
      1. Hyporeninemia-hypoaldosteronism, most commonly from early diabetic nephropathy

    2. ACE inhibitor (ACE I) or Angiotensin receptor blocker (ARB) therapy; combination of both drug classes, especially dangerous in diabetic kidney disease

    3. NSAID therapy

    4. Cyclosporine therapy

C. Decreased cell uptake/increased cell release

    1. Insulin deficiency as in diabetic hyperglycemia

    2. Cellular disruption

      a. Intravascular hemolysis

      b. Rhabdomyolysis in muscle ischemia or crush injury

      c. Tumor lysis syndrome after chemotherapy

    3. Pseudohyperkalemia: occurs in venipuncture tube only

      a. Hemolysis using small needle or excess venous occlusion

      b. Thrombocytosis, platelet count greater than $500,000/mm^3$

      c. Leukocytosis, WBC count greater than $100,000/mm^3$

    4. Metabolic acidosis: usually hyperchloremic variety

    5. Digitalis toxicity

D. Increased intake

    1. Oral: potassium supplements or dietary salt substitutes

    2. Intravenous: overly aggressive replacement with potassium salts of drugs

III. Subjective findings

A. Muscle weakness to paralysis

B. Symptoms of underlying disorder often dominate

IV. Physical examination findings

A. Muscle weakness

B. Signs of underlying disorder

V. Laboratory/diagnostic findings

A. Serum potassium greater than 5.5 mEq/L

B. ECG: progression of peaked T waves, widened QRS complex, disappearance of P wave, fusion of QRS and T to form sine wave

C. Elevated BUN and serum creatinine identify renal failure

D. Paired serum renin and aldosterone levels identify primary or secondary hypoaldosteronism

E. Plasma potassium: measured in heparinized tube; normal in pseudohyperkalemia

VI. Management

A. Urgency and level of intervention based on absence or severity of ECG changes

B. All cases

    1. Repeat serum (or plasma) potassium

    2. Seek and limit sources of potassium intake

    3. Discontinue drugs that limit potassium excretion

    4. Obtain ECG

C. ECG normal

1. Furosemide (Lasix), 40–80 mg IV, to increase renal potassium excretion
2. Sodium polystyrene resin (Kayexalate), 15–45 grams with osmotic cathartic (33% sorbitol or lactulose) to increase GI potassium excretion; must establish bowel activity by abdomen exam (bowel necrosis or perforation complications, especially in post-operative period); slow-acting (greater than 4 hr) as resin must reach colon and be excreted to be effective
3. Hemodialysis or peritoneal dialysis to remove potassium in renal failure

D. ECG abnormal; monitor ECG until normal
   1. Absent P wave, QRS widening, or sine waves
      a. Calcium gluconate 10%: 1 gram IV infusion over 1–2 min to antagonize hyperkalemic effect
         i. Immediate onset; repeat in 3–5 min if needed to normalize ECG
         ii. Does not lower serum K; effect lasts for minutes only
      b. Calcium chloride may also be used, but the dose needs to be adjusted to prevent calcium toxicity because this drug contains about 3 times the amount of calcium per 10-mL dose.
      c. Regular insulin (10 units) IV over 2–5 min to increase cellular potassium uptake;
         i. Add glucose (D50%) 25–50 grams if euglycemic
         ii. Effect in 15–30 min; lasts for 30–60 min
         iii. Does not lower serum potassium
      d. Albuterol (10–20 mg) via inhalation over 10 min to increase cellular potassium uptake; effect in 15–30 minutes
         i. Does not lower serum potassium; effect lasts for 60–120 min
      e. Sodium bicarbonate (50 mEq) IV over 1–2 min
         i. Variable efficacy in acidosis only
         ii. May cause dangerous hypernatremia with repeat doses
         iii. Does not lower serum potassium; effects lasts for 2–6 hr
      f. Diuretic, resin, dialysis as above to enhance removal after above measures
   2. Peaked T waves alone
      a. Insulin/glucose or albuterol as above to increase cellular potassium uptake
      b. Diuretic, resin, dialysis as above to enhance removal

HYPOCALCEMIA

I. **Definition**
- **A.** Decreased serum calcium (Ca) concentration: Ca less than 8.6 mg/dl
  - **1.** Normal is 8.6–10.2 mg/dl
  - **2.** Portion of total calcium binds to serum albumin
    - **a.** Correct serum calcium upward by 0.8 mg/dl for each 1 gram/dl decrease in serum albumin
- **B.** The fraction of serum calcium not bound to albumin, ionized calcium (Ca^{++}_i), is physiologically active
  - **1.** Hypocalcemia can also be revealed by ionized calcium less than 4.5 mg/dl or 1.1 mmol/L
  - **2.** Normal sub ionized calcium is 4.6–5.3 mg/dl, or 1.12–1.30 mmol/L

II. **Etiology/incidence/predisposing factors**
- **A.** Hypoparathyroidism, usually surgical; post thyroidectomy or parathyroidectomy
- **B.** Hypomagnesemia, especially with serum magnesium less than 1 mEq/L
- **C.** Pancreatitis (40%–70% incidence in acute pancreatitis)
- **D.** Vitamin D deficiency
  - **1.** Malnutrition, especially in infants and the elderly
  - **2.** Fat malabsorption
    - **a.** Pancreatic: exocrine insufficiency (chronic pancreatitis)
    - **b.** Intestinal: regional enteritis, jejunoileal bypass
  - **3.** Chronic renal failure
- **E.** Chronic alcoholism
- **F.** Drugs
  - **1.** Phenytoin
  - **2.** Cisplatin
  - **3.** Estrogen therapy

III. **Subjective findings**
- **A.** Mental changes: depression, anxiety, confusion
- **B.** Extrapyramidal changes: tremors, ataxia, dystonia
- **C.** Tetany
- **D.** Seizures
- **E.** Weakness

IV. **Physical examination findings**
- **A.** Chvostek's sign: facial twitch on tapping ipsilateral facial nerve
- **B.** Trousseau's sign: carpal spasm on inflation of BP cuff to occlude brachial artery for 3 minutes
- **C.** Proximal muscle weakness
- **D.** Integument; dry skin, brittle hair and nails

V. **Laboratory/diagnostic findings**
- **A.** Serum calcium corrected for serum albumin; serum ionized calcium if necessary

    B. Serum albumin (normal, 3.5–4.6 grams/dl) to correct serum calcium level (above)

    C. Serum magnesium (normal, 1.6–2.2 mg/dl) for hypomagnesemia, seen in about 20% of hypocalcemic patients

    D. ECG

        1. Prolonged QTc interval

        2. Nonspecific T wave changes

VI. Management

    A. Symptomatic, acute (tetany or seizures), or if NPO

        1. Calcium chloride: 1 gram 10% solution IV injection over 3–5 min

        2. Calcium gluconate: 1 gram 10% solution IV injection over 3–5 min for 2 doses

        3. Follow with 1 gram/hr calcium gluconate in 500 ml D5W or NS over 3 hr

    B. Asymptomatic, chronic

        1. Calcium carbonate or other calcium salt

            a. 2–3 grams elemental calcium/day in divided doses

            b. Starting regimen (calcium carbonate [$CaCO_3$] 500 mg PO, 3–4 times daily) of 1.5–2 grams per day

            c. Adjunct therapy: Docusate 250 mg PO BID +/- Senokot 8.8–17.6 mg PO daily

            d. Adequate fluid intake

        2. Vitamin D oral preparations

            a. Ergocalciferol (Drisdol) 50,000–200,000 units orally or IM once a day

            b. Calcitriol (Rocaltrol), 0.5–2 mcg/day

HYPERCALCEMIA

I. Definition

    A. Increased total and ionized serum calcium

    B. Total serum calcium corrected for serum albumin greater than 10.2 mg/dl, or ionized calcium greater than 5.3 mg/dl

        1. Normal range for ionized calcium: 1.12–1.30 mmol/L

        2. Hypercalcemia: greater than 1.30 mmol/L

II. Etiology/incidence/predisposing factors

    A. Hyperparathyroidism

        1. 10%–20% of hypercalcemia

        2. Most common cause

    B. Malignancy

        1. Most common in hospitalized patients; lung, renal, or breast cancer

        2. Circulating parathyroid hormone-related peptide (PHRP)

        3. Local bone resorption of metastatic disease

    C. Vitamin D excess

        1. Exogenous intake: high dose vitamin D plus calcium supplements

   2. Endogenous production: granulomatous diseases such as sarcoidosis (15%–20% of patients develop hypercalcemia)
   D. Vitamin A intoxication, high dose therapy
   E. Hyperthyroidism: 10%–20% of patients develop hypercalcemia
   F. Immobilization: paralysis or body cast, especially in young people
   G. Thiazide diuretic therapy
III. **Subjective findings**
   A. Neurologic
      1. Lethargy progressing to coma
      2. Depression or memory impairment
      3. Personality changes
   B. Gastrointestinal
      1. Nausea and vomiting
      2. Constipation
   C. Musculoskeletal
      1. Proximal muscle weakness
      2. Bone pain
   D. Renal
      1. Polyuria or nocturia (form of nephrogenic diabetes insipidus)
      2. Renal colic (complication of renal calculi)
IV. **Physical examination findings**
   A. Global CNS dysfunction
   B. Depressed deep tendon reflexes
   C. Hypertension: usually in moderate, chronic hypercalcemia
   D. Hypotension: in severe hypercalcemia with volume depletion
V. **Laboratory/diagnostic findings**
   A. Serum calcium corrected for serum albumin; serum ionized calcium if necessary
   B. Parathyroid hormone (PTH) level
   C. Thyroid panel
      1. Thyroid-stimulating hormone (TSH)
      2. Free T_4 level
   D. Vitamin D levels: $25-OH\ D_3$ and $1,25-(OH)_2\ D_3$
   E. Radiographic bone survey: changes in hyperparathyroidism or metastases
   F. PHRP level, if appropriate
   G. ECG: shortened QTc interval
VI. **Management**
   A. Severe hypercalcemia, typically in malignancy
      1. Intravenous 0.9% NS to restore volume and induce diuresis of more than 200 ml/hr
      2. Calcitonin (Calcimar, Miacalcin), 4–8 international units/kg every 12 hr subcutaneously or IM; effective only for few days
      3. Intravenous bisphosphonates (caution in renal insufficiency)

        a. Pamidronate (Aredia), 60–90 mg IV infused over 24 hr, repeat after 7 days

        b. Etidronate (Didronel), 7.5 mg/kg in 250 ml NS over 2–3 hr for 3 days

        c. Zoledronic acid (Zometa), 4 mg IV infused over 15 min; may repeat after 7 days

    4. Furosemide (Lasix), 40–80 mg IV every 8–12 hr to maintain urine output of 150–200 ml/hr (with constant NS [0.9% NS] or ½ NS [0.45% NS] infusion)

    5. Hemodialysis with low-calcium dialysis bath

  B. Chronic hypercalcemia

    1. Prednisone, 40–80 mg/day orally: best for hypercalcemia of sarcoidosis, hypervitaminosis D, or lymphoma

    2. Furosemide (Lasix), 40–80 mg oral BID, plus 6- to 8-gram sodium diet

    3. Reduced calcium diet, 750–1000 mg/day

HYPOMAGNESEMIA

I. **Definition**

  A. Decreased serum magnesium concentration

    1. Mg less than 1.5 mg/dL

    2. Normal is 1.5–2.5 mg/dL

II. **Etiology/incidence/predisposing factors**

  A. Renal magnesium loss

    1. Diuretics

        a. Especially loop diuretics and thiazides

        b. 20%–45% incidence of hypomagnesemia

    2. Chronic alcohol use: 30% incidence of hypomagnesemia

    3. Renal drug toxicity

        a. Aminoglycosides

        b. Amphotericin B

        c. Cisplatin

  B. Gastrointestinal magnesium loss

    1. Persistent diarrhea or laxative abuse

    2. Malabsorption and inflammatory bowel disease

  C. Deficient magnesium intake

    1. Chronic alcohol use

    2. Protein-calorie malnutrition

  D. Cellular uptake

    1. Alcohol withdrawal: 80%–85% incidence of hypomagnesemia

    2. Acute insulin therapy, as in diabetic ketoacidosis

III. **Subjective findings**

  A. Muscle weakness

  B. Neurologic symptoms of tremors to seizures

IV. **Physical examination findings**
  A. Trousseau's sign and Chvostek's sign (See Hypocalcemia)
  B. Muscle fasciculations or tremors
V. **Laboratory/diagnostic findings**
  A. Serum Mg less than 1.5 mg/dL
  B. Serum Ca and serum K decreased in severe hypomagnesemia
  C. Urinary Mg excretion less than 3 mEq/24 hr denotes body deficiency
  D. ECG
    1. Prolonged QTc interval
    2. Ventricular arrhythmias
VI. **Management**
  A. Discontinue drugs that enhance magnesium excretion
  B. Parenteral route preferred if patient symptomatic or has hypocalcemia
    a. Mild symptoms
      i. 4 grams magnesium sulfate ($MgSO_4$) IV in 1 L D5W over 3–6 hr
      ii. Then, 2–4 grams in D5W over next 12–24 hr
      iii. Goal: serum Mg to exceed 1.5 mg/dL
        (a) Patients at risk for arrhythmias may be required to have a goal of greater than 2.0 mg/dL
    b. Severe symptoms (seizure, ventricular arrhythmia)
      i. 2 grams IV in 30–50 ml D5W over 5–10 min; may be administered as IV push for patients with arrhythmias
      ii. Then, infusions as above
  C. Oral
    1. Magnesium chloride (Mag−L−100), 2 tablets 3 times a day
    2. Magnesium oxide (Mag−Ox 400), 400 mg PO BID
    3. Magnesium lactate (Magtab SR), 84 mg PO BID

HYPERMAGNESEMIA

I. **Definition**
  A. Increased serum magnesium concentration: serum magnesium greater than 2.5 mg/dL
  B. Clinical consequences unusual at serum magnesium less than 4.0 mEq/L
II. **Etiology/incidence/predisposing factors**
  A. Decreased renal function; almost always in severe hypermagnesemia
  B. Ongoing magnesium intake with renal insufficiency
    1. Antacids: magnesium hydroxide (Maalox and others)
    2. Cathartics; common cause in elderly
      a. Magnesium sulfate (Epsom salt)
      b. Magnesium hydroxide (Milk of Magnesia)
      c. Magnesium citrate

    C. Massive magnesium intake
        1. Intravenous magnesium sulfate in eclampsia
        2. Oral Epsom salt

III. **Subjective findings**
    A. Weakness progressing to paralysis; difficulty swallowing early
    B. Lethargy
    C. Nausea and emesis

IV. **Physical examination findings**
    A. Hypotension
    B. Diminished or absent deep tendon reflexes (serum magnesium, 4–5 mEq/L)
    C. Weakness to flaccid paralysis, including respiratory muscle paralysis (serum magnesium 8–10 mEq/L)

V. **Laboratory/diagnostic findings**
    A. Serum magnesium greater than 2.2 mEq/L
    B. BUN and serum creatinine to identify renal insufficiency
    C. ECG
        1. Lengthening PR interval
        2. Widening of QRS
        3. Complete heart block

VI. **Management**
    A. All cases: stop magnesium intake
    B. ECG changes
        1. 10% calcium gluconate 1–3 grams
        2. Calcium chloride 500–1000 mg
        3. Furosemide (Lasix) 40 mg IV plus ½ NS (0.45% NS) 50–100 ml/hr
    C. Hemodialysis: ECG changes; consider for any serum magnesium greater than 4 mEq/L

HYPOPHOSPHATEMIA

I. **Definition**
    A. Decreased serum phosphorus to less than 2.5 mg/dl
    B. Severe when serum phosphorus less than 1.5 mg/dl (normal is 2.5–4.5 mg/dl)

II. **Etiology/incidence/predisposing factors**
    A. Loss of urinary phosphorus
        1. Diuretics
        2. DKA
        3. Hyperparathyroidism
        4. Renal tubule defects
            a. Fanconi's syndrome
            b. Amphotericin B toxicity
    B. Cellular uptake
        1. Increased glucose utilization

        a. Treatment of DKA or alcohol withdrawal

        b. Total parenteral nutrition

    2. Acute respiratory alkalosis

    3. Burns

  C. Deficient GI intake or absorption

    1. Chronic alcohol use

    2. Use of oral phosphate binders

        a. Calcium salts (PhosLo, Os–Cal, and others)

        b. Polymer gels (Renagel)

        c. Lanthanum chloride (Fosrenol)

    3. Malabsorption syndromes

III. **Subjective findings**

  A. Irritability, confusion, paresthesias

  B. Weakness

IV. **Physical examination findings**

  A. Muscle weakness

V. **Laboratory/diagnostic findings**

  A. Serum phosphorus less than 2.5 mg/dl

  B. Hemolysis due to severe hypophosphatemia; CBC, increased serum free hemoglobin, and decreased haptoglobin

  C. Rhabdomyolysis due to severe hypophosphatemia (especially alcoholics): increased creatine kinase (CK) level, and positive urinary myoglobin

  D. Metabolic acidosis: decreased serum bicarbonate and arterial pH

VI. **Management**

  A. Oral: tablets of sodium or potassium neutral phosphorus (Neutra phos, K–Phos Neutral), 1–2 grams PO daily in divided doses

  B. Intravenous: solution of sodium or potassium phosphate 2 mg phosphorus/kg in ½ NS infused over 6 hr, or 5 mg/kg over 12 hr

HYPERPHOSPHATEMIA

I. **Definition**

  A. Increased serum phosphorus

  B. Serum phosphorus greater than 5 mg/dl in adults

  C. Normal level in adults is 2.5–4.5 mg/dl

II. **Etiology/incidence/predisposing factors**

  A. Deficient renal phosphate excretion

    1. Acute or chronic renal failure

        a. Usually, glomerular filtration rate (GFR) less than 25 ml/min

        b. Most common cause of persistent hyperphosphatemia

    2. Decreased PTH effect: primary hypoparathyroidism or pseudohypoparathyroidism

  B. Redistribution of phosphorus from cell to extracellular fluids

    1. Tumor lysis syndrome: post chemotherapy for leukemia or lymphoma

  2. Rhabdomyolysis or crush injury
  3. Acute respiratory acidosis
 C. Increased intestinal absorption
  1. Use of phosphate-containing salts or cathartics
  2. Vitamin D therapy, especially in renal insufficiency
III. Subjective findings
 A. None, or related to secondary hypocalcemia
IV. Physical examination findings
 A. Ectopic tissue calcification: (serum phosphorus [P] × serum Ca) greater than 55
 B. Sites
  1. Cornea or acute conjunctivitis
  2. Skin
   a. Grainy feeling of skin
   b. Pruritus
  3. Vascular calcification identified on plain film or CT radiography
  4. Cardiac tissue
   a. Valvular and arterial calcification
   b. Conduction defects on ECG
   c. Increased cardiac mortality
V. Laboratory/diagnostic findings
 A. Serum phosphorus greater than 5 mg/dl in adults, greater than 6 mg/dl in children
 B. BUN, serum creatinine, or creatinine clearance for renal insufficiency
 C. Serum PTH and vitamin D levels
 D. Serum calcium to calculate phosphorus × Ca product; danger above 55
 E. Arterial pH (hypoventilation), WBC (leukemia), and serum CK (crush injury)
VI. Management
 A. Peritoneal dialysis or hemodialysis in acute and chronic renal failure
 B. Dietary restriction on phosphorus (800–1000 mg/day)
 C. Oral phosphate binders
  1. Calcium acetate 667–1334 mg PO TID with meals
  2. Sevelamer 800–3200 mg PO TID with meals
  3. Lanthanum 500–1000 mg PO TID with meals

ACID-BASE DISORDERS

I. Definition
 A. Disturbances in the processes that, collectively, maintain a nearly constant body hydrogen ion concentration (H^+) or pH throughout all body fluids
 B. Primary disorder
  1. Pathologic change that, unchecked, would displace H^+ from normal value
  2. Compensatory process

        a. Reactive change to primary disorder that allows complementary factors to move hydrogen ions back toward normal (i.e., metabolic alkalosis [kidney] compensates for respiratory acidosis [lung])

        b. Arterial pH points to primary disorder (e.g., acid pH indicates primary acidosis)

    3. Duration

        a. For respiratory abnormalities, the body compensates metabolically with changes in serum bicarbonate through renal regulation, which may take 3–5 days to begin and up to a week to see the full compensation.

        b. For metabolic disorders, the compensation through pulmonary regulation of partial pressure of carbon dioxide (pCO_2); occurs more rapidly than metabolic compensation, taking minutes to being with full compensation seen in hours.

C. Mixed disorder

    1. More than one primary disorder occurring simultaneously

    2. pH points to dominant disorder (e.g., acid pH indicates dominant acidosis)

II. **Laboratory/diagnostic findings**

A. $pH = \log [H^+]$

    1. pH $7.40 = 10^{-7.4}$ Eq/L, or $H^+ = 40$ mEq/L

B. $H^+ = 24 \times pCO_2/HCO_3$

    1. pCO_2 and HCO_3 determine the pH

C. Arterial blood gas (ABG) measures pH and pCO_2

    1. Normal pH $= 7.35$–7.45

        a. In acidemia, pH less than 7.35

        b. In alkalemia, pH greater than 7.45

    2. Normal $pCO_2 = 35$–45 mmHg

D. Serum electrolytes measure HCO_3 and anion gap (AG)

    1. $AG = Na^+ - ([Cl^-] + [HCO_3^-])$

    2. Normal $HCO_3 = 22$–26 mEq/L

    3. Normal AG $= 8$–10 mEq/L

METABOLIC ACIDOSIS

I. **Definition**

A. Nonventilatory process that increases H^+; pH less than 7.35

    1. Identified by a decrease in HCO_3, usually to less than 22 mEq/L

    2. Respiratory alkalosis (decreased pCO_2) seen as compensating process

B. Normal AG metabolic acidosis

    1. AG less than 12 mEq/L

    2. Indicates primary HCO_3^- loss, or H^+ plus Cl^- gain

C. High AG metabolic acidosis

    1. AG greater than 15 mEq/L

      2. Indicates addition to serum of non-chlorine acid anion (e.g., lactate from lactic acid)

II.   **Etiology/incidence/predisposing factors**
  A. Normal AG metabolic acidosis
    1. GI bicarbonate loss
      a. Diarrhea
      b. Pancreatic drainage
    2. Insufficient renal acid excretion
      a. Renal tubule acidosis, types I, II, and IV
      b. Mild/moderate kidney failure (glomerular filtration rate [GFR] greater than 20–30 ml/min)
    3. Hydrogen chloride (HCl) intake of acidifying salts: ammonium chloride (NH_4Cl) or arginine HCl
  B. High AG metabolic acidosis
    1. Endogenous acids
      a. Lactic acidosis: hypoxia, sepsis, circulatory shock
      b. Diabetic ketoacidosis: lack of insulin
      c. Alcoholic ketoacidosis: drinking binge ending in nausea and vomiting with poor nutrition
      d. Advanced renal insufficiency: GFR less than 15–20 ml/min
    2. Exogenous acids
      a. Salicylate poisoning: aspirin or salicylic acid
      b. Methanol: formic acid metabolite
      c. Ethylene glycol: glycolic and oxalic acid metabolites

III.   **Subjective findings**
  A. Anorexia and nausea
  B. Weakness, lethargy to coma
  C. Symptoms of underlying disorder

IV.   **Physical examination findings**
  A. Kussmaul breathing: rapid, regular, deep breathing
  B. Hypotension
  C. Signs of underlying disorder (e.g., sweet breath in ketoacidosis)

V.   **Laboratory/diagnostic findings**
  A. Arterial blood gases
    1. pH
    2. pCO_2
    3. Calculated HCO_3
  B. Serum sodium, bicarbonate, and chlorine Cl; calculate AG
  C. BUN and serum creatinine to identify renal failure
  D. Urine pH
    1. If greater than 5.5, suspect renal acidifying defect
    2. If less than 5.5, suspect GI bicarbonate loss or anion gap acidosis (above)
  E. Serum and urine ketones: positive in ketotic states
  F. Serum salicylate, methanol, or ethylene glycol levels

VI.   Management

    A. $NaHCO_3$ therapy; intravenous $NaHCO_3$ infusion controversial

        1. Rarely indicated when pH is 7.10 or greater

        2. Diabetic ketoacidosis: not required or recommended

        3. Lactic acidosis: $NaHCO_3$ may actually increase lactate levels

        4. $NaHCO_3$ injection

            a. Very hypertonic

            b. Limit to 50 mEq (1–2 ampules)

        5. $NaHCO_3$ isotonic infusion

            a. Example: HCO_3 required = 0.5 × body wt (kg) × (20 − serum HCO_3)

            b. Add 3 ampules $NaHCO_3$ (150 mEq) to 1 liter of D5W; infuse over 6–12 hr

        6. Shohl's solution (Bicitra and others): 1 ml (1 mEq)/kg body weight daily

            a. Start with 30 ml PO

        7. $NaHCO_3$ tablets: 650 mg tablet ≈ 8 mEq HCO_3

            a. Start with 650 mg PO TID

    B. Primary disorder treatment

        1. Stop or limit GI HCO_3^- losses

        2. Methanol or ethylene glycol ingestion

            a. Infuse ethanol to maintain blood level at 100–150 mg/day; limits acid metabolites

            b. Fomepizole 15 mg initial infusion then 10 mg q 12 hr; limits acid metabolites

            c. Dialysis indicated for severe intoxications, toxic levels greater than 50 mg/dl

        3. Salicylate poisoning

            a. Alkalinize urine with isotonic $NaHCO_3$ infusion (above) to maintain urine pH at 8 or above

            b. Dialysis indicated for severe intoxications, levels greater than 100 mg/dl acute or greater than 40 mg/dl chronic

        4. Diabetic ketoacidosis: intravenous NS (0.9% NS) and insulin infusions (see Diabetic Emergencies chapter)

        5. Alcoholic ketoacidosis: IV glucose (D5W or 5% dextrose in 0.9% NS at 100–150 ml/hr) plus thiamine (100 mg)

        6. Lactic acidosis

            a. Maintain tissue perfusion

            b. Intravenous 0.9% NS more effective than intravenous $NaHCO_3$

METABOLIC ALKALOSIS

I.   Definition

    A. Nonventilatory process that decreases H^+; pH greater than 7.45

        1. Identified by an increase in HCO_3, usually exceeding 28 mEq/L

    2. Respiratory acidosis (increased pCO_2) seen as a compensating process

II. **Etiology/incidence/predisposing factors**

  A. GI hydrogen loss

    1. Vomiting

    2. Nasogastric aspiration

  B. Renal hydrogen loss

    1. Secondary hyperaldosteronism from volume contraction

      a. Diuretic therapy

      b. Vomiting or nasogastric aspiration

      c. Potassium depletion with or without magnesium deficiency

    2. Hyperaldosteronism with normal or expanded volume

      a. Primary aldosteronism

      b. Cushing's syndrome

      c. Renal artery stenosis

  C. Bicarbonate gains; only occur in renal insufficiency

    1. $NaHCO_3$ administration

    2. Massive organic anion infusion

      a. Citrate (blood or fresh frozen plasma transfusion)

      b. Acetate (parenteral nutrition or dialysis solutions)

III. **Subjective findings**

  A. CNS symptoms

    1. Headache

    2. Lethargy to coma

  B. Tetany or seizure: may be associated with decreased Ca^{2+}

  C. Cardiac arrhythmias, especially with sympathetic nerve stimulation

IV. **Physical examination findings**

  A. Postural hypotension or tachycardia

  B. Respiratory depression

  C. Signs of primary disorder

V. **Laboratory/diagnostic findings**

  A. Arterial blood gases

    1. pH

    2. pCO_2

    3. Calculated HCO_3

  B. Serum electrolytes, for decreased potassium, magnesium, and ionized calcium

  C. Urine C: marker of volume status

    1. Urine Cl less than 20 mEq/L

      a. Vomiting

      b. Low NaCl intake

      c. Diuretic use after drug stopped

    2. Urine Cl greater than 40 mEq/L

      a. Aldosterone excess (primary or secondary)

      b. Active diuretic use

VI. **Management**
  A. Volume-depleted states: IV 0.9% NS at 100–150 ml/hr
  B. KCl replacement for all potassium-depleted or losing states
  C. Acetazolamide (Diamox), 250–500 mg IV or PO BID; especially useful in volume-expanded states
  D. Metabolic alkalosis caused/induces by excess aldosterone states may require spironolactone or eplerenone
  E. Hemodialysis against low $[HCO_3^-]$ bath

RESPIRATORY ACIDOSIS

I. **Definition**
  A. Ventilatory process that increases hydrogen; pH less than 7.35
     1. Identified by an increase in arterial pCO_2 greater than 45 mmHg
     2. Metabolic alkalosis seen as compensating process
II. **Etiology/incidence/predisposing factors**
  A. Acute hypoventilation
     1. CNS depression: opiates major cause, sedatives additive effect to opiates
     2. CNS injury: brain stem injury, CVA
     3. Neuromuscular disease
        a. Myasthenia gravis
        b. Guillain-Barré syndrome
        c. Poliomyelitis
     4. Airway obstruction
        a. Mucus/foreign body
        b. Severe bronchospasm of status asthmaticus
        c. Bronchitis
        d. Emphysema
     5. Chest disorders
        a. Flail chest
        b. Pneumothorax
        c. Kyphoscoliosis
  B. Chronic hypoventilation
     1. COPD
     2. Obesity—Pickwickian hypoventilation syndrome
     3. Diaphragmatic weakness/paralysis
III. **Subjective findings**
  A. Acute respiratory acidosis
     1. Decreased level of consciousness: drowsiness to coma
     2. Mental changes
        a. Headache
        b. Anxiety
        c. Confusion
        d. Hallucinations
     3. Dyspnea

    B. Chronic respiratory acidosis

       1. CNS symptoms

          a. Sleep disturbances

          b. Memory loss

       2. Neuromuscular changes

          a. Impaired coordination

          b. Tremor

IV. **Physical examination findings**

    A. Acute respiratory acidosis

       1. Blood pressure usually elevated

       2. CNS signs

          a. Altered level of consciousness

          b. Papilledema

       3. Neuromuscular signs

          a. Tremor

          b. Abnormal deep tendon reflexes

    B. Chronic respiratory acidosis

       1. CNS signs: no findings to mild tremor

       2. Cardiovascular: signs of cor pulmonale

          a. Right ventricular heave

          b. Pulmonary diastolic murmur

          c. Cyanosis

       3. Pulmonary: signs of COPD

          a. Increased anterior-posterior chest diameter

          b. Expiratory wheeze

          c. Accessory respiratory muscle use

V. **Laboratory/diagnostic findings**

    A. ABG: pH, pCO_2, pO_2, and calculated HCO_3

    B. Pulmonary function tests

       1. Decreased forced expiratory volume in 1 second (FEV_1)

       2. Increased residual volume

VI. **Management**

    A. Acute respiratory acidosis

       1. Assist ventilation

          a. Facemask for continuous positive airway pressure

          b. Airway intubation with mechanical ventilation

       2. Reverse CNS depression if appropriate

          a. Naloxone (Narcan), 0.4–2 mg IV for opioid overdose

          b. Flumazenil (Romazicon), 0.2 mg (2 ml) IV over 30 seconds for benzodiazepine overdose (observe for seizures)

       3. Reverse airway obstruction

          a. Bronchodilator therapy for bronchospasm

             i. Albuterol (Ventolin, Proventil), 180 mcg inhaled aerosol every 6 hr

ii. Ipratropium (Atrovent), 36 mcg inhaled aerosol every 6 hr

b. Mechanical extraction of secretions, foreign bodies

B. Chronic respiratory acidosis

1. Avoid respiratory depression (e.g., sedatives, O_2 therapy exceeding 3 L/min)

2. Nocturnal continuous positive airway pressure

3. Vigorous treatment underlying disorder

RESPIRATORY ALKALOSIS

I. Definition

A. Ventilatory process that decreases hydrogen; pH greater than 7.45

1. Identified by a decrease in arterial pCO_2 to below 35 mmHg

2. Metabolic acidosis (decreased HCO_3) seen as compensating process

II. Etiology/incidence/predisposing factors

A. Acute hyperventilation

1. CNS disorders

a. Anxiety, pain

b. Fever

c. Head trauma

d. Salicylates

2. Pulmonary diseases: decreased lung compliance

a. Pulmonary edema/congestive heart failure

b. Pneumonia

c. Pulmonary embolism

d. Asthma

e. Sepsis

f. Acute salicylate toxicity

B. Chronic hyperventilation

1. Residence at high altitude

2. Pregnancy

3. Chronic hepatic insufficiency/cirrhosis

III. Subjective findings

A. Acute respiratory alkalosis

1. CNS symptoms

a. Light-headedness

b. Confusion

2. Neurological symptoms

a. Paresthesias, especially around the mouth

3. Muscular symptoms

a. Chest tightness

b. Muscle cramps

B. Chronic respiratory alkalosis: generally none

IV.   Physical examination findings
  A. Acute respiratory alkalosis
    1. Hyperactive deep tendon reflexes
    2. Carpopedal spasm (tetany): flexed wrist/ankle with hyperextended digits
  B. Chronic respiratory alkalosis: generally none
V.   Laboratory/diagnostic findings
  A. ABG: pH, pCO_2, pO_2, and calculated HCO_3
  B. ECG: tachyarrhythmias, ischemic-like ST wave to T wave changes
VI.   Management
  A. Acute respiratory alkalosis
    1. Treatment of underlying cause
    2. Anxiety/hyperventilation
      a. Assurance
      b. Rebreathing into paper bag
  B. Chronic respiratory alkalosis: generally none required

INTRAVENOUS FLUID MANAGEMENT

I.   Principles of body fluid spaces
  A. TBW
    1. Volume
      a. 50%–60% of body weight (kg)
      b. Lower percentage in women and obese individuals
      c. Higher percentage in men and lean individuals
    2. Composition
      a. Solute composition varies among compartments, but total solute concentration (osmolality) is equal (isotonic) among compartments.
  B. Intracellular fluid
    1. Volume approximately 60% of TBW
    2. Composition
      a. High concentrations of potassium and phosphate ions
      b. Low concentrations of sodium and bicarbonate ions
  C. ECF
    1. Volume approximately 40% of TBW
    2. Composition
      a. Primarily sodium salts ($NaCl$, $NaHCO_3$)
      b. Low concentrations of potassium and phosphate
    3. Extravascular (interstitial) compartment of ECF
      a. Volume approximately 80% of ECF volume
      b. Composition: protein-poor electrolyte solution of ECF
    4. Intravascular compartment of ECF
      a. Volume approximately 20% of ECF volume
      b. Composition: protein-enriched electrolyte solution of ECF

      c. The compartment whose volume most closely reflects, and best determines, cardiovascular function

      d. Usefulness

         i. Compartment into which all therapeutic fluids are administered

         ii. Distribution to all other body fluid spaces occurs by diffusion or transport into those compartments

II. **Purposes of intravenous fluid administration**

  A. ECF volume repletion and maintenance

    1. Signs of ECF volume depletion

      a. Physical

         i. Hypotension

         ii. Tachycardia

         iii. Postural fall in blood pressure or rise in heart rate

         iv. Decreased internal jugular vein filling

      b. Invasive

         i. Decreased central venous pressure (CVP)

         ii. Decreased pulmonary capillary wedge pressure (PCWP)

    2. Signs of ECF volume excess

      a. Physical

         i. Hypertension

         ii. Internal jugular vein distention

         iii. Edema: peripheral, pulmonary, ascites

      b. Invasive: increased central venous pressure or pulse capillary wedge pressure

  B. Body water (osmolality) adjustment or maintenance

    1. Signs of water deficit: hypernatremia or serum hyperosmolality

    2. Signs of water excess: hyponatremia with serum hyposmolality

  C. Delivery of therapeutic agents

    1. Electrolytes: specific adjustment of potassium, magnesium, calcium, bicarbonate, phosphate, etc.

    2. Nutrition

      a. Calories

         i. Glucose

         ii. Lipids

      b. Nitrogen (amino acids)

      c. Water-soluble vitamins

      d. Trace elements (zinc [Zn], manganese [Mn])

    3. Drugs: multiple water-soluble agents

III. **Composition of common intravenous fluids**

  A. NS (0.9% NaCl) approximately isotonic to plasma

    1. Distribution: ECF volume

    2. ECF volume expansion; approximately one third of infused volume remains in vascular space at full distribution to support circulatory function

3. Drug delivery: for drugs stable only in saline solution

B. D5W approximately isotonic to plasma

   1. Distribution: intracellular and extracellular body water spaces
   2. Repletion or maintenance of body water (osmolality): equivalent to giving pure water once dextrose has metabolized
   3. Drug delivery: for compatible drugs when ECF volume expansion undesirable (less than 10% remains in vascular space at full distribution)

C. Lactated Ringer's solution (LR); containing NaCl, KCl, CaC_{12}, Na Lactate approximately isotonic to plasma

   1. Distribution
      a. ECF compartment
      b. Similar to NS
   2. Usage
      a. Mostly as repletion or resuscitation fluid in the face of actual or ongoing blood loss
      b. Lactate ion metabolized in liver to generate HCO_3
      c. Repletion or maintenance fluid in trauma or surgical patients

D. ½NS, 0.45% NaCl: hypotonic to plasma

   1. Distribution
      a. Half of volume equivalent to pure water distributes into total body water
      b. Half of volume equivalent to NS distributes into ECF compartment
      c. About 1/6 of volume remains in vascular space
   2. Maintenance fluid (most common use)
      a. Saline component replaces ongoing NaCl losses, maintains ECF volume
      b. Free water component replaces insensible free water losses, maintains osmolality
   3. Replacement fluid
      a. Saline component restores ECF volume deficit
      b. Free water component restores water deficit in hyperosmolar (hypernatremic) state

E. Dextrose in saline (D5 NS, D5 ½ NS, and D5 1/4 NS)

   1. Equivalent to corresponding saline solution plus supplying 200 kcal energy per liter of solution

F. Colloid solutions

   1. Solutions of large molecular weight particles that are substantially retained in the vascular volume and are used for selective vascular volume expansion and hemodynamic support
   2. 25% human albumin
      a. Expensive
      b. Best given in bolus (25 m/100 ml) in hypoalbuminemic patients

   3. 5% albumin in saline
      a. Expensive
      b. Comparable with NS alone
   4. Fresh frozen plasma
      a. Expensive
      b. Should not be used in fluid therapy, but only when depleted clotting factors are replaced
G. Electrolyte solutions
   1. Solutions used for specific replacement therapy
   2. Sodium bicarbonate: see acid base disorders
   3. $NaHCO_3$ potassium chloride: added to any dextrose or saline solution in final K concentration of 10–60 mEq/L

BIBLIOGRAPHY

Anderson, D., Knight, M. S., Spaniol, C. J. R., & Zeblet, J. L. (2012). Fluid resuscitation therapy for hemorrhagic shock. *Journal of Trauma Nursing, 14*(3), 152–160.

Assadi, F. (2010). Hypophophatemia: An evidence-based problem solving approach to clinical cases. *Iranian Journal of Kidney Disease, 4*(3), 195–201.

Brunton, L., Chabner, B., & Knollman, B. (2011). *Goodman & Gilman's the pharmacological basis of therapeutics* (12th ed.). New York, NY: McGraw-Hill.

Coleman, R. (2011). The use of biophosphonates in cancer treatment. *Annals of the New York Academy of Sciences*, 1218, 3–14.

Crawford, A., & Harris, H. (2011). Balancing act: Hypomagnesemia and hypermagnesemia. Nursing2014, 41(10), 52–55.

Dellinger, R. P., Levy, M. M., Rhodes, A., Annane, D., Gerlach, H., Opal, S. M., . . . Moreno, R. (2013). Surviving Sepsis Campaign: International guidelines for management of severe sepsis and septic shock, 2012. *Intensive Care Medicine, 39*(2), 165–228.

Duke, G., & Harley, I. (2012). Fluids and electrolytes. *Anesthesia: An introduction* (5th ed.). Melbourne: AU: IP Communications.

Eddington, H., Hoefield, R., Sinha, S., Chrysochou, C., Lane, B., Foley, R. N., . . . Kalra, P. A. (2010). *Clinical Journal of the American Society of Nephrology, 5*(12), 2251–2257.

Elliot, M. J., Ronksley, P. E., Clase, C. M., Ahmed, S. B., & Hemmelgarn, B. R. (2010). Management of patients with acute hyperkalemia. *Canadian Association Medical Journal, 182*(15), 1631–1635.

Garth, D. (2014). *Hypokalemia*. Retrieved from http://www.emedicine.com/emerg/topic273.htm

Gennari, F. J. (2012). Metabolic alkalosis. In D. Mount, M. H. Sayegh, & A. K. Singh (Eds.), *Core concepts in the disorders of fluid, electrolytes, and acid-base balance* (pp.275–296). New York, NY: Springer.

Halperin, M. L., Goldstein, M. B., & Kamel, K. S. (2010). *Fluid, electrolyte, and acid-base physiology: A problem based approach*. Amsterdam: Elsevier Health Sciences.

Kraut, J. A., & Madias, N. E. (2010). Metabolic acidosis: Pathophysiology, diagnosis, and management. *Nature Reviews Nephrology, 6*, 274–285.

LeGrand, S. B. (2011). Modern management of malignant hypercalcemia. *American Journal of Hospice & Palliative Medicine*. doi:10.1177/1049909111414164

Longo, D., Fauci, A., Kasper, D., Hauser, S., Jameson, J., & Loscalzo, J. (2012). *Harrison's principles of internal medicine* (18th ed.). New York, NY: McGraw Hill.

Marcocci, C., & Cetani, F. (2011). *Primary hyperparathyroidism*. New England Journal of Medicine, 365, 2389–2397.

Martin, K. J., Gonzalez, E. A., & Slatopolsky, E. (2009). Clinical consequences and management of hypomagnesemia. *Journal of the American Society of Nephrology, 20*(11), 2291–2295.

McPhee, S. J., Papadakis, M. A., Rabow, M. W. (2014). *Current medical diagnosis & treatment*. New York, NY: McGraw Hill/Lange.

Noritomi, D. T., Soriano, F. G., Kellum, J. A., Cappi, S. B., Biselli, P. J., Paolo, J. C., . . . Park, M. (2009). Metabolic acidosis in patients with severe sepsis and septic shock: A longitudinal quantitative study. *Critical Care Medicine, 37*(10), 2733–2739.

Palmer, B. F. (2012). Evaluation and treatment of respiratory alkalosis. *American Journal of Kidney Disease, 60*(5), 834–838.

Peacock, M. (2010). Calcium metabolism in health and disease. *Clinical metabolism in health and disease, 5*(Suppl 1), S23-S30.

Persey, V. P., Behets, G. J., DeBroe, M. E., & D'Haese, P. C. (2009). Management of hyperphosphatemia in patients with end-stage renal disease: Focus on lanthanum carbonate. *International Journal of Nephrology and Renovascular Disease*, 1–9.

Reddi, A. S. (2014). *Fluid, Electrolyte and Acid-Base Disorders* (pp. 289–299). SpringerLink.

Salem, C. B., Badreddine, A., Fathallah, N., Slim, R., & Hmouda, H. (2014). Drug-induced hyperkalemia. *Drug Safety, 37*, 677–692.

Unwin, R. J., Luft, F. C., & Shirley, D. G. (2011). Pathophysiology and management of hypokalemia: A clinical perspective. *Nature Reviews Nephrology, 7*, 75–84.

Vaidya, C., Ho, W., & Freda, B. J. (2010). Management of hyponatremia: Providing treatment and avoiding harm. *Cleveland Clinical Journal of Medicine, 77*(10), 715–726.

Yee, A. H., & Rabinstein, A. A. (2010). Neurologic presentations of acid-base imbalance, electrolyte abnormalities, and endocrine emergencies. *Neurologic Clinics, 28*(1), 1–16.

Youn, J. H., & McDonough, A. A. (2009). Recent advances in understanding integrative control of potassium homeostatis. *Annual Review of Physiology, 71*, 381–401.

CHAPTER 79

Poisoning and Drug Toxicities

ELIZABETH A. VANDE WAA • THOMAS W. BARKLEY, JR.

I. Regional poison control center consultation is highly recommended in cases of suspected poisoning and to help guide management in confirmed cases.

II. All facilities, health care providers, as well as patients/caregivers should have the local poison control center telephone number: 1–800–222–1222

ACETAMINOPHEN TOXICITY

I. Examples
  A. Anacin-3
  B. Liquiprin
  C. Panadol
  D. Tylenol

II. Subjective findings
  A. Usually asymptomatic early
  B. Nausea and vomiting at 24–48 hr
  C. Right upper quadrant pain
  D. Hypotension, hypothermia

III. Physical examination findings
  A. Hepatotoxicity, including jaundice, prolonged bleeding time, and hepatic encephalopathy (altered mental status, stupor, delirium, coma, asterixis, flapping tremor)

IV. Laboratory/diagnostic findings
  A. Draw for blood levels at 4 hr after ingestion
    1. Toxicity and liver injury seen with doses greater than 7.5 grams (adult) or 140 mg/kg (children)

2. Increased risk for hepatic injury at lower doses in the chronic alcoholic, those with preexisting liver disease, or those taking hepatotoxic medications

B. The following findings should be monitored every 24 hr until treatment is complete:

1. Elevated aspartate transaminase
2. Elevated alanine transaminase
3. Elevated blood urea nitrogen
4. Elevated creatinine
5. Prolonged prothrombin time
6. Elevated bilirubin
7. Metabolic acidosis

C. The following levels should be monitored every 24 hr until treatment is complete:

1. Lactic acid
2. Alkaline phosphatase
3. Phosphate
4. Blood pH

V. Management

A. Activated charcoal given in a dose of 25–100 grams diluted in water if patient presents within 4 hr of ingestion

1. Use 10 grams activated charcoal per 1 gram acetaminophen ingested (or 1 gram per kg body weight)
2. Charcoal should be removed by gastric lavage prior to acetylcysteine administration, as this may prevent its absorbance. Insert large bore OG or NG tube to facilitate the administration of activated charcoal

B. N-Acetylcysteine (Mucomyst), 140 mg/kg loading dose given PO within 8–10 hr of overdose; maintenance doses of 70 mg/kg every 4 hr for a total of 17 doses are indicated for as many doses as the acetaminophen stays in the toxic range (above 20 mcg/ml)

1. Check blood levels every 4 hr

C. Acetylcysteine may also be given IV as Acetadote; in this form, it is diluted in 5% dextrose and is given as 3 doses:

1. The first dose is 150 mg/kg in 200 ml 5% dextrose infused over 15 min–1 hr
2. The second dose is 50 mg/kg in 500 ml 5% dextrose infused over 4 hr
3. The third dose is 100 mg/kg in 100 ml 5% dextrose infused over 16 hr
4. Monitor the patient for allergic reactions (reduce these by slowing the infusion rate)

ALCOHOL (ETHANOL) TOXICITY

I.   **Subjective findings**
    A. Emotional lability
    B. Impaired coordination
    C. Nausea
    D. Vomiting
    E. Facial flushing
    F. Diaphoresis

II.   **Physical examination findings**
    A. Respiratory depression
    B. Electrolyte and acid-base imbalances
    C. Stupor
    D. Mydriasis
    E. Nystagmus
    F. Diplopia
    G. Seizures
    H. Coma
    I. Tachycardia
    J. Hypotension
    K. Hypoglycemia

III.   **Laboratory/diagnostic findings**
    A. Blood levels ranging from 50%–100% (mild toxicity), 100%–300% (moderate toxicity), to more than 300% (severe toxicity)

IV.   **Management**
    A. ABCs (airway, breathing, circulation)
    B. Hemodialysis may be used to reduce ethanol levels in severe toxicity.
    C. IV glucose, 200–500 mg/kg/dose as D50%W or 50% dextrose in patients with suspected hypoglycemia
    D. Alcoholics require pretreatment with thiamine (100 mg IV/IM/PO daily for at least 3 days), multivitamin (1 tablet PO/NGT daily), folic acid (1 mg PO daily), fluids, and electrolytes PRN

ANTIDYSRHYTHMIC DRUG OVERDOSE

I.   **Examples**
    A. Class I antiarrhythmics
        1. Flecainide
        2. Lidocaine
        3. Procainamide
        4. Quinidine

II.   **Subjective/physical examination findings**
    A. Nausea
    B. Vomiting
    C. Diarrhea
    D. Dizziness

    E. Blurred vision
    F. Bradycardia
    G. Hypotension
    H. Cardiovascular collapse
    I. Tinnitus
    J. Hearing loss
    K. Confusion
    L. Delirium
    M. Psychosis
    N. Seizures
    O. Coma

III.   **Laboratory/diagnostic findings**
    A. Serum levels may confirm overdose and the need for monitoring
    B. Bradycardia with atrioventricular (AV) block
    C. Prolonged QRS complex, PR interval, and QTC interval
    D. Ventricular arrhythmias
        1. Torsade de pointes
    E. Hypotension
    F. Respiratory depression
    G. Acute lung injury
    H. Thrombocytopenia
    I. Leukopenia
    J. Hemolytic anemia
    K. Hepatotoxicity
    L. Drug-induced lupus with procainamide overdose

IV.   **Management**
    A. 12-lead ECG, electrolytes, and continuous ECG monitoring
    B. Charcoal administration
        1. 30 grams charcoal in 240 ml water (25–100 grams total in adults)
        2. Whole bowel irrigation if sustained-release preparations are involved
        3. Insert large bore OG or NG tube to facilitate the administration of activated charcoal
    C. For bradycardia:
        1. Atropine, 1 mg IV, repeat every 5 minutes if necessary (consider isoproterenol)
        2. Overdrive pacing
        3. Isoproterenol, 2 mg/250 ml continuous infusion: 2–10 mcg/min. Initiate at 2 mcg/min and increase/decrease by 2 mcg/min to maintain HR greater than 60. Titration parameter: HR

BARBITURATE OVERDOSE

I.   **Examples**
    A. Amobarbital
    B. Meprobamate

      C. Pentobarbital

      D. Phenobarbital

      E. Secobarbital

II.   **Subjective findings**

      A. Confusion

      B. Slurred speech

      C. Ataxia

      D. Impaired coordination

      E. CNS depression

      F. Stupor

III.   **Physical examination findings**

      A. CNS depression

      B. Drowsiness

      C. Confusion

      D. Coma

      E. Hypothermia

      F. Respiratory depression

      G. Respiratory acidosis

      H. Absent deep tendon, gag, and corneal reflexes

      I. Miosis

IV.   **Management**

      A. Maintenance of airway and ventilation is essential

      B. A single dose of activated charcoal should be given to cooperative, clinically stable patients who present within 1 hr of acute oral overdose. Insert large bore OG or NG tube to facilitate the administration of activated charcoal

      C. Hemodynamic support, including administration of dopamine or norepinephrine, may be necessary to correct hypotension (see Table 76.2)

BENZODIAZEPINE OVERDOSE

I.   **Examples**

      A. Clonazepam

      B. Clorazepate

      C. Diazepam

      D. Flurazepam

      E. Prazepam

II.   **Subjective findings**

      A. Drowsiness

      B. Ataxia

      C. Confusion

      D. Slurred speech

      E. Unsteady gait

III.   **Physical examination findings**

      A. Respiratory depression

B. Hypoactive reflexes

IV. **Management**

A. Monitor blood pressure and support respiration

B. Flumazenil (Romazicon)

1. Initial dose 0.2 mg IV over 30 seconds, if desired level of consciousness not obtained after an additional 30 seconds then further doses of 0.5 mg over 30 seconds may be given at 1 min intervals (max 3 mg)

2. Not recommended for patients who have been given a benzodiazepine for control of a potentially life-threatening condition (e.g., control of intracranial pressure or status epilepticus) or patients who are showing signs of serious cyclic antidepressant overdose

C. Gastric lavage with 0.9% sodium chloride or activated charcoal, 1 gram/kg PO via 36–40 French tube every 2–6 hr, may also be used. Insert large bore OG or NG tube to facilitate the administration of activated charcoal

1. Activated charcoal (1 gram/kg) binds effectively to benzodiazepines and may be considered

2. Check stomach for pill fragments and send these for toxicological confirmation and analysis

3. Continue lavage until return runs clear

BETA BLOCKER OVERDOSE

I. **Examples**

A. Propranolol

B. Timolol

C. Atenolol

D. Labetalol

E. Metoprolol

F. Nadolol

G. Pindolol

II. **Subjective findings**

A. Nausea

B. Vomiting

C. Diarrhea

III. **Physical examination findings**

A. Bradycardia

B. Hypotension

C. CNS depression

D. Delirium

E. Coma

F. Seizures

G. Bronchospasm

H. Respiratory depression

      I. Myocardial depression

      J. Cardiogenic shock

      K. Heart failure

IV.   **Laboratory/diagnostic findings**

      A. Blood levels not very helpful or available

      B. Hyperkalemia

      C. Hypoglycemia

      D. Atrioventricular block

      E. Prolonged QRS complex

      F. QT prolongation

      G. Asystole

V.   **Management**

      A. Assess ABCs

      B. Glucagon, bolus dose of 5 or 10 mg over 2 minutes, can be repeated PRN. If a beneficial effect is seen from the glucagon bolus, a continuous infusion of 1–10 mg/hr can be titrated to maintain effect.

      C. Activated charcoal, 1 gram/kg PO repeated every 2–6 hr. Insert large bore OG or NG tube to facilitate the administration of activated charcoal

          1. May consider whole bowel irrigation if sustained-release preparations were used

      D. Calcium (10% calcium chloride at a dose of 0.2 ml/kg body weight IV over 5 min) to reverse negative inotropic effects

      E. Monitor patient for hyperkalemia, treat seizures, if they occur, and monitor blood glucose

      F. Treat hypotension with β-adrenergic agonists (norepinephrine, epinephrine, or dopamine) or isoproterenol (see Table 79.1)

          1. Isoproterenol, 2 mg/250 ml continuous infusion: 2–10 mcg/min. Initiate at 2 mcg/min and increase/decrease by 2 mcg/min to maintain HR greater than 60. Titration parameter: HR

      G. May consider temporary transvenous pacing, intra-aortic balloon pump, or cardiopulmonary bypass

CALCIUM CHANNEL BLOCKER OVERDOSE

I.   **Examples**

      A. Amlodipine

      B. Bepridil

      C. Diltiazem

      D. Felodipine

      E. Nicardipine

      F. Nifedipine

      G. Nisoldipine

      H. Verapamil

II.   **Subjective findings**

      A. Mental status changes (confusion)

  B. Light-headedness

  C. Headache

III. **Physical examination findings**

  A. Bradycardia

  B. Conduction disturbances

  C. Hypotension

  D. Cyanosis

  E. Seizures

  F. Coma

  G. Death

IV. **Laboratory/diagnostic findings**

  A. Atrioventricular block

  B. Prolonged QRS complex

  C. Asystole

  D. Metabolic acidosis

  E. Hyperglycemia

V. **Management**

  A. IV calcium chloride or gluconate (10%) at 1–3 gram boluses

   1. Patients who do not respond to calcium administration or who require repeated administration may be treated with an adrenergic agonist (norepinephrine, epinephrine, or dopamine) (see Table 79.1 for dosing)

  B. Glucagon, bolus dose of 5 or 10 mg over 2 minutes, can be repeated PRN. If a beneficial effect is seen from the glucagon bolus, a continuous infusion of 1–10 mg/hr can be titrated to maintain effect.

  C. Atropine, 0.5–1 mg IV; repeat PRN every 5 min or isoproterol, 2 mg/250 ml continuous infusion: 2–10 mcg/min; initiate at 2 mcg/min and increase/decrease by 2 mcg/min to maintain HR greater than 60.

  D. Aggressive GI decontamination with polyethylene glycol solution (1–2 L/hr via orogastric or nasogastric tube until clear) when sustained-release medications are suspected

  E. Activated charcoal 1 gram/kg, then multiple doses of 0.5 gram/kg

  F. High dose insulin therapy utilizing 1unit/kg bolus followed by 0.5–1 unit/kg/hr infusion is being utilized with success. Glucose (50 ml of D50%, followed by D10% infusion, at a rate to maintain blood glucose 150–300) to maintain euglycemia.

  G. Continuous cardiac monitoring, 12-lead ECG every 1–2 hr for the first 6 hr

CARBON MONOXIDE POISONING

I. **Subjective findings**

  A. Shortness of breath

  B. Headache

  C. Confusion

    D. Clumsiness

    E. Mental status changes

    F. Nausea

    G. Vomiting

    H. Diarrhea

    I. Dizziness

    J. Weakness

    K. Chest pain

    L. Blurred vision

    M. Psychosis

    N. Parkinsonism

    O. Paralysis

II. **Physical examination findings**

    A. Dysrhythmias

    B. Cardiac arrest

    C. Heart failure

    D. Respiratory depression

    E. Hypoxia

III. **Laboratory/diagnostic findings**

    A. Elevated carboxyhemoglobin level (10%–50%)

    B. Sinus tachycardia

    C. ST depression

    D. Premature ventricular contractions

    E. Metabolic acidosis

IV. **Management**

    A. 100% oxygen by mask/positive-pressure mask or endotracheal tube

    B. With significant exposure, hyperbaric oxygen if carboxyhemoglobin levels are greater than 25%, or if patient is pregnant or has altered mental status

DIGOXIN TOXICITY

I. **Subjective findings**

    A. Nausea

    B. Vomiting

    C. Diarrhea

    D. Blurred vision

    E. Green halos

    F. Anorexia

    G. Abdominal pain

    H. Fatigue

    I. Dizziness

    J. Confusion

    K. Headache

    L. Occasional hallucinations

II. Laboratory/diagnostic findings

A. Atrioventricular block with
1. Supraventricular tachydysrhythmias
2. Supraventricular bradydysrhythmias
3. Atrial tachydysrhythmias
4. Ventricular tachycardia
5. Ventricular dysrhythmias
6. Hypotension

B. Hyperkalemia in acute overdose

C. Digoxin level greater than 2.4 ng/ml

III. Management

A. Continuous ECG monitoring
1. Monitor and correct serum potassium levels; maintain in the high normal range
2. Dysrhythmias may be managed with lidocaine

B. Administer activated charcoal, 1 gram/kg PO. Insert large bore OG or NG tube to facilitate the administration of activated charcoal.

C. Digoxin immune Fab (DigiFab)
1. Acute ingestion of known amount of digoxin: dose (in vials) = (digoxin ingested [mg] X bioavailability)/0.5 mg of digoxin bound per vial
   a. Bioavailability of digoxin tablets: 0.8, capsules: 1
2. Acute ingestion of unknown amount of digoxin: 20 vials (800 mg) IV; start with 10 vials (400 mg) IV, observe response; repeat with 10 vials PRN
3. Chronic digoxin toxicity: 6 vials (240 mg) IV or dose (in vials) = (serum digoxin concentration in nanograms/ml x weight in kg)/100
4. Digoxin levels obtained after administering DigiFab have little correlation with clinical toxicity. Because laboratory assays do not distinguish between Fab-bound and unbound digoxin, total serum levels following administration may increase 10- to 20-fold; this does not correlate with clinical toxicity

LITHIUM TOXICITY

I. Examples

A. Eskalith

B. Lithobid

II. Subjective findings

A. Nausea

B. Vomiting

C. Diarrhea

D. Muscle weakness

E. Tremor

F. Rigidity

      G. Ataxia

      H. Dementia

      I. Delirium

III.   **Laboratory/diagnostic findings**

      A. Lithium levels greater than 1.5 mEq/L

      B. Hyperglycemia

      C. Atrioventricular block

      D. Prolonged QT interval

      E. Nephrogenic diabetes insipidus

      F. Leukocytosis

      G. Seizures

      H. Stupor

      I. Coma

      J. 10% risk of permanent neurologic sequelae

IV.   **Management**

      A. IV saline, 0.9% bolus of 1 liter followed by 100–200 ml/hr

      B. Activated charcoal is ineffective

      C. Gastric lavage or whole bowel irrigation may be used for acute ingestion in cases where ingestion occurred within one hour, or if large quantities of sustained-release products were ingested. Insert large bore OG or NG tube, to facilitate the administration of activated charcoal.

      D. Supportive care

      E. Diuretics for lithium serum levels greater than 2–3 mEq/L

          1. Once fluid losses replaced, diuretic-induced diuresis does not enhance lithium elimination and can be potentially dangerous because they promote sodium and water loss

      F. Hemodialysis in acute intoxication (serum levels greater than 4 mEq/L)

      G. Benzodiazepines IV used for seizure management

SALICYLATE TOXICITY

I.   **Subjective findings**

      A. Nausea

      B. Vomiting

      C. Fever

      D. Tinnitus

      E. Headache

      F. Dizziness

II.   **Physical examination findings**

      A. Tachypnea

      B. Cyanosis

      C. Metabolic acidosis

      D. Respiratory alkalosis

      E. Dehydration

      F. Hyperthermia

III. Management

A. Monitor serum salicylate concentrations as well as electrolytes

B. Volume replacement (0.9% saline at 100 ml/hr)

C. Give activated charcoal 1 gram/kg PO

D. Sodium bicarbonate (1–1.5 mEq/kg IV over 10 min) to correct severe acidosis (pH less than 7.2) or 150 mEq sodium bicarbonate/1000 ml D5W and infuse at 100–150 ml/hr to maintain urine pH greater than 7.5

E. Consider hemodialysis in patients who have acid-base and electrolyte abnormalities that are not responding

OPIOID TOXICITY

I. Examples

A. Codeine

B. Heroin

C. Hydrocodone

D. Meperidine

E. Methadone

F. Morphine

G. Opium

H. Oxycodone

I. Oxymorphone

II. Subjective findings

A. Hypothermia

B. Drowsiness

C. Mental status changes

III. Laboratory/diagnostic findings

A. Evaluate toxicology screen and urine screen

B. Monitor blood glucose and serum creatine phosphokinase

IV. Physical examination findings

A. Shallow respirations

B. Respiratory depression

C. Pinpoint pupils (miosis)

D. Coma

V. Management

A. Continuous ECG monitoring

B. Ensure adequate ventilation, and provide respiratory support

C. Naloxone (Narcan, Evzio Autoinjector), 0.4–2 mg every 2–3 min PRN IV/IM or intranasally; may need to repeat doses every 20–60 min

   1. Continuous infusion (0.4–0.8 mg/hr) should be considered only if the patient responded to the naloxone bolus and required repeat administration

D. In patients with no spontaneous respirations, orotracheal intubation should be initiated.

E. Decontamination with 1 gram/kg PO single-dose activated charcoal; should be initiated in all patients with PO overdose. Protection of airway is essential to prevent aspiration. Insert large bore OG or NG tube to facilitate the administration of activated charcoal

ORGANOPHOSPHATE (INSECTICIDE) POISONING

I.   Examples
  A. Malathion
  B. Parathion
II.   Subjective findings
  A. Nausea
  B. Vomiting
  C. Cramping
  D. Diarrhea
  E. Excessive salivation
  F. Diaphoresis
  G. Headache
  H. Blurred vision (miosis)
  I. Mental confusion
  J. Slurred speech
  K. Anxiety
  L. Drowsiness
  M. Urinary incontinence
  N. Muscle fasciculations
III. Physical examination findings
  A. Miosis
  B. Seizures
  C. Paralysis
  D. Coma
  E. Bradycardia
  F. Conduction defects
  G. Respiratory depression/paralysis
IV.   Management
  A. Maintain airway and assist ventilation
  B. Wash skin thoroughly (to avoid self-contamination, medical personnel should wear neoprene or nitrile gloves)
  C. Activated charcoal if the insecticide was ingested; give 1 gram/kg of activated charcoal PO. Insert large bore OG or NG tube, to facilitate the administration of activated charcoal.
  D. Atropine is the drug of choice for organophosphate toxicity
    1. Administer atropine, 2 mg (6 mg IV for life-threatening cases) in initial dose, then 2 mg IV every 15 min until atropinization occurs
      a. Flushing
      b. Dry mouth
      c. Dilated pupils

> **d.** Tachycardia)
>
> **2.** Doses up to 40 mg/day are not uncommon

E. Administer pralidoxime, 1–2 grams IV over 10 min, then a constant infusion of 250–500 mg/hr to reverse nicotinic signs such as muscle weakness and respiratory depression

  1. Not recommended for asymptomatic patients or for patients with known carbamate exposure presenting with minimal symptoms

F. Place urinary catheter to prevent urinary retention

ANTIPSYCHOTIC TOXICITY

I. Examples
  - **A.** Clozapine
  - **B.** Haloperidol
  - **C.** Loxapine
  - **D.** Olanzapine
  - **E.** Quetiapine
  - **F.** Risperidone
  - **G.** Sertindole
  - **H.** Thioridazine
  - **I.** Ziprasidone

II. Subjective findings
  - **A.** Lethargy
  - **B.** Deep sleep
  - **C.** Dystonias and extrapyramidal symptoms
    - **1.** Rigidity
    - **2.** Stiff neck
    - **3.** Hyperreflexia
  - **D.** Neuroleptic malignant syndrome (increased temperature, rigidity)
  - **E.** Cardiovascular alterations
  - **F.** Urinary retention
  - **G.** Decreased bowel sounds

III. Physical examination/laboratory findings
  - **A.** Hypotension
  - **B.** Atrioventricular block
  - **C.** Atrial and ventricular arrhythmias
  - **D.** Widened QRS complex
  - **E.** Prolonged QT interval
  - **F.** Tachycardia

IV. Management
  - **A.** Activated charcoal, 1 gram/kg PO; insert large bore OG or NG tube to facilitate the administration of activated charcoal
  - **B.** Benztropine mesylate (Cogentin), 2 mg PO/IV four times a day for extrapyramidal signs (may titrate dose by 1 mg/dose to symptom relief)

C. For neuroleptic malignant syndrome (NMS), dantrolene sodium (Dantrium), 1 mg/kg IV push and continue (starting at 1 mg/kg) until symptoms subside or until maximum cumulative dose of 10 mg/kg is reached

D. Supportive care, including cooling blankets for neuroleptic malignant syndrome

E. Vasopressors (norepinephrine, vasopressin) for hypotension (see Table 79.1)

ANTIDEPRESSANT TOXICITY

I. **Examples**
  A. Amitriptyline
  B. Bupropion
  C. Citalopram
  D. Fluoxetine
  E. Imipramine
  F. Nortriptyline
  G. Protriptyline
  H. Sertraline
  I. Venlafaxine

II. **Subjective findings**
  A. Hallucinations
  B. Confusion
  C. Blurred vision
  D. Altered mental status
  E. Urinary retention

III. **Physical examination findings**
  A. Tachycardia
  B. Hypotension
  C. Arrhythmias
  D. Seizures
  E. Hypothermia
  F. Hyperthermia
  G. Anticholinergic effects

IV. **Management**
  A. Evidence of CNS or cardiac toxicity within 6 hr of antidepressant ingestion is an indication for admission to the intensive care unit
  B. Activated charcoal, 1 gram/kg; avoid emesis if risk of seizures. Insert large bore OG or NG tube, to facilitate the administration of activated charcoal
  C. Sodium bicarbonate IV (1–2 mEq/kg); additional boluses every 5 min or 1000 ml D5W with 150 mEq sodium bicarbonate and infuse at 100–150 ml/hr until QRS interval narrows or serum pH exceeds 7.55
    1. Target pH between 7.5 and 7.55

Table 79.1	Vasopressor Agents						
Drug	**Dose**	**HR**	**MAP**	**PCWP**	**CO**	**SVR**	**Adverse Effects/ Comments**
Norepinephrine	2–40 mcg/min (0.01–0.5 mcg/kg/min) Increase/decrease rate by minimum of 1 mcg/min at intervals no longer than Q 30 minutes Titration parameter: MAP; SBP Usual target: MAP greater than 65 OR SBP: 80–100	+	+	+	+	++	arrhythmias, tissue/ myocardial ischemia Most potent vasoconstrictor Drug of first choice for most types of shock
Epinephrine	1–10 mcg/min (0.01–0.2 mcg/kg/min) Increase/decrease rate by minimum of 1mcg/min at intervals no longer than Q 5 minutes Titration parameter: MAP; SBP Usual target: MAP greater than 65 OR SBP: 80–100	+	+	+	++	+	tachyarrhythmias, tissue ischemia, myocardial ischemia, hyperglycemia Second line or adjunct agent for refractory hypotension First-line for cardiopulmonary resuscitation and anaphylactic shock
Vasopressin	0.04 units/min	0	+	0	0	+	myocardial ischemia, tissue necrosis and end organ ischemia (doses greater than 0.04 units/ minute) Primary use is adjunct therapy Doses greater than 0.04 units/min may lead to cardiac arrest

Table 79.1	Vasopressor Agents						
Drug	Dose	HR	MAP	PCWP	CO	SVR	Adverse Effects/Comments
Dopamine	5–10 mcg/kg/min	+	+	0	+	0	tachycardia, arrhythmias, myocardial ischemia
	greater than 10–20 mcg/kg/min Increase/decrease rate by minimum of 1 mcg/kg/min at intervals no longer than Q 30 minutes Titration parameter: MAP; SBP Usual target: MAP greater than 65 OR SBP: 80–100	+	+	+	+	++	Dosage-dependent effects vary by individual and have not been reproduced in critically ill patients May be considered first line agent for select patients (i.e. depressed LV function, bradycardia)
Phenylephrine	50–400 mcg/min (0.5–5 mcg/kg/min) Increase/decrease rate by minimum of 10 mcg/min at intervals no longer than Q 15 minutes Titration parameter: MAP; SBP Usual target: MAP greater than 65 OR SBP: 80–100	0	+	0/+	0	++	reflex bradycardia, decreased renal perfusion Second-line agent Uses: Non-cardiogenic hypotension Vasoconstrictor effect similar to norepinephrine Caution use in renal impairment

Note. + = increase; - = decrease; 0 = no change; HR = heart rate; MAP = mean arterial pressure; PCWP = pulmonary capillary wedge pressure; CO = cardiac output; SVR = systemic vascular resistance

*Administration through a central line is preferred for all vasopressor agents

D. Benzodiazepine (e.g., diazepam [Valium], 5–10 mg IV PRN up to 20-mg dose; or lorazepam [Ativan], 4 mg IV) to control seizures

E. Lorazepam (Ativan) is used to treat rigor (0.5 mg PO three times a day)

F. Supportive measures such as cooling blankets are used to control temperature

G. If patient still demonstrates signs of delirium, agitation, and enhanced skeletal muscle tone or hyperreflexia, cyproheptadine may be used.

    1. An initial dose of 12 mg PO is recommended, followed by 2 mg PO every 4 hr PRN if symptoms continue

H. Patient should be monitored for hypotension and should be treated with vasopressors (see Table 79.1)

STIMULANT TOXICITY

I. **Examples**
    A. Amphetamine
    B. Cocaine
    C. Dextroamphetamine
    D. Methylphenidate

II. **Subjective findings**
    A. Increased talkativeness
    B. Insomnia
    C. Irritability
    D. Dry mouth
    E. Anorexia

III. **Physical examination findings**
    A. Arrhythmias
    B. Anginal chest pain
    C. Heart block
    D. Hypertension
    E. Tachycardia
    F. Dilated pupils (mydriasis)
    G. Seizures
    H. Hyperthermia
    I. Metabolic acidosis
    J. Rhabdomyolysis

IV. **Management**
    A. Activated charcoal 1 gram/kg PO. Insert large bore OG or NG tube to facilitate the administration of activated charcoal
    B. Reduce external stimuli
    C. Administer diazepam (Valium), 5 mg IV or lorazepam (Ativan), 2 mg IV and repeat every 15 minutes until patient is calm (monitor airway)

D. For hypertension, administer nitroprusside (Nipride), 0.2–8 mcg/kg/min, increase/decrease rate by 0.1 mcg/kg/min every 10 minutes to maintain SBP less than 140 or nicardipine, 2.5–15 mg/hr, increase/decrease by 0.5 mg every 15 minutes to maintain SBP less than 140

E. Treat for seizures (lorazepam [Ativan], 4 mg IV, or diazepam [Valium], 5–10 mg IV)

F. Use a cooling blanket for hyperthermia and vasodilators for hypertension. Monitor for wide-complex tachydysrhythmias and QRS-complex prolongation

THEOPHYLLINE TOXICITY

I. Subjective/physical examination findings

   A. Vomiting

   B. Sometimes hematemesis

   C. Restlessness

   D. Agitation

   E. Irritability

   F. Tachycardia

   G. Premature ventricular contractions

   H. Atrial arrhythmias

   I. Seizures in severe overdose

II. Laboratory/diagnostic findings

   A. Theophylline levels of 20–60 mg/L in chronic overdose

   B. Levels of 60–100 mg/L in acute overdose are associated with seizures

   C. Hypokalemia

   D. Hyperglycemia

   E. Metabolic acidosis

III. Management

   A. Maintain airway, support ventilation and circulation

   B. Treat arrhythmias

   C. Multiple doses of activated charcoal 1 gram/kg (50–100 grams PO), followed by 20 grams every 2–6 hr, until theophylline level is less than 20 mg/L

   D. Consider whole bowel irrigation

   E. Charcoal hemoperfusion is indicated in acute ingestion with levels higher than 100 mg/L (serum levels greater than 40 mg/L), or in patients with seizures or serious arrhythmias. Insert large bore OG or NG tube to facilitate the administration of activated charcoal.

   F. Monitor patient for seizures

      1. Can be treated with lorazepam (Ativan), 4 mg IV, or diazepam, (Valium), 5–10 mg IV)

      2. Use phenobarbital only when escalating dose of a benzodiazepine is ineffective

ANTICOAGULANT OVERDOSE

I. **Examples**
   A. Heparin
   B. Warfarin
   C. Low Molecular Weight Heparins
      1. Enoxaparin (Lovenox)
      2. Dalteparin (Fragmin)
      3. Tinzaparin (Innohep)
   D. Factor Xa Inhibitors
      1. Fondaparinux (Arixtra)
      2. Rivaroxaban (Xarelto)
      3. Apixaban (Eliquis)
   E. Direct Thrombin Inhibitors
      1. Lepirudin (Refludan)
      2. Argatroban (Acova)
      3. Bivalirudin (Angiomax)
      4. Dabigatran (Pradaxa)
      5. Desirudin (Iprivask)

II. **Subjective/physical examination findings**
   A. Severe hemorrhage

III. **Laboratory/diagnostic findings**
   A. Heparin: increased activated partial thromboplastin time to 1.5–2.5 times control
   B. Warfarin: increased prothrombin time to 1.3–2 times control; international normalized ratio higher than 3

IV. **Management**
   A. Heparin overdose
      1. Give protamine sulfate IVPB given over 15–30 minutes, 1 mg/100 units heparin; use 0.5 mg/100 units heparin if given more than 30 min after heparin. Maximum: 50 mg IVPB, given over 15–30 minutes
         a. Monitor signs/symptoms of bleeding until activated partial thromboplastin time is normal
         b. Must be administered slowly to prevent anaphylaxis and hypotension
   B. Warfarin overdose
      1. Give vitamin K (phytonadione) IM, PO, SC, or IVPB in doses of 2.5–10 mg until international normalized ratio is normal
      2. Give fresh frozen plasma or whole blood if needed
   C. Other Anticoagulants (Factor Xa Inhibitors, Direct Thrombin Inhibitors, and Fondaparinux)
      1. No treatment or reversing agent exists for these agents. In cases of intentional overdose with PO agents, activated charcoal may be considered.

METHANOL TOXICITY

I. Examples
  A. Toxic alcohol form, found in
    1. Automobile washer solvent
    2. Automobile gas line antifreeze solutions
    3. Copy machine fluid
    4. Paint strippers
    5. Fuel for small stoves
    6. Industrial solvent preparations

II. Subjective findings
  A. Drowsiness
  B. Ataxia
  C. Confusion
  D. Weakness
  E. Headache
  F. Abdominal pain
  G. Blurred vision

III. Physical examination findings
  A. Metabolic acidosis
  B. Pupillary dilatation
  C. Decreased papillary reflex
  D. Hypotension
  E. Rapid pulse
  F. Cyanosis

IV. Management
  A. Correct acidosis with fomepizole, 15 mg/kg IV loading dose (slow IV infusion over 30 minutes), followed by 10 mg/kg IV (slow IV infusion over 30 minutes) every 12 hr for 4 doses, then 15 mg/kg IV (slow IV infusion over 30 minutes) every 12 hr until methanol concentrations are below 20 mg/dl.
    1. Bicarbonate infusion may improve metabolic acidosis, but buffer therapy has not been shown to improve outcome
  B. Administer folic acid, 1 mg/kg (up to 50 mg) IV every 6 hr
  C. Perform hemodialysis in severe cases
    1. Greater than 30 ml methanol ingested
    2. Serum methanol greater than 20 mg/dL
    3. Visual complications
    4. No improvement following sodium bicarbonate therapy

ETHYLENE GLYCOL TOXICITY

I. Examples
  A. Sweet-tasting chemical, found in many household products such as:
    1. Antifreeze
    2. De-icing products

   3. Detergents
   4. Paints
   5. Cosmetics
II. **Subjective/physical examination findings**
   A. Euphoria
   B. Nausea
   C. Vomiting (1–4 hr after ingestion)
   D. CNS depression
   E. Seizures
   F. Coma
   G. Tachycardia
   H. Hypertension
   I. Progressive metabolic acidosis
   J. Flank pain
   K. Tubular necrosis
   L. Renal failure (beginning at 12 hr post ingestion)
III. **Management**
   A. Maintain ABCs
   B. Fomepizole, 15 mg/kg IV loading dose (slow IV infusion over 30 minutes), followed by 10 mg/kg IV (slow IV infusion over 30 minutes) every 12 hr for 4 doses, then 15 mg/kg IV (slow IV infusion over 30 minutes) every 12 hr until methanol concentrations are below 20 mg/dl
   C. Bicarbonate infusion may improve metabolic acidosis, but buffer therapy has not been shown to improve outcome
   D. Adjunctive therapy can be given to facilitate ethylene glycol metabolism to nontoxic products by administering pyridoxine, 50 mg IV every 6 hr for 2 days, and thiamine, 100 mg IV every 6 hr for 2 days; magnesium sulfate, 2 grams IV for one day
   E. In severe toxicity, perform hemodialysis

OTHER INTOXICANTS

I. **Examples**
   A. Bath salts
   B. MDMA (ecstasy or Molly)
   C. Spice
II. **Subjective/physical examination findings**
   A. Agitation
   B. Paranoia
   C. Seizures
   D. Hostility
   E. Elevated body temperature (Molly, ecstasy)
   F. Tachycardia
   G. Dysrhythmias
   H. Altered level of consciousness

III. Management

A. Mephedrone, MDPV, and MDMA are central nervous stimulants and produce effects similar to those of amphetamines, cocaine, and ecstasy (sympathetic hyper-stimulation and psychiatric effects); therefore management should be similar

B. Single dose of activated charcoal, 1 gram/kg for ingestions less than 1 hr. Insert large bore OG or NG tube to facilitate the administration of activated charcoal

C. Monitor for dysrhythmias
   1. Manage according to ACLS protocol, including defibrillation and use of lidocaine, if needed

D. Treat for seizures (lorazepam, 4 mg IV, or diazepam, 5–10 mg IV)

E. Use a cooling blanket for hyperthermia and vasodilators for hypertension
   1. Nicardipine, continuous infusion, 2.5–15 mg/hr; titrate by 2.5 mg/hr every 5–15 min to maximum dose of 15 mg/hr; titration parameter: SBP
   2. Nitroglycerin, continuous infusion, 5–300 mcg/min, titrate by 10 mcg/min every 5 min to maximum of 300 mcg/min; titration parameter: SBP, angina
   3. Nitroprusside, continuous infusion, 0.1–5 mcg/kg/min to maximum dose of 10 mcg/kg/min); increase/decrease rate by minimum of 0.5 mcg/kg/min at intervals no longer than every 15 minutes; titration parameter: SBP

F. Confirm presence of intoxicants with toxicology screen

BITES AND STINGS

I. Hymenoptera

A. Bees, hornets, wasps, yellow jackets, stinging ants

B. Immunoglobulin (Ig)E-mediated painful wheal or hive from the venom is usually apparent

C. Anaphylaxis possible but rare
   1. Severe urticaria
   2. Bronchospasm
   3. Laryngospasm
   4. Nausea
   5. Vomiting
   6. Hypotension

D. Management of local reactions:
   1. Remove any remaining stinger
      a. Flick with a fingernail
      b. Do not squeeze/pinch, because more venom will be exposed to the area
   2. Oral antihistamines
      a. Diphenhydramine, 25 mg PO every 6 hr PRN for pain

        3. Steroid

          a. Taper for severe cases of extensive swelling and erythema

   E. Management of anaphylaxis

        1. Constrict the area with a band a few inches above the sting (do not occlude arterial flow)

        2. Ice to the area is appropriate

        3. Position the patient flat with legs elevated

        4. For respiratory symptoms/compromise, epinephrine, 0.5–1 mg (0.5–1 ml) repeated every 15 min

        5. Antihistamines (e.g., diphenhydramine 50 mg IV once) may relieve itching, flushing, urticaria, angioedema, and nasal and eye symptoms

        6. Corticosteroids, 250 mg, IV if symptoms persist

II. Widow spiders

   A. Bite is often "pinprick"

   B. Site may be slightly red

   C. Symptoms begin to occur approximately 1 hr post bite

   D. Spasmodic muscle pain—most common complaint, spreads regionally

   E. Other signs or symptoms may include:

        1. Respiratory distress

        2. Tachycardia

        3. Hypertension

        4. Headache

        5. Diaphoresis

        6. Nausea

        7. Vomiting

        8. Anxiety

   F. Management includes ice to the site and ABCs; muscle spasm treatment remains controversial

   G. Hydromorphone to manage pain and lorazepam to manage muscle spasms

   H. Antivenin may be used in cases of severe pain. Its use is controversial, as it may induce anaphylaxis.

III. Brown spiders

   A. Bite is relatively painless—may go unnoticed

   B. 2–8 hr post bite: becomes red, pruritic, painful, localized swelling

   C. 12–18 hr post bite: small, central vesicle develops surrounded by an irregular border or erythema or edema

   D. Blister ruptures and erythema darkens, spreading downward

   E. After 5–7 days of progressive aseptic necrosis, the center becomes depressed and is covered with black eschar.

   F. Eventually sloughs, leaving an open ulcer that heals over weeks

   G. Although rare, systemic hemolysis may be severe, especially in children

        1. Fever

   2. Chills
   3. Headache
   4. Malaise
   5. Weakness
   6. Anemia
   7. Coagulopathy
   8. Renal failure
   9. Shock
   10. Seizures
   11. Coma
   12. Death
H. CBC (including platelets) and urinalysis are the most important initial tests
I. Management:
   1. Ice may reduce the severity of necrosis
   2. Standard, local, daily wound care with tetanus prophylaxis is usually sufficient

IV.   Scorpion stings
A. Allergic reactions are rare; no deaths have been reported since 1968.
B. Immediate, intense pain that worsens with light pressure and radiates along the affected extremity
C. Swelling and bruising are uncommon
D. Systemic signs and symptoms may include:
   1. Restlessness
   2. Hypersalivation
   3. Dysphagia
   4. Visual changes
   5. Rolling eye movements
   6. Respiratory distress
   7. Hypertension
   8. Fever
   9. Arrhythmias
   10. Muscle spasms
   11. Paralysis
E. Management
   1. Ice, analgesics, tetanus, PRN
   2. For severe reactions:
      a. ABCs
      b. Respiratory management
      c. IV benzodiazepines (lorazepam 2 mg IV) for sedation
      d. β blockers for supraventricular tachycardia
      e. Antihypertensives PRN
      f. Supportive care
      g. An antivenin (Scorpion Immune F[ab]2) is available for patients with severe symptoms.

      i. 3 vials by IV infusion over 10 minutes as soon as possible after scorpion sting in patients who display clinically important signs of scorpion envenomation

V. Dog, cat, and human bites

A. All bites can obviously lead to infection, particularly cat bites

B. Timely, copious high-pressure irrigation with normal saline or Ringer's lactate (using 18- to 19-gauge needle) given to reduce the rate of infection is warranted

C. For animal bites, ascertain rabies status

D. X-rays PRN (e.g., skull X-ray if bite occurs to the head)

E. Primary closure of some wounds—remains controversial

F. Wounds to the hands or lower extremities should be left open

G. Any wound older than 6 hr is generally left open to heal by secondary intention

H. Plastic surgery consult as appropriate

I. For human and animal bites, administer a 3- to 7-day course of prophylactic PO antibiotics, with coverage provided for staphylococci and anaerobes (e.g., amoxicillin/clavulanate, 875 mg PO BID)

GERONTOLOGICAL CONSIDERATIONS

I. Subjective findings

A. Mental status changes in overdose and toxicity may be more pronounced, including:

    1. Drowsiness

    2. Ataxia

    3. Decreased alertness

    4. Confusion

    5. Weakness

    6. Agitation

    7. Irritability

B. Differentiate between delirium due to drug overdose and dementia

II. Physical examination findings

A. Altered liver function

B. Altered renal function; monitor creatinine clearance

C. Presence of multiple pathologies

III. Management

A. Treat as discussed above

B. Assess compliance with drug regimens

C. Monitor for polypharmacy, use of high risk drugs

D. Medication reconciliation should be incorporated

BIBLIOGRAPHY

Alapat, P. M., & Zimmerman, J. L. (2008). Toxicology in the critical care unit. *Chest, 133,* 1006–1013.

Barkley, T. W., Jr. (2012). *Acute care nurse practitioner certification review manual.* West Hollywood, CA: Barkley & Associates.

Barkley, T. W., Jr. (2012). *Pediatric nurse practitioner—Acute care certification review manual.* West Hollywood, CA: Barkley & Associates.

Barrett, J., Revis, D. R., Jr., & Brusch, J. L. (2014). *Human bites clinical presentation.* Retrieved from http://emedicine.medscape.com/article/218901-clinical#a0256

Berkow, R., & Fletcher, A. J. (2011). *The Merck manual of diagnosis and therapy* (19th ed.). Whitehouse Station, NJ: Merck Publishing Group.

Body, R., Bartram, T., Azam, F., & Mackway-Jones, K. (2011). Guidelines in emergency medicine network (GEMNet): Guideline for the management of tricyclic antidepressant overdose. *Emergency Medicine Journal, 28*(4), 347–368.

Cole, J. B., Stellpflug, S. J., Ellsworth, H., Anderson, C. P., Adams, A. B., Engebretsen, K. M., . . . Holger. J. S. (2013). A blinded, randomized, controlled trial of three doses of high-dose insulin in poison-induced cardiogenic shock. *Clinical Toxicology, 51*(4), 201–207.

Cushing, T. A., Kim, H., Benzer, T. I., & Tarabar, A. (2014). *Selective serotonin reuptake inhibitor toxicity.* Retrieved from http://emedicine.medscape.com/article/821737-overview

Dipiro, J. T., Talbert, R. L., Yee, G. C., Matzke, G. R., Wells, B. G., & Posey, L. M. (2011). *Pharmacotherapy: A pathophysiologic approach* (8th ed.). New York, NY: McGraw-Hill.

Engebretsen, K. M., Kaczmarek, K. M., Morgan, J., & Holger, J. S. (2011). High-dose insulin therapy in beta-blocker and calcium channel-blocker poisoning. *Clinical Toxicology, 49*(4), 277–283.

Evans, R. W., Tepper, S. J., Shapiro, R. E., Sun-Edelstein, C., & Tietjen, G. E. (2010) The FDA alert on serotonin syndrome with use of triptans combined with selective serotonin reuptake inhibitors or selective serotonin-norepinephrine reuptake inhibitors: American Headache Society position paper. *Headache: The Journal of Head and Face Pain, 50*(6), 1089–1099.

Ferri, F. F. (2013). *Ferri's clinical advisor.* St. Louis, MO: Mosby.

Garth, A. P., Harris, N. S., & Spanierman, C. (2012). *Animal bites in emergency medicine.* Retrieved from http://emedicine.medscape.com/article/768875-overview

Keyes, D. C., & Tarabar, A. (2012). *Ethylene glycol toxicity*. Retrieved from http://emedicine.medscape.com/article/814701-overview

Klotz, J. H., Klotz, S. A., & Pinnas, J. L. (2009). Animal bites and stings with anaphylactic potential. *Journal of Emergency Medicine, 36*(2), 148–156.

Liisanantti, J. (2012). *Acute drug poisoning: Outcome and factors affecting outcome* (Unpublished doctoral dissertation). University of Oulu, Finland.

Longo, D. L., Fauci, A. S., Kasper, D. L., Hauser, S. L., Jameson, J. L, & Loscalzo, J. (2011). *Harrison's Principles of Internal Medicine: Volumes 1 and 2* (18th ed.). New York, NY: McGraw-Hill Professional.

Nelson, L. S., Lewin, N. A., Howland, M. A., Hoffman, R. S., Goldfrank, L. R., & Flomenbaum, N. E. (2011). *Goldfrank's toxicologic emergencies* (9th ed.). New York, NY: McGraw-Hill Professional.

Pagana, K. D., & Pagana, T. J. (2012). *Mosby's diagnostic and laboratory test reference*. Amsterdam, UK: Elsevier.

Perry, P. J., & Wilborn, C. A. (2012). Serotonin syndrome vs. neuroleptic malignant syndrome: A contrast of causes, diagnoses, and management. *Annals of Clinical Psychiatry, 24*(2), 155–162.

Preston, J., O'Neal, J., & Talaga, M. (2013). *Handbook of clinical psychopharmacology for therapists* (7th ed.). Oakland, CA: New Harbinger Publishing.

Sheehy, S. B. (2013). *Manual of emergency care* (7th ed.). St. Louis, MO: Mosby.

Tintinalli, J., Stapczynski, J., Ma, O. J., Cline, D., Cydulka, R., & Meckler, G. (2011). *Tintinalli's emergency medicine: A comprehensive study guide* (7th ed.). New York, NY: McGraw-Hill.

Turkoski, B. B. (2011). *Drug information handbook for advanced practice nursing: 2011–2012*. Cleveland, OH: Lexi-Comp.

CHAPTER 80

Wound Management

CATHERINE BLACHE • THOMAS W. BARKLEY, JR. • CHARLENE M. MYERS

TYPES OF WOUNDS—DEFINITIONS

I. **Acute**
    A. Acute surgical: clean or contaminated after surgery
    B. Traumatic wound: clean or contaminated
II. **Chronic ulcers**
    A. Arterial: ischemia associated with various types of arterial occlusive disease
    B. Venous: related to disorders that affect venous blood return to the central circulation
    C. Diabetic: associated with excessive and prolonged elevations in glucose levels and peripheral neuropathy in diabetic patients
    D. Pressure: underlying tissue damage due to prolonged pressure or shearing that results in decreased blood and oxygen to capillaries of soft tissue beds

KEY FACTORS IN DELAYED HEALING

I.   **Excessive tissue load/pressure**
II.   **Decreased tissue perfusion and oxygenation**
III. **Urinary or bowel incontinence**
IV.   **Infection**
V.   **Systemic diseases such as diabetes mellitus**
VI.   **Inadequate or poor nutrition**
VII. **Necrotic tissue**
VIII. **Immunosuppression**
IX.   **Drugs such as steroids**
X.   **Deficiencies such as proteins, vitamins, and minerals**
XI.   **Aging**

SUBJECTIVE FINDINGS

I. **Specific to diminished arterial or venous flow or varying combinations, depending on areas involved**
  A. Pain and tenderness
    1. Arterial: claudication
    2. Venous: lower legs and feet "heavy" and "sore" after prolonged standing
  B. Neuropathy
    1. Arterial and diabetic ulcers: "numbness and tingling"
  C. Arterial, venous, and diabetic ulcers: patient report of poor wound healing
  D. Stated "foot problems" or trauma

II. **Applicable pressure ulcer risk assessment tools, such as the Braden or Norton tools (subjective and objective combinations)**

GENERAL PHYSICAL EXAMINATION GUIDELINES FOR WOUND ASSESSMENT

I. **Acute or chronic etiologic factors as underlying cause**
II. **Specific anatomic location (see Wound-Specific Physical Examination Findings section)**
III. **Length and width in centimeters**
IV. **Depth of tissue destruction**
  A. Superficial
  B. Partial thickness
    1. Extension through epidermis and partially into dermis
  C. Full thickness
    1. Extension through epidermis and dermis and some subcutaneous layer involvement
    2. Muscle and bone may be involved
  D. Undermining and tunneling
    1. Depth and direction
  E. Sinus tracts

V. **Color of wound: red-yellow-black classification system for wound healing by secondary intention**
  A. Red
    1. Wound bed is clean and healthy
    2. Color is pink to beefy red
  B. Yellow
    1. Exudate present
    2. Debridement and cleaning needed
    3. Color is beige, creamy, whitish-yellow, or yellow-greenish
  C. Black
    1. Eschar present, indicating necrotic tissue
    2. Debridement and cleaning needed

    D. Mixed combination of two or more colors

        1. Identify predominant color (treatment is geared toward predominant color)

VI. **Color, amount, and consistency of drainage**

VII. **Presence of foul odor, indicating infection**

VIII. **Appearance and temperature of surrounding skin and tissue**

    A. Presence of erythema, maceration, induration, or edema

IX. **Calluses (typically on plantar surface of foot)**

X. **Wound classification system, such as the Wagner Ulcer Grade Classification System of Staging or the National Pressure Ulcer Advisory Panel**

XI. **Presence of pain**

WOUND-SPECIFIC PHYSICAL EXAMINATION FINDINGS

I. **Arterial and diabetic ulcers**

    A. Typical locations:

        1. Toes and below ankles (general arterial disease)

        2. Plantar surfaces of feet (diabetic ulcers)

    B. Pulse volume is diminished or absent

    C. Shiny, cool lower extremities

    D. Leg hair is sparse or absent

    E. Feet and lower legs near ankle are cool

    F. Ankle-brachial index of less than 0.5 (arterial); may exceed 1.0 for diabetic patients and can be unreliable in this group

    G. Toenails are thickened

    H. Deep ulcers with smooth wound margins, small amount of drainage, cellulitis, and necrosis (large amount of callus surrounding ulcer [diabetic ulcer])

        1. Wound classification system, such as the Wagner Ulcer Grade Classification System of Staging or the University of Texas Classification System

II. **Venous ulcers**

    A. Typical location

        1. Lower legs, above ankle

    B. Varicosity noticeable

    C. Edema of lower legs or feet

    D. Warm lower extremities and feet

    E. Superficial, ruddy, and granulating ulcer with irregular margins; moderate to heavy drainage

    F. Brawny discoloration

III. **Pressure ulcers**

    A. Typical locations: bony prominences (sacrum, heels, and occiputs)

B. Ulcer description in terms of general assessment of wound and a wound classification system for pressure ulcers, for example, the classification description by stages according to the National Pressure Ulcer Advisory Panel
  1. Stage I
     a. Skin intact with non-blanchable erythema
     b. Heralding lesion of skin ulceration
  2. Stage II
     a. Partial-thickness loss
  3. Stage III
     a. Full-thickness loss
     b. Clinically appears deep, craterlike, with or without underlying adjacent tissue
  4. Stage IV
     a. Full-thickness loss and extensive destruction
     b. Tissue necrosis or muscle/bone/supporting structure damage (tendon and joint capsule)

LABORATORY/DIAGNOSTIC FINDINGS

I. **Findings conclusive of absent or diminished arterial or venous flow dynamics**
  A. Doppler pressure studies, reduced PVR waveforms
     1. Normal: pressure gradients less than 30 mmHg between cuffs
  B. Digital plethysmography: measures systolic toe pressure
     1. Normal toe pressure is 80% to 90% of brachial systolic pressure
  C. Transcutaneous oxygen measurements ($TcpO_2$): measures O_2 delivery to skin tissue
     1. $TcpO_2$ values higher than 30 mmHg indicate a wound area that will heal
     2. $TcpO_2$ values lower than 20 mmHg indicate a wound area that will not heal
  D. Venous Doppler ultrasonography
     1. Conclusive findings may indicate clots or incompetent venous valves

II. **Guidelines for referral to vascular specialist (surgeon or vascular laboratory)**
  A. Urgent vascular appointments
     1. Presence of gangrene
     2. Visible tendon or bone at ulcer base
     3. Cellulitis
     4. Severe infection
     5. Ankle-brachial index less than 0.5; indicator of perfusion and measure of systolic pressure in ankles
     6. New ischemia
  B. Semi-urgent vascular appointments

      1. TcpO$_2$ measurement higher than 30 mmHg and ankle-brachial index higher than 1

      2. Weak or absent pulses with ankle-brachial index lower than 1

      3. Ankle-brachial index between 0.5 and 0.8

      4. Poor wound healing in presence of normal pulses and aggressive wound care protocols

    C. Routine/standard vascular appointment

      1. Ankle-brachial index higher than 0.8

III. Complete blood count: leukocytosis, decreased red cells or hemoglobin

IV. Abnormal clotting times: prothrombin time less than 11 seconds, activated partial thromboplastin time less than 30 seconds, and partial thromboplastin time less than 60 seconds

V. Elevated glucose levels (greater than 150 mg/dl)

VI. Decreased albumin levels (greater than 3 grams/dl)

VII. Low vitamin D level

VIII. Quantitative culture and wound culture and sensitivity (specific to organism)

MANAGEMENT

I. Arterial ulcers

    A. Wet-to-moist dressings (saline) 3–4 times a day

    B. Enzymatic agents (no surgical debridement)

      1. Collagenase (Santyl), apply directly to the ulcer daily (or more frequently if dressing is soiled)

    C. Calcium alginates

    D. Nonocclusive/nonadherent dressing (no occlusive dressings)

    E. Evaluation and treatment of underlying condition

    F. Analgesics PRN

II. Venous ulcers

    A. Evaluation of and possibly treatment of underlying condition

    B. Elevate leg

    C. Nonadherent dressing under compression

    D. Sharp debridement if cellulitis or infection is present

    E. Enzymatic debridement

      1. Collagenase (Santyl), apply directly to the ulcer daily (or more frequently if dressing is soiled)

    F. Initial empiric therapy should be based on severity of infection and available microbiological data (recent cultures; local prevalence of pathogens, especially antibiotic-resistant strains). Adjust/de-escalate treatment to defined therapy when culture and susceptibility data is available

      1. Oral: cephalexin, 500 mg PO every 6 hr; dicloxacillin, 250 or 500 mg PO four times a day

        a. Penicillin allergic: erythromycin, 250 mg PO four times a day; erythromycin ethylsuccinate 400 mg PO four times a day; clindamycin 300 mg PO four times a day

    2. Intravenous: cefazolin, 1 gram IV every 8 hr; clindamycin, 600 mg IV every 8 hr

    3. MRSA Suspicion

        a. Oral: linezolid, 600 mg PO twice a day; clindamycin, 300 mg or 450 mg PO four times a day; trimethoprim/sulfamethoxazole, 1 or 2 tablets PO twice a day

        b. Intravenous: Vancomycin, consult pharmacy for dose/frequency to achieve vancomycin level of 10–15 µg/ml; clindamycin 600 mg IV every 8 hr; linezolid, 600 mg IV every 12 hr

    4. Avoid prescribing antibiotics for clinically uninfected wounds

  G. Compression therapy, in presence of normal pulses

  H. Analgesics PRN

III. **Diabetic ulcers**

  A. Increase insulin PRN (routine and sliding scale) or oral hypoglycemic dosage to control glucose levels

  B. No weight bearing

  C. Incision and drainage as indicated

  D. Topical antimicrobial PRN

    1. Limited data to support using topical antimicrobial therapy for mildly infected open wounds with minimal cellulitis

  E. Nonocclusive/nonadherent dressings

  F. Enzymatic debridement

    1. Collagenase (Santyl), apply directly to the ulcer daily (or more frequently if dressing becomes soiled)

    2. Becaplermin (Regranex), apply daily

  G. Systemic antibiotics if evidence of osteomyelitis, cellulitis, or septicemia; bactericidal antibiotics specific to microbiologic findings and wound appearances

    1. Initial empiric therapy based on severity of infection and available microbiological data (recent culture results; local prevalence of pathogens, especially antibiotic-resistant strains). Most diabetic ulcer infections can be polymicrobial.

    2. Mild:

        a. Cephalexin, 500 mg PO every 6 hr

        b. Dicloxacillin, 250 or 500 mg PO four times a day

        c. Augmentin, 500 mg PO three times a day or 875 mg PO twice a day

        d. Clindamycin, 300 or 450 mg PO four times a day

        e. MRSA suspicion: doxycycline, 100 mg PO twice a day or trimethoprim/sulfamethoxazole, 1 or 2 DS tablets PO twice a day

    3. Moderate:

      a. Moxifloxacin, 400 mg PO/IV daily

      b. Levofloxacin, 750 mg PO/IV daily with clindamycin 450 mg PO four times a day or 600 mg IV every 8 hr

      c. MRSA suspicion: vancomycin, consult pharmacy for dose/frequency to achieve vancomycin level of 10–15 µg/ml; linezolid, 600 mg PO/IV every 12 hr; daptomycin, 4 mg/kg IV every 24 hr

    4. Severe:

      a. Vancomycin, consult pharmacy for dose/frequency to achieve vancomycin level of 10–15 µg/ml, plus piperacillin-tazobactam, 3.375 grams IV every 6 hr

      b. Cefepime, 1 gram IV every 12 hr, plus metronidazole, 500 mg IV every 8 hr

      c. Carbapenem (imipenem-cilastatin), 500 mg IV every 6 hr

      d. Meropenem, 1 gram IV every 8 hr

    5. Adjust/de-escalate treatment to define therapy when culture/susceptibility data is available. Avoid prescribing antibiotics for clinically uninfected wounds. Successfully treating a diabetic foot infection also requires appropriate wound care

    6. Aerobic Gram-positive cocci coverage for ulcers limited in extent

    7. Polymicrobic (aerobes and anaerobes) coverage for recurrent, chronic, and limb-threatening lesions

    8. Septic and chronic, limb-threatening

  H. Analgesics, PRN

  I. Wet-to-moist saline dressings 3–4 times a day

  J. Wet gangrene—Do not debride; call surgeon

IV. **Pressure ulcers**

  A. Positioning: order turning of patient to relieve pressure on ulcer every 2 hr

  B. Support surfaces: consider ordering air-fluidized beds for wounds

  C. Skin barrier products (Stage I and II ulcers)

    1. Polyurethane, such as Tegaderm or OpSite, per manufacturer's instructions

    2. Hydrogel, such as IntraSite or Vigilon, per manufacturer's instructions

    3. Hydrocolloids, such as Duoderm or Restore, per manufacturer's instructions

  D. Debridement

  E. Cleansing

    1. Normal saline for most pressure ulcers

    2. Cleanse wound initially and with each dressing change

    3. Avoid cytotoxic skin cleansers and antiseptic agents, such as povidone-iodine, iodophor, sodium hypochlorite solution (Dakin solution), hydrogen peroxide, and acetic acid

4. Irrigation
   a. Discontinue when wound is clean
F. Dressing
   1. Select to keep ulcer bed continuously moist while maintaining dry surrounding skin and controlling exudate without desiccating ulcer bed
G. Topical antibiotics PRN
   1. Should be effective against Gram-negative, Gram-positive, and anaerobic organisms, such as silver sulfadiazine or triple antibiotic, with each dressing change
H. Systemic antibiotics as appropriate—limited data support using topical antimicrobial therapy for mildly infected open wounds with minimal cellulitis (refer to Management sections above [IIF, IIIG] and Cellulitis Management chapter)
   1. For bacteremia, sepsis, advancing cellulitis, or osteomyelitis
I. Nutrition
   1. Increased protein, high caloric diet
   2. Ascorbic acid supplement, 500 mg BID
      a. Although used quite commonly for "wound healing," at present there is no evidence to suggest that oral ascorbic acid accelerates wound healing in patients with normal nutritional status
   3. Zinc sulfate, 220 mg daily
      a. Although used quite commonly for "wound healing," there is no data to support its use for arterial and venous leg ulcers in people with adequate zinc levels
J. Analgesics, PRN

SELECTED TREATMENT OPTIONS

I.　See Table 80.1 for selected treatment options for chronic ulcers

Table 80.1	Treatment options for chronic ulcers			
	Type of ulcer			
	Arterial	Venous	Diabetic	Pressure
Cleaning	Saline preferred	Saline preferred	Saline preferred	Saline preferred
Antibiotic	As indicated by culture and sensitivity of wound	As indicated by culture and sensitivity of wound Topical: silver sulfadiazine Systemic: oral, IV	As indicated by culture and sensitivity of wound Topical: ointment, cream, amorphous hydrogels, antimicrobial Oral: Use for localized soft tissue IV: Use for systemic, bone, osteomyelitis	As indicated by culture and sensitivity of wound Topical: Use for clean, non-healing ulcers or exudate after 2- to 4-week period Effective against Gram-negative, Gram-positive, and anaerobic organisms Systemic: Use for bacteremia, cellulitis, osteomyelitis
Compression therapy	None	In presence of normal pulses, no infection, heart failure, or concurrent arterial disease: Elastic bandages, Unna boot, anti-embolytic hose, sequential compression device	None	None

Table 80.1	Treatment options for chronic ulcers			
	Type of ulcer			
	Arterial	**Venous**	**Diabetic**	**Pressure**
Cleaning	Saline preferred	Saline preferred	Saline preferred	Saline preferred
Debridement	Wet-to-moist saline dressing	Sharp--if cellulitis, infection or necrotic	Wet-to-moist saline	Wet-to-dry saline
	Enzymatic, no surgical debridement	Wet-to-moist, sharp or whirlpool to remove moderate amount of debris from fibrotic tissue or eschar	Sharp, aggressive—if nonischemic Enzymatic, whirlpool, nonaggressive sharp, if ischemic	
	Calcium alginates	Enzymatic debridement	Do not debride if wet gangrene	
Dressing	Nonocclusive, nonadherent Wet-to-moist saline	Wet-to-moist saline	Nonocclusive, nonadherent dressing Gauze dressing to plantar area Occlusive dressing to dorsal area	Depending on amount of debris and drainage: collagen, foams, hydrocolloids, hydrogels, moist and impregnated packing, wound fillers per manufacturer's guide

BIBLIOGRAPHY

American Medical Directors Association. (2011). *Common infections in the long-term care setting*. Columbia, MD: Author.

Association for the Advancement of Wound Care. (2010). *Association for the Advancement of Wound Care guideline of pressure ulcer guidelines*. Malvern, PA: Author.

Ayello, E. A., & Sibbald, R. G. (2012). Preventing pressure ulcers and skin tears. In M. Boltz, E. Capezuti, T. Fulmer, & D. Zwicker (Eds.), *Evidence-based geriatric nursing protocols for best practice* (4th ed., pp. 298–323). New York, NY: Springer Publishing Company.

Beitz, J. M. (2012, June). Management of complex wounds. *Critical Care Nursing Clinics of North America, 24*(2), 239–253.

Brady, A., McCabe, C., & McCann, M. (2013). *Fundamentals of Medical-Surgical Nursing*. Hoboken, NJ: John Wiley & Sons.

Centre for Clinical Practice. (2011, March). *Diabetic foot problems. Inpatient management of diabetic foot problems*. London, UK: National Institute for Health and Clinical Excellence.

Dumville, J. C., Deshpande, S., O'Meara, S., & Speak, K. (2013). Hydrocolloid dressings for healing diabetic foot ulcers. *Cochrane Database of Systematic Reviews, 8*, CD009099. doi:10.1002/14651858.CD009099.pub3

Dumville, J. C., O'Meara, S., Deshpande, S., & Speak, K. (2013). Alginate dressings for healing diabetic foot ulcers. *Cochrane Database of Systematic Reviews, 6*, CD009110. doi:10.1002/14651858.CD009110.pub3

Edwards, J., & Stapley, S. (2010). Debridement of diabetic foot ulcers. *Cochrane Database of Systematic Reviews, 1*, CD003556. doi:10.1002/14651858. CD003556.pub2

European Pressure Ulcer Advisory Panel and National Pressure UlcerAdvisory Panel. (2009). *Prevention and treatment of pressure ulcers: Quick reference guide*. Washington, DC: National Pressure Ulcer Advisory Panel.

Greer, N., Forman, N. A., McDonald, R., Dorrian, J., Fitzgerald, P. . . . Wilt, T. J. (2013) Advanced wound care therapies for nonhealing diabetic, venous, and arterial ulcers: A systematic review. *Annals of Internal Medicine, 159*(8), 532–542.

Institute for Clinical Systems Improvement. (2012, January). *Pressure ulcer prevention and treatment protocol. Health care protocol*. Bloomington, MN: Author.

Korzendorfer, H., Scarborough, P., & Hettrick, H. (2013). Tissue destruction classification systems. *Advances in Skin & Wound Care, 26*(11), 499–503. doi:10.1097/01.ASW.0000434296.70617.6a

Lipsky, B. A., Berendt, A. R., Cornia, P. B., Pile, J. C., Peters, E. J., Armstrong, D. G., . . . Senneville, E. (2012, June). 2012 Infectious Diseases Society of America clinical practice guideline for the diagnosis and treatment of diabetic foot infections. *Clinical Infectious Diseases, 54*(12), e132-e173.

Liu, C., Bayer, A., Cosgrove, S. E., Daum, R. S., Fridkin, S. K., Gorwitz, R. J., . . . Chambers, H. F. (2011, February). Clinical practice guidelines by the Infectious Diseases Society of America for the treatment of methicillin-resistant staphylococcus aureus infections in adults and children. *Clinical Infectious Diseases, 52*, 1–38.

Moore, Z. E. H., & Webster, J. (2013). Dressings and topical agents for preventing pressure ulcers. *Cochrane Database of Systematic Reviews, 8*, CD009362. doi:10.1002/14651858.CD009362.pub2

Moore, Z. E. H., & Cowman, S. (2013). Wound cleansing for pressure ulcers. *Cochrane Database of Systematic Reviews, 3*, CD004983. doi:10.1002/14651858.CD004983.pub3

National Clinical Guideline Centre. (2012, August). *Lower limb peripheral arterial disease: Diagnosis and management.* London, UK: National Institute for Health and Clinical Excellence.

Nelson, E. A., Mani, R., Thomas, K., & Vowden, K. (2011). Intermittent pneumatic compression for treating venous leg ulcers. *Cochrane Database of Systematic Reviews, 2*, CD001899. doi:10.1002/14651858.CD001899.pub3

Stevens, D. L., Bisno, A. L., Chambers, H. F., Dellinger, E. P., Goldstein, E. J., Gorbach, S. L., . . . Wade, J. C. (2014). Practice guidelines for the diagnosis and management of skin and soft tissue infections: 2014 update by the Infectious Diseases Society of America. *Clinical Infectious Diseases, 59*(2), e10-e52.

Thomas, D. R., & Burkemper N. M. (2013). Aging skin and wound healing. *Clinics in Geriatric Medicine, 29*(2), xi-xx.

Trans Tasman Dietetic Wound Care Group. (2011). *Evidence based practice guidelines for the nutritional management of adults with pressure injuries.*

Wicke, C., Bachinger, A., Coerper, S., Beckert, S., Witte, M. B., & Königsrainer, A. (2009). Aging influences wound healing in patients with chronic lower extremity wounds treated in a specialized wound care center. *Wound Repair and Regeneration, 17*(1), 25–33.

Wound, Ostomy, and Continence Nurses Society. (2010, June 1). *Guideline for prevention and management of pressure ulcers.* Mount Laurel, NJ: Author.

Wound, Ostomy, and Continence Nurses Society. (2011, June 1). *Guideline for management of wounds in patients with lower-extremity venous disease.* Mount Laurel, NJ: Author.

CHAPTER 81

Infections

ALISON FORBES • THOMAS W. BARKLEY, JR.

HOSPITAL-ACQUIRED INFECTIONS

I. **Nosocomial urinary tract infection**

    A. Definition

        1. Infection of the bladder or upper urinary tract

        2. Most nosocomial urinary tract infections are catheter associated; these are the most common hospital-acquired infections

    B. Incidence/predisposing factors

        1. Duration of catheterization is the most important risk factor

        2. Incidence is 3% to 10% per catheterization day

        3. Perineal flora and catheter/drainage bags are the sources of infecting organisms

        4. Common pathogens include

            a. *Escherichia coli*

            b. *Klebsiella pneumoniae*

            c. *Proteus mirabilis*

            d. *Pseudomonas aeruginosa*

            e. *Enterobacter* spp.

            f. *Enterococci* spp.

            g. *Staphylococcus aureus* and coagulase-negative Staphylococci

            h. Yeast

    C. Subjective findings

        1. Most cases are asymptomatic and do not require any treatment except discontinuation of catheter

        2. Fever, abdominal fullness, urinary urgency, or urethral irritation may be reported

    D. Physical examination findings

        1. Usually none or nonspecific; may have suprapubic tenderness

2. Urethral purulence may be present around the catheter at the entry site

E. Laboratory/diagnostic findings

1. Urinalysis usually reveals pyuria, increased leukocyte esterase, and hematuria

2. Urine culture usually shows 100,000 colony-forming units/ml of urine; however, fewer than 100,000 colony-forming units/ml may not be an indication of significant infection

F. Management

1. Discontinue catheterization if possible

2. Change to a new catheter

3. Switch to a condom catheter when appropriate

4. Use intermittent catheterization

5. Symptomatic bacteriuria: oral antibiotic therapy is usually sufficient to treat most cases; intravenous therapy is necessary in selected severely ill patients

   a. Antibiotic choice is dependent on the organism identified and the susceptibilities determined.

   b. For empiric therapy, knowledge of organisms in the medical unit is imperative; organisms vary from hospital to hospital and are likely to vary from unit to unit

   c. Recommended duration of therapy is 3–7 days in uncomplicated cases and 10–14 days in complicated cases

   d. Examples:

      i. Oral trimethoprim-sulfamethoxazole, 160/800 mg every 12 hr, or equivalent IV, or if sulfa allergic:

         (a) Ciprofloxacin, 500 mg PO or IV, every 12 hr

      ii. For urosepsis, when empiric coverage for nosocomial pathogens is needed, a combination of a β-lactam and an aminoglycoside is often prudent, such as ceftazidime, 1–2 grams IV every 8 hr, cefepime, 1–2 grams IV every 12 hr, or piperacillin, 3–4 grams IV every 6 hr, plus gentamicin 5 mg IV every 24 hr and adjusted for renal function

6. Symptomatic candiduria: change the catheter and treat with amphotericin B bladder irrigation, oral fluconazole, IV caspofungin (Cancidas) or IV amphotericin B, depending on the species of yeast, the azole susceptibilities in the medical unit, and the severity of the patient's illness. For example:

   a. Fluconazole, 100–200 mg PO every day

   b. Amphotericin B, 50 mg/L in dextrose 5% in water (D5W), 1 L/day bladder irrigation over 24 hr;

   c. Amphotericin B, 0.3–0.5 mg/kg/day IV for 5–7 days; or

   d. Cancidas, 70 mg loading dose on the first day, then 50 mg/day IV per day for 5–7 days

II. **Nosocomial and ventilator-associated pneumonia**
  A. Definition
     1. Most nosocomial infections of the lower respiratory tract are ventilator associated and are defined as onset of pneumonia 48 hr after endotracheal intubation
     2. Nosocomial pneumonia is the second most common hospital-acquired infection
  B. Etiology/incidence/predisposing factors
     1. Highest mortality rate of all the nosocomial infections
     2. Incidence ranges from 7% to 20%, depending on the intensive care unit setting
     3. Colonization of the upper respiratory tract and of endotracheal tubing by bacterial pathogens precedes infection
     4. Organisms usually reach the lower respiratory tract by aspiration into the distal airways
     5. Risk factors include the following:
        a. Intubation
        b. Intensive care unit setting
        c. Antibiotics
        d. Prolonged surgery
        e. Chronic lung disease
        f. Advanced age
        g. Immunosuppression
     6. Most common pathogens are predominantly Gram-negative bacilli and include the following:
        a. *P. aeruginosa*
        b. *Enterobacter* spp.
        c. *Klebsiella* spp.
        d. *E. coli*
        e. *Haemophilus influenzae*
        f. *Serratia marcescens*
        g. *Acinetobacter* spp.
     7. Most common Gram-positive pathogen
        a. *S. aureus*-methicillin-resistant and methicillin-sensitive species
  C. Subjective findings
     1. Fever
     2. Cough (usually productive)
     3. Shortness of breath
  D. Physical examination findings
     1. Rales or dullness to percussion on chest examination
     2. New onset or change in character of sputum
     3. Tachypnea
  E. Laboratory/diagnostic findings
     1. Purulent sputum

2. Isolation of a pathogen from the following:
   a. Sputum
   b. Transbronchial aspirate
   c. Bronchial brush
   d. Bronchoalveolar lavage
   e. Biopsy specimen
3. Organism isolated from blood culture
4. Deterioration in oxygenation or ventilation
5. Chest x-ray shows new or progressing
   a. Infiltrate
   b. Consolidation
   c. Cavitation
   d. Pleural effusion
6. Leukocytosis, often with a left shift

F. Management
   1. Hand washing by health care workers (prevention)
   2. Elevate the head of the patient's bed 30° to 45° (prevention)
   3. Discontinue nasogastric tubes when possible (prevention)
   4. Give sucralfate for stress ulcer prophylaxis (frequently recommended but remains controversial)
   5. Promote sputum clearance with incentive spirometry, chest physical therapy, and frequent suctioning
   6. Empiric antibiotics
      a. It is very important to know the susceptibilities of nosocomial pathogens in the medical unit
      b. Typically, antibiotic coverage is targeted broadly to include resistant Gram-negative pathogens (e.g., *P. aeruginosa*) at onset
      c. Once organisms have been identified by diagnostic means, narrower-spectrum antibiotic therapy usually can be used. For combination antipseudomonal coverage,
         i. Antipseudomonal β-lactam
            (a) Piperacillin, 3–4 grams IV every 4–6 hr;
            (b) Ceftazidime, 1–2 grams IV every 8–12 hr; or
            (c) Cefepime, 1–2 grams IV every 12 hr plus
         ii. Aminoglycoside
            (a) Gentamicin or tobramycin, 1.7–2 mg/kg IV every 8 hr, or 5 mg/kg IV every 24 hr or
         iii. Quinolone
            (a) Ciprofloxacin, 400 mg IV every 12 hr; or
            (b) Levofloxacin, 500 mg IV every 24 hr
      d. For patients with suspected aspiration pneumonia, anaerobic coverage should be considered
         i. Through the addition to the preceding regimen of clindamycin, 300–900 mg IV every 6–8 hr; or

   ii. With the use of a β-lactam/β-lactamase inhibitor such as piperacillin/tazobactam, 3.375 grams IV every 6 hr

  e. For critically ill patients and those at risk for methicillin-resistant Staphylococci, coverage with vancomycin, 1 gram IV every 12 hr, should be added.

  f. Duration of therapy for nosocomial pneumonia is 14–21 days

III. **Nosocomial bacteremia**

 A. Definition

  1. Laboratory-confirmed bloodstream infection with a pathogen recognized from blood culture or a skin colonizer isolated from multiple blood cultures on separate occasions

 B. Etiology/incidence/predisposing factors

  1. Third most common hospital-acquired infection

  2. Mortality ranges from 2% to 60%

  3. Most bacteremias are associated with intravascular catheters

  4. Sources of microbes include skin and intravascular fluids

  5. Pneumonia, urinary tract infection, and wound infection are usually the other sources of bacteremia

  6. Risk factors include the following:

   a. Bacterial colonization at the catheter site

   b. Longer duration of catheter insertion

   c. Older age

   d. Severe underlying illness

   e. Parenteral nutrition

   f. Loss of skin integrity

   g. Use of nonpermeable dressings

  7. Common organisms include the following:

   a. Coagulase-negative Staphylococci

   b. *S. aureus* (including methicillin-resistant *S. aureus*)

   c. Enterococci

   d. *Enterobacter* spp.

   e. *P. aeruginosa*

   f. *Candida* spp.

  8. Complications include the following:

   a. Cellulitis or abscess at the site of catheter insertion

   b. Septic phlebitis

   c. Endocarditis

 C. Subjective findings

  1. The patient may be asymptomatic

  2. Fever or chills

  3. Pain at the catheter insertion site

 D. Physical examination findings

  1. Local erythema, edema, tenderness, and warmth at the catheter site

  2. Exit site may be purulent

  3. Fever, tachycardia, or hypotension may be present

    4. May have a heart murmur and embolic/septic sequelae

E. Laboratory/diagnostic findings

    1. A recognized pathogen isolated from a blood culture (and not related to another site) or

    2. A symptomatic patient with a skin colonizer (e.g., a coagulase-negative *Staphylococcus*) identified in two blood cultures on separate occasions (and not related to another site)

F. Management

    1. It is of paramount importance that the source of the bacteremia/candidemia be identified (i.e., rule out pneumonia, urinary tract infection, wound infection, or endocarditis as the source of infection, as opposed to an intravenous catheter/device); choice and duration of therapy depend entirely on the diagnosis.

    2. Removal of the catheter is nearly always required

    3. Antibiotic therapy

        a. Gram stain results (Gram-positive compared with Gram-negative compared with yeast) from the blood culture will become available before identification and determination of susceptibilities and can be used as a guide for empiric antibiotic selection in cases of serious infection

        b. Once the organism has been identified and susceptibilities determined, a narrower-spectrum antibiotic regimen should be prescribed.

        c. Gram-positive cocci

            i. Nafcillin, 1–2 grams IV every 4 hr;

            ii. Cefazolin, 1–2 grams IV every 8 hr; or

            iii. Vancomycin, 1 grams IV every 12 hr, when methicillin resistance is suspected

        d. If methicillin-resistant *S. aureus* has been identified, the patient must be placed in contact isolation (gloves and gown if soiling is likely)

        e. If vancomycin-resistant *Enterococcus* is isolated, the patient must be placed in contact isolation.

            i. Optimal therapy for vancomycin-resistant *Enterococcus* has yet to be determined.

            ii. Possibly effective: ampicillin (*Enterococcus faecalis*); quinupristin/dalfopristin (Synercid) (*Enterococcus faecium*), 7.5 mg/kg IV every 8 hr; linezolid (Zyvox), 600 mg IV every 12 hr; or daptomycin (Cubicin), 4 mg/kg IV every 24 hr

            iii. An infectious disease consultation is critical for appropriate management of these infections under most circumstances

    f. Vancomycin is not recommended as treatment in response to a single positive blood culture for coagulase-negative Staphylococci.

    g. Gram-negative bacilli

        i. Antipseudomonal β-lactam

           (a) Piperacillin, 3–4 grams IV every 4–6 hr;

           (b) Ceftazidime, 2 grams IV every 8–12 hr; or

           (c) Cefepime, 2 grams IV every 12 hr plus

        ii. Aminoglycoside

           (a) Gentamicin or tobramycin, 1.7–2 mg/kg IV every 8 hr, or 5 mg/kg IV every 24 hr or

        iii. Quinolone

           (a) Ciprofloxacin, 400 mg IV every 12 hr; or

           (b) Levofloxacin, 500–750 mg IV every 24 hr

    h. Yeasts

        i. Echinocandins are first line antifungal treatment for *Candida* before species is identified and even used as antifungal broad-spectrum prophylaxis in severely ill or immunosuppressed patients.

           (a) Used most often as an alternative antifungal agent due to multiple drug interactions in azole class and nephrotoxic side effects of polyene class

           (b) Micafungin, 100 mg IV daily for 14–21 days

        ii. Azoles are preferred if *Candida* species is identified and susceptible to drug because it is inexpensive, not nephrotoxic, and available in PO or IV generic forms

           (a) Fluconazole, loading dose 800 mg PO or IV, then 400–800 mg PO or IV daily

        iii. Polyene antibiotics

           (a) Used less frequently due to significant nephrotoxicity

           (b) Amphotericin B, 0.5 mg/kg IV every 24 hr

  4. Duration of therapy is usually 14 days

IV. **Miscellaneous nosocomial infections**

  A. *Clostridium difficile* colitis (pseudomembranous colitis)

    1. Diagnosis: fever, abdominal pain, heme-positive stool, and diarrhea in a patient currently or recently receiving antibiotics, and a stool specimen positive for *C. difficile* toxin

    2. Treatment

      a. Discontinuation of implicated antibiotic when possible

      b. Patient should be placed in contact isolation

      c. Metronidazole, 500 mg PO every 8 hr for 10–14 days or

      d. Vancomycin, 125 mg PO every 6 hr for 10–14 days, if infection is severe

e. When oral treatment is not possible, metronidazole, 500 mg IV every 8 hr

f. For relapses (frequency, 5% to 50%), repeat above treatment

B. Surgical wound infections

1. Diagnosis

   a. Purulence within the surgical wound site

   b. May be associated with fever, leukocytosis, and sepsis (other nosocomial sources ruled out)

2. Rates of infection are related to the level of contamination (e.g., clean, clean-contaminated, or contaminated wound)

3. Source of contamination is dependent on multiple factors, including but not limited to skin flora and the surgical procedure or trauma site involved.

4. Common pathogens in surgical wound infections include the following:

   a. *S. aureus*

   b. *Enterococcus*

   c. Coagulase-negative *Staphylococcus*

   d. *E. coli*

   e. *P. aeruginosa*

   f. *Enterobacter* spp.

   g. *Klebsiella* spp.

   h. *Proteus* spp.

   i. *Streptococcus* spp.

   j. *Bacteroides fragilis*

5. Treatment

   a. For most clean procedures/wounds (e.g., cholecystectomy, cardiothoracic, vascular surgery, orthopedic surgery, and cesarean section), cefazolin is indicated for prophylaxis and for treatment.

   b. For clean-contaminated procedures/wounds (e.g., colon surgery and penetrating abdominal/pelvic trauma), cefoxitin is indicated for prophylaxis and treatment.

   c. For postoperative sepsis, broad coverage for nosocomial pathogens is indicated, and it is critical to determine the source.

      i. Empiric coverage for nosocomial pneumonia or bacteremia as described in the preceding sections is usually appropriate

      ii. If an abdominal contaminated wound may be a source of infection, then coverage for Gram-negatives and anaerobes is prudent, with piperacillin/tazobactam, 3.375 grams IV every 6 hr plus an aminoglycoside

COMMUNITY-ACQUIRED INFECTIONS

I. **Table 81.1 provides a limited selection of common community-acquired infections in adults that practitioners frequently encounter; it is by no means a definitive resource but rather an abbreviated guide for some of the most common organisms and appropriate empiric antibiotic treatment regimens for adults**

Table 81.1	Empiric Therapy for Selected Community-Acquired Infections	
Infection	**Organism**	**Recommended pharmacological treatment**
Pharyngitis	Primary concern about group A *Streptococcus* with possible acute rheumatic fever sequelae. Other pathogens include viral, *Neisseria*, *Corynebacterium diphtheriae*, and upper respiratory tract pathogens	If *Streptococcus* screen or throat cultures are positive for group A *Streptococcus*, then oral penicillin, cephalosporin, or erythromycin for 10 days; consider other pathogens if group A *Streptococcus* is not found.
Sinusitis	*Streptococcus pneumoniae* and *Haemophilus influenzae* are most common, but viral, *Staphylococcus aureus, Moraxella catarrhalis*, Gram-negatives, and anaerobes also may be responsible	Topical and systemic decongestants plus Augmentin, 875 mg PO BID, or Bactrim, DS PO BID for 10–14 days, are usually recommended empirically; broader-spectrum antibiotics (e.g., cefuroxime, 500 mg PO BID; Levaquin, 500 mg PO daily) and sinus x-rays are suggested for refractory cases
Pneumonia	See Chapter 32	See Chapter 32
Meningitis	See Chapter 5	See Chapter 5
Urinary tract infection	See Chapter 42	See Chapter 42

Table 81.1	Empiric Therapy for Selected Community-Acquired Infections	
Infection	**Organism**	**Recommended pharmacological treatment**
Skin and soft tissue furunculosis	Primary concern about *Staphylococcus* with a profound increase nationwide in methicillin-resistant *S. aureus*	Most important therapy is incision and drainage; oral clindamycin 300–450 mg PO 4 times a day or, if serious, vancomycin 1 gram IV every 12 hr is usually started empirically
Cellulitis	Primary concern about *S. aureus*, *Streptococcus pyogenes*, and other Gram-positives in immunocompetent hosts, but Gram-negatives and anaerobes are occasionally responsible	Cephalexin, 500 mg PO 4 times a day or, if serious, cefazolin, 1–2 grams IV every 8 hr, is usually started empirically for most skin and soft tissue infections; failure to quickly improve with these agents requires aggressive imaging and tissue and blood cultures for evaluation; surgical and infectious disease consultations if infection is severe and is limb or life threatening
In diabetes or the immunocompromised	Same Gram-positive organisms as above, but also Gram-negatives, including *Pseudomonas* and anaerobes	Same as above, but add a quinolone or, if infection is limb or life threatening, piperacillin/tazobactam, 3.375 grams IV every 6 hr
Bite wounds	*Staphylococcus*, *Streptococcus*, *Eikenella*, *Pasteurella*, and anaerobes are usually responsible	Cleaning and debridement of the wound and a tetanus shot are essential. Augmentin, 875 mg PO BID or, if severe, ampicillin/sulbactam, 3 grams IV every 6 hr
Surgical wounds	Gram-positives more than Gram-negatives or polymicrobial, dependent on injury	See chapter text
Gastrointestinal problems, simple diarrhea	Most cases of diarrhea are self-limiting and do not require antibiotics	Adequate oral hydration is usually sufficient

Table 81.1	Empiric Therapy for Selected Community-Acquired Infections	
Infection	**Organism**	**Recommended pharmacological treatment**
Endocarditis	Gram-positive more than Gram-negative	Nafcillin, 2 grams IV every 4 hr, plus gentamicin, 1 mg/kg IV every 8 hr, and follow-up on blood and tissue cultures; ampicillin, 2 grams IV every 4 hr, added if *Streptococcus viridans* is suspected; infectious disease consultation is highly recommended
Dysentery	*Shigella*, *Salmonella*, enterotoxigenic *Escherichia coli*, *Campylobacter*, *Clostridium difficile*, and *Entamoeba histolytica*; stool cultures, stains, ova and parasites (O&P), and toxins for these pathogens are often helpful for identification	Hydration is critical and may require intravenous therapy; in patients who appear toxic or who are immunocompromised, treat with a quinolone such as ciprofloxacin, 500 mg PO or IV every 12 hr; if *E. histolytica* or *C. difficile colitis* is suspected, add metronidazole, 750 mg PO or IV every 8 hr, and follow-up on stool studies to confirm
Sepsis, source unknown	Gram-positive and Gram-negative	Ceftriaxone, 2 grams IV every 24 hr; ampicillin/sulbactam, 3 grams IV every 6 hr; or piperacillin/tazobactam, 3.375 grams IV every 6 hr, usually with an aminoglycoside (gentamicin or tobramycin, 1 mg/kg IV every 8 hr)
Neutropenia with fever	Gram-positive and Gram-negative primarily; serious fungal infections are also to be considered	Ceftazidime, 2 grams IV every 8 hr, or cefepime, 2 grams IV every 8–12 hr plus an aminoglycoside or quinolone (dose as in nosocomial infections in this chapter); infectious disease consultation is highly recommended
If vascular device present	Primarily for Gram-positives, including methicillin-resistant *Staphylococcus*	Add vancomycin 1 gram IV every 12 hr, and follow-up on blood cultures; usually requires the removal of a vascular catheter when present (see section on Nosocomial Bacteremia)

Note. PO = administered orally; DS = double strength.

A. Empiric antibiotic therapy is not a substitute for a required diagnostic workup and treatment plan for a patient with a suspected infection.

B. For all infections, it is imperative for the clinician to identify in the most prudent way which organisms are responsible for the infection and their specific antibiotic susceptibilities.

C. On the basis of these results, confirmed effective and usually narrower-spectrum antibiotics should be used.

D. A patient's history and infectious disease risks may dramatically alter the organisms and presentation of infection in an individual; these are very important when one is considering empiric antibiotic regimens beyond the scope of this handbook.

E. Consequently, for any seriously or critically ill patient in whom infection may be present or suspected, these risks must be considered, and an infectious disease consultation is highly recommended.

II. **All antibiotics have the potential for serious allergic reactions and toxicities, and this potential is critical in selection of an antibiotic regimen.**

A. It is essential that the clinician know the possible allergic reactions and toxicities of an antibiotic before prescribing it.

B. Please refer to the package inserts of these medications, and ask the pharmacist at your facility or hospital any additional questions

III. **When vancomycin and aminoglycosides (gentamicin, tobramycin, and amikacin) are used, serum concentration monitoring (peaks and troughs) is required.**

A. Please refer to the package inserts and your pharmacist regarding specific recommendations

BIBLIOGRAPHY

DiCocco, J. M., & Croce, M. A. (2009). Ventilator-associated pneumonia: An overview. *Expert Opinion Pharmacotherapy, 10*(9), 1461–1467. doi:10.1517/14656560903007922

Havey, T. C., Fowler, R. A., & Daneman, N. (2011). Duration of antibiotic therapy for bacteremia: A systemic review and meta-analysis. *Critical Care, 15*(6), 1–11. doi:10.1186/cc10545

Hooten, T., Bradley, S., Cardenas, D., Colgan, R., Geerlings, S., Rice, . . . Nicolle, L. (2010). Diagnosis, prevention, and treatment of catheter-associated urinary tract infection in adults: 2009 International Clinical Practice Guidelines from the Infectious Diseases Society of America. *Clinical Infectious Diseases, 50*(5), 625–663.

Ksycki, M. F., & Namias, N. (2009). Nosocomial urinary tract infection. *Surgical Clinics of North America, 89*(2), 475–481. doi:10.1016/j.suc.2008.09.012

Lorente, L., Blot, S., & Rello, J. (2010). New issues and controversies in the prevention of ventilator-associated pneumonia. *American Journal of Respiratory and Critical Care Medicine, 182,* 870–876.

Mikulska, M., Del Bono, V., & Viscoli, C. (2012). Occurrence, presentation, and treatment of candidemia. *Expert Review of Clinical Immunology, 8*(8), 755–765. doi:10.1586/eci.12.52

Newman, D. (2010). Prevention and management of catheter-associated urinary tract infections. *Infectious Disease, 1,* 13–20.

Trautner, B. (2010). Management of catheter-associated urinary tract infection (CAUTI). *Current Opinion of Infectious Disease, 23*(1), 76–82. doi:10.1097/QCO.0b013e328334dda8

Van Hal, S. J., Jensen, S. O., Vaska, V. L., Espedido, B. A., Paterson, D. L., & Gosbell, I. B. (2012). Predictors of mortality in *Staphylococcus aureus* bacteremia. *American Society for Microbiology, 25*(2), 362–386.

CHAPTER 82

Chest, Abdominal, and Eye Trauma:
Trauma Considerations

ALISON FORBES • THOMAS W. BARKLEY, JR.

INITIAL ASSESSMENT AND MANAGEMENT

I. **Advanced Trauma Life Support**
    A. Developed in 1980 by the American College of Surgeons
    B. Standardized assessment and management of trauma patients using an evidence-based approach
    C. Multidisciplinary and an international program

II. **Primary survey**
    A. Airway maintenance with cervical spine protection
        1. Assess airway patency for signs of obstruction using chin-lift or jaw-thrust maneuvers
        2. While assessing the airway, prevent excessive movement of the cervical spine
            a. Do not hyperextend, hyperflex, or rotate the patient's head and neck to establish the airway
            b. Stabilize the patient's head and neck if immobilization devices are removed temporarily
    B. Breathing and ventilation
        1. Inspect and palpate the neck and chest for signs of injury, percuss and auscultate the chest bilaterally
        2. Administer high flow oxygen, ventilate with a bag-valve-mask device if necessary, and identify any life-threatening ventilation problems (i.e., tension pneumothorax)
    C. Circulation with hemorrhage control
        1. Identify sources of hemorrhage, assess pulses, evaluate skin color, and measure blood pressure

2. Apply direct pressure to sites with external bleeding, insert two large bore IVs, initiate warm intravenous fluid therapy, and consider surgical consult if you suspect internal hemorrhage

D. Disability: neurologic status
   1. Determine the level of consciousness using the Glasgow Coma Scale, check pupil size and reaction, and assess for focal neurologic deficits and spinal cord injury

E. Exposure and environment
   1. Completely undress the patient for a quick assessment, and then cover the patient with warm blankets to prevent hypothermia

III.   Adjuncts to primary survey

A. Adjuncts
   1. Obtain a full panel of labs including a Chem-10, complete blood count, coagulants, arterial blood gas (ABG), lactate, and type/screen
   2. Attach an electrocardiogram monitor to patient
   3. Insert urinary catheter for strict intake and output
   4. Insert a gastric catheter for gastric decompression
   5. Consider x-ray plain films such as a chest and pelvic x-ray
   6. Consider a bedside diagnostic peritoneal lavage or focused assessment with sonography in trauma (FAST) exam
   7. Reexamination of ABCs before beginning secondary survey

IV.   Secondary survey

A. Perform a head-to-toe evaluation of the trauma patient
   1. Take a complete history using the mnemonic AMPLE: allergies, medications, past illnesses/pregnancy, last meal, and events that led up to injury or environment related to the injury
   2. Physical examination follows in sequence of head, maxillofacial structures, cervical spine and neck, chest, abdomen, perineum/rectum/vagina, musculoskeletal system, and neurologic system

CHEST TRAUMA

I.   Rib fracture

A. Definition
   1. Fracture of one or more ribs
   2. Possibly resulting in severe damage to underlying structures
      a. Lungs (e.g., pneumothorax and pulmonary contusion)
      b. Subclavian artery
      c. Subclavian vein

B. Etiology/incidence
   1. Eighty-five percent of patients with blunt chest trauma experience rib fractures
   2. Associated with motor vehicle crashes (MVCs), assaults, and falls

C. Subjective/physical examination findings

1. Pain that worsens with breathing, coughing, movement, and on palpation
2. Shallow respirations
3. Splinting of region
4. Crepitus
5. Decreased breath sounds on the affected side

D. Laboratory/diagnostic findings
   1. Chest x-ray may reveal fracture, atelectasis
   2. ABG analysis
      a. ABGs may reveal respiratory acidosis (increased $PaCO_2$ greater than 45 mmHg) if the patient is hypoventilating
      b. If the patient is hyperventilating, respiratory alkalosis (decreased $PaCO_2$ less than 35 mmHg) may be seen
      c. Also, hypoxemia may be observed (PaO_2 less than 90 mmHg) if severe pulmonary contusion is present
   3. Complete blood count if hemothorax is suspected

E. Management
   1. Rule out underlying structural damage (e.g., lacerated subclavian artery or subclavian vein, pneumothorax, and lacerated liver or spleen) by ordering arteriography, x-rays, CT scan
   2. Pain medications (refer to Pain chapter)
      a. For minor injuries, outpatient management options such as aspirin, acetaminophen, and nonsteroidal anti-inflammatory drugs (e.g., Ibuprofen, 600 mg PO/NGT every 8 hr or every 8 hr PRN for pain)
      b. For acute injuries, consider ketorolac (Toradol), 30 mg IV every 6 hr PRN for pain, with opioid options such as morphine sulfate, 2 mg IV initially, then titrated PRN until pain is relieved (watch out for respiratory depression), or hydromorphone (Dilaudid), 0.2 mg IV every 15 minutes for 3 doses, then 0.5 mg IV/SQ every 4 hr PRN for pain
      c. Intercostal nerve blocks (such as lidocaine 1%), patient-controlled analgesia, or epidural anesthesia options should be considered for severe pain management
      d. Consult to pain service/anesthesia for orders
   3. Aggressive pulmonary toilet, such as turn, cough, deep breathe, and chest physiotherapy, should be used on unaffected side, along with incentive spirometry; encourage resting on affected side if tolerable to promote expansion of the unaffected lung.
   4. Consider aerosol therapy with albuterol (Ventolin), 2.5 mg via HHN every 4 hr or every 4 hr PRN for shortness of breath/wheezing to prevent atelectasis and pneumonia
   5. Monitor oxygen saturation; consider giving O_2 at 2 L per nasal cannula, with oxygen saturation (SaO_2) maintained above 92%

II. **Flail chest**
   A. Definition
      1. Fracture of at least two adjacent ribs at two sites
      2. Results in a "floating" segment or sternum
   B. Etiology/incidence
      1. Most serious chest wall injury
      2. High likelihood of underlying structural injury
      3. Caused by blunt force/trauma
   C. Subjective/physical examination findings
      1. Pain
      2. Shortness of breath
      3. Paradoxical chest wall movement—opposite from normal on inspiration/expiration
      4. Shallow respirations
      5. Tachypnea
      6. Decreased level of consciousness (LOC) related to hypoxia
      7. Cyanosis
      8. Tachycardia
      9. Splinting of chest wall
      10. Crepitus
      11. Decreased breath sounds on affected side
   D. Laboratory/diagnostic findings
      1. ABGs: hypoxia, possible respiratory acidosis
      2. Chest x-ray: reveals rib fractures
   E. Management
      1. Administer O_2, correct possible respiratory acidosis, and consider ventilatory support with positive end-expiratory pressure and pressure support
      2. Administer crystalloids, such as lactated Ringer solution or normal saline 2 L IV bolus, then 100 ml/hr
      3. Consider supporting/stabilizing flail segment with sandbags, although controversy is expressed in the current literature regarding the effectiveness of this treatment; if ventilatory restriction is severe, provide operative stabilization
      4. Pain medications
         a. Morphine sulfate, 2 mg IV initially, then titrate PRN until pain is relieved (watch out for respiratory depression)
         b. Hydromorphone (Dilaudid), 0.2 mg IV every 15 minutes for 3 doses; then 0.5 mg IV/SQ every 4 hr PRN for pain
      5. If lung contusion occurs, the patient may require long-term ventilation
      6. Ventilation with induced paralysis may also be provided
III. **Collapsed lung**
   A. Pneumothorax

    1. Occurs when air is introduced into the pleural space, causing complete or partial collapse of the lung

    2. May be caused by blunt trauma, mechanical ventilation, central venous access devices, rib fracture, and bleb rupture

B. Hemothorax

    1. Occurs when blood accumulates in the pleural space; considered massive when drainage exceeds 1.5 L

    2. May be caused by blunt or penetrating trauma, lung cancer, or anticoagulant therapy complications

C. Open pneumothorax

    1. Sometimes referred to as "sucking chest wound"

        a. Air flows from atmosphere to pleural space and back again

        b. Can lead to tension pneumothorax if covered with an occlusive dressing or if skin flap does not allow air to escape

    2. May be caused by penetrating trauma, such as gunshot wounds or knife wounds

D. Tension pneumothorax

    1. Collapse of the lung caused by one-way entrance of air flow into the pleural space

        a. Results in increased pressure on the heart, mediastinal shift to the unaffected side, and eventual circulatory collapse

        b. Tension pneumothorax is a life-threatening condition

    2. May be caused by blunt or chest trauma, open pneumothorax, fractured rib, mechanical ventilation, and clamped chest tube

E. General subjective/physical examination findings of the collapsed lung

    1. Respiratory distress

    2. Hypoxia

    3. Tachypnea

    4. Decreased LOC

    5. Hypotension

    6. Cyanosis

    7. Tachycardia

    8. Shallow respirations

    9. Chest pain

    10. Decreased or absent breath sounds on affected side

    11. Deviation of the trachea to the unaffected side

    12. Tension pneumothorax may cause severe respiratory distress, leading to circulatory collapse (i.e., decreased cardiac output and decreased blood pressure)

    13. Open pneumothorax: sucking sound may be heard on inspiration

F. Laboratory/diagnostic findings

    1. ABGs may reveal respiratory acidosis

    2. Chest x-ray reveals collapsed lung and possible mediastinal shift

    3. Electrocardiogram may show heart strain

G. Management

1. Pneumothorax smaller than 15% to 20% requires only observation, serial chest x-rays, pigtail catheters, Heimlich valves or chest tube at the fourth to the fifth intercostal space, midaxillary line, PRN
2. If tension pneumothorax, rapid insertion of large-bore (14- to 16-gauge) needle into the second intercostal space, midclavicular line of the affected side
3. Chest tube insertion to low wall suction (-20 cm) for a pneumothorax or hemothorax
4. Consider mechanical ventilation with a positive end-expiratory pressure of +5, a pressure support of 10, and a tidal volume set at 6 ml/kg
5. Open pneumothorax: apply a three-sided dressing, leaving one side unsecured to allow air to escape
6. Massive hemothorax: fluid resuscitation with lactated Ringer solution should be considered before thoracostomy owing to loss of tamponade effect; consider autotransfusion

IV. **Cardiac tamponade (refer to chapter on Angina and Myocardial Infarction)**

V. **Aortic rupture**
   A. Definition
      1. An interruption of the wall of the aorta caused by blunt traumatic deceleration injuries
   B. Etiology
      1. MVC (most often without use of seat belt)
      2. Falls
      3. Pedestrian struck by automobile
      4. High mortality rate; most die before reaching the hospital
   C. Subjective/physical examination findings
      1. Shortness of breath
      2. Weakness
      3. Blood pressure and pulse amplitude are greater in upper extremities
      4. Chest or back pain
      5. Circulatory collapse
   D. Laboratory/diagnostic findings
      1. Chest x-ray may reveal a widened mediastinum, deviation of trachea to the right, obliteration of aortic knob, and fractures of first or second rib or scapula
      2. Aortogram may reveal a widened mediastinum
   E. Management
      1. Thoracotomy to repair the rupture, with cardiopulmonary bypass
      2. Adequate fluid resuscitation with crystalloids (e.g., normal saline and lactated Ringer solution)
      3. Packed red blood cells

4. Consider nitroprusside (Nipride), 0.2–8 mcg/kg/min, increase/decrease rate by 0.1 mcg/kg/min every 10 minutes to maintain SBP less than 100–110 for aortic rupture until patient can be taken to surgery or esmolol 50–300 mcg/kg/min, increase/decrease rate by 50 mcg/kg/min every 15 minutes to maintain SBP less than 100–110
5. Mechanical ventilation

ABDOMINAL TRAUMA

I. **Lacerated liver**
A. Definition
1. Laceration or tear of the liver caused by blunt or penetrating injury that typically results in profuse bleeding
2. Classified according to disruption of the organ as grades I through VI defined by the American Association for the Surgery of Trauma; grade VI is incompatible with survival
a. Grade I: capsular tear smaller than 1 cm
b. Grade II: 1- to 3-cm parenchymal depth, less than 10 cm in length
c. Grade III: greater than 3 cm parenchymal depth
d. Grade IV: parenchymal disruption of 25% to 75%
e. Grade V: parenchymal disruption of greater than 75%
f. Grade VI: hepatic avulsion
B. Etiology
1. Blunt trauma: MVC, falls, and assaults
2. Penetrating injury: stab wounds and gunshot wounds
3. Mortality is usually due to hemorrhage
C. Subjective/physical examination findings
1. Right upper quadrant pain
2. Guarding
3. Signs and symptoms of hypovolemic shock
a. Decreased blood pressure
b. Increased heart rate
c. Decreased LOC
d. Decreased urinary output
4. Possible hypoactive or absent bowel sounds
D. Laboratory/diagnostic findings
1. FAST ultrasound or positive diagnostic peritoneal lavage
2. Positive abdominal CT scan
3. Decreased hematocrit
4. Decreased hemoglobin
5. Elevated liver enzymes
6. Increased prothrombin time
E. Management

1. Stabilize impaled objects and wrap; do not remove (e.g., knife sticking out of abdomen)
2. Fluid resuscitation (see chapter on Management of the Patient in Shock)
3. Insert nasogastric tube
4. Insert Foley catheter
5. Peritoneal lavage
6. Surgery to ligate tears in hepatic artery or to perform resection
7. Hemodynamic monitoring
8. Hemodynamically stable patients may be managed nonoperatively and observed in the ICU unless a presence of a blush on the CT scan, then angiography is the treatment of choice
9. Hemodynamically unstable patients receive an exploration laparotomy
10. Antibiotic administration for penetrating abdominal trauma
    a. Single agent regimen:
       i. Imipenem-cilastatin, 500 mg IV every 6 hr
       ii. Meropenem, 1 gram IV every 8 hr
       iii. Piperacillin-tazobactam, 3.375 grams IV every 6 hr
    b. Combination regimen:
       i. Cefepime, 2 grams IV every 12 hr or ceftazidime, 2 grams IV every 8 hr plus
       ii. Metronidazole, 500 mg IV every 8 hr

II. **Ruptured spleen**
   A. Definition
      1. Tear to the spleen caused by blunt or penetrating injury
      2. Most commonly injured organ in blunt abdominal trauma cases
      3. Classified according to disruption of the organ
         a. Grade I: capsular tear smaller than 1 cm
         b. Grade II: 1- to 3-cm parenchymal depth
         c. Grade III: greater than 3 cm parenchymal depth
         d. Grade IV: greater than 25% of spleen
         e. Grade V: completely shattered spleen
   B. Etiology
      1. Most often caused by MVCs, gunshot wounds, or stab wounds
      2. May be due to rib fracture
   C. Subjective/physical examination findings
      1. Pain
      2. Kehr's sign—acute pain in the tip of the shoulder when a person is lying down with legs elevated
      3. Hypovolemic shock (increased heart rate and decreased blood pressure)
      4. Guarding
   D. Laboratory/diagnostic findings
      1. FAST exam or positive peritoneal lavage

2. Decreased hematocrit
3. Decreased hemoglobin
4. Increased WBC count (more than 10,000/mm)
5. Positive CT scan

E. Management
1. Stabilize impaled objects, and wrap sterile dressing around site; do not remove foreign object—tamponade effect may be lost
2. Fluid resuscitation (with lactated Ringer's) for prevention of hypovolemic shock
3. Insert nasogastric tube
4. Insert Foley catheter
5. Peritoneal lavage
6. Hemodynamic monitoring: hemodynamically stable patients may be managed nonoperatively and observed in the ICU. If the presence of contrast extravasation is present on the CT scan, angiography is the treatment of choice and admission to the ICU is warranted
7. Hemodynamically unstable patients receive an exploration laparotomy with pelvic packing

III. **Renal injuries**
A. Definition
1. Injuries to the kidneys that result in fragmentation; caused by blunt or penetrating trauma
2. Also may be caused by rib fracture
B. Subjective/physical examination findings
1. Pain—abdominal or flank
2. Flank bruising (Grey Turner's sign)
3. Hematuria
4. Palpable mass in flank region
5. Possible hemodynamic instability
C. Laboratory/diagnostic findings
1. Intravenous pyelogram
2. CT scan
3. Kidneys, ureters, and bladder x-ray
4. Urinalysis may reveal hematuria
D. Management
1. Depends on extent of injury (i.e., observation versus surgery)
2. Maintain hemodynamic stability.
3. Possible nephrectomy (ensure functioning of the remaining kidney)
4. Insert nasogastric tube
5. Insert Foley catheter
6. Monitor for renal failure

IV. **Pelvic trauma**
A. Definition

      1. Fractures of the pelvis including the hip bone, sacrum, and coccyx
      2. Classified based on mechanism of injury
          a. Anterior posterior compression, lateral compression, vertical shear, and complex
          b. Commonly caused by auto-pedestrian collision or fall from a height
      3. Associated injuries with pelvic trauma include venous hemorrhage, visceral injury, genitourinary injury, nerve deficits, and thoracic aortic rupture

B. Subjective/physical examination findings
      1. Pain present in the abdomen, thigh, or buttock
      2. Numbness or tingling in groin or legs
      3. Bleeding from urethra, vagina, or rectum: caution when performing rectal or vaginal exams as fractured bones can protrude into vault
      4. Manual palpation revealing crepitus or unstable pelvis

C. Laboratory or diagnostic findings
      1. Pelvic x-ray illustrating a disruption of the pelvic ring, widened sacroiliac joints, widened pubic symphysis, and rami fractures
      2. CT scan of the abdomen and pelvis to assess for fractures of bones and presence of contrast extravasation or blush

D. Management
      1. Insert Foley unless blood at the urethra or high-riding prostate is present. Otherwise, a urology consult is needed
      2. Consider transfer to a higher level of care for definitive management and orthopedic consult
      3. Pelvic stabilization and hemorrhage control
          a. Apply a pelvic binder, sheet, or external fixation device to wrap around until definitive orthopedic management (note this could cause increased bleeding; monitor vitals carefully)
      4. Hemodynamically stable patients with a venous injury are managed best by angiography for ligation
      5. Hemodynamically unstable patients with active bleeding go to operating room for a laparotomy to undergo pelvic packing, ligation of venous or arterial vessels actively bleeding, and internal fixation.

PENETRATING EYE TRAUMA

I. **Definition**
    A. Impalement of objects into the globe of the eye
II. **Etiology**
    A. Industrial accidents, failure to use protective eyewear
    B. Gunshot wounds and stab wounds
III. **Subjective/physical examination findings**
    A. Decreased visual acuity or complete vision loss
    B. Pain

    C. The patient may visualize foreign objects

    D. If retinal detachment occurs, the patient may experience light flashes, blurred vision, and severe eye pain

    E. Small, shrunken eyeball

IV.   **Diagnostic/laboratory findings**

    A. Decrease in intraocular pressure (normal, 10–20 mmHg)

V.   **Management**

    A. Ophthalmology consultation

    B. Immobilize the impaled object

    C. To decrease intraocular pressure (if greater than 21 mmHg), raise the head of the bed

    D. Patch or bandage both eyes

    E. Use no medications in the affected eye to avoid possible perforation of the eye

    F. Surgery

BIBLIOGRAPHY

American College of Surgeons. (2012). *Initial assessment and management. Advanced trauma life support* (9th ed., pp. 10–26). Chicago, IL: Author.

American College of Surgeons. (2012). *Thoracic trauma. Advanced trauma life support* (9th ed., pp. 96–106). Chicago, IL: Author.

American College of Surgeons. (2012). *Abdominal and pelvic trauma. Advanced trauma life support* (9th ed., pp. 125–137). Chicago, IL: Author.

Ferrada, P., Vanguri, P., Anand, R., Whelan, J., Duane, T., Aboutanos, M., . . . Ivatury, R. (2013). A, B, C, D, echo: Limited transthoracic echocardiogram is a useful tool to guide therapy for hypotension in the trauma bay. *Journal of Trauma and Acute Care Surgery, 74*(1), 220–223. doi:10.1097/TA.0b013e318278918a

Figler, B., Hofler, C. E., Reisman, W., Carney, K. J., Moore, T., Feliciano, D., & Master, V. (2012). Multi-disciplinary update on pelvic fracture associated bladder and urethral injuries. *Injury, 43*(8), 1242–1249. doi:10.1016/j.injury.2012.03.031

Mattox, K., Moore, E., & Feliciano, D. (2012) *Trauma* (7th ed.). New York, NY: McGraw Hill.

McCormack, R., Strauss, E. J., Alwattar, B. J., & Tejwani, N. C. (2010). Diagnosis and management of pelvic fractures. *Joint Disease, 68*(4), 281–291.

Smith, B. P., Fox, N., Fakhro, A., LaChant, M., Pathak, A., Ross, S., & Seamon, M. (2012). "SCIP" ping antibiotic prophylaxis guidelines in trauma: The consequences of noncompliance. *Journal of Trauma and Acute Care Surgery, 73*(2), 452–456.

Velmahos, G. C., Degiannis, E., & Doll, D. (2013) *Penetrating trauma: A practical guide on operative technique and peri-operative management.* New York, NY: Springer.

CHAPTER 83

Solid Organ Transplantation

HONORE GARRIN KOTLER • THOMAS W. BARKLEY, JR.

SOLID ORGAN TRANSPLANTATION

I. **Overview**
    A. Transplantation is the process by which the tissues or organs of one human being are grafted into another human being for the purpose of prolonging and improving quality of life.
    B. United Network for Organ Sharing is a private, nonprofit organization; it is a federal government contractor that oversees the procurement and distribution of organs and maintains the national wait-list.
    C. A total of 63 organ procurement organizations have been established in the United States; these groups oversee the procurement of organs.

II. **Incidence**
    A. The number of individuals waiting for an organ transplant exceeds 120,000; the kidney is the most frequently sought organ (98,881).
    B. Although the number of waiting recipients continues to rise, the number of deceased donors has remained stagnant for the past 10 years, at approximately 8,000.

III. **Types of transplants**
    A. Deceased donor
        1. Brain-dead donor
        2. Non-heartbeating donor
    B. Living donor
        1. Related (parent or sibling)
        2. Unrelated (spouse or friend)
        3. Paired exchange
        4. Altruistic

IV. **Absolute and relative contraindications to receive organs**
    A. Malignancy

B. Active infection
C. Active drug, tobacco, or illicit substance use
D. Inability to comply with medical regimen
E. Acquired immune deficiency syndrome
F. Human immunodeficiency virus (relative contraindication)
G. Morbid obesity (relative contraindication)

IMMUNOSUPPRESSION AND ORGAN REJECTION

I. **Overview of the immune response**
  A. Cell-mediated immunity (activated T lymphocytes are triggered by the cytokine interleukin-2)
     1. Cytokines are proteins that induce cell-mediated and humoral responses.
  B. Humoral or antibody immunity (production of antibodies from B lymphocytes)
     1. B cell recognizes matching antigen and digests it, binds to MHC molecule, then attracts matching T cell that helps B cell multiply and form into antibodies
  C. Cytokines are proteins that induce cell-mediated and humoral responses
  D. The major histocompatibility complex is a group of genetic loci located on the short arm of chromosome 6 that creates the human leukocyte antigens (HLAs), which recognize self and nonself; a total of six HLA genes are inherited and are identified via tissue typing.
  E. Panel reactive antibody (PRA) is a measurement of preformed HLA antibodies; elevated PRA may render a positive crossmatch and may limit a recipient's chance of transplantation
  F. The crossmatch is the final test undertaken to evaluate the reactivity of the donor to the recipient. Crossmatching is performed on all renal transplant recipients prior to surgery. Retrospective crossmatching is performed for heart, lung, liver, and pancreas recipients.

II. **Organ rejection**
  A. Allograft rejection occurs when the recipient's immune system recognizes that the graft is "nonself"; rejection involves local and systemic immune responses that may lead to local inflammation, deterioration of graft function, and eventual necrosis
  B. Types of rejection
     1. Hyperacute: rare, occurs within minutes, humorally mediated, rapid tissue necrosis
     2. Accelerated acute: occurs 1–5 days postoperatively; cellularly and humorally mediated; difficult to treat
     3. Acute: cellularly mediated in 90%; typically occurs within first few months but may occur at any time; amenable to treatment

Table 83.1	Signs and symptoms of rejection	
Organ	**Subjective**	**Objective**
Kidney	Decreased urine output (UOP), chills, arthralgias/myalgias, graft tenderness; may be asymptomatic	Elevated BUN and creatinine, increased resistive indices on ultrasonography
Liver	Fatigue, pruritus, graft tenderness	Elevated liver enzymes, elevated bilirubin, dark-colored urine, jaundice, ascites
Lung	Cough, dyspnea, fatigue	Fever, pulmonary effusions and infiltrates, decrease in spirometry, hypoxemia
Heart	Fatigue, exercise intolerance, dyspnea	Atrial arrhythmias, new S3, friction rub, jugular venous distention (JVD), edema, pulmonary edema
Pancreas	Graft tenderness	Elevated serum amylase/lipase, hyperglycemia (late), elevated creatinine (if kidney/pancreas recipient)
Intestine	Malaise, abdominal pain, change in stools, nausea, vomiting	Endoscopic evaluation may reveal edema, erythema, and reduced peristalsis; serum citrulline may be marker for rejection

4. Chronic: cell-mediated and humorally-initiated injury to the endothelium and vascular sclerosis; occurs slowly and leads to eventual graft loss; no definitive treatment

C. Subjective/objective findings (Table 83.1)

D. Diagnosis: the gold standard is biopsy of the allograft; alternative tests are organ-specific

E. Treatment: high-dose corticosteroids, optimizing immunosuppressant regimen, and antilymphocytic therapy

III. **Immunosuppression**

A. Overview

1. Immunosuppression is the pharmacological manipulation of the immune system performed to prevent or suppress rejection.

2. Induction therapy is administered before or after transplantation for up to 2 weeks to delay the onset of the first rejection episode or to help limit the initial quantity of calcineurin inhibitors. Induction therapy typically consists of monoclonal or polyclonal antilymphocyte antibodies.

3. Maintenance therapy consists typically of a calcineurin inhibitor, a corticosteroid, and an antimetabolite, but this varies by center. Maintenance therapy must be provided for the life of the allograft.

B. Medications (Table 83.2 & 83.3)

C. General considerations

Table 83.2	Immunosuppressive medications			
Drug class	**Indication**	**Dosage**	**Monitoring**	**Common Adverse effects**
Calcineurin inhibitors				
Tacrolimus (Prograf)	Prophylaxis of rejection	0.1–0.30 mg/kg PO/NG q 12 hr	Trough level, renal function	Tremor, renal dysfunction, hyperglycemia
Cyclosporine (Neoral)	Prophylaxis of rejection	8–18 mg/kg/day PO/NG q 12 hr	Trough level, renal function	Tremor, renal dysfunction, hypertension, hirsutism, gingival hyperplasia
mTOR Inhibitors				
Everolimus (Zortress)	Prophylaxis of rejection	0.75 mg PO q12h	Trough level, renal function, CBC, LFT's, lipid panel	Hypertension, peripheral edema, rash, hyperlipidemia, hypophosphatemia, hyperglycemia, decreased appetite, elevated LFT's, thrombocytopenia, fatigue, fever
Sirolimus (Rapamune)	Prophylaxis of rejection	Weight based 1–10 mg PO/NG daily	Trough level, renal function, CBC, lipid panel	Edema, peripheral edema, rash, hyperlipidemia, abdominal pain, nausea, diarrhea, thrombocytopenia, arthralgia, fever
Antimetabolites				
Azathioprine (Imuran)	Prophylaxis of rejection	1–3 mg/kg/day	Monitor CBC and liver function tests (LFTs)	Leukopenia, hepatotoxicity, neoplasia
Mycophenolate (Cellcept)	Prophylaxis of rejection	1000–1500 mg IV/PO/NG q 12 hr.	Monitor CBC	Diarrhea, leukopenia, sepsis
Monoclonal Antibodies				
Basiliximab (Simulect)	Induction	20 mg IV Day 0 and 4	Monitor for signs of infection	Fever, chills, malaise, hypertension
Rituximab (Rituxan)	Desensitization and Treatment of rejection	375 mg/m^2 IV once	CBC, renal function, infusion related reactions	Hypotension, peripheral edema, rash, abdominal pain, arthralgia, infection, shivering, cardiac dysrhythmia

Table 83.2	Immunosuppressive medications			
Drug class	**Indication**	**Dosage**	**Monitoring**	**Common Adverse effects**
Alemtuzumab (Campath)	Induction	No longer commercially available However, to ensure continued access to the drug for appropriate patients, it may be provided free of charge via the Campath Distribution Program		Hypotension, rash, urticaria, musculoskeletal pain, bronchospasm, fever, fatigue, cardiac dysrhythmia, toxic optic neuropathy
Polyclonal Antibodies				
Antithymocyte Globulin (ATG, Thymoglobulin)	Induction and Treatment of rejection	1.5 mg/kg/day x 4–10 days Premedicate prior to each administration	WBC and platelet counts	Fever, leukopenia, thrombocytopenia, anaphylaxis, dyspnea
IV Immuneo-globulin (Gamunex, Carimune)	Treatment of rejection	2 mg/kg/day IV Premedicate prior to each administration	CBC, renal function, BP	Headache, itching, hypo/hypertension, thrombotic complications, acute renal failure
Corticosteroids				
Prednisone	Prophylaxis of rejection	0.1–2 mg/kg/day	Monitor glucose and watch for infection	Fluid retention, hyperglycemia, impaired wound healing, aseptic necrosis of the femoral head, peptic ulcer
Solumedrol	Induction, Treatment and Prophylaxis of rejection	250–1000 mg		
Immunological Agents				
Belatacept (Nulojix)	Treatment of rejection EBV seropositive, in combination with basiliximab, mycophenolate, and corticosteroids	Initial: 10 mg/kg IV on day 1, day 5, and end of weeks 2, 4, 8 & 12 Maintenance: 5 mg/kg IV at end of week 16 and every 4 weeks thereafter		Headache, peripheral edema, infection, cough, nausea, vomiting, diarrhea, constipation, hypertension, fever, anemia, leukopenia

Table 83.3	Transplant Drug Level Monitoring			
Transplant	**Tacrolimus (ng/ml) (Prograf®)**	**Cyclosporine (ng/ml) (Neoral®, Gengraf®)**	**Sirolimus (ng/ml) (Rapamune®)**	**Everolimus (ng/ml) (Zortress®)**
Heart	1 month: 10–15 2–3 months: 8–12 greater than 3 months: 5–10	1 month: 250–350 2–3 months: 200–300 greater than 3 months: 100–200	1 month: Not used 2–3 months: Not used greater than 3 months: 4–8	1 month: Not used 2–3 months: Not used greater than 3 months: 3–8
Lung	0–3 months: 15–20 greater than 3 months: 10–15	0–3 months: 250–350 greater than 3 months: 200–300	0–3 months: Not used greater than 3 months: 8–12	0–3 months: Not used greater than 3 months: Range not established
Kidney	0–3 months: 8–10 3–6 months: 7–9 6–12 months: 5–7 greater than 12 months: 4–6	0–3 months: 225–275 3–6 months: 150–225 6–12 months: 125–175 greater than 12 months: 75–125	When given with CSA 0–3 months: 10–12 3–6 months: 8–10 6–12 months: 7–9 greater than 12 months: 5–7 When given with tacrolimus (total combined trough) 0–3 months: 10–12 3–6 months: 8–10 6–12 months: 7–9 greater than 12 months: 5–7	3–8
Liver	0–30 days: 5–15 31–90 days: 5–10 greater than 90 days: 2–10	0–30 days: 200–400 31–90 days: 200–300 greater than 90 days: 150–250 50–200	Not used	3–8

1. Conversion between generic and brand forms of cyclosporine requires careful trough monitoring.
2. Calcineurin inhibitors are metabolized via the cytochrome P450 enzyme; thus, other medications metabolized via this route may alter drug concentrations.
3. It is recommended that grapefruit juice be avoided by patients on calcineurin inhibitors because of interference with pharmacokinetics and pharmacodynamics that increase plasma drug levels.

COMMON MEDICAL COMPLICATIONS IN SOLID ORGAN TRANSPLANTATION

I. **Hypertension**
    A. Hypertension is a very common complication after solid organ transplantation; it may be caused by preexisting disease, calcineurin inhibitors, or corticosteroids.
    B. Optimize pharmacologic therapy for blood pressure management as defined by the guidelines put forth in the Eighth Report of the Joint National Committee on Prevention, Detection, Evaluation, and Treatment of High Blood Pressure (JNC VIII)
    C. Calcium channel blockers are frequently used because of their ability to decrease renal vascular resistance, which may offset calcineurin-induced vasoconstriction
    D. Single-agent therapy is typically not effective; relative hypotension should be avoided postoperatively in the kidney recipient.

II. **Posttransplant diabetes mellitus (PTDM)**
    A. The incidence of PTDM is estimated at quite a variable range of 4%–20%
    B. PTDM may be directly related to corticosteroids that enhance glyconeogenesis and to calcineurin inhibitors that decrease insulin resistance; they may directly affect the release of insulin from β cells.
    C. PTDM is associated with a higher incidence of graft loss
    D. Tight glycemic control is indicated
    E. Optimize medical/pharmacologic therapy for glycemic management as defined by current evidenced based/guideline-recommended therapy.

III. **Renal insufficiency**
    A. May be seen in all solid organ transplant recipients due to nephrotoxicity associated with calcineurin inhibitors
    B. May be treated by reducing the calcineurin dose, prudently managing diabetes and hypertension, and limiting other medications that may be nephrotoxic (e.g., nonsteroidal anti-inflammatory drugs, diuretics, certain antibiotics)

IV. **Hyperlipidemia**
   A. Hyperlipidemia is estimated to occur in greater than 50% of transplant recipients because of the effects of immunosuppressive agents on lipid levels.
   B. May contribute to cardiovascular disease and chronic allograft nephropathy because of chronically elevated lipid levels over time
   C. The pathogenesis of hyperlipidemia has been found to be associated with immunosuppressive agents, most notably sirolimus
   D. Optimize pharmacologic therapy for cholesterol management as defined by current evidence-based/guideline-recommended therapy
   E. An increased incidence of myopathy has been reported in cardiac recipients who were taking cyclosporine and an HMG-CoA reductase inhibitor

V. **Bone disease**
   A. Osteoporosis is a common complication after solid organ transplantation
   B. It is directly related to corticosteroids; the maximum amount of bone loss occurs during the first 3 months after surgery.
   C. Baseline and annual bone scans are indicated
   D. Treatment includes minimization of corticosteroids, supplemental calcium, bisphosphonates, and hormone replacement when indicated

VI. **Malignancy**
   A. An increased incidence of lymphoma, skin cancer, and Kaposi's sarcoma has been reported in the posttransplant population
   B. Lymphomas, which are primarily B-cell non-Hodgkin's type, are related to infection with the Epstein-Barr virus, most notably in seronegative recipients who receive positive organs
   C. Posttransplant lymphomas have also been associated with higher doses of cyclosporine and tacrolimus and with repeated anti-lymphocyte antibody therapy
   D. Treatment consists of minimization or cessation of immunosuppression, chemotherapy, and radiation therapy
   E. The prognosis is poor

COMMON INFECTIONS

I. **Overview**
   A. Infection is one of the leading causes of death in solid organ recipients
   B. Transplant recipients are at highest risk for infection during the first 6 months posttransplant.
   C. Immunosuppressive medications may alter the inflammatory response; thus, fever and increased white blood cell count may not be as pronounced as in the non-transplant patient. Fever in the transplant recipient may also signal rejection rather than infection; regardless, a high index of suspicion is warranted.

Table 83.4	Common infections in the transplant recipient		
Viral	**Fungal**	**Bacterial**	**Protozoal**
Cytomegalovirus	*Candida*	*Mycobacterium*	*Cryptosporidium*
Epstein-Barr	*Aspergillus*	Tuberculosis	*Toxoplasma gondii*
Hepatitis B, C	*Cryptococcus*	*Pseudomonas aeruginosa*	*Strongyloides*
Herpes	*Pneumocystis jiroveci*	Legionella	
BK polyoma		*Listeria*	
Varicella		*Nocardia asteroides*	
		Gram-negative bacteria	

II. **Viral**
   A. Viral infections cause high incidences of morbidity and mortality among posttransplant patients; they may be newly acquired or may result from reactivation of latent infection
   B. Cytomegalovirus is of particular concern in the transplant recipient because it may cause substantial morbidity and has been associated with allograft rejection
   C. Serologic testing is done prior to transplantation to determine the status of the donor and of the recipient
   D. Negative recipients who receive organs from positive donors carry the greatest risk for de novo infection
   E. Frequent monitoring via antigenemia or polymerase chain reaction is routinely done at all centers
   F. Prophylaxis with ganciclovir or valganciclovir is recommended (see Table 83.4 for other common infections)

III. **Fungal**
   A. The incidence of fungal infection in solid organ recipients varies widely, depending on the organ transplanted. The highest reported incidence of *Candida* is in liver transplant recipients; post-lung transplant patients have the highest incidence of *Aspergillus*.
   B. Oral fluconazole or itraconazole is frequently prescribed for fungal prophylaxis. Trimethoprim-sulfamethoxazole (Bactrim) is given for *Pneumocystis jiroveci* prophylaxis (see Table 83.4 for a list of common fungal infections)

IV. **Bacterial**
   A. Bacterial infections are the most commonly found infection in posttransplant recipients.
   B. The types and causes of bacterial infection in these patients differ according to the organ transplanted.
      1. Intra-abdominal infections are typically seen in liver, pancreas, and intestinal transplant recipients.

2. Pneumonia, typically nosocomially-acquired, is the most common infection in heart and lung recipients

3. In the renal recipient and the pancreas recipient with urinary drainage of exocrine secretions, urinary tract infections are most frequently encountered (see Table 83.4 for a list of common bacterial pathogens)

C. Vaccinations

1. Evidence-based guidelines have been established for transplant recipients. It is recommended that vaccinations be updated prior to transplantation, if possible, and include recommendation for the annual influenza vaccine. Transplant centers differ in their protocols for this vaccine. Transplant recipients should not receive live vaccinations and should avoid exposure to household members who have received a live vaccination.

KIDNEY TRANSPLANTATION

I. **Incidence/indications**

A. Kidney failure is defined as creatinine clearance less than 15 ml/min

B. Patients are listed for transplant on the basis of their ABO type, panel reactive antibody (PRA) test (to determine the percentage of risk of reaction due to existing antibodies), and accrued wait time

C. Preemptive transplantation, performed before the start of dialysis, may be possible, especially if a living donor is available

D. The most common causes of end-stage renal disease are diabetes mellitus, hypertension, and glomerular diseases.

II. **Complications**

A. Surgical

1. Graft thrombosis
   a. Thrombosis typically occurs 2–3 days postoperatively
   b. Arterial and venous thrombosis present with sudden cessation of urine output
   c. Venous thrombosis presents with graft swelling and gross hematuria
   d. Diagnosis is confirmed by Doppler ultrasound
   e. The prognosis is poor, and the condition usually results in graft loss

2. Urine leak
   a. Urine leaks occur 2–3 days postoperatively and may be caused by either surgical technique or necrosis of the ureteral anastomosis to the bladder
   b. Urine leaks present as abdominal fullness or pain and as elevated serum creatinine
   c. Diagnosis is made by needle aspiration and analysis of the fluid, which reveals creatinine

    d. Treatment consists of placement of a Foley catheter, use of a nephrostomy tube, or surgical repair.

  3. Lymphocele

    a. A lymphocele is a collection of lymph fluid that surrounds the allograft as a result of severed lymphatics around the iliac vessels.

    b. Lymphoceles may cause ureteral obstruction, compression of the iliac vein, scrotal edema, and abdominal pain.

    c. Ultrasound-guided needle aspiration of clear, protein-containing fluid is diagnostic

    d. Treatment includes percutaneous aspiration, marsupialization of fluid into an internal cavity, or use of povidone-iodine (Betadine), tetracycline, or fibrin glue for sclerosis

  4. Bleeding

  5. Ureteral obstruction

    a. Ureteral obstruction presents as a decline in allograft function

    b. Obstruction may be due to a blood clot, surgical technique, stricture, rejection, or infection

    c. Ultrasonography may reveal hydronephrosis

    d. Treatment consists of nephrostomy tube placement, dilatation of the stricture, removal of the clot, or surgical correction

B. Nonsurgical

  1. Delayed graft function

    a. Delayed graft function or inability of the newly transplanted kidney to function may occur in 10%–50% of transplanted kidneys

    b. Its source includes acute tubular necrosis, accelerated acute rejection, and ischemia-reperfusion injury

    c. Treatment includes dialysis and modification of the immunosuppressive regimen

  2. Rejection

  3. Infection

    a. Urinary tract infections are common in the renal transplant recipient

    b. Antibiotic treatment is guided by urine culture and sensitivity

    c. BK-type polyoma virus is found primarily in renal transplant recipients; it presents with elevated serum creatinine and possible hematuria, which may be confused with acute rejection. Diagnosis is made with quantitative polymerase chain reaction assays of the blood and urine or by biopsy. BK nephropathy may be treated with intravenous cidofovir (Vistide) and by reduction in immunosuppression.

LIVER TRANSPLANTATION

I. **Incidence/indications**
 A. The most common indications for liver transplant include chronic hepatitis, alcoholic liver disease, cholestatic disease, hepatocellular carcinoma, Wilson's disease, and genetic disorders such as Crigler-Najjar syndrome and hemochromatosis.
 B. Survival rates are 80% at 1 year and approximately 65% at 5 years
 C. Liver transplantation is the standard of care for irreversible end-stage liver disease, but many patients die while waiting for a liver. New treatments on the horizon currently under investigation include extracorporeal liver perfusion, bioartificial livers, and hepatocyte transplants that may bridge the gap for these patients until an organ becomes available.

II. **Complications**
 A. Surgical
  1. Hepatic artery thrombosis (HAT)
   a. Hepatic artery stenosis may occur in 5%–10% of liver transplant recipients but may vary depending on the transplant center; HAT may occur at any time posttransplant and is associated with bile leaks, graft necrosis, and intrahepatic abscesses.
   b. Diagnosis is made by ultrasonography or CT scan
   c. Treatment may include thrombectomy, thrombolytic therapy, and regrafting
  2. Portal vein thrombosis
   a. Occurs infrequently but may lead to development of portal hypertension and esophageal varices
   b. Treatment is geared toward management of portal hypertension
  3. Biliary leaks
   a. Treated with either percutaneous or surgical drainage
  4. Anastomotic bile duct strictures
   a. Bile duct strictures are corrected surgically by reanastomosis to a Roux loop of jejunum
 B. Nonsurgical
  1. Primary graft dysfunction
   a. Primary graft dysfunction is the failure of the graft to function within the first week posttransplant
   b. Acidosis, elevated liver enzymes, encephalopathy, and poor bile production may be observed
   c. Prognosis may be poor
   d. Treatment is supportive; N-acetylcysteine and prostaglandins may be of some value
   e. Patients may be placed back on the transplant list with a higher priority score due to this indication

2. Rejection
3. Infection
4. Biliary cast syndrome
   a. Biliary cast syndrome is associated with bile duct stricture and clogging of the biliary trees with cast sludge; it manifests as severe, intractable pruritus
   b. Treatment consists of percutaneous cholangiography and retransplantation
5. Recurrence of disease

LUNG TRANSPLANTATION

I. **Incidence/indications**
   A. The most common indications for lung transplantation include primary pulmonary hypertension, cystic fibrosis, chronic obstructive pulmonary disease, sarcoidosis, idiopathic pulmonary fibrosis, and Eisenmenger syndrome.
   B. Typically, the transplant is a single lung, except in patients with cystic fibrosis and, in some centers, primary pulmonary hypertension.
   C. Patients are referred for transplantation when life expectancy is estimated to be 24–36 months. Lung transplants are allocated according to wait time on the United Network for Organ Sharing list Prioritization is not based on disease acuity.

II. **Complications**
   A. Surgical
      1. Bronchial anastomotic complications
         a. Bronchial anastomotic complications include ischemia and necrosis of the anastomosis, bronchial strictures, and total dehiscence
         b. These complications may be treated with silastic endobronchial stents, dilatation via bronchoscope, and retransplantation
      2. Bleeding
      3. Ischemia-reperfusion injury
         a. This syndrome, which manifests as alveolar damage, pulmonary edema, and hypoxemia, usually occurs 72 hr postoperatively and is a major cause of mortality
         b. The syndrome is similar to acute respiratory distress syndrome and is managed by ventilatory management.
         c. Nitric oxide and extracorporeal membrane oxygenation may be beneficial
   B. Nonsurgical
      1. Sepsis
      2. Bronchiolitis obliterans syndrome (BOS)
         a. BOS is a manifestation of chronic rejection

      b. It presents as a decrease in forced expiratory volume in 1 second (FEV_1) and histologically as dense fibrosis.

      c. Progressive exertional dyspnea and cough are characteristic

      d. Therapeutic options are limited and include addition of high-dose corticosteroids and antilymphocytic therapy

   3. Rejection

HEART TRANSPLANTATION

I.   **Incidence/indications**

   A. The most common indications for heart transplantation include cardiomyopathy, cardiac tumor, congenital defect, and valvular heart disease.

II.   **Complications**

   A. Bleeding

   B. Rejection

   C. Cardiac allograft vasculopathy (CAV)

      1. CAV is the leading cause of death in heart recipients

      2. It is an accelerated form of coronary artery disease that affects the epicardial and intramyocardial arteries, along with the veins.

      3. The incidence at 1 year posttransplant is 11%

      4. It presents as heart failure, ventricular arrhythmias, or sudden death

      5. Diagnosis is made by angiography, and treatment consists of angioplasty, revascularization, and retransplantation

   D. Denervation

      1. The transplanted heart is denervated and, thus, has an altered response to cardiovascular drugs.

      2. The most commonly used inotropic agents are dobutamine and milrinone.

      3. Digoxin and atropine have little or no effect on the transplanted heart

PANCREAS TRANSPLANTATION

I.   **Incidence/indications**

   A. The only indication for pancreas transplantation is diabetes mellitus type 1.

   B. Patients may undergo pancreas or simultaneous kidney/pancreas transplantation if renal failure is present.

   C. The pancreas is anastomosed to the bladder or the small intestine for the purpose of draining exocrine secretions.

   D. Islet cell transplantation may provide an alternative to pancreas transplantation

II.   **Complications**

   A. Surgical

      1. Anastomotic leaks

       a. Anastomotic leaks occur within the first few months posttransplant

       b. Patients present with abdominal pain and elevated serum amylase

       c. Surgical correction is required

    2. Bleeding

    3. Bladder-drained pancreas transplants: hematuria, cystitis, balanitis, urethritis, urine leak, and metabolic acidosis related to drainage of large quantities of alkaline pancreatic secretions

    4. Enteric-drained pancreas transplant: intra-abdominal abscess, gastrointestinal bleeding

  B. Nonsurgical

    1. Pancreatitis

       a. Mild pancreatitis may be seen early posttransplant as a result of handling of the organ and preservation

       b. Serum amylase must be monitored closely because an increase may be a sign of rejection

       c. Pancreatitis resolves spontaneously

    2. Sepsis

       a. Sepsis is the leading cause of death among pancreas recipients; sepsis is most prevalent in the pancreas and occurs in the pancreas more frequently than in any other transplanted organ.

       b. Sepsis presents as peritonitis that is thought to occur in association with erosion of the anastomosis by pancreatic enzymes.

    3. Rejection

INTESTINAL TRANSPLANTATION

I. **Incidence/indications**

  A. The most common indications are necrotizing enterocolitis, Crohn's disease, gastroschisis, radiation enteritis, stenosis of the small bowel, and chronic intestinal pseudo-obstruction syndrome.

  B. Complications

    1. Surgical

       a. Bleeding

       b. Bowel obstruction

       c. Chylous ascites

       d. Perforation

       e. Biliary leaks

  C. Nonsurgical

       a. Hypermotility

          i. Hypermotility is seen early in the posttransplantation course and is attributed to denervation of the intestinal graft.

   ii. It is controlled with antidiarrheals and fiber
  b. Rejection
  c. Infection

BIBLIOGRAPHY

Benitez, C. E., Puig-Pey, I., Lopez, M., Martinez-Llordella, M., Lozano, J. J., Bohne, F., . . . Sanchez-Fueyo, A. (2010). A TG-Fresenius treatment and low-dose tacrolimus: Results of a randomized controlled trial in liver transplantation. *American Journal of Transplantation, 10*(10), 2296–2304.

Berglund, D., Bengtsson, M., Biglarnia, A., Berglund, E., Yamamoto, S., von Zur-Mühlen, B., . . . Tufveson, G. (2011). Screening of mortality in transplant patients using an assay for immune function. *Transplant Immunology, 24*(4), 246–250.

Bodziak, K. A., & Kricik, D. E. (2009). New-onset diabetes mellitus after solid organ transplantation. *Transplant International, 22*(5), 519–530.

Danziger-Isakov, L., & Kumar, D. (2009). Guidelines for vaccination of solid organ transplant candidates and recipients. *American Journal of Transplantation, 9,* S258-S262.

DeMeyer, E. S. (2009). Emerging immunology of stem cell transplantation. *Seminars in Oncology Nursing, 25*(2), 100–104.

Diamond, J. M., Lee, J. C., Kawut, S. M., Shah, R. J., Localio, A. R., Bellamy, S. L., . . . Christie, J. D. (2013). Clinical risk factors for primary graft dysfunction after lung transplantation. *American Journal of Respiratory and Critical Care Medicine, 187*(5), 527–534.

Eberhard, W., Olbricht, C. J., Susal, C., Gurragchaa, P., Bohler, T., Israeli, M., . . . Oellerich, M. (2010). Biomarkers as a tool for management of immunosuppression in transplant patients. *Therapeutic Drug Monitoring, 32*(5), 560–572.

Ebeling, P. R. (2009). Approach to the patient with transplantation-related bone loss. *The Journal of Clinical Endocrinology & Metabolism, 94*(5).

Garcia-Prado, M. E., Cordero, E., Cabello, V., Pereira, P., Torrubia, F. J., Ruiz, M., & Cisneros, J. M. (2009). Infectious complications in 159 consecutive kidney transplant recipients. *Enferm Infec Microbio Clin, 27*(1), 22–27.

Geissler, E. K., & Schlitt, H. J. (2010). The potential benefits of rapamycin on renal function, tolerance, fibrosis, and malignancy following transplantation. *Kidney International, 78,* 1075–1079.

Gentry, S. E., Montgomery, R. A., & Segev, D. L. (2010). Kidney paired donation: Fundamentals, limitations, and expansions. *American Journal of Kidney Diseases, 57*(1), 144–151.

Gillis, K. A., Patel, R. K., Jardine, A. G. (2014). Cardiovascular complications after transplantation: Treatment options in solid organ recipients. *Transplantation Reviews*, *28*(1), 47–55.

Koreth, J., Matsuoka, K., Kim. H. T., McDonough, S. M., Bindra, B., Alyea, E. P., ... Soiffer, R. J. (2011). *New England Journal of Medicine, 365*, 2055–2066.

Kumar, R., Brar, J., Yacoub, R., Khan, T., Zachariah, M., & Venuto, R. (2012). Assessment of cardiovascular risk factors after renal transplantation: A step towards reducing graft failure. *Transplantation Proceedings*, *44*(5), 1270–1274.

Leventhal, J. S., & Schroppel, B. (2012). Toll-like receptors in transplantation: Sensing and reacting to injury. *Kidney International, 81,* 826–832.

Levey, A., & Coresh, J. (2012). Chronic kidney disease. *Lancet, 379,* 165–180.

Lyu, D. M., & Zamora, M. R. (2009). Medical complications of lung transplantation. *Proceedings of the American Thoracic Society*, *6*(1), 101–107.

Mazariegos, G. V. (2009). Intestinal transplantation: Current outcomes and opportunities. *Current Opinion in Organ Transplantation, 14*(5), 515–521.

Neofytos, D., Fishman, J. A., Horn, D., Anaissie, E., Chang, C.-H., Olyaei, A., ... Marr, K. A. (2010). Epidemiology and outcome of invasive fungal infections in solid organ transplant recipients. *Transplant Infectious Disease, 12*(3), 220–229.

Neidlinger, N., Singh, N., Klein, C., Odorico, J., Munoz del Rio, A., Becker, Y., ... Pirsch, J. (2010). Incidence of and risk factors for posttransplant diabetes mellitus after pancreas transplantation. *American Journal of Transplantation*, *10*(2), 398–406.

Organ procurement and transplantation network. Retrieved December 2, 2013, from http://optn.transplant.hrsa.gov

Pallet, N., Burgard, M., Quamouss, O., Rabant, M., Bererhi, L., Martinez, F., ... Legendre, C. (2010). Cidofovir may be deleterious in BK virus-associated nephropathy. *Transplantation, 89*(12), 1542–1544.

Ponticelli, C., Cucchiari, D., & Graziani, G. (2011). Hypertension in kidney transplant patients. *Transplant International*, *24*(6), 523–533.

Razonable, R. R., Findlay, J. Y., O'Riordan, A., Burroughs, S. G., Ghobrial, R. M., Agarwal, B., ... Gropper, M. (2011). Critical care issues in patients after liver transplantation. *Liver Transplantation, 17*(5), 511–527.

Ruiz, P., Tryphonopoulos, P., Island, E., Selvaggi, G., Nishida, S., Moon, J., ... Tzakis, A. G. (2010). Citrulline evaluation in bowel transplantation. *Transplantation Proceedings, 42*(1), 54–56.

Salvalaggio, P. R., Dzebisashvili, N., MacLeod, K. E., Lentine, K. L., Gheorghian, A., Schnitzler, M. A., ... Alexrod, D. A. (2011). *Liver Transplantation, 17*(3), 233–242.

Shabanzadeh, A. P., Sadr, S. S., Ghafari, A., Nozari, B. H., & Toushih, M. (2009). Organ and tissue donation knowledge among intensive care unit nurses. *Transplantation Proceedings, 41*(5), 1480–1482.

Shahid, H., Kashif, R., Pilewski, J. M., Zaldonis, D., Crespo, M., Toyoda, Y., ... Zeevi, A. (2009). Experience with immune monitoring in lung transplant recipients: Correlation of low immune function with infection. *Transplantation, 87*(12), 1852–1857.

Terrault, N. A., Roland, M. E., Schiano, T., Dove, L., Wong, M. T., Poordad, F., ... Stock, P. G. (2012). Outcomes of liver transplant recipients with hepatitis C and human immunodeficiency virus coinfection. *Liver Transplantation, 18*(6), 716–26.

United Network for Organ Sharing. Retrieved December 2, 2013, from www.unos.org

White, S. A., Shaw, J. A., & Sutherland, D. (2009). Pancreas transplantation. *The Lancet, 373*(9677), 1808–1817.

Widmaier, E. P., Raff, H., Strang, K. T. (2011). *Vander's human physiology: The mechanisms of body function.* New York, NY: McGraw Hill.

Wilkinson, A. (2010). The "first quarter": The first three months after transplant. In G. M. Danovitch (Ed.), *Handbook of kidney transplantation* (5th ed.). Philadelphia, PA: Lippincott Williams & Wilkins.

CHAPTER 84

Burns

CATHERINE BLACHE • THOMAS W. BARKLEY, JR.

I.   **Definition/general comments**
   A. Injury to skin or tissues caused by heat, radiation, electricity, or chemical toxins
   B. Approximately 450,000 individuals seek treatment for burn injuries per year
      1. 40,000 are hospitalized each year in the U.S., with 30,000 requiring admission to a burn center
      2. An estimated 3,400 deaths occur annually

II.   **Types of burn injury include the following:**
   A. Thermal
      1. Caused by flames, scalding, or other hot objects
      2. Most common type of burn
   B. Chemical
      1. Caused by necrotizing agents
      2. Most commonly caused by acids
   C. Electrical
      1. Caused by heat from electrical current
      2. Results in damage to nerves and tissues
   D. Inhalation injury
      1. Caused by smoke or hot air, resulting in respiratory tissue damage
      2. Includes carbon monoxide poisoning and injuries above and below the glottis
   E. Cold thermal injury (frostbite)

III. **Categories of burns**
   A. First degree (superficial partial thickness) (e.g., sunburn)
      1. Painful

        2. Dry, red, no blisters but mild swelling possible

        3. Involves epidermis only

        4. Infection barrier not destroyed

  B. Second degree (partial thickness)

        1. Severely painful

        2. Moist blisters

        3. Extends beyond epidermis

        4. Mild to moderate edema

        5. Infection barrier destroyed

  C. Third degree (full thickness)

        1. Not painful because nerve supply destroyed

        2. Dry, leathery, black/white, pearly, waxy

        3. Extends from epidermis to dermis to underlying tissues, fat, muscle, or bone

IV. **Measuring extent of burn injury**

  A. Approximately 1% of total body surface area (TBSA) may be depicted by the planar surface of the patient's hand including fingers

  B. Rule of nines

        1. Each arm = 9%

        2. Each leg = 18%

        3. Thorax = 18% front + 18% back

        4. Head = 9%

        5. Perineum/genitals = 1%

  C. Lund and Browder chart—most commonly used in burn centers because it takes into consideration TBSA according to age, with specific calculations (percentages) for each body part burned

V. **Fluid resuscitation**

  A. Various common formulas, including the Brooke and Parkland formulas, are used

  B. Overall requirements range from 2–4 ml/kg × TBSA during the first 24 hr

  C. Lack of fluid is frequently a major error in management (i.e., under-resuscitating the patient); more times than not, the patient needs more fluid

  D. Fluid resuscitation begins as soon as possible (in the field), not when the patient reaches the hospital or burn center. Requirements are calculated from time of injury

  E. As a general rule, half of all fluids required during the first 24 hr are administered within the first 8 hr of injury, with the remaining fluid given over the next 16 hr of care (i.e., half in the first 8 hr, one fourth in the next 8 hr, and one fourth in the remaining 8 hr of the first 24-hr period). Example: burn injury occurs at 0800, patient arrives at hospital at 1000; the first 8 hr of required fluid based on calculation must be infused by 1600

  F. Examples of first 24-hr fluid resuscitation:

1. Parkland formula = 4 ml/kg/TBSA % burn—crystalloid; no colloids
2. Modified Brooke = 2 ml/kg/TBSA % burn—crystalloid; no colloids

G. Urinary output general goal = 30–50 ml/hr; the formulas are used to calculate fluid requirements
   1. If the patient is not putting out enough urine, then fluid should be adjusted

H. Monitor for metabolic acidosis—expected during the early resuscitation phase

I. Monitor for hyperkalemia during the first 24–48 hr after burn injury, and then monitor for hypokalemia after fluid resuscitation/diuresis around 3 days postburn

VI. **Emergent burn management considerations**

A. Rinse chemical injuries in copious amounts of clean water as soon as possible

B. Do not use ice, lotions, toothpaste, lard, butter, or other products. Do not use specific neutralizing agents because this may produce an exothermic reaction causing more damage to the tissue

C. Wrap the area in a clean, dry towel (do not use wet coverings in order to preserve body temperature) and transport to the nearest hospital ASAP

D. If dressing the burn injury before transport, sterile normal saline is used in initial treatment (no Betadine, peroxide, or other products, as these will have to be removed at the hospital for evaluation of the burn injury by the medical staff).

E. Affected areas are wrapped or covered with sterile towels

F. Maintain normal temperature 98°F–99.5°F (37°C–37.5°C) with warming blankets, head coverings, warming lights/shields, etc.

G. After stabilization, pain management with intravenous agents (morphine is the most common) and anxiolytics may be used in small doses. Never use intramuscular or subcutaneous routes because of uncertain absorption.

H. Topical antibiotic options
   1. Silver sulfadiazine (Silvadene)
      a. Indicated for Gram-positive and Gram-negative organisms, as well as *Candida*
   2. Mafenide acetate (Sulfamylon)
      a. Indicated for Gram-positive and Gram-negative organisms, most anaerobes, electrical burns, and burns to the ear; monitor for acidosis as this is a carbonic anhydrase inhibitor
   3. Bacitracin
      a. Indicated for superficial burns, facial burns, and staphylococcal organism coverage
   4. Mupirocin (Bactroban)

    a. Indicated for Gram-positive organisms and is most commonly used as a secondary agent

  5. Enzymatic debridement agents

    a. Collagenase (Santyl) only one approved in U.S. for use

  6. Other surface agents/dressings commonly used in initial treatment of burn injuries

    a. Meta honey

    b. Silver impregnated barrier dressings

    c. Biologic dressings

    d. Advanced composite dressings/biologic synthetics

VII. Intubation

A. Laryngeal edema is a common and serious complication of some burns; intubation may be required to prevent airway obstruction

B. Clinical history of burn injury and signs/symptoms associated with laryngeal edema

  1. Burns to the face

  2. Singed nares or eyebrows

  3. Dark soot/mucus from nares or mouth

  4. Hoarseness

  5. Drooling

  6. Difficulty swallowing

  7. Suspicion of inhalation injury (e.g., burn that occurred in a closed space)

C. Indications for timely intubation

  1. Presence of any one or more of B1–7 in section VII above after machidascopic/bronchoscopic/direct or indirect laryngoscopic evidence of laryngeal edema

VIII. American Burn Association criteria for transport to a burn center

A. Partial thickness burn injury greater than 10% TBSA

B. Burn injury involving the face, hands, feet, genitalia, perineum, or major joints due to functional issues

C. Full thickness (third degree burn injury in any age-group)

D. Electrical burn injury (including those caused by lightning)

E. Chemical burn injury

F. Inhalation injuries

G. Burned children when the local hospital does not have appropriate burn management capabilities (personnel or equipment)

H. Patients with preexisting medical conditions that could result in complications for management, prolong the recovery, or affect mortality

I. Any burn patient with concomitant trauma in which the burn injury creates the greatest risk of morbidity/mortality; if the trauma poses the great risk, the patient should be held in the trauma center then transferred to burn center once stabilized

J. Burn-injured patients who require or will require special, emotional, social, or rehabilitative intervention

IX. **Carbon monoxide exposure/poisoning**

A. Home furnaces/gas stoves with poor ventilation and car exhaust are the most common causes

B. Spectrum of signs and symptoms—headache, dyspnea, confusion, loss of attention span, irritability, dim/loss of peripheral vision, nausea, vomiting, tachycardia, seizures, coma, and death

C. Hyperbaric oxygen therapy is used for severe cases (e.g., acidosis, carboxyhemoglobin [HbCO] level higher than 40%, shock, neurologic deterioration)

1. Hyperbaric oxygen chamber is used while the patient breathes 100% oxygen at a pressure higher than atmospheric

2. Complications include oxygen toxicity and barotrauma

3. Specialist referral

BIBLIOGRAPHY

American Burn Association. (2014). *Factsheet*. Retrieved from http://www. ameriburn.org/resources_factsheet.php

Cheek, D. J., Martin, L. L., & Morris, S. E. (2010). Shock, multiple organ dysfunction syndrome, and burns in adults. In K. McCance, S. Huether, V. Brashers, & N. Rote (Eds.), *Pathophysiology: The biologic basis for disease in adults and children*. St. Louis, MO: Mosby Elsevier.

Lloyd, E. C. O., Rodgers, B. C., Michener, M., & Williams, M. S. (2012). Outpatient burns: Prevention and care. *American Family Physician, 85*(1), 25–32.

Nemer, J. A. (2013). Disorders related to environmental emergencies. In M. A. Papadakis & S. J. McPhee (Eds.), *Current Medical Diagnosis and Treatment 2014* (53rd ed., pp. 1497–1501). McGraw-Hill Medical.

Storm-Versloot, M. N., Vos, C. G., Ubbink D. T., & Vermeulen H. (2010). Topical silver for preventing wound infection. *Cochrane Database of Systematic Reviews, 3*. Art. No.: CD006478. doi:10.1002/14651858.CD006478.pub2

Wasiak, J., Cleland, H., Campbell, F., & Spinks, A. (2013). Dressings for superficial and partial thickness burns. *Cochrane Database of Systematic Reviews, 3*. Art. No.: CD002106. doi:10.1002/14651858.CD002106.pub4

CHAPTER 85

Hospital Admission Considerations

JUDI KURIC • THOMAS W. BARKLEY, JR.

HISTORY AND PHYSICAL EXAMINATION

I. **General considerations**
   A. Should be concise, thorough, and focused on the individual patient
   B. Information may be obtained from previous histories and physicals (H&Ps) (e.g., if the adult-gerontology acute care nurse practitioner [AGACNP] is seeing the patient in a "consult" capacity), but one should always confirm information obtained from the patient's chart with the patient or with the person giving pertinent information (e.g., significant other) if able, or note that the information is from another source and is unverifiable.
   C. The AGACNP should remember to always include his/her own physical findings, impressions, and differential diagnoses, even if these are different from those previously ascertained from the chart or medical records (for a sample H&P, see Box 85.1).

II. **Identifying data**
   A. Patient's name
   B. Age
   C. Race
   D. Gender
   E. Informant
      1. Self
      2. Relative
      3. Friend
      4. Significant other
   F. Reliability of informant

Box 85.1	History and Physical Note Example

Identifying Data: John Doe, 72, Caucasian male, information obtained from patient who appears to be reliable.

Chief Complaint: Chest pain for 2 days.

HPI: Mr. Doe is a 72-year-old gentleman with a history of myocardial infarction (MI) 5 years ago; a subsequent cardiac stent was placed at the LAD at that time. He has been asymptomatic until recently, when he complained of intermittent, substernal pressure that was nonradiating. He first noticed the pain 2 days ago after mowing the lawn; it lasted 1–2 min, the patient rated the intensity of pain as 6–7/10. The pain was described as a "squeezing pressure" around the middle of the chest, with relief of symptoms after resting for a few minutes. He denies dyspnea, orthopnea, and paroxysmal nocturnal dyspnea. Since that time, he has experienced the same symptoms 2–3 times, usually in association with some sort of exertional activity. In the emergency department, the patient experienced an episode of chest pain that was relieved with 1 SL nitroglycerin. ECG shows ST changes in the inferior leads. Current labs are pending.

PMH: History of MI 2000 status post (S/T) stent, HTN, hyperlipidemia, and non-insulin-dependent diabetes mellitus (NIDDM). Patient denies history of CVA, PUD, and renal disease.

PSH: Coronary stent 2000, hernia repair 1997

Medications: ASA, 81 mg daily; Atenolol, 50 mg bid; Altace, 5 mg bid; Glucophage, 500 mg bid; Glyburide, 5 mg bid; Lipitor, 20 mg daily; multivitamin daily. Taking no herbal remedies.

Allergies: PCN (rash) and codeine (severe nausea/vomiting)

Immunizations: Pneumococcal vaccine 3 years ago

Family history: Father expired at age 50 of MI, and mother expired at age 72 with breast cancer. He has two brothers (living), both of whom had CAD/MI before age 50.

Social history: 50 pack-year smoker (quit 5 years ago), 1–2 beers on weekends, denies illicit drug use. Patient is a retired engineer. Hobbies include gardening and woodwork.

Review of systems: Negative unless otherwise indicated
General: Recent fatigue due to HPI
Head/Eyes/Ears/Nose/Throat (HEENT): Wears glasses, no recent dental work
Respiratory: Treated successfully for pneumonia 2 years ago. Last CXR 6 months ago was clear.
Cardiovascular: See HPI
Endocrine: Diabetes controlled with medication
All other review of systems negative

Note. HPI = history of present illness; ECG = elektrocardiogram; PMH = past medical history; LAH = ;PSH = ; PCN = penicillin; ASA = acetylsalicylic acid; CAD = coronary artery disease; CVA = cerebrovascular accident; PUD = peptic ulcer disease; PSH = past surgical history; CXR = chest x-ray; CBC = complete blood count; BNP = brain natriuretic peptide; PT = prothrombin time; PTT = partial thromboplastin time; CCU = critical care unit; ICS = intercostal space; MCL = midclavicular line.

Box 85.1	History and Physical Note Example

Physical exam:

General: Height, 6'1"; weight, 190 lbs. Patient is a well-developed, Caucasian gentleman who is alert, oriented, and in no current distress.

Vitals: Temperature, 98.6°F (37°C) (orally); HR, 88 (regular rate and rhythm [RRR]); Resp, 12; BP, 130/70

Skin: Warm, dry, and intact

HEENT: Unremarkable

Neck: Without evidence of jugular venous distention (JVD), carotid bruits, or lymphadenopathy

Chest: Within normal limits, equal lung expansion, breath sounds with bibasilar crackles

Breast: Within normal limits

Heart: Monitor shows sinus rhythm without ectopy, point of maximal impulse (PMI) 5th ICS, MCL. No extra heart sounds or murmurs noted.

Abdomen: Soft, nontender, without organomegaly; positive bowel sounds x 4

Genitourinary: Normal circumcised male, currently with Foley catheter in place that is draining adequate amounts of clear yellow urine.

Genital/rectal: Deferred because of recent chest pain

Musculoskeletal: No evidence of joint deformities/swelling.

Peripheral vascular: 1+ to 2+ pretibial edema noted bilaterally; 2+ pedal pulses palpated bilaterally.

Neurologic: Alert/oriented x 4, strong, equal strength x all 4 extremities. Face symmetrical. Cranial nerves intact.

Assessment: Chest pain—given patient's history of previous MI and ECG changes, this is most likely cardiac in nature. Could also be cholelithiasis, but in light of symptoms, this would not be likely.

HTN currently under control with medications.

Diabetes good control on medications.

Hyperlipidemia.

Plan:

Standard nitroglycerin drip—titrate to chest pain relief.

O_2 at 2 L N/C—Keep sat below 92%

STAT CBC, BNP, troponins now and every 8 hr x 3

BMP, PT/PTT, lipase, amylase, and CXR

STAT Chewable ASA 81 mg and 4 tablets now

Admit to CCU.

Cardiology consult STAT for probable urgent angiogram/PTCA.

III. **Chief complaint**
  A. Current problem
    1. Why is the patient being seen by the AGACNP?
  B. Should be written in patient's own words with quotations (if possible, based on the patient's condition)

IV. **History of present illness (HPI)**
  A. Describe the patient's complaint
    1. Use the "OLD CARTS" or "PQRST + the 3 As" mnemonics

2. OLD CARTS
  a. Onset
    i. When did this start?
    ii. What brings on the pain/complaint?
  b. Location of pain/complaint
  c. Duration of pain/complaint
  d. Characteristics
    i. Is the pain stabbing, gnawing, etc.?
  e. Aggravating factors
    i. What makes things worse?
  f. Relieving factors
    i. What makes things better?
  g. Treatment
    i. What has relieved the pain/complaint?
  h. Severity of pain/complaint (preferably, on a 1–10 scale)
3. PQRST + 3 As
  a. Provocative factors
    i. What brings on the pain/complaint?
  b. Quality of pain/complaint
  c. Radiation of pain/complaint
  d. Severity of pain/complaint (preferably, on a 1–10 scale)
  e. Timing of pain/complaint
    i. When does it occur?
  f. Alleviating factors
    i. What makes things better?
  g. Associated factors
    i. What other conditions/feelings/life events/factors happen at the same time?
  h. Aggravating factors
    i. What makes things worse?
4. Arrange events in chronological order
B. Related history
  1. Previous treatments
  2. Previous diagnostics (include pertinent positives/negatives)
  3. Risk factors
C. Family/psychosocial history (pertinent only to chief complaint)
D. Other significant ongoing health, medical, or psychosocial problems
V. **Past medical history (PMH)**
A. Major past diseases/medical conditions not related to HPI include the following:
  1. Hypertension
  2. Myocardial infarction
  3. Peptic ulcer disease
  4. Diabetes mellitus
  5. Asthma

      6. Cancer

      7. Cerebrovascular accident/transient ischemic attack

      8. Bleeding

      9. Others

   B. Past hospitalizations (be sure to include whether patient had a complicated course and specifics regarding such)

VI.   **Past surgical history (PSH)**

   A. Past surgeries; include approximate dates

VII.   **Medications**

   A. Include all medications that the patient is currently taking

      1. Prescribed medications

      2. Over-the-counter/herbal remedies

      3. Vitamins/supplements

VIII. **Allergies**

   A. What medications caused any problems? What reactions were observed?

IX.   **Immunizations**

   A. Last influenza, pneumococcal, pertussis, and tetanus toxoid vaccine

   B. Hepatitis series, meningococcal, and other immunizations

X.   **Family history**

   A. Medical problems of blood relatives

   B. List whether alive or expired (if expired, note cause of death)

XI.   **Social history**

   A. ETOH (ethyl alcohol) (number of drinks/day; current/quit, and number of years)

   B. Smoking (ever smoked; current/quit, number of years, pack-years)

   C. Marital status

      1. Is home support available?

   D. Employment status/situation

XII.   **Review of systems—listed by symptoms, not diagnoses**

   A. General

      1. Weight gain/loss

      2. Fatigue

      3. Weakness

      4. Fever/chills

      5. Night sweats

   B. Skin

      1. Rashes

      2. Skin discolorations (bruising)

      3. Lesions

      4. Hair

      5. Nails

   C. HEENT (head, ears, eyes, nose, and throat)

      1. Headaches

      2. Dizziness

    3. Seizures
    4. Syncope
    5. Visual changes
    6. Cataracts/glaucoma
    7. Hearing changes
    8. Tinnitus
    9. Vertigo
   10. Nosebleeds
   11. Sinus problems
   12. Dental disease
   13. Hoarseness
   14. Throat pain
   15. Lymph node enlargement/tenderness

D. Respiratory
    1. Cough
    2. Sputum production (note color)
    3. Dyspnea
    4. Recent pneumonia or influenza
    5. Positive purified protein derivative (PPD) test

E. Cardiovascular
    1. Chest pain
    2. Orthopnea
    3. Paroxysmal nocturnal dyspnea (PND)
    4. Dyspnea on exertion (DOE)
    5. Murmurs
    6. Palpitations
    7. Claudication
    8. Peripheral edema

F. Hematology
    1. Anemias
    2. Bleeding tendencies
    3. Easy bruising

G. Gastrointestinal
    1. Dysphagia
    2. Abdominal pain
    3. Nausea
    4. Vomiting
    5. Hematemesis
    6. Diarrhea
    7. Constipation
    8. Melena
    9. Hematochezia
   10. Recent change in bowel habits

H. Genitourinary
    1. Dysuria

2. Frequency
3. Hesitancy
4. Hematuria
5. Incontinence
6. Unusual discharge
7. Sexual history
   a. Number of partners
   b. Sexual orientation
   c. History of sexually transmitted infections (STIs)
8. History of renal disease (failure/insufficiency)

I. Gynecologic
   1. Gravida/para
   2. Abortions
   3. Last menstrual period
   4. Dysmenorrhea
   5. Age of menopause (if applicable)

J. Endocrine
   1. Polyuria
   2. Polydipsia
   3. Polyphagia
   4. Temperature intolerance
   5. Skin/hair changes
   6. History of hormone therapy

K. Musculoskeletal
   1. Arthralgias
   2. Arthritis
   3. Joint swelling
   4. Redness
   5. Tenderness
   6. Limitations in range of motion (ROM)
   7. Gout
   8. Trauma

L. Neurologic
   1. Seizures
   2. Weakness or paralysis
   3. Altered sensation/coordination
   4. Memory changes
   5. Tremors

M. Psychiatric
   1. Depression
   2. Anxiety
   3. Mood changes
   4. Suicidal thoughts
   5. Sleep disturbances

XIII. Physical examination—should be performed as appropriate for the patient population

  A. General appearance

    1. Age

    2. Gender

    3. Race

    4. Height and weight

      a. Note whether patient appears ill, well, or malnourished

  B. Vital signs

    1. Temperature

    2. Pulse

    3. Respirations

    4. Blood pressure (BP)

  C. Skin

    1. Rashes

    2. Scars

    3. Moles

    4. Tattoos

  D. HEENT

    1. Head

      a. Bruising/masses

    2. Eyes

      a. Pupils equal, round, reactive to light, and accommodation (PERRLA)

      b. Extraocular movements (EOMs)

      c. Funduscopic examination (if applicable)

      d. Visual acuity

    3. Ears

      a. Hearing acuity

      b. Tenderness

      c. Discharge

      d. Tympanic membrane appearance

    4. Nose

      a. Symmetry

      b. Palpate over sinuses

      c. Inspect nares for obstructions, lesions, and inflammation

    5. Throat

      a. Mucous membranes

      b. Oral lesions

      c. Dentition

      d. Pharynx

      e. Tonsils

  E. Neck

    1. ROM

    2. Tenderness

3. Jugular venous distention (JVD)
4. Bruits
5. Lymphadenopathy
6. Thyromegaly present

F. Chest
   1. Expansion
   2. Tactile fremitus
   3. Percussion (include diaphragmatic excursion)
   4. Breath sounds (including adventitious sounds)
      a. Include egophony, whispered pectoriloquy, if indicated (found with consolidation)

G. Heart
   1. Point of maximal impulse (PMI)
   2. Thrills
   3. Rhythm
   4. Extra heart sounds (S3, S4, gallops, and murmurs)
      a. Note grade and area auscultated

H. Breast
   1. Dimpling
   2. Tenderness
   3. Masses
   4. Discharge
   5. Axillary masses

I. Abdomen
   1. Contour
   2. Scars
   3. Bowel sounds
   4. Tenderness/guarding
   5. Suprapubic tenderness
   6. Masses
   7. Organomegaly (liver/spleen)
   8. Percussion findings

J. Genitourinary
   1. Inguinal masses
   2. Hernias
   3. Scrotum
   4. Testicles
   5. Genital lesions
   6. Pelvic examination

K. Rectal
   1. Hemorrhoids
   2. Sphincter tone
   3. Masses
   4. Prostate examination
   5. Test for occult blood

  L. Musculoskeletal
   1. Amputations
   2. Deformities
   3. Joint swelling
   4. Tenderness
   5. Warmth
   6. Crepitus
  M. Peripheral vascular
   1. Hair pattern
   2. Color changes in skin
   3. Pulses
   4. Calf tenderness
  N. Neurologic
   1. Mental status
   2. Cranial nerves
   3. Motor/sensory
   4. Deep tendon reflexes (DTRs)

XIV. **Assessment/diagnoses**
 A. List assessment/diagnoses in order of priority
 B. Include possible/relevant differential diagnosis with reasons that support/exclude

XV. **Plan**
 A. Describe the therapeutic plan for each problem listed from the Assessment/Diagnoses section
 B. Include planned laboratory tests, radiologic tests, studies, medications, and consults

ADMISSION ORDERS

I. Use mnemonic: "A.D.C. VAAN DISSL" (admit/attending, diagnosis, condition, vital signs, activity, allergies, nursing procedures, diet, intake/output, specific medications, symptomatic medications, laboratory/diagnostic procedures)

II. **Admit**
 A. What level of care?
 B. What service?

III. **Diagnosis**
 A. List admitting diagnosis and procedure (if patient is postoperative)

IV. **Condition**
 A. Stable
 B. Critical
 C. Other

V. **Vital signs**
 A. Frequency and specific parameters to be documented (e.g., pulmonary artery catheter readings, intracranial pressure measurements)

VI.   Activity
   A. Bed rest
   B. Up with assistance
   C. Bathroom privileges

VII.   Allergies
   A. Any known or perceived allergies

VIII.   Nursing procedures
   A. Preparations (enema, scrubs)
   B. Respiratory care (intermittent positive-pressure breathing [IPPB], incentive spirometry, and ventilator settings)
   C. Dressing changes/wound care
   D. Parameters to notify MD or AGACNP (e.g., systolic blood pressure greater than 170 mmHg, saturation less than 90%, urine output less than 30 ml/hr)

IX.   Diet
   A. NPO
   B. Clear liquid
   C. Soft, regular

X.   Intake/output (I/O)
   A. Record IV solution/rate and I/O every shift, including drains/tubes (e.g., Foley catheter, nasogastric tube to low intermittent suction, endotracheal tube, and arterial line/pulmonary artery catheters)

XI.   Specific medications
   A. Routine medications (include patient's home medications as appropriate)
   B. Medications to avoid

XII.   Symptomatic medications
   A. As needed medications (e.g., pain medications, sleeping pills, and laxatives)

XIII.   Laboratory/diagnostics
   A. Include blood work specific to specimens (e.g., lumbar puncture and urinalysis), and specify times as applicable
   B. Electrocardiograms (ECGs)
   C. X-rays
   D. Other diagnostic studies, consult requests, and so forth

PROGRESS NOTE

I.   **Should summarize developments during the patient's hospitalization, problems that remain active and plans to treat such problems, and discharge/transfer plans (as appropriate); "SOAP" note charting format:**

II.   **Date/time/service**

III.   **Subjective data (e.g., how the patient feels; include any complaints, preferably in direct quotations)**

IV.   **Objective data**
   A. General appearance
   B. Vital signs
   C. I/O
   D. Physical examination (emphasize changes from previous examinations)
   E. Laboratory/test results
   F. Current medications
   G. List other laboratory results as appropriate
      1. Prothrombin time (PT)
      2. Partial thromboplastin time (PTT)
      3. Amylase
      4. Albumin
      5. Calcium (Ca)
      6. Magnesium (Mg)
   H. If laboratory results are abnormal, it is a good idea to mark whether this is "up" (increased) or "down" (decreased) from the patient's previous results

V.   **Assessment/diagnosis (for each problem) including status (resolved)**
   A. Evaluation of the data and any conclusions that may be drawn

VI.   **Plan (for each problem)**
   A. Changes/additions to orders
   B. Any new laboratory results/tests/medications
   C. Disposition (discharge/transfer plans)

PRESENTATION OF PATIENT (During rounds with team facility)

   A. Be brief and concise; should take less than 23 min per patient
   B. Patient's name, age, gender, diagnosis, surgeries/procedures performed, and when
   C. Pertinent data (patient's current status; include abnormal laboratory results, tests, examinations, referrals, etc.)
   D. Diagnosis/differentials
   E. Plan

Box 85.2	Procedure Note Example

08/27/14 13:00   Procedure Note: Chest tube placement

Indications: Moderate–large pleural effusion noted on CXR; patient with increasing SOB

Informed of risks/benefits of procedure and agrees to above (signed consent in chart)

Labs: PT/INR 12.2/ 1, Hgb 16.2, Hct 50, Plt 352

Patient was placed in a left lateral decubitus position. The area was prepped and draped sterilely; 10 ml of 1% lidocaine was injected into the intercostal space midaxillary line per protocol. A 20 F trocar chest tube inserted with immediate 1500 ml clear yellow drainage returned. Chest tube connected to Pleur-evac system with 20 cm H_2O suction. No air leak noted. Specimens sent for cytology, pH, cell count, culture, Gram stain, lactate dehydrogenase (LDH), protein, and glucose. No complications noted. Patient tolerated procedure well. CXR post-procedure pending.

Nancy Nurse, MSN, APRN, BC, ACNP

PROCEDURE NOTE

I.   **Should be written in the chart whenever an invasive procedure (e.g., lumbar puncture, thoracentesis, and chest tube placement) is performed (Box 85.2)**

II.   **Date/time**
    A. Specify time of procedure

III.   **Procedure**
    A. List procedure performed

IV.   **Indications**
    A. Reason procedure necessary

V.   **Patient consent**
    A. Document that the patient/representative was informed of risks/benefits (most hospitals require that a separate consent must be signed)

VI.   **Laboratory tests**
    A. List relevant results (e.g., international normalized ratio [INR]/ complete blood count [CBC])

VII.   **Description of procedure**
    A. Briefly describe procedure, including the following:
       1. Sterile preparation
       2. Patient position
       3. Devices used
       4. Anesthesia/sedation used
       5. Location of procedure
       6. Drains
       7. Outcome

VIII.   **Complications and estimated blood loss (EBL)**
    A. Note complications (if any); if EBL is more than "minimal," estimate the actual amount lost

IX.   Disposition

   A. Describe how well the patient tolerated the procedure

X.   Specimens/findings obtained

   A. Describe findings, opening pressures, appearance of specimens obtained, method of collection, and time sent to laboratory

DISCHARGE SUMMARY

I.   Date of admission

   A. Specify date

II.   Date of discharge

   A. Specify date

III.   Admitting diagnosis

   A. Specify main reason for initial admission

IV.   Discharge diagnosis

   A. Specify primary diagnosis and any secondary diagnoses

V.   Attending physician/ACNP/referrals

   A. List names

VI.   Procedures

   A. Include surgery and invasive diagnostic procedures (e.g., lumbar puncture, angiogram)

VII.   Brief history, pertinent physical examination, and laboratory data

   A. Summarize the most important points about the patient's admission

      1. Brief history of findings in the H&P

      2. Admission laboratory findings

VIII.   Hospital course

   A. Briefly summarize the evaluation, treatment, and progress of the patient's hospitalization

      1. Include treatments, medications, and the patient's response to all of the above

IX.   Discharge condition

   A. Describe whether the patient's condition has improved, has deteriorated, or is unchanged

X.   Disposition

   A. Detail the location where the patient is being discharged

      1. Home

      2. Skilled nursing facility

      3. Other hospital

   B. Identify who will be assuming care (if possible)

XI.   Discharge medications

   A. List medications, dosages, scheduling, and refill parameters

XII.   Instructions and follow-up

   A. Office appointment follow-up date

   B. Dietary instructions

   C. Activity requirements/restrictions

XIII. **Problem list**
  A. List active and past medical problems (if different from discharge diagnosis)
XIV. **List of consultants and names of primary care providers who should be copied to discharge summary**

Box 85.3	Dangerous Abbreviations
Some "DON'Ts" to remember when writing prescriptions/orders:	
Don't use trailing zeros (e.g., use 1 mg, not 1.0 mg)	
Don't use a naked decimal point (e.g., use 0.5 ml, not .5 ml)	
Don't abbreviate drug names	
Don't use U; instead, spell out units	
Don't use IU; instead, spell out international units	
Don't use QD; instead, spell out once a day or daily	
Don't use QOD; instead, spell out every other day	

PRESCRIPTIONS (Box 85.3)

I. **Follow state law for required elements to be preprinted on prescription pads**
II. **Prescriptions for scheduled drugs must be written and signed on the day they are issued**
III. **Providers writing for scheduled drugs must have a Drug Enforcement Agency (DEA) number, and in some states, additional controlled substance registrations are required**
IV. **Prescriptions for scheduled drugs must include the prescriber's DEA number either written or printed on the prescription. Some states require that the DEA of collaborating physicians also be included on the prescription.**
  A. Patient's full name/date of birth/current date
  B. Rx
    1. Drug name
    2. Strength
    3. Form
    4. Route (if ordering only a brand name preparation, state or sign: "no substitution")
  C. Dispense
    1. Amount/number (ml/tabs) or time period (e.g., 1-month supply)
    2. Indicate whether any refills are allowed
  D. Sig
    1. Patient instructions (transcribed by a pharmacist on the label of the dispensed medication)
  E. Signature
    1. Sign name and title, and include DEA number if the medication is a controlled substance

GENERAL GUIDELINES FOR ADMISSION TO AN INTENSIVE CARE UNIT (ICU)

A. Keep in mind that these are only guidelines. It is important to note that common sense and good clinical assessment should always guide your decision of whether to admit a patient to the ICU. Examples of commonly occurring, reasonable conditions by system category that warrant ICU admission include the following:

I. **Cardiac**
  A. Acute myocardial infarction with complications
  B. Cardiogenic shock
  C. Complex arrhythmias requiring close monitoring and intervention
      1. Ventricular tachycardia
      2. Ventricular fibrillation
      3. Supraventricular tachycardia
      4. Atrial fibrillation
  D. Acute congestive heart failure with respiratory failure or requiring hemodynamic support
  E. Hypertensive emergencies
  F. Unstable angina, particularly with arrhythmias, hemodynamic instability, or persistent chest pain
  G. Status post cardiac arrest
  H. Cardiac tamponade or constriction with hemodynamic instability
  I. Dissecting aortic aneurysm
  J. Complete heart block requiring temporary or permanent pacemaker
  K. Others

II. **Pulmonary**
  A. Acute respiratory failure requiring ventilatory support
  B. Pulmonary emboli with hemodynamic instability
  C. Any patient in a lower level of care unit who exhibits respiratory deterioration or the need for close observation/treatment by nursing/respiratory care services
  D. Massive hemoptysis
  E. Respiratory failure with imminent need for intubation

III. **Neurologic**
  A. Acute stroke with altered mental status
  B. Coma
      1. Metabolic
      2. Toxic
      3. Anoxic
  C. Intracranial hemorrhage with potential for herniation
  D. Acute subarachnoid hemorrhage
  E. Meningitis with altered mental status or respiratory compromise
  F. CNS or neuromuscular disorders with deteriorating neurologic or pulmonary function

G. Status epilepticus

H. Brain damaged or potentially brain dead patients who are aggressively managed while organ donation status is being determined

I. Vasospasm

J. Severely head injured patients

K. Spinal cord injury

IV. **Drug ingestion and drug overdose**

A. Hemodynamically unstable drug ingestion

B. Drug ingestion with significantly altered mental status and inadequate airway protection

C. Seizures after drug ingestion

V. **Gastrointestinal**

A. Life-threatening gastrointestinal bleeding, including hypotension, angina, continued bleeding, or other comorbid conditions

B. Fulminant hepatic failure

C. Severe pancreatitis

D. Esophageal perforation with or without mediastinitis

VI. **Endocrine**

A. Diabetic ketoacidosis complicated by hemodynamic instability, altered mental status, respiratory insufficiency, or severe acidosis

B. Thyroid storm or myxedema coma with hemodynamic instability

C. Hyperosmolar hyperglycemic nonketotic state

D. Other endocrine problems such as adrenal crises with hemodynamic instability

E. Severe hypercalcemia with altered mental status requiring hemodynamic monitoring

F. Hyponatremia or hypernatremia with seizures, altered mental status

G. Hypomagnesemia or hypermagnesemia with hemodynamic compromise or arrhythmias

H. Hypokalemia or hyperkalemia with arrhythmias or muscular weakness

I. Hypophosphatemia with muscular weakness

VII. **Surgical**

A. Postoperative patients requiring hemodynamic monitoring/ventilatory support or extensive nursing care

VIII. **Miscellaneous**

A. Septic shock with hemodynamic instability

B. Frequent hemodynamic monitoring requirements

C. Clinical conditions requiring frequent assessments, monitoring procedures, or ICU level nursing care

D. Environmental injuries (e.g., lightning, near-drowning, hypothermia/hyperthermia)

E. New/experimental therapies with potential for complications

GENERAL GUIDELINES FOR DISCHARGE FROM AN ICU

I.   **Common sense and good clinical assessment should always guide the decision of whether to discharge a patient from the ICU. The status of patients admitted to an ICU should be continuously revised so that those patients who may no longer need ICU care are identified. Examples of reasonable conditions that warrant ICU discharge include the following:**

   A.   The patient's physiologic status has stabilized, and ICU monitoring and care are no longer necessary.

   B.   The patient's physiologic status has deteriorated, and active interventions are no longer planned; thus, discharge to a lower level of care is appropriate.

GENERAL GUIDELINES FOR ELECTRONIC MEDICAL RECORDS (EMR)

I.   **EMRs include templates for each type of documentation (H&P, SOAP, and procedure)**

   A.   AGACNPs should edit note templates to only include elements that are pertinent to their own practice (i.e., a neuro nurse would exclude PA catheter readings). Data included in a template and signed by practitioner indicates review and responsibility for addressing parameter. In lieu of deleting information from a document, comment that management of these problems will be done by a specific provider or service.

   B.   Prefilled data should be reviewed, verified, or corrected if needed. Some EMR systems have boxes to be checked indicating you have reviewed the information.

II.   **Evidence-based practice can be enhanced by incorporation of standard order sets for frequent diagnosis.**

   A.   Use of these order sets can improve outcomes and decrease complications

   B.   Periodic review and update are essential

III.   **Computerized order entry reduces errors, monitors interactions, and highlights labs for review prior to ordering medications.**

   A.   Review and sign off of these flagged orders, improves patient safety

IV.   **Automatic date and time stamps provide auditing capabilities to ensure hospital policy is followed related to cosigning of notes, medications, or evaluation of patients within a prescribed time frame.**

V. **Providers that were studied felt like their productivity decreased when EMRs were implemented. Strategies to maintain productivity include the following:**
   A. Customizing order sets
   B. Customizing note templates
   C. Saving routine orders to favorite lists
   D. Providing access training
   E. Seeking information from other providers on ways to maximize use of the system

VI. **Computerized prescription generation is convenient, but potential for inadvertent quantities exist (i.e., 150 tablets instead of 15 due to typing error).**
   A. AGACNPs can work with the software vendor to flag large numbers of tablets to prevent errors of this kind.

VII. **Most EMRs provide critical results to be reported to the clinician as they sign onto the system. This is a useful setting that allows you to prioritize patients to be seen.**

VIII. **Ensure the system is set to allow you to access patient lists for providers you are covering. Developing a backup method of communicating patient lists is strongly recommended in case of system maintenance, system failure, access errors, or list errors.**

BIBLIOGRAPHY

Bowman, S. (2013). Impact of electronic health record systems on information integrity: Quality and safety implications. *Perspectives in Health Information Management, 10*(Fall).

Buppert, C. (2011). 10 habits to adopt to avoid prescribing errors. *Journal for Nurse Practitioners, 7*(7), 600–601.

Chan, P. D. (2012). *Medicine.* Laguna Hills, CA: Current Clinical Strategies.

Edmunds, M. W., & Mayhew, M. S. (2014). *Pharmacology for the primary care provider* (4th ed.). St Louis, MO: Mosby.

El-Kareh, R., Gandhi, T. K., Poon, E. G., Newmark, L. P., Ungar, J., Lipsitz, S., & Sequist, T. D. (2009). Trends in primary care clinician perceptions of a new electronic health record. *Journal of General Internal Medicine, 24*(4), 464–468.

Gomella, L. G., Haist, S. A., & Adams, A. G. (2014). *Clinician's pocket reference 2014* (5th ed.). New York, NY: McGraw-Hill Medical.

Hamid, F., & Cline, T. (2013). Providers' acceptance factors and their perceived barriers to electronic health record (EHR) adoption. *Online Journal of Nursing Informatics (OJNI), 17*(3).

Jarvis, C. (2011). *Physical examination and health assessment* (6th ed.). St. Louis, MO: WB Saunders.

Klein, T., & Kaplan, L. (2010). Prescribing competencies for advanced practice registered nurses. *The Journal for Nurse Practitioners, 6*(2), 115–122.

Maxwell, R. W. (2011). *Maxwell quick medical reference* (6th ed.). New York, NY: Maxwell Publishing Co.

Seidel, H. M., Ball, J. W., Dains, J. E., Flynn, J. A., Solomon, B. S., & Stewart, R. W. (2010). *Mosby's guide to physical examination* (6th ed.). St. Louis, MO: Mosby.

Wells, M., & Wade, M. (2013). Physical performance measures: An important component of the comprehensive geriatric assessment. *The Nurse Practitioner, 38*(6), 48–53.

CHAPTER 86

Managing the Surgical Patient

BIMBOLA F. AKINTADE • THOMAS W. BARKLEY, JR.

PREOPERATIVE ASSESSMENT

I. **History and physical examination—special emphasis on identification of undiagnosed cardiopulmonary disease**
   A. Past medical history
   B. Past surgical history
   C. Family history
   D. Psychosocial history
   E. Allergies
   F. Review of systems
   G. Current medications, including over-the-counter and herbal supplements
   H. Head-to-toe physical examination

II. **Laboratory and diagnostic screening**
   A. Urinalysis
   B. Complete blood count
   C. Posteroanterior and lateral chest radiographs
   D. Patients older than 40 years
      1. Electrocardiogram
      2. Stool for occult blood
      3. Blood chemistry screening battery
   E. Pulmonary function testing
      1. Not routinely obtained
      2. Should be ordered for the following:
         a. Patients having lung surgery
         b. Patients with a history of smoking of more than 10 pack-years who are having coronary artery bypass grafting or upper or lower abdominal surgery

F. Appropriate specific laboratory/diagnostic evaluation of complaints or abnormal physical findings identified during the history and physical examination

III. **Assessment of surgical risk**
A. Nutritional status
1. Dietary history
2. Serum albumin below 3 grams/dl correlates with prolonged recovery and increased mortality
3. Serum transferrin below 150 mg/dl correlates with prolonged recovery and increased mortality
4. Weight loss over 20% caused by illness correlates with prolonged recovery and increased mortality
B. Immune competence
1. Total lymphocyte count
2. Cell-mediated immunity measured by serology
3. Known immunodeficiency, such as HIV
4. Others factors that increase risk of infection:
   a. Corticosteroid use
   b. Immunosuppressive agents
   c. Cytotoxic drugs
   d. Prolonged antibiotic therapy
   e. Renal failure
   f. Irradiation
   g. Hyperglycemia
C. Bleeding risk factors
1. Patient history
   a. Prolonged bleeding after procedure or injury
   b. Bleeding 1 day after tooth extraction
   c. Spontaneous bruising
   d. Liver or kidney disease
   e. Recent thrombolytics, anticoagulants, non-steroidal anti-inflammatory drugs, acetylsalicylic acid, or other drugs that prolong bleeding
   f. Personal (moral, ethical, and religious) contraindication to transfusion of blood products
2. Physical examination—consider the presence of the following:
   a. Hepatosplenomegaly
   b. Petechiae
   c. Ecchymoses
   d. Findings consistent with anemia
3. Diagnostic findings
   a. Anemia
   b. Prolonged prothrombin time or partial thromboplastin time
   c. Thrombocytopenia
   d. Elevated liver function tests

D. Thromboembolic risk increases with the following:
  1. Cancer
  2. Obesity
  3. Age older than 45 years
  4. Myocardial dysfunction
  5. History of thrombosis
  6. Use of oral contraceptives
  7. History of peripheral vascular disease
E. Patients with coronary artery disease
  1. Reduce systolic BP to below 140 mmHg and diastolic BP to below 90 mmHg
  2. In low-risk patients:
      a. Exercise tolerance test should be conducted when history is unreliable.
      b. Dipyridamole thallium scintigraphy, stress echocardiography, or ambulatory ischemia monitoring should be performed in patients unable to exercise.
  3. High-risk patients:
      a. Postpone surgery unless there is an emergency; obtain clearance from specialists (cardiologist, etc.)
  4. Patient should be at least 3 months, and preferably 6 months, post-myocardial infarction
F. Patients with congestive heart failure
  1. Should receive medications up to and including day of surgery
  2. Document objective assessment of left ventricular function (echocardiography)
G. Assessment of pulmonary risk
  1. Chronic lung disease (obstructive or restrictive)
  2. Morbid obesity
  3. Tobacco use

IV. Control of chronic illness
A. Diabetes mellitus (DM)
  1. Patients who require insulin
      a. Type 1 DM
      b. Type 2 DM managed with insulin
      c. Type 2 DM managed with oral agents who are having major procedures
      d. Methods of insulin administration
          i. One-half to two-thirds usual dose subcutaneously
          ii. Regular insulin, 5–15 units, in 5% to 10% glucose at the rate of 100 ml/hr (maintain serum glucose below 200 mg/dl)
          iii. Infuse insulin via intravenous drip at 0.5–1.5 units/hr; infuse glucose separately to maintain serum glucose below 200 mg/dl

         iv. Portland Protocol

         v. Monitor serum glucose every 2–4 hr

   2. Patients not requiring insulin

     a. Diet-controlled diabetics

         i. Avoid glucose solutions on the day of surgery

         ii. Monitor serum glucose every 4–6 hr during surgery

     b. Type 2 DM controlled with oral agents

         i. Discontinue oral agents on the day before surgery

         ii. Infuse 5% glucose at 100 ml/hr

         iii. Monitor glucose every 4–6 hr

         iv. Maintain glucose at below 200 mg/dl with subcutaneous insulin injection every 6 hr

         v. Return to oral treatment when baseline diet is resumed

B. Cardiovascular conditions

   1. Coronary artery disease

     a. Continue aspirin unless concerns about hemostasis are overriding

     b. β-adrenergic blockers, calcium channel blockers, and nitrates should be continued throughout the perioperative period

C. Anemia

   1. Hemoglobin below 8 mg/dl is associated with increased perioperative complications

   2. Transfuse preoperatively as indicated by low hemoglobin, presence of cardiopulmonary disease, type of surgery, and anticipated blood loss

D. Renal disease

   1. Patients with chronic failure not requiring maintenance: glomerular filtration rate below 15 mg/min; serum creatinine over 6 mg/dl

     a. Ensure adequate preoperative hydration: preoperative BUN and creatinine should be at patient's baseline

     b. If no contraindications, transfuse to hematocrit over 32 ml/dl

   2. Patients maintained on dialysis

     a. If no contraindications, transfuse to hematocrit over 32 ml/dl

     b. Dialyze on the morning of surgery

   3. Increased risk of bleeding because platelets are inactive in uremic plasma

E. Pulmonary disease

   1. Cessation of smoking

   2. Administer antibiotics for purulent sputum

   3. Administration of bronchodilators if patient has a history of pulmonary disease (e.g., albuterol metered-dose inhaler, two puffs before anesthesia); in severe disease, may be intravenously administered intraoperatively

V. Physical readiness

    A. Nutritional status

        1. Preoperative supplementation if indicated by physical examination or diagnostic evaluation

        2. Preoperative supplementation if prolonged NPO status is anticipated postoperatively

    B. Fluid and electrolyte status

        1. Fluid supplementation/diuresis preoperatively as indicated by physical examination/diagnostic studies

        2. Correction of Na^+, K^+, $Ca2^+$, $Mg2^+$, and phosphorus to as normal as possible

    C. Acid-base balance

        1. Correction of acid–base imbalance as indicated by preoperative condition

        2. Correction of abnormal anion gap to below 20

            a. $Na^+ - (Cl^- + HCO_3^-)$

    D. Anxiety

        1. Accelerates physiologic stress response

        2. Keep patient well informed—answer questions

        3. Nonpharmacological and pharmacological anxiety reduction measures as indicated

            a. Guided imagery

            b. Relaxation exercises

            c. Medium-length-acting benzodiazepine, such as oxazepine (Serax), to promote sleeping on the night before surgery (avoid in geriatric patients, may cause delirium)

VI. Morning of surgery

    A. Answer patient/family questions, and ensure that informed consent is signed

    B. Ensure that patient has remained NPO since at least 10:00 p.m. on the preceding evening

    C. Ensure that preoperative medications are administered

        1. Antibiotics

        2. Analgesics, sedatives, and other medications ordered by anesthesia provider

        3. Other medications, fluids, and blood products as indicated by preoperative assessment

    D. Prepare patient for postoperative period

        1. Anticipation of the following:

            a. Ventilator support: possible use of soft wrist restraints

            b. Noninvasive oxygen: facemask and nasal cannula

            c. Pulmonary artery monitoring, triple-lumen catheter, peripherally inserted central catheter line, arterial line monitoring

            d. Continuous cardiac monitoring

      e. Nasogastric tube
      f. Chest tube or drains
      g. Incisions/dressings
      h. Foley catheter
      i. Other drains/monitoring equipment
      j. Pain
      k. Hospital noise/lights
   2. Answer questions and reinforce teaching

POSTOPERATIVE CARE

I.   **Fluid and electrolytes**

   A. Postoperative fluid replacement—D5NS (5% dextrose in normal saline) solution or lactated Ringer's solution

      1. Maintenance requirements: 1,500–2,500 ml per 24-hr period

      2. Increased needs caused by hypercatabolism

      3. Consider losses from drains

      4. Consider third space losses

      5. Estimate replacement needs: 30 ml × weight in kilograms per 24-hr period; for example, a 70-kg patient would need 2,100 ml of fluid per 24-hr period (30 × 70 = 2,100)

   B. Electrolyte replacement

      1. Electrolyte measurements are indicated for complicated cases

      2. K^+ should not be added to intravenous fluids for the first 24 hr after surgery because an intracellular shift occurs during surgery; postoperatively, K^+ returns to the extracellular space, and serum measurements rise without supplementation.

         a. Exception is replacement fluids lost via nasogastric or gastric drainage

         b. Replace 20 mEq for every liter of fluid lost

      3. Other electrolytes are replaced as assessed on an individual case basis

II.   **Pulmonary care**

   A. Encourage deep breathing every hr

   B. Incentive spirometry every 2 hr

   C. Mobilization out of bed to chair by postoperative day 1; walking on postoperative day 1 or as soon as tolerated by patient, physical therapy or occupational therapy PRN

   D. Adequate pain control

   E. Instruction regarding splinting with pillows for decreased pain and increased lung expansion

III.   **Wound care/assessment**

   A. Removal of dressing and handling of wound should be aseptic for the first 24 hr

   B. Dressings may be removed from dry wounds

   C. Any drainage should be cultured

D. Skin staples and sutures may be removed on postoperative day 5 or 6; leave in for 2 weeks over creased areas or those closed under tension

E. Assess for signs of infection

1. Erythema
2. Edema
3. Heat
4. Increased pain
5. Drainage

IV. Management of drains

A. External portion should be handled with aseptic technique

B. Attach bag if more than 50 ml drainage anticipated in an 8-hr period

C. Do not leave Penrose drain in for more than 2 weeks; if continued drainage, replace with rubber catheter such as a Foley catheter

D. Remove all invasive lines (e.g., Foley catheter, central line, and arterial line) as soon as possible to prevent infection; if unable to remove, document why

V. Deep vein thrombosis prophylaxis

A. Early ambulation

B. Anticoagulation as indicated by procedure

C. Thromboembolic stockings until patient is ambulating, or lower extremity edema is no longer present

D. Sequential boots until patient is ambulating

VI. Fever

A. Postoperative fever is most often noninfectious

1. Increase lung inflation via turning, coughing, deep breathing, and incentive spirometry provided every 2 hr because decreased lung expansion is a major cause of fever during the postoperative course
2. Ensure adequate hydration by using assessment of vital signs, urine output, BUN/creatinine, and physical examination as indicators
3. Rule out reaction to drugs
4. Rule out deep vein thrombosis via physical examination

B. Suspect infectious fever if:

1. Patient feels subjectively unwell
2. Pain is worsening

C. Rule out infection if indicated

1. CBC with differential to evaluate leukocytosis/neutrophilia
2. Culture any purulent drainage
   a. Incision
   b. Intravenous lines
   c. Foley catheter
   d. Drains
   e. Chest/mediastinal tube drainage
   f. Sputum

   g. Stool
   3. Obtain blood cultures
   4. Begin empiric antibiotic therapy
VII. **Bleeding**
   A. Assess for signs of internal bleeding, such as the following:
      1. Change in vital signs: tachycardia and hypotension
      2. Localized pain (e.g., abdomen)
      3. Grey Turner sign
      4. Hematoma
      5. Change in mental status
      6. Low or dropping hemoglobin/hematocrit level
      7. Elevated reticulocyte count
   B. Management of bleeding
      1. External bleeding usually responds to pressure; may need to apply firm pressure for 20 min
      2. Internal bleeding
         a. Drain hematoma
         b. Transfuse as indicated
         c. Consider reoperation
VIII. **Infection (refer to Infections chapter)**
IX. **Pain**
   A. Must be managed aggressively
   B. Limitation of movement associated with pain can increase risks for the following:
      1. Venous stasis
      2. Thrombosis
      3. Atelectasis/pneumonia
   C. Release of stress hormones can promote the following:
      1. Vasospasm
      2. Hypertension
   D. Pharmacological management (refer to Pain chapter)
      1. Patient-controlled analgesia with a variety of medications (e.g., morphine sulfate); delivering appropriate basal rate and patient-controlled boluses to total an hourly dose appropriate for weight and tolerance
         a. The goal for pain management is to transition from intravenous patient-controlled analgesia to a combination of oral medications and intravenous medications for breakthrough pain once the patient is able to tolerate oral medications.
      2. Consider epidural or other nerve blocks, as appropriate, per anesthesia consultation
      3. Other agents
         a. Parenteral ketorolac tromethamine (Toradol) has analgesic efficacy equivalent to that of morphine sulfate

       i. May be contraindicated in select post-operative patients and, depending on the surgery, many surgeons may not agree with ketorolac administration

X. **Psychosocial**
- **A.** Advise patient of surgical outcomes; answer questions regarding condition
- **B.** Communicate with family members and significant others

BIBLIOGRAPHY

Brunicardi, F. C., Andersen, D. K., Billiar, T. R., Dunn, D. L., Hunter, J. G., Matthews, J. B., & Pollock, R. E. (Eds.). (2014). *Scharwtz's principles of surgery* (10th ed.). New York, NY: McGraw-Hill.

Cameron, J. L., & Cameron, A. M. (Eds.). (2014). *Current surgical therapy* (11th ed.). Baltimore, MD: Mosby.

Chernecky, C. C., & Berger, B. J. (2012). *Laboratory tests and diagnostic procedures* (6th ed.). Philadelphia, PA: Elsevier Saunders.

Doherty, G. M. (Ed.). (2009). *Current diagnosis and treatment surgery* (13th ed.). New York, NY: McGraw-Hill/Appleton & Lange.

Godara, H., Hirbe, A., Nassif, M., Otepka, H., & Rosenstock, A. (Eds.). (2014). *The Washington manual of medical therapeutics* (34th ed.). Philadelphia, PA: Wolters Kluwer Health/Lippincott, Williams, & Wilkins.

Justinger, C., Slotta, J. E., Ningel, S., Gräber, S., Kollmar, O., & Schilling, M. K. (2013). Surgical-site infection after abdominal wall closure with triclosan-impregnated polydioxanone sutures: Results of a randomized clinical pathway facilitated trial (NCT00998907). *Surgery, 154*(3), 589–595. doi:10.1016/j.surg.2013.04.011

Lau, W. C., & Eagle, K. A. (2012). Medical evaluation of the surgical patient. In D. L. Longo, A. S. Fauci, D. L. Kasper, S. L. Hauser, J. L. Jameson, & J. Loscalzo (Eds.), *Harrison's principles of internal medicine* (18th ed., pp. 62–66).

Mottram, C. D. (2012). *Ruppel's manual of pulmonary function testing* (10th ed.). Maryland Heights, MO: Elsevier Mosby.

Papadakis, M. A., McPhee, S. J., & Rabow, M. W. (Eds.). (2014). *Current medical diagnosis and treatment* (54th ed.). New York, NY: McGraw-Hill/Appleton and Lange.

Swartz, M. H. (2014). *Textbook of physical diagnosis* (7th ed.). Philadelphia, PA: WB Saunders.

SECTION THIRTEEN

Health Promotion

CHAPTER 87

Guidelines for Health Promotion and Screening

HELEN MILEY • THOMAS W. BARKLEY, JR. • CHARLENE M. MYERS

VISIONARY PLAN FOR HEALTH

I. **"Health" is defined as an optimal state of well-being**
   A. In 1958, the World Health Organization expanded the traditional description of health as the absence of disease holistically to include mental, physical, and social realms of completeness.
   B. Today, most "health" professions, including nursing, embrace a tri- or quad-dimensional weltanschauung, or a broad view of wellness that includes mental, physical, spiritual, and sociologic domains.
   C. When the body, mind, and spirit are at peak function, it is said that one is in optimal health.
II. **In contrast, human life from inception is vulnerable to illness, injury, and deterioration.**
   A. Threats to health/life may be predictable in some instances
   B. Generally, an American may anticipate about eight decades of life if not significantly affected by genetic predisposition to disease or by an actual interruption in health caused by illness or injury.
      1. Actual and potential threats to life and health include the following:
         a. Intrinsic and extrinsic
         b. Multifactorial
            i. Genetic
            ii. Environmental
            iii. Ergonomic
            iv. Stress and violence related

  c. Status data inform the determination of personal risk for disease and injury.
   i. Age
   ii. Gender
   iii. Residence (i.e., urban or rural)
   iv. Socioeconomic status
   v. Ethnicity
   vi. Culture and language
   vii. Lifestyle, described here as the behaviors that encapsulate one's life choices

C. For most patients, lifestyle combined with genetic influences predominantly shapes health risk

D. With the use of screening, awareness, and educational methods, advanced practice nurses (APNs) can help prevent disease and injury and promote health by identifying risk factors and supporting patients in recognizing and choosing healthy lifestyles individualized to their unique profiles.

III. **Foundational to the capacity of the APN to promote health and to screen for unhealthy conditions or risk factors is a personal belief system that encompasses the uniqueness and diversity of each individual, including a distinct, albeit juxtapositional, view of health.**

A. Willingness to collaborate within the bounds of the patient's belief system remains integral to achieving "healthy people for all"

B. Further, health care and social justice are intertwined; the two issues must be reconciled
  1. With approximately 46 million uninsured persons in the United States having the ability to have insurance, every APN must become an advocate for every patient. Acquiescence involves distortion of the title of "health care provider" into an oxymoron. APNs represent a potential force for major change in health care services—a shift to primary prevention and health promotion that is not only economically feasible but is morally reasonable.

IV. **Healthy People 2020**

A. What began as the U.S. Public Health Service disease prevention and health promotion model in 1979 is today our nation's health promotion framework, known as Healthy People 2020.

B. National health promotion and disease prevention efforts involve implementing the 42 specific focus areas of the Healthy People 2020 document and its specific, detailed objectives. These objectives are accessible at www.health.gov/healthypeople and are published in the text, Healthy People 2020, Volumes I and II.

C. The 42 focus areas found in the 2020 update of the original World Health Organization (WHO) conceptual framework include the following:

1. Access to health services
2. Adolescent health (new)
3. Arthritis, osteoporosis, and chronic back conditions
4. Blood disorders and blood safety (new)
5. Cancer
6. Chronic kidney disease
7. Dementia, including Alzheimer's disease (new)
8. Diabetes
9. Disability health
10. Early and middle childhood (new)
11. Educational and community-based programs
12. Environmental health
13. Family planning
14. Food safety
15. Genomics (new)
16. Global health (new)
17. Health communication and health information technology
18. Health-associated infections (new)
19. Health-related quality of life and well-being (new)
20. Hearing and other sensory or communication disorders (new)
21. Heart disease and stroke
22. Human immunodeficiency virus
23. Immunization and infectious diseases
24. Injury and violence prevention
25. Lesbian, gay, bisexual, and transgender health
26. Maternal, infant, and child health
27. Medical product safety
28. Mental health and mental disorders
29. Nutrition and weight status
30. Occupational safety and health
31. Older adults (new)
32. Oral health
33. Physical activity
34. Preparedness (new)
35. Public health infrastructure
36. Respiratory disease
37. Sexually transmitted diseases
38. Sleep health (new)
39. Social determinants of health (new)
40. Substance abuse
41. Tobacco use
42. Vision

D. The Healthy People 2020 campaign, which has been adopted by the WHO, outlines two overreaching goals for all people:
   1. To increase the quality and years of a healthy life

Table 87.1	Health People 2020 Twelve Indicators
Indicator	**Health strategies framework**
Access to Health Services	• Person with medical insurance • Persons with a usual primary care providers
Clinical preventative services	• Adults who receive a colorectal cancer (under recent guidelines) • Adults with hypertension whose BP is under control • Adults diabetic population with an A1c greater than 9% • Children aged 19–35 months who received recommended vaccinations
Environmental quality	• Air quality Index exceeding 100 (EH-1) • Children aged 3–11 years exposed to secondhand smoke
Injury and violence	• Fatal injuries • Homicides
Maternal, Infant, and Child Health	• Infant deaths • Preterm births
Mental health	• Suicides • Adolescents who experience major depressive episodes
Nutrition, physical activity, and obesity	• Adult who meet current federal physical activity guidelines • All patients who are obese • Total vegetable intake for persons 2 years and older
Oral health	• Persons 2 years and older who used the oral health care system in past 12 months
Reproductive and sexual health	• Sexually active females aged 5–14 years who received reproductive health services in the past 12 months • Persons living with HIV who know their serostatus
Social determinants	• Students who graduate with a regular diploma 4 years after starting ninth grade
Substance abuse	• Adolescents using alcohol or any illicit drugs during the past 30 years • Adults engaging in binge drinking during the past 30 days
Tobacco	• Adults who are current cigarette smokers • Adolescents who smoked cigarettes in the past 30 days

   2. To eliminate health disparities
E. Healthy People 2020 lists 12 leading health indicators that may serve as a framework for the APN in developing health strategies with the patient (see Table 87.1)
   1. These indicators, underpinned by theory and clinical data, are useful to the APN and the patient in achieving health and preventing illness and injury.

2. These indicators provide the cornerstone for targeted health promotion and preventive practices and should be incorporated, at least theoretically, into care at all levels—primary, secondary, and tertiary.

PREVENTION

I. **Prevention is essential to health maintenance and is a component of health promotion at all ages.**
   A. Research supports the purpose and significance of prevention in primary care, as well as in other settings
   B. The leading authority on prevention guidelines is the U.S. Preventive Services Task Force (USPSTF), which engages a complex risk-to-benefit analysis of research-based clinical interventions aimed at preventing disease and injury.
      1. The task force grades recommendations via an A through D scale.
         a. A is strongly recommended; D is not recommended
         b. This scale includes one category indicating that data are insufficient to recommend for or against an intervention.
      2. The task force scores the quality of the evidence on a three-point scale as good, fair, or poor.
   C. Using the Healthy People 2020 framework integrated into all three levels of prevention, and in accordance with a careful risk-to-benefit analysis, the APN together with the patient can individualize a holistic health promotion plan
   D. The role of the clinician in prevention and health promotion as outlined in the USPSTF report includes the following professional markers:
      1. Intervention in lifestyle behaviors that place individuals at risk and that can be modified
      2. Mutuality in the establishment of individualized plans of care for prevention and health promotion
      3. Judicious use of preventive healthcare services and screening tests
      4. Shared impetus in the delivery of preventive care to patients
      5. Selective use of community intervention
   E. A more in-depth description of the integral role of APNs in patients' achieving wellness, health promotion, and disease prevention specifically includes the following:
      1. Holistic assessment of the individual
      2. Age-appropriate screening for disease
      3. Mutually planned and implemented intervention
      4. Continued monitoring
      5. Social advocacy

PREVENTION AND HEALTH PROMOTION IN CLINICAL PRACTICE

I. **Components**
   A. Primary prevention
      1. Defined as health promotion that precedes disease or onset of symptoms
      2. Methods of primary prevention include general health promotion practices aimed at influencing positive lifestyle choices and specific protective strategies that combat disease. Interventions include the following:
         a. Immunizations
         b. Health education
         c. Blood pressure measurements
         d. Genetic screening for sex-linked disorders
         e. Use of seat belts
         f. Smoking cessation and avoidance of secondhand smoke and other environmental pollutants
         g. Community disaster preparedness planning and education
         h. Age 10–24, fair-skinned individuals to minimize exposure to UV radiation
   B. Secondary prevention
      1. Identification and diagnosis, early intervention, and limitation of disability in disease and injury encompassing secondary response to illness
      2. The goals of secondary prevention are to either shorten or halt the disease process, and arrest or prevent complications and further disability. Examples of secondary interventions include the following:
         a. Case finding
         b. Screening for specific disease (e.g., cervical cancer by Pap smear, dyslipidemia by measurement of total cholesterol and its components, diabetes by blood glucose, and blood pressure screening to identify cardiovascular risk [i.e., hypertension], one time HIV screening in age 15–65)
         c. Isolation to prevent the transmission of communicable diseases (e.g., varicella and active tuberculosis)
         d. In addition, the general screening guidelines for cancer, heart disease, and diabetes for average-risk adults are outlined in a joint recommendation by the American Heart Association; the American Cancer Society; the National Heart, Lung and Blood Institute; the Centers for Disease Control; and the American Diabetes Association, summarized briefly here as follows:

i. All patients should be advised of healthy diet, exercise, and smoking cessation benefits

ii. Assessment between 18–20 years of age should include the following:

(a) Body mass index (BMI) at every regular health care visit (USPSTF B recommendation)

(b) If BMI exceeds 25 kg/m², the APN should measure waist-to-hip ratio and assess for visceral obesity. If the waist circumference is greater than 40 inches in males and 35 inches or more in females, risk for metabolic syndrome is increased.

(c) Pediatric patients should minimally receive height, growth, and BMI measurements annually as advised by the AAP, although the USPSTF grants the intervention with only a rating of 1.

(d) Blood pressure at every health care visit and at least once every 2 years if less than 120/80 mmHg (recommendation: good evidence); according to the Seventh Report of the Joint National Committee on Prevention, Detection, Evaluation, and Treatment of High Blood Pressure (JNC 7), the hypertension diagnosis is updated as follows:

1. Normal: BP less than 120 mmHg/less than 80 mmHg

2. Prehypertension: 120–139 mmHg/80–89 mmHg

3. Stage 1: 140–159 mmHg/90–99 mmHg

4. Stage 2: 160 mmHg or greater/100 mmHg or greater

5. Additional stages are added to emphasize the risk of systolic hypertension and the need for early diagnosis and treatment, with lifestyle management for prehypertension and lifestyle and antihypertensive agents for stages 1 and 2.

(e) Beginning at age 20, a fasting lipoprotein profile is recommended, including total cholesterol, low-density lipoprotein (LDL), high-density lipoprotein (HDL), and triglycerides (if a nonfasting lipoprotein profile is used, only total cholesterol and HDL are usable). If total cholesterol is greater than or equal to 200 mg/dl or HDL is less than or equal to 40 mg/dl, a follow-up fasting lipoprotein panel is needed; cardiovascular disease risk factor screening is also indicated, including a 10-year risk assessment using the Framingham scoring system.

(f) Clinical breast examination every 3 years for females younger than 40 years of age, then annually thereafter

(g) Papanicolaou test in females should begin 3 years after beginning vaginal intercourse or by age 21 years. Screening should be done every year with the regular Pap test or every 2 years using the newer liquid-based Pap test. At age 30 years, with three consecutive negative PAP results, screening may occur every 2–3 years. Higher-risk women should continue to be screened annually. At age 70 years, with three consecutive negative Pap results and no abnormal Pap results in the last 10 years, screening may be discontinued.

iii. Assessment at age 45 years should include all gender- and non-gender-specific interventions noted previously, along with

(a) Blood glucose test every 3 years

iv. Assessment at age 50 years should include all of those steps described earlier as specified by gender and the following:

(a) Colorectal screening

(b) A recommendation (good evidence) by the USPSTF (frequency dependent on history and type of test used): if in doubt, screen

(c) The American Cancer Society recommends annual fecal occult blood testing and flexible sigmoidoscopy every 5 years after age 50 years, or a double-contrast barium enema or colonoscopy every decade after age 50 years.

(d) Prostate-specific antigen (PSA) with digital rectal examination annually for males

3. Age- and risk-specific cancer screening is an effective means of reducing morbidity and mortality.

   a. According to the National Cancer Institute, screening for breast and cervical cancers alone may reduce total cancer deaths by 3% annually.

   b. Although an evidence-based approach to screening should be taken by the practitioner, general guidelines for cancer screening are as follows:

      i. Breast

         (a) Regular mammography every 1–2 years for females before age 50 years (baseline at age 40 years or soon after) with increased frequency of examination during the fifth decade of life and beyond as determined by risk factors such as first-degree relatives with history of breast cancer; generally, minimally every 1–2 years, noting that the greatest benefit occurs between ages 40 and 70 years.

         (b) MRI may be indicated in women who have a positive history of gene mutations for breast cancer

         (c) Women with limited life expectancy may not benefit from mammography, especially after age 70 years. Risk of unnecessary biopsy to benefit of early detection should be discussed, and an informed decision of whether to continue to screen or not should be documented.

         (d) Clinical breast exam and teaching breast self-examination have a rating of 1, indicating that the evidence is insufficient to recommend. Whether or not to perform these procedures should be discussed with the patient and a mutual decision should be reached.

         (e) Colorectal

      a. Annual digital rectal examination (DRE) after age 50 years (consider history of polyps and heritable risk factors at age 40 years), with fecal occult blood testing

      b. Flexible sigmoidoscopy every 5 years after age 50 years as screening for rectal precancerous polyps; colorectal cancer is easy to treat and carries a good prognosis when diagnosed early

      c. Colonoscopy every 10 years

      d. The advent of DNA marker testing and virtual colonoscopy may change the recommendation in the near future.

      e. Earlier screening is indicated when the family history is positive for colon cancer and other bowel diseases correlated with colon cancer risk, such as inflammatory bowel disease

    (f) Prostate: the AAFP found insufficient evidence on whether or not to recommend annual DRE/PSA testing for prostate cancer. However, the subject should be addressed with the patient and a mutual informed decision to screen or not should be reached and documented. The following facts should be discussed:

        1. DRE and PSA test can help identify prostate cancer

        2. Men at increased risk, such as those with positive family history of prostate cancer in first-degree relatives, may choose screening as early as age 40 years. However, early diagnosis has not been shown to decrease mortality, and there are risks of the procedures.

        3. When in doubt, screen

    (g) Other: screening for oral, lung, liver, ovarian, gastric, endometrial, and testicular cancers should be guided by a detailed patient history of heredity, use of tobacco, exposure to infectious disease and carcinogens, and other pertinent factors. Note that testicular exams in asymptomatic males are not recommended in adults or adolescents.

  4. Women at age 65 years should undergo the following:

    a. Screening for osteoporosis according to the USPSTF (B recommendation)

    b. Screening should begin at age 60 years for women with increased risk factors

      i. Weight less than 70 kg

Table 87.2	Screening Recommendations		
Topic	**Description**	**Grade**	**Current recommendation date**
Abdominal aortic screening: men only	One time screen by ultrasound in men who have ever smoked between ages 65 and 75 years	B	February 2005
Alcohol misuse: screening and counseling	Adults 18 years and older; provide brief behavioral counseling interventions if screen is +	B	May 2013
Anemia screening: pregnant women	Routine for iron deficiency anemia in asymptomatic pregnant women	B	May 2006
ASA to prevent DV disease in men	ASA age 49–79 years when the potential benefit due to a reduction in MI outweighs the harm due to an increased risk in GI hemorrhage	A	March 2009
ASA to prevent DV disease in women	Recommends the use of ASA women 55–79 years	A	March 2009
Bacteriuria screening: pregnancy women	Recommends at 12–16 weeks gestation or the first prenatal visit	A	July 2008
BP	Adults 18+	A	July 2008
VRCA screening counseling	Women with an FH associated with an increased risk for mutations in BRCA1 or BRCA2 should be referred	B	September 2005
Breast cancer preventive medication	Discuss chemoprevention with women at high risk for breast cancer and low risk for adverse effects of chemoprevention	B	July 2002
Breast cancer screening	Age 40 every 1–2 years	B	September 2002
Cervical cancer screening	Screening for women ages 21–65 with cytology every 3 years or for women age 30–65 years who want to lengthen the screening interval	A	March 2012
Cholesterol abnormalities screening: men younger than 35 years; women younger than 45 years	Screening age 20–35 years if they are at increased risk for CHD	B	June 2008

Table 87.2	Screening Recommendations		
Topic	**Description**	**Grade**	**Current recommendation date**
Cholesterol abnormalities screening: men older than 35 years; women 45 years and older	Age 45 years and older if they are at increased risk of CHD	A	June 2008
Colorectal cancer screening	FOBT; sigmoidoscopy, or colonoscopy in adults at age 50–75 years	A	October 2008
Depression screening: adults	Screening adult for depression when staff assisted depression care supports are in place to assure accurate dx, effective treatment, and follow-up	B	December 2009
Diabetes screening	Asymptomatic adults with sustained BP (either treated or untreated) greater than 135/80	B	June 2008
Fall prevention in older adults	Exercise or physical therapy	B	May 2012
Fall prevention in older adults	Vitamin D	B	May 2012
Healthy diet counseling	Intensive behavioral dietary counseling for adults with hyperlipidemia and other known risk factors for CV and diet-related chronic disease	B	January 2003
Hepatitis C virus infection screening: adults	Recommends in person at high risk for infection one time screening for HCV to adults born between 1945 and 1965	B	June 2013
HIV screening: adults	Screen for HIV infection in adolescents and adults age 15–65 years. Younger adolescents and older adults who are at increased risk should also be screened	A	April 2013
Intimate partner violence screening: women of child bearing years	Screen women and provide or refer women who screen positive to intervention services	B	January 2013

Table 87.2	Screening Recommendations		
Topic	**Description**	**Grade**	**Current recommendation date**
Obesity screening and counseling: adults	Clinic should offer or refer patient with a BMI greater than 30 kg/m² or higher to intensive multicomponent behavioral interventions	B	June 2012
Osteoporosis: women	Women age 65 years and older and in younger women whose fracture risk is equal to or greater than that of a 64 year old white woman who has no additional risk factors	B	January 2012
Sexually transmitted infections counseling	Recommends high-intensity behavioral counseling to prevent STIs in all sexually active adolescents and for adults at increased risk of STIs	B	October 2008
Skin cancer behavioral	Recommends counseling children, adolescents, and young adults age 10–24 years who have fair skin about minimizing their exposure to ultraviolet radiation to reduce risk for skin cancer	B	May 2012
Tobacco use counseling and intervention: nonpregnant adults	Recommends that clinicians as all adults about tobacco use and provide tobacco cessation intervention for those who use tobacco products	A	April 2009

Note. Recommendations from the U.S. preventative service task force (2013).

     ii. No estrogen replacement

     iii. Family history

     iv. Smoking

     v. Sedentary lifestyle

     vi. Alcohol or caffeine use

     vii. Low calcium and vitamin D ingestion

C. Tertiary prevention

  1. The hallmark of tertiary care is the provision of services aimed at restoring or arresting disability.

  2. The objective of tertiary prevention is to return the patient to optimal health within the constraints of the impairment, preventing further decline or arresting the progression of complications.

  3. The use of specialized health care teams (e.g., occupational therapy, speech therapy, and rehabilitative services) and the appropriate referrals for injury or illness, such as head and neck injury and cerebrovascular accident, are examples of tertiary prevention.

  4. The use of an interdisciplinary team is the superior format for prevention at the tertiary level.

II. **Periodic health history and examination**

 A. The recommended interval of assessment varies in the literature but should be judiciously individualized to the patient's age, risk, and state of health or illness; further, most research today indicates that women are more likely to participate in screening programs.

  1. APNs should remain cognizant of the overall health of population aggregates and individuals, and should know that socioeconomic and educational status is directly linked to the health of populations and of individuals for virtually all indicators.

  2. Although specific guidelines for frequency remain controversial, the periodic health examination is commonly administered by APNs to asymptomatic patients in three major age groups (Table 87.3):

   a. 11–24 years

   b. 25–64 years

   c. 65 years and older

 B. Additional preventive services

  1. Select screening tests (see Table 87.2)

  2. Immunizations (see Table 87.3)

Table 87.3	Age-Specific Suggestions for Prevention, Screening, and Counseling
Ages 11–24	

Immunization/ Preventative Care	• HBV series if not done
	• Varicella and rubella by age 11 or 12 years
	• Td booster once by age 11 or 12 years and every 10 years thereafter
	• MMR by age 11 or 12 years (also given during preschool years)
	• Consider meningococcal vaccination if college age and living in dormitory or communal setting
	• Influenza annually if at risk
	• Treat diseases such as diabetes, hypertension, and scoliosis before complications; for example, for early treatment of hyperlipidemia, three indications require pharmacological intervention:
	
	    a. LDL higher 160 mg/dl and fewer than two CHD factors
	    b. LDL higher 130 mg/dl and two or more CHD factors
	    c. Diagnosed CHD and LDL higher than 100 mg/dl
	
	• Suggest chemoprevention against neural tube defect with folic acid for females of childbearing age capable of becoming pregnant

Screening tests	• Height and weight • Blood pressure • Anemia (CBC) • Urinalysis • TB • Hearing and vision • Dental • Cancer (breast, testicular, and cervical if sexually active or age 20 years) • Chlamydia screening if sexually active • Rubella serology if female older than 12 years (or vaccinate) • The American Academy of Pediatrics (www.aap.org) recommends a total cholesterol level for children after age 2 years if indicated by risk (parent with total cholesterol higher than 240 mg/dl) and a full lipid panel, including triglyceride level, if family history of cardiac disease younger than age 55 years; random total cholesterol/HDL and CHD risk factors after age 20 years every 5 years (total cholesterol less than 200 mg/dl, desirable; 200–239 mg/dl, moderate more than 239 mg/dl, high); HDL less than 40 is an independent coronary risk factor; ATP III guidelines recommend a complete lipoprotein profile as the initial screening; if fasting levels are high and triglycerides are higher than 200, diet is not likely to lower levels acceptably; consider all risk factors in determining treatment course

Table 87.3	Age-Specific Suggestions for Prevention, Screening, and Counseling		

Ages 11–24

	LDL/HDL		
	Age	Male	Female
	10–11	45–149/ 34–81	56–140/30–74
	12–13	55–135/ 30–82	58–138/33–73
	14–15	48–143/ 26–72	47–140/29–73
	16–17	53–134/ 25–66	44–147/27–78
Developmental/ Age related counseling	• Injuries • STIs (including HIV) and sexual behaviors • Substance abuse • School gang or domestic violence • Physical activity • Smoking • Family planning, pregnancy prevention, contraception, or abstinence • Folic acid supplements during childbearing years • Oral/dental health • Sun exposure • Nutrition/obesity • Suicide inventory (The HEADDSSS [home, education, activities, drugs, driving, seat belts, sex, and suicide] survey instrument is a lifestyle questionnaire that is commonly used to identify high-risk teens.) • Career guidance support • Family history and other specific health-related risk factors • Occupational/environmental/travel outside the United States		

Ages 25–64 years

Immunization, Preventative Care	• Td every 10 years • MMR, HBV, and IPV if needed • Influenza annually at age 50 years and after • Multivitamin with folic acid for women of childbearing age • Treatment of hypertension, hyperlipidemia, anemia, and depression, as indicated • Hormone prophylaxis (perimenopausal and postmenopausal women) • USPSTF strongly recommends the screening of men older than 35 years and women older than 45 years for lipid disorders and treatment of lipid disorders in those who are at high risk for coronary artery disease (A recommendation)

Table 87.3	Age-Specific Suggestions for Prevention, Screening, and Counseling

Ages 25–64 years

Screening/tests	• Height and weight (annually)
	• Blood pressure (annually)
	• Total serum cholesterol (men, ages 35–64 years; women, ages 45–64 years) every 4–5 years
	• Pap smear yearly (once sexually active or 21 years of age)
	• Mammogram annually after age 50 years (baseline at 40 years unless high risk)
	• Clinical breast examination annually after 18 years or at time of Pap smear
	• Breast self-examination (female)/testicular (male) examination monthly after age 18 years
	• Fecal specimen for occult blood annually after age 50 years
	• Sigmoidoscopy or colonoscopy at age 50 years and every 5 years or as indicated
	• Alcohol and substance abuse inventory (i.e., CAGE questionnaire)
	• Women only:
	  a. Folic acid 4 mg daily if considering pregnancy
	  b. Rubella titer or immunization if of childbearing age
	• Tonometry (glaucoma) screening in both genders beginning at age 40 years
	• Men only:
	  a. Clinical testicular examination annually
	  b. Digital prostate examination annually after age 50 years (40 years if at high risk)

Counseling	• Injury identification (occupational, environmental, and domestic violence) • Injury prevention: lap/shoulder belts, helmet use (bicycles, skateboarding, in-line skating, motorcycle, and ATV use), water sports safety, smoke and carbon monoxide detectors, and storage and use of firearms • Screening sexual history for high-risk behaviors, STIs, and unplanned pregnancy • Other high-risk areas (exposure to TB, chemicals, biohazards, and genetic or familial risk for illness) • Tobacco, alcohol, illicit drug, and other abuse of substances (including caffeine) • Diet, stress, and exercise: adopt healthy nutritional habits, limit fat and processed starches and sugars, maintain ideal BMI, emphasize food pyramid, consider calcium supplementation for women, discuss effective coping mechanisms, and encourage regular (daily) aerobic exercise • Smoking cessation intervention • Substance dependency or abuse • STI prevention, use of condoms or other forms of contraception. High-risk behavior avoidance • Dental hygiene (effective brushing and flossing, regular examinations, and need for immediate follow-up)

Table 87.3	Age-Specific Suggestions for Prevention, Screening, and Counseling

Ages 65 years and older

Immunization, Preventive care	• Td booster (every 10 years) • Influenza annually • Pneumococcal vaccine • Hepatitis B, if at risk • MMR in susceptible adults • Varicella in susceptible adults • Consider ASA, vitamin E, folic acid, and multivitamin daily • Women only: consider calcium supplementation

Screening/tests	• Blood pressure
	• Height and weight
	• Fecal occult blood test or sigmoidoscopy
	• Women only:
	  a. Pelvic exam/Pap smear (if sexually active and cervix/uterus in situ) every 1–3 years. Note: Difficulty in detecting ovarian neoplasm; screening history recommended annually, pelvic examination and diagnostics discretionary
	  b. Mammogram and clinical breast examination annually
	• Hearing and vision
	• Activities of daily living
	• Risk for falls
	• Mental examination (depression, suicide, alcohol and other substance abuse, polypharmacy, and memory changes)
	• Signs of elder abuse

Counseling	• Injury prevention (smoke/CO detector, stairs in home, use of seat belts, helmets, and other protective sports gear) • Safe storage of firearms • Fall prevention • BCLS education for caregiver or family members • Hot water heater set at 120°F (48.9°C) • Diet and exercise • STI, including HIV prevention • Dental health (regular examinations, fluoride toothpaste, and flossing)

Note. ASA = aspirin; ATP III = Adult Treatment Panel III; ATV = all-terrain vehicle; BCLS = basic cardiac life support; BMI = body mass index; CAGE = alcohol abuse questionnaire; CHD = coronary heart disease; CBC = complete blood count; CO = carbon monoxide; HBV = hepatitis B virus; HDL = high-density lipoprotein; HIV = human immunodeficiency virus; IPV = inactivated polio vaccine; LDL = low-density lipoprotein; MMR = measles-mumps-rubella; STI = sexually transmitted infection; TB = tuberculosis; Td = tetanus-diphtheria; USPSTF = U.S. Preventive Services Task Force.

a. Immunization status should be ascertained at every patient encounter and should be updated as necessary.

b. Tetanus-diptheria (Td) series in all adults not previously immunized, and/or boosters every 10 years or at least by age 50 years; single dose Tdap is indicated once as an adult.

3. Chemoprophylaxis or chemoprevention is the use of medications or biologicals for the preservation of health or the prevention of disease (e.g., vitamin therapy, folic acid supplements for female reproductive health, aspirin [acetylsalicylic acid; ASA] for cardioprotective effects, chemoprevention of breast cancer, and postmenopausal hormone replacement therapy [HRT]).

   a. The USPSTF recommends that chemoprevention for breast cancer should be considered for high-risk women (B recommendation), and against the routine use of agents such as tamoxifen and raloxifene for women at low risk (D recommendation).

   b. The USPSTF recommends against estrogen and progestin hormone replacement for all women because of the mixed benefit-to-harm ratio.

      i. The USPSTF concluded that hormone replacement may be linked with harmful effects (risk of breast cancer, venous thromboembolism, coronary heart disease, stroke, and cholecystitis).

      ii. Possible benefits (i.e., improved cognition, protection from dementia, bone health, and other long-term effects) were supported by less than conclusive data to guide the recommendation for its use.

      iii. The USPSTF did not evaluate HRT prescribed for symptoms of menopause alone

      iv. For women who have undergone hysterectomy, an I recommendation is assigned (insufficient data to recommend for or against)

      v. In concluding that harm likely outweighed the benefits, USPSTF states that the absolute increased risk from HRT is modest.

4. Counseling regarding specific health risk and prevention of disease

   a. Tobacco and controlled substance avoidance

      i. USPSTF strongly recommends counseling to prevent tobacco use and tobacco-caused disease, and assigns an A recommendation (strong evidence to support)

      ii. USPSTF recommends that all pregnant women should be screened for tobacco use and provided counseling on smoking cessation structured for, and specific to, pregnancy (A recommendation)

        iii. Screening of children and adolescents for tobacco use received an I recommendation (inconclusive data to support)

  b. Disease prevention and stress management linked with regular physical exercise

        i. Lack of physical activity is a huge risk factor for cardiovascular disease, diabetes, obesity, osteoporosis, cancer, and depression. A tenet of Healthy People 2010 is that Americans should engage in regular physical exercise, that is, 30 min of moderate activity on 5 or more days each week, or 20 min of vigorous exercise 3 times a week.

        ii. Since 1996, the USPSTF has recommended that clinicians counsel patients, including children, in primary health care to engage in regular exercise because of methodological limitations in research examining the effectiveness of counseling in promoting exercise. The recommendation is not rated.

  c. Dietary counseling based on BMI and patient history

        i. Generally, a diet low in saturated fats is advised

        ii. For patients at high risk or with diagnosed coronary artery disease, diabetes, hypertension, obesity, or dyslipidemia, intensive diet counseling in a structured manner is recommended.

  d. Promoting breastfeeding

        i. Structured education and behavioral counseling programs receive a USPSTF recommendation B (fair evidence to support the intervention)

        ii. Scientific evidence for promoting breastfeeding includes the following data:

            (a) Breast-fed infants have fewer otitis media and respiratory infections and less gastroenteritis and atopic eczema than their bottle-fed counterparts

            (b) The practice has benefits for the mother, such as improved uterine recovery and lower breast and ovarian cancer rates.

        iii. Contraindications to breastfeeding, although rare, include HIV infection and the use of some medications

  e. Preventing skin cancer

        i. Regular self-examination of skin

        ii. Avoidance of tanning and sun exposure

        iii. Use of sunscreen

        iv. Periodic early clinical evaluation of any suspicious mole or lesion

    f. Crisis intervention for mental and behavioral acute needs as determined by history or depression screening

        i. Early referral to mental health specialists and appropriate agencies for possible abuse, potential for suicide or homicide, or need for specialized care

    g. Age- and development-specific safety counseling (see age-specific areas of focus below)

C. Categories of regular surveillance of health risks include the following:

    1. Physical activity

    2. Overweight and obesity

    3. Tobacco use

    4. Substance abuse

    5. Responsible sexual behavior

    6. Mental health

    7. Injury and violence

    8. Environmental quality

    9. Immunization

    10. Access to health care

    11. Underuse of known prevention strategies (e.g., breast, cervical, and colorectal cancer screening)

D. Age- or gender-related areas of focus

    1. Adolescents

        a. Sexually transmitted infections (STIs); although approximately 25% of adults will be affected by an STI at some point in their lives, teen females are disproportionately affected, particularly by chlamydial infection rates.

        b. Unwanted pregnancy

        c. Substance abuse

        d. Depression or suicide

        e. Scoliosis

        f. Family- or school-related violence

    2. Elderly

        a. Peripheral vascular disease

        b. Thyroid disease

        c. Inability to perform activities of daily living

        d. Safety risks (e.g., falling)

        e. STIs

            i. Older Americans represent one of the fastest growing groups of newly diagnosed HIV infection, possibly owing to the development of erectile dysfunction treatment modalities.

    3. Women

        a. Hormone replacement therapy

        b. Osteoporosis

        c. Mental health and its relationship to cardiac risk

         i. Particularly between ages 25 and 74 years, cardiac risk is lower if mental health is good

         ii. The presence of depression (major or minor) or other comorbidities negatively affects cardiac risk, especially after age 45 years

         iii. The incidence of depression in women is 2–3 times greater than in males.

         iv. Data indicate that women are more vulnerable to mental health illness triggered by social stressors and exhibit greater signs of stress from relationship problems.

      d. Women who are pregnant or are considering pregnancy

         i. Thyroid disorders

         ii. Blood pressure

         iii. Anemia

         iv. STIs, including HIV

         v. Rubella

         vi. Hepatitis B

         vii. Urinary tract infections

         viii. Rh typing

         ix. Daily folic acid

         x. Alcohol, tobacco, and other substance use

III. The CDC's behavioral Risk Factor Surveillance System (DATA 2010) is a standardized tracking mechanism that allows health care providers and patients access to current morbidity and risk factor data; it may be accessed at www.cdc.gov/nccdphp/brfss.

IV. The Healthy People 2020 website, which offers regular status reports regarding the nation's progress on meeting specific goals of health, may be accessed at www.health.gov/healthypeople.

    A. Although improvements in insurance coverage for clinical preventive services such as Pap smears, mammograms, and immunizations have occurred, many Americans remain uninsured and unaffected by these changes.

    B. Continued research concerning preventive care and implementation of methods to improve access, reduce barriers, and increase the appropriate use of clinical preventive health services remains the impetus for APNs in the provision of screening, prevention, and health promotion services.

    C. Routine screening, although recommended by numerous distinguished clinical entities, remains a mutual decision agreed upon by the provider and the patient.

      1. Many third-party payers do not reimburse for preventive and health promotion interventions.

      2. The APN should educate and inform the patient about the need for testing and about associated costs, benefits, and risks.

      3. Ultimately, the choice of undergoing testing/examination, as with lifestyle decisions, lies with the patient.

BIBLIOGRAPHY

Adams, P. F., Kirzinger, W. K., & Martinez, M. E. (2013). Summary health statistics for the U.S. population: National Health Interview Survey, 2012. National Center for Health Satistics. Vital and Health Statistics, 10(259).

Agency for Healthcare Research and Quality. (2011). *Screening for cardiovascular disease and risk factors*. Retrieved from http://www.guideline. gov/content.aspx?id=39338

Alters, S., & Schiff, W. (2012). *Essential concepts for healthy living* (6th ed.). Sudbury, MA: Jones and Bartlett Publishing.

American Cancer Society. (2013). *American Cancer Society guidelines for the early detection of cancer*. Retrieved from http://www.cancer.org/healthy/ findcancerearly/cancerscreeningguidelines/american-cancer-society-guidelines-for-the-early-detection-of-cancer

American Cancer Society. (2014). *Cancer facts and figures 2014*. Atlanta, GA: American Cancer Society. Retrieved from http://www.cancer.org/acs/groups/ content/@research/documents/webcontent/acspc-042151.pdf

Buttaro, T. M., Trybulski, J., Polgar-Bailey, P., & Sandberg-Cook, J. (2012). *Primary care: A collaborative practice* (4th ed.). St. Louis, MO: Mosby.

Croswell, J. M., Brawley, O. W., & Kramer, B. S. (2012). Prevention and early detection of cancer. In D. L. Longo, A. S. Fauci, D. L. Kasper, S. L. Hauser, J. L. Jameson, & J. Loscalzo (Eds.), *Harrison's principles of internal medicine* (18th ed., pp. 655–662). New York, NY: McGraw-Hill.

DeNavas-Walt, C., Proctor, B. D., & Smith, J. C. (2013). *Income, poverty, and health insurance coverage in the United States: 2012*. Washington, D.C.: US Census Bureau. Retrieved September 26, 2014 from http://www.census.gov/ prod/2013pubs/p60–245.pdf

Edelman, C. L., Mandle, C. L., & Kudzma, E. C. (2012). *Health promotion throughout the lifespan* (8th ed.). St. Louis, MO: Elsevier/Mosby.

Hamric, A. B., Hanson, C. M., Tracy, M. F., O'Grady, E. T. (2013). *Advanced practice nursing: An integraive approach* (5th ed.). Philadelphia, PA: WB Saunders.

Hay, W. W., Levin, M. J., Deterding, R. R., Abzug, M. J., & Sondheimer, J. M. (2012). *Current diagnosis and treatment pediatrics* (21st ed.). New York, NY: Lange Medical Books/McGraw-Hill.

James, P. A., Oparil, S., Carter, B. L., Cushman, W. C., Dennison-Himmelfarb, C., Handler, J., Lackland, D. T., . . . Ortiz, E. (2014). 2014 evidence-based guidelines for the management of high blood pressure in adults: Report from the panel members appointed to the Eighth Joint National Committee (JNC 8). *Journal of the American Medical Association, 311*(5), 507–520. doi:10.1001/ jama.2013.284427

Legal Advisor. (2010). The case of the elusive breast lump. *Clinical Advisor,* October 2004. Retrieved September 26, 2014 from http://www.clinicaladvisor. com/the-case-of-the-elusive-breast-lump/article/162064/

Nicoll, C. D., Pignone, M., & Lu, C. M. (2014). Diagnostic testing & medical decision making. In Papadakis, M. A., McPhee, S. J., & Rabow, M. W. (Eds.), *Current medical diagnosis and testing* (53rd ed.). Retrieved from http://accessmedicine.mhmedical.com/content. aspx?bookid=1019&sectionid=56908840

O'Connor, A. M., Bennett, C. L., Stacey, D., Barry, M., Col, N. F., Eden, K. B., . . . Rovner, D. (2009). Decision aids for people facing health treatment or screening decisions. *The Cochrane Library.* doi:10.1002/14651858.CD001431. pub2

Prospective Studies Collaboration. (2009). Body-mass index and cause-specific mortality in 900,000 adults: Collaborative analyses of 57 prospective studies. *Lancet, 373*(9669), 1083–1096. doi:10.1016/S0140–6736(09)60318–4

Uphold, C. R., & Graham, M. V. (2013). *Clinical guidelines in family practice* (3rd ed.). Gainesville, FL: Barmarrae Books.

U.S. Department of Health and Human Services. *2020 topics & objectives.* Retrieved November 2013 from http://www.healthypeople.gov/2020/ topicsobjectives2020/default.aspx

US Preventive Services Task Force (2014). *Guide to clinical preventive services.* Retrieved from http://www.ahrq.gov/professionals/clinicians-providers/ guidelines-recommendations/guide/

Webster's New World College Dictionary (5th ed.). (2014). Boston, MA: Houghton Mifflin Harcourt.

CHAPTER 88

Major Causes of Mortality in the United States

BARBARA A. S. BROOME

LEADING CAUSES OF DEATH IN THE UNITED STATES

I.   **Male and female, all ages (see Tables 88.1–88.4)**
   A. Diseases of the heart
   B. Malignant neoplasms
   C. Chronic lower respiratory disease
   D. Cerebrovascular disease
   E. Accidents (unintentional injuries)
   F. Alzheimer's disease
   G. Diabetes mellitus
   H. Influenza and pneumonia
   I. Nephritis, nephritic syndrome, and nephrosis
   J. Intentional self-harm (suicide)

Table 88.1	Leading Causes of Death		
Rank	**Hispanic**	**Caucasian**	**Black**
1	Diseases of the heart such as rheumatic fever and hypertension	Diseases of the heart such as rheumatic fever and hypertension	Diseases of the heart such as rheumatic fever and hypertension
2	Malignant neoplasms	Malignant neoplasms	Malignant neoplasms
3	Accidents (unintentional injuries)	Chronic lower respiratory diseases	Cerebrovascular diseases: hypertension
4	Cerebrovascular diseases	Cerebrovascular disease	Accidents (unintentional injuries)
5	Diabetes mellitus	Accidents (unintentional injuries)	Diabetes mellitus

Table 88.1	Leading Causes of Death		
Rank	Hispanic	Caucasian	Black
6	Chronic liver disease and cirrhosis	Alzheimer's disease	Assault (homicide)
7	Assault	Diabetes mellitus	Chronic lower respiratory diseases
8	Chronic lower respiratory diseases	Influenza and pneumonia	Nephritis, nephrotic syndrome, and nephrosis
9	Influenza and pneumonia	Nephritis, nephritic syndrome, and nephrosis	HIV
10	Certain conditions originating during the perinatal period	Intentional self-harm (suicide)	Septicemia

Table 88.2	Leading Cause of Death, Females		
Rank	Hispanic	Caucasian	Black
1	Malignant neoplasms	Diseases of the heart	Diseases of the heart
2	Diseases of heart	Malignant neoplasms	Malignant neoplasms
3	Cerebrovascular diseases	Chronic lower respiratory diseases	Cerebrovascular diseases
4	Diabetes mellitus	Cerebrovascular diseases	Diabetes mellitus
5	Accidents (unintentional injuries)	Alzheimer's disease	Nephritis, nephritic syndrome, and Nephrosis
6	Alzheimer's disease	Accidents (unintentional injuries)	Chronic lower respiratory diseases
7	Chronic lower respiratory disease	Diabetes mellitus	Accidents (unintentional injuries)
8	Nephritis, nephrotic syndrome, and nephrosis	Influenza and pneumonia	Alzheimer's disease
9	Influenza and pneumonia	Nephritis, nephrotic syndrome, and nephrosis	Septicemia
10	Chronic liver disease and cirrhosis	Septicemia	Essential hypertension and hypertensive renal disease

Table 88.3	Leading Cause of Death, Males		
Rank	**Hispanic**	**Caucasian**	**Black**
1	Malignant neoplasms	Diseases of the heart	Diseases of the heart
2	Diseases of heart	Malignant neoplasms	Malignant neoplasms
3	Accidents (unintentional injuries)	Accidents (unintentional injuries)	Accidents (unintentional injuries)
4	Cerebrovascular diseases	Chronic lower respiratory disease	Cerebrovascular diseases
5	Diabetes mellitus	Cerebrovascular diseases	Homicide
6	Chronic liver disease and cirrhosis	Diabetes mellitus	Diabetes mellitus
7	Homicide	Intentional self-harm (suicide)	Chronic lower respiratory disease
8	Chronic lower respiratory diseases	Alzheimer's disease	Nephritis, nephritic syndrome, and nephrosis
9	Suicide	Influenza and pneumonia	HIV
10	Nephritis, nephrotic syndrome, and nephrosis	Nephritis, nephrotic syndrome, and nephrosis	Septicemia

Table 88.4	Leading Causes of Death, All Races/Sexes		
Rank	Ages 15–19 years	Ages 20–24 years	Ages 25–29 years	Ages 30–34 years
1	Accidents (unintentional injuries)	Accidents (unintentional injuries)	Accidents (unintentional injuries)	Accidents
2	Assault (homicide)	Assault (homicide)	Intentional self-harm (suicide)	Intentional self-harm (suicide)
3	Intentional self-harm (suicide)	Malignant neoplasms	Assault	Malignant neoplasms)
4	Malignant neoplasms	Malignant neoplasms	Malignant neoplasms	Diseases of the heart
5	Diseases of the heart	Diseases of the heart	Diseases of the heart	Assault (homicide)
Rank	Ages 15–19 years	Ages 20–24 years	Ages 25–29 years	Ages 30–34 years

Table 88.4	Leading Causes of Death, All Races/Sexes		
6	Congenital malformations, deformations, and chromosomal abnormalities	Congenital malformation, deformations, and chromosomal abnormalities	HIV	HIV
7	Cerebrovascular diseases	Influenza and pneumonia	Diabetes mellitus	Diabetes mellitus
8	Chronic lower respiratory diseases	HIV	Congenital malformation, deformations, and chromosomal abnormalities	Chronic liver disease and cirrhosis
9	Influenza and pneumonia	Pregnancy, childbirth, and the puerperium	Pregnancy, childbirth, and the puerperium	Cerebrovascular disease
10	In situ neoplasms, benign neoplasms of uncertain or unknown behavior	Diabetes mellitus	Influenza and pneumonia	Influenza and pneumonia
Rank	Ages 35–39 years	Ages 40–45 years	Ages 45–49 years	Ages 50–54 years
1	Accidents (unintentional injuries)	Accidents (Unintentional injuries	Malignant neoplasms	Malignant neoplasms
2	Malignant neoplasms	Malignant neoplasms	Diseases of the heart	Diseases of the heart
3	Intentional self-harm (suicide)	Diseases of the heart	Accidents (unintentional injuries)	Accidents (unintentional injuries)
4	Intentional self-harm (suicide)	Intentional self-harm (suicide)	Intentional self-harm (suicide)	Chronic liver disease and cirrhosis
5	Assault (homicide)	Chronic liver disease and cirrhosis	Chronic liver disease and cirrhosis	Intentional self-harm (suicide)
6	Chronic liver disease and cirrhosis	Cerebrovascular disease	Cerebrovascular disease	Cerebrovascular disease
Rank	Ages 35–39 years	Ages 40–45 years	Ages 45–49 years	Ages 50–54 years

Table 88.4	Leading Causes of Death, All Races/Sexes			
7	HIV	HIV	Diabetes mellitus	Diabetes mellitus
8	Diabetes mellitus	Diabetes mellitus	HIV	Chronic lower respiratory disease
9	Cerebrovascular disease	Assault (homicide)	Chronic lower respiratory diseases	Viral hepatitis
10	Septicemia	Influenza and pneumonia	Assault (homicide)`	HIV
Rank	Ages 55–59 years	Ages 60–64 years	Ages 65–69 years	Ages 70–74 years
1	Malignant neoplasms	Malignant neoplasms	Malignant neoplasms	Malignant neoplasms
2	Diseases of heart	Diseases of heart	Diseases of heart	Diseases of heart
3	Accidents (unintentional injuries)	Chronic lower respiratory diseases	Chronic lower respiratory disease	Chronic lower respiratory diseases
4	Chronic liver disease and cirrhosis	Diabetes mellitus	Cerebrovascular diseases	Cerebrovascular disease
5	Chronic lower respiratory diseases	Cerebrovascular diseases	Diabetes mellitus	Diabetes mellitus
6	Diabetes mellitus	Accidents (unintentional injuries)	Accidents (unintentional injuries)	Nephritis, nephrotic syndrome, and nephrosis
7	Cerebrovascular diseases	Chronic liver disease	Nephritis, nephrotic syndrome, and nephrosis	Accidents (unintentional injuries)
8	Intentional self-harm (suicide)	Nephritis, nephrotic syndrome, and nephrosis	Chronic liver disease and cirrhosis	Influenza and pneumonia
9	Nephritis, nephrotic syndrome, and nephrosis	Intentional self-harm (suicide)	Septicemia	Septicemia
10	Septicemia	Septicemia	Influenza and pneumonia	Alzheimer's disease
Rank	Ages 75–79 years	Ages 80–84 years	Ages 85–89 years	Age 90–95 years

Table 88.4	Leading Causes of Death, All Races/Sexes		
1	Malignant neoplasms	Diseases of heart	Diseases of heart	Diseases of heart
2	Diseases of heart	Malignant neoplasms	Malignant neoplasm	Malignant neoplasms
3	Chronic lower respiratory disease	Chronic lower respiratory disease	Cerebrovascular diseases	Alzheimer's disease
4	Cerebrovascular disease	Cerebrovascular disease	Alzheimer's disease	Cerebrovascular disease
5	Diabetes mellitus	Alzheimer's disease	Chronic lower respiratory disease	Chronic lower respiratory disease
6	Alzheimer's disease	Diabetes mellitus	Influenza and pneumonia	Influenza and pneumonia
7	Nephritis, nephrotic syndrome, and nephrosis	Nephritis, nephrotic syndrome, and nephrosis	Nephritis, nephrotic syndrome, and nephrosis	Nephritis, nephrotic syndrome, and nephrosis
8	Accidents (unintentional injuries	Influenza and pneumonia	Accidents (unintentional injuries)	Accidents (unintentional injuries)
9	Influenza and pneumonia	Accidental (unintentional injuries)	Diabetes mellitus	Diabetes mellitus
10	Septicemia	Parkinson's disease	Parkinson's disease	Essential hypertension and hypertensive renal disease

Tables adapted with permission from:

U. S. Department of Health and Human Services, National Center for Health Statistics (2012). LCWK1. Deaths, percent of total deaths, and death rates for the 15 leading causes of death in 5-year age groups, by race and sex: United States, 2010. Retrieved November 2013 from http://www.cdc.gov/nchs/data/dvs/LCWK1_2010.pdf

U.S. Census Bureau. (2011). Section 2: Births, Deaths, Marriages and Divorces. Retrieved September 26, 2014 from http://www.census.gov/prod/2011pubs/12statab/vitstat.pdf

U.S. Department of Health and Human Services, National Center for Health Statistics. (2013). Table 23: Leading Causes of Death and Numbers of Death by Age, United States, 1980 and 2010. Retrieved November 2013 from http://www.cdc.gov/nchs/data/hus/2013/023.pdf

tRISK ASSESSMENT

I. **Cardiac and cerebrovascular diseases**
   A. Obesity (20%–40% over ideal weight) is a risk factor for hypertension, stroke, myocardial infarction, and diabetes
   B. Hypertension (gold standard, greater than 120/80 mmHg)
   C. High triglycerides (goal: less than 150 mg/dl)
   D. Elevated cholesterol level (desirable: less than 200 mg/dl)
   E. Sedentary lifestyle
   F. Lower socioeconomic group; poverty is associated with increased health risk
   G. African American race increases cardiovascular risk
   H. Assess risk profile by stratifying risk and quantifying prognosis
   I. Smoking
   J. Diabetes
   K. Family history of cardiac or respiratory disease
II. **Malignant neoplasms**
   A. Use of tobacco
   B. Diet high in fat
   C. Extended exposure to sun
   D. Diet low in servings of fruits and vegetables (five servings recommended)
   E. Infection (especially associated with cervical cancer and human papillomavirus)
   F. Family history
   G. Exposure to toxins in environment/workplace
   H. Minorities are at greater risk for morbidity/mortality
III. **Chronic lower respiratory diseases**
   A. Smoking, tobacco use
   B. Passive exposure to smoke
   C. Occupational toxins (air pollution)
   D. Environmental toxins (air pollution)
   E. Poor nutrition
   F. Frequent lower respiratory infection during childhood
IV. **Accidents**
   A. Alcoholism
   B. Drug use
   C. Occupational hazards
   D. Environmental hazards
   E. Assess use of car safety equipment (seat belts)
   F. Assess use of helmets (for all cyclists)
   G. Assess fatigue (shift workers)
V. **Alzheimer's disease**
   A. Increased age (ages 65 years and older)
   B. Family history of Alzheimer's disease
   C. Altered blood circulation is hypothesized to be related

VI.   Diabetes
  A. Obesity (more than 20% over ideal body weight)
  B. Ages 45 years and older
  C. Higher in non-Caucasian race
  D. Low high-density lipoproteins (35 mg/dl) or triglyceride level higher than 250 mg/dl
  E. Hypertension
  F. Family history
  G. History of gestational diabetes or delivery of babies weighing more than 9 pounds

VII.   Influenza and pneumonia
  A. Assess vaccination yearly for influenza
  B. Assess pneumonia vaccination
  C. Risk increases with age

VIII.   Nephritis, nephritic syndrome, and nephrosis
  A. History of autoimmune disease
  B. Family history (Alport syndrome)
  C. History of streptococcal infection
  D. Diabetes mellitus
  E. HIV

IX.   Intentional self-harm (suicide)
  A. Substance abuse
  B. Gender and age
    1. Female, 45–54 years of age
    2. Male, 75 years and older
  C. American Indian/Alaskan Native

BIBLIOGRAPHY

Heron, M. (2012). Deaths: Leading causes for 2008. *National Vital Statistics Reports, 60*(6). Retrieved November 2013 from http://www.cdc.gov/nchs/data/nvsr/nvsr60/nvsr60_06.pdf

Hoyert, D. L., & Xu, J. (2012). Deaths: Preliminary Data for 2011. *National Vital Statistics Reports, 61*(6). Retrieved November 2013 from http://www.cdc.gov/nchs/data/nvsr/nvsr61/nvsr61_06.pdf

Kochanek, K. D., Arias, E., & Anderson, R. N. (2013). How did cause of death contribute to racial differences in life expectancy in the United States in 2010? *NCHS Data Brief (125)*. Retrieved November 2013 from http://health-equity.pitt.edu/id/eprint/4148

Murphy, S. L., Xu, J., & Kochanek, K. D. (2013). Deaths: Final data for 2010. *National Vital Statistics Reports, 61*(4). Retrieved November 2013 from http://www.cdc.gov/nchs/data/nvsr/nvsr61/nvsr61_04.pdf

U.S. Department of Health and Human Services, National Center for Health Statistics. (2012). *LCWK1. Deaths, percent of total deaths, and death rates for the 15 leading causes of death in 5-year age groups, by race and sex: United States, 2010.* Retrieved November 2013 from http://www.cdc.gov/nchs/data/dvs/LCWK1_2010.pdf

U.S. Census Bureau. (2011). *Section 2: Births, deaths, marriages and divorces.* Retrieved September 26, 2014 from http://www.census.gov/prod/2011pubs/12statab/vitstat.pdf

U.S. Department of Health and Human Services, National Center for Health Statistics (2013). *Table 23. Leading causes of death and numbers of deaths, by age: United States, 1980 and 2010.* Retrieved November 2013 from http://www.cdc.gov/nchs/data/hus/2013/023.pdf

CHAPTER 89

Immunization Recommendations

ALICIA HUCKSTADT • THOMAS W. BARKLEY, JR. • CHARLENE M. MYERS

IMMUNIZATION

I.   Definition

A. A mechanism to help prevent morbidity and mortality from infectious diseases

B. Immunizations help develop immunity by imitating an infection by causing the immune system to produce T-lymphocytes and antibodies.

C. Immunity is defined as resistance of a host that is developed in response to a stimulus by a foreign antigen or pathogen.

D. An antigen is a foreign or self-molecule that is recognized by the adaptive and innate immune system, resulting in immune cell triggering.

E. Antibodies are made up of immunoglobulin proteins produced by B lymphocytes; they have the property of recognizing unique antigenic molecular structures and help eliminate the antigen.

F. Immunization and vaccination are often used interchangeably; however, vaccination is the action of administering a vaccine, and immunization is the process of inducing or providing immunity that is active or passive.

G. Active immunity is achieved through the introduction of a specific agent to induce antibody formation; this process involves the use of live-attenuated agents or inactivated agents.

H. Live-attenuated agents contain a version of the living virus or bacteria that has been weakened so it does not cause serious disease in healthy people with normal immune systems.

I. Inactivated agents are made by inactivating or killing the virus or bacteria during the making of the vaccine.

J. Often multiple doses are necessary to build or maintain adequate immunity. Toxoid vaccines prevent diseases caused by bacteria that produce toxins in the body by using weakened toxins (toxoids), and the immune system alters itself to resist the natural toxin.

K. Passive immunity is achieved through transfer of antibody proteins such as maternal immunity to the fetus or administration of gamma globulin injections to immunodeficient patients or after accidental exposure to a known infectious substance.

L. Types
  1. Live-attenuated virus
     a. Measles
     b. Mumps
     c. Parainfluenza virus
     d. Poliovirus (oral)
     e. Respiratory syncytial virus
     f. Rubella
     g. Varicella
     h. Yellow fever
     i. Herpes zoster
  2. Live-attenuated bacteria
     a. Bacillus Calmette-Guérin (BCG)
     b. Tulare
     c. Typhoid (oral)
  3. Inactivated virus
     a. Hepatitis A
     b. Hepatitis B
     c. Human papillomavirus
     d. Influenza
     e. Poliovirus (subcutaneous)
     f. Rabies
  4. Inactivated bacteria
     a. Anthrax
     b. Cholera
     c. Diphtheria (toxoid)
     d. Gonococcus
     e. *Haemophilus influenzae* type b (polysaccharide/protein conjugate)
     f. Lyme disease
     g. Meningococcus (polysaccharide)
     h. Pertussis (acellular)
     i. Pertussis (inactivated whole bacteria)
     j. Plague
     k. Pneumococcus (polysaccharide)
     l. Pneumococcus (polysaccharide/protein conjugate)
     m. Tetanus (toxoid)
     n. Typhoid (subcutaneous)
     o. Inactivated rickettsiae: Q fever (*Coxiella burnetii*)

II. **Initiation of active immunity is not without risk when live-attenuated preparations are used; the most important factor involved in contraindications to a vaccine is the recipient's immunocompetence.**

    A. Severely immunocompromised patients usually should not receive live-attenuated vaccines because of the potentially lethal risk.

    B. Although killed vaccines may be given to immunocompromised persons, the immune response may be inadequate and no protective efficacy is clearly evident.

III. **Consult manufacturer's recommendations in the package insert for specific doses, schedules, routes of administration, and potential adverse effects.**

IV. **Education regarding the specific vaccination and consent for administration of vaccines must be obtained before administration.**

V. **Documentation on patients' records should include dose, route of administration, manufacturer, and lot number.**

VI. **Instructions for reporting adverse events to the Vaccine Adverse Event Reporting System are available at http://www.vaers.hhs. gov, or by telephone at 800–822–7967 or FAX at 877–721–0366.**

VII. **International travelers may encounter risks when visiting other countries; specific vaccinations are required by different countries.**

    A. Recommendations from the Centers for Disease Control and Prevention can be accessed at the following Internet address: www. cdc.gov/travel/

    B. Recommendations and information on disease outbreaks by country and region are available at the above web site

VIII. **Current information on immunizations and vaccines can be accessed from the Centers for Disease Control National Centers for Immunization and Respiratory Diseases (NCIRD) at the following internet address: http://www.cdc.gov/ncird/**

IX. **Immunization schedules (see Tables 89.1 and 89.2) are available for health care professions and are available at http://www. cdc.gov/vaccines/schedules/ and available in various printable formats, download as an interactive tool or download to a smartphone. Vaccine recommendations of the Advisory Committee for Immunization Practices (ACIP) are available at http://www.cdc.gov/vaccines/hcp/acip-recs/index.html and updates are provided.**

Table 89.1

2014 Recommended Immunizations for Adults by Age

	19–21 years	22–26 years	27–49 years	50–59 years	60–64 years	65+ years
Influenza (Flu)	Get a flu vaccine every year					
Tetanus, diphtheria, pertussis (Td/Tdap)	Get a Tdap vaccine once, then a Td booster vaccine every 10 years					
Varicella (Chickenpox)	2 doses					
HPV vaccine (women)	3 doses					
HPV vaccine (men)	3 doses	3 doses				
Zoster (Shingles)					1 dose	
Measles, mumps, rubella (MMR)	1 or 2 doses					
Pneumococcal (PCV13)	1 dose					
Pneumococcal (PPSV23)	1 or 2 doses					1 dose
Meningococcal	1 or more doses					
Hepatitis A	2 doses					
Hepatitis B	3 doses					
***Haemophilus influenza* type b (Hib)**	1 or 3 doses					

Boxes this color show that the vaccine is recommended for all adults who have not been vaccinated unless healthcare provider tells them that they can safely receive the vaccine or that it is not needed

Boxes this color show that the vaccine is recommended for adults with certain risks related to their health, job, or lifestyle that put them at higher risk for certain diseases.

No recommendation

Note. Modified from "2014 Recommended Immunizations for Adults by Age" by the U.S. Department of Health and Human Services, Centers for Disease Control and Prevention, 2014. Retrieved from http://www.cdc.gov/vaccines/schedules/downloads/adult/adult-schedule-easy-read-bw.pdf. See website for more information regarding each immunization.

Table 89.2 2014 Recommended Immunizations for Adults by Medical Condition

Vaccine	Pregnancy	Weakened immune system (not HIV)	HIV infection CD4 < 200	HIV infection CD4 ≥ 200	Kidney disease or poor kidney function	Asplenia	Heart disease, chronic lung disease, chronic alcoholism	Diabetes (Type 1 and 2)	Chronic liver disease
Influenza (Flu)	Get a flu vaccine every year	Get a flu vaccine every year	Get a flu vaccine every year	Get a flu vaccine every year	Get a flu vaccine every year	Get a flu vaccine every year	Get a flu vaccine every year	Get a flu vaccine every year	Get a flu vaccine every year
Tetanus, diphtheria, pertussis (Td/Tdap)	1 dose Tdap each pregnancy	Get Tdap vaccine once, then a Td booster every 10 years	Get Tdap vaccine once, then a Td booster every 10 years	Get Tdap vaccine once, then a Td booster every 10 years	Get Tdap vaccine once, then a Td booster every 10 years	Get Tdap vaccine once, then a Td booster every 10 years	Get Tdap vaccine once, then a Td booster every 10 years	Get Tdap vaccine once, then a Td booster every 10 years	Get Tdap vaccine once, then a Td booster every 10 years
Varicella (Chickenpox)	Should not get vaccine	Should not get vaccine	Should not get vaccine	2 doses	2 doses	2 doses	2 doses	2 doses	2 doses
HPV vaccine (women)		3 doses through age 26 years	3 doses through age 26 years	3 doses through age 26 years	3 doses through age 26 years				
HPV vaccine (men)		3 doses through age 21 years	3 doses through age 21 years	3 doses through age 21 years	3 doses through age 21 years				
Zoster (Shingles)	Should not get vaccine	Should not get vaccine	Should not get vaccine	Should not get vaccine	1 dose for those 60 years and older	1 dose for those 60 years and older	1 dose for those 60 years and older	1 dose for those 60 years and older	1 dose for those 60 years and older
Measles, mumps, rubella (MMR)	Should not get vaccine	Should not get vaccine	Should not get vaccine	1 or 2 doses	1 or 2 doses	1 or 2 doses	1 or 2 doses	1 or 2 doses	1 or 2 doses
Pneumococcal (PCV13)		1 dose	1 dose	1 dose	1 dose	1 dose			
Pneumococcal (PPSV23)		1 or 2 doses	1 or 2 doses	1 or 2 doses	1 or 2 doses	1 or 2 doses	1 dose	1 dose	1 dose
Meningococcal		1 or more doses	1 or more doses	1 or more doses	1 or more doses	1 or more doses	1 or more doses		
Hepatitis A		2 doses	2 doses	2 doses	2 doses	2 doses	2 doses	2 doses	2 doses
Hepatitis B		3 doses	3 doses	3 doses	3 doses	3 doses	3 doses	3 doses	3 doses
Haemophilus influenza type b (Hib)		Post HSCT recipients only	Post HSCT recipients only	Post HSCT recipients only	1 or 3 doses	1 or 3 doses			

Table 89.2	2014 Recommended Immunizations for Adults by Medical Condition		
	Boxes this color show that the vaccine is recommended for all adults who have not been vaccinated unless healthcare provider tells them that they can safely receive the vaccine or that it is not needed	Boxes this color show that the vaccine is recommended for adults with certain risks related to their health, job, or lifestyle that put them at higher risk for certain diseases.	Boxes this color indicate that the adult should not get the vaccine	No recommendation

Note. Modified from "2014 Recommended Immunizations for Adults by Medical Condition" by the U.S. Department of Health and Human Services, Centers for Disease Control and Prevention, 2014. Retrieved from http://www.cdc.gov/vaccines/schedules/downloads/adult/adult-schedule-easy-read-bw.pdf. See website for more information regarding each immunization.

BIBLIOGRAPHY

Chin-Hong, P. V., & Guglielmo, B. J. (2013). Common problems in infectious diseases and antimicrobial therapy. In M. A. Papadakis, S. J. McPhee, & M. W. Rabow (Eds.), *Current medical diagnosis & treatment* (53rd ed., pp. 1276–1318). New York, NY: McGraw-Hill/Appleton & Lange.

Cohn, A. C, & Harrison, L. H. (2013). Meningococcal vaccines: Current issues and future strategies. *Drugs, 73*(11), 1147–1155. doi:10.1007/s40265–013–0079–2

Grossman, S. C., & Porth, C. M. (Eds.) (2014). *Porth's pathophysiology: Concepts of altered health states* (9th ed.). Philadelphia, PA: Wolters Kluwer Health/Lippincott Williams & Wilkins.

Immunization Action Coalition. (2014). *Handouts for patients & staff.* Retrieved December 10, 2013, from http://www.immunize.org/handouts/?f=8

Immunization Action Coalition. (2014). *Diseases and vaccines.* Retrieved December 10, 2013, from http://www.immunize.org/vaccines/

Longo, D. L., Fauci, A. S., Kasper, D. L., Hauser, S. L., Jameson, J. L., & Loscalzo, J. (Eds.). (2012). *Harrison's principles of internal medicine* (18th ed.). New York, NY: McGraw-Hill.

U.S. Department of Health and Human Services, Centers for Disease Control and Prevention. (2013). Advisory Committee on Immunization Practices (ACIP) recommended immunization schedules for persons aged 0 through 18 years and adults aged 19 years and older—United States, 2013. *Morbidity and Mortality Weekly Report, 62*(Supplement). Retrieved December 11, 2013, from http://www.cdc.gov/mmwr/pdf/other/su6201.pdf. And errata http://www.cdc.gov/mmwr/preview/mmwrhtml/mm6213a6.htm?s_cid=mm6213a6_w

U.S. Department of Health and Human Services, Centers for Disease Control and Prevention. (2013). *Combined Tdap vaccine.* Retrieved February 17, 2014, from http://www.cdc.gov/vaccines/vpd-vac/combo-vaccines/DTaP-Td-DT/tdap.htm

U.S. Department of Health and Human Services, Centers for Disease Control and Prevention. (2013). *Travelers' health: Yellow book* (Health information for international travel). Retrieved December 10, 2013, from http://wwwnc.cdc.gov/travel/page/yellowbook-home-2014

U.S. Department of Health and Human Services, Centers for Disease Control and Prevention. (2013). *Vaccines and immunizations: Mumps vaccination.* Retrieved December 10, 2013, from http://www.cdc.gov/vaccines/vpd-vac/mumps/default.htm

U.S. Department of Health and Human Services, Centers for Disease Control and Prevention. (2013). *Vaccine recommendations of the Advisory Committee for Immunization Practices (ACIP).* Retrieved December 11, 2013, from http://www.cdc.gov/vaccines/hcp/acip-recs/index.html

U.S. Department of Health and Human Services, Centers for Disease Control and Prevention. (2014). *Emergency preparedness and response*. Retrieved September 26, 2014, from http://www.bt.cdc.gov//

U.S. Department of Health and Human Services, Center for Disease Control and Prevention. (2014). *Human Papillomavirus vaccination*. Retrieved September 26, 2014, from http://www.cdc.gov/vaccines/vpd-vac/hpv/

U.S. Department of Health and Human Services, Centers for Disease Control and Prevention. (2014). *Immunization schedules*. Retrieved February 17, 2014, from http://www.cdc.gov/vaccines/schedules/index.html

U.S. Department of Health and Human Services, Centers for Disease Control and Prevention. (2014). *Shingles (herpes zoster) vaccination*. Retrieved September 26, 2014, from www.cdc.gov/vaccines/vpd-vac/shingles/default.htm#vacc

U.S. Department of Health and Human Services, Centers for Disease Control and Prevention. (2014). *Travelers' health*. Retrieved September 26, 2014, from www.cdc.gov/travel/

U.S. Department of Health and Human Services, Centers for Disease Control and Prevention. (2014). *Vaccines and immunizations*. Retrieved July 28, 2014, from http://www.cdc.gov/vaccines/default.htm

U.S. Department of Health and Human Services, Centers for Disease Control and Prevention. (2014) *Vaccines & immunizations: Meningococcal vaccination*. Retrieved September 26, 2014, from http://www.cdc.gov/vaccines/vpd-vac/mening/default.htm

U.S. Department of Health and Human Services, Centers for Disease Control and Prevention. (2014). *Viral hepatitis*. Retrieved February 17, 2014, from http://www.cdc.gov/hepatitis/index.htm

U.S. Department of Health and Human Services, National Center for Immunization and Respiratory Diseases (NCIRD). (2014). Retrieved July 28, 2014, from http://www.cdc.gov/ncird/

U.S. Department of Health and Human Services, National Institute of Allergy and Infectious Diseases. (2013, November 27). *FDA study helps provide an understanding of rising rates of whooping cough and response to vaccination*. Retrieved December 10, 2013, from http://www.niaid.nih.gov/news/newsreleases/2013/Pages/FDApertussis.aspx#

U.S. Department of Health and Human Services, National Institute of Allergy and Infectious Diseases. (2014). *Home page*. Retrieved September 26, 2014, from http://www.niaid.nih.gov/Pages/default.aspx

Walsh, S. R., & Dolin, R. (2011). Vaccinia viruses: Vaccines against smallpox and vectors against infectious diseases and tumors. *Expert Review of Vaccines, 10*(8), 1221–1240. doi:10.1586/erv.11.79

World Health Organization. (2014). *Infectious diseases*. Retrieved September 26, 2014, from http://www.who.int/topics/infectious_diseases/en/

Woo, T. M., & Wynne, A. L. (2011). *Pharmacotherapeutics for nurse practitioner prescribers* (3rd ed.). Philadelphia, PA: F. A. Davis Company.

APPENDIX

Appendix A. ICD-9 Codes		
Chapter	**Condition/Topic**	**ICD-9 Code**
Section 1. Management of Patients with Neurological Disorders		
Cerebrovascular Accidents: Brain Attack	Hemorrhagic stroke	431
	Ischemic stroke	434.91
	Stroke/brain attack	434.91
	Transient ischemic attack	436
Structural Abnormalities	Aneurysm	442.9
	Hydrocephalus	331.4
Peripheral Neuropathies	Guillain-Barre syndrome	357.0
	Myasthenia gravis	358.00
Neurologic Trauma	Head trauma/traumatic brain injury	959.01
	Spinal cord trauma	952.9
Central Nervous System Disorders	Cerebral abscess	324.0
	Encephalitis	323.9
	Encephalopathy	348.30
	Meningitis	322.9
Seizure Disorders	Seizure disorders	780.39
Dementia	Dementia	290.8
Multiple sclerosis	Multiple sclerosis	340
Parkinson's Disease	Parkinson's disease	332.0
Amyotrophic Lateral Sclerosis	Amyotrophic lateral sclerosis	335.20
Section 2. Management of Patients with Cardiovascular Disorders		
Cardiovascular Assessment	Cardiovascular disorders	306.2
Hypertension	Hypertension	401.9
Coronary Artery Disease and Hyperlipidemia	Coronary artery disease	414.00
	Hyperlipidemia	272.4
Angina and Myocardial Infarction	Angina	413.9
	Myocardial infarction	410.9
Adjunct Equipment/ Devices		
Peripheral Vascular Disease	Deep vein thrombosis	453.8
	Occlusive arterial disease	444.22
	Peripheral vascular disease	443.9
	Thromboangiitis obliterans (Buerger's disease)	443.1
	Venous disease	459.9
Inflammatory Cardiac Diseases	Endocarditis	424.90
	Pericarditis	423.9
Heart Failure	Heart failure	428.9

Valvular Disease	Aortic regurgitation	424.1
	Aortic stenosis	424.1
	Mitral regurgitation	424.0
	Mitral stenosis	394.0
	Mitral valve prolapse	424.0
	Valvular disease	459.9
Cardiomyopathy	Cardiomyopathy	425.4
Arrhythmias	Agonal rhythm	427.89
	Asystole	427.5
	Atrial fibrillation	427.31
	Atrial flutter	427.32
	Cardiac rhythms/arrhythmias	427.9
	First-degree AV block	426.11
	Idioventricular rhythm	426.89
	Junctional/nodal	427.89
	Premature atrial contractions	427.61
	Premature ventricular contractions	427.69
	Pulseless electrical activity	427.89
	Second-degree block (Mobitz type I) (Wenckebach)	426.13
	Second-degree block (Mobitz type II)	426.12
	Sinus arrhythmia	427.9
	Sinus bradycardia	427.89
	Sinus tachycardia	427.89
	Supraventricular tachycardia	427.89
	Third-degree AV block (complete heart block)	426.0
	Ventricular fibrillation	427.41
	Ventricular tachycardia	427.1

Section 3. Management of Pulmonary Disorders

Diagnostic Concepts of Oxygenation and Ventilation	Respiratory measurement	89.38
Measures of Oxygen and Ventilation	Respiratory measurement	89.38
The Chest X-Ray	Congestive heart failure	428.0
	Emphysema	492.8
	Pericardial effusions	423.9
	Pneumonia	486
	Pulmonary nodules (also called coin lesions)	793.1

Pulmonary Function Testing	Abnormal results of pulmonary function studies	794.2
Obstructive (Ventilatory) Lung Diseases	Asthma	493.9
	Bronchiectasis	494.0
	Chronic bronchitis	491.9
	Chronic obstructive pulmonary disease	496
	Emphysema	492.8
	Obstructive airway lesions	519.8
Restrictive (Inflammatory) Lung Diseases	Acute lung injury	861.20
	Acute respiratory distress syndrome	518.5
	Cardiogenic pulmonary edema	514
	Congestive heart failure	428.0
	Idiopathic pulmonary fibrosis	515
	Pneumonia	486
	Pulmonary edema	514
	Restrictive (inflammatory) lung diseases	518.89
	Sarcoidosis	135
	Tuberculosis	011.90
Pulmonary Hypertension and Pulmonary Vascular Disorders	Pulmonary hypertension	416.0
Chest Wall and Secondary Pleural Disorders	Pleural disorders	511.0
	Chest wall disorders	306.2
Respiratory Failure	Acute respiratory failure	518.81
	Chronic respiratory failure	518.83
	Shock	785.50
Pneumothorax	Pneumothorax	512.8
Lower Respiratory Tract Pathogens	Acute tracheobronchitis	466.0
	Chronic obstructive pulmonary disease	496
	Pneumonia, community-acquired	486
Obstructive Sleep Apnea	Obstructive sleep apnea	327.23
Oxygen Supplementation	Dependence on supplemental oxygen	V46.2
Mechanical Ventilatory Support	Dependence on respiratory ventilator	V46.11
Section 4. Management of Patients with Gastrointestinal Disorders		
Peptic Ulcer Disease	Gastroesophageal reflux disease	530.81
	Peptic ulcer disease	533.9

Liver Disease	Hepatic failure	572.8
	Hepatitis	573.3
Biliary Dysfunction	Acute pancreatitis	577.0
	Cholecystitis	575.10
Inflammatory Gastrointestinal Disorders	Appendicitis	541
	Diverticulitis	562.11
	Peritonitis	567.9
	Ulcerative colitis	556.9
Anatomic Intestinal Disorders	Mesenteric ischemia	557.9
	Small-bowel obstruction	560.9
Gastrointestinal Bleeding	Esophageal varices	456.1
	Lower gastrointestinal bleeding	578.9
	Upper gastrointestinal bleeding	578.9

Section 5. Management of Patients with Genitourinary Disorders

Urinary Tract Infections	Urinary tract infections	599.0
Renal Insufficiency and Failure	Acute renal failure	584.9
	Chronic renal failure	585.9
Benign Prostatic Hyperplasia	Benign prostatic hypertrophy	600.00
Renal Artery Stenosis	Renal artery stenosis	440.1
Nephrolithiasis	Renal calculi-nephrolithiasis	592.0

Section 6. Management of Patients with Endocrine Disorders

Diabetes Mellitus	Diabetes mellitus	250.00
	Type 1 diabetes mellitus	250.01
	Type 2 diabetes mellitus	250.02
Diabetic Emergencies	Diabetic ketoacidosis	250.30
	Hyperosmolar hyperglycemic non-ketosis	250.20
	Hypoglycemia	251.2
Thyroid Disease	Hyperthyroidism (thyrotoxicosis)	242.90
	Hypothyroidism (myxedema coma)	244.9
	Thyroid storm (thyrotoxic crisis)	242.91
Cushing's Syndrome	Cushing's syndrome	255.0
Primary Adrenocortical Insufficiency (Addison Disease) & Adrenal Crisis	Addison disease	359.5
	Addisonian crisis	255.41
	Primary adrenocortical insufficiency	255.41
Pheochromocytoma	Pheochromocytoma	194.0

Syndrome of Inappropriate Antidiuretic Hormone	Syndrome of inappropriate antidiuretic hormone	253.6
Diabetes Insipidus	Diabetes insipidus	253.5

Section 7. Management of Musculoskeletal Disorders

Arthritis	Gout	274.9
	Osteoarthritis	715.9
	Rheumatoid arthritis	714.0
Subluxations and Dislocations	Dislocation of ankle	718.37
	Dislocation of shoulder	718.31
	Dislocation of hand	718.34
	Dislocation of hip	835
	Dislocation of shoulder joint	831
	Subluxation of unspecified scapula	831.09
	Subluxation of wrist and hand	833
Soft Tissue Injury	Disorders of soft tissue	729.90
	Soft tissue disorder related to use, overuse, and pressure	729.90
Fractures	Closed fracture	924.8
	Open fracture	924.8
	Stress fracture	733.95
Compartment syndrome	Compartment syndrome	958.8
Back Pain Syndromes	Herniated disk	722.2
	Low back pain	724.2

Section 8. Management of Patients with Hematologic Disorders

Anemias	Anemia of chronic disease (ACD)	285.29
	Anemias	285.9
	Folic acid deficiency	281.2
	Iron deficiency	280.9
	Pernicious anemia	281.0
	Thalassemia	282.49
	Vitamin B12 deficiency	281.1
Sickle Cell Disease/Crisis	Sickle cell disease/crisis	282.60
Coagulopathies	Disseminated intravascular coagulation	286.6
	Heparin-induced thrombocytopenia	287.4
	Idiopathic thrombocytopenic purpura	287.3

Section 9. Management of Patients with Oncologic Disorders

Leukemias	Acute lymphocytic leukemia	204.0
	Acute myelogenous leukemia	205.0
	Chronic lymphocytic leukemia	204.1
	Chronic myelogenous leukemia	205.1
Lymphoma	Hodgkin's disease	201.9
	Lymphoma	202.8
	Non-Hodgkin's lymphoma	202.8
Other Common Cancers	Bladder cancer	188.9
	Breast cancer	174.9
	Cervical cancer	180.0
	Colorectal cancer	154.0
	Endometrial cancer	182.0
	Lung cancer	162.9
	Ovarian cancer	183.0
	Prostate cancer	185

Section 10. Management of Patients with Immunologic Disorders

HIV/AIDS and Opportunistic Infections	Contact with or exposure to viral diseases	V01.79
	HIV infection	042
	Immunodeficiency	279.3
Autoimmune Diseases	Giant cell arteritis	446.5
	Systemic lupus erythematosus	710.0

Section 11. Management of Patients with Miscellaneous Health Problems

Integumentary Disorders	Cellulitis	682.9
	Dermatitis medicamentosa (drug eruption)	693.0
	Herpes zoster (shingles)	053.9
	Integumentary disorders	709.9
Ectopic Pregnancy and STIs	*Chlamydia trachomatis* infection	079.98
	Ectopic pregnancy	633.90
	Gonorrhea	098.0
	Herpes	054.9
	Pelvic inflammatory disease (PID salpingitis)	614.9
	Syphilis	097.9

Eye, Ear, Nose, and Throat Disorders	Allergic rhinitis	477.9
	Bell's palsy	351.0
	Central and branch retinal artery obstruction	362.30
	Conjunctivitis	372.30
	Corneal abrasion	918.1
	Diabetic retinopathy	362.01
	Epiglottitis	464.30
	Epistaxis	784.7
	Glaucoma	365.9
	Otitis externa	380.10
	Otitis media	382.9
	Pharyngitis	462.0
	Retinal detachment	361.9
	Sinusitis	473.9
	Temporomandibular joint disorder	524.60
	Trigeminal neuralgia (tic douloureux)	350.1
	Vertigo	780.4
Headache	Headache	784.0

Section 12. Common Problems in Acute Care

Fever	Fever	780.6
Pain	Acute pain	338.11
	Chronic pain	338.29
	Neoplasm related pain	338.3
	Unspecified pain	780.96
Psychosocial Problems in Acute Care	Anxiety	300.00
	Delirium	780.09
	Depression	311
	Substance abuse	305.90
	Psychosis	293.81
	Violence	300.9
Management of the Patient in Shock	Anaphylactic shock	995.0
	Cardiogenic shock	785.51
	Hypovolemic shock	785.59
	Septic shock	785.52
	Shock	785.50
Nutritional Considerations	Encounter for screening for nutritional disorder	V77.99
	Nutritional deficiency	269.9

Fluid, Electrolyte, and Acid-Base Imbalances	Acid-base disorders	276.4
	Hypercalcemia	275.42
	Hyperkalemia	276.7
	Hypermagnesemia	275.2
	Hypernatremia	276.0
	Hyperphosphatemia	275.3
	Hypocalcemia	275.41
	Hypokalemia	276.8
	Hypomagnesemia	275.2
	Hyponatremia	276.1
	Hypophosphatemia	275.3
	Metabolic acidosis	276.2
	Metabolic alkalosis	276.3
	Respiratory acidosis	276.2
	Respiratory alkalosis	276.3
Poisoning and Drug Toxicities	Acetaminophen toxicity	965.4
	Alcohol (ethanol) toxicity	980.0
	Antiarrhythmic drug overdose	972.0
	Anticoagulant overdose	964.2
	Antidepressant toxicity	969.0
	Antipsychotic toxicity	969.3
	Barbiturate overdose	967.0
	Benzodiazepine overdose	969.4
	Beta-blocker overdose	972.0
	Calcium channel blocker overdose	972.0
	Carbon monoxide poisoning	986
	Digoxin toxicity	972.1
	Lithium toxicity	985.8
	Organophosphate (insecticide) poisoning	989.3
	Salicylate toxicity	976.4
	Stimulant toxicity	970.9
	Theophylline toxicity	974.1
Wound Management	Pressure ulcer	707.0
	Type 1 diabetes mellitus with foot ulcer	250.81
	Type 2 diabetes mellitus with foot ulcer	250.80

Infections	Cellulitis	682.9
	Clostridium difficile colitis	008.45
	Dysentery	009.0
	Endocarditis	424.90
	Meningitis	322.9
	Neutropenia	288.0
	Nosocomial and ventilator-associated pneumonia	507.0
	Nosocomial bacteremia	790.7
	Nosocomial urinary tract infection	599.0
	Pharyngitis	462
	Pneumonia	486
	Simple diarrhea	787.91
	Sinusitis	473.9
	Skin and soft tissue furunculosis	680.9
	Sepsis	995.91
	Urinary tract infection	599.0
Trauma Considerations	Angina	413.9
	Aortic rupture	441.5
	Cardiac tamponade	423.9
	Collapsed lung	518.0
	Flail chest	807.4
	Lacerated liver	864.05
	Myocardial infarction	410.8
	Penetrating eye trauma	871.7
	Renal injuries	866.00
	Rib fractures	807.0
	Ruptured spleen	289.59
Solid Organ Transplantation	Complication of transplanted intestine	996.87
	Complication of transplanted kidney	996.81
	Complication of transplanted liver	996.82
	Complication of transplanted lung	996.84
	Complication of transplanted pancreas	996.86
	Heart transplantation	V50.0
	Intestinal transplantation	V42.84
	Kidney transplantation	V42.0
	Lung transplantation	V42.6
	Pancreas transplantation	V42.83

Burns	Burns	949.0
Hospital Admission Considerations		
Managing the Surgical Patient	Pre-operative examination	V72.84

Section 13. Health Promotion

Guidelines for Health Promotion and Screening	Screening for unspecified condition	V82.9
Major Causes of Mortality in the U.S.	Alzheimer's disease	331.0
	Cerebrovascular diseases	437.0
	Chronic lower respiratory diseases	519.9
	Diabetes mellitus	250.00
	Diseases of the heart	414.9
	Influenza	487.1
	Nephritic syndrome	581.9
	Nephritis	583.9
	Nephrosis	581.9
	Pneumonia	486
	Septicemia	638, 995.9
Immunization Recommendations	Diptheria	V03.5
	Hepatitis A	V05.3
	Hepatitis B	V05.3
	Influenza	V04.81
	Measles	V04.2
	Mumps	V04.6
	Polio	V04.0
	Rabies	V04.5
	Rubella	V04.3
	Smallpox	V04.1
	Tetanus	V03.7
	Varicella	V05.4

Note. Appendix A. International Classification of Diseases (2010). *ICD9data.com: The Web's free 2015 medical coding reference* [Data file]. Retrieved from icd9data.com

Appendix B. ICD-10 Codes

Chapter	Condition/Topic	ICD-10 Code
Section 1. Management of Patients with Neurological Disorders		
Cerebrovascular Accidents: Brain Attack	Nontraumatic intracerebral hemorrhage	I61.9
	Transient ischemic attack	G45.9
	Unspecified sequela of cerebrovascular accident	I69.90
Structural Abnormalities	Cerebral aneurysm	I67.1
	Malignant neoplasm of brain	C71
	Obstructive hydrocephalus	G91.1
Peripheral Neuropathies	Guillain-Barre syndrome	G61.0
	Myasthenia gravis	G70.0
Neurologic Trauma	Other specified injuries of head, initial encounter	S09.8XXA
	Unspecified injury of head, initial encounter	S09.90XA
	Unspecified injury to sacral spinal cord, initial encounter	S34.139A
	Unspecified injury to unspecified level of cervical spinal cord, initial encounter	S14.109A
	Unspecified injury to unspecified level of lumbar spinal cord, initial encounter	S34.109A
	Unspecified injury to unspecified level of thoracic spinal cord, initial encounter	S24.109A
Central Nervous System Disorders	Encephalitis and encephalomyelitis	G04.90
	Encephalopathy	G93.40
	Intracranial abscess and granuloma	G06.0
	Meningitis	G03.9
	Meningococcus, meningococcal	A39.0
Seizure Disorders	Seizure disorders	R56.9
Dementia	Dementia without behavioral disturbance	F03.90
Multiple sclerosis	Multiple sclerosis	G35
Parkinson's Disease	Parkinson's disease	G20
Amyotrophic Lateral Sclerosis	Amyotrophic lateral sclerosis	G12.21
Section 2. Management of Patients with Cardiovascular Disorders		
Cardiovascular Assessment	Abnormalities of heartbeat	R00
	Cardiac murmurs	R01

Hypertension	Essential hypertension	I10
	Other secondary hypertension	I15.8
	Secondary hypertension	I15
Coronary Artery Disease and Hyperlipidemia	Atherosclerotic heart disease of native coronary artery without angina pectoris	I25.10
	Hyperlipidemia	E78.5
Angina and Myocardial Infarction	Angina pectoris	I20
	Angina pectoris with documented spasm	I20.1
	Cardiac tamponade	I31.4
	Coronary atherosclerosis of unspecified bypass graft	I25.810
	Percutaneous transluminal coronary angioplasty status	Z98.61
	ST elevation (STEMI) myocardial infarction of unspecified site	I21.3
	Unstable angina	I20.0
Adjunct Equipment/ Devices		
Peripheral Vascular Disease	Deep vein thrombosis	I82.619
	Occlusive arterial disease	I714.3
	Peripheral vascular disease	I73.9
	Thromboangiitis obliterans (Buerger's disease)	I73.1
	Venous disease	I87.9
Inflammatory Cardiac Diseases	Acute and subacute endocarditis	I33
	Acute pericarditis, unspecific	I30.9
	Chronic pericarditis	I31.1
	Disease of pericardium, unspecified	I31.9
	Endocarditis	I38
Heart Failure	Heart failure, unspecified	I50.9
	Heart failure due to hypertension	I11.0
	Heart failure due to hypertension and chronic kidney disease	I13
	Heart failure following surgery	I97.13
	Rheumatic heart failure	I09.81

Valvular Disease	Disorder of vein, unspecified	I87.9
	Nonrheumatic aortic valve disorder, unspecified	I35.9
	Nonrheumatic aortic valve insufficiency	I35.1
	Nonrheumatic aortic valve stenosis	I35.0
	Nonrheumatic aortic valve stenosis with insufficiency	I35.2
	Nonrheumatic mitral valve insufficiency	I34.0
	Other nonrheumatic aortic valve disorders	I35.8
	Other nonrheumatic mitral valve disorders	I34.8
	Rheumatic mitral stenosis	I05.0
	Unspecified disorder of circulatory system	I99.9
Cardiomyopathy	Dilated cardiomyopathy	I42.0
	Hypertrophy cardiomyopathy	I42.1
	Restrictive cardiomyopathy	I42.5
Arrhythmias	Atrial premature depolarization	I49.1
	Atrioventricular block, complete	I44.2
	Atrioventricular block, first degree	I44.0
	Atrioventricular block, second degree	I44.1
	Bradycardia	R00.1
	Cardiac arrest	I46.9
	Cardiac arrhythmia, unspecified	I49.9
	Other premature depolarization	I49.49
	Other specified cardiac arrhythmias	I49.8
	Other specified conduction disorders	I45.89
	Unspecified atrial fibrillation	I48.91
	Unspecified atrial flutter	I48.92
	Ventricular fibrillation	I49.01
	Ventricular premature depolarization	I49.3
	Ventricular tachycardia	I47.2

Section 3. Management of Pulmonary Disorders

Diagnostic Concepts of Oxygenation and Ventilation	Respiratory measurement	4A09
	Respiratory monitoring	4A19
Measures of Oxygen and Ventilation	Respiratory measurement	4A09
	Respiratory monitoring	4A19

The Chest X-Ray	Disease of pericardium, unspecified	I31.9
	Emphysema, unspecified	J43.9
	Heart failure, unspecified	I50.9
	Pericardial effusion	I31.3
	Pneumonia, unspecified organism	J18.9
	Solitary pulmonary nodule	R91.1
Pulmonary Function Testing	Abnormal results of pulmonary function studies	R94.2
Obstructive (Ventilatory) Lung Diseases	Asthma	J45
	Bronchiectasis	J47
	Chronic bronchitis	J42
	Chronic obstructive pulmonary disease	J44.9
	Emphysema	J43.9
	Obstructive airway lesions	J44.9
Restrictive (Inflammatory) Lung Diseases	Acute lung injury	S27.309A
	Acute respiratory distress syndrome	J80
	Cardiogenic pulmonary edema	J81.1
	Congestive heart failure	I50.9
	Idiopathic pulmonary fibrosis	J84.10
	Pneumonia	J18.9
	Pulmonary edema	J81.1
	Restrictive (inflammatory) lung diseases	J98.4
	Sarcoidosis	D86.9
	Tuberculosis	A15.0
Pulmonary Hypertension and Pulmonary Vascular Disorders	Primary pulmonary hypertension	I27.0
	Pulmonary embolism	I26
	Secondary pulmonary hypertension	I27.2
	Wegener granulomatosis without renal involvement	M31.30
Chest Wall and Secondary Pleural Disorders	Chest wall disorders	F45.8
	Pleural condition, unspecified	J94.9
	Pleural effusion	J90
	Pleuritis	R09.1
Respiratory Failure	See Appendix C for respiratory failure ICD codes	

Pneumothorax	Chronic pneumothorax	J93.81
	Pneumothorax and air leak	J93
	Spontaneous pneumothorax	J93.0
	Tension pneumothorax	J93.0
	Traumatic pneumothorax	S27.0
Lower Respiratory Tract Pathogens	See Appendix C for list of lower respiratory tract infections	
Obstructive Sleep Apnea	Hypoxemia	R09.02
	Obstructive sleep apnea	G47.33
	Sleep apnea	G47.3
Oxygen Supplementation	Dependence on supplemental oxygen	Z99.81
Mechanical Ventilatory Support	Dependence on respiratory ventilator	Z99.11

Section 4. Management of Patients with Gastrointestinal Disorders

Peptic Ulcer Disease	Gastroesophageal reflux disease	K21.9
	Gastrointestinal mucositis	K92.81
	Peptic ulcer, site unspecified	K27.9
	Personal history of peptic ulcer disease	Z87.11
Liver Disease	Acute hepatitis	B17.9
	Alcoholic liver disease	K70.9
	Biliary cirrhosis	K74.3
	Cholangitis	K83.0
	Hereditary hemochromatosis	E83.110
	Liver disease, unspecified	K76.9
	Wilson disease	E83.01
Biliary Dysfunction	Acute pancreatitis	K85.9
	Cholecystitis	K81.9
Inflammatory Gastrointestinal Disorders	Appendicitis	K37
	Diverticulitis	K57.32
	Peritonitis	K65.9
	Ulcerative colitis	K51.90
Anatomic Intestinal Disorders	Intestinal obstruction	K56.60
	Paralytic ileus and intestinal obstruction	K56.0
	Traumatic ischemia of muscle	T79.6XXS
	Vascular disorder of the intestine, unspecified	K55.9
Gastrointestinal Bleeding	Esophageal varices	I85.00
	Lower gastrointestinal bleeding	K92.2
	Upper gastrointestinal bleeding	K92.2

Section 5. Management of Patients with Genitourinary Disorders

Urinary Tract Infections	History of urinary tract infections	Z87.440
	Urinary tract calculus	N21
	Urinary tract infection, site not specified	N39.0
Acute Kidney Injury and Chronic Kidney Disease	Acute kidney injury	S37.0
	Chronic kidney disease	N18.9
Benign Prostatic Hyperplasia	Enlarged prostate without lower UTI symptoms	N40.0
	Enlarged prostate with lower UTI symptoms	N40.1
Renal Artery Stenosis	Atherosclerosis of renal artery	I70.1
	Congenital renal artery stenosis	Q27.1
	Fibromuscular dysplasia	I77.3
Nephrolithiasis	Calculus of kidney	N20.0
Section 6. Management of Patients with Endocrine Disorders		
Diabetes Mellitus	Other specified diabetes mellitus	E13
	Type 1 diabetes mellitus	E10
	Type 2 diabetes mellitus	E11
Diabetes-Related Emergencies	Diabetes mellitus with ketoacidosis	E13.1
	Diabetes mellitus with hyperosmolarity with coma	E11.01
	Hypoglycemia	E16.2
Thyroid Disease	Hyperthyroidism	E05
	Hypothyroidism	E03.9
	Myxedema coma	E03.5
	Thyroid storm (thyrotoxic crisis)	E05.81
Cushing's Syndrome	Cushing's syndrome	E24.9
Primary Adrenocortical Insufficiency (Addison Disease) & Adrenal Crisis	Addison disease	G73.7
	Addisonian crisis	E27.2
	Primary adrenocortical insufficiency	E27.1
Pheochromocytoma	Pheochromocytoma	C74.10
Syndrome of Inappropriate Antidiuretic Hormone	Syndrome of inappropriate antidiuretic hormone	E22.2
Diabetes Insipidus	Diabetes insipidus	E23.2
	Nephrogenic diabetes insipidus	N25.1
Section 7. Management of Musculoskeletal Disorders		
Arthritis	Gout	M10.9
	Osteoarthritis	M19.91
	Rheumatoid arthritis	M06.9

Subluxations and Dislocations	Dislocation of ankle	M24.473
	Dislocation of shoulder	M24.419
	Dislocation of hand	M24.443
	Dislocation and subluxation of hip	S73.0
	Dislocation and subluxation of shoulder joint	S43.0
	Subluxation of unspecified scapula	S43.313A
	Subluxation of wrist and hand	S63.003
Soft Tissue Injury	Disorders of soft tissue	M79.9
	Soft tissue disorder related to use, overuse, and pressure	M70.99
Fractures	Closed fracture	T14.8
	Open fracture	T14.8
	Stress fracture	M84.3
Compartment syndrome	Compartment syndrome	T79.80
	Early complications of trauma, initial encounter	T79.8XXA
Back Pain Syndromes	Herniated disk	M51.9
	Low back pain	M54.5

Section 8. Management of Patients with Hematologic Disorders

Anemias	Anemia of chronic disease (ACD)	D63.8
	Anemias	D64.9
	Folic acid deficiency	D50.9
	Iron deficiency	D50.9
	Pernicious anemia	E61.1
	Thalassemia	D56.9
	Vitamin B12 deficiency	D51.0
Sickle Cell Disease/Crisis	Sickle cell disease/crisis	D57.819
	Sickle cell disease without crisis	D57.1
Coagulopathies	Disseminated intravascular coagulation	D65
	Heparin-induced thrombocytopenia	D75.82
	Idiopathic thrombocytopenic purpura	D69.3

Section 9. Management of Patients with Oncologic Disorders

Leukemias	Acute lymphocytic leukemia	C91.0
	Acute leukemia of unspecified cell	C95.02
	Acute myeloblastic leukemia	C92.0
	Chronic lymphocytic leukemia	C91.1
	Chronic myelogenous leukemia	C93.11, C93.12
	Refractory anemia with excess of blasts not in transformation	D46.2

Lymphoma	Hodgkin's disease	C81.9
	Lymphoma	C81.90
	Non-Hodgkin's lymphoma	C85.90
Other Common Cancers	Bladder cancer	C67.9
	Breast cancer	C50.919
	Cervical cancer	C53.0
	Colorectal cancer	C19
	Endometrial cancer	C54.1
	Lung cancer	C34.90
	Ovarian cancer	C56.9
	Prostate cancer	C61

Section 10. Management of Patients with Immunologic Disorders

HIV/AIDS and Opportunistic Infections	Contact with or exposure to viral diseases	Z20.6
	HIV infection	B20-B24
	Immunodeficiency	D84.9
Autoimmune Diseases	Giant cell arteritis	M31.6
	Systemic lupus erythematosus	M32.10

Section 11. Management of Patients with Miscellaneous Health Problems

Integumentary Disorders	Cellulitis	L03.90
	Dermatitis medicamentosa (drug eruption)	L27.0
	Herpes zoster (shingles)	B02.9
	Integumentary disorders	L98.9
	Skin disorders	C44.90
	Melanoma	C73.9
Ectopic Pregnancy and STIs	*Chlamydia trachomatis* infection	A74.9
	Ectopic pregnancy	O00.9
	Gonorrhea	A54.00
	Herpes	B00.9
	Pelvic inflammatory disease (PID salpingitis)	N73.9
	Syphilis	A53.9
	Vaginitis	N76.0
Eye, Ear, Nose, and Throat Disorders	See appendix E for ICD-10 codes for common eye, ear, nose, and throat disorders	

Headache	Chronic tension type headache	G44.229
	Cluster headaches syndrome	G44.001
	Episodic cluster headache	G44.019
	Episodic tension-type headache	G44.211
	Headache	R51
	Migraine	G43

Section 12. Common Problems in Acute Care

Fever	Fever	R50.9
Pain	Acute pain	G89.11
	Chronic pain	G89.29
	Neoplasm related pain	G89.3
	Unspecified pain	R52
Psychosocial Problems in Acute Care	Anxiety	F41.9
	Delirium	F05
	Depression	F32.9
	Psychosis	F06.0
	Substance Use Disorder (Alcohol)	F10.20
	Violence	R45.6
Management of the Patient in Shock	Anaphylactic shock	T78.2XXA
	R57.0	785.51
	Hypovolemic shock	R57.1
	Septic shock	R65.21
	Shock	R57.9
Nutritional Considerations	Encounter for screening for nutritional disorder	Z13.21
	Nutritional deficiency	E63.9

Fluid, Electrolyte, and Acid-Base Imbalances	Acid-base disorders	E87.4
	Hypercalcemia	E83.52
	Hyperkalemia	E87.5
	Hypermagnesemia	E83.41
	Hypernatremia	E87.0
	Hyperphosphatemia	E83.30
	Hypocalcemia	E83.51
	Hypokalemia	E87.6
	Hypomagnesemia	E83.42
	Hyponatremia	E87.1
	Hypophosphatemia	E83.30
	Metabolic acidosis	E87.3
	Metabolic alkalosis	E87.3
	Respiratory acidosis	E87.2
	Respiratory alkalosis	E87.3
Poisoning and Drug Toxicities	Acetaminophen toxicity	T39.1X2A
	Alcohol (ethanol) toxicity	T51.0X4A
	Antiarrhythmic drug overdose	T46.2X3A
	Anticoagulant overdose	T45.514A
	Antidepressant toxicity	T43.011A
	Antipsychotic toxicity	T433504A
	Barbiturate overdose	T42.3X4A
	Benzodiazepine overdose	T42.4X4A
	Beta-blocker overdose	T46.2X4A
	Calcium channel blocker overdose	T46.2X4A
	Carbon monoxide poisoning	T58.94XA
	Digoxin toxicity	T46.0X4A
	Lithium toxicity	T56.4X4A
	Organophosphate (insecticide) poisoning	T60.0X4A
	Salicylate toxicity	T49.4X4A
	Stimulant toxicity	T50.991A
	Theophylline toxicity	T50.2X1A
Wound Management	Non-pressure chronic ulcer	L98.4
	Pressure ulcer	L89
	Type 1 diabetes mellitus with foot ulcer	E10.621
	Type 2 diabetes mellitus with foot ulcer	E11.621

Infections	Cellulitis	L03.90
	Clostridium difficile colitis	A04.7
	Dysentery	A09
	Endocarditis	I38
	Meningitis	G03.9
	Neutropenia	D70
	Nosocomial and ventilator-associated pneumonia	J69.0
	Nosocomial bacteremia	R78.81
	Nosocomial urinary tract infection	J69.0
	Pharyngitis	J02.9
	Pneumonia	J18.9
	Simple diarrhea	R19.7
	Sinusitis	J32.9
	Skin and soft tissue furunculosis	L02.92
	Sepsis	R65.2
	Urinary tract infection	N39.0
Trauma Considerations	Angina	I20.9
	Aortic rupture	I71.8
	Cardiac tamponade	I31.9
	Collapsed lung	J98.11
	Flail chest	S22.5XXA
	Lacerated liver	S36.113A
	Myocardial infarction	I25.2
	Penetrating eye trauma	S05.60XA
	Renal injuries	S37.009A
	Rib fractures	S22.39XA
	Ruptured spleen	D73.3
Solid Organ Transplantation	Complication of transplanted intestine	T86.850
	Complication of transplanted kidney	T86.10
	Complication of transplanted liver	T86.40
	Complication of transplanted lung	T86.819
	Complication of transplanted pancreas	T86.899
	Heart transplantation	V50.0
	Intestinal transplantation	V42.84
	Kidney transplantation	V42.0
	Lung transplantation	V42.6
	Pancreas transplantation	V42.83

Burns	Burns of unspecified body region	T30.0
	First degree burn	T21.10XS
	Second degree burn	T21.20XS
	Third degree burn	T21.30XS
Hospital Admission Considerations		
Managing the Surgical Patient	Pre-operative examination	Z01.818
	Encounter for post procedural aftercare	Z48

Section 13. Health Promotion

Guidelines for Health Promotion and Screening	Encounter for general adult medical examination	Z00.0
	Encounter for screening, unspecified	Z13.9
Major Causes of Mortality in the U.S.	Alzheimer's disease	G30.9
	Cerebral atherosclerosis	I67.2
	Chronic ischemic heart disease, unspecified	I25.9
	Influenza due to other identified influenza virus with other respiratory manifestations	J10.1
	Nephritic syndrome	N04.9
	Pneumonia	J18.9
	Respiratory disorder	J98.9
	Systemic inflammatory response syndrome of non-infectious origin without acute organ dysfunction	R65.10
	Type 2 diabetes without complications	E11.9
	Unspecified nephritic syndrome with unspecified morphologic changes	N05.9
Immunization Recommendations	Encounter for immunization	Z23

Note. Appendix B. International Classification of Diseases (2014). *ICD10data.com: The Web's free 2015 medical coding reference* [Data file]. Retrieved from icd10data.com

Appendix C. ICD-10 Coding, Respiratory Failure (CMS, 2013)	
ICD-10 Code	**Disorder**
J96	Respiratory failure not otherwise specified Excludes: acute respiratory distress syndrome (J80) Cardiorespiratory failure (R09.2) Post-procedural respiratory failure (J95.82-) Respiratory arrest (R09.2)
J96	Acute respiratory failure
J96.00	Acute respiratory failure unspecified whether with hypoxia or hypercapnia
J96.01	Acute respiratory failure with hypoxia
J96.02	Acute respiratory failure with hypercapnia
J96.1	Chronic respiratory failure
J96.10	Chronic respiratory failure unspecified whether with hypoxia or hypercapnia
J96.11	Chronic respiratory failure with hypoxia
J96.12	Chronic respiratory failure with hypercapnia
J96.2	Acute and chronic respiratory failure (or acute or chronic respiratory failure)
J96.20	Acute and chronic respiratory failure unspecified whether with hypoxia or hypercapnia
J96.21	Acute and chronic respiratory failure with hypoxia
J96.22	Acute and chronic respiratory failure with hypercapnia
J96.9	Respiratory failure unspecified
J96.90	Respiratory failure unspecified whether with hypoxia or hypercapnia
J96.91	Respiratory failure unspecified with hypoxia
J96.92	Respiratory failure unspecified with hypercapnia

Note. Appendix C. International Classification of Diseases (2014). *ICD10data.com: The Web's free 2015 medical coding reference* [Data file]. Retrieved from icd10data.com

Appendix D. Former ICD-9 and ICD-10 Coding, Lower Respiratory Tract Infections (see Lower Respiratory Tract Pathogens chapter), for 2014 (CMS, 2013)

Former ICD-9 Coding (2013):

466.0	Acute tracheobronchitis
496	Chronic obstructive pulmonary disease
486	Pneumonia, community-acquired

ICD-10 Code (2014):

J09	Influenza due to certain identified influenza viruses
J09.X	Influenza due to identified novel influenza A viruses, including: •Avian influenza •Bird influenza •Influenza A/H5N1 •Influenza of other animal origin, not bird or swine •Swine influenza virus
J09.X1	Influenza due to identified novel influenza A virus with pneumonia
J10	Influenza due to other identified influenza virus
J10.0	Influenza due to other identified influenza virus with pneumonia
J10.00	Influenza due to other identified influenza virus with unspecified type of pneumonia
J10.01	Influenza due to other identified influenza virus with the same other identified influenza virus pneumonia
J10.08	Influenza due to other identified influenza virus with other specified pneumonia
J11	Influenza due to unidentified influenza virus
J11.0	Influenza due to unidentified influenza virus pneumonia
J11.00	Influenza due to unidentified influenza virus with unspecified type of pneumonia
J11.08	Influenza due to unidentified influenza virus with specified pneumonia
J12	Viral pneumonia, not elsewhere classified
J12.0	Adenoviral pneumonia
J12.1	Respiratory syncytial virus pneumonia
J12.2	Parainfluenza virus pneumonia
J12.3	Human metapneumovirus pneumonia
J12.8	Other viral pneumonia
J12.81	Pneumonia due to SAS-associated coronavirus
J12.89	Other viral pneumonia
J12.9	Viral pneumonia, unspecified
J13	Pneumonia due to *Streptococcus pneumoniae*
J14	Pneumonia due to *Hemophilus influenzae*
J15	Bacterial pneumonia, not elsewhere classified

J15.0	Pneumonia due to *Klebsiella pneumoniae*
J15.1	Pneumonia due to *Pseudomonas*
J15.2	Pneumonia due to *Staphylococcus*
J15.20	Pneumonia due to *Staphylococcus*, unspecified
J15.21	Pneumonia due to *Staphylococcus aureus*
J15.211	Pneumonia due to methicillin-susceptible *Staphylococcus aureus*
J15.212	Pneumonia due to methicillin-resistant *Staphylococcus aureus*
J15.3	Pneumonia due to *Streptococcus*, group B
J15.4	Pneumonia due to other streptococci
J15.5	Pneumonia due to *Escherichia coli*
J15.6	Pneumonia due to other Gram-negative bacteria, including *Serratia marcescens*
J15.7	Pneumonia due to *Mycoplasma pneumoniae*
J15.8	Pneumonia due to other specified bacteria
J15.9	Unspecified bacterial pneumonia due to Gram-positive bacteria
J16	Pneumonia due to other infectious organisms, not elsewhere classified
J16.0	Chlamydial pneumonia
J16.8	Pneumonia due to other specified infectious organisms
J18	Pneumonia, unspecified organism
J18.0	Bronchopneumonia
J18.1	Lobar, pneumonia, unspecified organism
J18.2	Hypostatic pneumonia, unspecified organism
J18.8	Other pneumonia, unspecified organism
J18.9	Pneumonia, unspecified organism
J20	Acute bronchitis
J20.0	Acute bronchitis due to *Mycoplasma pneumoniae*
J20.1	Acute bronchitis due to *Hemophilus influenzae*
J20.2	Acute bronchitis due to *Streptococcus*
J20.3	Acute bronchitis due to Coxsackie virus
J20.4	Acute bronchitis due to parainfluenza virus
J20.5	Acute bronchitis due to respiratory syncytial virus
J20.6	Acute bronchitis due to rhinovirus
J20.7	Acute bronchitis due to echovirus
J20.8	Acute bronchitis due to other specified organisms
J20.9	Acute bronchitis, unspecified
J21	Acute bronchiolitis
J21.0	Acute bronchiolitis due to respiratory syncytial virus
J21.1	Acute bronchiolitis due to human metapneumovirus

J21.8	Acute bronchiolitis due to other specified organisms
J21.0	Acute bronchiolitis, unspecified
J22	Unspecified acute lower respiratory infection

Note. Appendix D. International Classification of Diseases (2014). *ICD10data.com: The Web's free 2015 medical coding reference* [Data file]. Retrieved from icd10data.com

ICD-9 Code (2013) Category	Disorder

Appendix E. ICD-9 and ICD-10 Codes for Common Eye, Ear, Nose, and Throat Disorders (see Common Eye, Ear, Nose, and Throat Disorders chapter)

ICD-9 Code (2013) Category	Disorder
477.9	Allergic rhinitis
351.0	Bell palsy
362.30	Central and branch retinal artery obstruction
372.30	Conjunctivitis
918.1	Corneal abrasion
362.01	Diabetic retinopathy
464.30	Epiglottitis
784.7	Epistaxis
365.9	Glaucoma
380.10	Otitis externa
382.9	Otitis media
462.0	Pharyngitis
361.9	Retinal detachment
473.9	Sinusitis
524.60	Temporomandibular joint disorder
350.1	Trigeminal neuralgia (tic douloureux)
ICD-10 Code (2014) Category	**Disorder**
Disorders of the eye	
E11 (see also E08)	Type 2 diabetes mellitus (Diabetes mellitus due to underlying conditions)
E11.31	Type 2 diabetes mellitus with unspecified retinopathy
G45	Transient cerebral ischemic attacks and related syndromes
G45.3	Amaurosis fugax
H00.0	Hordeolum (externum) (internum) of eyelid
H00.01	Hordeolum externum (stye)
H00.02	Hordeolum internum (infection of meibomian gland)
H00.1	Chalazion (cyst of meibomian gland)
H01.0	Blepharitis
H01.00	Unspecified blepharitis
H01.1	Noninfectious dermatoses of eyelid
H01.11	Allergic (contact) dermatitis of eyelid

H01.13	Eczematous dermatitis of eyelid
H01.9	Unspecified inflammation of eyelid
H02.0	Entropion and trichiasis of eyelid
H02.00	Unspecified entropion of eyelid
H02.03	Senile entropion of eyelid
H02.1	Ectropion of eyelid
H02.10	Unspecified ectropion of eyelid
H02.13	Senile ectropion of eyelid
H02.4	Ptosis of eyelid
H02.40	Unspecified ptosis of eyelid
H02.6	Xanthelasma of eyelid
H02.60	Xanthelasma of unspecified eye
H04.1	Other disorders of lacrimal gland
H04.12	Dry eye syndrome
H04.3	Acute and unspecified inflammation of lacrimal passages
H04.30	Unspecified Dacryocystitis
H04.4	Chronic inflammation of lacrimal passages
H04.41	Chronic dacryocystitis
H05.0	Acute inflammation of orbit
H05.00	Unspecified acute inflammation of orbit
H05.01	Cellulitis (including abscess) of orbit
H05.20	Unspecified exophthalmos
H10.0	Mucopurulent conjunctivitis
H10.01	Acute follicular conjunctivitis
H10.02	Other mucopurulent conjunctivitis
H11.0	Pterygium of eye
H11.00	Unspecified pterygium of eye
H11.3	Conjunctival (subconjunctival) hemorrhage
H11.30	Conjunctival hemorrhage unspecified eye
H25.0	Age-related incipient cataract
H25.01	Cortical age-related cataract
H25.1	Age-related nuclear cataract
H25.10	Age-related nuclear cataract unspecified eye
H33	Retinal detachments and breaks
H33.00	Unspecified retinal detachment with retinal break
H33.8	Other retinal detachment
H34	Retinal vascular occlusions
H34.0	Transient retinal artery occlusion

H34.1	Central retinal artery occlusion
H40.0	Glaucoma suspect
H40.00	Preglaucoma unspecified
S05.0	Injury of conjunctiva and corneal abrasion without foreign body
S05.00	Injury of conjunctiva and corneal abrasion without foreign body unspecified eye

Disorders of the Ear

H60	Otitis externa
H60.33	Swimmer's ear
H60.50	Unspecified acute noninfective otitis externa
H65	Nonsuppurative otitis media (acute)
H65.0	Acute serous otitis media
H66.0	Suppurative and unspecified otitis media
H66.00	Acute suppurative otitis media without spontaneous rupture of ear drum
H81	Disorders of vestibular function
H81.0	Ménière disease
H81.1	Benign paroxysmal vertigo
R42	Dizziness and giddiness; vertigo, NOS

Disorders of the Face (nerve-related)

G50	Disorders of trigeminal nerve
G50.0	Trigeminal neuralgia (Tic douloureux)
G51	Facial nerve disorders
G51.0	Bell's palsy

Disorders of the Nose and Sinuses

J01	Acute sinusitis
J01.00	Acute maxillary sinusitis unspecified
J01.10	Acute fontal sinusitis
J30	Vasomotor and allergic rhinitis unspecified
J30.0	Vasomotor rhinitis
J30.1	Allergic rhinitis due to pollen (hay fever)
R04	Hemorrhage from respiratory passages
R04.4	Epistaxis

Disorders of the Temporomandibular Joint

M26.6	Temporomandibular joint disorders
M26.60	Temporomandibular joint disorder unspecified
M26.62	Arthralgia of temporomandibular joint

Disorders of the throat and larynx

J02	Acute pharyngitis

J02.0	Streptococcal pharyngitis
J02.9	Acute pharyngitis unspecified
J03	Acute tonsillitis
J03.0	Streptococcal tonsillitis
J03.9	Acute tonsillitis unspecified
J04	Acute laryngitis and tracheitis
J04.0	Acute laryngitis
J04.3	Supraglottitis unspecified
J05	Acute obstructive laryngitis [croup] and epiglottitis
J05.0	Acute obstructive laryngitis {croup]
J05.1	Acute epiglottitis
J05.10	Acute epiglottitis without obstruction
J05.11	Acute epiglottitis with obstruction
J06	Acute upper respiratory infections of multiple and unspecified sites
J06.0	Acute laryngopharyngitis
J06.9	Acute upper respiratory infection unspecified

Note. ICD 9 codes (2013) and ICD-10 (2014) codes for disorders of the eye and adnexa (CDC, 2013). Please note that there are 85 pages of coding for these ocular disorders. Codes provided are only for those disorders likely to be encountered in an acute care nurse practitioner role, while caring for elderly patients. Furthermore, there are also codings for right or left eye, which eyelid is involved, and other descriptors. The reader is directed to the following URL for additional information under Chapter 7 of the ICD-10 coding. Additional coding to specify whether the disorder affects the right eye, the left eye, or both is available, especially if the coding below states "unspecified."

Appendix E. International Classification of Diseases (2014). *ICD10data.com: The Web's free 2015 medical coding reference* [Data file]. Retrieved from icd10data.com

Index